Principles and Practice of Pulmonary Rehabilitation

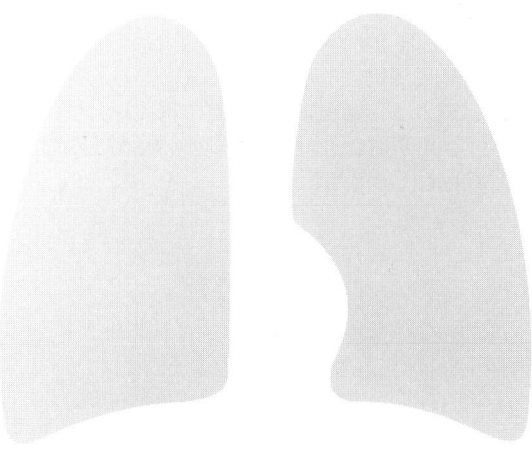

RICHARD CASABURI, PhD, MD
Associate Professor of Medicine
Department of Medicine
UCLA School of Medicine
Director
Pulmonary Physiology Laboratories
Associate Chief
Division of Respiratory and Critical
  Care Physiology and Medicine
Harbor-UCLA Medical Center
Torrance, California

THOMAS L. PETTY, MD
Professor of Medicine
University of Colorado
Health Sciences Center
Professor of Medicine
Rush University Medical Center
Associate Dean
Rush-Presbyterian-St. Luke's Medical Center
Denver Campus
President for the Presbyterian/St. Luke's Center
  for Health Sciences Education
Director of Academic and Research Affairs
Presbyterian/St. Luke's Medical Center
Denver, Colorado

Principles and Practice of Pulmonary Rehabilitation

W.B. SAUNDERS COMPANY
A Division of Harcourt Brace & Company
Philadelphia London Toronto Montreal Sydney Tokyo

W.B. SAUNDERS COMPANY
A Division of
Harcourt Brace & Company

The Curtis Center
Independence Square West
Philadelphia, Pennsylvania 19106

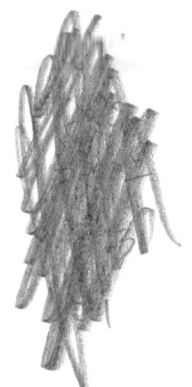

Library of Congress Cataloging-in-Publication Data

Principles and practice of pulmonary rehabilitation/
[edited by] Richard Casaburi, Thomas L. Petty.
   p.   cm.
ISBN 0-7216-3304-8
1. Lungs—Diseases—Patients—Rehabilitation.
  I. Casaburi, Richard.   II. Petty, Thomas L.
  [DNLM: 1. Lung Diseases, Obstructive—rehabilitation.
  WF 600 P957]
RC756.P75 1993
616.2′403—dc20
DNLM/DLC   92-13386

PRINCIPLES AND PRACTICE OF PULMONARY REHABILITATION   ISBN 0-7216-3304-8

Copyright © 1993 by W. B. Saunders Company

All rights reserved. No part of this publication may be reproduced or transmitted in any form or by any means, electronic or mechanical, including photocopy, recording, or any information storage and retrieval system, without permission in writing from the publisher.

Printed in Mexico.

Last digit is the print number: 9   8   7   6   5   4   3   2   1

TO OUR PATIENTS, OUR TEACHERS

Contributors

THOMAS K. ALDRICH, M.D.
Associate Professor of Medicine, Albert Einstein College of Medicine; Adjunct Attending in Pulmonary Medicine, Montefiore Medical Center, Bronx, New York
  Acute and Chronic Respiratory Failure

WILLIAM M. ANDERSON, M.D.
Associate Professor of Medicine, Louisiana State University School of Medicine; Chief, Section of Pulmonary and Critical Care Medicine, Overton Brooks Veterans Affairs Medical Center, Shreveport, Louisiana
  Pharmacologic Therapy

MONICA A. AVENDANO, M.D., F.R.C.P.(C)
Assistant Professor of Medicine, University of Toronto; Associate Director, Respiratory Programme, West Park Hospital, Toronto, Ontario, Canada
  Candidate Evaluation

KENNETH AXEN, Ph.D.
Associate Professor of Rehabilitation Medicine, New York University School of Medicine, New York, New York
  Desensitization to Dyspnea in Chronic Obstructive Pulmonary Disease

THOMAS J. BARSTOW, Ph.D.
Adjunct Assistant Professor of Medicine, Harbor-UCLA Medical Center, Torrance, California
  Ventilatory Control in Lung Disease

MICHAEL J. BELMAN, M.D.
Associate Professor of Medicine, UCLA School of Medicine, Torrance, California; Associate Director, Pulmonary Division, and Director, Pulmonary Physiology Laboratory, Cedars-Sinai Medical Center, Los Angeles, California
  Ventilatory Muscle Training and Unloading

DOROTHY G. BIGGAR, M.S.N., R.N.
Respiratory Nurse Coordinator, Barnes Hospital, St. Louis, Missouri
  Pulmonary Rehabilitation Before and After Lung Transplantation

MARY BURNS, R.N., B.S.
Assistant Clinical Professor, UCLA School of Nursing; Supervisor, Pulmonary Rehabilitation, Little Company of Mary Hospital, Torrance, California
  Continuing Care Programs

RICHARD CASABURI, Ph.D., M.D.
Associate Professor of Medicine, Department of Medicine, UCLA School of Medicine; Associate Chief, Division of Respiratory and Critical Care Physiology and Medicine, Harbor-UCLA Medical Center, Torrance, California
  Ventilatory Control in Lung Disease; Exercise Training in Chronic Obstructive Lung Disease

MARGARET CHAIKA-MEDEIROS, R.C.P.
Pulmonary Rehabilitation Coordinator, Washington Hospital, Fremont, California
  Reimbursement for a Community Hospital-Based Program

CHRISTOPHER J. CLARK, M.D., F.R.C.P.
Honorary Senior Lecturer in Medicine, University of Glasgow; Consultant Physician, Hairmyres Hospital, East Kilbride, Glasgow, Scotland
  Evaluating the Results of Pulmonary Rehabilitation Treatment; The Role of Physical Training in Asthma

CHRISTOPHER B. COOPER, M.D.
Assistant Professor of Medicine, UCLA School of Medicine, Division of Respiratory and Critical Care Physiology and Medicine, Harbor-UCLA Medical Center, Torrance, California
Long-term Oxygen Therapy

JOEL D. COOPER, M.D.
Professor of Surgery, Washington University School of Medicine; Attending Physician, Barnes Hospital, St. Louis, Missouri
Pulmonary Rehabilitation Before and After Lung Transplantation

THOMAS CORBRIDGE, M.D.
Assistant Professor of Medicine, University of Colorado Health Sciences Center; Director, Adult Special Care Unit, and Staff Physician, Department of Medicine, National Jewish Center for Immunology and Respiratory Medicine, Denver, Colorado
Pathophysiology of Chronic Obstructive Pulmonary Disease with Emphasis on Physiologic and Pathologic Correlations

ANDRÉ DE TROYER, M.D., Ph.D.
Professor of Medicine, and Director, Laboratory of Cardiorespiratory Physiology, Brussels School of Medicine; Professor of Medicine, Chest Service, Erasme University Hospital, Brussels, Belgium
Respiratory Muscle Function in Chronic Obstructive Pulmonary Disease

MICHAEL DONAHOE, M.D.
Assistant Professor of Medicine, University of Pittsburgh School of Medicine; Director, Medical Intensive Care Unit, Presbyterian-University Hospital, University of Pittsburgh Medical Center, Pittsburgh, Pennsylvania
Nutritional Assessment and Therapy

CLAUDIO FERDINANDO DONNER, M.D., F.C.C.P.
Professor of Medicine, School of Medicine, University of Turin; Chief, Division of Pulmonary Disease, and Director, Medical Center of Rehabilitation, Clinica del Lavoro Foundation, Veruno, Italy
Exercise Prescription

NEIL J. DOUGLAS, M.D., F.R.C.P.E.
Reader in Medicine and Respiratory Medicine, University of Edinburgh; Consultant Physician, City Hospital; Director, Scottish National Sleep Laboratory, Edinburgh, Scotland
Sleep Disordered Breathing

DONALD L. DUDLEY, M.D.
President, Washington Institute of Neurosciences, Inc., Seattle, Washington
Psychobiologic Evaluation and Rehabilitation in Pulmonary Disease

ELIZABETH G. EAKIN, B.A.
Joint Doctoral Program in Clinical Psychology, University of California, San Diego, and San Diego State University, San Diego, California
Psychosocial Issues in the Rehabilitation of Patients with Chronic Obstructive Pulmonary Disease

L. JACK FALING, M.D.
Associate Professor of Medicine, Tufts University School of Medicine; Associate Chief of Medicine, Veterans Administration Medical Center, Boston, Massachusetts
Controlled Breathing Techniques and Chest Physical Therapy in Chronic Obstructive Pulmonary Disease and Allied Conditions

RONALD B. GEORGE, M.D.
Professor of Medicine, and Chief, Pulmonary and Critical Care Medicine, Louisiana State University School of Medicine; Acting Chairman, Department of Medicine, Louisiana State University Medical Center, Shreveport, Louisiana
Pharmacologic Therapy

ROGER S. GOLDSTEIN, M.B., Ch.B., F.R.C.P.(C), F.R.C.P.(UK), F.C.C.P.
Associate Professor of Medicine, University of Toronto; Director, Respiratory Programme, West Park Hospital, Toronto, Ontario, Canada
Candidate Evaluation

IGOR GRANT, M.D.
Professor of Psychiatry, School of Medicine, University of California at San Diego, La Jolla, California; Staff Psychiatrist, Department of Veterans Affairs Medical Center, San Diego, California
Neurocognitive Aspects of Chronic Obstructive Pulmonary Disease

FRANCOIS HAAS, Ph.D.
Associate Professor of Rehabilitation Medicine, New York University School of Medicine; Director, Pulmonary Function Laboratory, New York University Medical Center, New York, New York
Desensitization to Dyspnea in Chronic Obstructive Pulmonary Disease

MARGARET CAMPBELL HAGGERTY, R.N.C., M.S.N.
Assistant Clinical Professor, Yale University School of Nursing, New Haven, Connecticut; Pulmonary Clinical Nurse Specialist, Norwalk Hospital, Norwalk, Connecticut
Relaxation and Biofeedback: Coping Skills Training

CONTRIBUTORS

ROBERT K. HEATON, Ph.D.
Professor of Psychiatry, University of California at San Diego, San Diego, California
Neurocognitive Aspects of Chronic Obstructive Pulmonary Disease

MILLICENT HIGGINS, M.D., D.P.H.
Associate Director, National Heart, Lung and Blood Institute, Bethesda, Maryland; Professor Emeritus of Epidemiology and Internal Medicine, University of Michigan, Ann Arbor, Michigan
Epidemiology of Obstructive Pulmonary Disease

FRANCESCO IOLI, M.D.
Chief Assistant, Division of Pulmonary Disease, Medical Center of Rehabilitation, Clinica del Lavoro Foundation, Veruno, Italy
Exercise Prescription

CHARLES G. IRVIN, Ph.D.
Associate Professor of Medicine, University of Colorado Health Sciences Center; Associate Director, Pulmonary Physiology Unit, National Jewish Center for Immunology and Respiratory Medicine, Denver, Colorado
Pathophysiology of Chronic Obstructive Pulmonary Disease with Emphasis on Physiologic and Pathologic Correlations

ANNE JERMAN, R.N., M.S., C.S.
Clinical Faculty, Department of Psychiatry, University of Vermont; Psychiatric/Mental Health Clinical Specialist, Medical Center Hospital of Vermont, Burlington, Vermont
Relaxation and Biofeedback: Coping Skills Training

ROBERT M. KACMAREK, Ph.D., R.R.T.
Assistant Professor, Department of Anesthesiology, Harvard Medical School; Director of Respiratory Care, Massachusetts General Hospital, Boston, Massachusetts
Home Ventilator Care

ROBERT M. KAPLAN, Ph.D.
Professor of Community and Family Medicine, and Chief, Division of Health Care Sciences, University of California, San Diego, San Diego, California
Psychosocial Issues in the Rehabilitation of Patients with Chronic Obstructive Pulmonary Disease

KIERAN J. KILLIAN, M.D., F.R.C.P.(C)
Professor of Medicine, Ambrose Cardiorespiratory Department, McMaster University Department of Medicine, Hamilton, Ontario, Canada
Dyspnea: Implications for Rehabilitation

GERARD H. KOËTER, M.D.
Professor in Pulmonology, Department of Pulmonology, University Hospital, Groningen, The Netherlands
Course and Prognosis in Patients with Chronic Airflow Obstruction: Possible Implications for Therapy

HOWARD M. KRAVETZ, M.D., F.C.C.P.
Codirector, Respiratory Care Department, Pulmonary Function Laboratory, Yavapai Regional Medical Center, Prescott, Arizona
How the Office-based Pulmonary Rehabilitation Program Works

R. WAYNE MALL, M.D.
Staff Physician, Washington Hospital, Fremont, California
Reimbursement for a Community Hospital-Based Program

JILL FELDMAN MALEN, M.S., N.S., R.N.
Thoracic/Pulmonary Clinical Nurse Specialist, Barnes Hospital, St. Louis, Missouri
Pulmonary Rehabilitation Before and After Lung Transplantation

JULIET M. MANCINO, M.S., R.D.
Coordinator, COPD Enteral Nutrition Project, University of Pittsburgh School of Medicine, Division of Pulmonary, Allergy and Critical Care Medicine, Pittsburgh, Pennsylvania
Nutritional Assessment and Therapy

DOUGLASS A. MORRISON, M.D., F.A.C.C.
Associate Professor of Medicine, University of Colorado Health Sciences Center; Director, Cardiac Catheterization Laboratory, Veterans Administration Medical Center, Denver, Colorado
Cardiovascular Consequences of Chronic Obstructive Pulmonary Disease

LOUISE M. NETT, R.N., R.R.T.
Clinical Research Associate, Presbyterian/St. Luke's Center for Health Sciences Education, Denver, Colorado
Nicotine Addiction Treatment

RICHARD S. NOVITCH, M.D.
Instructor in Medicine, Cornell University Medical College, New York, New York; Assistant Director, Pulmonary Medicine, Burke Rehabilitation Center, White Plains, New York; Assistant Attending Physician, New York Hospital, New York, New York
Rehabilitation of Patients with Chronic Ventilatory Limitation from Nonobstructive Lung Diseases

BLAKESLEE E. NOYES, M.D.
Assistant Professor of Pediatrics, University of Pitts-

burgh School of Medicine; Codirector, Cystic Fibrosis Center, Pittsburgh, Pennsylvania
Cystic Fibrosis

DAVID M. ORENSTEIN, M.D.
Associate Professor of Pediatrics, School of Medicine, and Associate Professor of Instruction and Learning, School of Education, University of Pittsburgh; Director, Cystic Fibrosis Center, and Director, Pediatric Pulmonology, Children's Hospital of Pittsburgh, Pittsburgh, Pennsylvania
Cystic Fibrosis

MICHAEL W. OWENS, M.D.
Assistant Professor of Medicine, Louisiana State University School of Medicine; Medical Director of Respiratory Therapy, Overton Brooks Veterans Affairs Medical Center, Shreveport, Louisiana
Pharmacologic Therapy

ANTONIO PATESSIO, M.D.
Chief Assistant, Division of Pulmonary Disease, Medical Center of Rehabilitation, Clinica del Lavoro Foundation, Veruno, Italy
Exercise Prescription

THOMAS L. PETTY, M.D.
Professor of Medicine, University of Colorado Health Sciences Center, and Presbyterian-St. Luke's Medical Center, Denver, Colorado; Professor of Medicine, Rush Presbyterian-St. Luke's Medical Center, Chicago, Illinois
Pulmonary Rehabilitation: A Personal Historical Perspective; Chronic Obstructive Pulmonary Disease: Treatment of Advanced Stages of Disease; The Ventilator-Dependent Patient

DAVID J. PIERSON, M.D.
Professor, Division of Pulmonary and Critical Care Medicine, Department of Medicine, University of Washington School of Medicine; Medical Director, Respiratory Care Department, Harborview Medical Center, Seattle, Washington
Home Ventilator Care

DIRKJE S. POSTMA, M.D.
Associate Professor, Department of Pulmonology, University Hospital, Groningen, The Netherlands
Course and Prognosis in Patients with Chronic Airflow Obstruction: Possible Implications for Therapy

ANDREW L. RIES, M.D., M.P.H.
Associate Professor of Medicine, University of California, San Diego; Medical Director, Pulmonary Rehabilitation Program, UCSD Medical Center, San Diego, California
Psychosocial Issues in the Rehabilitation of Patients with Chronic Obstructive Pulmonary Disease

ROBERT M. ROGERS, M.D.
Professor of Medicine and Anesthesiology, and Chief, Division of Pulmonary, Allergy and Critical Care Medicine, University of Pittsburgh School of Medicine; Director, Comprehensive Lung Center, Pittsburgh, Pennsylvania
Nutritional Assessment and Therapy

SEAN B. ROURKE, B.Sc., Hons. B.A.
Research Assistant, Department of Psychiatry, University of California at San Diego, San Diego, California
Neurocognitive Aspects of Chronic Obstructive Pulmonary Disease

JOHN SALAZAR-SCHICCHI, M.D.
Research Fellow, Department of Rehabilitation Medicine, Rusk Institute, New York University School of Medicine, New York, New York; Specialist in Respiratory Diseases and Intensive Care Medicine, Buenos Aires University, Buenos Aires, Argentina
Desensitization to Dyspnea in Chronic Obstructive Pulmonary Disease

PAUL A. SELECKY, M.D.
Associate Clinical Professor of Medicine, UCLA School of Medicine, Los Angeles, California; Medical Director, Pulmonary Department, Hoag Memorial Hospital Presbyterian, Newport Beach, California
Sexuality and the Patient with Lung Disease

JUDITH SITZMAN, R.N., D.N.Sc., Ph.D.
Comprehensive Psychiatric Centers, Santa Rosa, California
Psychobiologic Evaluation and Rehabilitation in Pulmonary Disease

FRANK D. SUTTON, M.D.
Clinical Professor of Medicine, University of Alabama Medical College; Baptist Medical Center, Division of Pulmonary Diseases, Birmingham, Alabama
The Proprietary Pulmonary Rehabilitation Program

HENRY M. THOMAS III, M.D.
Professor of Clinical Medicine, Cornell University Medical College; Lecturer in Medicine, Columbia University; Attending Physician, New York Hospital, New York, New York; Director, Pulmonary Medicine, Burke Rehabilitation Center, White Plains, New York
Rehabilitation of Patients with Chronic Ventilatory Limitation from Nonobstructive Lung Diseases

BRIAN L. TIEP, M.D.
Staff, Pulmonary Rehabilitation Department, Casa Colina Hospital, Pomona, California
Pulmonary Rehabilitation Program Organization

JUDITH A. TIETSORT, R.N., R.R.T.
Director, Respiratory Care Services, Lutheran Medical Center, Wheat Ridge, Colorado
A Storefront Program for Pulmonary Rehabilitation

E. P. TRULOCK, M.D.
Associate Professor of Medicine, Washington University School of Medicine; Medical Director, Lung Transplant Program, Barnes Hospital, St. Louis, Missouri
Pulmonary Rehabilitation Before and After Lung Transplantation

KARLMAN WASSERMAN, M.D., Ph.D.
Professor of Medicine, UCLA School of Medicine; Chief, Division of Respiratory and Critical Care Physiology and Medicine, Harbor-UCLA Medical Center, Torrance, California
Exercise Tolerance in the Pulmonary Patient

PETER J. WIJKSTRA, M.D.
Postdoctoral Fellow, Beatrixoord Asthma Center, Groningen, The Netherlands
Course and Prognosis in Patients with Chronic Airflow Obstruction: Possible Implications for Therapy

BRAM D. ZUCKERMAN, M.D.
Assistant Professor of Medicine, University of Colorado Health Sciences Center, Denver, Colorado
Cardiovascular Consequences of Chronic Obstructive Pulmonary Disease

Preface

> "Some books are to be tasted, others to be swallowed, and some few to be chewed and digested."
>
> Francis Bacon (1561–1626)

In the United States alone, more than 10 million people have chronic obstructive pulmonary disease. A smaller, but still large, number suffer from a range of restrictive lung diseases. Although cigarette smoking, the major cause of chronic obstructive pulmonary disease, seems to be declining in the Western world, we will be dealing with its consequences for decades to come. These pulmonary disorders are frustrating and debilitating and their influence permeates every aspect of the patient's life. Unfortunately, medical science seems to be nowhere near devising a way to reverse the disease process.

The goal of pulmonary rehabilitation is to alleviate the symptoms of lung disease and to encourage the patient to lead a full life. We seem to be perched on the threshold of the third era in pulmonary rehabilitation. In the first era, which lasted until the 1950s, rest and the avoidance of stress were the main strategies. The late Alvan Barach ushered in the second era of pulmonary rehabilitation, pioneering a more active approach that stressed a progressive increase in the patient's level of activity. The last 30 years have seen widespread application of this approach, with trained therapists interacting with patient groups in a supportive environment.

The third era promises to see the extensive multidisciplinary application of scientific principles to the therapy of lung disease patients. The art and the science of pulmonary rehabilitation will harmonize, and the empiric approach will be replaced by modes of therapy that are calibrated to benefit the individual patient.

A major purpose of this book is to facilitate a transition to a scientific basis for pulmonary rehabilitation. It is intended not only to convey a sense of the current status of pulmonary rehabilitation, but also to point out those areas that need further study. The authors of this book are among the vanguard of those fostering this approach. Most are actively conducting research in this field. We hope that the readers of this book will be encouraged to participate in the emergence of improved rehabilitative programs. Our target audience is broad. Pulmonologists directing rehabilitative programs and pulmonologists in training are this work's most natural audience. Researchers in specialized aspects of pulmonary rehabilitation should find the multidisciplinary approach broadening. Finally, a new generation of rehabilitation therapists is needed to apply this emerging approach to patient care; this volume should help in their education and serve as a practical reference.

This book is divided into four parts. Part I explores the causes of lung disease and the impact of lung disease on the body's function. Applied pulmonary pathophysiology is, of course, a major focus. However, several other organ systems are also affected, and separate consideration of ventilatory control as well as of respiratory muscle, cardiovascular, and neuropsychiatric function is provided. The genesis of the mysterious sensation of dyspnea and its contribution to disability is explored. Lung disease predisposes to respiratory failure, exercise intolerance, and sleep abnormalities; these problems are also addressed individually. Finally, the current state of knowledge concerning the factors that determine the prognosis of both obstructive and restrictive lung diseases is described.

In Part II, established and emerging modes of therapy are explored. Controversial aspects are examined, and areas for future research are identified. Therapy aimed at bronchodilation, the control of secretions, and the decrease of the inflammatory response is reviewed. The scientific basis of chest physical therapy and breathing retraining is defined. Long-term oxygen therapy has demonstrated benefits; however, since its financial costs are substantial, finding the proper indications for oxygen therapy is an important pursuit. The current controversy concerning the value of achieving a physiologic training response of either the muscles of respiration or the muscles of ambulation is addressed. Techniques specifically designed to desensitize the patient to the sensation of dyspnea have only recently begun to be systematically evaluated. Long-term disability leads to depression, and programs of psychologic and pharmacologic treatment are often indicated. The special problems of the patient who requires nocturnal or around-the-clock ventilator support are considered. Smoking cessation is often considered a prerequisite of pulmonary rehabilitation; therefore, the scientific basis of smoking cessation programs is discussed.

Part III of this book explores practical aspects of conducting a multidisciplinary pulmonary rehabilitation program. A well-organized program and good criteria for candidate selection are necessary ingredients for a successful program. Preprogram patient evaluation, including both clinical (history and physical examination) and laboratory (pulmonary function, radiologic, blood gas, and exercise testing) aspects are important in individualizing therapy. The methods used by the rehabilitation team for exercise, nutritional, psychosocial, and sexual therapy are discussed in detail. Therapeutic considerations for the rehabilitation candidate with end-stage disease are considered. The role of continuing care programs in maintaining the benefits of rehabilitation is analyzed. The results of pulmonary rehabilitation are explored, both with regard to the benefits that accrue to the individual patient and with regard to its impact on the health care delivery system.

In Part IV, we attempt to provide the reader with guidelines for individualizing therapy for patients with less typical manifestations of lung disease. These patients become better candidates for pulmonary rehabilitation if their requirements are better understood. Restrictive disease, asthma, and cystic fibrosis are discussed. Only recently have we begun to consider rehabilitation for patients who undergo lung transplantation. We also attempt to define strategies for dealing with the ventilator-dependent patient. Finally, in Part V we describe how pulmonary rehabilitation programs function in specific environments and the innovative ways in which they are funded.

It is our firm conviction that pulmonary rehabilitation should be the standard of care for most patients with debilitating pulmonary disease. We hope that this book will give the reader new insight into the rationale, details, and practices of pulmonary rehabilitation and that this new vision will in turn aid more of the millions who desperately need this care.

Richard Casaburi, Ph.D., M.D.
Thomas L. Petty, M.D.

Acknowledgments

We would like to thank Judy Fletcher, Editor at W.B. Saunders Co., and her staff for shepherding this project from its conception to its completion. Bill Preston in Production and Frank Messina in Editing and their staffs did an outstanding job in editing and typesetting the text.

Mrs. Maclovia Wallace contributed expert secretarial support for Dr. Casaburi, facilitating the large volume of correspondence needed for this project. Mrs. Kay Bowen assisted Dr. Petty in his writing and editing.

Finally, we acknowledge the enthusiasm, ideas, and expertise that all of the chapter authors contributed to this undertaking.

Contents

CHAPTER ONE
Pulmonary Rehabilitation: A Personal Historical Perspective 1
THOMAS L. PETTY, M.D.

1 Causes and Consequences of Chronic Pulmonary Disease

CHAPTER TWO
Epidemiology of Obstructive Pulmonary Disease 10
MILLICENT HIGGINS, M.D., D.P.H.

CHAPTER THREE
Pathophysiology of Chronic Obstructive Pulmonary Disease with Emphasis on
Physiologic and Pathologic Correlations 18
THOMAS CORBRIDGE, M.D., AND CHARLES G. IRVIN, Ph.D.

CHAPTER FOUR
Respiratory Muscle Function in Chronic Obstructive Pulmonary Disease 33
ANDRÉ DE TROYER, M.D., Ph.D.

CHAPTER FIVE
Ventilatory Control in Lung Disease 50
THOMAS J. BARSTOW, Ph.D., AND RICHARD CASABURI, Ph.D., M.D.

CHAPTER SIX
Cardiovascular Consequences of Chronic Obstructive Pulmonary Disease 66
DOUGLASS A. MORRISON, M.D., F.A.C.C., AND BRAM D. ZUCKERMAN, M.D.

CHAPTER SEVEN
Neurocognitive Aspects of Chronic Obstructive Pulmonary Disease 79
SEAN B. ROURKE, B.Sc., Hons. B.A., IGOR GRANT, M.D., AND ROBERT K. HEATON, Ph.D.

CHAPTER EIGHT
Sleep Disordered Breathing 92
NEIL J. DOUGLAS, M.D., F.R.C.P.E.

CHAPTER NINE
Dyspnea: Implications for Rehabilitation 103
KIERAN J. KILLIAN, M.D., F.R.C.P.(C)

CHAPTER TEN
Exercise Tolerance in the Pulmonary Patient 115
KARLMAN WASSERMAN, M.D., Ph.D.

CHAPTER ELEVEN
Acute and Chronic Respiratory Failure 124
THOMAS K. ALDRICH, M.D.

CHAPTER TWELVE
Course and Prognosis in Patients with Chronic Airflow Obstruction: Possible Implications
for Therapy 138
DIRKJE S. POSTMA, M.D., GERARD H. KOËTER, M.D., AND PETER J. WIJKSTRA, M.D.

2   Therapeutic Modalities in Pulmonary Rehabilitation

CHAPTER THIRTEEN
Pharmacologic Therapy 152
MICHAEL W. OWENS, M.D., WILLIAM M. ANDERSON, M.D., AND RONALD B. GEORGE, M.D.

CHAPTER FOURTEEN
Controlled Breathing Techniques and Chest Physical Therapy in Chronic Obstructive
Pulmonary Disease and Allied Conditions 167
L. JACK FALING, M.D.

CHAPTER FIFTEEN
Long-term Oxygen Therapy 183
CHRISTOPHER B. COOPER, M.D.

CHAPTER SIXTEEN
Exercise Training in Chronic Obstructive Lung Disease 204
RICHARD CASABURI, Ph.D., M.D.

CHAPTER SEVENTEEN
Ventilatory Muscle Training and Unloading 225
MICHAEL J. BELMAN, M.D.

CHAPTER EIGHTEEN
Desensitization to Dyspnea in Chronic Obstructive Pulmonary Disease 241
FRANCOIS HAAS, Ph.D., JOHN SALAZAR-SCHICCHI, M.D., AND KENNETH AXEN, Ph.D.

CHAPTER NINETEEN
Psychobiologic Evaluation and Rehabilitation in Pulmonary Disease 252
DONALD L. DUDLEY, M.D., AND JUDITH SITZMAN, R.N., D.N.Sc., Ph.D.

CHAPTER TWENTY
Home Ventilator Care 274
DAVID J. PIERSON, M.D., AND ROBERT M. KACMAREK, Ph.D., R.R.T.

CHAPTER TWENTY-ONE
Nicotine Addiction Treatment 289
LOUISE M. NETT, R.N., R.R.T.

3 Components of the Pulmonary Rehabilitation Program

CHAPTER TWENTY-TWO
Pulmonary Rehabilitation Program Organization 302
BRIAN L. TIEP, M.D.

CHAPTER TWENTY-THREE
Candidate Evaluation 317
ROGER S. GOLDSTEIN, M.B., Ch.B., F.R.C.P.(C), F.R.C.P.(UK), F.C.C.P.,
AND MONICA A. AVENDANO, M.D., F.R.C.P.(C)

CHAPTER TWENTY-FOUR
Exercise Prescription 322
ANTONIO PATESSIO, M.D., FRANCESCO IOLO, M.D.,
AND CLAUDIO FERDINANDO DONNER, M.D., F.C.C.P.

CHAPTER TWENTY-FIVE
Nutritional Assessment and Therapy 336
JULIET M. MANCINO, M.S., R.D., MICHAEL DONAHOE, M.D., AND ROBERT M. ROGERS, M.D.

CHAPTER TWENTY-SIX
Psychosocial Issues in the Rehabilitation of Patients with Chronic Obstructive Pulmonary
Disease 351
ROBERT M. KAPLAN, Ph.D., ELIZABETH G. EAKIN, B.A., AND ANDREW L. RIES, M.D., M.P.H.

CHAPTER TWENTY-SEVEN
Relaxation and Biofeedback: Coping Skills Training 366
ANNE JERMAN, R.N., M.S., C.S., AND MARGARET CAMPBELL HAGGERTY, R.N.C., M.S.N.

CHAPTER TWENTY-EIGHT
Sexuality and the Patient with Lung Disease 382
PAUL A. SELECKY, M.D.

CHAPTER TWENTY-NINE
Chronic Obstructive Pulmonary Disease: Treatment of Advanced Stages of Disease 392
THOMAS L. PETTY, M.D.

CHAPTER THIRTY
Continuing Care Programs 398
MARY BURNS, R.N., B.S.

CHAPTER THIRTY-ONE
Evaluating the Results of Pulmonary Rehabilitation Treatment 405
CHRISTOPHER J. CLARK, M.D., F.R.C.P.

4 Special Considerations in Pulmonary Rehabilitation

CHAPTER THIRTY-TWO
Rehabilitation of Patients with Chronic Ventilatory Limitation from Nonobstructive Lung Diseases 416
RICHARD S. NOVITCH, M.D., AND HENRY M. THOMAS III, M.D.

CHAPTER THIRTY-THREE
The Role of Physical Training in Asthma 424
CHRISTOPHER J. CLARK, M.D., F.R.C.P.

CHAPTER THIRTY-FOUR
Cystic Fibrosis 439
DAVID M. ORENSTEIN, M.D., AND BLAKESLEE E. NOYES, M.D.

CHAPTER THIRTY-FIVE
Pulmonary Rehabilitation Before and After Lung Transplantation 459
DOROTHY G. BIGGAR, M.S.N., R.N., JILL FELDMAN MALEN, M.S., N.S., R.N., E. P. TRULOCK, M.D., AND JOEL D. COOPER, M.D.

CHAPTER THIRTY-SIX
The Ventilator-Dependent Patient 468
THOMAS L. PETTY, M.D.

5 Special Environments for Pulmonary Rehabilitation, and Aspects of Care Reimbursement

CHAPTER THIRTY-SEVEN
A Storefront Program for Pulmonary Rehabilitation 474
JUDITH A. TIETSORT, R.N., R.R.T.

CHAPTER THIRTY-EIGHT
The Proprietary Pulmonary Rehabilitation Program 478
FRANK D. SUTTON, M.D.

CHAPTER THIRTY-NINE
How the Office-based Pulmonary Rehabilitation Program Works 483
HOWARD M. KRAVETZ, M.D., F.C.C.P.

CHAPTER FORTY
Reimbursement for a Community Hospital-Based Program **487**
R. WAYNE MALL, M.D., AND MARGARET CHAIKA-MEDEIROS, R.C.P.

INDEX **495**

Chapter 1

Pulmonary Rehabilitation: A Personal Historical Perspective

THOMAS L. PETTY, M.D.

Pulmonary rehabilitation is the art and method of systematized, multidisciplinary care. It is now established as beneficial in the management of large numbers of patients with advanced chronic obstructive pulmonary disease (COPD). The purpose of this perspective is to trace some of the origins of the present practices of pulmonary rehabilitation.

The roots of pulmonary rehabilitation extend back to the period when tuberculosis was quite prevalent before the turn of this century. Figures 1–1 and 1–2, reproduced from a monograph by the pioneer Denver pulmonologist Dr. Charles L. Denison, for whom the University of Colorado Health Sciences Center Library is named, begin to tell the story. A systematic program of exercise for pulmonary invalids suffering from the residual effects of tuberculosis and a crude approach to breathing exercises are cited in the 1895 monograph. Earlier, Denison had left his home in Hartford, Connecticut, because he was suffering from pulmonary hemorrhages. After a brief sojourn in Texas, he moved to Colorado to initiate climate therapy for his tuberculosis, from which he eventually recovered. During his recuperation, he noticed a feeling of well-being whenever he exercised. He also recognized the value of good nutrition to help combat the ravages of tuberculosis and the resultant respiratory insufficiency. His first book, *Rocky Mountain Health Resorts, an Analytical Study of Chronic Pulmonary Disease,* was published in Boston in 1880.

Two of the greatest pioneers and, indeed, true heroes in the field of pulmonary rehabilitation in the 20th century were the late Dr. Alvan Barach of New York (Fig. 1–3) and Dr. Albert Haas, who is now retired but who also did his pioneering work in New York (Fig. 1–4). Barach was fascinated by dyspnea. This was largely because of the fact that his mother suffered episodic dyspnea due to laryngeal spasm. Barach discovered that the "leaning forward posture" relieved dyspnea. He also learned that breathing training, including pursed-lip breathing and certain other breathing exercises, could improve exercise tolerance in patients with advanced stages of emphysema.[1-5] Barach was also the first in this country to recognize the value of ambulatory oxygen therapy.[4] J. E. Cotes independently pioneered the use of portable oxygen supplies for the treatment of advanced respiratory insufficiency in the United Kingdom at the same time.[6] I had the pleasure of knowing Dr. Barach for nearly 20 years, and during that time we had many warm and friendly visits together in New York. I dedicated the first edition of my book, *Dedication in COPD,* to Dr. Barach following his death in 1977.[7] This book contained his last writings on "Physiotherapy of Advanced Disease States" (Chapter 5) and "Adaptive Function of Hypercapnia" (Chapter 6). They continue to serve as excellent resources for the contemporary student of pulmonary rehabilitation.

As with Denison, Haas's interest in rehabilitation can be traced to his own tuberculosis, which he first contracted in 1932 during his medical school training in Budapest. Although standard convalescent treatment of the era required months or years of prolonged inactivity and bed rest and included exposure to fresh air and a good diet, the boredom that resulted from this treatment became intolerable for Haas. He asked to return to his medical studies, and his family brought him his books. He observed that lifting and carrying his heaviest books did not tire him, and he began to recognize that physical

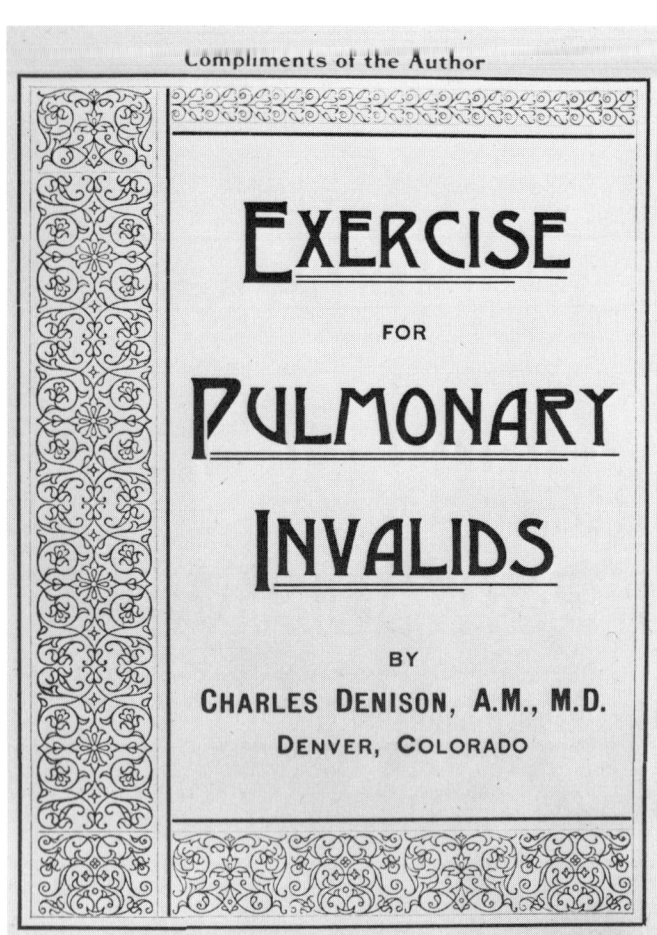

FIGURE 1–1. A monograph entitled *Exercise for Pulmonary Invalids* authored by Dr. Charles Denison in 1895.

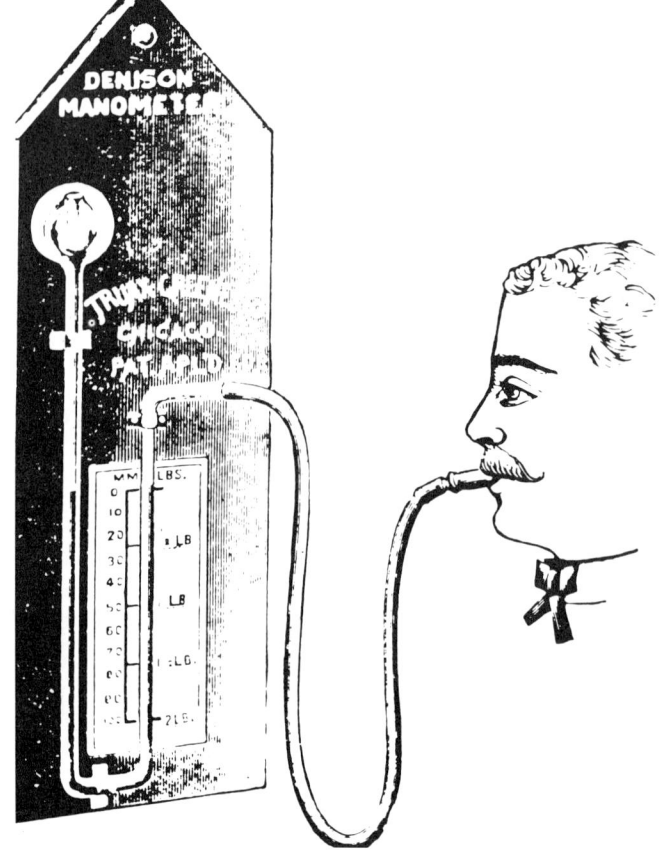

FIGURE 1–2. An illustration of a crude approach to breathing exercises appearing in Dr. Denison's book is shown.

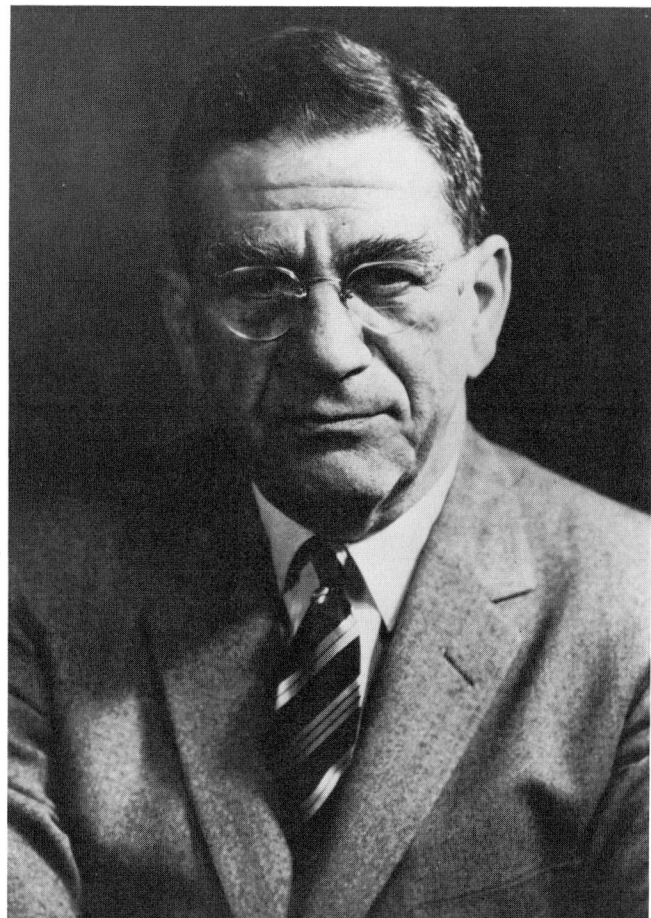

FIGURE 1-3. A photograph of the late Dr. Alvan Barach of New York.

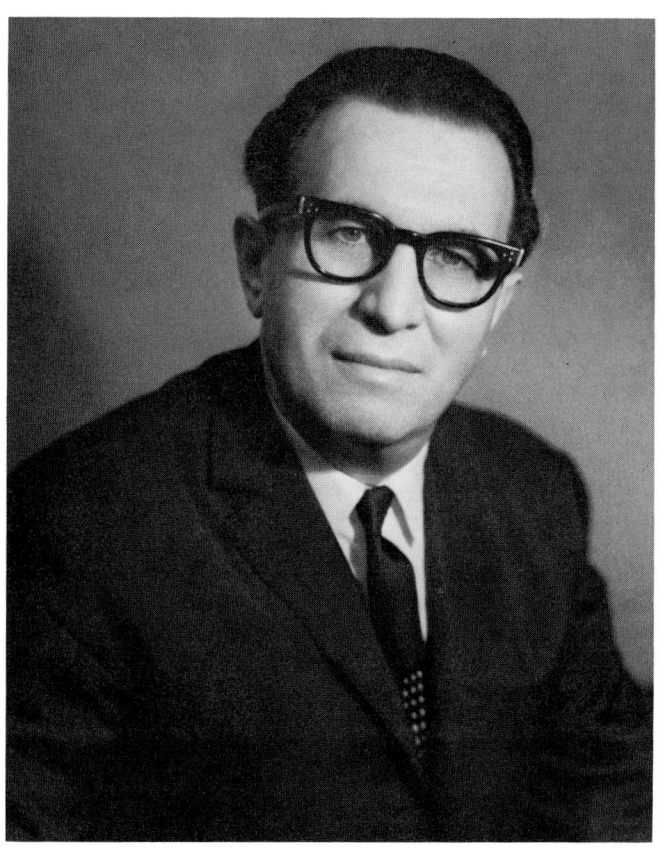

FIGURE 1-4. A photograph of Dr. Albert Haas, who is still living in New York. Dr. Haas and Dr. Oscar Balchum were Cochairmen of the Human Interaction Research Institute Conference in 1968.

activity was associated with weight gain and a feeling of well-being. He hypothesized that at least in his case exercise was good, not harmful. After immigrating to this country, Haas designed breathing exercises to deal with the pain and physical limitations of thoracoplasty, which was the first effective form of surgical collapse therapy for tuberculosis. Still later, Haas realized that breathing exercises were helpful for other tuberculosis patients and not just those who had undergone thoracoplasty. Later, Haas began to work with emphysema patients at the Rusk Institute in New York.[3, 8] Thus, Haas, along with Barach, were early contributors to a growing body of clinical observations and science that laid the groundwork for the pulmonary rehabilitation programs that followed.

Dr. William F. Miller, who still practices in Dallas, applied many of Barach's techniques to his own innovations and was an earlier contributor to the study of oxygen use during exercise in patients with advanced COPD.[9]

The Eighth Aspen Emphysema Conference (now known as the Thomas L. Petty Aspen Lung Conference) was the first to deal with evolving methods of treatment for advanced COPD.[10] The previous seven conferences had addressed only the scientific basis of emphysema and related disorders. I was concerned that there had never been a conference on treatment, and my mentor Dr. Roger Mitchell provided me the first major opportunity of my budding academic career by asking me to organize and chair a conference on the therapy of advanced COPD. The mid-1960s was the era of the intensive care unit, and pulmonary care specialists were learning new methods of ventilator applications. This was also the year that we began our oxygen studies in patients with advanced COPD and hypoxemia, the first of which was published in 1967.[11] Many leaders participated in the Eighth Conference, including William F. Miller of Dallas, Ben V. Branscomb of Birmingham, and Reuben Cherniack, at that time of Winnipeg, Canada. Theodore Noehren (now retired in Salt Lake City) was the summarizer of the conference. Everyone left this conference thrilled over the possibilities of improving the length and quality of life of emphysema patients by using various modalities of therapy that included the systematic application of pharmacologic therapy, oxygen therapy in selected patients, mechanical ventilation for acute respiratory failure, and home care for patients with the most advanced disease. In fact, we were so excited about the possibilities of studying the outcome of systematized care for chronic respiratory patients that we applied for and received a contract to develop a research-oriented pulmonary rehabilitation program funded by the Chronic Respiratory Disease Control Program of the Public Health Service. Two pilot projects were funded, one in Denver and one in Minneapolis, under the direction of the late Sumner Cohen. The purpose of these two demonstration projects was to learn the outcome of what was defined as "comprehensive and rehabilitative care." At that time, our developing approach to pulmonary rehabilitation included patient and family education, certain pharmacologic strategies, breathing retraining, physical reconditioning, and oxygen therapy in selected patients. Our program began in May of 1966, and between May of 1966 and March of 1968 182 consecutive patients were enrolled.[12] This series of patients has been followed to the present, and numerous reports on them have formed the basis of extensive additional studies by many investigators.

Probably the most important stimulus for the expanded development and instruction of concepts concerning comprehensive care for respiratory patients came from the Human Interaction Research Institute, directed by Edward Glaser of Los Angeles. In 1967, Glaser (Fig. 1–5) visited our group in Denver and proposed a conference that was intended to bring together as many of the major contributors in the field as possible. The cochairmen of this unique conference were Oscar Balchum of Los Angeles (Fig. 1–6) and Albert Haas of New York. The participants, along with myself, included Ben V. Branscomb of Birmingham, Donald L. Dudley (a psychiatrist from Seattle), Edward Glaser (president of the Human Interaction Committee), John Hodgkin (chief of the Pulmonary Section at Loma Linda Hospital, Loma Linda, California), Irving Kass (chief of the Pulmonary Section at the University of Nebraska Hospital, Nebraska and a recipient of a major grant from Social Services of the Public Health Service to study pulmonary rehabilitation), Phil Kimbel (chief of the Pulmonary Disease Center at Albert Einstein Medical Center, Philadelphia), William F. Miller (a professor and the director of the Pulmonary Division at Methodist Hospital of Dallas), Louise M. Nett (a respiratory care nurse specialist from Denver), Harold S. Novey (chief of the Allergy and Immunology Section at Orange County Medical Center, Anaheim, California), and D. Barry Shaw of the Eisenhower Medical Center, Palm Springs, California. After a 2-day interactive session, we decided to develop an up-to-date document intended to reflect "the consensus of well-informed researchers and practitioners." A report, "A Pilot Study to Determine the Feasibility of Promoting the Use of Systematized Care Program for Patients With Chronic Obstructive Pulmonary Disease," was published by the Public Health Service of the Department of Health, Education, and Welfare in that same year.[13] Key participants in the conference were encouraged by Edward Glaser to undertake a revision and further development of this consensus concept. Numerous writing sessions and revisions of a paper intended to be submitted to the *Journal of the American Medical Association (JAMA)* followed. Since the fifth draft, John E. Hodgkin served as editor, synthesizer, and integrator of the advice and suggestions that were received from 29 other contributors. Finally, an up-to-date paper on COPD was published in the *JAMA* in 1975.[14] This comprehensive article contained an explicit invitation from the authors for additional feedback from its readers. Approximately 8500 reprints of this paper were requested.

Many valuable suggestions and criticisms were received following publication of the *JAMA* article. Many of those who replied suggested the preparation of an even more comprehensive document that could best address the additional concerns of primary care physicians. Accordingly, following the publication of the

FIGURE 1–5. A photograph of Dr. Edward Glaser of Pasadena. Dr. Glaser was the organizer of the Human Interaction Research Institute Conference in 1968.

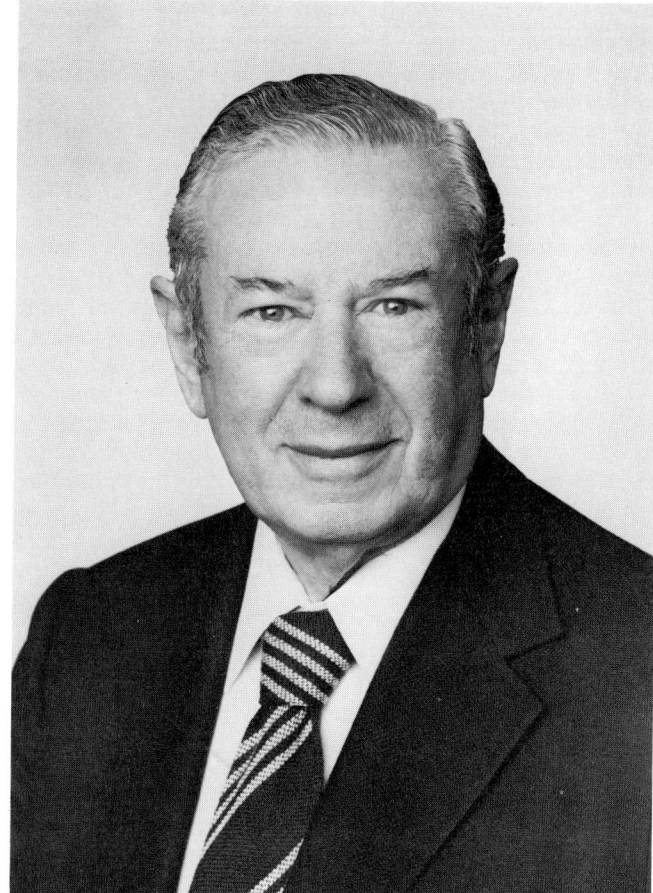

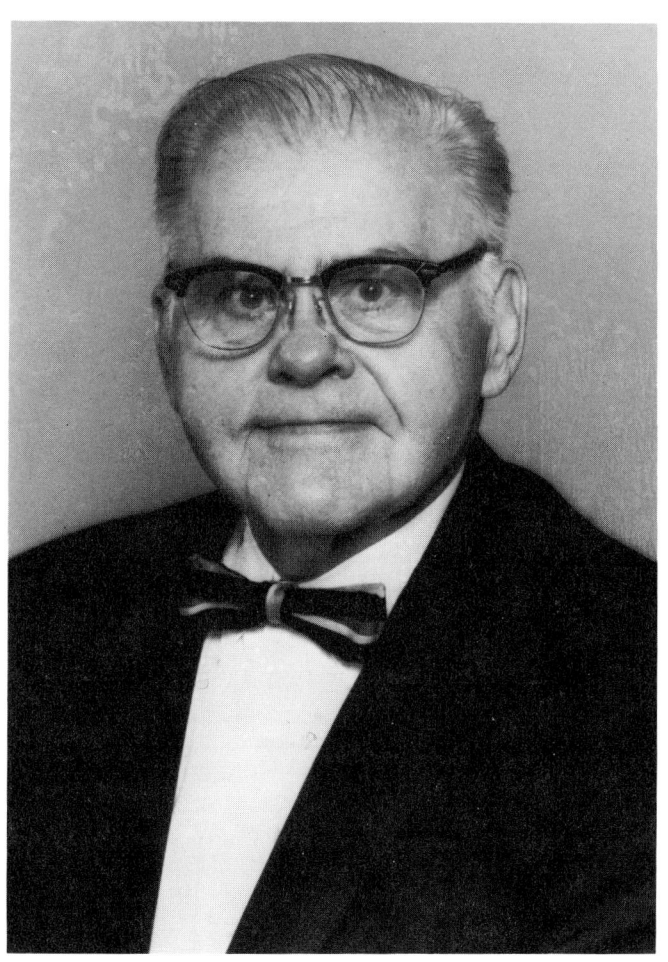

FIGURE 1–6. A photograph of Dr. Oscar Balchum of Los Angeles. Dr. Balchum was Cochairman of the Human Interaction Research Institute Conference in 1968 along with Dr. Albert Haas.

JAMA paper, the team began to work on a definitive monograph that would include the further suggestions and criticisms received concerning the most recent advances in the field. John E. Hodgkin led this writing committee as well, and, finally, a full-length monograph was published in 1979 by the American College of Chest Physicians.[15] This organization distributed nearly 10,000 copies of this monograph, which was very well received.

From 1969 to 1978 I had the privilege of being chairman of the Pulmonary Rehabilitation Committee of the American College of Chest Physicians. From 1969 to 1974, this Committee worked on a definition of pulmonary rehabilitation as well as the presentation of various scientific studies. The final statement of this Committee, made in 1974, was as follows: "Pulmonary rehabilitation is 'an art of medical practice wherein an individually tailored, multidisciplinary program is formulated which, through accurate diagnosis, therapy, emotional support, and education, stabilizes or reverses both the physiology and psychopathology of pulmonary disease and attempts to return the patient to the highest possible function level allowed by his pulmonary handicap and overall life situation.'" This definition has become the standard for pulmonary rehabilitation therapy. Another statement from the Intersociety Commission on Heart Disease Resources addressing pulmonary rehabilitation was also published in 1974.[16]

Two additional major stimuli for the study of pulmonary rehabilitation were provided by conferences sponsored by the National Heart, Lung, and Blood Institute. The first, the Conference on the Scientific Basis of Respiratory Therapy, was held in Sugarloaf, Pennsylvania, from May 2 to 4, 1974. This conference considered the scientific basis for oxygen therapy, aerosol therapy, physical therapy, and intermittent positive-pressure breathing. *The Conference Report,* published as a supplement in the *American Review of Respiratory Diseases* in December of that year, summarized the scientific basis for much of what is done in the field of pulmonary rehabilitation.[17] A second conference on the scientific basis of inpatient therapy was held in Atlanta, Georgia, from November 14 to 16th, 1979.[18] Pulmonary rehabilitation was specifically addressed at this conference. On that occasion, I had the privilege of reporting 8 years of survival data from our pulmonary rehabilitation program as compared with the survival data of patients with similar degrees of emphysema in the Denver metropolitan area who had not participated in a rehabilitation program. Although this was by no means a randomized, controlled clinical trial, the survival curves (Fig. 1–7) suggested that a small survival benefit could be attained from pulmonary rehabilitation.

Another crucial stimulus for pulmonary rehabilitation came from the Nocturnal Oxygen Therapy Trial pub-

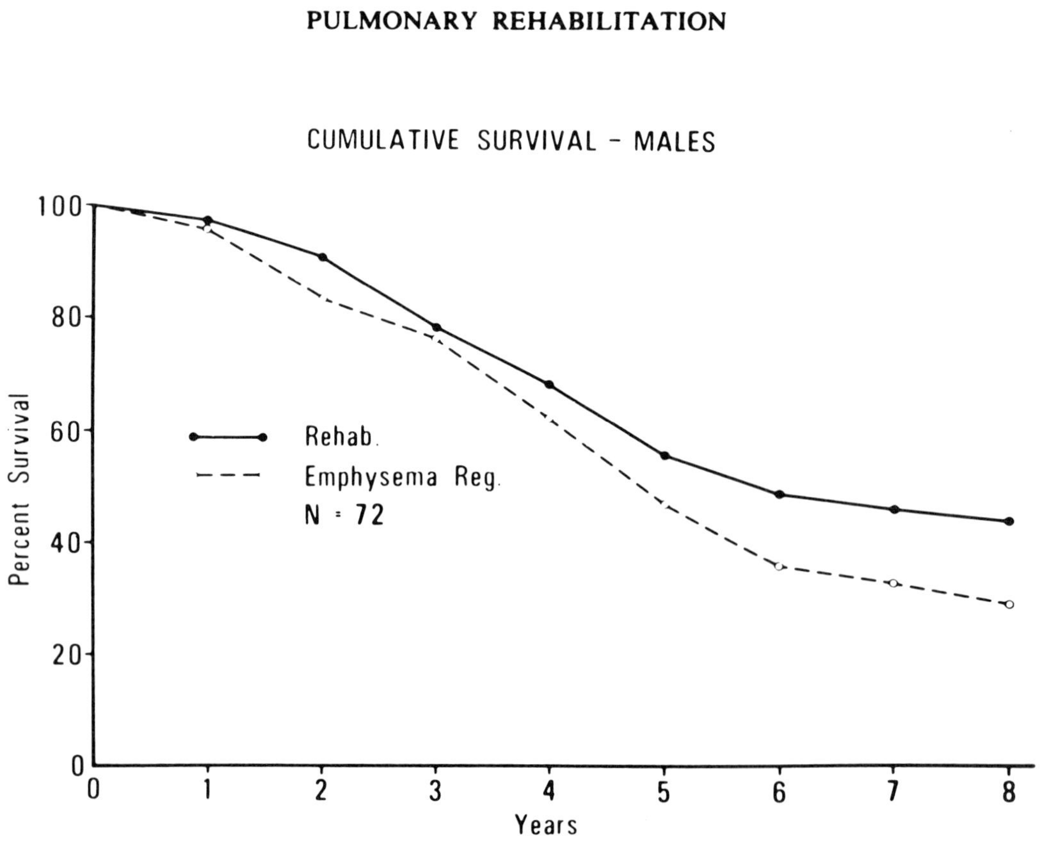

PULMONARY REHABILITATION

FIGURE 1–7. This graph suggests an improved survival rate for males receiving pulmonary rehabilitation in the Colorado program compared with that for matched patients included in an emphysema registry. (Reproduced from Glaser EM. A pilot study to determine the feasibility of promoting the use of a systematized care program for patients with chronic obstructive pulmonary disease. Final report, Social and Rehabilitation Services, Department of Health, Education, and Welfare. Project No. RD-2571-6-67. Los Angeles Human Interaction Research Institute, 1968.)

lished more than a decade ago.[19] This study, which was proposed at the Sugarloaf conference, was the first rigorous controlled clinical trial of the application of ambulatory versus stationary oxygen in patients with advanced COPD and chronic stable hypoxemia. Almost simultaneously a second study was being conducted by the British Medical Research Council that compared the administration of oxygen 15 hours per day with no oxygen supplementation in similar patients with advanced COPD.[20] Systematized therapy was given to all participants in the Nocturnal Oxygen Therapy Trial. All patients received education about their disease, were encouraged to exercise, and received systemic pharmacologic therapy. Participation in the study also provided the patients with a certain degree of social support. The outcome of the Nocturnal Oxygen Therapy Trial showed that patients who received continuous oxygen (approximately 19.4 h/day) had a far better survival rate than those patients who only received stationary oxygen therapy for approximately 12 hours per day (including during the hours of sleep). The companion Medical Research Council Study showed a very poor survival rate in advanced COPD patients with hypoxemia and cor pulmonale who received no oxygen; a much better survival rate was observed in those patients who received oxygen approximately 15 hours per day (including during the hours of sleep). Since the background factors in these patients were similar, it is possible to compare outcomes. Survival rates in advanced COPD are poor when oxygen is not administered and when chronic stable hypoxemia is present. Survival rates are better when some oxygen is administered (e.g., 12–15 h/day from a stationary source), but the survival rate is far better in patients who receive nearly continuous oxygen therapy from an ambulatory source (see Chapter 15).

Although the Nocturnal Oxygen Therapy Trial and the Medical Research Council Study focused on oxygen as a major therapeutic variable, these studies were performed against a background of comprehensive ancillary care. Thus, these studies gave further momentum to the emerging concept that systematized care, including the use of oxygen in selected patients, could improve survival in advanced COPD.

Two international conferences, the first World Congress on Oxygen Therapy and Home Care (February 1987) and the first International Conference on Pulmonary Rehabilitation and Home Mechanical Ventilation (March 1988), brought together pulmonologists, respiratory therapists, and other researchers from more than 20 countries to consider newer developments in respiratory care. Nearly 1000 participants attended each of these Denver conferences, which I had the privilege of organizing, along with my colleagues and my friend, the late David Flenley of Edinburgh, Scotland. Together we were the summarizers of these two landmark conferences. Numerous exhibitors from the pulmonary healthcare industry were also present. These major events are cited because they also contributed to the dissemination of knowledge and enthusiasm concerning pulmonary rehabilitation around the world.

Three books should be cited as summarizing the newest developments of pulmonary rehabilitation in the 1980s. *Pulmonary Rehabilitation from Hospital to Home* by Jerry O'Ryan and Donald G. Burns (Year Book Medical Publishers, Inc., Chicago, 1984) and *Pulmonary Rehabilitation (Guidelines to Success)* by John E. Hodgkin, Ellen G. Zorn, and Gwenolyn Connors (Butterworth's, London, 1984) provided the most recent information available at that time. Finally, John E. Hodgkin and I updated the Human Interaction Research Institute consensus document originally published by the American College of Chest Physicians. The resultant book, *Chronic Obstructive Pulmonary Disease: Current Concepts* (W.B. Saunders Co., Philadelphia, 1987), represented the latest update of our knowledge in the mid-1980s.

In the years that have followed, pulmonary rehabilitation has become widely accepted in many community hospitals. Indeed, the California Thoracic Society has recently issued the following statement: "A program of rehabilitation has become an important part of the care for many patients with debilitating chronic pulmonary disease." The history of pulmonary rehabilitation is fascinating. It has been a rich experience to participate in some of the various developments that have led to the present state of our understanding of the scientific basis for pulmonary rehabilitation and its many applications. It is my hope that the chapters that follow will set the stage for further advancement in our knowledge of the methods in pulmonary rehabilitation and in their improved application on behalf of the millions of patients who require more comprehensive care than they are currently receiving.

REFERENCES

1. Barach AL. Principles and Practices of Inhalational Therapy. Philadelphia: J.B. Lippincott Co., 1944.
2. Barach AL. Physiologic Therapy in Respiratory Diseases. Philadelphia: J.B. Lippincott Co., 1958.
3. Barach AL. Breathing exercises in pulmonary emphysema and allied chronic respiratory disease. Arch Phys Med Rehabil 1955; 36:379–390.
4. Barach AL. Ambulatory oxygen therapy: Oxygen inhalation at home and out of doors. Dis Chest 1957; 35:229–241.
5. Barach AL. A Treatment Manual for Patients with Emphysema. New York: Grune & Stratton, Inc., 1969.
6. Cotes JE, Gilson JC. Effect of oxygen in exercise ability in chronic respiratory insufficiency: Use of a portable apparatus. Lancet 1956; 1:822–876.
7. Petty TL (ed). Dedication in COPD. New York: Marcel Dekker, Inc., 1978.
8. Haas A, Cardon H. Rehabilitation in chronic obstructive pulmonary disease: A five-year study of 252 male patients. Med Clin North Am 1969; 53:593–606.
9. Miller WF. Rehabilitation of patients with chronic obstructive lung disease. Med Clin North Am 1967; 51:349–361.
10. Petty TL (ed). Principles of management of chronic obstructive lung diseases. In: Proceedings of the Eighth Aspen Emphysema Conference. Washington, DC, 1966. U.S. Department of Health, Education, and Welfare publication (PHS) 1457.
11. Levine BE, Bigelow PB, Hamstra RP, et al. The role of long-term continuous oxygen administration in patients with chronic airway obstruction with hypoxemia. Ann Intern Med 1967; 66:639–650.
12. Petty TL, Nett LM, Finigan MM, et al. A comprehensive care

program for chronic airway obstruction: Methods and preliminary evaluation of symptomatic and functional improvement. Ann Intern Med 1969; 70:1109–1120.
13. Glaser EM. A pilot study to determine the feasibility of promoting the use of a systematized care program for patients with chronic obstructive pulmonary disease. Final Report. Los Angeles Human Interaction Research Institute; 1968. Social and Rehabilitation Service, Department of Health, Education, and Welfare. Project RD–2571–6–67.
14. Hodgkin JE, Balchum OJ, Kass I, et al. Chronic obstructive airway diseases: Current concepts in diagnosis and comprehensive care. JAMA 1975; 232:1243–1260.
15. Hodgkin JE (ed). Chronic Obstructive Pulmonary Disease: Current concepts in Diagnosis and Comprehensive Care. Park Ridge, IL: American College of Chest Physicians, 1979.
16. Intersociety Commission on Heart Disease (Petty TL, Chairman). Pulmonary Rehabilitation Study Group. Community resources for rehabilitation of patients with chronic obstructive pulmonary disease and cor pulmonale. Circulation 1974; 49(Suppl 1):A1–A20.
17. Proceedings of the Conference on the Scientific Basis of Respiratory Therapy. Am Rev Respir Dis 1974; 110(Suppl):1–202.
18. Proceedings of the Conference on the Scientific Basis of In-Hospital Respiratory Therapy. Am Rev Respir Dis 1980; 122(Suppl):1–161.
19. Nocturnal Oxygen Therapy Trial Group: Continuous or nocturnal oxygen therapy in hypoxemic chronic obstructive lung disease. A clinical trial. Ann Intern Med 1980; 93:391–398.
20. Report of the Medical Research Council Working Party: Long-term domiciliary oxygen therapy in chronic hypoxic cor pulmonale complicating chronic bronchitis and emphysema. Lancet 1981; 1:681–685.

1

Causes and Consequences of Chronic Pulmonary Disease

Chapter 2

Epidemiology of Obstructive Pulmonary Disease

MILLICENT HIGGINS, M.D., D.P.H.

Chronic obstructive pulmonary diseases (COPDs) and allied conditions command attention as the fifth leading cause of death and as a major cause of morbidity and disability in the United States. Between 1979 and 1989, the number of deaths attributed to COPD and allied conditions increased from 49,933 to 84,350 (a 69% increase), and the death rate increased from 22.3 to 34.0 per hundred thousand (a 52% increase). Growth in the total population and increasing life expectancy are partly responsible for these trends, which are projected to continue and to lead to increasing numbers of patients in need of pulmonary rehabilitation.

EPIDEMIOLOGY

The epidemiology of obstructive pulmonary diseases integrates biomedical and demographic information and uses biostatistical techniques to describe, analyze, and interpret data on these conditions in the population. The primary interest of epidemiologists is in making biologic inferences about the causes, natural history, and course of disease and in assessing effects of medical interventions or changes in lifestyle. Descriptive information about the frequency and distribution of disease indicates the magnitude of the problem by age, sex, and race, and socioeconomic, occupational, and other characteristics as well as according to geographic location and over time. In addition to its applications in suggesting or evaluating hypotheses about the determinants of morbidity and mortality, this information is used by clinicians in their management of individual patients. It influences decisions about the use of preventive, diagnostic, and therapeutic procedures that are determined, in part, by the probabilities of the presence of specific diseases as well as by the presenting symptoms, signs, and family history, as well as any harmful behavior or exposure reported by the patient. Epidemiologic data are also used by policy makers, planners, and administrators to set priorities and allocate resources.

In this chapter, the definitions of obstructive pulmonary disease with which the epidemiologist works are considered, and information on the frequency and distribution of morbidity and mortality in the United States, including trends over time, is presented. The risk factors for COPD as well as the predictors of its onset and course, which can be used to identify individual patients at high risk of morbidity and mortality, are also addressed. Strategies to deal with high-risk individuals and approaches aimed at the general population are needed to reduce the burden of obstructive pulmonary disease in the future.

DEFINITION OF OBSTRUCTIVE PULMONARY DISEASE

Imprecise and variable definitions and incomplete ascertainment of obstructive pulmonary diseases have hindered the accurate description of its epidemiology and have impaired recognition and assessment of their determinants. Estimates of morbidity and mortality available from national statistics are based on information recorded on death certificates and medical records by individual physicians (who use their own definitions and diagnostic labels) and on reports made by individ-

TABLE 2–1. MORBIDITY AND MORTALITY FOR COPD AND ASTHMA AMONG THE UNITED STATES POPULATION (248 MILLION) IN 1989*

	ICD/9 Codes	Deaths (Thousands)	Hospitalizations (Thousands)	Physician Office Visits† (Thousands)	Prevalence (Millions)	%
Chronic bronchitis	490, 491	3,720	70	8,220	12.0	4.9
Emphysema	492	15,520	26	430	2.0	0.8
Other chronic airways obstruction	494–496	59,960	133	2,620	—	—
COPD (total)‡	490–492 and 494–496	79,200	229	11,270	—	—
Asthma‡	493	5,150	475	6,500	11.6	4.8
COPD and allied conditions	490–496	84,350	704	17,770	19.6§	8.0§

*Data from World Health Organization. Manual of the International Classification of Diseases, Injuries, and Causes of Death. Geneva, 1977, and Annual Summary of Births, Marriages, Divorces, and Deaths: United States, 1989. Monthly Vital Statistics Report. Hyattsville, MD: National Center for Health Statistics; 1990. US Department of Health and Human Services (PHS). 13(13).
†1985.
‡Estimated direct costs for COPD and asthma equaled $10.4 billion in 1988.
§Estimate for 1983–1985.

uals in response to standard questions. Published mortality data also reflect nosologists' practice of using the World Health Organization's International Classification of Disease (ICD) codes to reflect the physicians' entries on death certificates (Table 2–1).[1,2] Physicians' discharge diagnoses are reflected in the information about hospitalizations, which is also shown in Table 2–1 for first listed diagnoses only.[3] Physicians' office visit reports use the diagnoses made by a variety of practitioners providing primary care.[4] However, prevalence data are based on what individuals report about their own health in response to standard questions asked in the National Health Interview Survey (NHIS).[5] In epidemiologic studies, the definitions in general use are those proposed by the American College of Chest Physicians–American Thoracic Society in 1975.[6] Despite their shortcomings, these definitions permit comparisons to be made within and between studies using the same standardized approaches. Agreement with clinical diagnoses by physicians is not very good.[7] Several efforts at developing newer and better criteria have not proved successful so far.[8] Nevertheless, understanding of the epidemiology, natural history, and course of COPD and asthma has been advanced in recent years. This chapter, therefore, makes use of the data that are available; variations in terminology and diagnostic criteria are mentioned as needed.

FREQUENCY AND DISTRIBUTION

In this chapter, *COPD and allied conditions* is the term used for ICD codes 490–496, whereas unqualified COPD excludes asthma (code 493). Codes 494–496 for other COPDs and allied conditions are the codes for terms used most frequently by physicians in the United States when completing death certificates and hospital discharge records for this group of diseases (see Table 2–1). However, physicians in their offices and patients responding to health interview questions report chronic bronchitis, asthma, and emphysema in decreasing order of frequency. In 1989, there were over 84,000 deaths from COPD and allied conditions and 704,000 hospital discharges for which these conditions were recorded as the primary cause of hospitalization. In 1985, there were 17.5 million physician's office visits, and 19.5 million men and women were estimated to have chronic bronchitis, emphysema, asthma, or more than one of these conditions.[2-6] The frequency with which people report having one, two, or all three conditions is shown in Figure 2–1. The National Heart, Lung and Blood Institute estimates that the direct costs for COPD and asthma amounted to 10.4 billion dollars in 1988.

Death rates by age, sex, and race are shown for COPD in Figure 2–2 and for asthma in Figure 2–3.[9] Death rates for COPD are very low at ages under 45 years but then rise steeply with increasing age, especially among white men for whom the rate at ages 75 to 84 years is 60 times that at ages 45 to 54 years. The rise with age is least for black women, amounting to an 11-

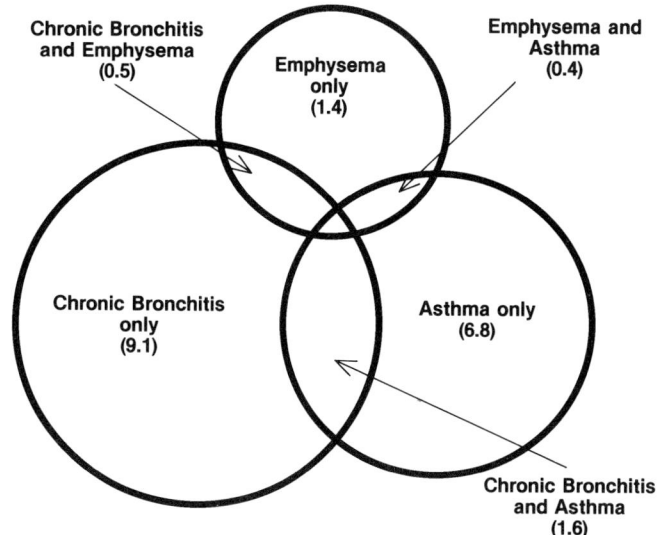

FIGURE 2–1. Estimates of the prevalence of lung disease (in millions of patients). (From the National Health Interview Survey, 1983–1985. National Center for Health Statistics. Unpublished data.)

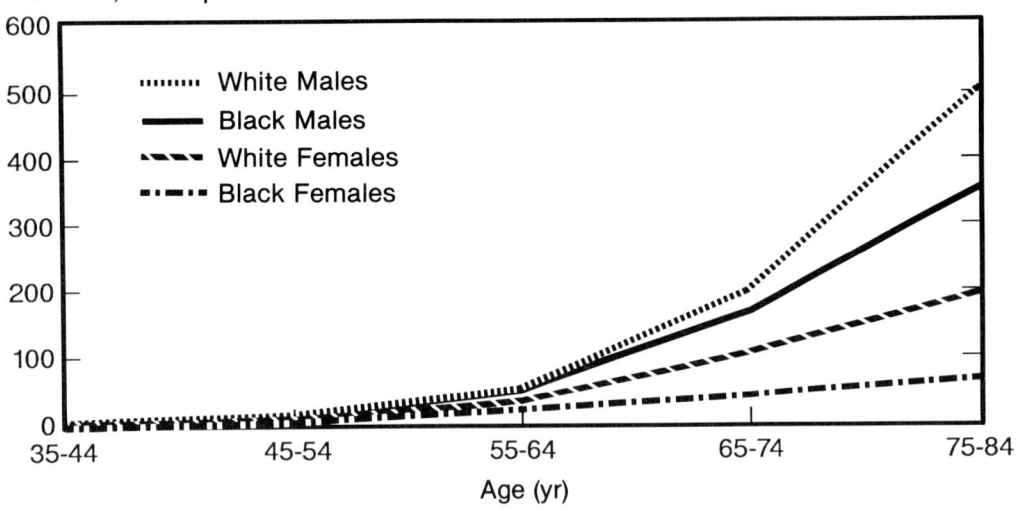

FIGURE 2–2. Death rates for COPD by age, sex, and race in the United States in 1988. (From Vital Statistics of the United States, 1988, Vol 2, Mortality, Part A. Hyattsville, MD: National Center for Health Statistics; 1990. US Department of Health and Human Services publication [PHS] 90-110, pp 490–492, 494–496.)

fold increase between these two age ranges. The death rates for COPD are higher in men than women and higher in white persons than in black persons. The male-to-female ratio is 2.1, and the white-to-black ratio is 1.4 for age-adjusted rates. Death rates for asthma are much lower than those for COPD (1.9 versus 31.8 per 100,000), and the distribution by age, sex, and race is different (Table 2–2). The rise with age is less steep for asthma, and rates are higher in blacks than in whites but are similar in men and women of both races. The ratios of age-adjusted rates for males to females and blacks to whites are 0.8 and 3.2, respectively.

Prevalence rates of chronic bronchitis and asthma based on NHIS data are higher for women than for men, but, as expected, the prevalence of emphysema is higher among males (Table 2–3).[5] Prevalence rates of reported chronic bronchitis and emphysema are higher for whites than for blacks. The reported prevalence of asthma was highest for ages under 45 years in men but increased with age in women; rates were generally higher for the black population than for the white population.[5]

Differences in the distributions for self-reported disease by sex, race, and age compared with those for physician-diagnosed disease and causes of death illustrate some of the problems inherent in using readily available statistics for epidemiologic purposes. Although all the data presented in Table 2–1 are estimates based on representative national samples or on the total population, estimates from people questioned by lay interviewers cannot provide accurate information about COPD, which is poorly and variably defined and which may be asymptomatic or confused with other diseases. The deficit is undoubtedly greater for emphysema and obstructive airways disease than for chronic bronchitis or asthma. Deficiencies in death certificate information are well known, especially for conditions such as COPD that are predominantly causes of death in old age and that are cited more often as contributory than as underlying causes of death. Autopsies were reported for only

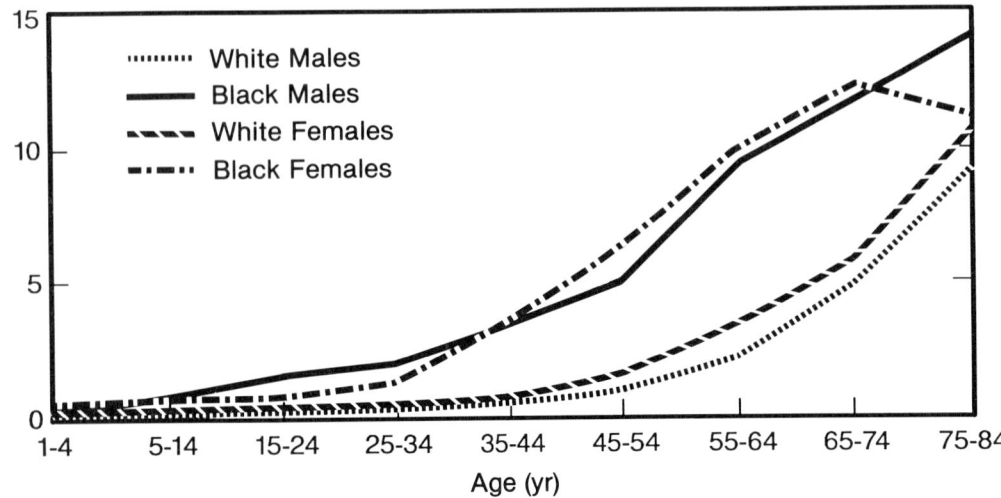

FIGURE 2–3. Death rates for asthma by age, sex, and race in the United States in 1988. (From Vital Statistics of the United States, 1988, Vol 2, Mortality, Part A. Hyattsville, MD: National Center for Health Statistics; 1990. US Department of Health and Human Services publication [PHS] 90-110, p 48.)

TABLE 2–2. AGE-ADJUSTED DEATH RATES FOR COPD AND ALLIED CONDITIONS IN THE UNITED STATES FOR 1988* (RATE/100,000 POPULATION†)

Cause of Death	Male			Female		
	Total	White	Black	Total	White	Black
COPD and allied conditions	27.5	27.8	26.0	14.0	14.5	10.0
Bronchitis	1.1	1.1	0.8	0.7	0.7	0.4
Emphysema	5.5	5.7	4.6	2.5	2.7	0.9
Asthma	1.2	1.0	3.5	1.5	1.2	3.4
Other COPDs	19.6	20.1	17.0	9.3	9.8	5.3
COPD (excluding asthma)	26.2	26.9	22.4	12.5	13.2	6.6

*From Vital Statistics of the United States, 1988, Vol II, Mortality, Part A. Hyattsville, MD: National Center for Health Statistics; 1990. Department of Health and Human Services publication (PHS) 90-1101.
†Adjusted to the United States population for 1940.

5% of deaths attributed to COPD and allied conditions in 1988.[9] Comparison of conditions detected by examination of the Tecumseh study population with information on death certificates showed that there was no mention of COPD and allied conditions on the death certificates of more than 80% of the persons who had chronic bronchitis or obstructive airways disease as a study diagnosis.[10]

Information on disability associated with obstructive lung diseases and on their prevalence by level of family income is available from the NHIS.[5] In general, rates of reporting chronic bronchitis, emphysema, and asthma are highest among those with the lowest family incomes and lowest among those with the highest incomes. The gradients are most consistent for chronic bronchitis and emphysema below age 65 years and for emphysema above age 65 years (Fig. 2–4). Similar inverse relationships with respect to socioeconomic status are apparent in mortality data.[11]

The proportion of persons who say their activity is limited by their disease is 46% for emphysema, 19% for asthma, and 3% for chronic bronchitis (see Table 2–3). These estimates are subjective and related to a person's perception of whether his or her activity is reduced either in the long term or the short term. Nevertheless, emphysema, although reported by fewer people, is clearly the most important chronic lung disease causing chronic disability.

Unfortunately, there are no objective measures of impairment resulting from these disorders available for a representative sample of the population of the United States. However, such data are being collected in the National Health and Nutrition Examination Survey; the Survey will provide prevalence data for symptoms, diagnosed disease, and impaired pulmonary function.

TIME TRENDS

The upward trends in COPD and asthma death rates are in marked contrast to the downward trends for heart disease, stroke, and most causes of death other than lung cancer and acquired immune deficiency syndrome. Between 1979 and 1989, the age-adjusted death rate for COPD rose 31%, the asthma death rate rose 56%, and the lung cancer death rate rose 15%, whereas the death rate for all causes combined declined 9% and that for coronary heart disease declined 30%.[2,12] Trends over the last 20 years for COPD combined with asthma, all causes, and a few selected causes are shown in Figure 2–5. Trends in COPD and asthma have not equally affected all ages, races, and sexes. For COPD, recent increases have been greater in women than in men and greater in blacks than in whites. At younger ages, death rates have declined, whereas they are still increasing among the oldest members of our population.[13] Patterns by sex and race are shown in Figure 2–6. Trends in asthma death rates are less certain because the number of deaths is smaller, but deaths appear to have increased most in black males and in those aged under 35 years in both black and white male populations. Among women, especially among black women, the increase has been greater at ages 5 to 14 years and over 35 years. Hospital discharge rates for asthma have also increased

TABLE 2–3. ESTIMATED PREVALENCE (IN THOUSANDS) OF SELECTED LUNG DISEASES IN THE UNITED STATES FROM 1986 TO 1988*

Condition	Men				Women			
	Prevalence		Limited Activity		Prevalence		Limited Activity	
	Number	Rate†	Number	%	Number	Rate†	Number	%
Chronic bronchitis	4918	42.6	152	3.1	7096	57.6	235	3.3
Emphysema	1259	10.9	596	47.3	722	5.9	327	45.3
Asthma	4645	40.2	904	19.5	5090	41.3	985	19.4

*Adams PF, Benson V. Current Estimates from the National Health Interview Survey, 1989. Hyattsville, MD: National Center for Health Statistics, Vital and Health Statistics; 1990. US Department of Health and Human Services publication (PHS) 10-176.
†Number of patients per 1000.

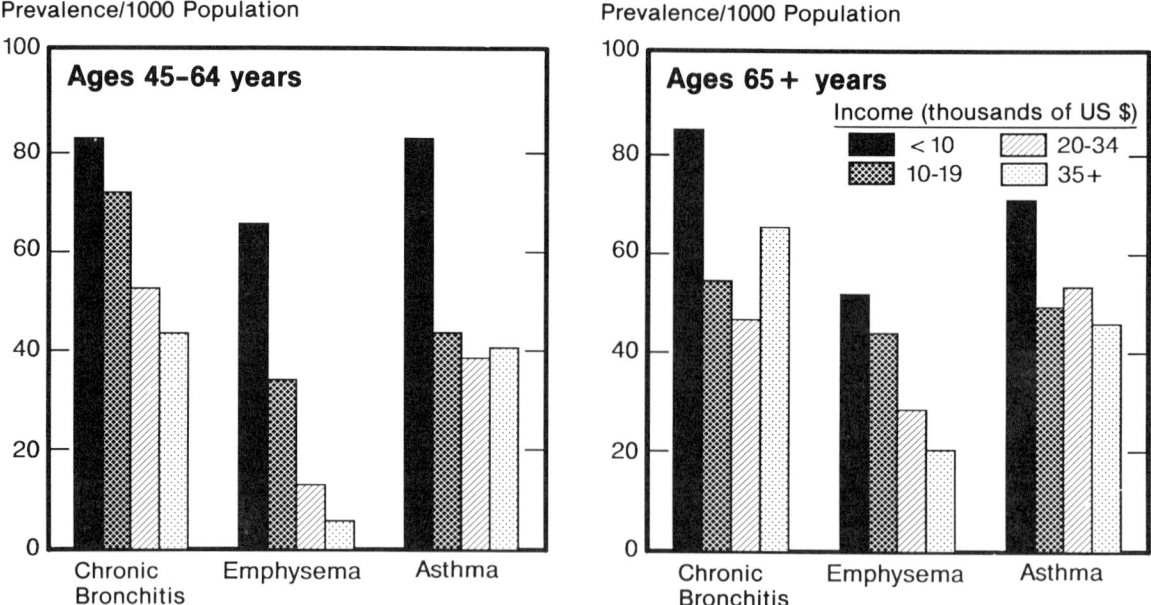

FIGURE 2–4. Prevalence of chronic bronchitis, emphysema, and asthma by age and family income in the United States in 1989. (From Adams PF, Benson V. Current Estimates from the National Health Interview Survey, 1989. Hyattsville, MD: National Center for Health Statistics; 1990. US Department of Health and Human Services publication [PHS] 10-176, pp 90, 92.)

among children and adolescents, and self-reported prevalence rates have increased at all ages.[2, 3, 5, 9, 12]

REGIONAL PATTERNS

Within the United States, age-adjusted death rates for COPD and allied conditions among males ages 55 to 74 years varied from a high of 178 per 100,000 in Kentucky to a low of 64 per 100,000 in Hawaii in 1986. The states with rates over 160 per 100,000 were Kentucky, Colorado, Idaho, West Virginia, Montana, Tennessee, and Wyoming, and those with rates below 100 per 100,000 were Alaska, New York, Minnesota, Massachusetts, New Jersey, Connecticut, and Hawaii. Utah, which has the lowest reported prevalence of cigarette smoking, ranked 13th among the 50 states and the District of Columbia. The correlation between mortality and the prevalence of smoking by state was only 0.13.[14] The prevalence of self-reported chronic bronchitis was higher for the southern and midwestern geographic regions than for the Northeast and the West. Asthma and emphysema were reported more frequently in the South than in any of the other regions, but the rates are not age-adjusted and their interpretation is uncertain because of the many factors influencing ascertainment by the NHIS.

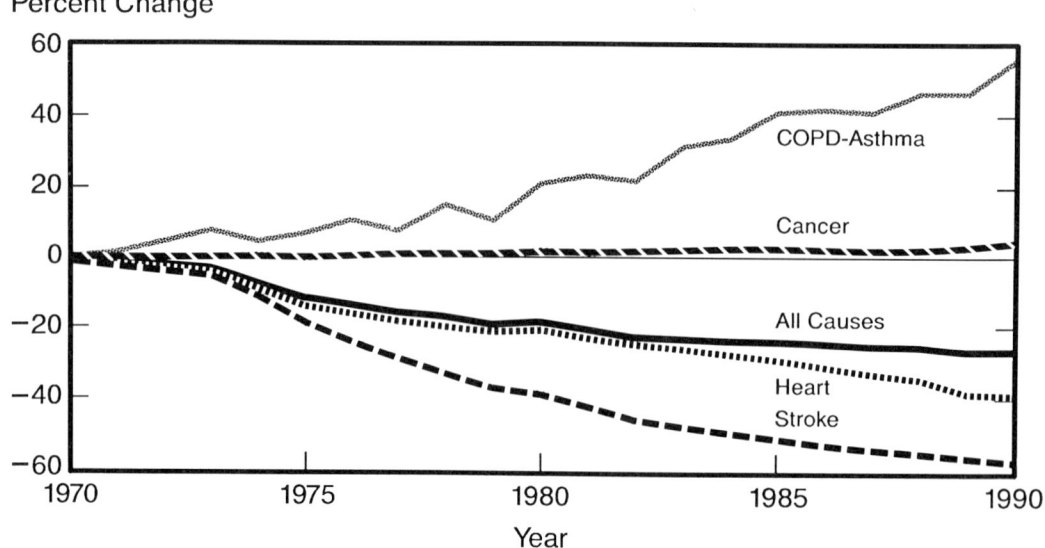

FIGURE 2–5. Percentage of change in age-adjusted death rates for selected causes in the United States from 1970 to 1990. (COPD: Chronic obstructive pulmonary disease.) (From Vital Statistics of the United States, 1970–1990.)

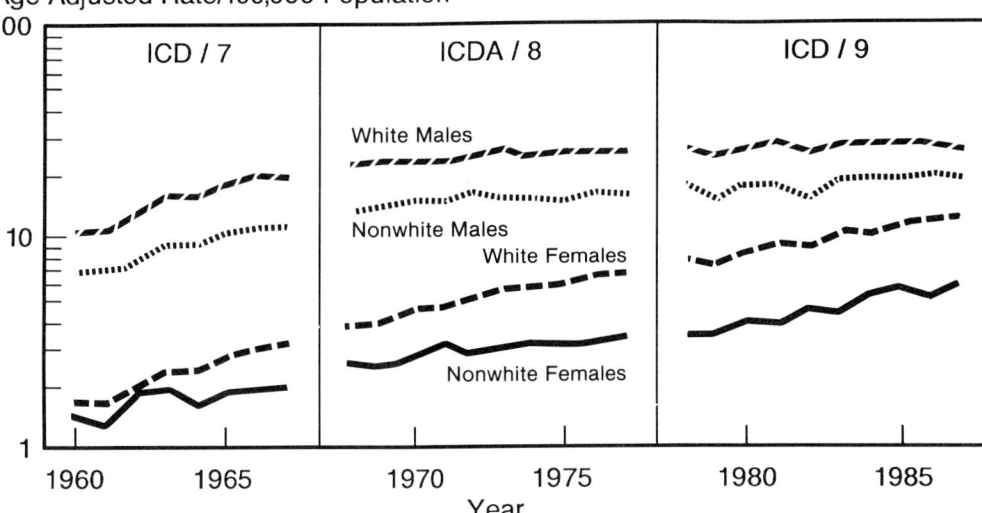

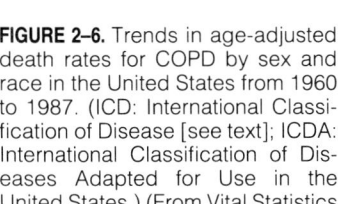

FIGURE 2-6. Trends in age-adjusted death rates for COPD by sex and race in the United States from 1960 to 1987. (ICD: International Classification of Disease [see text]; ICDA: International Classification of Diseases Adapted for Use in the United States.) (From Vital Statistics of the United States, 1970–1990.)

RISK FACTORS FOR OBSTRUCTIVE PULMONARY DISEASE

A large number of genetic, constitutional, familial, behavioral, sociodemographic, and environmental factors have been associated with the development of obstructive pulmonary disease. Only cigarette smoking and ventilatory lung function are considered in any detail in this chapter, since the evidence implicating these factors is incontrovertible and relevant to both individual and population-based approaches to prevent or reduce the burden of obstructive pulmonary disease. The extensive literature on smoking and pulmonary disease and pulmonary function has been reviewed and discussed in the reports of the United States Surgeon General on smoking and health, to which readers are referred for overviews of this information.[15,16]

The salient facts are that 80% or more of COPD cases in the United States are attributable to cigarette smoking and that risks of developing disease vary among smokers. Criteria for judging the association between smoking and COPD to be causal have been satisfied for more than 20 years. Although the evidence for a dose-response relationship is strong, the extent and duration of exposure to cigarette smoke are not the only determinants of COPD among smokers. Thus, although abolition of smoking would result in a massive reduction in the public health burden of morbidity and mortality from smoking-related diseases, including COPD, practical considerations require that counseling of high-risk individuals be combined with community intervention strategies. Individual counseling is likely to be more effective and efficient if it takes into account personalized estimates of susceptibility and if it targets those at greatest risk.

Several longitudinal prospective studies have identified baseline level of pulmonary function as a risk factor in addition to sex, age, and cigarette smoking. Probabilities of developing COPD over intervals of 10 or more years can be estimated using information easily obtained by questioning individuals and measuring forced expiratory volume in 1 second (FEV_1) according to standardized methods. Figures 2–7 and 2–8 illustrate the gradient of risk for 50-year-old men and women according to their smoking habits and levels of FEV_1 (expressed as a per cent of predicted values derived from values in asymptomatic nonsmokers and corrected for height).[17] Risks vary from .02 to .5 and from .01 to .68 in men and women, respectively. Among nonsmokers, risks are greater in men, but among smokers of 20 cigarettes per day, they are about the same for both sexes. Risks appear to be greater for women than for men who smoke more heavily. However, estimates for women are based on a small sample and are, therefore, less reliable, especially at the extreme of the observations. The risks of continuing and the benefits of quitting smoking are clear.

These estimated probabilities for groups of men and women were calculated from multiple logistic regression equations developed from the Tecumseh population[17] and validated in other population-based studies.[18] The equations for estimating risks of developing obstructive airways disease within 10 years, assuming no change in cigarette use, are as follows:

For men,

$$P = [1 + \exp - (2.793 + .089 \text{ age} + .039 \text{ cigs/day} - .117 \text{ } FEV_1\%Pr)]^{-1}$$

For women,

$$P = [1 + \exp - (3.004 + .078 \text{ age} + .069 \text{ cigs/day} - .118 \text{ } FEV_1\%Pr)]^{-1}$$

A system of estimating risk by summing points for specific ages, levels of FEV_1, %Pr, and numbers of cigarettes per day is available,[19] and graphic presentations such as Figures 2–7 and 2–8 can be used to aid patients in understanding the risks and benefits of continuing or quitting smoking. Although other risk factors did not make statistically significant improvements to the predictions for the Tecumseh population as a whole, they may be important for individual patients and should be evaluated and influence advice and medical manage-

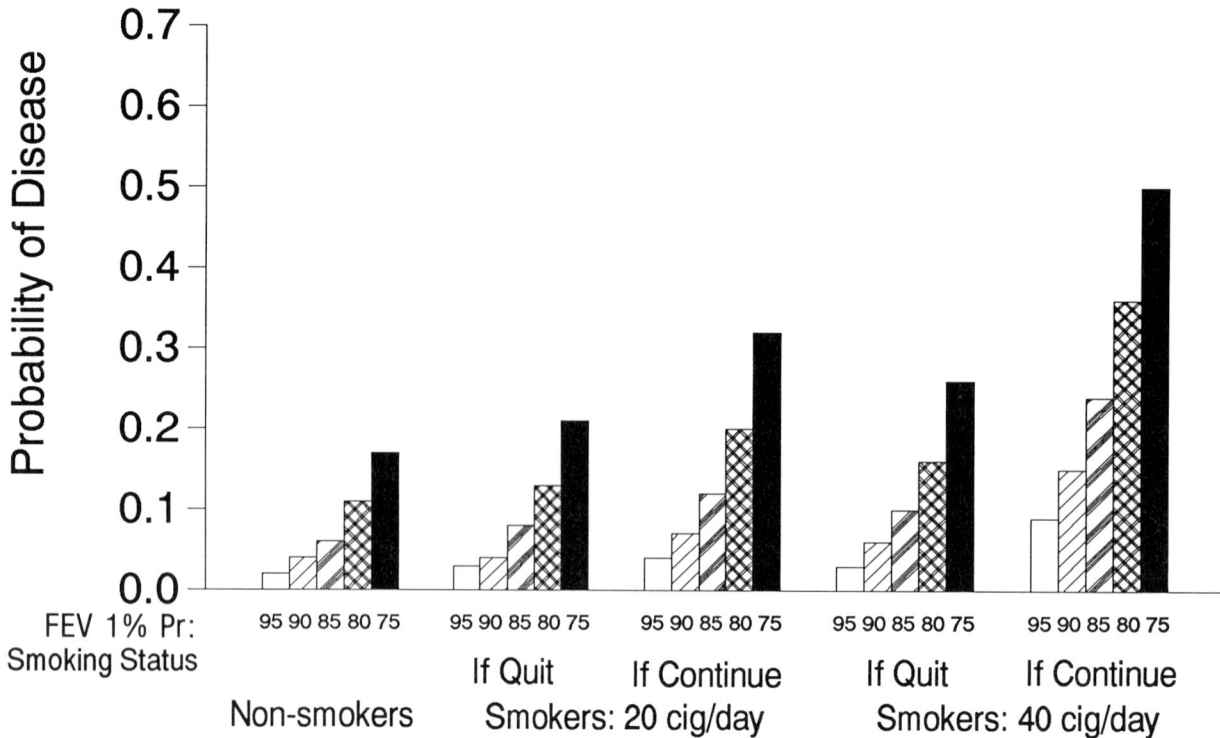

FIGURE 2–7. The estimated probability for the onset of obstructive pulmonary disease in 50-year-old men in a 10-year period. (cig-cigarettes; FEV 1% Pr: forced expiratory volume at 1 second, per cent predicted.) (From Higgins MW, Keller JB, Becker M, et al. An index of rise for obstructive airways disease. Am Rev Respir Dis 1982; 125:144–151.)

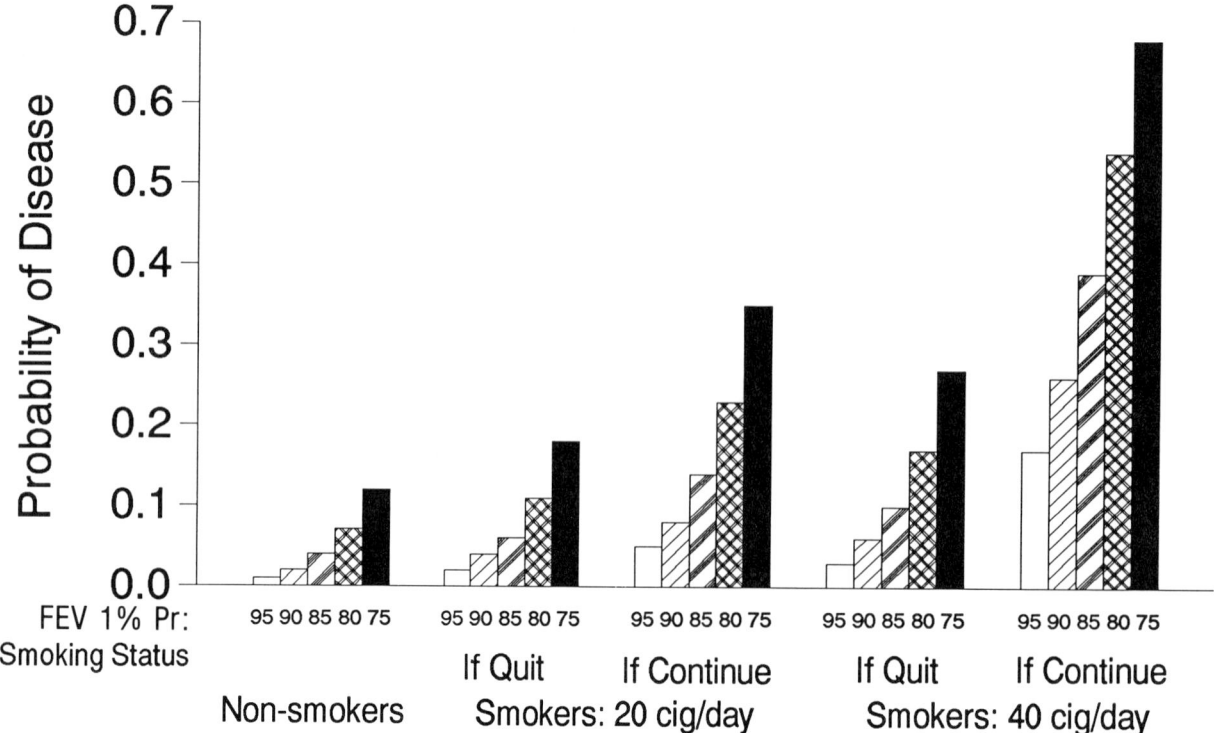

FIGURE 2–8. The estimated probability for the onset of obstructive pulmonary disease in 50-year-old women in a 10-year period. (From Higgins MW, Keller JB, Becker M, et al. An index of risk for obstructive airways disease. Am Rev Respir Dis 1982; 125:144–151.)

ment. In particular, the presence of respiratory symptoms, including cough, the presence of phlegm, wheezing, and breathlessness as well as histories and diagnoses of pneumonia, recurrent bronchitis, asthma, or emphysema and measurements of bronchial hyperreactivity may lead to specific recommendations, investigations, or treatments for individual patients. Reports of the late 1980s suggest that elevated white blood cell counts are associated with increased rates of decline in pulmonary function, but it is unclear whether this applies to nonsmokers as well as smokers.[20]

Hazardous occupational or environmental exposures can be identified and reduced as appropriate, and detailed genetic and family studies, including alpha$_1$-antitrypsin phenotyping and measurements, can be performed if indicated. Medical management, including the rehabilitation of patients with established disease, is discussed extensively in subsequent chapters.

REFERENCES

1. World Health Organization. Manual of the International Classification of Diseases, Injuries, and Causes of Death. Geneva, 1977.
2. Annual Summary of Births, Marriages, Divorces, and Deaths: United States, 1989. Monthly Vital Statistics Report. Hyattsville, MD: National Center for Health Statistics; 1990. US Department of Health and Human Services (PHS). 38(13).
3. Detailed Diagnoses and Surgical Procedures for Patients Discharged from Short-Stay Hospitals: United States, 1989. Hyattsville, MD: National Center for Health Statistics; 1992. US Department of Health and Human Services publication (PHS) 91–1769.
4. National Heart, Lung, and Blood Institute. Morbidity and Mortality Chartbook on Cardiovascular, Lung, and Blood Diseases, 1990. Bethesda, MD: National Institutes of Health; 1990. US Department of Health and Human Services.
5. Adams PF, Benson V. Current Estimates from the National Health Interview Survey, 1989. Hyattsville, MD: National Center for Health Statistics, Vital and Health Statistics; 1990. US Department of Health and Human Services publication (PHS) 10-176.
6. American College of Chest Physicians–American Thoracic Society. Pulmonary terms and symbols. Chest 1975; 67:583–593.
7. Burrows B, Lebowitz MD. Characteristics of chronic bronchitis in a warm, dry region. Am Rev Respir Dis 1975; 112:365–370.
8. Samet JM. Definitions and methodology in COPD research. In: Hensley MJ, Saunders NA (eds). Clinical Epidemiology of Chronic Obstructive Pulmonary Disease. New York: Marcel Dekker, Inc., 1989.
9. Vital Statistics of the United States, 1988, Vol II, Mortality, Part A. Hyattsville, MD: National Center for Health Statistics; 1990. Department of Health and Human Services publication (PHS) 90-1101.
10. Higgins MW, Keller JB. Trends in COPD morbidity and mortality in Tecumseh, Michigan. Am Rev Respir Dis 1989; 140:S42–48.
11. Rogot E, Sorlie PD, Johnson NJ, et al. A Mortality Study of One Million Persons by Demographic, Social, and Economic Factors: 1979–1981 Follow-Up. U.S. Longitudinal Mortality Study. Bethesda, MD; 1988. NIH 88-2896.
12. Vital Statistics of the United States, 1979, Vol II, Mortality, Part A. Hyattsville, MD: National Center for Health Statistics; 1984. Department of Health and Human Services publication (PHS) 84-1101.
13. Higgins MW. Risk factors associated with chronic obstructive lung disease. Ann NY Acad Sci 1991; 624:7–17.
14. Thom, Thomas. Personal communication.
15. The Health Consequences of Smoking: Chronic Obstructive Lung Disease. A Report of the Surgeon General. Washington, DC: Public Health Service; 1984. Department of Health and Human Services publication (PHS) 84-50205.
16. The Health Benefits of Smoking Cessation. A Report of the Surgeon General. Atlanta, GA: Centers for Disease Control, Center for Chronic Disease Prevention and Health Promotion, Office on Smoking and Health; 1990. Department of Health and Human Services publication 90-8416.
17. Higgins MW, Keller JB, Becker M, et al. An index of risk for obstructive airways disease. Am Rev Respir Dis 1982; 125:144–151.
18. Higgins MW, Keller JB, Landis JR, et al. Risk of chronic obstructive pulmonary disease: Collaborative assessment of the validity of the Tecumseh Index of Risk. Am Rev Respir Dis 1984; 130:380–385.
19. Higgins MW, Keller JB. Estimating your patient's risk of COPD. Am J Respir Dis 1983; 4:97–108.
20. Chan-Yeung M, Abboud R, Buncio AD, Vedal S. Peripheral leucocyte count and longitudinal decline in lung function. Thorax 1988; 43:462–466.

Chapter 3

Pathophysiology of Chronic Obstructive Pulmonary Disease with Emphasis on Physiologic and Pathologic Correlations

THOMAS CORBRIDGE, M.D.
CHARLES G. IRVIN, Ph.D.

Before the pathophysiology of chronic obstructive pulmonary disease (COPD) and the correlations between physiology and pathology can be considered, some disease definitions are needed. For purposes of this chapter, we will use the definitions established by the American Thoracic Society (ATS) in 1986.[1] The ATS defines COPD as a "disorder characterized by abnormal tests of expiratory flow that do not change markedly over periods of several months of observation." That is, COPD refers only to patients with chronic airflow limitation. COPD does not refer to patients (even heavy smokers) with chronic productive cough and normal airflow. Chronic bronchitis, emphysema, and peripheral airways disease are included in the more generic term COPD. Other causes of chronic airflow obstruction, such as bronchiectasis and localized disease of the upper airways, are excluded. Chronic bronchitis is defined as chronic "excess mucus secretion into the bronchial tree," which is present on most days for at least 3 months of the year and for at least 2 consecutive years. This term applies whether excess sputum is expectorated or is swallowed. Emphysema is defined as a "condition of the lung characterized by abnormal permanent enlargement of the airspaces distal to the terminal bronchiole, accompanied by destruction of their walls, and without obvious fibrosis." Patients with emphysema are almost always significantly hyperinflated. Alveolar destruction decreases the vascular markings on the radiograph and is associated with a low diffusing capacity. A variety of abnormalities have been seen in the peripheral airways of patients with COPD, including inflammation of the terminal and respiratory bronchioles.[1] These lesions may represent early COPD and may precede the development of emphysema, although such a progression has yet to be proved. Peripheral airways disease results in abnormalities in pulmonary function tests and contributes to chronic airflow obstruction.[1] A history of cigarette smoking increases the chance that a patient with chronic airflow limitation has chronic bronchitis or emphysema (since almost all such patients have smoked). A negative smoking history, however, does not rule out these diagnoses. For example, chronic bronchitis may result from industrial exposures, and emphysema occurs in nonsmokers with alpha$_1$-antitrypsin deficiency.

The above definition of COPD was intended to distinguish COPD from asthma. The ATS defines asthma as a "clinical syndrome characterized by increased responsiveness of the tracheobronchial tree to a variety of stimuli." However, as is apparent in clinical practice, considerable overlap exists between asthma and COPD. Patients with chronic severe asthma may develop irreversible airflow limitation, and patients with COPD may have airways hyperresponsiveness (although marked hyperresponsiveness is rare) and often exhibit significant improvement in airflow after the inhalation of a bronchodilator.

With these definitions, the major physiologic abnormalities of COPD and the correlations between these abnormalities and the pathologic alterations of this disorder can be considered.

LUNG VOLUMES

One of the hallmarks of patients with COPD is lung hyperinflation. In the most severely hyperinflated patients, this finding is obvious on physical inspection of the thorax. In others, hyperinflation is evident only on pulmonary function testing or on the chest radiograph. To understand the causes of lung hyperinflation in COPD, we will first consider the determinants of static lung inflation by studying the relationship between pressure and volume. Next, we will address the determinants of dynamic hyperinflation and the frequency-dependent behavior of a branching network of airways. For a more in-depth analysis of the concepts put forth in this section we direct the reader to the *Handbook of Physiology*.[2, 3]

Pressure-Volume Curve. Considerable insight into the determinants of lung volumes can be gathered from the study of the static pressure-volume (P-V) relationships of the chest wall (cw), lung (L), and their sum, the respiratory system (RS) (Fig. 3–1A). The static P-V curve of the lung is obtained by simultaneously measuring airway opening pressure (Pao), lung volume, and pleural pressure (Ppl) as estimated by an esophageal balloon positioned in the lower third of the esophagus. During a slow exhalation from total lung capacity (TLC) to residual volume (RV), the airway is occluded for 1 to 2 seconds at periodic intervals to stop flow. Under static conditions of zero flow, Pao is measured and assumed to equal alveolar pressure (P_A). The distending pressure of the lung, or transpulmonary pressure (Ptm = P_A − Ppl), can then be measured and plotted against lung volume to obtain the static P-V curve of the lung. Lung compliance (C_L, the reciprocal of elastance) is calculated by dividing the change in lung volume by the change in Ptm. Compliance is a measure of the distensibility of the lung. The easier it is to inflate or deflate the lungs (that is, the greater the change in volume per change in pressure), the greater the compliance. Compliance is decreased and elastic recoil increased in pulmonary fibrosis (P-V curve shifted downward and to the right; see Fig. 3–1B), whereas compliance is increased and elastic recoil decreased in emphysema (P-V curve shifted upward and to the left). Identifying an exact value for compliance is problematic because lung compliance decreases (elastance increases) in a curvilinear fashion as lung volume increases. Therefore, comparisons of compliance must include some consideration of lung volume. This is commonly done by reporting "specific compliance," which is compliance divided by the lung volume at which it was measured (e.g., functional residual capacity [FRC]). Exponential curve fitting analysis also deals with the effects of lung volume in a more rigorous way. Another convenient measure of lung elasticity is the "coefficient of elastic retraction," which is the ratio of the maximum Ptm (Ptmmax) to the TLC.

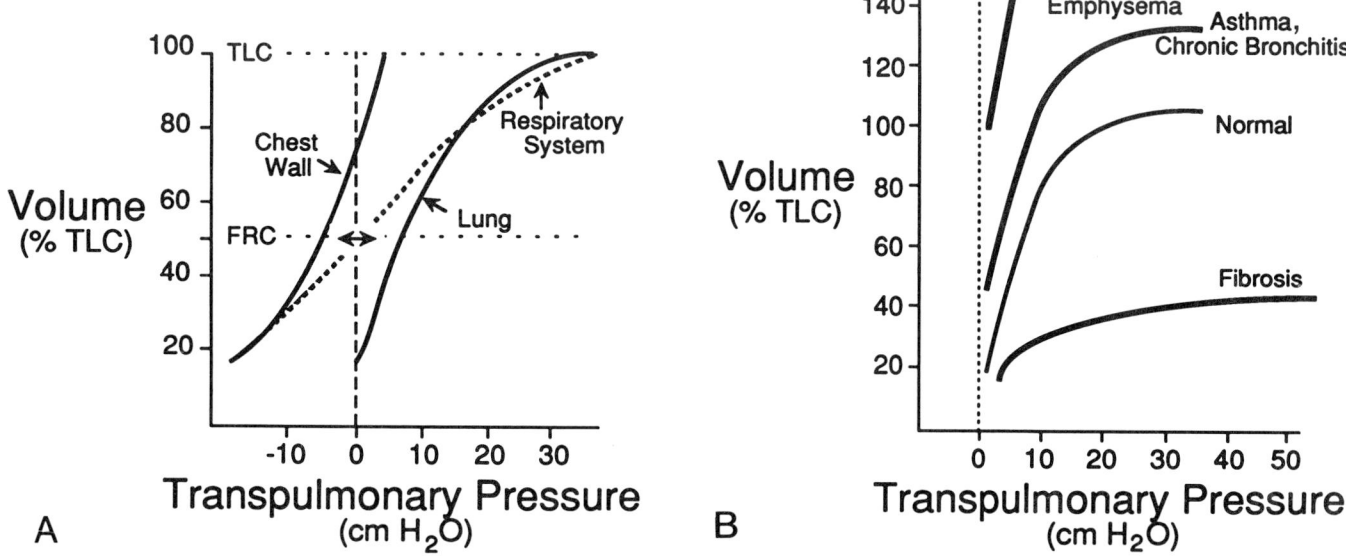

FIGURE 3-1. Pressure-volume (P–V) relationships for the respiratory system. *A*, P–V relationships for the component parts of the respiratory system. At lung volumes below approximately 70% TLC, the chest wall presents an outward force (negative transpulmonary pressure), which tends to inflate the lung. At all lung volumes, the lung presents an inward force (positive transpulmonary pressure). At functional residual capacity (FRC), these forces are equal but opposite, and as a result recoil of the respiratory system equals zero. Compliance is the slope of these curves. *B*, P–V relationships of the lung for different lung disorders.

Normally, the coefficient of elastic retraction is between 2.5 and 8.5 cm H_2O/L, whereas in emphysema it is generally less than 2.5 cm H_2O/L.[4]

To obtain the P-V curve of the respiratory system (the lung and the chest wall), the distending pressure across this system (PRS, which is PA minus barometric pressure [PB]) is plotted against lung volume. The P-V curve of the chest wall is determined by subtracting the P-V curve of the lung from the P-V curve of the respiratory system; however, here complete relaxation of the muscles of the chest wall, a state rarely achieved, must be assumed.

Frequency Dependence of Compliance. C_L measured during breathing is called "dynamic" compliance (Cdyn). It is obtained by dividing the tidal volume (VT) by the difference in Ptm between the brief instances of zero-flow at end-expiration and at end-inspiration. In normal subjects, C_L measured over a tidal breath does not change much with increased breathing frequency. However, in patients with airway obstruction, C_L falls as breathing frequency increases, a phenomenon called the *frequency dependence of compliance*. To understand the fall in Cdyn with increasing breathing frequency, the concept of the *time constant* (Fig. 3–2) must be considered. When a system (in this case the lung) is subjected to a sudden, instantaneous step-change in pressure, the time required for the lung to inflate to 63% of its eventual new volume is termed the time constant. An alternative means to calculate the time constant is to multiply the resistance times the compliance (cm H_2O/L/sec × L/cm H_2O = sec). In the diseased lung, if resistance is increased, the time required for the lung to inflate or deflate is prolonged (i.e., the value of the time constant is high). Now consider a lung with two units, one with a normal time constant and one with a high time constant owing to airflow obstruction. At low breathing frequencies, both units contribute to compliance because there is time for the diseased unit to respond. However, at high breathing frequencies, the diseased unit cannot respond (inflate or deflate) to the pressure changes in the pleural space because its time constant is too great. As a result, the lung appears to be less compliant. In addition, higher respiratory rates decrease the time available for expiration, resulting in dynamic lung hyperinflation and a further decrease in C_L. Since lung units have not fully deflated in this situation, PA remains positive at end-expiration, a state referred to as *intrinsic positive end-expiratory pressure* (PEEPi). The finding of frequency dependence of compliance or PEEPi may identify patients with early disease, such as those with peripheral airways disease.

Definitions, Determinants, and Measurement of Lung Volumes. Clinically, it is difficult to measure P-V characteristics or the frequency dependence of compliance. However, lung volumes are easily measured in a body plethysmograph or by gas dilution techniques and provide indirect information about C_L and Ccw as well as respiratory muscle strength and airway function. In particular, measurement of the crucial boundaries of lung volume, FRC, TLC, and RV wherein breathing takes place provides the most information about the physiology of the lung.[4]

The FRC is the volume of gas present in the lungs at the end of a normal tidal breath. It is normally 40 to 50% of TLC (Figs. 3–3 and 3–4). In normal subjects, the FRC is determined by the point at which the outward recoil pressure of the relaxed chest wall equals the inward elastic recoil pressure of the lung (see Fig. 3–1A) and is thus a point of equilibrium. Because FRC is an effort-independent measurement, and since both RV and TLC require its determination, FRC is the most

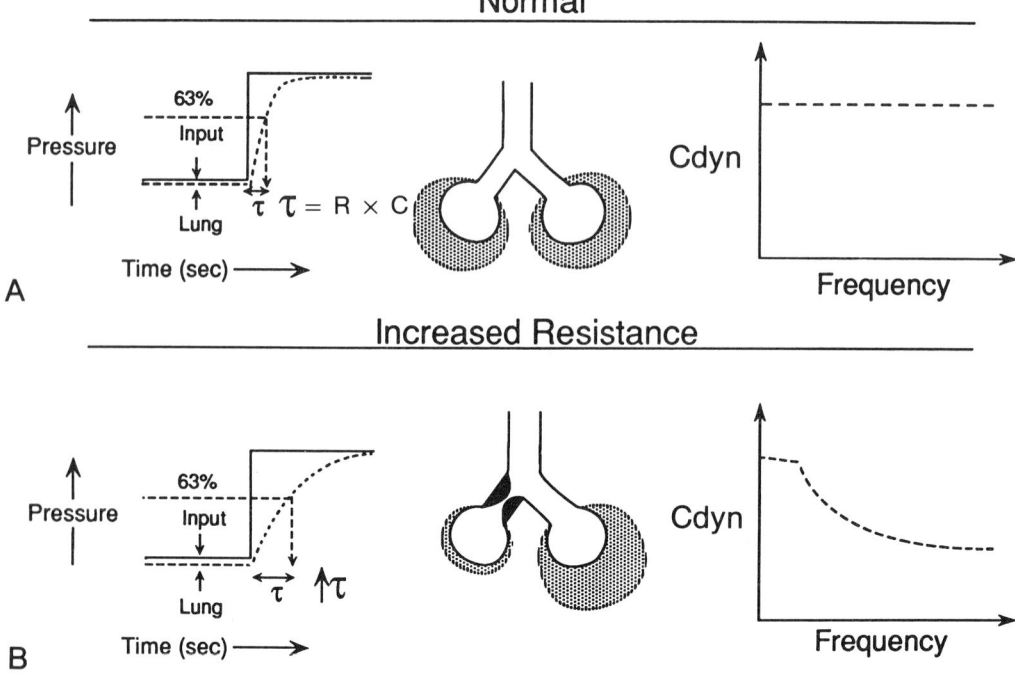

FIGURE 3–2. The concept of the time constant (τ) for a normal (A) and a diseased (B) lung with increased airways resistance of one lobe. In the lung, the response to an input step change in pressure (*left plot*) can be described by τ of the response of the lung (*dashed line*). The value of τ is the time in seconds required by the lung to reach 63% of the maximum response, or the product of resistance (R) times compliance (C). For a normal lung, in which the inflation (*dotted area*) is normal and uniform, the value of τ is small. As a result, dynamic compliance (Cdyn) is independent of frequency (*right plot*). However, for a diseased lung with increased resistance (B), the response of the lung is now slower, and τ is greater. Since the increase in resistance is rarely uniform, the inflation of the lung is uneven (*center diagram*). As a result, Cdyn is frequency-dependent (*right diagram*).

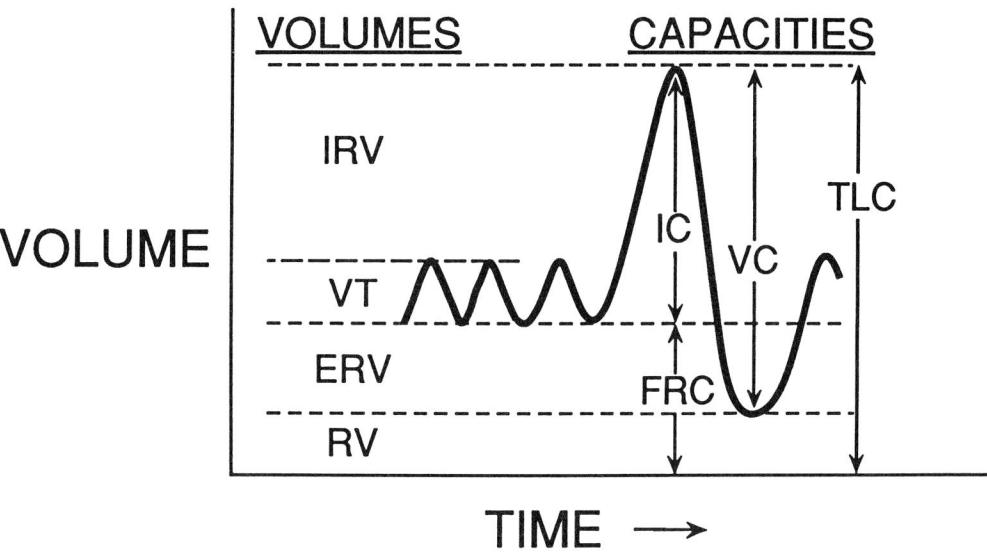

FIGURE 3-3. A plot of lung volume versus time is termed a *spirogram*. The thick line is an example of a patient's effort, first during tidal breathing and then during maximum inhalation and maximum exhalation. Lung capacities are combinations of more than one lung volume, that is, a lung volume cannot be further divided. (Volumes—IRV: inspiratory reserve volume; VT: tidal volume; ERV: expiratory reserve volume; RV: residual lung volume. Capacities—IC: inspiratory capacity [IRV + VT]; FRC: functional residual capacity [ERV + RV]; VC: vital capacity [IRV + VT + ERV]; TLC: total lung capacity [IRV + VT + ERV + RV].) Note that TLC, FRC, and RV represent the important boundaries that yield insight into lung function, but since RV cannot be determined by simple spirometry, the measurement of FRC by another technique is required.

reliable and important volume indicator. The FRC increases when either lung elastic recoil pressure is decreased (as in emphysema) or the outward recoil pressure of the chest wall is increased. The latter may occur in patients with airways disease caused by persistent activity of inspiratory muscles throughout respiration. It may also occur with muscle "splinting" after rib fracture. Additionally, if the time constant (resistance times compliance) is prolonged, inspiration occurs before the equilibrium point is reached, and substantial increases in FRC can occur. The FRC is best measured in a body plethysmograph when the shutter is closed at end-expiration and with the application of Boyle's law, although a number of gas dilution techniques are also used, of which the dilution of helium within a closed-circuit apparatus is the most common.[5,6] In bullous emphysema, the value of FRC by helium (FRC_{He}) and by body plethysmograph (FRC_{BP}) can be markedly different. Since FRC_{He} measures communicating gas spaces and FRC_{BP} measures gas spaces that compress whether or not they communicate, FRC_{BP} can measure liters higher than FRC_{He}. This difference is termed *trapped gas*.

TLC is the volume of gas present after a full inflation (see Fig. 3-3). In common practice, TLC is measured by adding FRC and the inspiratory capacity (IC). In health, it is determined by the ability of patients to inspire (strength and effort) and by the P-V characteristics of the lung (see Fig. 3-1A). It should be noted that when there is adequate inspiratory muscle strength, TLC occurs when the P-V curve of the lung reaches a plateau.

Inspiratory muscle strength is commonly assessed by measuring the maximum inspiratory pressure (P_{Imax}) that can be generated at the mouth against a closed airway starting at RV or FRC. P_I is inversely related to the lung volume at which it was measured; therefore, values obtained at RV are greater than those at FRC. In patients with COPD, P_{Imax} is significantly decreased at RV and FRC. However, when patients with COPD inspire from lung volumes comparable (in per cent of predicted TLC) to normal subjects, P_{Imax} normalizes, suggesting that the mechanical disadvantage caused by lung hyperinflation was the major cause of inspiratory muscle weakness.[7]

RV is the volume of gas remaining in the lungs after maximum exhalation, which in normal subjects is usually 25% of TLC; that is, the ratio of RV to TLC (RV/TLC) is 25% (see Fig. 3-4). In common clinical practice, RV equals FRC minus expiratory reserve volume (ERV; see Fig. 3-3). The RV is determined by a patient's ability

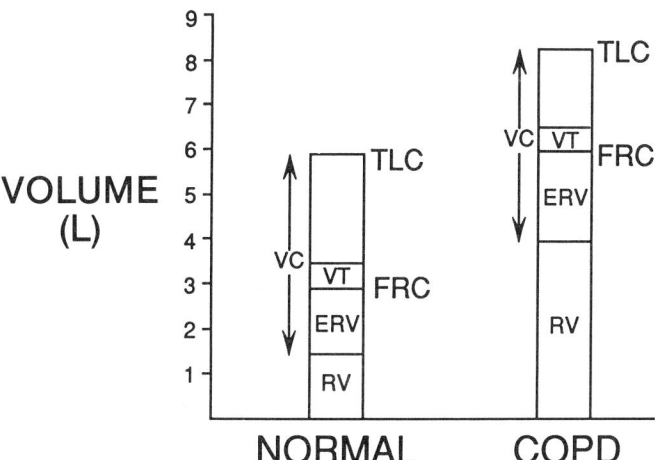

FIGURE 3-4. The lung division of a normal subject (*left column*) and of a patient with COPD. For the normal person, RV is about 20% of TLC, and FRC is about 50% of TLC. In patients with COPD, RV has risen with little change in VC. Now RV/TLC and FRC/TLC are increased, indicating hyperinflation. Note how simple spirometry (with which only VC is measured) would probably not detect this change, since VC is nearly the same in both the normal subject and the COPD patient.

to exhale maximally (strength and effort) and by closure of airways (closing volume). In young patients pain may determine RV, but in older patients RV is determined by closure of airways or airflow limitation due to compression of airways (amplified in emphysema by a loss of tethering of the airways). It is perhaps not surprising that in COPD RVs of greater than 70% of the predicted TLC are common. However, the determination of RV is highly variable, and as such it has limited clinical usefulness.

Only the vital capacity (VC) and its subdivisions can be measured with a spirometer (see Fig. 3–3). These include VT and the inspiratory reserve volume (IRV), which is the additional amount of air that can be inspired from end-inspiration during tidal breathing; their sum is the IC (the amount of air that can be inspired from FRC). Spirometry can also determine the ERV, which is the volume of air that can be maximally exhaled from FRC. However, none of these indices yield the insight into lung function that can be gained by measuring RV, FRC, and TLC. Hence, it is useful to include measurement of FRC by body plethysmography or helium dilution when interpreting the VC and its subdivisions.

Abnormalities of Lung Volumes in Obstructive Diseases. Figure 3–4 contains a schematic drawing of the lung volumes in healthy individuals and in a typical patient with COPD. By contrast with normal subdivisions of plethysmographic gas volumes (TLC, FRC, RV) and spirometric capacities (IC and VC), obstructive lung disease increases TLC, FRC, and RV and decreases IC and VC. In emphysema, the P-V curve of the lung may shift upward and to the left (see Fig. 3–1B), and the slope may increase, indicating a loss of elastic recoil pressure. The P-V curve of the chest wall in hyperinflated patients may also shift upward, but it maintains a normal slope. The exact reason for the change in the P-V curve of the chest wall is unclear, but it may be a result of chronic hyperinflation. The result of these changes is an increase in FRC, TLC, and RV (Fig. 3–5). Additionally, high time constants cause dynamic hyperinflation.

In chronic bronchitis or asthma, the P-V curve of the lung is classically shifted upward and to the left, but the slope of the curve is normal; the coefficient of elastic retraction is also normal. Note that theoretically one of the best separations between bronchitis and emphysema is achieved by measuring P-V relationships. Unfortunately, the correlation between in vivo measurement of elastic recoil and the amount of emphysema is poor (see further on).

AIRFLOW OBSTRUCTION

In addition to hyperinflation, COPD is characterized by irreversible or fixed expiratory airflow obstruction. Patients demonstrate delayed lung emptying, which can be identified easily at the bedside by timing a patient's forced expiration during auscultation of the chest. Although fixed airways obstruction is present, many patients demonstrate some reversibility after the adminis-

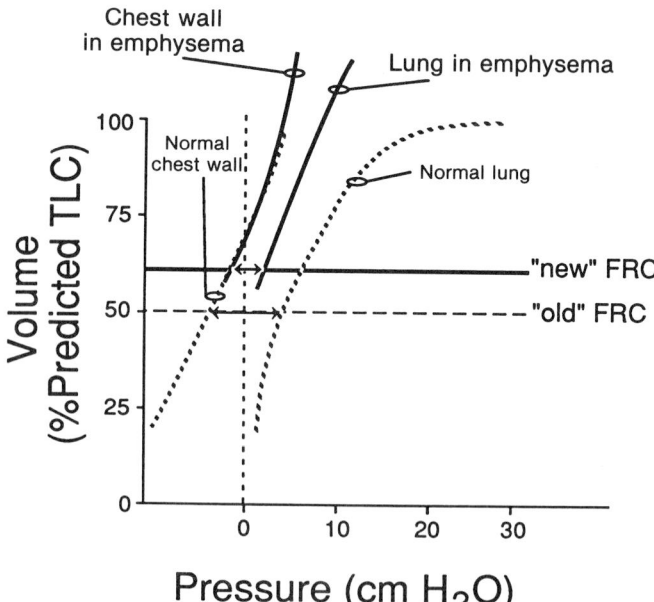

FIGURE 3–5. The P–V relationship in a normal subject and in a patient with emphysema. For the normal subject, the equilibrium point for the respiratory system is about 50% of predicted TLC. However, for the patient with emphysema, FRC rises because the equilibrium point has shifted to a higher lung volume. The "new" FRC is now higher owing to the loss of elastic recoil.

tration of bronchodilators. Forced expired volumes obtained before and after the use of bronchodilators can be used to assess the reversibility of airflow obstruction; however, it should be cautioned that bronchodilation may attenuate lung hyperinflation without changing forced expired volumes or flows, yet they significantly improve airflow at any given lung volume (isovolume flow; see later discussion). Therefore, unless lung volumes are measured before and after bronchodilator use, patients may be diagnosed incorrectly as having only irreversible airflow obstruction. Still, repeating spirometric study after the administration of a bronchodilator identifies most patients with reversible airflow obstruction.

Volume-Time Curve. Measurements from the volume-time curve include the forced expiratory volume in 1 second (FEV_1), which measures flow starting at TLC, and the forced vital capacity (FVC), the change in lung volume from TLC during a maximum, sustained expiratory effort to RV. The equipment specifications and procedure for delivering the FEV_1 and FVC have been extensively investigated, since they are the most common tests of pulmonary function performed.[8] The FEV_1 and FVC are consistently reproducible measurements (typically ±5%). The results obtained are comparable among laboratories and probably reflect the most preferred measurements of lung function.

In the absence of a restrictive ventilatory defect, an FEV_1 or FVC less than 80% of that predicted is suggestive of obstructive disease. When measured after the inhalation of a bronchodilator, the FEV_1 has also proved to be the best predictor of mortality in patients with COPD.[9] Normally, FEV_1 falls about 30 ml per year. In "susceptible" smokers, however, decreases in FEV_1 averaging 80 ml per year are not uncommon.[10, 11] The FVC is a relatively nonspecific measurement affected by changes in TLC, RV, and the time of exhalation. Whereas normal subjects can deliver the FVC in less than 4 seconds, older patients and patients with obstructive lung disease require much more time. Consequently, these patients should exhale for at least 10 seconds to ensure accurate measurement of FVC, and any apparent changes in FVC should be checked against the duration of exhalation to ensure similar effort. In severely obstructed patients, the volume-time curve rarely plateaus (Fig. 3–6); that is, RV is never reached despite exhalations in the range of 15 seconds, and the "real" FVC is underestimated. The time required to exhale the complete VC during forceful exhalation is called the *forced exhalation time* (FET). As alluded to previously, FET is also a measure of airflow obstruction. The FEV_1 expressed as a percentage of FVC (or $FEV_{1\%}$) is determined as $FEV_1/FVC \times 100$. In health, the $FEV_{1\%}$ is typically 80%, although it declines slowly with age. In obstructive diseases or processes characterized by airflow limitation, $FEV_{1\%}$ is low (less than 70%) because FEV_1 is reduced more than FVC. The $FEV_{1\%}$ may be misleadingly normal if an obstructed patient fails to reach RV and if FVC is artificially low. Similarly, in patients with severe disease who fail to deliver the entire FVC, there can be a false stabilization of this ratio despite the presence of progressive disease. The usefulness of the $FEV_{1\%}$ as a measure of airway obstruction is therefore limited to the evaluation of patients with mild disease. A high $FEV_{1\%}$ suggests a restrictive process that is best assessed by the measurement of lung volumes. The forced expiratory flow over the middle half (25–75%) of FVC ($FEF_{25-75\%}$), like the $FEV_{1\%}$, is of limited use in patients who fail to deliver the entire FVC. In these patients, $FEF_{25-75\%}$ is falsely elevated and results in underestimation of the degree of airway obstruction. The $FEF_{25-75\%}$ largely reflects flows at low lung volumes. On rare occasions it may identify patients with mild or early COPD before FEV_1 drops, such as in patients with peripheral airways disease. For all practical purposes, however, the $FEF_{25-75\%}$ provides no more information than the FEV_1, and the variability and poor reproducibility of this measure further limit its usefulness.

Flow-Volume Loop. Another approach to measuring lung function is to plot flow against volume. Note that when time markers are added to the standard flow-volume loop, most of the information available from the volume-time curve, including FEV_1, is retained (Fig. 3–7). Figure 3–7 provides a visual representation of the influence of volume on flow and is particularly useful in evaluating certain types of obstruction (e.g., fixed narrowing of the central airway) and in evaluating effort. A "scooped" or concave flow-volume curve is characteristic of airflow obstruction (see Fig. 3–10), although a high peak expiratory flow rate (PEFR) relative to other normal flows may produce a similar appearance.

At TLC, expiratory flow rate is initially limited by effort, muscle strength, and airways resistance. This is because at high lung volumes airways are pulled open by the elasticity of the surrounding lung parenchyma, which allows for high flow rates and, thus, no airflow limitation (see following). Therefore, measurements of expiratory flow rate near full inflation, such as PEFR or the $FEV_{0.5}$ (the forced expired volume in one half of a second of exhalation) are very effort-dependent. At lower lung volumes, however, airways resistance increases, and the phenomenon of *airflow limitation* occurs. In other words, expiratory airflow does not increase despite increasing effort. Figure 3–8 shows the

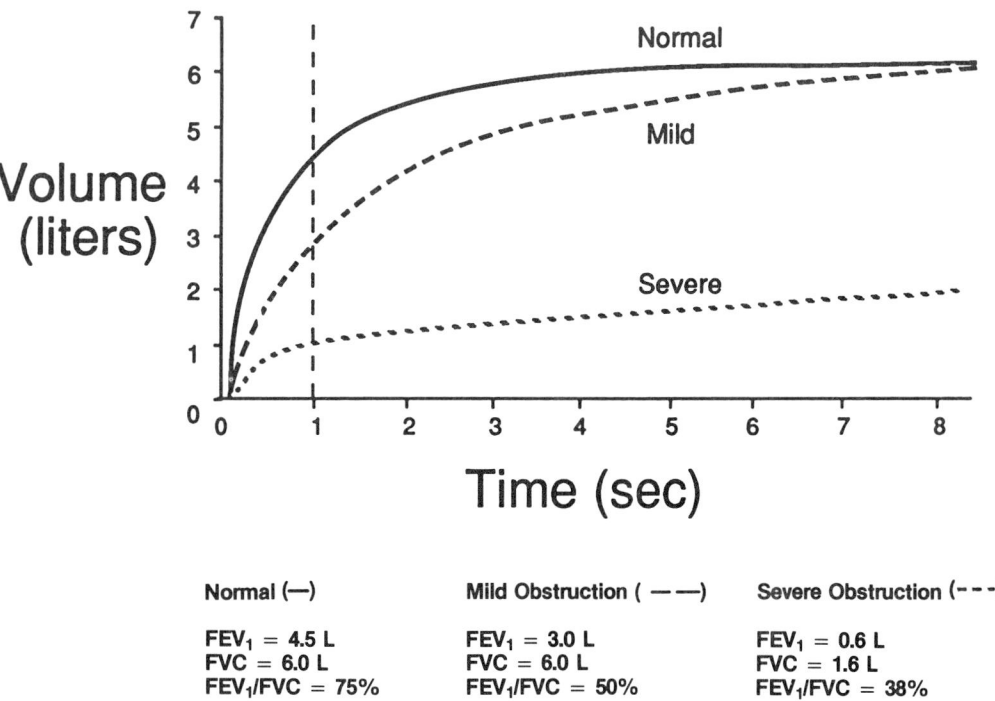

FIGURE 3–6. Volume-time relationships (spirogram) for three subjects. The normal curve represents an example of a well-performed spirogram with a clear, sharp start. The patient did not cough, hesitate, or terminate breathing prematurely. The mild obstruction curve represents a good effort put forth by a patient with mild airflow limitation. Note the fall in FEV_1, which is greater than the fall in FVC (i.e., a decrease in FEV_1/FVC). The severe obstruction curve describes the effort of a patient with very severe COPD. Note the failure to totally reach a "plateau," which indicates that FVC is underestimated.

Normal (—)
FEV_1 = 4.5 L
FVC = 6.0 L
FEV_1/FVC = 75%

Mild Obstruction (— —)
FEV_1 = 3.0 L
FVC = 6.0 L
FEV_1/FVC = 50%

Severe Obstruction (- - -)
FEV_1 = 0.6 L
FVC = 1.6 L
FEV_1/FVC = 38%

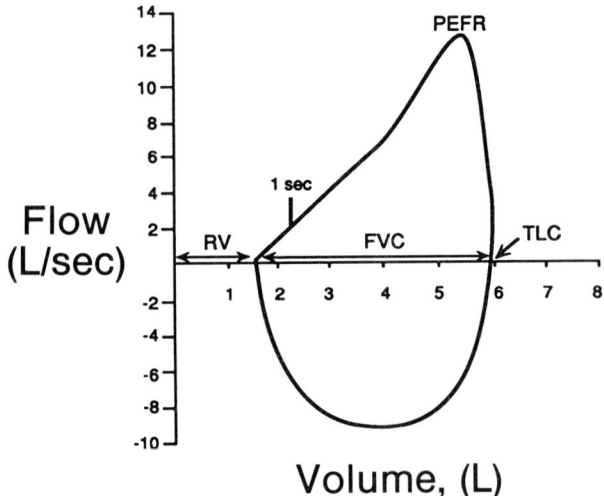

FIGURE 3–7. Flow-volume relationship of a normal subject. Since a separate measurement of FRC was performed, flow is plotted against absolute lung volume. The subject initially exhales to RV (not shown), then inhales maximally to TLC and exhales maximally to RV. The pulse on the flow-volume loop indicates volume exhaled from TLC in 1 second, i.e., the FEV$_1$. (PEFR: peak expiratory flow rate.)

is the principal cause of airflow limitation (Fig. 3–9). At the onset of maximum expiratory airflow, the contraction of muscles of expiration raises Ppl. Since they are physically linked in a series, the Ppl vector sums with the elastic recoil pressure (Pel) vector to produce alveolar pressure (P$_A$ = Ppl + Pel), which is the driving pressure for expiratory airflow. On expiration, airway pressure falls down the length of the airway to where pressure is atmospheric (Patm = 0), following the pressure gradient formed between the alveolus and the mouth. At some point along the airway, intraluminal pressure falls to a point where it equals Ppl. This *equal pressure point* (EPP) typically occurs in the segmental bronchi of normal subjects and divides the bronchus into an upstream component (toward the alveolus) and a downstream component (toward the mouth). Downstream from the EPP, Ppl exceeds intraluminal pressure, and airways are subject to dynamic compression. If this occurs in an unsupported airway, the airway starts to close.

Maximum airflow ($\dot{V}$max) during forced expiration at any lung volume where airflow limitation occurs is determined by the pressure gradient upstream from the EPP (P$_A$ − P$_{EPP}$) and by the upstream resistance (Rus) analogously to Ohm's law of electricity:

$$I = (E1 - E2)/R \text{ (Ohm's law)} \quad \text{Equation 1}$$

where I is current, E1 − E2 is the electrical potential difference between two points along a wire, and R is resistance. In the lung, where $\dot{V}$ is analogous to current and P is analogous to voltage:

$$\dot{V}\text{max} = (P_A - P_{EPP})/\text{Rus} \quad \text{Equation 2}$$

Since P$_{EPP}$ = Ppl, and P$_A$ = Pel + Ppl, $\dot{V}$max = [(Pel + Ppl) − Ppl]/Rus, or when simplified:

$$\dot{V}\text{max} = \text{Pel/Rus} \quad \text{Equation 3}$$

Note that maximum expiratory airflow is effort-independent at lung volumes where there is airflow limitation (provided patients generate enough Ppl to "flow limit").

effects of increasing expiratory effort as measured by P$_A$ on airflow at three different lung volumes, the so-called *isovolume pressure-flow curves*.[12] Note how expiratory flow remains relatively constant after a threshold expiratory effort despite increasing P$_A$; that is, in spite of increasing effort, there is no further increase in flow. It is for this reason that expiratory flow is described as "effort-independent." Dynamic compression of airways

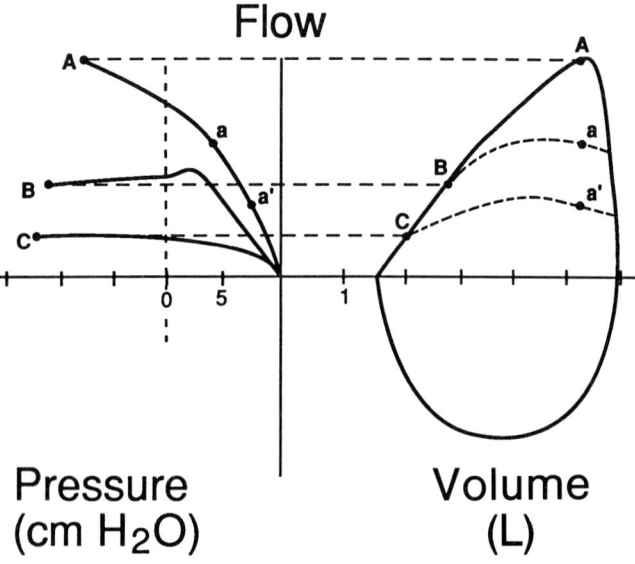

FIGURE 3–8. The relationship between pleural pressure, flow, and volume during maximum expiratory flow. The *left side* of this graph is the flow-pressure relationship at isovolumes. For example, to generate curve A, flow-pressure points from A, a, and a' are plotted. Points ABC on the isovolume-flow curves relate to the same points on the flow-volume curve. After the initial generation of pressure, the isovolume-flow curves flatten, and flow is independent of effort. For example, as pressure is increased for isovolume C, there is no further increase in flow.

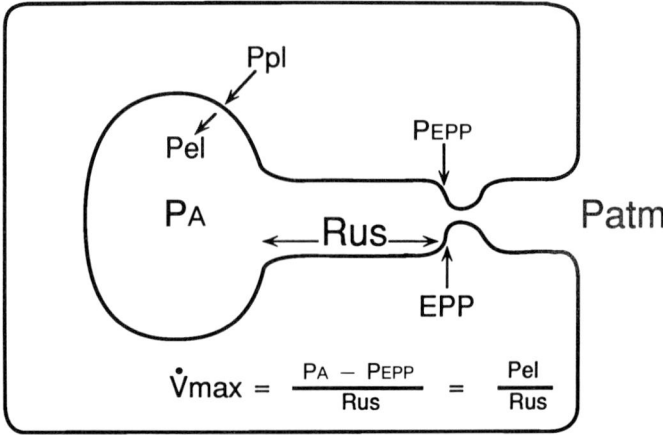

FIGURE 3–9. The equal pressure point (EPP) concept of flow limitation during expiration. The driving pressure for maximum airflow ($\dot{V}$max) is alveolar pressure (P$_A$), which is the sum of pleural pressure (Ppl) and elastic pressure (Pel) minus the pressure at the equal pressure point (P$_{EPP}$). The resistance offered by the system is upstream to the EPP.

Increased expiratory airflow limitation (i.e., decreased $\dot{V}$max) results from either decreased Pel (as in emphysema[13]) or increased Rus (as occurs in emphysema and chronic bronchitis).[13] The relative contributions of Pel and Rus to the reduction in airflow can be further partitioned by plotting maximum expiratory airflow against lung elastic recoil pressure to measure Rus. It should be further noted that maximum expiratory flow rates determine the shape of the flow-volume loop (see Fig. 3–8), and when they are low, as in COPD, the flow-volume loop takes on a characteristic "scooped" appearance (Fig. 3–10). Severely affected patients may demonstrate expiratory flow limitation even during quiet breathing.

By contrast, inspiratory flow is not "flow limited" under normal situations because airway compression does not occur. Rather, during inspiration, intrathoracic airways dilate, and flow is enhanced. Maximum inspiratory flow depends primarily on the force generated by the inspiratory muscles and less on flow resistance during inspiration. Increased flow resistance during inspiration is more characteristic of chronic bronchitis and asthma than of emphysema, but this finding is relatively nonspecific. The most important use of the maximum inspiratory flow-volume loop comes in the evaluation of upper airway (extrathoracic) obstruction, in which the inspiratory flow-volume loop may characteristically flatten. Upper airway obstruction is rare but may be a complication of previous intubation in patients with COPD. When present, it can be detected with spirometry[14] or bronchoscopy in patients with COPD, and it adds to the resistive load to breathing.

Whereas PEFR and $FEV_{0.5}$ measure expiratory airflow at lung volumes where airways are widely open and airflow limitation does not occur, FEV_1 measures airflow over a larger range of lung volumes, including volumes at which airflow limitation is present. Thus, FEV_1 is influenced by Pel and Rus. Still, like PEFR and $FEV_{0.5}$, patients must inspire to TLC and exhale maximally to obtain interpretable values for FEV_1. Because FEV_1 reflects alterations in several mechanical properties of the lung (and is easy to record), it has emerged as a preferred measure of functional impairment. Its measurement is essential to the assessment of the patient with pulmonary disease and for screening purposes.

Maximum Voluntary Ventilation. Another measure of dynamic lung function is maximum voluntary ventilation (MVV). The MVV is the maximum volume of air that a patient can breathe in and out in 1 minute as predicted by 12 to 15 seconds of maximum hyperventilation. During this maneuver, respiratory rate should approach 90 breaths per minute. When patient cooperation or other factors preclude direct measurement, MVV is estimated as $FEV_1 \times 40$ in healthy individuals and in patients with obstructive disease. However, this estimate often gives erroneously low values because of airways compression, which is more likely to occur during the maximum forced expiratory flow-volume maneuver than the MVV maneuver. The difference between MVV and the maximum minute ventilation during exercise measures the ventilatory reserve (see Chapter 10).

Airway Resistance. In addition to measuring delayed lung emptying with spirometry, obstruction can be evaluated by measuring airway resistance (Raw) or specific airway conductance. Direct measurements of Raw do not provide information about changes in lung elastic recoil pressure and therefore provide less information (as a single measurement) about the severity of functional impairment than does forced spirometry.[15] The larger, central airways are responsible for 90% of total Raw, whereas the smaller, peripheral airways contribute nominally to total Raw because of their much greater cross-sectional area. Thus, significant airway obstruction can occur in the peripheral airways without much change in total Raw. Nevertheless, specific pulmonary conductance can be quite sensitive to changes in resistance, especially when the central airways are involved (e.g., in centrilobular emphysema).

Raw is determined by measuring the pressure drop along the airway ($P_A - P_{ao}$) required to achieve a certain flow ($\dot{V}$). When P_{ao} is atmospheric (0 cm H_2O), $P_A - P_{ao} = P_A$ and

$$Raw = (P_A - P_{ao})/\dot{V} = P_A/\dot{V} \quad \text{Equation 4}$$

Raw is most often measured in a body plethysmograph, though other methods are available. Patients pant through an open shutter while $\dot{V}$ and plethysmographic volume (V_{BP}) are measured. The shutter is then closed while panting continues to measure P_{ao} and V_{BP}. Under these conditions of zero flow, P_{ao} is assumed to equal P_A, P_A can be plotted against V_{BP}, and $\dot{V}$ against V_{BP}. Raw is calculated by dividing the slope (P_A/V_{BP}) of the first plot by the slope ($\dot{V}/V_{BP}$) of the second plot:

$$Raw = (P_A/V_{BP})/(\dot{V}/V_{BP}) = P_A/\dot{V} \quad \text{Equation 5}$$

Normal Raw from the alveolus to the mouth is about 1.5 cm H_2O/L/sec.

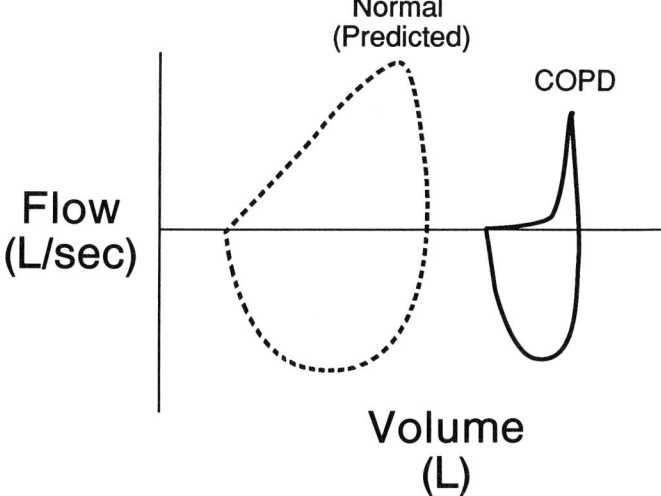

FIGURE 3–10. A flow-volume curve for a patient with severe airflow limitation. The curve shows hyperinflation (increased lung volume) and airflow limitation (reduced airflow). Note the "scooped" appearance of the expiratory part of the flow-volume loop, but also note the preservation of an ability to generate inspiratory flow. The *dashed loop* is the flow-volume loop for a normal subject.

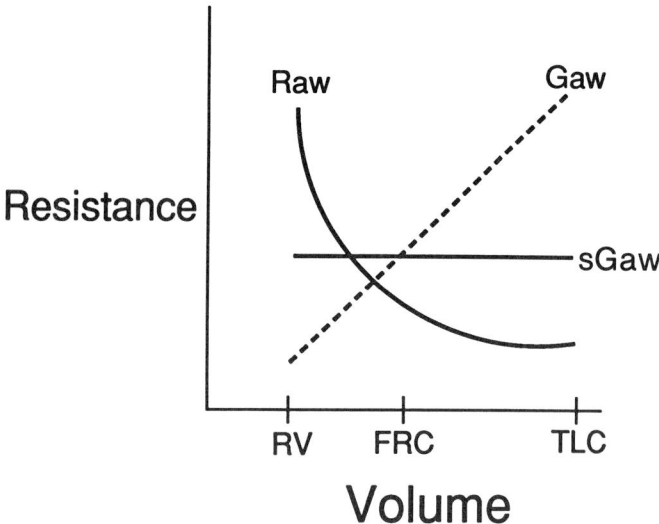

FIGURE 3–11. Effect of lung volume on airway resistance (Raw), airway conductance (Gaw = 1/Raw), and specific airway conductance (sGaw = Gaw/thoracic gas volume [Vtg]). As lung volume increases from RV to TLC, resistance falls. Conversely, its inverse conductance rises. Dividing Gaw by the lung volume at which it was determined renders this measurement independent of lung volume.

linear with respect to lung volume. In practice, Gaw is normalized to lung volume by dividing it by thoracic gas volume (TGV) or FRC (the volume at which it is measured) to give the specific airway conductance (sGaw). As such, sGaw provides one of the only common approaches to measuring airway function that accounts for changes in lung volume.

WORK OF BREATHING

For inspiratory gas flow to occur, the inspiratory muscles (mainly the diaphragm) must generate enough negative pleural pressure to overcome the resident resistive and elastic pressures. In other words, strength must be greater than load. Patients with COPD have a precarious combination of decreased inspiratory muscle strength (see Chapter 4) and increased elastic and resistive loads. Not surprisingly, relatively small insults affecting either may precipitate acute respiratory failure.[16] Conversely, one goal of therapeutic management is to increase strength and decrease load.

Work of breathing is the sum of the elastic and the resistive loads to breathing. It is increased in patients with COPD because Raw is high and Cdyn is low. Most of the increase in the work of breathing (which may be five times the norm in stable COPD) is done by the inspiratory muscles on the lung parenchyma and airways. Common estimates of the work of breathing, therefore, are made by examining the work done solely on the lung and do not take into account work done on the chest wall.

Raw is influenced by a number of factors, including lung volume, bronchomotor tone, secretions, airway edema, phase of respiration, and loss of support from the surrounding lung tissue. Figure 3–11 shows the nonlinear, exponential relationship between lung volume and Raw. Resistance rises considerably as the lungs deflate and the airways narrow. At high lung volumes, resistance falls as airways are pulled open by the elasticity of the surrounding lung tissue. Emphysema results in a loss of lung elastic recoil pressure. Airways are therefore narrower and resistance is higher, a phenomenon diminished somewhat by lung hyperinflation.

Airway conductance (Gaw), the reciprocal of Raw, is

Work is calculated as the product of pressure and volume (P × V); thus work done on the lung is the area "under" the P-V relationship of the lung. Figure 3–12 shows a P-V curve of the lung in a normal subject (A) and in a patient with airflow obstruction (B) during tidal breathing. Area *ABHDFA* represents the work

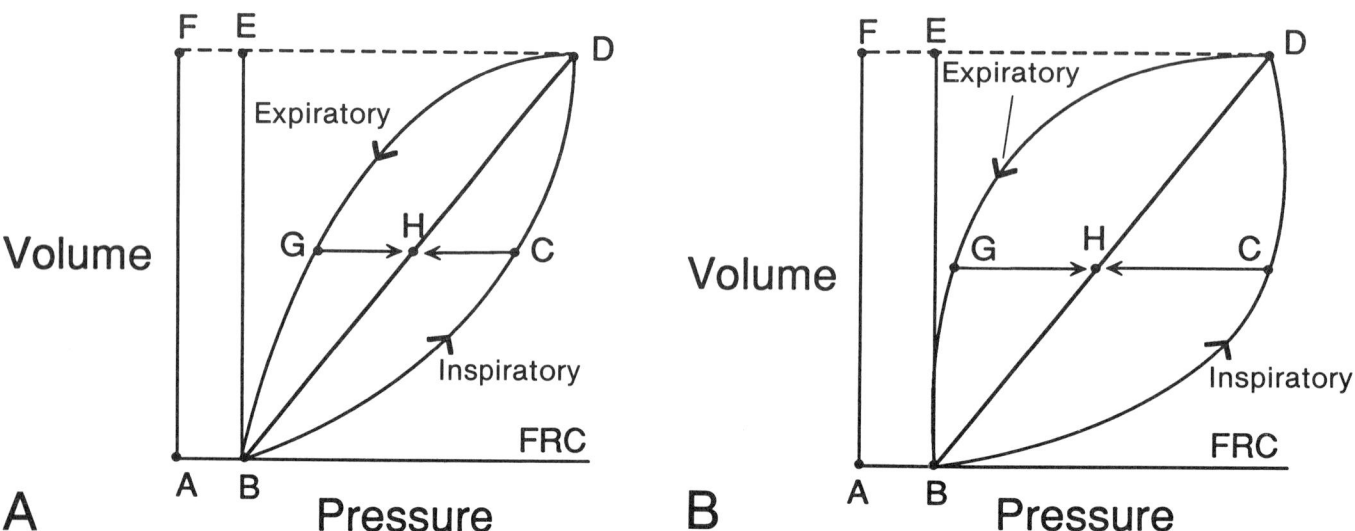

FIGURE 3–12. Volume-pressure relationship (work of breathing) for a person with normal lungs (A) and a patient with COPD (B). Work is defined as the product of pressure and volume, and components of work are described as different areas of the volume-pressure relationship (see text for explanation). The *arrows* represent the tracking of pressure when flow is stopped.

done to overcome the static elastic properties of the lung. It can be divided into the work required to maintain the lung at FRC (*ABEFA*) and the elastic work required to take a tidal breath (*BHDEB*). Area *BCDHB* represents the additional work required to overcome frictional Raw during inspiration. Likewise, area *DGBHD* is the work required to overcome frictional Raw during exhalation. Note that if flow were interrupted during inspiration at point *C*, Ppl would fall to point *H*. The difference in pressure from point *C* to point *H* represents flow resistance. Similarly, if flow were interrupted during exhalation at point *G*, Ppl would increase to point *H*. The total work of breathing done on the lung during inspiration is the sum of elastic work and flow-resistive work, or area *ABCDFA*.

In patients with airflow obstruction, increased Raw adds to the total work of breathing (see Fig. 3–12*B*). Work of breathing also increases in patients with airflow obstruction because Cdyn is low owing to PEEPi. Though static CL is high in emphysema, compliance falls during tidal breathing in the presence of airflow obstruction (see previous discussion on the frequency dependence of compliance). Additional elastic loads include atelectasis, pulmonary edema, infection, and tumor.[16]

In an intubated, sedated, and muscle-relaxed patient, the load on the respiratory system during tidal breathing can be estimated based on the resistive and static pressures generated by a VT that is similar to that of the patient's spontaneous breath (often about 300 ml). Resistive pressure is calculated by subtracting static pressure from peak pressure. Static pressure is determined using an end-inspiratory hold maneuver. PEEPi can be measured by an end-expiratory hold maneuver.

AIRWAY RESPONSIVENESS

Airway responsiveness is defined for purposes of this discussion as either the response to inhaled bronchodilators or the response to inhaled bronchoconstrictors.

Response to Inhaled Bronchodilators. A large percentage of patients with COPD have some degree of reversible airways obstruction. Reversible components of the pathologic alterations observed in COPD include mucosal edema, secretions, inflammation, and smooth muscle dysfunction (i.e., bronchospasm). Typically, reactive airways disease is demonstrated by repeating spirometry after the inhalation of a beta$_2$ agonist (e.g., albuterol 2.5 mg). Improvement in either FVC or FEV$_1$ by more than 15% suggests reactive airways disease.[17] It must be kept in mind, however, that significant improvement in airflow can occur at any given lung volume (isovolume flow) without a change in FEVs (Fig. 3–13). This occurs when administration of a bronchodilator attenuates lung hyperinflation without changing FEVs. Therefore, unless lung volumes are measured before and after bronchodilator use, improvement in isovolume flows can be missed in some patients, and such patients may be labeled incorrectly as having only irreversible airflow obstruction. Also, the lack of an apparent response to an inhaled bronchodilator does not exclude reactive airways disease, since bronchodilator response can vary with the time, duration, and dose of therapy as well as the type of bronchodilator used. Conversely, a false improvement in FEV$_1$ can occur if the patient inhaled more air, that is, if the TLC was greater.

Although conflicting data exist, the presence of a bronchodilator response appears to be positively correlated with survival. This relationship disappears, however, when postbronchodilator FEV$_1$ is substituted for prebronchodilator FEV$_1$,[9] indicating that the degree of fixed obstruction is the important factor.

Response to Bronchial Challenge. Bronchial challenge with methacholine or histamine is rarely performed in patients with COPD or with grossly abnormal spirograms to avoid precipitating severe airflow obstruction. In addition, it is known that the degree of reactivity to nonspecific bronchial challenge is directly correlated with baseline FEV$_1$. Accordingly, assessment of FEV$_1$ usually suffices in patients with abnormal spirograms at

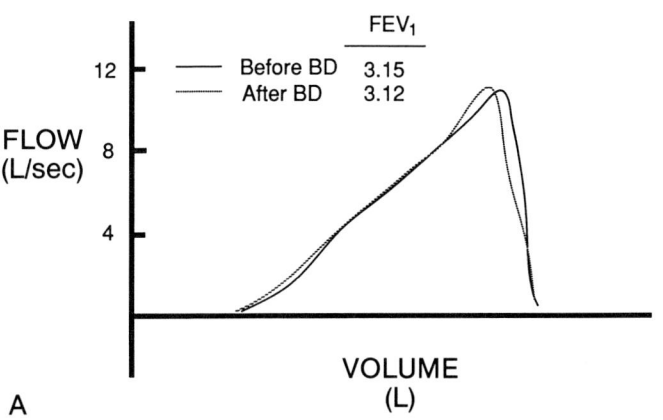
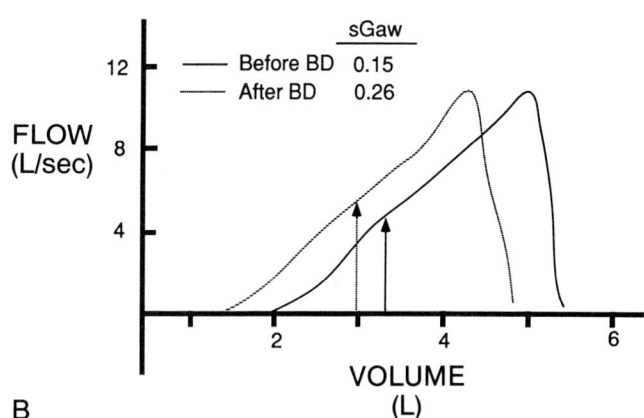

FIGURE 3–13. Flow-volume relationships before (*solid line*) and after (*dashed line*) the inhalation of a bronchodilator (BD). *A*, When these two flow-volume curves are superimposed at TLC (assuming TLC did not change), there is no apparent improvement. *B*, However, when the curves are plotted at absolute lung volume, there is a shift to the left owing to a decrease in lung volume. The *solid and dashed vertical arrows* indicate flow at FRC for both situations. There is an increase in airflow at any absolute lung volume (isovolume). Note the increase in sGaw, another volume-corrected index of airflow limitation. (From Irvin CG, Cherniak RM. Pathophysiology and physiologic assessment of the asthmatic patient. Semin Respir Med 1987, 8:212.)

first presentation. However, if the spirogram is normal, as may be the case in the early stages of chronic bronchitis, the identification of airway hyperresponsiveness may prove useful. Airway hyperresponsiveness is demonstrated by a greater than 20% decrease in FEV_1 ($PC_{20\%}$-FEV_1), a greater than 35% increase in sGaw ($PC_{35\%}$-sGaw), or both of these features in response to lower doses of inhaled methacholine or histamine than is seen in normal individuals. Using published guidelines for their administration, most normal subjects require doses of methacholine or histamine greater than 8 mg/ml to produce a 20% decrease in FEV_1 ($PC_{20\%}$-FEV_1 > 8 mg/ml).[18–20] Marked airway hyperresponsiveness ($PC_{20\%}$-FEV_1 < 2 mg/ml) is characteristic of unstable asthma. Patients with stable asthma and those with chronic bronchitis may have mild to moderate hyperresponsiveness ($PC_{20\%}$-FEV_1 > 2 < 8 mg/ml).[21, 22] Airway hyperresponsiveness may be overestimated in patients with COPD if reduced airway caliber causes inhaled particles to deposit in larger, central airways responsible for most of the total airway resistance.[23] Some authors have suggested that further information can be gained from the shape of the dose-response curve for methacholine.[21, 24] In unstable asthma, the dose-response curve does not plateau even though the FEV_1 has been reduced more than 50%. In healthy subjects and in patients with COPD the dose-response curve usually plateaus after the administration of a certain dose.

The mechanisms responsible for airway hyperresponsiveness in patients with COPD are unclear. Hypothesized causes include airway inflammation (allergic and nonallergic), neural reflexes, abnormalities in airway smooth muscle, alterations in the bronchial circulation,[25] and, most probably, fixed airways narrowing. However, it is clear that airway hyperresponsiveness contributes to the symptoms of cough, wheezing, and shortness of breath, and that it is a risk factor for further decline in FEV_1.[26]

GAS EXCHANGE

Oxygenation. The principal causes of arterial hypoxemia in patients with COPD are ventilation-perfusion mismatch ($\dot{V}A/\dot{Q}$ mismatch), alveolar hypoventilation, and low mixed venous PO_2 ($P\bar{v}O_2$). Shunt is uncommon unless a separate alveolar filling process is present, such as pneumonia or pulmonary edema. Thus, correction of arterial hypoxemia in these patients usually requires only slight enrichment of inspired air (e.g., 1–2 L/min of oxygen delivered by nasal cannula). Interestingly, the degree of arterial hypoxemia correlates poorly with other measures of severity in COPD, such as FEV_1.[27]

The multiple inert gas elimination technique and, more recently, positron-emission tomography (PET) have added considerably to our understanding of the relationship between ventilation and perfusion. The multiple inert gas technique involves infusing inert gases of different solubility into a peripheral vein, from where they travel to the pulmonary circulation. Under normal conditions, gases of low solubility escape readily into alveolar gas, whereas gases of high solubility are retained in the circulation. When lung units are perfused but not ventilated, gases with low solubility are retained in the circulation to a greater degree than under normal conditions. Computer analysis of retention-excretion patterns of these gases and measurement of blood flow make it possible to characterize the relationship between ventilation and perfusion. Data obtained from this method agree well with recent data collected from PET imaging.[28]

Under normal conditions ventilation and perfusion are closely matched (i.e., $\dot{V}A/\dot{Q}$ almost equals 1). In COPD different patterns exist. In patients with few gas exchange abnormalities, areas of normal to high $\dot{V}A/\dot{Q}$ ratios can be observed.[28, 29] High $\dot{V}A/\dot{Q}$ regions appear to result from ventilation of areas of alveolar wall destruction where blood flow is low.[28, 29] These patients often fit the description of the type A patient ("pink puffer"), a thin patient who maintains adequate gas exchange by maintaining a high minute ventilation ($\dot{V}E$). A more variable pattern of $\dot{V}A/\dot{Q}$ inequality, including areas of low $\dot{V}A/\dot{Q}$ ratios, is seen in type B patients ("blue bloaters").[27–29] These patients are typically hypoxemic, hypercarbic, and much more likely to develop cor pulmonale and peripheral edema. Low $\dot{V}A/\dot{Q}$ areas appear to result from secretions and wall thickening (which decrease ventilation to perfused lung units) and not from dynamic compression.[27] Formerly, type A patients with emphysema were equated with type B patients with chronic bronchitis. It is now known that both patient groups have airway inflammation and loss of alveolar walls, and that the major differences between these groups of patients are the responsiveness of the respiratory center to derangements in blood gases and the pattern of $\dot{V}A/\dot{Q}$ mismatch. Type A patients tend to be patients who maintain alveolar ventilation and have normal to high $\dot{V}A/\dot{Q}$ regions, whereas type B patients fail to maintain adequate alveolar ventilation and have areas of low $\dot{V}A/\dot{Q}$ ratios.

To understand how low $\dot{V}A/\dot{Q}$ may cause arterial hypoxemia, consider a lung with two units (Fig. 3–14). Under the normal conditions of uniform ventilation and perfusion each unit receives about 50% of the ventilation and 50% of the cardiac output, mixed venous blood is fully oxygenated, and a normal amount of CO_2 is eliminated.[30] When ventilation to unit 2 is decreased without a change in perfusion, mixed venous blood is not fully oxygenated and less CO_2 is removed. The desaturated blood leaving unit 2 mixes with the blood leaving unit 1 to form arterial blood. Because of the sigmoidal shape of the oxyhemoglobin dissociation curve, hemoglobin saturations (or oxygen contents), and not the partial pressures of oxygen, are averaged to calculate the composition of arterial blood. PaO_2 is set by the hemoglobin saturation of the mixture of units 1 and 2 as well as by the shape of the oxyhemoglobin dissociation curve. Since the CO_2 dissociation curve is more linear than the oxyhemoglobin dissociation curve, averaging the PCO_2 of each effluent provides a close estimate of $PaCO_2$. Note further that low $\dot{V}A/\dot{Q}$ causes CO_2 retention as well as hypoxemia, a situation usually masked by hyperventilation.

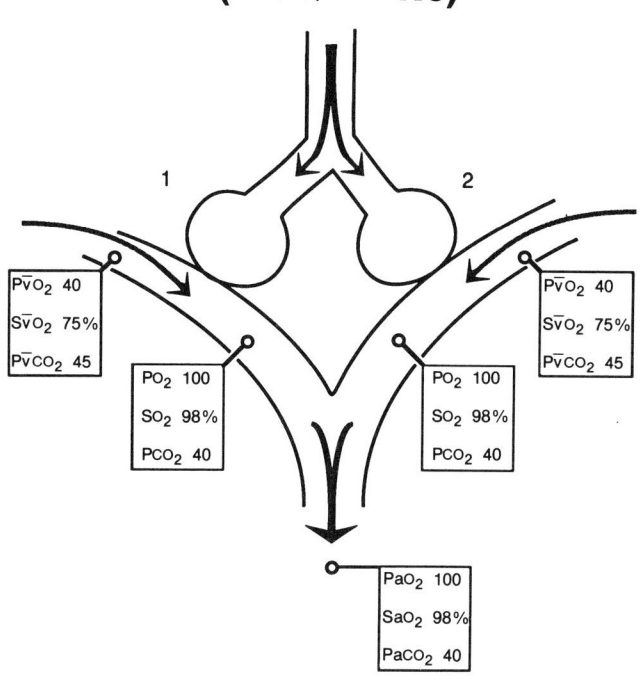
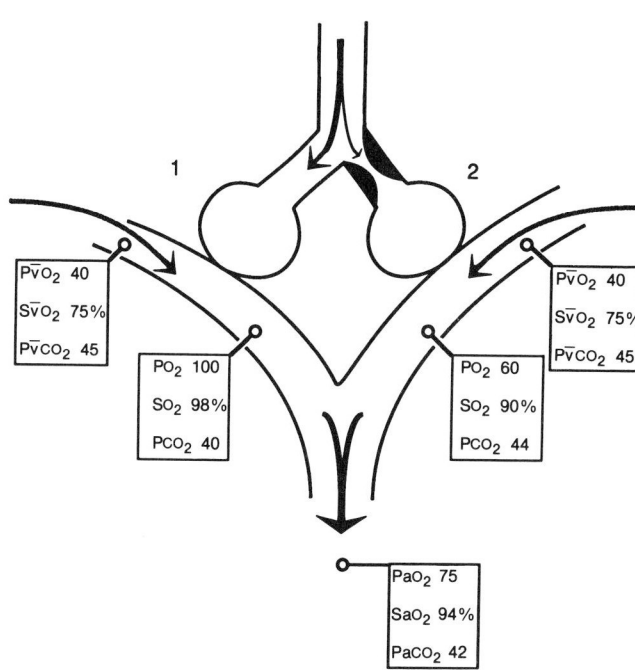

FIGURE 3–14. Ventilation-perfusion relationships for a normal (A, $\dot{V}_A/\dot{Q}$ ~1.0 and a diseased (B, $\dot{V}_A/\dot{Q}$ <1.0) lung that consist of two exchange units (1 and 2), each receiving 50% of the cardiac output. ($P\bar{v}_{O_2}$: partial pressure of oxygen, mixed venous blood; $S\bar{v}_{O_2}$: oxygen saturation, mixed venous blood; $P\bar{v}_{CO_2}$: partial pressure of carbon dioxide, mixed venous blood.) Three points along the transit of the blood are noted: the mixed venous entry point (upper open circles, left and right), the end capillary point (middle open circles, left and right), and arterial blood (last open circle). In COPD (B), airways of unit 2 narrow, and the ventilation of this unit falls; however, perfusion to unit 2 is maintained. The poorly oxygenated blood mixes with that of unit 1, and hypoxemia results.

Although most patients with type B COPD have areas of low $\dot{V}_A/\dot{Q}$ ratios, and since low $\dot{V}_A/\dot{Q}$ causes hypoxemia, there is little correlation between the $\dot{V}_A/\dot{Q}$ distribution pattern (high, low, or mixed) and arterial blood gas values.[27] Reductions in $\dot{V}_A/\dot{Q}$ are still expected to result in hypoxemia,[27] but this observation calls attention to the other causes of hypoxemia in patients with COPD, namely, hypercapnia and low $P\bar{v}_{O_2}$. Thus, in any given patient a combination of these factors determines Pa_{O_2}.[27]

To understand how hypercapnia causes hypoxemia, consider the simplified alveolar gas equation (Equation 6). This equation predicts alveolar P_{O_2} (P_{AO_2}) for a given barometric pressure (P_B), alveolar water vapor pressure (P_{AH_2O}), fraction of inspired oxygen (F_{IO_2}), alveolar CO_2 (P_{ACO_2}, assumed to equal Pa_{CO_2}), and respiratory quotient (RQ = CO_2 production/O_2 consumption):

$$P_{AO_2} = (P_B - P_{AH_2O}) F_{IO_2} - P_{ACO_2}/RQ$$
Equation 6

In a normal subject breathing ambient air at sea level, P_B is 760 mm Hg, P_{AH_2O} is 47 mm Hg, F_{IO_2} is 0.21, Pa_{CO_2} is 40 mm Hg, and RQ is 0.8. The predicted P_{AO_2} under these conditions is 100 mm Hg. If we assume a normal alveolar-arterial P_{O_2} difference (e.g., 5 mm Hg), then Pa_{O_2} equals 95 mm Hg. When the blood of a hypercapnic patient equilibrates with alveolar gas, the elevated alveolar CO_2 level dilutes the inspired oxygen and lowers P_{AO_2}. In the above example, increasing Pa_{CO_2} from 40 mm Hg to 55 mm Hg under the same conditions would decrease P_{AO_2} from 100 mm Hg to 81 mm Hg.

Arterial hypoxemia also results from perfusing lung units having very low $\dot{V}_A/\dot{Q}$ with a low $P\bar{v}_{O_2}$, a frequent finding in patients with pulmonary hypertension and low cardiac output. In these patients, increasing venous saturation by raising cardiac output or hemoglobin or by decreasing oxygen consumption increases arterial saturation.

Ventilation. Chronic respiratory acidosis is common in patients with COPD. To understand why this acid-base disturbance occurs, what determines Pa_{CO_2}, that is, the ratio of CO_2 production ($\dot{V}_{CO_2}$) to CO_2 elimination, should first be considered:

$$Pa_{CO_2} = K \times CO_2 \text{ production}/CO_2 \text{ elimination}$$
Equation 7

where K = 863, a constant necessary to convert CO_2 elimination in the gas phase (measured in BTPS) to STPD and to convert fractional concentration to partial pressure

Elimination of CO_2 is synonymous with alveolar ventilation ($\dot{V}_A$), which is the amount of minute ventilation ($\dot{V}_E$ = respiratory rate [RR] $\times V_T$) that participates in gas exchange. In other words, $\dot{V}_A$ is equal to $\dot{V}_E$ minus wasted or dead space ventilation ($\dot{V}_{DS}$):

$$\dot{V}_A = \dot{V}_E - \dot{V}_{DS} \quad \text{Equation 8}$$

Therefore, "CO_2 elimination" can be replaced by $\dot{V}_E - \dot{V}_{DS}$ in Equation 7:

$$Pa_{CO_2} = K \times \dot{V}_{CO_2}/ (\dot{V}_E - \dot{V}_{DS}) \quad \text{Equation 9}$$

Since $\dot{V}_E - \dot{V}_{DS} = \dot{V}_E (1 - V_{DS}/V_T)$, Equation 9 can be rewritten into an equation that is useful in the clinical setting:

$$Pa_{CO_2} = K \times \dot{V}_{CO_2}/[\dot{V}_E (1 - V_{DS}/V_T)],$$
$$\text{where } K = 863 \quad \text{Equation 10}$$

For example, in a normal 70-kg patient with $\dot{V}_{CO_2}$ of 190 ml/min, RR of 12/min, V_T of 500 ml, and V_{DS} of 150 ml, Pa_{CO_2} equals 39 mm Hg. In normals individuals, V_{DS} (in milliliters) can be estimated based on a patient's weight in pounds, and the ratio of dead space to tidal volume (V_{DS}/V_T) is usually less than 0.3.

Values of V_{DS}/V_T in the range of 0.4 to 0.5 are common in patients with COPD because alveolar wall destruction and hyperinflation reduce blood flow to ventilated units. Additionally, a breathing pattern characterized by fast and shallow breaths (as is typical of acute exacerbations of COPD) further elevates V_{DS}/V_T by lowering V_T.[31] Increasing V_{DS}/V_T from 0.4 to 0.6 requires an increase in minute ventilation of 50% to maintain a constant Pa_{CO_2} (see Equation 9). Greater minute ventilation in turn increases PEEPi, $\dot{V}_{CO_2}$, and work of breathing, and is associated with the development of hypercapnic respiratory failure.[16] To make matters worse, progressive hypercapnia may increase respiratory muscle weakness.[32]

The breathing pattern in stable patients with COPD and eucapnia is usually characterized by an increase in respiratory rate and a normal V_T.[33] Failure to maintain adequate minute ventilation is typical of hypercapnic type B patients. Whereas a eucapneic type A patient may have a $\dot{V}_E$ of 12 L/min, a hypercapnic patient may have a $\dot{V}_E$ of only 8 L/min.[34] Note that even hypercapnic patients tend to have values for $\dot{V}_E$ that are higher than normal. Failure to maintain adequate minute ventilation most likely results from decreased responsiveness of the respiratory center to derangements in blood gases and respiratory muscle weakness.

DIFFUSING CAPACITY

The diffusing capacity of a gas across the alveolocapillary membrane depends on the amount of gas that can cross the alveolocapillary barrier per unit time and on the alveolocapillary partial pressure difference of the gas. In common clinical practice, the diffusing capacity for carbon monoxide (D_{LCO}) is determined, although oxygen can be used as well. Thus:

$$D_{LCO} = \dot{V}_{CO}/(Pa_{CO} - Pc_{CO}) \quad \text{Equation 11}$$

where $\dot{V}_{CO}$ is the carbon monoxide uptake per minute, Pa_{CO} is alveolar carbon monoxide tension, and Pc_{CO} is the partial pressure of carbon monoxide in the capillary.

Because practically all carbon monoxide is bound by hemoglobin, Pc_{CO} is trivial and usually ignored; thus, Equation 10 reduces to:

$$D_{LCO} = \dot{V}_{CO}/Pa_{CO} \quad \text{Equation 12}$$

The D_{LCO} is most often determined by the single-breath test, in which patients are required to inhale a low concentration of carbon monoxide and hold their breath for 10 seconds. Analyses of the inspired gas, expired gas, lung volume, and breath hold time are all that is required to measure D_{LCO}. This does not mean, however, that this is an easy measurement to take. Measuring D_{LCO} is difficult in dyspneic patients, who find it hard to hold their breath the required 10 seconds. The measurement of D_{LCO} is also very dependent on technique and may not be comparable among laboratories. Despite these limitations, the D_{LCO} is one of the most useful measurements available to assess the severity of emphysema.

In order to diffuse from the alveolus to hemoglobin, carbon monoxide must overcome the resistances of two major components. The first is called the *membrane component* ($1/D_{mCO}$), which represents the resistance to diffusion offered by the alveolocapillary membrane, plasma, and red blood cell membrane. The second component is *red blood cell resistance,* which depends on the volume of blood in the pulmonary capillaries (V_c) and on the rate at which carbon monoxide binds to hemoglobin (Θ). The total resistance ($1/D_{LCO}$) can be expressed as the sum of these two component resistances:

$$1/D_{LCO} = 1/D_{mCO} + 1/\Theta V_c \quad \text{Equation 13}$$

Of the two components of total resistance to diffusion, $1/\Theta V_c$ is the most important. When there is loss of pulmonary capillary bed, as in emphysema, D_{LCO} falls. Similarly, when there is an increase in pulmonary blood volume, as during exercise, or more substantially during pulmonary hemorrhage, D_{LCO} is elevated. The D_{LCO} is particularly useful in differentiating emphysema from chronic severe asthma where diffusing capacity may be normal or slightly elevated. Slight increases in D_{LCO} are common in asthma; this is presumably the result of greater negative intrapleural pressure during breathing, which increases venous return to the chest and intracapillary blood volume.

PHYSIOLOGIC AND PATHOLOGIC CORRELATIONS

A question that must be asked concerning all of the physiologic tests performed on patients is what, if any, is the correlation of each of these tests to the pathologic alterations of the disease? For patients with COPD, we are most interested in the correlation between pulmonary function tests, arterial blood gases, and radiographs, and the degree of tissue loss. It should be pointed out that no single test other than autopsy proves or disproves the presence and extent of emphysema, although some tests are better predictors of emphysema than others. A general principle is that in the right clinical setting the more abnormal the pulmonary function test findings and radiographs, the better the prediction of the amount of emphysema.[35, 36] Clearly, an integrated approach to each patient is desirable. In this section, the structural correlates of the P-V curve, lung volumes, airflow obstruction, and diffusing capacity are briefly discussed.

In general, the correlation between loss of elastic recoil and emphysema has been closer in lungs examined at autopsy than in lungs examined in vivo.[35, 37] Autopsy studies have found a statistically significant relationship between loss of elastic recoil measured post mortem and the extent of emphysema[38, 39]; however, this relationship is difficult to show when the P-V curve is performed in a living patient and then compared with the extent of emphysema found in a surgically excised specimen.[40] The reasons for this poor correlation include the variability of emphysema in surgically excised lobes (which may not reflect what occurs in the rest of the lung) and the inaccuracies of in vivo measurements of esophageal pressure, which, among other factors, are affected by chest wall mechanics.[35] In fact, as many as one third of emphysematous lungs may have normal elastic recoil.[35]

Abnormalities of the subdivisions of lung volumes are better predictors of the amount of emphysema than elastic recoil. In general, as emphysema gets worse, RV, FRC, and TLC all increase. Early studies found the best predictor was RV/TLC.[34] In other words, large increases in RV are strongly suggestive of emphysema. The TLC was initially thought to be a poor predictor of emphysema, but in these studies the gas dilution technique was used to measure TLC, and hence the increase in TLC was probably underestimated.[37] When TLC is measured in a body plethysmograph, a good correlation between TLC and emphysema results,[36] even in patients with a mild degree of disease. Large increases in FRC, as with RV and TLC, are also predictive of emphysema.[41]

It has been known for quite some time that the frequency of airflow obstruction increases as the severity of emphysema increases and that most patients with severe emphysema have severe chronic airflow obstruction.[35] Conversely, mild emphysema may not be associated with airflow limitation.[38] In one retrospective study,[42] two thirds of patients with severe emphysema had severe chronic airflow obstruction. Patients were determined to have severe chronic airflow obstruction if they died from chronic airflow obstruction or if they died from other causes but had an FEV_1 of less than 40% of that predicted and an $FEF_{25-75\%}$ of less than 25% of that predicted. One third of the patients with the worst emphysema, however, did not have evidence of severe airflow limitation. These patients had either mild chronic airflow obstruction (FEV_1 between 40% and 80% of that predicted), or no identifiable chronic airflow obstruction. The reasons for this disparity are not entirely clear, although some patients may have been underdiagnosed.[41]

Diffusing capacity is perhaps the single best laboratory measurement of the severity of emphysema. Whereas the correlation coefficients found for other pulmonary function tests range between 0.3 and 0.5, the correlation coefficients for the relationship between D_{LCO} and severity of emphysema are typically between 0.6 and 0.8.[35, 40, 43]

To establish better radiographic and pathologic correlations, recent studies have compared computed tomography with pathologic specimens. Chest computed tomography has emerged as the best imaging technique to evaluate emphysema, and there is a good correlation between computed tomography findings and pathology (correlation coefficients between 0.6 and 0.8).[44, 45] However, current computed tomography techniques are not sufficiently sensitive for detecting early lesions.[44]

SUMMARY

Lung hyperinflation in patients with COPD is a result of abnormalities of both the static and dynamic properties of the respiratory system. The dominant physiologic abnormality in these patients is chronic expiratory airflow obstruction, which is not completely reversible. Work of breathing is increased in COPD patients because airway resistance is high and dynamic compliance is low.

Gas exchange abnormalities in COPD are characterized by arterial hypoxemia and normal or increased Pa_{CO_2}. Hypoxemia results from $\dot{V}_A/\dot{Q}$ mismatch, alveolar hypoventilation, and low $P\bar{v}_{O_2}$. Chronic respiratory acidosis results from increases in V_{DS}/V_T and a failure to maintain adequate minute ventilation either because of decreased responsiveness of the respiratory control center to derangements in blood gases, respiratory muscle weakness, or both.

The diffusing capacity is one of the most useful measurements available to differentiate emphysema from chronic severe asthma and to assess the severity of emphysema. When TLC is measured in a body plethysmograph, there is a good correlation between TLC and emphysema. Large increases in FRC and RV are also predictive of emphysema. Chest CT has emerged as the best imaging technique available to evaluate emphysema.

REFERENCES

1. American Thoracic Society. Standards for the diagnosis and care of patients with chronic obstructive pulmonary disease (COPD) and asthma. Am Rev Respir Dis 1986; 136:225–244.
2. Agonstoni E, Hyatt RE. Static behavior of the respiratory system. In: Fishman AP, Macklem PT, Mead J (eds). Handbook of Physiology. Section 3, The Respiratory System. Vol 3. The Mechanics of Breathing, Part 1. Bethesda, MD: American Physiological Society, 1986, pp 113–130.
3. Anthonisen NR. Tests of mechanical function. In: Fishman AP, Macklem PT, Mead J (eds). Handbook of Physiology. Section 3, The Respiratory System. Vol 3. The Mechanics of Breathing, Part 2. Bethesda, MD: American Physiological Society, 1986, pp 753–784.
4. Irvin CG, Cherniack RM. Pathophysiology and physiologic assessment of the asthmatic patient. Semin Respir Med 1987; 8:201–215.
5. Zarins LP. Closed-circuit helium dilution method of lung volume measurement. In: Clausen JL (ed). Pulmonary Function Testing Guidelines and Controversies. New York: Academic Press, Inc., 1982, pp 129–140.
6. Zarins LP, Clausen JL. Body plethysmography. In: Clausen JL (ed). Pulmonary Function Testing Guidelines and Controversies. New York, Academic Press, Inc., 1982, pp 141–153.

7. Decramer M, Demedts M, Rochette F, et al. Maximal transrespiratory pressures in obstructive lung disease. Bull Eur Physiopathol Respir 1980; 16:479–490.
8. American Thoracic Society. Standardization of spirometry: 1987 update. Am Rev Respir Dis 1987; 136:1285–1298.
9. Traver GA, Cline MG, Burrows B. Predictors of mortality in chronic obstructive pulmonary disease. Am Rev Respir Dis 1979; 119:895–902.
10. Burrows B. Course and prognosis in advanced disease. In: Petty TL (ed). Chronic Obstructive Pulmonary Disease. 2nd ed. New York: Marcel Dekker, Inc., 1985, pp 31–42.
11. Hodgkin JE. Pulmonary rehabilitation. Clin Chest Med 1990; 2:7 447–460.
12. Hyatt RE. Forced expiration. In: Fishman AP, Macklem PT, Mead J (eds). Handbook of Physiology. Section 3, The Respiratory System. Vol 3. The Mechanics of Breathing, Part 1. Bethesda, MD: American Physiological Society, 1986, pp 295–314.
13. Duffell MG, Marcus JH, Ingram RH. Limitation of expiratory flow in chronic obstructive pulmonary disease: Relation of clinical characteristics, pathophysiological type, and mechanisms. Ann Intern Med 1970; 72:365–374.
14. Rotman HH, Liss HP, Weg JG. Diagnosis of upper airway obstruction by pulmonary function testing. Chest 1975; 68:796–799.
15. Pride NB. The assessment of airflow obstruction: Role of measurements of airways resistance and of tests of forced expiration. Brit J Dis Chest 1971; 65:135–169.
16. Schmidt GA, Hall JB. Acute or chronic respiratory failure: Assessment and management of patients with COPD in the emergent setting. JAMA 1989; 261:3444–3453.
17. Ries AL. Response to bronchodilators. In: Clausen JL (ed). Pulmonary function testing guidelines and controversies. New York: Academic Press, Inc., 1982, pp 215–221.
18. Guidelines for bronchial inhalation challenges with pharmacologic and antigenic agents. Am Thor Soc News 1980; 6:11–19.
19. Guidelines for standardization of bronchial challenges with (nonspecific) bronchoconstricting agents. Bull Eur Physiopathol Respir 1983; 19:495–514.
20. Yan K, Salome C, Woolcock AJ. Rapid method for measurement of bronchial responsiveness. Thorax 1983; 38:760–765.
21. Woolcock AJ. Asthma. In: Murray JE, Nadel JA (eds). Textbook of Respiratory Medicine. Philadelphia: W.B. Saunders Co., 1988, pp 1030–1068.
22. Woolcock AJ, Permutt S. Bronchial hyperresponsiveness. In: Fishman AP, Macklem PT, Mead J (eds). Handbook of Physiology. Section 3, The Respiratory System. Vol 3. The Mechanics of Breathing, Part 2. Bethesda, MD: American Physiological Society, 1986, pp 727–736.
23. Dolovich MB, Sanchis J, Rossman C, et al. Aerosol penetrance: A sensitive index of peripheral airways obstruction. J Appl Physiol 1976; 40:468–471.
24. Woolcock AJ, Anderson SD, Peat JK, et al. Characteristics of bronchial hyperresonsiveness in chronic obstructive pulmonary disease and in asthma. Am Rev Respir Dis 1991; 143:1438–1443.
25. McFadden ER. Airway responsivity and chronic obstructive lung disease. In: Cherniack NS (ed). Chronic Obstructive Pulmonary Disease. Philadelphia: W.B. Saunders Co., 1991, pp 90–96.
26. Postma DS, deVries K, Koëter GH, et al. Independent influence of reversibility of air-flow obstruction and nonspecific hyperreactivity on the long-term course of lung function in chronic air-flow obstruction. Am Rev Respir Dis 1986; 134:276–280.
27. Wagner PD. Effects of COPD on gas exchange. In: Cherniack NS (ed). Chronic Obstructive Pulmonary Disease. Philadelphia: W.B. Saunders Co., 1991, pp 73–79.
28. Wagner PD, Rodriguez-Roisin R. Clinical advances in pulmonary gas exchange. Am Rev Respir Dis 1991; 143:883–888.
29. Wagner PD, Dantzker DR, Dueck R, et al. Ventilation-perfusion inequality in chronic obstructive pulmonary disease. J Clin Invest 1977; 59:203–216.
30. Murray JF. Gas exchange and oxygen transport. In: Murray JF (ed). The Normal Lung: The Basis for Diagnosis and Treatment of Pulmonary Disease. Philadelphia: W.B. Saunders Co., 1976, pp 171–197.
31. Sharp JT. The respiratory muscles in chronic obstructive pulmonary disease. Am Rev Respir Dis 1986; 134:1089–91.
32. Juan G, Calverley P, Talamo C, et al. Effect of carbon dioxide on diaphragmatic function in human beings. N Engl J Med 1984; 310:874–879.
33. Loveridge B, West P, Anthonisen NR, et al. Breathing patterns in patients with chronic obstructive pulmonary disease. Am Rev Respir Dis 1984; 130:730–737.
34. Rochester DF. Effects of COPD on the respiratory muscles. In: Cherniack NS (ed). Chronic Obstructive Pulmonary Disease. Philadelphia: W.B. Saunders Co., 1991, pp 134–157.
35. Thurlbeck WM. Chronic airflow obstruction, correlation of structure and function. In: Petty TL (ed). Chronic Obstructive Pulmonary Disease. 2nd ed. New York: Marcel Dekker, Inc., 1985, pp 129–203.
36. West WW, Nagai A, Hodgkin JE, et al. The National Institutes of Health intermittent positive-pressure breathing trial-pathology studies. III. The diagnosis of emphysema. Am Rev Respir Dis 1987; 135:123–129.
37. Thurlbeck WM. Pathology of chronic airflow obstruction. In: Cherniack NS (ed). Chronic Obstructive Pulmonary Disease. Philadelphia: W.B. Saunders Co., 1991, pp 3–20.
38. Petty TL, Silvers GW, Stanford RE. Mild emphysema is associated with reduced elastic recoil and increased lung size but not with air-flow limitation. Am Rev Respir Dis 1987; 136:867–871.
39. Berend N, Skoog C, Thurlbeck WM. Pressure-volume characteristics of excised human lungs: Effects of sex, age, and emphysema. J Appl Physiol 1980; 49:558–65.
40. Berend N, Woolcock AJ, Marlin GE. Correlation between the function and structure of the lung in smokers. Am Rev Respir Dis 1979; 119:695–705.
41. Thurlbeck WM. Chronic airflow obstruction. In: Thurlbeck WM (ed). Pathology of the Lung. Stuttgart: Thieme Medical Publishers Inc., 1988, pp 551–554.
42. Thurlbeck WM. Aspects of chronic airflow obstruction. Chest 1977; 72:341–349.
43. Thurlbeck WM, Henderson JA, Fraser RG, et al. Chronic obstructive lung disease. A comparison between clinical, roentgenologic, functional and morphologic criteria in chronic bronchitis, emphysema, asthma and bronchiectasis. Medicine (Baltimore) 1970; 49:81–145.
44. Miller RR, Muller NL, Vedal S, et al. Limitations of computed tomography in the assessment of emphysema. Am Rev Respir Dis 1989; 139:980–983.
45. Bergin C, Muller N, Nichols DM, et al. The diagnosis of emphysema. A computed tomographic-pathologic correlation. Am Rev Respir Dis 1986; 133:541–546.

Chapter 4

Respiratory Muscle Function in Chronic Obstructive Pulmonary Disease

ANDRÉ DE TROYER, M.D., Ph.D.

The obvious airway and pulmonary abnormalities of chronic obstructive pulmonary disease (COPD) have for many years distracted attention from the importance of the respiratory muscles in this condition. The increased airflow resistance characteristic of COPD, however, makes the respiratory muscles work chronically against an increased load; this requires that the inspiratory muscles generate more force (or pressure) than normal to move air into the lungs. Furthermore, even though the emphysematous alterations in the lung usually produce an increase in static pulmonary compliance, the increased inequality of time constants is such that as breathing frequency increases, dynamic pulmonary compliance falls markedly below the value of static compliance. This increased frequency dependence of dynamic compliance implies that in COPD patients, the effective pulmonary compliance operating during spontaneous breathing may be substantially lower than static compliance. Hence, the elastic load imposed on the inspiratory muscles may be greater than normal as well. In addition, the emphysematous changes in the lung also cause a loss of lung recoil pressure, such that the neutral position of the respiratory system (i.e., functional residual capacity [FRC]) is displaced toward higher lung volumes. Such a displacement induces substantial geometric changes in the chest wall and the respiratory muscles.

As pointed out by Younes,[1] the increased load resulting from the increased airflow resistance and the decreased dynamic pulmonary compliance in COPD patients are fairly small relative to the load that the respiratory muscles can compensate for and sustain. When normal subjects are given external resistances of the magnitude encountered in COPD patients, the alterations in maximum breathing capacity and maximum exercise tolerance are small.[2] On the other hand, the increase in FRC dictates that the inspiratory muscles operate at shorter than normal lengths, and this places a severe stress on the respiratory muscle pump. Consequently, in this review the effects of acute hyperinflation on the respiratory muscles are analyzed first. How the chest wall and the respiratory muscles respond to chronic, isolated hyperinflation, such as that observed in animal models of emphysema, is then examined. Next, the abnormalities that have been observed in the chest wall and the individual respiratory muscles in patients with COPD are summarized. Finally, how these different abnormalities affect the activation of the respiratory muscles and the pattern of chest wall motion during breathing is explored.

THE RESPIRATORY MUSCLES DURING ACUTE HYPERINFLATION

The Length-Tension Relationship

Although a detailed discussion of the mechanisms of skeletal muscle contraction is beyond the scope of this

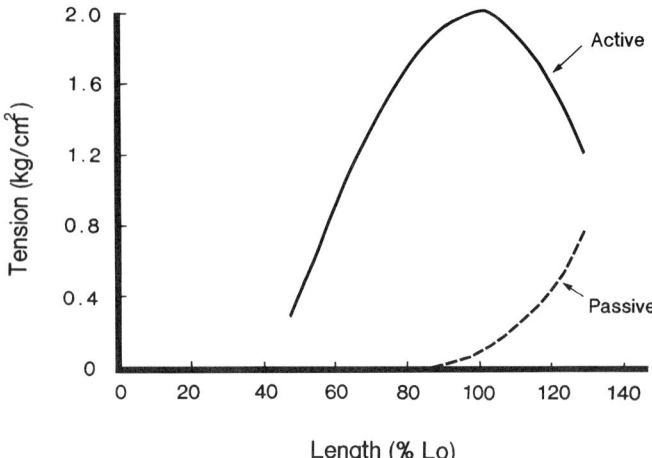

FIGURE 4-1. In vitro active *(solid line)* and passive *(broken line)* length-tension relationships of a typical skeletal muscle. Length is expressed as a percentage of the optimum force-generating length (Lo), and tension is expressed as kilograms per square centimeter of muscle cross-sectional area (kg/cm^2).

review, understanding respiratory muscle function in COPD requires a clear understanding of the length-tension relationship. This relationship, which is well known from studies of single fibers from amphibian muscles[3] and from studies of excised bundles from mammalian limb muscles,[4] describes that property whereby the isometric tension developed by a muscle bundle in vitro varies as a function of the resting, precontractile muscle length (Fig. 4-1). Thus, when the resting length of the muscle is increased before stimulation, the tension developed during the contraction, called *active* tension, increases progressively. Beyond a certain length, resting tension develops in the muscle before contraction takes place; this *passive* tension results mostly from the elastic forces of the connective tissue, the sarcolemma, and the blood vessels. Active tension, however, continues to increase up to a maximum level; the muscle length at which maximum active tension is recorded is usually referred to as Lo. If the resting muscle is lengthened beyond Lo, then active tension decreases gradually.

The Diaphragm

The diaphragm is a skeletal muscle, and as such it shares in the length-tension relationship. McCulley and Faulkner[5] have measured the length-tension properties of excised bundles of diaphragmatic muscle fibers from five animal species (rats, cats, rhesus monkeys, dogs, and pigs), and they have established that the relationship between length and active muscle tension for the diaphragm is similar to that for limb muscles. Thus, diaphragmatic muscle fibers in vitro produce progressively less force as their length is gradually decreased below their optimum length. Active force actually becomes zero when the muscle is shortened to approximately 50% of Lo.

This relationship plays a major role in determining the influence of hyperinflation on the behavior of the diaphragm as a pressure generator. The recent introduction of sonomicrometric techniques has made possible the direct assessment of diaphragm length in animals. In supine anesthetized dogs, increasing lung volume above FRC causes progressive shortening of the diaphragm, such that at total lung capacity (TLC) the diaphragm is about 30% shorter than at FRC.[6, 7] Conversely, decreasing lung volume from FRC to residual volume (RV) lengthens the diaphragm by about 5%. The use of sonomicrometry has also established that in supine dogs the diaphragm at FRC is somewhat shorter than its in vitro optimum force-producing length (Lo).[7, 8] On this basis, one would expect that the force or pressure-generating ability of the diaphragm in vivo decreases markedly as lung volume is increased above FRC; indeed, when the phrenic nerves in supine dogs and cats are selectively stimulated in the neck, the pressure generated for a given stimulation decreases progressively as lung volume is increased.[9–13] This decrease is such that near TLC the pressure generated by the contracting diaphragm is almost zero. Minh and coworkers[12] and Sant'Ambrogio and Saibene[14] have even observed that when the respiratory system in dogs and rabbits is inflated to a lung volume greater than 104% of TLC, stimulation of the phrenic nerves induces a rise rather than a fall in airway pressure; at such very high lung volumes, the diaphragm has thus ceased to be inspiratory and has become expiratory to the lung.

The response of the normal human diaphragm to hyperinflation is not different from that in animals. Although there have been no direct measurements of diaphragmatic muscle fiber length in humans, Braun and associates[15] have combined posteroanterior and lateral chest radiographs taken at different lung volumes and autopsy measurements to demonstrate that the human diaphragm muscle shortens by 30 to 40% when lung volume is increased from RV to TLC. These values are very close to those found in supine dogs. In addition, Danon and colleagues[16] have provided unequivocal evidence that the pressure-generating ability of the human diaphragm is closely dependent on lung volume. These investigators measured the decrease in airway pressure and the pressure difference across the diaphragm (i.e., transdiaphragmatic pressure [Pdi]) in subjects with transection of the upper cervical cord in whom bilateral pacing of the phrenic nerves in the neck made it possible to maintain the degree of diaphragmatic activation at a constant level. When these subjects were supine at FRC and when a valve was occluded at the mouth, the unassisted paced diaphragm was able to generate an adequate fall in airway pressure (40–60 cm H_2O) and an adequate Pdi. However, the pressures produced by phrenic pacing decreased almost linearly when the respiratory system of the subjects was passively inflated above FRC; at a volume of FRC + 2.5 L, the fall in airway pressure was only 8 to 17 cm H_2O. A similar decline in the pressure-generating ability of the diaphragm with increasing lung volume has been found during bilateral stimulation of the phrenic nerves in normal subjects.[17] As in animals, the human diaphragm ceases to act as an inspiratory pressure generator at TLC.

It has long been thought that the dome of the diaphragm becomes flatter at or near TLC and that this increase in the radius of curvature contributes to the decreased pressure-generating ability of the diaphragm at high lung volumes (Laplace's equation). Several lines of evidence, however, have recently indicated that this mechanism plays little or no role over the range of a normal vital capacity. Indeed, Kim and coworkers[13] have found that the relationship between active diaphragmatic tension and Pdi during phrenic nerve stimulation in supine dogs was linear between RV and TLC; if the increase in the radius of curvature was an important determinant of the decrease in Pdi at high lung volumes, then the ratio of active tension to Pdi should have increased near TLC. Furthermore, radiographic measurements of diaphragmatic curvature in normal human subjects have failed to detect any significant shape change in diaphragmatic silhouette from RV to TLC.[15] Finally, Smith and Bellemare[17] have pointed out that the relationship between lung volume and Pdi obtained during bilateral stimulation of the phrenic nerves in normal human subjects is similar to the length-tension relationship observed for diaphragmatic muscle bundles in vitro. It appears, therefore, that the effect of hyperinflation on the pressure-generating ability of the diaphragm in normal human subjects is primarily, if not exclusively, related to the reduction in diaphragmatic length.

Acute increases in lung volume affect not only the pressure-generating ability of the diaphragm but also its action on the rib cage. When the diaphragm contracts alone at FRC, as in subjects with tetraplegia caused by low cervical cord transection, it produces a rise in abdominal pressure and an increase in abdominal dimensions associated with a decrease (paradoxical motion) in the dimensions of the upper portion of the rib cage[16, 18–20]; this inspiratory contraction of the upper rib cage results from the fall in pleural pressure.[21, 22] At the same time, however, contraction of the diaphragm causes expansion of the lower rib cage. Experimental and theoretic work has shown that this expansion results from two mechanisms.[23, 24] The muscle fibers of the diaphragm originate from the upper margins of the lower six ribs and from the xyphoid process of the sternum and then run cranially such that they are directly apposed to the inner aspect of the rib cage (Fig. 4–2). Hence, when these fibers contract, they exert a force on the lower ribs, and provided that the abdominal visceral mass effectively opposes the descent of the diaphragmatic dome, this force is oriented cranially. It thus has the effect of lifting the lower ribs and rotating them outward. In addition, the direct apposition of the diaphragm to the inner aspect of the rib cage makes the lower rib cage, in effect, part of the abdominal container.[25] In standing human subjects at rest, this "zone of apposition" of the diaphragm to the rib cage represents about 30% of the total surface area of the rib cage. Consequently, the rise in abdominal pressure that takes place during inspiration is transmitted through the apposed diaphragm so as to push the lower rib cage outward.[26]

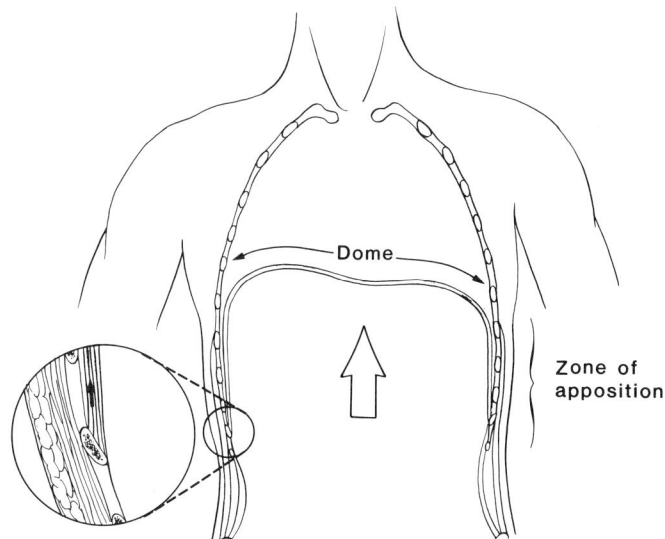

FIGURE 4–2. Frontal section of the chest wall at end-expiration in a normal subject. Note the orientation of the costal diaphragmatic fibers (inset); these fibers run cranially and are directly apposed to the inner aspect of the lower rib cage (zone of apposition). Thus, as these fibers contract and shorten, they exert a force on the lower ribs; if the abdominal visceral mass effectively opposes the descent of the diaphragmatic dome (open arrow), this force is oriented cranially (bold arrow). In addition, the zone of apposition allows the rise in abdominal pressure to be transmitted to the lower rib cage, pushing it outward. (Adapted from De Troyer A, Estenne M. Functional anatomy of the respiratory muscles. Clin Chest Med 1988; 9:175–193.)

As lung volume increases above FRC, however, the dome of the diaphragm descends relative to its costal insertions. As a result, the zone of apposition decreases in size while the fraction of the rib cage exposed to pleural pressure increases. Hence, the diaphragm's expanding action on the lower rib cage decreases progressively.[21, 23, 24, 27] When lung volume approaches TLC, the zone of apposition disappears, such that the diaphragmatic muscle fibers at their insertions on the ribs become oriented transversally inward. In these conditions, the increase in abdominal pressure can no longer operate to expand the lower rib cage; furthermore, the insertional force is expiratory rather than inspiratory in direction. Hence, when contracting alone the diaphragm deflates the entire (lower and upper) rib cage.

The Other Respiratory Muscles

The diaphragm is not the only important contracting muscle employed during resting breathing. Normal individuals at rest also contract the internal intercostal muscles of the parasternal region of the rib cage (also called the "parasternal intercostals") and the scalene muscles during inspiration.[28–32] The primary action of these muscles is to displace the ribs cranially and to expand the rib cage.[32–34]

Studies in dogs have shown that, like all skeletal muscles, the parasternal intercostal muscles have active length-tension properties such that active force decreases as the muscles are made shorter than Lo.[35] When compared with the diaphragm, however, the length-tension relationship of the parasternal intercostal muscles is such that a given reduction in resting precontractile length below Lo is associated with a much larger reduction in force (Fig. 4–3). This would suggest that with hyperinflation, as both muscle groups shorten, the decrement of force would be greater for the parasternal intercostal muscles than for the diaphragm. However, whereas passive inflation from FRC to TLC results in a 30 to 40% shortening in the canine diaphragm, it causes the parasternal intercostal muscles to shorten by only 10%.[36] In addition, in contrast to the diaphragm whose resting FRC length in supine dogs is close to or a little bit shorter than Lo, the parasternal intercostal muscles at FRC are about 15% longer than Lo.[35] Consequently, in supine dogs, increasing lung volume above FRC causes the parasternal intercostal muscles to move toward rather than away from Lo (see Fig. 4–3). Hence, the force-generating ability of the parasternal muscles should be well maintained with hyperinflation, and indeed measurements of force and intramuscular pressure at different lung volumes suggest that in supine dogs the force-generating capacity of the parasternal intercostal muscles remains unchanged or slightly increases as lung volume is increased from FRC to TLC.[37]

The scalene muscles differ from the parasternal intercostal muscles in that their length-tension relationship is similar to that of the diaphragm.[38] In addition, the resting FRC length of the scalene muscles in supine dogs is somewhat shorter than Lo.[38] Consequently, the scalene muscles resemble the diaphragm in that they move away from Lo when the respiratory system is inflated passively. The amount of shortening of the scalene muscles during passive inflation, however, is considerably smaller than the amount of diaphragmatic shortening. In supine dogs, inflating the system from FRC to TLC causes the scalene muscles to shorten by only 6%.[38] Therefore, as is the case for the parasternal intercostal muscles, the force-generating ability of the scalene muscles should be better preserved than that of the diaphragm during hyperinflation.

Although external measurements with calipers have shown that the scalene muscles in normal humans also shorten by only 4.5% from RV to TLC,[31] most of these observations in the dog cannot be extended to the human respiratory system without caution. Indeed, the changes in length of the parasternal intercostal muscles in humans have not been determined, and the lung volume corresponding to the Lo of these muscles is not known. The finding that the resting length of the parasternal intercostal muscles at FRC is above Lo pertains to dogs in the supine posture; this might not be true in the prone position (which is more physiologic for the dog) or in humans. In addition, it must be appreciated that the relationship between the force produced by a given set of intercostal muscles in situ and the change in airway or pleural pressure that this set of muscles can elicit is not a simple one. More specifically, the fall in pleural pressure produced by the contracting parasternal intercostal muscles depends on both the force developed by the muscles and the ability of the ribs to be displaced in the cranial direction. Measurements in dogs have shown that the impedance of the ribs to cranial displacement increases as lung volume is increased above FRC,[39] thus implying that during hyperinflation, as the ribs become more horizontal, the load imposed on the contracting parasternal intercostal muscles increases. Hence, the fall in pleural pressure might well decrease even though the force generated might be greater. In agreement with this prediction, Di Marco and associates[40] have observed in dogs that the fall in airway (pleural) pressure induced by supramaximum stimulation of the parasternal and external intercostal muscles in the six or seven cranial interspaces decreases progressively as lung volume is increased above FRC.

Whereas acute hyperinflation causes shortening of all of the inspiratory muscles, it induces lengthening of the expiratory muscles of the abdominal wall. This lengthening appears to be particularly pronounced for the transversus abdominis and internal oblique muscles. Measurements with sonomicrometry in supine dogs have shown that during passive inflation, these two muscles lengthen by 15 to 25% of their resting FRC length.[41] On the other hand, the rectus abdominis and external oblique muscles lengthen by only 1 to 3%.[41] This is fortunate, since the transversus abdominis is the most important abdominal expiratory muscle employed during breathing in quadrupeds.[42, 43] So, even though the resting FRC length of this muscle in relation to Lo has not yet been determined, presumably its force-generating ability increases as lung volume is increased above FRC.

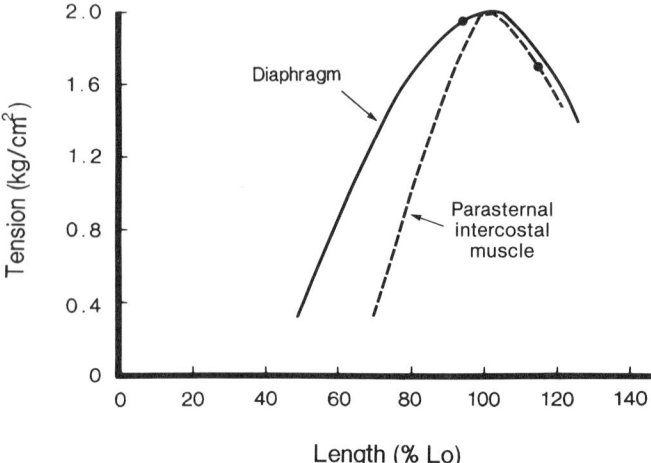

FIGURE 4–3. Active length-tension relationships of the diaphragm (solid line) and a parasternal intercostal muscle (broken line) in the dog. Note that the parasternal intercostal muscle has a shorter effective length range than the diaphragm. Note also that in the supine dog at FRC (closed circles), the diaphragm is somewhat shorter than Lo, whereas the parasternal intercostal muscle is longer than Lo. As a result, the diaphragm moves away from Lo when the system is inflated above FRC, and the parasternal intercostal muscle moves toward Lo.

Chest Wall Motion and Respiratory Muscle Use

The importance of the length-tension relationship of the individual respiratory muscle groups is illustrated by the effect of hyperinflation on the pattern of chest wall motion during breathing. When supine dogs breathe quietly at resting lung volume, the inspiratory intercostal muscles (in particular the parasternal muscles) contract in concert with the diaphragm during inspiration, and this causes simultaneous expansion of the rib cage and abdominal compartments of the chest wall together with a rise in abdominal pressure. The relative expansion of the two chest wall compartments in this circumstance is, in fact, very close to that observed when the system is passively inflated in the paralyzed animal. However, when the animal is forced to breathe near TLC, the rib cage continues to expand during inspiration, but abdominal pressure falls and the abdomen frequently moves paradoxically inward.[37, 44] A similar alteration in thoracoabdominal motion during hyperinflation has been observed in normal human subjects.[45, 46] Thus, during breathing at high lung volumes, the chest wall behaves as though the diaphragm were paralyzed. Yet, activation of the diaphragm in this condition is maintained or increased.[37, 44] This observation has been interpreted as reflecting the dramatic reduction in the mechanical effectiveness of the diaphragm at high lung volumes and the relative preservation of the effectiveness of the inspiratory rib cage muscles.

In view of the fact that the parasternal intercostal muscles in the dog are longer than Lo at FRC[35] and shorten little from FRC to TLC,[36] this interpretation appears reasonable. As previously discussed, however, the preserved or improved force-generating capacity of the parasternal muscles at high lung volumes does not necessarily translate into pleural pressure.[40] Therefore an alternative possibility is that hyperinflation elicits a marked increase in the inspiratory activation of the parasternal intercostal muscles so as to compensate for the increased resistance of the ribs to cranial displacement; during breathing near TLC, however, the inspiratory activity recorded from the canine parasternal muscles was observed to be slightly decreased.[37, 44] Still another possibility would be that hyperinflation is associated with a large increase in the inspiratory activation of the other rib cage inspiratory muscles. The effect of hyperinflation on the activation of these muscles, however, has not yet been evaluated.

Respiratory Muscle Strength

The importance of the length-tension relationships of the respiratory muscles in human subjects is also illustrated by the influence of lung volume on the pressures that a subject can generate at the mouth during maximum inspiratory and expiratory efforts against an occluded valve.[47] This is the most widely used test of respiratory muscle performance in clinical practice; maximum inspiratory pressure at the mouth (PImax) gives an index of global inspiratory muscle strength, whereas maximum expiratory mouth pressure (PEmax) reflects global expiratory muscle strength. The relationships between lung volume and maximum mouth pressure in a normal subject are illustrated in Figure 4–4 (solid curves). As can be seen, PImax and PEmax vary substantially with lung volume. The PImax is greatest at RV (when the inspiratory muscles are longest) and decreases progressively from RV through FRC toward TLC; at TLC (when the inspiratory muscles are shortest), PImax is zero. In contrast, PEmax is greatest at TLC (when the expiratory muscles are longest), decreases progressively from TLC to FRC, and becomes zero at RV (when the muscles are shortest).

It must be appreciated, however, that although PImax and PEmax depend primarily on the force generated by

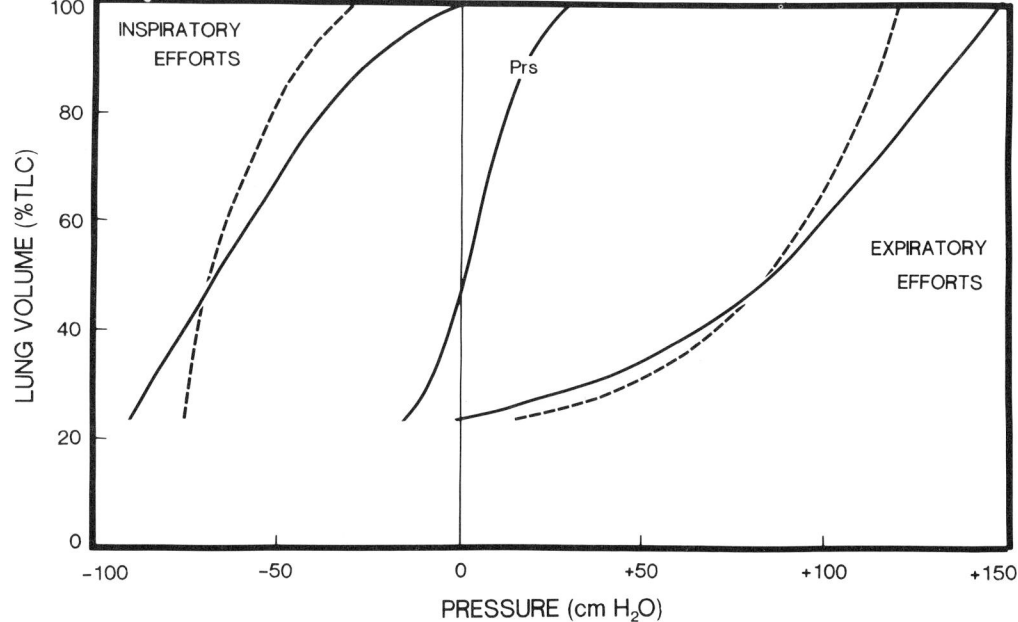

FIGURE 4–4. Volume-pressure curves of the respiratory system during relaxation (Prs) and during maximum static inspiratory and expiratory efforts (solid lines). The broken lines indicate the pressure contributed by the muscles (Pmus). Note that as lung volume increases, inspiratory Pmus decreases and expiratory Pmus increases.

the inspiratory and expiratory muscles, they are also related to the recoil pressure of the respiratory system. Thus, to assess the pressures really exerted by the contracting muscles, the pressures measured at the mouth must be corrected for the respiratory system recoil. The pressure-volume (P-V) curve of the respiratory system during relaxation is also shown in Figure 4–4 (Prs); at each lung volume, the net pressure exerted by the contracting inspiratory or expiratory muscles (Pmus) is thus given by the horizontal distance between Prs and Pimax or Pemax, respectively. The broken lines in Figure 4–4 are the relationship between volume and Pmus. The importance of correcting Pimax and Pemax values for Prs is explained more clearly later in the evaluation of respiratory muscle strength in patients with COPD.

THE CHEST WALL AND THE RESPIRATORY MUSCLES IN EXPERIMENTAL EMPHYSEMA

Acute hyperinflation has been widely used experimentally as a tool for evaluating the potential consequences of COPD on respiratory muscle function. There are definite similarities between the two conditions. However, there are striking differences as well. In particular, the time course of the alterations is very different; whereas acute increases in lung volume in anesthetized animals and in normal humans are induced in seconds, COPD develops slowly over many years.

To assess the influence of the time factor, investigators have used animal models of emphysema. A single intratracheal injection of papain or porcine pancreatic elastase in the rat or in the hamster produces after a few weeks anatomic lesions in the lung that are similar to those observed in severe panlobular emphysema in humans. The induced functional alterations in the lungs are also similar to those seen in severe human emphysema; FRC and TLC are markedly increased, static pulmonary compliance is increased, and lung recoil pressure is decreased. Airway resistance, however, is normal. Thus, experimental emphysema in the rat or in the hamster provides a model of isolated, chronic hyperinflation, and recent studies have shown that profound adaptive changes occur in both the chest wall and the respiratory muscles.

The Chest Wall: Statics

As shown by Thomas and colleagues,[48] experimental emphysema in the hamster induces alterations in the structural characteristics of the chest wall. Six months after the injection of elastase, the ribs and the sternum are longer than those in control animals. As a result, the resting circumference of the rib cage and its dorsoventral and transverse dimensions are increased. The angles at the sternochondral junctions in the cranial portion of the rib cage are also altered, such that the upper ribs are in a more cranial position. Thus, the configuration of the relaxed rib cage in emphysematous animals is close to that of a normal rib cage inflated above FRC. It is worth noting, however, that the angles of articulation of the lower ribs with the vertebrae are reduced, rather than increased, thus indicating that the lower ribs are displaced in a more caudal position. This caudal displacement of the lower ribs combined with the cranial displacement of the upper ribs contributes to the increase in the rostrocaudal dimension of the rib cage in emphysematous animals.

In view of these structural alterations, the effects of experimental emphysema on the elastic properties of the relaxed chest wall can be understood. Indeed, the P-V curve of the chest wall in emphysematous animals is shifted upward, such that the volume of the chest wall at any given pressure is increased. The slope of the curve (chest wall compliance), however, remains unchanged.[48]

The Diaphragm

Skeletal muscle fibers are made of numerous sarcomeres placed in series; hence, muscle fiber length depends both on the number of sarcomeres and on the length of each individual sarcomere. Acute reductions in muscle fiber length, as occurs in the diaphragm during acute increases in lung volume, decrease the length of all sarcomeres placed in series; this decrease in sarcomere length accounts for the reduction in muscle contractile force (length-tension relationship). Landmark experiments on limb muscles by Tabary, Goldspink, and their colleagues,[49–51] however, have shown that skeletal muscles are extremely adaptable. Thus, when a limb muscle is immobilized for a few weeks in a lengthened position, sarcomeres are added on; conversely, when a muscle is immobilized in a shortened position, sarcomeres are lost. As a result, the length of each individual sarcomere is virtually re-established to its initial length. The physiologic consequence of this adjustment is that the chronically shortened muscle has a leftward shift of its active length-tension relationship (the relationship is shifted toward shorter lengths) but retains normal maximum tension (Fig. 4–5).

Studies by Supinski and Kelsen[52, 53] and by Farkas and Roussos[54, 55] have shown that similar adaptive changes occur in the diaphragm in experimental emphysema. With chronic hyperinflation in the hamster, there is a 10 to 15% dropout of sarcomeres in the diaphragmatic muscle fibers. Therefore, although the length of the muscle fibers is decreased, their active length-tension relationship measured in vitro is shifted to the left (see Fig. 4–5), and the muscle's pressure-generating ability in vivo is better preserved than would be expected. At any comparable lung volume, the Pdi developed during spontaneous inspiratory efforts against an occluded valve or during selective stimulation of the phrenic nerves is thus substantially greater in emphysematous than in control animals.[56] In other words, emphysematous animals are able to generate Pdi at lung volumes at which Pdi is essentially zero in control animals. It must be pointed out, however, that the pressure-gener-

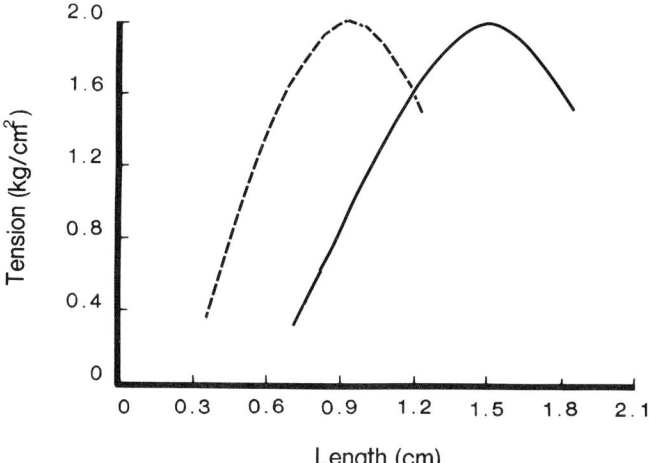

FIGURE 4–5. Diagram illustrating the effects of chronic shortening on the active length-tension relationship of a limb muscle. Note that muscle length is expressed as absolute values (cm). With chronic shortening, the curve is shifted to the left, and the optimum force-producing length (Lo) is decreased. The maximum tension, however, remains normal.

ating ability of the diaphragm in emphysematous animals is not fully restored. Although their diaphragm has a greater than normal ability to generate pressure at high lung volumes, the maximum Pdi that can be generated is lower than that in control animals.[56] The critical factor responsible for this reduction in maximum Pdi is probably a change in diaphragmatic configuration (increased radius of curvature) that is secondary to the very large increase in lung volume.

The Other Respiratory Muscles

The effects of experimental emphysema on the other inspiratory muscles have not been studied. Consequently, whether the parasternal intercostal muscles and the scalene muscles in emphysematous hamsters behave like the diaphragm and lose sarcomeres is not known. The structural alterations observed in the chest wall, including the cranial displacement of the upper ribs,[48] would suggest that the parasternal intercostal muscles and the scalene muscles are chronically shortened as well. The small changes in length of these muscles during acute hyperinflation would also suggest, however, that the amplitude of the sarcomere loss is small compared with that of the diaphragm.

The responses of the nondiaphragmatic respiratory muscles to chronic hyperinflation, however, might be more complex than one would expect. Arnold and coworkers[57] have studied the effects of experimental emphysema on two abdominal muscles in hamsters; namely, the external oblique and the transversus abdominis. These two muscles were found to respond differently. The external oblique showed essentially no change; the number of sarcomeres, the muscle fiber length, and the active length-tension relationship were similar in emphysematous and control animals, which is compatible with the observation that this muscle length-

ens by only 2 to 3% during acute hyperinflation in the dog.[41] On the other hand, acute hyperinflation in dogs causes substantial lengthening of the transversus abdominis[41] and hence one would expect that the changes in structure and in the length-tension curve associated with experimental emphysema would be opposite to those observed in the diaphragm. Emphysematous hamsters, however, were observed to have a reduction, rather than an increase, in sarcomere number in the transversus abdominis. Furthermore, the active length-tension relationship for this muscle was displaced toward shorter lengths, thus suggesting that the transversus abdominis, like the diaphragm, is chronically shortened.[57] The mechanisms of such a chronic shortening of the transversus abdominis are unclear, but it is worth noting that the bundles studied by Arnold and coworkers were removed from the portion of the muscle inserted onto the caudally displaced lower ribs. The more caudal portions of the muscle might have shown different structural changes.

THE CHEST WALL AND THE RESPIRATORY MUSCLES IN COPD

Although experimental emphysema in rodents causes chronic hyperinflation of the thorax in much the same way as COPD does, the clinical condition is much more complex for at least two reasons. First, in addition to chronic hyperinflation, COPD is associated with an increase in airway resistance and a decreased dynamic pulmonary compliance; the resulting increase in inspiratory load could have a training effect on the respiratory muscles and induce an increase in respiratory muscle strength and endurance. Second, COPD may introduce other confounding variables, such as denutrition, that are known to have a detrimental effect on the respiratory muscles. Thus patients with COPD are unlikely to be as homogeneous as a group as emphysematous hamsters are. In addition, hamsters continue to show increases in long bone growth after the onset of adulthood, but humans do not; it is not known whether adult or elderly humans retain mechanisms for adjusting sarcomere number in response to chronic muscle shortening. Consequently, observations made in emphysematous hamsters are not necessarily applicable to COPD patients.

The Chest Wall: Statics

Although it is well known from chest radiographs that patients with COPD and hyperinflation have a lower diaphragm than normal subjects, the mechanisms whereby the chest wall accommodates the increased lung volume in COPD have received little attention. Gilmartin and Gibson[58] have used pairs of magnetometers to measure precisely different rib cage diameters at FRC in 40 patients with varying degrees of airflow obstruction and hyperinflation and in 20 normal control subjects. The anteroposterior diameter of the rib cage was significantly greater in the patients, whereas the transverse diameters of the rib cage were not different. As a result, the ratio of rib cage's transverse diameter to its anteroposterior diameter was lower in the patients than in the control subjects. In another study, Sharp and associates[59] used lateral radiographs of the chest to measure the angles made by the fourth through the seventh ribs with the coronal plane in a group of 12 patients with severe COPD (mean forced expiratory volume in 1 second [FEV_1] = 37% of predicted) and hyperinflation (TLC = 121 to 149% of predicted) and in 12 healthy control subjects of similar age. The acute angles made by the ribs with the coronal plane were found, on average, to be greater in the patients, more markedly so for the cranial than for the more caudal ribs. These measurements thus confirm the clinical impression that the rib cage is more circular in cross-section and that the ribs are more horizontal in COPD patients than in normal subjects.

In spite of these structural alterations in the rib cage, the static elastic properties of the relaxed chest wall in COPD patients are relatively preserved.[60] Thus, as is the case in emphysematous hamsters, the P-V curve of the chest wall in these patients is shifted to the left, such that a given trans-chest wall pressure is associated with a larger thoracic volume, but the slope of the curve (i.e., chest wall compliance) is normal.

Pathology of the Diaphragm and Other Respiratory Muscles

A number of observers have examined the structure of the diaphragm at autopsy in patients with COPD. Steele and Heard[61] found that the diaphragm in 15 patients with COPD was reduced in thickness, volume, and area compared with that in 23 control subjects. Butler[62] similarly observed a reduction in the surface area of the diaphragm, particularly of the muscular portion of the diaphragm, in 95 patients with COPD; the reduction in diaphragm area was larger the more severe the emphysema. The thickness of the diaphragm in Butler's patients, however, was maintained. Thurlbeck[63] also observed a reduction in diaphragm weight in patients with COPD as well as a negative correlation between the amount of emphysema and diaphragm weight. On the other hand, Ishikawa and Hayes[64] observed that the diaphragms of 9 patients with COPD had the same area as those of their 14 control subjects, but the diaphragms of their patients were thicker. Histologically, two of their patients with COPD also had thicker muscle fibers in their diaphragms as compared with those of the control subjects. Scott and Hoy[65] also observed that the average cross-sectional area of the diaphragmatic muscle fibers was increased in patients with COPD, whereas Sanchez and colleagues[66] reported this cross-sectional area to be smaller in COPD patients than in control subjects.

The pathologic findings in the diaphragm in COPD are thus conflicting. Several reasons may account for this. In some series, COPD has been assessed based on the severity of emphysema, whereas in others it has been identified simply on the basis of a history of chronic bronchitis. Conceivably, the diaphragm might become hypertrophied in the patients whose disease is characterized primarily by a large increase in airflow resistance (increased work of breathing), whereas it might retain a more normal thickness in the patients who have a small increase in airflow resistance and severe hyperinflation. In addition, many series consist of relatively few cases, and the potential differences in body weight and sex between patients and controls have been ignored. It has been clearly established, however, that the diaphragm weighs more in men than in women.[63] Furthermore, diaphragm weight and thickness are related to body weight[63]; hence, diaphragm weight and thickness are decreased in underweight patients with chronic non-respiratory illnesses as compared with patients dying suddenly or from acute illnesses, whereas both are increased in muscular laborers.[67] Since severe COPD is commonly associated with a loss of body weight, the frequently observed loss of diaphragm weight and thickness in these patients could be only part of the general process of skeletal muscle wasting. Recent studies by Arora and Rochester[68] support this hypothesis. In comparing the diaphragms of 18 patients with COPD with those in 16 age-matched healthy male subjects, they found that the diaphragms of the patients were reduced in weight. The patient group, however, included several females and several underweight subjects, and when these subjects were excluded from the comparison, the differences in diaphragm weight essentially disappeared. Of interest, however, is the finding that, after exclusion of these underweight subjects, the ratio of diaphragm weight to body weight was still lower in the patients.[68] Steele and Heard[61] and Thurlbeck[63] had previously reached a similar conclusion.

Arora and Rochester[69] have also assessed the sternocleidomastoid muscle diameter in COPD patients. Using anthropometric techniques, they observed that the diameter of this muscle was reduced in such patients, particularly in underweight patients. As is the case for the diaphragm, however, the reduction in sternocleidomastoid muscle diameter was disproportionately greater than the loss of body weight, thus suggesting that the prominence of this muscle in many COPD patients is primarily related to a decrease in the overlying skin fold thickness and not to muscle hypertrophy as has been conventionally thought.

Although the parasternal intercostal muscles and the scalene muscles contribute actively to the act of breathing in normal individuals, the structure of these muscles in COPD patients has not been studied. Campbell and coworkers[70] have examined fragments of intercostal muscles taken from the fifth interspace in the midaxillary line in 17 patients undergoing thoracotomy for pulmonary masses. Variations in fiber size, splitting, and atrophy were observed in many patients, more markedly so in the internal interosseous (expiratory) than in the external (inspiratory) intercostal muscles. The authors felt that these alterations were multifactorial and related to malignancy and weight loss as well as to airflow obstruction. On the other hand, Sanchez and associates[71] have failed to detect any changes in the external or internal intercostal muscles in 12 patients with COPD, even though many of them had weight loss owing to lung cancer. These findings are thus inconclusive, and furthermore, they are of relatively limited interest because the patients in both studies had only moderate airflow obstruction (forced expiratory volume in 1 second [FEV_1] = 55–65% of predicted) without any significant hyperinflation (TLC = 103% of predicted).

In conclusion, the majority of observations indicate that many patients with COPD have a loss of diaphragm weight and thickness. This is due primarily to the associated loss of body weight, but several studies suggest that other factors may also play a role; these factors, however, have not yet been identified. In addition, it appears that some patients with COPD might have increased diaphragm weight; although this might be related to the chronically increased work of breathing, the particular associations of this increased diaphragm weight are unknown. The effects of COPD on the scalene, intercostal, and abdominal muscles are essentially unknown as well.

Length of the Diaphragm and Other Respiratory Muscles

Autopsy measurements of the surface area and diameters of the diaphragm have been made in an attempt to assess the changes in diaphragm muscle fiber length in COPD.[68] Death, however, as well as the excision of the muscle at autopsy is likely to influence muscle length. The significance of such measurements as indicators of diaphragm muscle fiber length in vivo is, therefore, questionable.

There have been no direct measurements of in vivo diaphragm muscle fiber length in humans, rather only indirect estimates based on chest radiographs. In studies of 21 men with moderately severe or severe COPD (the pulmonary function test results were not provided) and of 23 normal subjects, Sharp and colleagues[72] have found that the patients' diaphragms at FRC were about 40% shorter than normal; this value is close to the 30 to 40% shortening observed in healthy subjects on inspiration from RV to TLC.[15] Rochester and Braun[73] have also made radiographic comparisons of diaphragm muscle length in 32 patients with COPD (FEV_1 = 35% of predicted; TLC = 112% of predicted; RV = 70% of predicted TLC) and in 22 healthy subjects. In computing an index of diaphragmatic muscle fiber length in both groups of subjects, they found that this index, on average, was 28% lower (the diaphragm muscle was 28% shorter) in the patients than in the healthy subjects. As anticipated, the amount of diaphragm shortening was related to the degree of hyperinflation, that is, the more severe the hyperinflation, the shorter the diaphragm.

Sharp and colleagues[72] have also used radiographs of the chest and of the neck to estimate the length of the rib cage muscles in patients with severe COPD. They estimated that as occurs in the diaphragm, the scalene muscles, and the sternocleidomastoid muscles at both FRC and TLC are significantly shorter in these patients than in healthy subjects. However, whereas the diaphragms in their patients were 40% shorter than normal, the scalene muscles and sternocleidomastoid muscles were, respectively, only 5 and 8% shorter than normal. In a more recent study, Sharp and colleagues[59] also computed the length of the external and internal interosseous intercostal muscles in 12 patients with COPD and severe hyperinflation (FEV_1 = 37% of predicted; TLC = 121–149% of predicted) and in 12 age-matched normal subjects. The external intercostal muscles at RV, FRC, and TLC were approximately 5% shorter than normal, whereas the internal interosseous intercostal muscles were about 15% longer than normal.

Thus, patients with COPD and severe hyperinflation have shorter inspiratory muscles and probably longer expiratory muscles than normal subjects. On this basis, provided there is no weight loss and no adjustment in sarcomere number, one would predict that these patients have markedly reduced inspiratory muscle strength and maintained or increased expiratory muscle strength. However, in agreement with the observed effect of acute hyperinflation in normal humans and in animals, the length of the inspiratory intercostal and neck muscles in these patients is better preserved than is the length of the diaphragm. Therefore, one would also predict that the force or pressure-generating ability of the former muscles is less affected than that of the latter.

Respiratory Muscle Strength

Sharp and colleagues[60] were among the first to obtain measurements of respiratory muscle strength in patients with COPD and hyperinflation. Measuring PImax at FRC in 20 patients and in 19 age-matched normal subjects, they found lower (less negative) values among the patients; they attributed these values to the hyperinflation and the consequent shortening of inspiratory muscles. Byrd and Hyatt[74] also measured PImax and PEmax at FRC in a group of 31 patients with COPD and found that when the patients' increased lung volume was taken into account, most patients generated higher (more negative) PImax and higher PEmax than normal. Byrd and Hyatt also pointed out that many patients could develop inspiratory pressures at volumes greater than predicted TLC. They concluded, therefore, that inspiratory and expiratory muscle strength in their patients was greater than normal, probably owing to work hypertrophy.

However, as was discussed previously, the pressure developed by the inspiratory or expiratory muscles is the difference between mouth pressure and the static recoil pressure of the respiratory system (PRs), not simply mouth pressure. Since the P-V curve of the respiratory system in COPD is shifted to higher lung volumes, mouth pressure measurements tend to overestimate inspiratory muscle strength and underestimate expiratory muscle strength (Fig. 4–6). Rochester and coworkers[75] did correct for PRs the PImax values re-

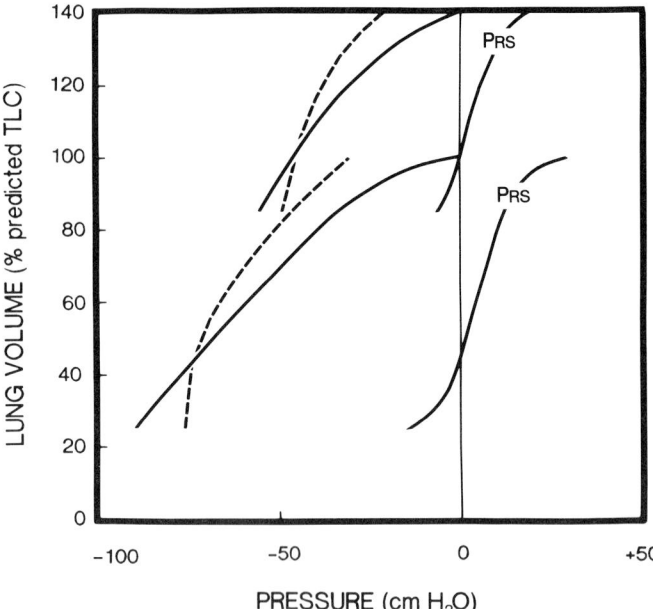

FIGURE 4–6. Volume-pressure curves of the respiratory system during relaxation (PRS) and during maximum static inspiratory efforts in a normal subject and in a hypothetic patient with COPD and hyperinflation whose FRC is equal to predicted TLC *(solid lines)*. The PRS curve in the patient is shifted toward higher volumes. As a result, measurements of mouth pressure during static inspiratory efforts (PImax) tend to overestimate the pressure contributed by the inspiratory muscles *(broken curves)*. The converse is true for PEmax relative to expiratory muscle strength.

ported by Byrd and Hyatt, and they concluded that these values were in fact scattered about the normal average value. More recent measurements of PImax at FRC and RV have confirmed that at these lung volumes, most patients with COPD and hyperinflation have essentially normal inspiratory muscle strength.[73, 76]

Notwithstanding the shift in the P-V curve of the respiratory system and its influence on PImax, the observations of Byrd and Hyatt[74] and those of Decramer and coworkers[76] indicate that patients with COPD and severe hyperinflation are able to generate negative pressures at volumes greater than predicted TLC. This would suggest that such patients adapt to hyperinflation in much the same way as emphysematous hamsters do; that is, they would lose sarcomeres in series in the inspiratory muscle fibers so as to maintain a reasonable inspiratory muscle strength at abnormally elevated lung volumes. The recent study of Similowski and associates[77] supports this conclusion. In order to determine the potential adaptation of the diaphragm in such patients, they measured Pdi during bilateral stimulation of the phrenic nerves to induce single twitches; neural activation of the diaphragm was thus controlled externally. Eight patients with COPD and hyperinflation (FRC = 130–180% of predicted) were studied, and their twitch Pdi at FRC was found to range between 10.9 and 26.6 cm H_2O. These values are lower than those found at FRC in normal subjects (34.6 ± 10.0 cm H_2O) but are higher than expected on the basis of the increased lung volume. Yet, these patients had a low, flat diaphragm, which might have caused further reduction in Pdi. Even though specific information about the pressure-generating ability of the inspiratory intercostal and neck muscles cannot be obtained in humans, it may be concluded, therefore, that patients with COPD and hyperinflation lose sarcomeres in the inspiratory muscles, at least in the diaphragm.

This conclusion, however, should be taken with caution for two reasons. First, FRC and TLC in most studies were measured in a body plethysmograph. In the presence of severe airway obstruction, however, swings in mouth pressure during panting are smaller than the swings in pleural or esophageal pressure, with the result that measurements of FRC and TLC may be artifactually elevated.[78–80] Second, values of PImax in patients with COPD show a wide range, and some patients have lower than normal values. Also of interest, some patients with COPD and hyperinflation show a reduction of PEmax.[73, 76] Yet, at high lung volumes, the expiratory muscles should have an advantage with respect to their length-tension relationship. Reduced PEmax values might be interpreted as indicating an addition of sarcomeres in the expiratory muscles in response to chronic hyperinflation; if such an adaptation occurred, then PEmax values would be normal before correcting for the increased lung volume but lower than normal after this correction is made. The observation by Rochester and Braun[73] that the COPD patients who have low PEmax also have low PImax, however, is a strong argument against this hypothesis. Rather, this observation suggests that some patients with COPD have generalized muscle weakness.

Several factors may contribute to generalized muscle weakness in patients with COPD. As was discussed previously, weight loss is a common occurrence in such patients, and severe weight loss in patients without pulmonary disease is associated with a reduction in diaphragm muscle mass and thickness[67] and causes a reduction in the strength of both the inspiratory and the expiratory muscles.[81] Similarly, it has been shown that increasing end tidal CO_2 to 7.5 or 9% (54–64 mm Hg) in normal subjects reduces Pdi for a given diaphragmatic electrical activity.[82] Hypoxemia has also been reported to decrease endurance times in healthy subjects engaged in exercise and breathing against high resistances[83]; however, in a recent study in which the experimental conditions were carefully controlled, moderate hypoxia (FIO_2 of 0.13) had no effect on respiratory muscle function in healthy subjects.[84] Corticosteroid treatment,[85] hypocalcemia,[86] hypophosphatemia,[87] hypokalemia, and hypomagnesemia[88] may be additional contributory factors acting in concert with malnutrition and hypercapnia to promote the generalized muscle weakness of these patients.

CHEST WALL MOTION AND RESPIRATORY MUSCLE USE IN CHRONIC OBSTRUCTIVE PULMONARY DISEASE

Resting Breathing

As shown in Figure 4–2, the normal human diaphragm at FRC inserts onto the lower ribs. From these insertions, its muscle fibers run cranially such that they are apposed to the inner aspect of the lower rib cage. When the diaphragm is activated during inspiration, shortening of its muscle fibers thus causes a descent of the diaphragmatic dome. This descent produces both a rise in abdominal pressure with an expansion of the ventral wall of the abdomen and an increase in lung volume. During resting inspiration in normal human subjects, the descent of the diaphragmatic dome is about 2.0 cm, whereas the increases in the transverse and dorsoventral dimensions of the lower rib cage are only about 0.3 and 0.5 cm, respectively. Thus, the primary mechanism of the diaphragmatic contribution to tidal volume is a piston-like axial displacement of the dome related to the shortening of the apposed muscle fibers.

In patients with COPD and hyperinflation, the diaphragm is lower and flatter than in normal subjects, and the zone of apposition is reduced in size. Therefore, when it contracts, the dome descends less than it does in normal subjects, and hence the increase in lung volume is smaller and the rise in abdominal pressure and the expansion of the ventral wall of the abdomen are weaker. Because of the reduction of the zone of apposition and the smaller rise in abdominal pressure, the expansion of the lower rib cage due to diaphragmatic contraction is also smaller than in normal subjects (see The Respiratory Muscles During Acute Hyperinflation, The Diaphragm, in this chapter). In some patients with severe hyperinflation, the normal curvature of the diaphragm is even everted (with concavity facing upward rather than downward), such that the zone of apposition has completely disappeared and the muscle fibers at their insertions on the ribs run transversely inward rather than cranially. In this condition, the contracting diaphragm can no longer increase lung volume or expand the abdomen and produces a decrease (paradoxical motion) in the transverse diameter of the lower rib cage.[58, 89] This inspiratory decrease in the transverse dimensions of the lower rib cage in COPD patients is conventionally associated with the name of Hoover.[90]

Patients with COPD and hyperinflation thus have a less effective diaphragm than normal subjects. One would expect, therefore, that to generate a reasonable tidal volume these patients contract the scalene muscles and parasternal intercostal muscles more vigorously than normal subjects do.[28-32] One would also expect that these patients may also contract some muscles that, like the sternocleidomastoid muscles, are not normally active.

Since technical factors play a major role in determining the amount of electrical activity that can be recorded from a muscle, it has not been possible to demonstrate directly that patients with COPD have greater inspiratory electrical activity in the scalene and parasternal intercostal muscles than normal subjects do. Several lines of evidence, however, indicate that the inspiratory rib cage muscles do indeed contract more vigorously in such patients. First, the scalene muscles feel tense on palpation during inspiration in many COPD patients but not in most normal subjects. Second, surface electromyographic recordings have shown that, unlike normal subjects, many patients with COPD contract the sternocleidomastoid muscles when breathing at rest.[91, 92] Third, Levine and coworkers[93] have recently measured the swings in abdominal and pleural pressure during resting breathing in 11 patients with moderately severe COPD ($FEV_1 = 1.0$ L) and 8 control subjects, and they found that for a given fall in pleural pressure, the rise in abdominal pressure is smaller in the patients. Martinez and associates[94] have made similar measurements in 45 patients with varying degrees of airflow obstruction and hyperinflation, and they also observed that as airflow obstruction and hyperinflation become more severe, the increase in abdominal pressure decreases relative to the decrease in pleural pressure (Fig. 4–7). In patients with severe disease, the inspiratory fall in pleural pressure is even associated with a decrease in abdominal pressure and with a reduction in abdominal dimensions. These observations altogether confirm that patients with COPD and hyperinflation have a diaphragm that becomes increasingly ineffective as the disease progresses and that an increased inspiratory activation of the inspiratory intercostal and neck muscles compensates for this decreased effectiveness.

The fact that patients with severe COPD may have rib cage expansion with an inward abdominal motion during resting inspiration had been recognized in earlier measurements of thoracoabdominal motion.[72, 95, 96] This abnormal pattern had initially been interpreted as indicating respiratory muscle discoordination[95] or diaphragmatic fatigue.[97] In agreement with Sharp and colleagues,[96] however, I believe it more likely that this pattern is, in fact, simply related to the ineffective diaphragm. Indeed, in spite of the strong inspiratory activation of the diaphragmatic muscle fibers,[98] the dome of a low, flat diaphragm is not able to descend. Therefore, as the inspiratory intercostal and neck muscles contract vigorously and cause a large expansion of the rib cage, the larger than normal decrease in pleural pressure (due to the increased airflow resistance) pulls the diaphragm cranially. As a result, abdominal pressure falls, and the abdomen moves paradoxically inward. In other words, the diaphragm in such patients would function essentially as a fixator, rather than as a piston.

Earlier electromyographic recordings from the abdominal muscles in COPD patients have failed to detect any electrical activity at rest.[91, 99-101] Hence, expiration in these patients has conventionally been considered a passive process. These earlier recordings, however, were obtained with surface electrodes attached to the skin overlying the external oblique and rectus abdominis muscles. These two muscles do not have a prominent expiratory function in the dog.[41-43] Similarly, when normal subjects are made to use the abdominal muscles during breathing, such as during hyperoxic hypercapnia or during breathing against inspiratory mechanical loads, the transversus abdominis muscle is recruited during expiration well before activity can be recorded from the external oblique or the rectus abdominis.[102] Electromyographic studies using concentric needle electrodes implanted in the different abdominal muscles have shown that when breathing at rest, patients with COPD have

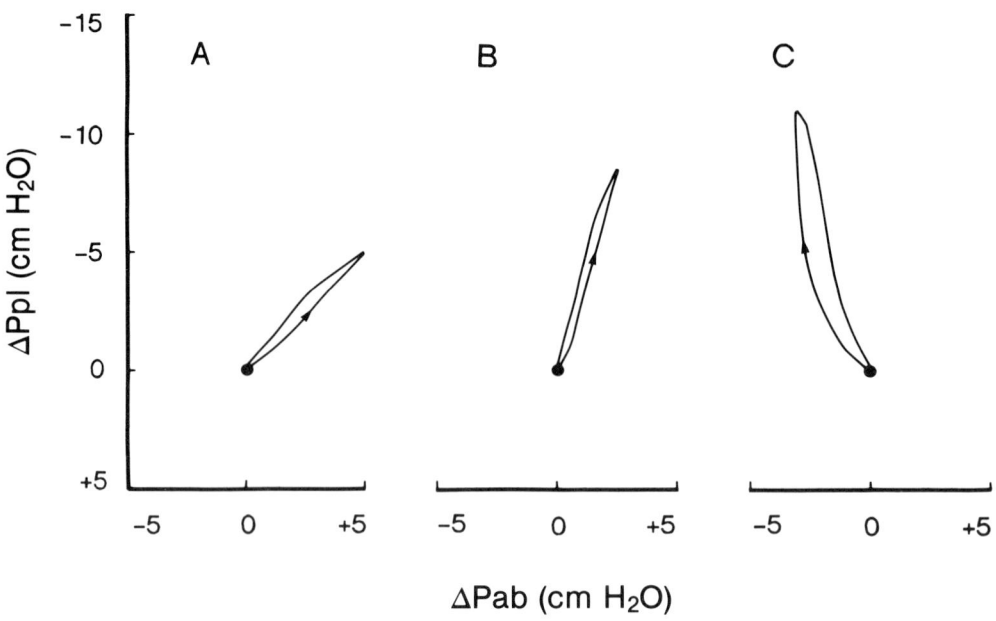

FIGURE 4-7. Inspiratory pressure generation during tidal breathing in a normal subject (panel A), in a patient with moderately severe COPD (panel B), and in a patient with severe COPD (panel C). The pleural pressure swing (ΔPpl) is on the ordinate, and the abdominal pressure swing (ΔPab) is on the abscissa. The *closed circle* in each panel corresponds to end-expiration, and the *arrow* indicates the inspiratory phase of the breathing cycle. In the normal subject, Pab increases during inspiration by about as much as Ppl decreases. In the patient with moderately severe COPD, however, ΔPpl is greater (owing to increased airflow resistance), whereas ΔPab is smaller; this indicates a smaller diaphragmatic contribution to tidal volume. The patient with severe COPD has a decrease (rather than an increase) in Pab during inspiration, which corresponds to a cranial displacement of the diaphragm and an inward displacement of the ventral abdominal wall. (Data from Martinez FJ, Couser JI, Celli BR. Factors influencing ventilatory muscle recruitment in patients with chronic airflow obstruction. Am Rev Respir Dis 1990; 142:276–282.)

a similar pattern of abdominal muscle activation. Thus, although the rectus abdominis and external oblique muscles are silent, many patients at rest experience expiratory contraction of the transversus abdominis, particularly when airflow obstruction is severe.[103] The mechanical correlate and the usefulness of this expiratory contraction, however, remain uncertain.

Contracting the abdominal muscles during expiration is conventionally regarded as being beneficial to the act of breathing because the consequent rise in abdominal pressure induces lengthening of the diaphragmatic muscle fibers, such that their force-generating ability during the subsequent inspiration is greater than it would be otherwise.[104–106] When active in COPD patients, however, the transversus abdominis muscle contracts only during expiration; it relaxes before the diaphragm begins to contract and remains silent throughout inspiration.[103] This suggests that when the diaphragm starts contracting, it is back to its neutral, relaxed length, and hence that its force-generating ability is not increased. Alternatively, Dodd and coworkers[107] have suggested that expiratory contraction of the abdominal muscles induces the storage of elastic and gravitational energy in the diaphragm and abdomen. By relaxing at the end of expiration, the transversus abdominis would allow this potential energy to be released, such that intrathoracic pressure would fall before the onset of diaphragmatic contraction. Patients with severe COPD, however, are flow-limited, even during breathing at rest.[108] Consequently, it is unlikely that expiratory contraction of the transversus abdominis muscle is able to increase expiratory flow and decrease lung volume below the neutral position of the respiratory system. In this condition, contracting the transversus during expiration would be somewhat analogous to performing a "belly-in" isovolume maneuver at FRC, and it is difficult to see how such a maneuver could be beneficial to the act of breathing.

Younes[109] has pointed out that expiratory contraction of the abdominal muscles is a natural (i.e., automatic) component of the response of the normal respiratory system to supranormal stimulation. When normal subjects increase their ventilation, such as during exercise or during hyperoxic hypercapnia, they recruit the abdominal muscles, and particularly the transversus abdominis, during expiration. Expiratory recruitment of the abdominal muscles also occurs when normal subjects are given inspiratory mechanical loads.[102, 110] In the absence of expiratory flow limitation, contracting the abdominal muscles during expiration is an appropriate response to these challenges, since it allows the work of breathing to be shared by the inspiratory and the expiratory muscles. It is possible that in patients with severe COPD, this "automatic" response to increased ventilatory stimulation is already triggered during breathing at rest, even though it might be useless or purposeless.

Influence of Body Position

Many patients with severe COPD claim relief of their dyspnea when they lean forward and support their arms on some fixed object, such as a piece of furniture.[111, 112] Some patients with severe COPD also report relief of their dyspnea when shifting from the seated to the supine position. Since these changes in body position do not alter pulmonary mechanics, this relief of dyspnea has been thought to result from an improvement in respiratory muscle mechanics. Sharp, Druz, and their colleagues[98, 113] studied the pattern of thoracoabdominal motion and the mechanics of the diaphragm in a group of seven patients who had relief of dyspnea when leaning forward, when assuming the supine position, or when performing both of these maneuvers. When breathing in the standing position and in the erect sitting posture, all patients had an inspiratory expansion of the rib cage associated with a decrease in abdominal dimensions. However, when breathing in the supine and the leaning forward positions, an inspiratory decrease in abdominal dimensions was no longer observed. Assuming the favored postures was also associated with an increased Pdi for a given amount of electrical activity in the diaphragm.[98] On this basis, Sharp, Druz, and colleagues[98, 113] have suggested that the postural relief of dyspnea was related to an improved efficiency of the diaphragm as a pressure generator. That is, the supine posture relieved dyspnea because the hydrostatic effect of the abdominal contents in this posture tends to push the diaphragm cranially, thus lengthening its muscle fibers and improving their force-generating ability. Likewise, leaning forward causes abdominal compression, which would also lengthen the diaphragmatic muscle fibers.

Since assuming the leaning forward or the supine position is associated with an improved mechanical efficiency of the diaphragm and causes relief of dyspnea, it is attractive to see a cause-and-effect relationship between the two phenomena. A number of observations, however, argue against such a causal relationship. In their investigations, Sharp and colleagues[98, 113] studied another group of 10 patients who had similar degrees of airflow obstruction but did not have postural relief of dyspnea. These patients, as the seven patients who claimed postural relief of dyspnea, had a decrease in gastric and transdiaphragmatic pressures in the standing and the sitting erect positions relative to the supine and the leaning forward positions. Kongragunta and coworkers[114] studied eight patients with severe COPD during exercise and also failed to find a relationship between the mechanical performance of the diaphragm and the severity of dyspnea. In more recent studies, Bradley and associates[115] and Ward and colleagues[116] have examined the sensation of inspiratory effort, probably the equivalent of dyspnea, in normal subjects breathing against inspiratory resistances with different patterns of inspiratory muscle contraction. Again, no relationship was found between the severity of the sensation and the level of diaphragm activation or the presence of diaphragmatic fatigue.

On the other hand, Ward and colleagues[116] noted a strong correlation between the level of activation of the inspiratory intercostal and neck muscles and the sense of effort. In his description of postural relief of dyspnea in COPD patients, Barach[111] also observed that relief of dyspnea in the leaning forward position coincided with the reduced use of the scalene and the sternocleidomastoid muscles. Sharp and colleagues[113] similarly reported that although all COPD patients had increased inspiratory activation of the scalene and the sternocleidomastoid muscles when assuming the standing and the sitting erect postures relative to the supine and the leaning forward positions, the increase was substantially greater in the patients who had postural relief of their dyspnea than in those who did not. We would speculate, therefore, in agreement with Barach, that the relief of dyspnea in COPD patients when leaning forward is primarily related to the decreased activation of the neck inspiratory muscles, rather than to the improved mechanical efficiency of the diaphragm.

Surely, the mechanism of dyspnea in COPD is complex, and further studies are needed to understand these phenomena. However, the observation by Banzett and coworkers[117] that normal volunteers leaning forward have a greater ventilatory capacity when their arms are braced on a table than when they are unsupported at their sides supports Barach's[111] and our hypothesis. This effect of bracing the arms is probably related to the improved function of the muscles of the neck and shoulder girdle. Indeed, some of the muscles that may contribute to the inspiratory expansion of the rib cage during strenuous ventilatory efforts originate on the pectoral girdle (for example, the pectoralis and the serratus). Thus when they contract, they tend to pull the pectoral girdle caudally. By the patient's leaning on elbows braced on a table, however, the pectoral girdle may be fixed, such that these muscles have an anchoring point; this should allow them to act more effectively on the rib cage while being less activated. Furthermore, when the arms are not braced, the muscles of the neck and shoulder girdle also must hold the arms and shoulders against gravity; they are thus compelled to perform two tasks simultaneously and may fatigue sooner.[117]

The dual postural and respiratory functions of the shoulder girdle muscles may also account for the inappropriate dyspnea that some patients with severe COPD manifest when performing seemingly trivial upper extremity activities (e.g., combing the hair, brushing the teeth). These muscles are inactive during resting breathing and probably remain so during upper extremity activities in normal subjects. However, they might contribute to resting inspiration in patients with severe COPD and be more active during such forms of mild exercise. During unsupported arm activities, however, some of these muscles also become engaged in the maintainance of the position of the upper torso and the extended arms; hence, they might be mechanically less effective, and their contribution to ventilation might decrease.[118, 119]

Exercise

When normal subjects are engaged in exercise, they show a reduction in end-expiratory lung volume due to increased expiratory activation of the abdominal and expiratory rib cage muscles (the triangularis sterni, and the internal interosseous intercostal muscles). Reductions of 200 to 400 ml already appear with the transition from rest to light or moderate exercise,[120–122] and most studies indicate that the reduction increases in magnitude as the intensity of exercise progresses to high levels. However, patients with COPD usually demonstrate an increase in end-expiratory lung volume during exercise.[107, 123, 124] This increase is primarily related to the increase in breathing frequency, that is, in the presence of expiratory airflow limitation, the increase in breathing frequency causes inspiration to begin before the respiratory system has had time to return to its neutral position. As a result, dynamic hyperinflation develops.

The exercise-induced increase in end-expiratory lung volume in COPD is particularly pronounced in patients with severe airflow obstruction. Average increases of 600 ml have been reported.[107, 125] Exercise, however, elicits a strong expiratory activation of the abdominal muscles and a marked reduction in the end-expiratory abdominal dimensions in these patients as it does in normal subjects.[107] The marked increase in the end-expiratory dimensions of the rib cage accounts for this apparent discrepancy.[107, 123] In other words, during exercise the rib cage compartment of the chest wall in these patients accommodates both the increase in end-expiratory lung volume and the volume by which the abdominal compartment is reduced. One would expect, therefore, that the inspiratory intercostal and neck muscles undergo marked shortening and, hence, that their force-generating ability is reduced relative to that during rest. Furthermore, to the extent that exercise, acting through hyperinflation, would cause further cranial displacement of the ribs at end-expiration, the load against which the inspiratory intercostal and neck muscles operate would be greater. This load would be further increased by exercise because of dynamic hyperinflation. Indeed, in the presence of dynamic hyperinflation, the inspiratory muscles must first offset the recoil pressure of the system before inspiratory flow can begin and lung volume can increase; this is equivalent to a threshold load. For all these reasons, the inspiratory intercostal and neck muscles would be at a major mechanical disadvantage during exercise. This might be an important factor in determining the patients' exercise limitation.

CONCLUSIONS

In this chapter, some physiologic concepts that relate specifically to the chest wall and the respiratory muscles in patients with COPD have been reviewed. As these patients develop hyperinflation, their diaphragms becomes flatter and shorter. Chronic shortening possibly causes the diaphragmatic muscle fibers to lose sarcomeres, such that the force-generating ability of these fibers might be better preserved than it would be otherwise. However, the low position of the diaphragm in the chest wall makes it less effective in its inspiratory action, and therefore as the disease progresses, the act of breathing becomes gradually more dependent on the inspiratory intercostal and neck muscles. These muscles are less affected by hyperinflation than is the diaphragm, and provided no malnutrition is present, they may ensure reasonable ventilation at rest. During exercise, however, these muscles are likely to operate at an additional mechanical disadvantage. They may also be overloaded when they have to ensure postural and ventilatory functions simultaneously, such as during activities with unsupported arms. Clearly, important questions regarding respiratory muscle function (or dysfunction) in COPD still need to be answered and these questions have been outlined in this chapter. Understanding these concepts and unanswered questions is essential if coherent, effective rehabilitation programs are to be designed.

ACKNOWLEDGMENTS

I wish to express my gratitude to Marc Estenne for his reading of the manuscript and to Gaetana Basile for her expert secretarial assistance. This work was supported in part by the Fonds National de la Recherche Scientifique (FNRS, Belgium), Grant No. 9-4583-90.

REFERENCES

1. Younes M. Load responses, dyspnea, and respiratory failure. Chest 1990; 97:59S–68S.
2. Demedts M, Anthonisen NR. Effects of increased external airway resistance during steady-state exercise. J Appl Physiol 1973; 35:361–366.
3. Gordon AM, Huxley AF, Julian FJ. The variation in isometric tension with sarcomere length in vertebrate muscle fibers. J Physiol (Lond) 1966; 184:170–192.
4. Rack PMH, Westbury DR. The effect of length and stimulus rate on tension in the isometric cat soleus muscle. J Physiol (Lond) 1969; 204:443–460.
5. McCully KK, Faulkner JA. Length-tension relationship of mammalian diaphragm muscles. J Appl Physiol 1983; 54:1681–1686.
6. Newman S, Road J, Bellemare F, et al. Respiratory muscle length measured by sonomicrometry. J Appl Physiol 1984; 56:753–764.
7. Farkas GA, Rochester DF. Functional characteristics of canine costal and crural diaphragm. J Appl Physiol 1988; 65:2253–2260.
8. Road J, Newman S, Derenne JP, Grassino A. In vivo length-force relationship of canine diaphragm. J Appl Physiol 1986; 60:63–70.
9. Marshall R. Relationships between stimulus and work of breathing at different lung volumes. J Appl Physiol 1962; 17:917–921.
10. Pengelly LD, Alderson AM, Milic-Emili J. Mechanics of the diaphragm. J Appl Physiol 1971; 30:797–805.
11. Evanich MJ, Franco MJ, Lourenço RV. Force output of the diaphragm as a function of phrenic nerve firing rate and lung volume. J Appl Physiol 1973; 35:208–212.
12. Minh VD, Dolan GF, Konopka RF, Moser KM. Effect of hyperinflation on inspiratory function of the diaphragm. J Appl Physiol 1976; 40:67–73.
13. Kim MJ, Druz WS, Danon J, et al. Mechanics of the canine diaphragm. J Appl Physiol 1976; 41:369–382.
14. Sant'Ambrogio G, Saibene F. Contractile properties of the diaphragm in some mammals. Respir Physiol 1970; 10:349–357.
15. Braun NMT, Arora NS, Rochester DF. Force-length relationship of the normal human diaphragm. J Appl Physiol 1982; 53:405–412.
16. Danon J, Druz WS, Goldberg NB, Sharp JT. Function of the isolated paced diaphragm and the cervical accessory muscles in C1 quadriplegics. Am Rev Respir Dis 1979; 119:909–919.
17. Smith J, Bellemare F. Effect of lung volume on in vivo contraction characteristics of human diaphragm. J Appl Physiol 1987; 62:1893–1900.
18. Mortola JP, Sant'Ambrogio G. Motion of the rib cage and the

abdomen in tetraplegic patients. Clin Sci Mol Med 1978; 54:25–32.
19. Estenne M, De Troyer A. Relationship between respiratory muscle electromyogram and rib cage motion in tetraplegia. Am Rev Respir Dis 1985; 132:53–59.
20. Strohl KP, Mead J, Banzett RB, et al. Effect of posture on upper and lower rib cage motion and tidal volume during diaphragm pacing. Am Rev Respir Dis 1984; 130:320–321.
21. D'Angelo E, Sant'Ambrogio G. Direct action of contracting diaphragm on the rib cage in rabbits and dogs. J Appl Physiol 1974; 36:715–719.
22. Jiang TX, Demedts M, Decramer M. Mechanical coupling of upper and lower canine rib cages and its functional significance. J Appl Physiol 1988; 64:620–626.
23. De Troyer A, Sampson M, Sigrist S, Macklem PT. Action of costal and crural parts of the diaphragm on the rib cage in dogs. J Appl Physiol 1982; 53:30–39.
24. Loring SH, Mead J. Action of the diaphragm on the rib cage inferred from a force-balance analysis. J Appl Physiol 1982; 53:756–760.
25. Mead J. Functional significance of the area of apposition of diaphragm to rib cage. Am Rev Respir Dis 1979; 119:31–32.
26. Urmey WF, De Troyer A, Kelly KB, Loring SH. Pleural pressure increases during inspiration in the zone of apposition of diaphragm to rib cage. J Appl Physiol 1988; 65:2207–2212.
27. Zocchi L, Garzaniti N, Newman S, Macklem PT. Effect of hyperinflation and equalization of abdominal pressure on diaphragmatic action. J Appl Physiol 1987; 62:1655–1664.
28. Taylor A. The contribution of the intercostal muscles to the effort of respiration in man. J Physiol (Lond) 1960; 151:390–402.
29. Delhez L. Contribution électromyographique à l'étude de la mécanique et du contrôle nerveux des mouvements respiratoires de l'homme. Liège, Belgium: Vaillant-Carmanne, 1974.
30. De Troyer A, Sampson MG. Activation of the parasternal intercostals during breathing efforts in human subjects. J Appl Physiol 1982; 52:524–529.
31. Raper AJ, Thompson WT Jr, Shapiro W, Patterson JL Jr. Scalene and sternomastoid muscle function. J Appl Physiol 1966; 21:497–502.
32. De Troyer A, Estenne M. Coordination between rib cage muscles and diaphragm during quiet breathing in humans. J Appl Physiol 1984; 57:899–906.
33. De Troyer A, Kelly S. Chest wall mechanics in dogs with acute diaphragm paralysis. J Appl Physiol 1982; 53:373–379.
34. De Troyer A, Kelly S. Action of neck accessory muscles on rib cage in dogs. J Appl Physiol 1984; 56:326–332.
35. Farkas GA, Decramer M, Rochester DF, De Troyer A. Contractile properties of intercostal muscles and their functional significance. J Appl Physiol 1985; 59:528–535.
36. Decramer M, De Troyer A. Respiratory changes in parasternal intercostal length. J Appl Physiol 1984; 57:1254–1260.
37. Jiang TX, Deschepper K, Demedts M, Decramer M. Effects of acute hyperinflation on the mechanical effectiveness of the parasternal intercostals. Am Rev Respir Dis 1989; 139:522–528.
38. Farkas GA, Rochester DF. Contractile characteristics and operating lengths of canine neck inspiratory muscles. J Appl Physiol 1986; 61:220–226.
39. De Troyer A, Kelly S, Macklem PT, Zin WA. Mechanics of intercostal space and action of external and internal intercostal muscles. J Clin Invest 1985; 75:850–857.
40. Di Marco AF, Romaniuk JR, Supinski GS. Mechanical action of the interosseous intercostal muscles as a function of lung volume. Am Rev Respir Dis 1990; 142:1041–1046.
41. Leevers AM, Road JD. Mechanical response to hyperinflation of the two abdominal muscle layers. J Appl Physiol 1989; 66:2189–2195.
42. Gilmartin JJ, Ninane V, De Troyer A. Abdominal muscle use during breathing in the anesthetized dog. Respir Physiol 1987; 70:159–171.
43. De Troyer A, Gilmartin JJ, Ninane V. Abdominal muscle use during breathing in unanesthetized dogs. J Appl Physiol 1989; 66:20–27.
44. Decramer M, Jiang TX, Demedts M. Effects of acute hyperinflation on chest wall mechanics in dogs. J Appl Physiol 1987; 63:1493–1498.
45. Camus P, Desmeules MJ. Chest wall movements and breathing pattern at different lung volumes (abstract). Chest 1982; 82:243.
46. Wolfson DA, Strohl KP, Di Marco AF, Altose MD. Effects of an increase in end-expiratory volume on the pattern of thoracoabdominal movement. Respir Physiol 1983; 53:273–283.
47. Rahn H, Otis AB, Chadwick LE, Fenn WO. The pressure-volume diagram of the thorax and lungs. Am J Physiol 1946; 146:161–178.
48. Thomas AJ, Supinski GS, Kelsen SG. Changes in chest wall structure and elasticity in elastase-induced emphysema. J Appl Physiol 1986; 61:1821–1829.
49. Tabary JC, Tabary C, Tardieu C, et al. Physiological and structural changes in the cat's soleus muscle due to immobilization at different lengths by plaster casts. J Physiol (Lond) 1972; 224:231–244.
50. Goldspink G, Tabary C, Tabary JC, et al. Effect of denervation on the adaptation of sarcomere number and muscle extensibility to the functional length of the muscle. J Physiol (Lond) 1974; 236:733–742.
51. Williams PE, Goldspink G. Changes in sarcomere length and physiological properties in immobilized muscle. J Anat 1978; 127:459–468.
52. Supinski GS, Kelsen SG. Effect of elastase-induced emphysema on the force-generating ability of the diaphragm. J Clin Invest 1982; 70:978–988.
53. Kelsen SG, Wolanski T, Supinski GS, Roessman U. The effect of elastase-induced emphysema on diaphragmatic muscle structure in hamsters. Am Rev Respir Dis 1983; 127:330–334.
54. Farkas GA, Roussos C. Adaptability of the hamster diaphragm to exercise and/or emphysema. J Appl Physiol 1982; 53:1263–1272.
55. Farkas GA, Roussos C. Diaphragm in emphysematous hamsters: sarcomere adaptability. J Appl Physiol 1983; 54:1635–1640.
56. Oliven A, Supinski GS, Kelsen SG. Functional adaptation of diaphragm to chronic hyperinflation in emphysematous hamsters. J Appl Physiol 1986; 60:225–231.
57. Arnold JS, Thomas AJ, Kelsen SG. Length-tension relationship of abdominal expiratory muscles: Effect of emphysema. J Appl Physiol 1987; 62:739–745.
58. Gilmartin JJ, Gibson GJ. Abnormalities of chest wall motion in patients with chronic airflow obstruction. Thorax 1984; 39:264–271.
59. Sharp JT, Beard GAT, Sunga M, et al. The rib cage in normal and emphysematous subjects: A roentgenographic approach. J Appl Physiol 1986; 61:2050–2059.
60. Sharp JT, Van Lith P, Nuchprayoon CV, et al. The thorax in chronic obstructive lung disease. Am J Med 1968; 44:30–46.
61. Steele RH, Heard BE. Size of the diaphragm in chronic bronchitis. Thorax 1973; 28:55–60.
62. Butler C. Diaphragmatic changes in emphysema. Am Rev Respir Dis 1976; 114:155–159.
63. Thurlbeck WM. Diaphragm and body weight in emphysema. Thorax 1978; 33:483–487.
64. Ishikawa S, Hayes JA. Functional morphometry of the diaphragm in patients with chronic obstructive lung disease. Am Rev Respir Dis 1973; 108:135–138.
65. Scott KWM, Hoy J. The cross sectional area of diaphragmatic muscle fibers in emphysema, measured by an automated image analysis system. J Pathol 1976; 120:121–128.
66. Sanchez J, Medrano G, Debesse B, et al. Muscle fiber types in costal and crural diaphragm in normal men and in patients with moderate chronic respiratory disease. Bull Eur Physiopathol Respir 1985; 21:351–356.
67. Arora NS, Rochester DF. Effect of body weight and muscularity on human diaphragm muscle mass, thickness, and area. J Appl Physiol 1982; 52:64–70.
68. Arora NS, Rochester DF. COPD and human diaphragm muscle dimensions. Chest 1987; 91:719–724.
69. Arora NS, Rochester DF. Effect of chronic obstructive pulmonary disease on sternocleidomastoid muscle (abstract). Am Rev Respir Dis 1982; 125:252.
70. Campbell JA, Hughes RL, Sahgal V, et al. Alterations in inter-

costal muscle morphology and biochemistry in patients with obstructive lung disease. Am Rev Respir Dis 1980; 122:679–686.
71. Sanchez J, Derenne JP, Debesse B, et al. Typology of the respiratory muscles in normal men and in patients with moderate chronic respiratory diseases. Bull Eur Physiopathol Respir 1982; 18:901–914.
72. Sharp JT, Danon J, Druz WS, et al. Respiratory muscle function in patients with chronic obstructive pulmonary disease: Its relationship to disability and to respiratory therapy. Am Rev Respir Dis 1974; 110:154–167.
73. Rochester DF, Braun NMT. Determinants of maximal inspiratory pressure in chronic obstructive pulmonary disease. Am Rev Respir Dis 1985; 132:42–47.
74. Byrd RB, Hyatt RE. Maximal respiratory pressures in chronic obstructive lung disease. Am Rev Respir Dis 1968; 98:848–856.
75. Rochester DF, Arora NS, Braun NMT, Goldberg SK. The respiratory muscles in chronic obstructive pulmonary disease (COPD). Bull Eur Physiopathol Respir 1979; 15:951–975.
76. Decramer M, Demedts M, Rochette F, Billiet L. Maximal transrespiratory pressures in obstructive lung disease. Bull Eur Physiopathol Respir 1980; 16:479–490.
77. Similowski T, Yan S, Gauthier AP, et al. Contractile properties of the human diaphragm during chronic hyperinflation (abstract). Am Rev Respir Dis 1990; 141:A166.
78. Shore SA, Huk O, Mannix S, Martin JG. Effect of panting frequency on the plethysmographic determination of thoracic gas volume in chronic obstructive pulmonary disease. Am Rev Respir Dis 1983; 128:54–59.
79. Stanescu DC, Rodenstein D, Cauberghs M, Van de Woestijne KP. Failure of body plethysmography in bronchial asthma. J Appl Physiol 1982; 52:939–948.
80. Rodenstein DO, Stanescu DC, Francis C. Demonstration of failure of body plethysmography in airway obstruction. J Appl Physiol 1982; 52:949–954.
81. Arora NS, Rochester DF. Respiratory muscle strength and maximal voluntary ventilation in undernourished patients. Am Rev Respir Dis 1982; 126:5–8.
82. Juan G, Calverley P, Talamo C, et al. Effect of carbon dioxide on diaphragmatic function in human beings. N Engl J Med 1984; 310:874–879.
83. Jardim J, Farkas G, Prefaut C, et al. The failing inspiratory muscles under normoxic and hypoxic conditions. Am Rev Respir Dis 1981; 124:274–279.
84. Ameredes BT, Clanton TL. Hyperoxia and moderate hypoxia fail to affect inspiratory muscle fatigue in humans. J Appl Physiol 1989; 66:894–900.
85. Janssens S, Decramer M. Corticosteroid-induced myopathy and the respiratory muscles: Report of two cases. Chest 1989; 95:1160–1162.
86. Aubier M, Viires N, Piquet J, et al. Effects of hypocalcemia on diaphragmatic strength generation. J Appl Physiol 1985; 58:2054–2061.
87. Aubier M, Murciano D, Lecocguic Y, et al. Effect of hypophosphatemia on diaphragmatic contractility in patients with acute respiratory failure. N Engl J Med 1985; 313:420–424.
88. Molloy DW, Dhingra S, Solven F, et al. Hypomagnesemia and respiratory muscle power. Am Rev Respir Dis 1984; 129:497–498.
89. Gilmartin JJ, Gibson GJ. Mechanisms of paradoxical rib cage motion in patients with chronic obstructive pulmonary disease. Am Rev Respir Dis 1986; 134:684–687.
90. Hoover CF. The diagnostic significance of inspiratory movements of the costal margin. Am J Med Sci 1920; 159:633–646.
91. Gronbaek P, Skouby AP. The activity pattern of the diaphragm and some muscles of the neck and trunk in chronic asthmatics and normal controls. A comparative electromyographic study. Acta Med Scand 1960; 168:413–425.
92. Skarvan K, Mikulenka V. The ventilatory function of sternomastoid and scalene muscles in patients with pulmonary emphysema. Respiration 1970; 27:480–492.
93. Levine S, Gillen M, Weiser P, et al. Inspiratory pressure generation: Comparison of subjects with COPD and age-matched normals. J Appl Physiol 1988; 65:888–899.
94. Martinez FJ, Couser JI, Celli BR. Factors influencing ventilatory muscle recruitment in patients with chronic airflow obstruction. Am Rev Respir Dis 1990; 142:276–282.
95. Ashutosh K, Gilbert R, Auchincloss JH Jr, Peppi D. Asynchronous breathing movements in patients with chronic obstructive pulmonary disease. Chest 1975; 67:553–557.
96. Sharp JT, Goldberg NB, Druz WS, et al. Thoracoabdominal motion in chronic obstructive pulmonary disease. Am Rev Respir Dis 1977; 115:47–56.
97. Cohen CA, Zagelbaum G, Gross D, et al. Clinical manifestations of inspiratory muscle fatigue. Am J Med 1982; 73:308–316.
98. Druz WS, Sharp JT. Electrical and mechanical activity of the diaphragm accompanying body position in severe chronic obstructive pulmonary disease. Am Rev Respir Dis 1982; 125:275–280.
99. Campbell EJM, Friend J. Action of breathing exercises in pulmonary emphysema. Lancet 1955; 1:325–329.
100. Skarvan K. The ventilatory function of abdominal muscles in normal subjects and in patients with chronic obstructive lung disease. Respiration 1971; 28:347–359.
101. Morris MJ, Madgwick RG, Frew AJ, Lane DJ. Breathing muscle activity during expiration in patients with chronic airflow obstruction. Eur Respir J 1990; 3:901–909.
102. De Troyer A, Estenne M, Ninane V, et al. Transversus abdominis muscle function in humans. J Appl Physiol 1990; 68:1010–1016.
103. Ninane V, Rypens F, Yernault JC, De Troyer A. Abdominal muscle use during breathing in patients with chronic airflow obstruction. Am Rev Respir Dis (in press).
104. Grimby G, Goldman M, Mead J. Respiratory muscle action inferred from rib cage and abdominal V-P partitioning. J Appl Physiol 1976; 41:739–751.
105. Goldman MD, Grimby G, Mead J. Mechanical work of breathing derived from the rib cage and abdominal V-P partitioning. J Appl Physiol 1976; 41:752–763.
106. Takasaki Y, Orr D, Popkin J, et al. Effect of hypercapnia and hypoxia on respiratory muscle activation in humans. J Appl Physiol 1989; 67:1776–1784.
107. Dodd DS, Brancatisano T, Engel LA. Chest wall mechanics during exercise in patients with severe chronic airflow limitation. Am Rev Respir Dis 1984; 129:33–38.
108. O'Donnell DE, Sanii R, Anthonisen NR, Younes M. Effect of dynamic airway compression on breathing pattern and respiratory sensation in severe chronic obstructive pulmonary disease. Am Rev Respir Dis 1987; 135:912–918.
109. Younes M. Determinants of thoracic excursions during exercise. In: Whipp BJ, Wasserman K (eds). Exercise. Pulmonary Physiology and Pathophysiology. New York: Marcel Dekker Inc., 1991, Vol 52, pp 1–65.
110. Martin JG, De Troyer A. The behavior of the abdominal muscles during inspiratory mechanical loading. Respir Physiol 1982; 50:63–73.
111. Barach AL. Chronic obstructive lung disease: Postural relief of dyspnea. Arch Phys Med Rehabil 1974; 55:494–504.
112. O'Neill S, McCarthy DS. Postural relief of dyspnea in severe chronic airflow limitation: Relationship to respiratory muscle strength. Thorax 1983; 38:595–600.
113. Sharp JT, Druz WS, Moisan T, et al. Postural relief of dyspnea in severe chronic obstructive pulmonary disease. Am Rev Respir Dis 1980; 122:201–211.
114. Kongragunta VR, Druz WS, Sharp JT. Dyspnea and diaphragmatic fatigue in patients with chronic obstructive pulmonary disease. Am Rev Respir Dis 1988; 137:662–667.
115. Bradley TD, Chartrand DA, Fitting JW, et al. The relation of inspiratory effort sensation to fatiguing patterns of the diaphragm. Am Rev Respir Dis 1986; 134:1119–1124.
116. Ward ME, Eidelman D, Stubbing DG, et al. Respiratory sensation and pattern of respiratory muscle activation during diaphragm fatigue. J Appl Physiol 1988; 65:2181–2189.
117. Banzett RB, Topulos GP, Leith DE, Nations CS. Bracing arms increases the capacity for sustained hyperpnea. Am Rev Respir Dis 1988; 138:106–109.
118. Celli BR, Rassulo J, Make BJ. Dyssynchronous breathing during arm but not leg exercise in patients with chronic airflow obstruction. N Engl J Med 1986; 314:1485–1490.
119. Martinez FJ, Couser JI, Celli BR. Respiratory response to arm

elevation in patients with chronic airflow obstruction. Am Rev Respir Dis 1991; 143:476–480.
120. Henke KG, Sharratt M, Pegelow D, Dempsey JA. Regulation of end-expiratory lung volume during exercise. J Appl Physiol 1988; 64:135–146.
121. Sharratt MT, Henke KG, Pegelow DF, et al. Exercise-induced changes in functional residual capacity (FRC). Respir Physiol 1987; 70:313–326.
122. Younes M, Kivinen G. Respiratory mechanics and breathing pattern during and following maximal exercise. J Appl Physiol 1984; 57:1773–1782.
123. Grimby G, Elgefors B, Oxhoj H. Ventilatory levels and chest wall mechanics during exercise in obstructive lung disease. Scand J Respir Dis 1973; 54:45–52.
124. Stubbing DG, Pengelly LD, Morse JLC, Jones NL. Pulmonary mechanics during exercise in subjects with chronic airflow obstruction. J Appl Physiol 1980; 49:511–515.
125. O'Donnell DE, Sanii R, Younes M. Improvement in exercise endurance in patients with chronic airflow limitation using continuous positive airway pressure. Am Rev Respir Dis 1988; 138:1510–1514.

Chapter 5

Ventilatory Control in Lung Disease

THOMAS J. BARSTOW, Ph.D.
RICHARD CASABURI, Ph.D., M.D.

The human lung faces a significant task in bringing ambient air down to the level of the alveoli for the extraction of oxygen and the elimination of carbon dioxide. Other functions of the respiratory system that must be coordinated with the primary function of gas exchange include the production of speech, the interruption for mastication, and a mechanism for the compensation of metabolic acid-base disturbances. Disease processes may affect either the flow of air in and out of the lung spaces (ventilation) or the diffusive process of gas transfer between the alveolar space and the blood (gas exchange).

PHYSIOLOGY OF RESPIRATORY CONTROL

Pulmonary respiration is fundamentally linked to maintaining the homeostasis of the arterial blood with regard to blood gases (O_2 and CO_2) and hydrogen ion concentration. To accomplish this with the dead-end lung structure inherent in the mammalian lung, the respiratory system must produce the biphasic expansion and contraction of the lungs that alternately draws in and forces out air. Initiation of the biphasic motions is accomplished by a group of cells in the central nervous system called the *central pattern generator*, which is thought to be located in the medulla. The effectiveness of the resultant ventilation in maintaining blood gases and pH is sensed by chemoreceptors, which feed back information that is used to alter the output of the CPG.

Structures Subserving Respiratory Control

Respiratory Center

The pattern of respiratory activity is governed by groups of neurons within the medulla and the pons.[1,2] These neurons are localized into three primary centers: (1) the dorsal respiratory group, (2) the ventral respiratory group, and (3) the pontine respiratory group. The dorsal respiratory group is located in the dorsomedial medulla in the region of the ventrolateral portion of the nucleus tractus solitarius. These neurons are active primarily during inspiration. Because the nucleus tractus solitarius is the primary neuronal pathway for afferent fibers from the ninth and tenth cranial nerves and includes afferents from the airways, the lungs, the heart, and the peripheral chemoreceptors, it seems likely that the dorsal respiratory group may be a processing center for peripheral feedback during inspiration. In addition to receiving rich afferent information, many of the cells of the dorsal respiratory group make monosynaptic excitation connections with phrenic motoneurons.[3]

The second group of neurons located in the nucleus retrofacialis, the ventral respiratory group, consists of three collections of neurons: the nucleus retroambiguous, parambiguous, and ambiguous (in order from caudal to rostral). The first and third nuclei are primarily expiratory in activity, whereas the second nucleus is active during inspiration. These nuclei contain motoneurons that directly innervate the pharyngeal and the laryngeal muscles as well as cells that indirectly synapse in the spinal cord with both phrenic and intercostal muscle motoneurons.[4]

Finally, the dorsal lateral region of the pons contains two bilateral nuclei of respiratory-related neurons in what is collectively called the *pneumotaxic center*. Lesions in this area in humans,[5] and in combination with vagotomy in the anesthetized cat,[4] lead to a pattern of breathing called *apneustic respiration*, which consists of breaths whose inspiratory phases are sustained for a very long duration. The role of the pneumotaxic center in respiration is unclear.[4] Lesions in this region alter the lung volume threshold for the cessation of inspiration, whereas stimulation may cause switching between the respiratory phases.

Three phases of the respiratory cycle can be identified: inspiration, expiration, and a postinspiratory period in which both inspiratory and expiratory neurons are silent. During inspiration, the firing rate of many of the cells within the dorsal respiratory group rises in a ramp fashion, paralleling the rise in phrenic nerve activity.[1,2] It has thus been hypothesized that the central pattern generator for inspiration either resides in the dorsal respiratory group or sends projections through this area to the phrenic nerve motoneurons.[2] However, no specific cells or nuclei have been found that can be identified as the central pattern generator. Inspiration is normally terminated by inhibitory feedback from lung stretch receptors traveling via the vagus nerves, by activation of a group of postinspiratory neurons found in the dorsal respiratory group, or by both of these mechanisms.[6] Expiration under normal resting conditions is passive, with air flow resulting from the recoil of the chest wall and lungs back to functional residual capacity (FRC), whereas the expiratory muscles (such as the abdominal and internal costal muscles) are electrically silent. When the respiratory drive is greater, the rate of rise in the ramp-like increase in inspiratory activity increases, the time of inspiration usually shortens, and the expiratory muscles are activated to assist in thorax deflation.[1]

Respiratory Chemoreceptors

Chemoreception for the respiratory center occurs at sites both outside the central nervous system (peripheral chemoreceptors) and within it (central chemoreceptors). The peripheral chemoreceptors are located in the carotid and aortic bodies. The carotid bodies are located bilaterally at the bifurcation of the common carotid arteries, whereas the aortic bodies lie in the cephalic portion of the aortic arch. Each body consists of packets of type I (glomus) cells that surround a blood vessel and are supplied by an afferent sensory nerve.[7] The type I cell–sensory nerve complex is surrounded by a sheath of type II (or sustentacular) cells. The type I cells are thought to be the primary receptor, whereas the type II cells are believed to act as support tissue. The sensory nerve fibers leave the carotid body as part of the carotid sinus nerve, join the glossopharyngeal nerve, and enter the brain stem. The ratio of blood flow to metabolic rate is very high for these bodies, and thus the arteriovenous O_2 difference is low.

In addition to the afferent sensory nerves, the carotid body is innervated with efferent sympathetic preganglionic and postganglionic nerve fibers originating from the superior cervical ganglion and with preganglionic parasympathetic fibers that synapse with ganglion cells within the carotid bodies.[8] One of the primary functions of this autonomic innervation of the carotid bodies is thought to be regulation of the blood flow within each body.[9] In fact, a general increase in sympathetic activity leads to increased carotid body chemoreceptor activity.[10]

The response of the peripheral chemoreceptors differs for hypoxia and hypercapnia. The discharge rate of the afferent nerve rises hyperbolically as P_{O_2} decreases, but when represented as a function of the per cent of O_2 saturation, the increase is linear.[12] The actual hypoxic stimulus is thought to be transduced intracellularly by a change in the adenylate charge (ratio of adenosine diphosphate to adenosine triphosphate) or by changes in intracellular calcium levels brought about by the hypoxia.[7,11] In turn, this leads to the release of neurotransmitters from the type I cells (including possibly acetylcholine and substance P). Compounds that interfere with the oxidative regeneration of ATP (such as oligomycin, which prevents the formation of ATP, or antimycin, which blocks electron transfer in the mitochondria) lead to blunted responses to hypoxia.

In contrast to the response to hypoxia, the output of the peripheral chemoreceptors rises linearly with increasing P_{CO_2}.[12] The response to CO_2 appears to be sensed by changes in intracellular (and possibly extracellular) hydrogen ion concentration and can be blocked by carbonic anhydrase inhibitors.[9]

The presence of central chemoreceptors has been deduced from the observation that ventilation is stimulated by inhaled CO_2 even in animals with resected carotid and aortic bodies.[12] One of the primary sites of this chemosensitivity appears to be the ventrolateral medullary surface.[13] When this area of the medulla is perfused with an artificial cerebral spinal fluid, the pH of which has been lowered, ventilation increases rapidly.[14] Cooling or the topical application of anesthetics to this region decreases or eliminates breathing and depresses the ventilatory responses to hypercapnia.[12] Several afferent inputs have been shown to stimulate neurons in this region, including those neurons that originate from limb flexion or extension, the inhalation of CO_2, the excitation of peripheral chemoreceptors, and the stimulation of midbrain locomotor centers.[13,15] In addition, ventilation is stimulated when neuroactive substances, such as acetylcholine, neurotensin, and substance P, all of which have been identified in these neurons, are applied to the ventrolateral medullary surface.[16-18] However, the notion that the ventrolateral medullary surface sites are the sole or even primary location of central chemoreception has recently been challenged by the observations that cells elsewhere in the medulla also respond to changes in CO_2[19] and pH.[20]

Respiratory Mechanoreceptors

There are several kinds of sensory receptors found within the airways, lungs, and chest wall, and these receptors perform a variety of functions. Some are mechanoreceptors, which are stimulated by mechanical distortion of their local environment; others respond to chemical changes in the surrounding tissue. Of interest to this discussion are the receptors within the pulmonary tree itself (slowly and rapidly adapting pulmonary stretch receptors and C-fiber endings) and receptors located within the surrounding chest wall (which includes the diaphragm, the intercostal muscles, and the ribs).

The precise location of the pulmonary stretch receptors has not been identified. Indirect evidence suggests that the slowly adapting receptors may be found predominantly among smooth muscle cells of both intrathoracic and extrathoracic airways and primarily in the airways outside of the lungs proper; however, some receptors are found in the intrapulmonary airways.[21] The rapidly responding receptors have been hypothesized to lie superficially in the airways and to be associated with the epithelial cells. This hypothesis is based on observations that these receptors respond rapidly to topically applied stimuli.[22] Both types of stretch receptors send afferent information via myelinated nerve fibers.

The slowly adapting receptors respond primarily to changes in lung volume and demonstrate little adaptation to constant levels of lung inflation. Indeed, many are active even at the end of normal exhalations.[22] The early cessation of inspiration with lung inflation (Hering-Breuer reflex) and the prolongation of expiratory time seen with increased lung volumes are likely mediated by these receptors. In addition, these receptors are sensitive to the airway concentration of CO_2; hypercapnia can inhibit their discharge, whereas hypocapnia increases it.[22, 23] The physiologic significance of this chemoreflex is unknown; it is conceivable that it may be useful as negative feedback to reduce respiratory drive and to prevent further falls in airway P_{CO_2},[24] but because the change in discharge is seen almost exclusively at unphysiologically low P_{CO_2}, this seems unlikely.

The rapidly responding pulmonary stretch receptors, also called *irritant receptors*, are sensitive to both mechanical and chemical stimulation. The early description of these receptors by Knowlton and Larrabee[25] included the observations that these receptors had a higher threshold of lung volume before becoming active and adapted more rapidly to constant lung volumes than did the slowly adapting receptors. Furthermore, these receptors are sensitive to the rate of change in lung volume, especially during deflation.[23] Both exogenous agents (e.g., ammonia and cigarette smoke) and endogenous compounds (e.g., histamine and prostaglandins) can also stimulate these rapidly responding receptors,[26] but in contrast to the response to lung volume the receptors do not rapidly adapt.[27] Although the precise role of these receptors in the control of normal breathing is uncertain, they have been implicated in several pulmonary reflexes. Stimulation of these receptors in the trachea and large bronchi results in cough, bronchoconstriction, and the production of mucus, whereas stimulation of receptors farther down the pulmonary tree may lead to hyperpnea with a shortening of expiratory time.[28, 29] They may also be the mediators of the periodic sigh breath. In contrast to slowly responding stretch receptor stimulation, which causes vasodepression, irritant receptor stimulation has a vasopressor effect.[30]

The third type of intrapulmonary receptor that has been identified is the C-fiber ending. These receptors are characterized by unmyelinated fibers with slow conduction velocities.[31] These receptors were originally thought to be predominantly or exclusively found in the lung parenchyma near the pulmonary capillaries and were named type J receptors by Paintal[30] (for juxtapulmonary capillary receptor). More recently, end-organ receptors with unmyelinated C-fibers have been identified throughout the lung parenchyma. The C-fiber endings are stimulated by a variety of endogenously produced substances, including histamine, some prostaglandins, bradykinin, and serotonin.[24] Furthermore, at least in animals (such as the dog), discharge generally starts at lung volumes significantly above FRC.[32] Activation of these receptors produces expiratory apnea, hypotension, bradycardia,[30] and bronchoconstriction.[32] Coleridge and Coleridge[32] have hypothesized that these receptors may contribute to bronchomotor tone and breathing rate through the modulation of inspiratory and expiratory times.

The chest wall receptors that have been the most studied are the muscle spindles and the Golgi tendon organs; these structures are common to other skeletal muscles as well. The muscle spindles are slowly adapting mechanoreceptors that are arranged parallel to the extrafusal muscle fibers and that respond to muscle stretch. The diaphragm is less endowed with these spindles than the intercostal muscles, where the density of receptors is similar to that in other postural skeletal muscles.[33] Intrafusal muscle fibers within the spindle are activated by their gamma motoneurons rhythmically and in phase with the extrafusal fibers within which the spindles are located.[24] This suggests that the spindles may play a role in compensation for changes in the load of the respiratory muscles. Stimulation of the muscle spindles generally increases ventilation.[34]

In contrast to the muscle spindles, more Golgi tendon organs are found in the diaphragm than in the intercostal muscles. The tendon organs are slowly adapting mechanoreceptors that are located at the point of insertion of the muscle into its tendon and that transduce muscle tension.[33] It now appears that the threshold for the activation of these receptors is low and similar to that for the muscle spindles.[24] Generally, stimulation of the Golgi tendon organs leads to an inhibition of the homonymous muscle, information that might be useful in the prevention of overloading that muscle. Stimulation of the Golgi tendon organs generally has an inhibitory effect on ventilation.[34] However, at present the precise role of these organs in normal respiratory control is unclear.

Responses to Respiratory Stimuli

Chemical Stimuli

Carbon Dioxide. Alveolar ventilation ($\dot{V}_A$), alveolar P_{CO_2} (P_{ACO_2}), and CO_2 output ($\dot{V}_{CO_2}$), are related by the following equation:

$$\dot{V}_A = 863 \times \dot{V}_{CO_2}/P_{ACO_2}$$

where the constant 863 is derived from the correction terms for temperature, pressure, and water vapor to convert $\dot{V}_{CO_2}$ (which is in units of standard temperature and pressure, dry) to units of body temperature, ambient pressures, saturated (for $\dot{V}_A$). When $\dot{V}_A$ is plotted as a function of P_{ACO_2}, the resulting graph is hyperbolic (Fig. 5-1, curve *DAE*). Thus, for a given metabolic rate, the change in ventilation required to produce a given change in P_{ACO_2} is not constant but rather depends on the initial P_{ACO_2}. Increases in inspired CO_2 lead to an increase in the steady-state relationship between $\dot{V}_A$ and P_{ACO_2}, resulting in a shift of the curve to the right, but with the same curvilinearity (curve *HCL*). Increases in metabolic rate, such as those that occur with exercise, raise the hyperbola (curve *FMG*). The points *AMN* thus represent the ventilatory requirements for different levels of exercise $\dot{V}_{CO_2}$.

Line *AB* in Figure 5-1 represents the response of ventilation to increases in inhaled CO_2. The rise is linear and has been called the *CO_2 responsiveness*. Traditionally, this response curve was obtained by allowing a subject to equilibrate to several different concentrations of inspired CO_2; as a result, several hours or days were required to complete the various protocols. Now, similar results are obtained in a few minutes in one session by utilizing the dynamic test developed by Read.[35] In this test, the subject rebreathes from a bag containing an initial concentration of CO_2 of about 7 to 8% mixed with O_2. The CO_2 concentration in the bag progressively increases owing to the subject's metabolism, and the associated ventilatory response can be described. Al-

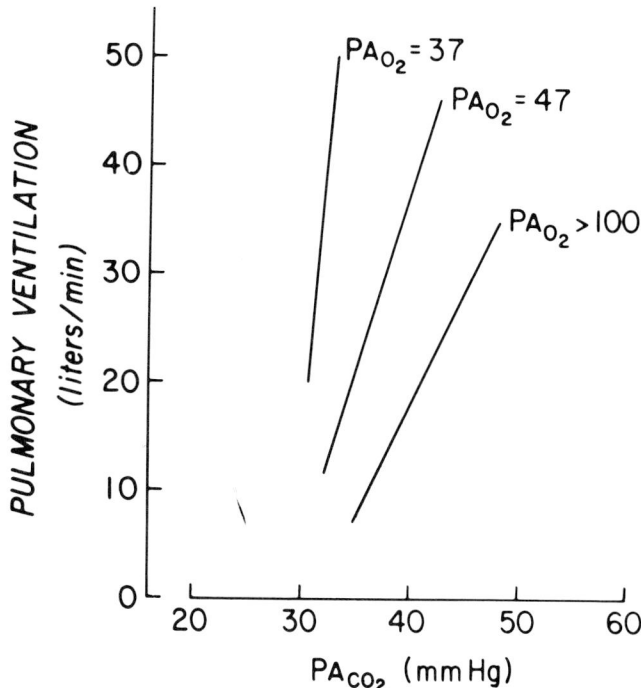

FIGURE 5-2. Influence of an inspired concentration of O_2 (P_{AO_2}) on the ventilatory response to inhaled CO_2 (P_{ACO_2}). (Data of Nielsen M, Smith H. Studies on the regulation of respiration in acute hypoxia. Acta Physiol Scand 1952; 24:293–313.)

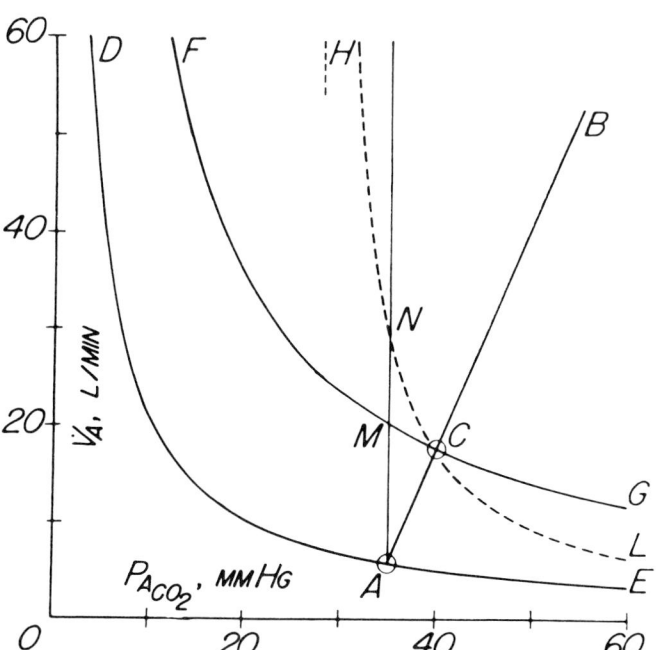

FIGURE 5-1. Schematic drawing showing the relationship between alveolar ventilation ($\dot{V}_A$) and alveolar P_{CO_2} (P_{ACO_2}). See text for details. (Reprinted from Fenn WO, Craig AB. Effect of CO_2 on respiration using a new method of administering CO_2. J Appl Physiol 1963; 18:1023–1024.)

though normal values for the slope of the ventilation ($\dot{V}_E$)/P_{ACO_2} response are fairly reproducible within any subject and range between 2 and 4 L/min/mm Hg[36] in most healthy subjects, there is considerable intersubject variability. A portion of this variability is associated with age, weight, and height as well as the presence and severity of pulmonary disease.[37] The clear implication is that, over a wide range, the magnitude of the $\dot{V}_E$/P_{ACO_2} slope is not crucial in determining breathing control at rest.[38]

The slope of the CO_2 sensitivity response is also affected by the background level of inspired O_2 (Fig. 5-2). Hypoxia dramatically steepens the slope, whereas hyperoxia (the condition in which the test is usually performed) results in a lower slope. Because hyperoxia substantially attenuates the response of the peripheral chemoreceptors, under these conditions the central chemoreceptors become the primary transducer of the rising CO_2 concentration.

The true, desired input of the CO_2 sensitivity test is P_{CO_2} at the chemoreceptors (as either P_{ACO_2} or P_{CO_2} of the CSF). However, these values are not easily obtained, certainly not at multiple times during a rebreathing test. Fortunately, during the rebreathing test an equilibrium is established between the mixed venous blood, arterial blood, and the gas in the rebreathing bag. Thus, monitoring of the bag P_{CO_2} (as end tidal P_{CO_2}, P_{ETCO_2}) can be easily accomplished and is indicative of the P_{CO_2} in the other compartments and chemoreceptors of interest (especially the brain tissue).

The output of interest for the CO_2 sensitivity test should reflect the output of the respiratory center.[38] This neural drive is best indicated by the phrenic neurogram but is usually estimated in humans based on $\dot{V}_E$. Ventilation is indicative of neural drive to the extent that the respiratory mechanics are normal. However, when a patient has abnormal mechanics, such as those seen with severe airflow obstruction or abnormally stiff lungs, $\dot{V}_E$ does not accurately reflect the neural drive.[38] A measure that is believed to more accurately reflect the neural drive in such circumstances is the mouth occlusion pressure (the pressure at the mouth at the very beginning [0.1 sec] of an occluded inspiration).[39]

Oxygen. Hypoxia, such as that observed at high altitudes, or in certain pulmonary diseases, leads to increased ventilation. It is important to differentiate the role of hypoxia per se from the concomitant changes in P_{CO_2} and pH that accompany hyperventilation under normal conditions. The concomitant hypocapnia and alkalosis tend to attenuate the overall hyperventilatory response, thus masking the true sensitivity to hypoxia.[40]

The ventilatory responses to varying levels of hypoxia, expressed as Pa_{O_2}, are shown in Figure 5-3 for different levels of Pa_{CO_2} (produced by different levels of inspired CO_2). Unlike the response to P_{CO_2}, which changes linearly from resting conditions, ventilation does not begin to rise appreciably until Pa_{O_2} falls to 50 to 60 mm Hg.[41] As noted above, when the maneuver is performed and P_{CO_2} is allowed to decrease naturally with the hyperventilation, the response shown in the lowest curve in Figure 5-3 is observed. However, when eucapnia is maintained by adding CO_2 to the inspired air, the response is magnified. The response can be further enhanced when the maneuver is performed against a background of elevated P_{CO_2}. It is interesting to note that although P_{O_2} is the signal transduced by the periph-

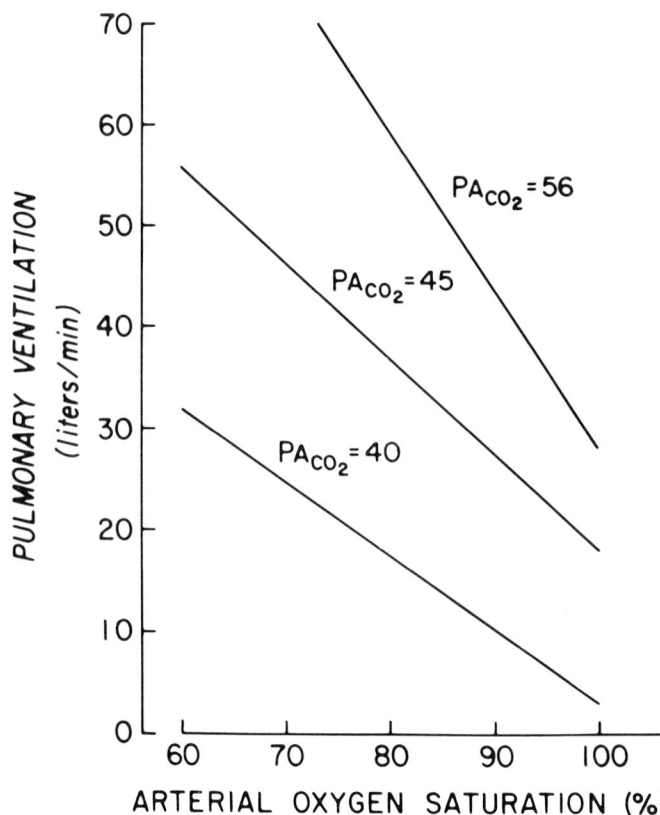

FIGURE 5-4. Responses of ventilation to different concentrations of O_2 as in Figure 5-3 but expressed as a function of the percentage of arterial hemoglobin saturation. Note the linearization of the responses for the percentage of saturation compared with P_{O_2} (see Fig. 5-3). (Data from Rebuck AS, Woodley WE. Ventilatory effects of hypoxia and their dependence on P_{CO_2}. J Appl Physiol 1975; 38:16-19.)

eral chemoreceptors and although the relationship between Pa_{O_2} and ventilation is nonlinear, the relationship becomes linear when ventilation is expressed as a function of arterial O_2 saturation or oxygen content (Fig. 5-4).[42] As with CO_2 sensitivity, the slope of the $\dot{V}_E$-O_2 saturation relationship shows wide interindividual variability, even among normal subjects. Interestingly, hypoxic sensitivity is positively correlated with CO_2 sensitivity[37] and declines with age,[36] not unlike CO_2 sensitivity.

Although the direct effects of P_{O_2} on respiratory control are mediated through the carotid bodies, there are secondary effects that must be considered when documenting O_2 sensitivity. The cerebral vasculature is sensitive to both P_{CO_2} and P_{O_2}. When hyperoxia is encountered, vasoconstriction of the cerebral vessels occurs; this slows the washout of endogenously produced CO_2. The consequence is central hypercapnia and metabolic acidosis, which stimulate the central chemoreceptors.[43] Thus, not only is the decrease in ventilation with hyperoxia reduced by this secondary mechanism, but the response to sustained hyperoxia is actually a slight hyperventilation. By a similar mechanism, marked hypoxia (Pa_{O_2} less than 50 mm Hg) leads to an initial hyperventilation that is caused by both carotid body stimulation and cerebral metabolic acidosis (due to the stimulation of anaerobic glycolysis).[44] Countering this is

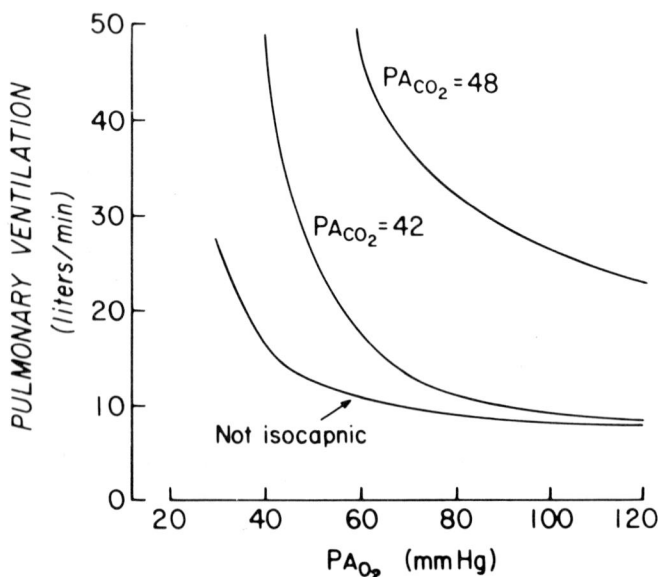

FIGURE 5-3. Ventilatory response to inspired concentrations of O_2 (as Pa_{O_2}) under nonisocapnic and two different backgrounds of isocapnic CO_2 concentrations. The hyperbolic nature of the relationship is shown. (Data of Loeschcke HH, Gertz KH. Einfluss des O_2-Druckes in der Einatmungsluft auf die Atemtätigkeit des Menschen, geprüft unter Konstanthaltung des alveolaren CO_2-Druckes. Pflugers Arch Ges Physiol 1958; 267:460-477.)

the observed depressor effect of sustained hypoxia on ventilation, which is possibly caused by cerebral hyperperfusion and the washout of CO_2 or possibly by the direct suppression of neural function by the hypoxia.[43]

The relative contribution of the peripheral chemoreceptors to ventilation under steady-state conditions has been assessed by inhibiting their neural activity transiently with the use of 100% inspired O_2. This technique is called the "Dejour switch" after the respiratory physiologist who first used it in anesthetized cats to show that 100% inspired O_2 silenced carotid body afferent neural activity.[45] Using this technique, Springer and coworkers[46] showed that the contribution of the carotid bodies to respiratory drive during exercise in humans was 23% during air breathing in adults, and it increased to 39% during hypoxic (FIO_2 = 0.15) exercise. In addition, maturational changes were found in the contribution of the carotid bodies; children demonstrated greater peripheral chemoreceptor input during hypoxic exercise than did adults.

Hydrogen Ion. Acute metabolic acidosis of either endogenous or exogenous origin leads to stimulated ventilation mediated via the carotid bodies, which are directly stimulated by increased H^+ concentrations.[47] The resultant hyperventilation leads to a reduction in CO_2 stores in the body, including those in the brain. This alkalinization of the brain in turn attenuates the ventilatory response to the acidosis.[48] If the metabolic acidosis is sustained for a few hours to several days, the bicarbonate levels in the brain fall. This reduces the alkalinization in the brain, which likely leads to restoration of some of the ventilatory response.[24] In addition to the direct stimulation of the carotid bodies by H^+, as H^+ increases an increase in the CO_2 sensitivity of ventilation occurs. This change is reflected primarily as a change in intercept (Fig. 5–5).[49]

Elastic and Resistive Loads

The work of breathing represents the work performed by the respiratory muscles to overcome three resistances to motion[50]: (1) elastic resistance of the tissues of the lungs and chest wall, (2) frictional resistance produced by the flow of air in the airways and by nonelastic deformation of tissue, and (3) inertial forces that are functions of the mass of tissues and gas. The last component is usually small and can be ignored. During inspiration, work must be performed to overcome the inward elastic recoil of the lungs. During passive expiration, part of the stored energy in the elastic components of the lungs is transferred to the chest wall, some is used to overcome the resistance to airflow in the airways, and some is used to overcome the continued contraction of the inspiratory muscles during at least the early phase of expiration.[50]

In healthy subjects, the metabolic cost of overcoming the resistive and the elastic elements of the respiratory system is small and represents only a small percentage of resting metabolism.[51] However, with increased ventilation, such as that observed with exercise, the cost of breathing dramatically rises and may exceed 15 to 20%

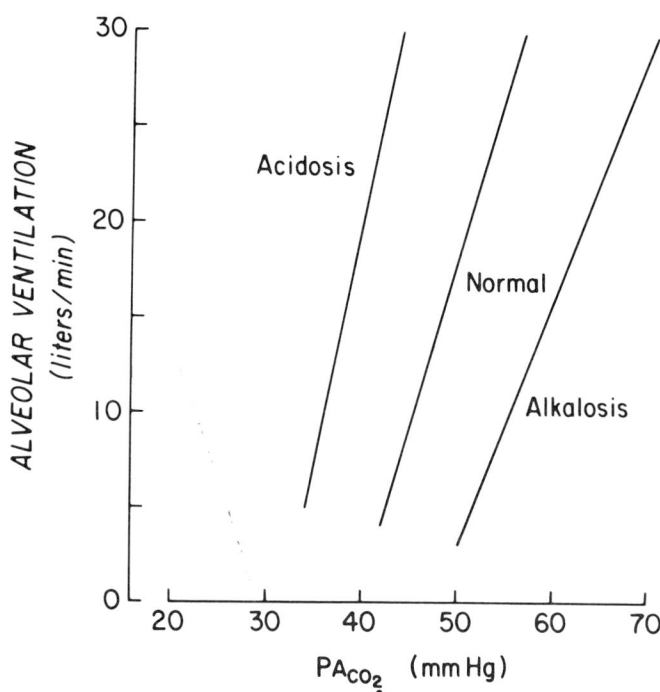

FIGURE 5–5. Effect of acid-base status on the ventilatory responses to changes in $PACO_2$. (From Fencl V, Vale JR, Broch JA. Respiration and cerebral blood flow in metabolic acidosis and alkalosis in humans. J Appl Physiol 1969; 27:67–76.)

of the metabolic rate for ventilation above 100 liters per minute. Many chronic respiratory pathologies (such as chronic obstructive pulmonary disease [COPD]) lead to changes in the mechanical properties of the lungs and chest wall that impact on the ability and efficiency of the respiratory system to ventilate the alveolar air spaces. In these patients, the work of breathing may be as high as 40% of the resting O_2 uptake.[51]

The respiratory adjustments to ventilatory loading significantly affect the relationship between tidal volume and breathing frequency. In both conscious and anesthetized human subjects, responses to respiratory loading are determined primarily by the mechanical characteristics of the chest wall and lungs and particularly of the diaphragm.[52] The responses at normal tidal respiration have little input from vagal reflexes owing to the weak Hering-Breuer reflex that occurs in this range of breathing in humans. Ventilatory loading may also inhibit ventilatory activity. Newsom Davis and Sears[53] found that the initial response to sudden changes in airway pressure and resistance led to inhibition of the electrical activity of the intercostal muscles. This initial inhibition was thought to be mediated by Golgi tendon organ stimulation. This same mechanism may be responsible for the observation that respiratory muscles do not increase their force of contraction during ventilatory loading in both conscious and anesthetized humans.[54]

Gas exchange may be compromised by the adjustments that are intended to decrease the work of breathing. Yamoshiro and colleagues[55] have tried to model the optimization strategies used to minimize the work of breathing during respiratory loading. They have suggested that the respiratory adjustments optimize gas exchange when ventilation and the work of breathing are low. In contrast, at higher ventilatory rates and work of breathing levels, the adjustments to mechanical loading seem designed to reduce the work of breathing.

Inspiratory work increases with increased tidal volume or hyperinflation because of the greater elastic recoil of the lung at higher volumes. In contrast, when the compliance of the chest wall or lung increases (as in emphysema), inspiratory elastic work decreases for a given tidal volume. Work to overcome resistive forces associated with airflow increases during hyperventilation or exercise and in conditions where increased pulmonary resistance is present (e.g., obstructive pulmonary disease).[50]

Over time the respiratory system adapts to chronic loading; this adaptation may partially compensate for the detrimental consequences of the loading. The respiratory muscles are one of the primary sites of adaptation. Hyperinflated lungs, such as those observed in COPD, lead to an initial shortening of the diaphragm and of the individual sarcomeres within each muscle fiber. Since force of contraction is determined by sarcomere length, this results in a reduced strength of contraction of the diaphragm.[54] Over time, a loss in muscle length and a reduction in the number of sarcomeres occur, such that the resting sarcomere length is restored.[57] This restores the contractile force to preinflation levels. In addition, in chronically loaded respiratory muscles, the number of fatigue-resistant fibers (type I, type IIa, or both) increases.[58]

Exercise

The responses to exercise, especially with regard to pulmonary disease, are covered in greater detail in Chapter 10. For the sake of this discussion, a brief summary of the normal responses is sufficient. With the increased metabolic rate associated with exercise, alveolar ventilation must rise in order to meet the requirement for greater gas exchange. During incremental exercise up to the anaerobic threshold (AT) (i.e., where there is little or no elevation in blood lactate level), ventilation appears tightly coupled with the metabolic production of CO_2 ($\dot{V}CO_2$), and both rise linearly with increasing work rate. For work rates that engender a low level of lactic acidosis (i.e., just above the AT), the hydrogen ions from the lactic acid can be buffered by bicarbonate to form CO_2 with little resultant decrease in pH. Both ventilation and $\dot{V}CO_2$ continue to rise, but more steeply than the linearly increasing $\dot{V}O_2$ (hyperventilation relative to oxygen uptake). As the work rate increases more above the AT, the further increased lactic acid production exceeds the ability of bicarbonate to completely buffer the hydrogen ions, and hence pH falls. For these heavy work rates, the progressively increasing lactic acidosis provides further stimulation to the peripheral chemoreceptors, and ventilation increases out of proportion to CO_2 production (hyperventilation relative to CO_2 production). The point at which the decrease in pH causes the additional stimulation of ventilation has been called the *respiratory compensation point*.[59] In normal subjects, up to the AT the increased ventilation is mainly accomplished by increasing tidal volume, but above the AT the further increases in ventilation are achieved primarily by increased breathing frequency.[60]

The adjustment of ventilation following the start of constant load exercise has been described for over 70 years, but there continues to be controversy regarding the underlying control mechanisms leading to the ventilatory response. Three components (or phases) have been described: (1) phase I, which represents an abrupt increase in ventilation within the first breath, (2) phase II, which starts 15 to 20 seconds after exercise onset and rises almost exponentially with a time constant usually for about 60 seconds in normal subjects, and (3) phase III, the new steady-state exercise level, which is obtained within about 4 minutes in normal subjects for work rates below the AT.[61] Earlier theories speculated that the rise in ventilation during phase I was attributable to neural feedback mechanisms originating from the exercising limbs or to feedforward mechanisms from higher brain centers.[62] The further rise during phase II was thought to be caused by humoral products of exercise metabolism reaching the central circulation. More recently, the ventilatory response during phase I has been termed a "cardiodynamic hyperpnea" because the increase correlates with estimated increases in cardiac output during the first few seconds of exercise.[63] The precise mechanism or mechanisms for the initial rise in ventilation during phase I are yet to be clarified.[64] During phases II and III of constant work rate exercise of moderate intensity (i.e., below the AT), ventilation is closely coupled with CO_2 production. The increased ventilation is primarily accomplished by increased tidal volume (Fig. 5–6). Following the initial adjustment, both tidal volume and breathing frequency remain constant over time. In contrast, for constant work rates above the AT, ventilation shows a secondary slow rise that delays the attainment of a steady state (see Fig. 5–6).[65] This slow "drift" in ventilation is likely the result of the decreasing pH from the accelerated lactic acidosis stimulating the carotid bodies; this leads to hyperventilation relative to CO_2 output, and thus $PaCO_2$ falls. This additional ventilation is usually the result of a slowly increasing breathing frequency, whereas tidal volume remains constant or decreases slightly after the initial adjustment.[61]

Altitude

Acute ascension to high altitude results in hyperventilation with subsequent arterial hypocapnia and respiratory alkalosis—ventilatory responses similar to those occurring with acute exposure to hypoxia. As noted above, the hypocapnia and alkalosis somewhat reduce the hyperventilatory response. Chronic exposure to altitude leads to adaptations that improve the efficiency of ventilation and oxygen delivery to the tissues.[66] Within several days, the pH of the cerebrospinal fluid is restored to normal values by the movement of bicarbonate out of the cerebrospinal fluid, and blood pH is restored as bicarbonate is excreted by the kidneys. The restoration

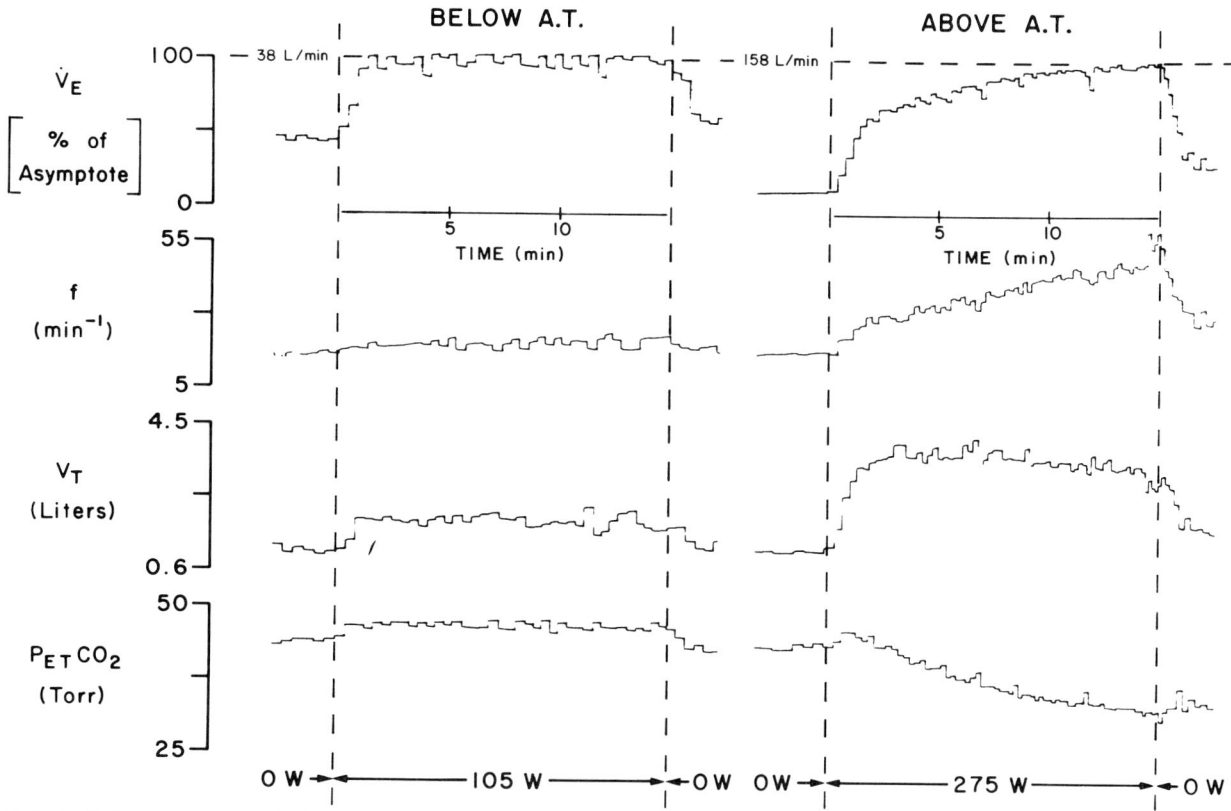

FIGURE 5-6. Ventilatory responses during exercise below (*left panel*) and above (*right panel*) the anaerobic (or lactic acid) threshold. The *baseline* represents the responses during unloaded cycling, and the work rate was started or stopped at the *dashed lines*. ($\dot{V}_E$: minute ventilation; V_T: tidal volume; $P_{ET}CO_2$: end-tidal partial pressure of CO_2; AT: anaerobic threshold.) (Reprinted from Wasserman K, Hansen JE, Sue DY, Whipp BJ. Principles of exercise testing and interpretation. Philadelphia: Lea & Febiger, 1987, p. 20.)

of pH then reduces the inhibition of ventilation, and ventilation increases. In addition, the hyperventilation helps to raise Pa_{O_2} by decreasing Pa_{CO_2}.

Another adaptation to altitude is polycythemia.[66] Red cell concentration, and thus hemoglobin concentration and O_2 carrying capacity, increase over a few days to several weeks. This effect means that although Pa_{O_2} and O_2 saturation are lower than at sea level, the O_2 content may be normal or even elevated. Also, polycythemia helps maintain the mixed venous P_{O_2}. The stimulus to the increased red blood cell production is the hypoxia; hypoxia stimulates the kidneys to release erythropoietin, which in turn stimulates bone marrow to increase erythrocyte production.

Chronic exposure to high altitude also results in a shift of the O_2 dissociation curve to the right, which facilitates the unloading of oxygen in the tissues. This is accomplished by the production of 2,3-diphosphoglycerate, which occurs in response to the hypoxemia. Other changes take place in the tissues (especially in skeletal muscle) that resemble the response to endurance exercise training, including an increase in capillarization and in the number of mitochondria with increased concentrations of oxidative enzymes. Because the air at high altitudes is less dense than at sea level, maximum breathing capacity is increased. Last, alveolar hypoxia leads to pulmonary vasoconstriction, which leads to elevated pulmonary artery pressure and subsequent hypertrophy of the right side of the heart. Occasionally, the pulmonary hypertension leads to pulmonary edema, even though the pulmonary venous pressure is normal.[66]

Interaction of Respiration and Circulation

Both ventilation and blood flow can be described as convective processes for the bulk transfer of O_2 and CO_2 between the environment and the tissues. It is thus intuitively sensible that control of both convections would at least in part share monitoring the sum total of the body's metabolic requirements for gas exchange. In fact, several reflex couplings between circulatory and ventilatory control have been described. Cardiac reflexes exist that relate to venous return and the output of the left side of the heart which in turn lead to the modification of ventilation. For instance, electrical stimulation of afferent cardiac fibers[67] and passive distention of either the right ventricle[68] or the pulmonary artery[69] increase ventilation. Ventilation has been shown to track the moving average of right ventricular pressure (an index of right ventricular strain) with changes in cardiac output.[70] Furthermore, distention of the left ventricle produces apnea.[68] Huszczuk and associates[71] utilized an anesthetized dog model in which they diverted a portion of the venous return from the right side of the heart into the systemic circulation, and utilized an extracorporeal gas exchanger to maintain arterial blood gas concentrations. They found that ventilation followed changes in the total flow of CO_2 into the lungs (blood flow multiplied by CO_2 concentration) and that bilateral cervical vagosympathectomy greatly reduced the ventilatory response at rest but not during electrically induced exercise.

Changes in the periphery have also been shown to modulate both ventilation and circulation. In both humans and anesthetized animals, electrical nerve stimulation leading to muscle contraction results in rapid increases in both heart rate[72, 73] and ventilation.[74, 75] Afferent information for these reflexes travels in the small myelinated and unmyelinated C-fibers. In the anesthetized cat, atropine or bilateral vagotomy eliminated the circulatory responses.[73] McCloskey and Mitchell[75] found that selective blockade of the small afferent fibers of contracting muscles eliminated both the exercise hyperpnea and the circulatory adjustments.

In addition to apparent common transduction of peripheral metabolic rate, ventilatory and circulatory control appear to share common, or at least intertwined, neural circuitry in the medulla. Pressor and depressor vasomotor neurons are located in the ventrolateral medullary surface in the same region as the respiratory neurons.[76] The significance of this proximity remains to be established.

ADAPTATIONS TO LUNG DISEASE

The Respiratory Chemostat

The ventilatory control system is one of several of the body's systems that facilitates adequate oxygen supply to the tissues. An additional goal is to prevent CO_2 build-up (and consequent tissue acidification). This is accomplished through closed-loop feedback of information from the arterial chemoreceptors (the arterial chemostat).[77, 78] Teleologically, the control strategy can be to regulate arterial P_{O_2}, P_{CO_2}, or pH at some "desired" value. Alternatively, all of these variables can be sensed, and the controller could attempt to effect some balance without necessarily achieving the precise "desired" value for any of the variables. Other systems are principally oriented to assure adequate oxygen transport and use oxygen sensors preferentially (e.g., most of cardiovascular control is oxygen-driven). However, the ventilatory control system is almost exclusively driven by the P_{CO_2} in the arterial blood under normal circumstances.

Examination of the relation between partial pressure and the content of CO_2 and O_2 in the blood reveals why CO_2 is the "better" controlled variable (Fig. 5–7). Small changes in arterial P_{CO_2} from the normal value of 40 mm Hg yield substantial changes in CO_2 content, whereas because of the shape of the oxyhemoglobin dissociation curve, small changes in arterial P_{O_2} from the normal value of about 90 mm Hg cause very little change in blood O_2 content. Thus, a "wise" control strategy would seek to keep P_{CO_2} near 40 mm Hg and only bring chemosensitivity for P_{aO_2} into play in the unusual situation when P_{aO_2} approaches the steep portion of the oxyhemoglobin dissociation curve (at 50 to

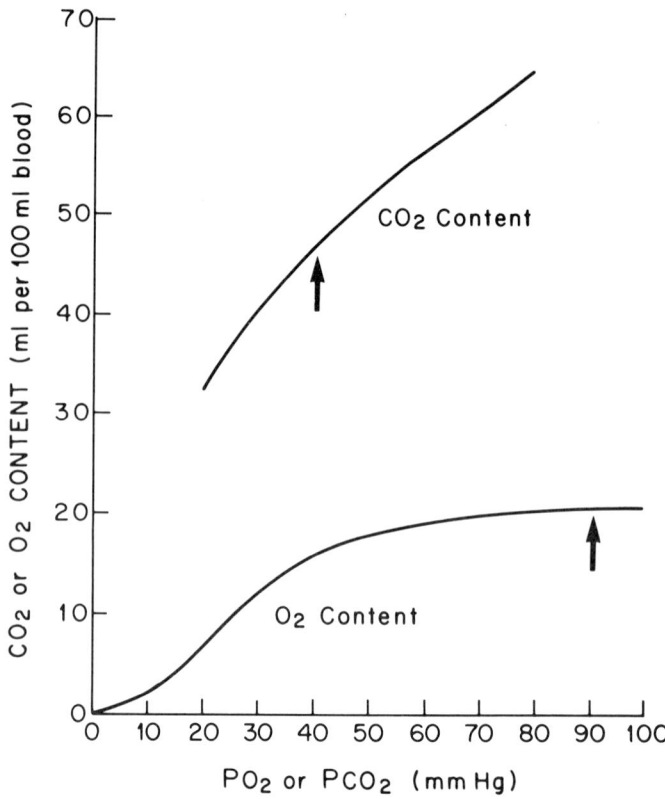

FIGURE 5–7. Small deviations from the normal Pa_{CO_2} cause substantial changes in CO_2 content, whereas small deviations from normal Pa_{O_2} cause little change in O_2 content. The dissociation curves for O_2 and CO_2 in the arterial blood are plotted; typical resting values for Pa_{CO_2} and Pa_{O_2} are indicated by the *vertical arrows*. The oxyhemoglobin dissociation curve is flat at a Pa_{O_2} of 90 mm Hg, whereas the dissociation curve for CO_2 is steep at 40 mm Hg.

60 mm Hg), such as at high altitudes or in lung disease. Not surprisingly, this "wise" strategy is just the one the ventilatory control system employs. An observable consequence of this strategy is that aging, exposure to modest altitude, and mild lung disease produce reductions in Pa_{O_2} but virtually no change in Pa_{CO_2}.

Ventilatory Control in Chronic Obstructive Pulmonary Disease

In lung disease, the maintenance of Pa_{CO_2} at 40 mm Hg carries a high cost. Because the COPD lung exchanges CO_2 inefficiently (i.e., V_D/V_T is high), more ventilation is required for any given level of Pa_{CO_2}. This is compounded by the fact that hyperinflation and increased airways resistance raise the work of breathing for any given level of ventilation. Under these circumstances, the patient with severe COPD faces two undesirable choices. The patient may maintain a Pa_{CO_2} of 40 mm Hg but consequently experience dyspnea and run the risk of respiratory muscle fatigue.[79] Alternatively, the patient may allow Pa_{CO_2} to drift upward. In this case, a lower level of ventilation is needed for a given rate of CO_2 production. In the acute situation, this latter strategy has a disadvantage in that pH decreases and that a number of metabolic processes are adversely impacted by acidosis (e.g., respiratory muscle function).[80] However, over a period of a few hours to several days renal mechanisms that promote the retention of sodium bicarbonate are activated. The higher blood bicarbonate level allows arterial pH to return to near normal levels despite the persistence of high $PaCO_2$.[81] Interestingly, hypercapnia by itself (i.e., not in combination with acidosis) does not seem to be detrimental to cell function. However, for unclear reasons patients who chronically retain CO_2 have a worse prognosis than those who do not.[82]

Just what makes some patients retain CO_2 while others do not has been intensely debated. The designations "pink puffer" and "blue bloater" imply a distinct division among COPD patients. The former are predominantly emphysemic and dyspneic; they fight to maintain a normal $PaCO_2$. The latter group is bronchitic, more comfortable, and retains CO_2 to the point of cyanosis (hence, the term "blue"). However, these designations are outmoded: COPD patients are seldom purely emphysemic or purely bronchitic. Emphysema patients are not always normocapnic, and bronchitic patients are not always CO_2 retainers. Several other theories to explain what causes some patients to retain CO_2 while others do not have been advanced.

Severity of Obstruction. A number of studies have shown what could have been logically predicted, that is, those with more severe COPD (as measured by a low forced expiratory volume in 1 second [FEV_1]) are more likely to retain CO_2 than those who are less obstructed.[83,84] Figure 5–8 shows the relationship between FEV_1 and the level of $PaCO_2$ at rest. Although it is apparent that CO_2 retention occurs most frequently at an FEV_1 below 1 L, the variability is impressive. A

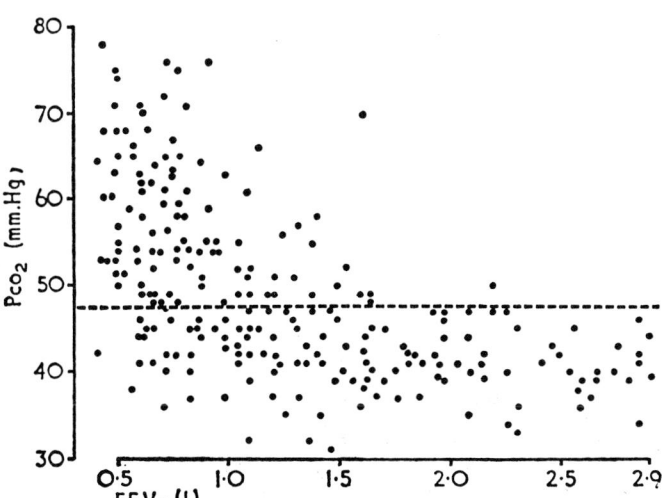

FIGURE 5–8. The relationship between FEV_1 and $PaCO_2$ in 13 patients with COPD studied serially over a period of 15 months to 5 years. The *broken horizontal line* represents the upper limit of normal values for $PaCO_2$ in this investigation. Although CO_2 retention is more common in those with FEV_1 less than 1 L, much variability among subjects occurs. (From Lane DJ, Howell JBL, Giblin B. Relation between airways obstruction and CO_2 tension in chronic obstructive airways disease. BMJ 1968; 3:707–709.)

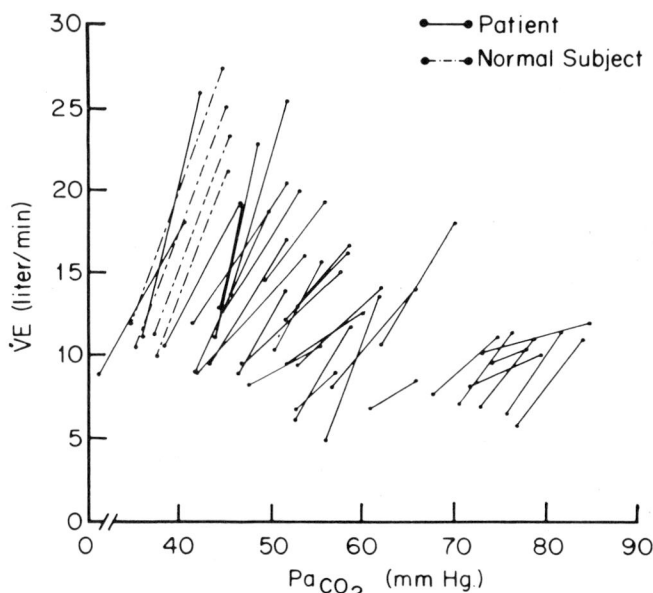

FIGURE 5–9. Ventilatory response to inhaled CO_2 in healthy subjects and patients with COPD with varying degrees of CO_2 retention. The *lower point* on each line represents the level of ventilation ($\dot{V}E$) and $PaCO_2$ as measured while the subjects were breathing 100% O_2. The *upper point* shows the $\dot{V}E$ and $PaCO_2$ observed while the subjects were inhaling 5% CO_2 in a hyperoxic gas mixture. The ventilatory response slope tends to be lower in patients who retain CO_2, although this tendency is not marked. (From Park SS. Factors responsible for carbon dioxide retention in chronic obstructive lung disease. Am Rev Respir Dis 1964; 92:245–254.)

number of patients with very severe obstruction do not retain CO_2. Other studies have shown an even weaker relationship between FEV_1 and the degree of CO_2 retention.[83,84] Therefore, although severe obstruction is usually present in those who retain CO_2, it cannot be the only factor.

Hypercapnic Sensitivity. A second reasonable supposition is that individuals who have a weak response to hypercapnia would be at risk to retain CO_2 under the stress of obstructive lung disease. Several studies have investigated the relationship between resting $PaCO_2$ and the slope of the ventilatory response curve to inhaled CO_2.[85–87] Such studies have inherent problems. First, the range of "normal" values of ventilatory sensitivity for inhaled CO_2 is very broad. Second, because patients with obstructive lung disease have a limited ability to increase ventilation, their ventilatory response to a given stimulus may underestimate the ventilatory "drive." Measurement of $P_{0.1}$ (the pressure generated during the first 0.1 seconds when an occlusion is imposed at the mouth) is thought to provide a better representation of ventilatory "drive" in such subjects.[39]

Figure 5–9 shows the results of an older study in which steady-state CO_2 inhalation responses were obtained and arterial blood was sampled.[85] Although the slope of the response curve might appear to be mildly lower in the patients who retain CO_2, the tendency is not marked. These results have been repeated with the noninvasive Read rebreathing technique[35] with similar results.[86,87] Those investigators who have quantitated ventilatory responsiveness with $P_{0.1}$ measurements have found little or no correlation between CO_2 responsiveness and the degree of CO_2 retention.[86]

Pattern of Breathing. There has been speculation that CO_2 retention is in some part related to an "unwise" pattern of breathing. A rapid shallow breathing pattern would yield a higher V_D/V_T and, thus, a higher Pa_{CO_2} for a given level of total ventilation. In studies of large groups of COPD patients, those with CO_2 retention tended to have a lower tidal volume at rest,[83, 84] which in turn leads to a lower alveolar ventilation. It has been supposed that chronic excitation of irritant receptors in the airways of "bronchitic" patients might be responsible for the rapid, shallow breathing pattern.[88] Also, a more shallow breathing pattern yields a lower maximum inspiratory pressure, which may help to avoid inspiratory muscle fatigue.[12] However, a rapid, shallow pattern is not employed by all patients with CO_2 retention,[87] and the possibility that the low tidal volumes may be the result of hypoventilation rather than its cause continues to exist.

Genetic Predisposition. An inherited tendency may exist for some individuals to defend a Pa_{CO_2} of 40 mm Hg poorly in the face of added work of breathing. Investigators have studied families of COPD patients. Significantly lower hypercapnic sensitivities, hypoxic sensitivities, or both, have been found in family members of those patients who retain CO_2.[89, 90] Deciding whether genetic predisposition plays a major role in determining which patients retain CO_2 and which do not must await study of larger populations.

Exercise Responses in Chronic Obstructive Pulmonary Disease

Mechanical factors limit the ventilation that patients with COPD can sustain during exercise. Inefficient gas exchange means that more ventilation is required for a given level of exercise. The sedentary lifestyle most patients adopt in combination with oxygen flow deficits imposed by concomitant pulmonary vascular disease results in the early onset of lactic acidosis, which adds to the ventilatory requirement. These factors, which are reviewed in detail in Chapters 10 and 16, are major determinants of the ventilatory response to exercise in COPD.

Patients with severe COPD (and many with moderate COPD as well) are distinctly ventilatorily limited; exercise tolerance is directly determined as the point at which the ventilatory requirement exceeds the mechanical ability to increase ventilation. But even in less severely impaired patients and even at submaximum rates of work, ventilatory control is often affected. The high work of breathing is considered in the overall ventilatory control strategy, and chemical control of ventilation is often sacrificed. In contrast to healthy subjects, in whom Pa_{CO_2} is maintained at 40 mm Hg despite manifold increases in metabolic rate that moderate exercise produces, patients with COPD often demonstrate increases in Pa_{CO_2}. Furthermore, the metabolic acidosis of heavy exercise, which produces hyperventilation leading to a reduction in Pa_{CO_2} in healthy subjects, fails to do so in many COPD patients. This is illustrated in Figure 5–10. These data were obtained from a group of COPD patients with disease severity ranging from mild to severe and who experienced lactic acidosis at the highest level of exercise tolerated.[91] In

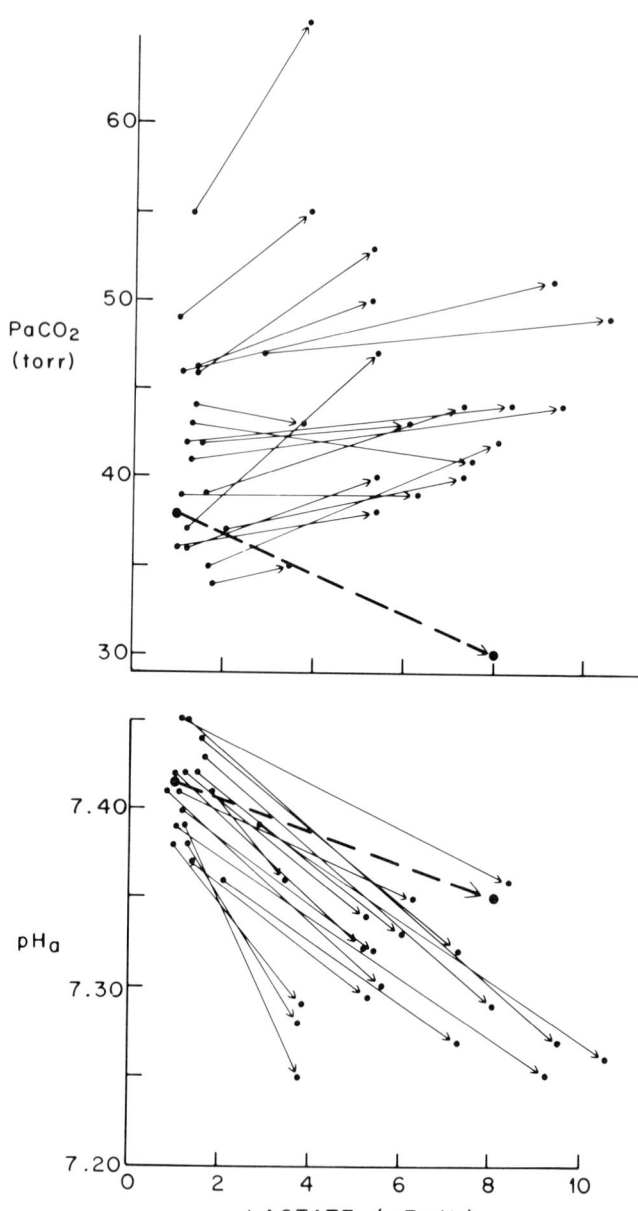

FIGURE 5–10. Changes in arterial P_{CO_2} and pH that take place in response to the lactic acidosis produced during heavy exercise in patients with COPD ranging in severity from mild to severe (*tail of arrow*: response to the unloaded pedaling; *head of arrow*: responses to highest tolerated work rate during an incremental exercise test; *heavy dashed arrows*: average response of 10 healthy subjects to exercise engendering a similar level of lactic acidosis). Healthy subjects lower Pa_{CO_2} in response to the lactic acidosis of exercise, but patients with COPD do not. As a result, patients with COPD experience a larger decrease in pH for a given rise in blood lactate level than do healthy subjects. (From Casaburi R, Patessio A, Ioli F, et al. Reductions in exercise lactic acidosis and ventilation as a result of exercise training in patients with obstructive lung disease. Am Rev Respir Dis 1991; 143:9–18.)

almost all patients, $Paco_2$ rises (rather than falls) in response to the metabolic acidosis of exercise, and the decrease in arterial pH is therefore accentuated. Note that these ventilatory control abnormalities occur even in those patients who do not retain CO_2 at rest. Perhaps CO_2 retention with exercise is an early marker for those who eventually retain CO_2 at rest when disease severity worsens.

THERAPY FOR RESPIRATORY CONTROL ABNORMALITIES

The respiratory control problems experienced by patients with chronic lung disease can only be properly remedied by curing the underlying lung disease. Since this is seldom possible, we are relegated to designing options for ameliorating symptoms. We might define a respiratory control "abnormality" as an adaptation that causes the patient to be more symptomatic than would another adaptation. Therapy is oriented toward forcing the patient to adopt a "wiser" ventilatory control strategy. Two conflicting sets of therapies have evolved. One set is for the hypoventilating patient who might benefit from a higher level of ventilation. The other set is for the very dyspneic patient who might be less dyspneic if the level of ventilation were depressed. As is apparent from the following discussion, neither set of therapies has yet been perfected.

Therapy for Hypoventilation

Long-term mechanical ventilation, either nocturnal or continuous, is an option for selected patients with hypoventilation. This therapy is discussed in detail in Chapter 20. The remainder of the therapies for hypoventilation are pharmacologic.

Progesterone

Increased blood levels of endogenous progesterone are responsible for the increased alveolar ventilation in pregnancy and in the progestational phase of the menstrual cycle. Progesterone administration has been studied for more than 30 years as a treatment for COPD patients with CO_2 retention.[92, 93] The precise mechanism of action is unclear, but it apparently acts diffusely on the central nervous system and may act by increasing the CO_2 sensitivity of central chemoreception.[94] The usual oral dose is 20 mg three times per day. In some patients, reduced $Paco_2$ results from chronic therapy (with consequent increase in Pao_2).[95, 96]. However, the improvements are often modest, and side effects, such as thromboembolism and male impotence, are occasionally observed.

Almatrine

Almatrine stimulates respiration primarily through stimulation of the carotid bodies. It appears that it also produces effects on pulmonary circulation that promote an improvement in ventilation-perfusion matching in the lung.[97] COPD patients treated chronically with oral almatrine generally experience modest reductions in $Paco_2$ and increases in Pao_2; the drug is usually well tolerated.[98, 99] Unfortunately, clinical trials were abandoned in the United States in the 1980s, and almatrine is not available for prescription in this country.

Acetazolamide

This drug is not actually a respiratory stimulant, but it can be used to "decompensate" compensated respiratory acidosis.[81, 100] This carbonic anhydrase inhibitor inhibits hydrogen ion secretion by the renal tubules and promotes, in effect, a bicarbonate diuresis. The resulting hyperchloremic metabolic acidosis increases the pH stimulation of ventilation. If the ventilatory system is able to respond to the relative acidemia, $Paco_2$ is reduced. This drug may be of use in COPD patients who have retained bicarbonate as a result of an acute exacerbation; restoration of their "usual" level of blood bicarbonate may be accelerated. The drug may be administered orally or intravenously in single doses of 250 to 500 mg. Subsequent doses depend on the arterial blood Pco_2 and pH response. Only a few investigators have attempted to treat COPD patients chronically with acetazolamide.[96]

Doxapram Hydrochloride

This is a respiratory stimulant that appears to act at both the central and the peripheral chemoreceptors. It also increases arousal and enhances the response to sensory stimulation. Seizures have been reported during its use. It is rapidly cleared from the blood following intravenous administration. Doxapram hydrochloride is not available for oral administration. It is generally administered by intravenous infusion (3–6 mg/min) and has been used occasionally in intensive care situations in hypoventilating patients.[101, 102]

Theophylline

This agent is a mild respiratory stimulant that acts on the central nervous system.[103] Its well-known side effects (nervousness, tremors, seizures) limit the dosage that can be used clinically. In COPD patients, its respiratory stimulant effect is usually overshadowed by its bronchodilator effect and perhaps by its ability to increase the contractility of the respiratory muscles.[104, 105]

Naloxone

This drug antagonizes opioids, which are known to depress breathing. Administered via intravenous bolus or infusion, it is useful in "reversing" the effects of opioid narcotic agents. Endogenous opioid secretion increases in times of stress, and blood levels are elevated in some COPD patients,[106] potentially contributing to depressed ventilatory responsiveness. Acute administration of naloxone to COPD patients with and without CO_2 retention has not been found to increase resting ventilation.[107-110] However, modest improvements in response to externally imposed increases in airways resistance,[107] in hypoxic responsiveness,[110] and in hypercapnic responsiveness[108] have been reported.

Therapy for Dyspnea

As explained above, some patients with lung disease choose a ventilatory control strategy in which they "fight" to maintain a $Paco_2$ of 40 mm Hg. The result is dyspnea on exertion and often at rest as well. There is a budding science that studies methods for desensitization to dyspnea. Ways are sought to reduce the sensation resulting from a given dyspneic stimulus. These methods are reviewed in Chapter 18. Another strategy is to attempt to reduce the dyspneic stimulus. In Chapters 16 and 17, methods for improving the fitness of muscles of the limbs and of the respiratory muscles in patients with lung disease are explored. Both methods hold promise for reducing dyspnea in selected patients.

An additional strategy is to interfere with the sensors or the integrating center that transduces dyspneic stimuli. This can be done with central respiratory depressants or with inhibitors of the peripheral chemoreceptors.

Central Respiratory Depressants

Several pharmacologic agents have been studied from two points of view. Does the agent reduce ventilation at a given level of metabolism (i.e., does $Paco_2$ increase)? Does the agent reduce the sensation of breathlessness? It can be argued that no centrally acting agent has yet been identified that provides adequate benefit from either point of view to justify the side effects engendered.

Diazepam was found to increase exercise tolerance in COPD patients,[111] but in another study patients became drowsy and unable to exercise after its administration.[112] The narcotic codeine has been found to increase exercise tolerance and decrease exercise ventilation in normal[113] and COPD patients,[114] but these benefits have been small. Promethazine mildly increased exercise tolerance in COPD patients[112] but not in normal subjects.[115] Chlorpromazine decreased breathlessness,[116] but it did not alter exercise ventilation.[115] Finally, indomethacin (an inhibitor of cyclooxygenase) had no effect on ventilation or breathlessness in COPD patients.[117]

Peripheral Receptor Inhibitors

Several investigators have sought to determine whether the blockade of pulmonary receptors might modify dyspnea. There is some evidence that the blockade of the vagus nerves reduces the sense of dyspnea.[116] However, inhalation of a local anesthetic aerosol does not seem to modify dyspnea,[118] either because the responsible receptors are not superficially located in the bronchi or because the aerosol does not penetrate far enough into the tracheobronchial tree.

Drugs to specifically inhibit peripheral chemoreceptor discharge have received little study. However, indirect evidence suggests that this approach might be fruitful. Supplemental oxygen is a prototype "drug" that improves exercise tolerance, even in patients who are not markedly hypoxemic.[119-121] Oxygen effectively attenuates carotid body discharge, but it is difficult to be sure that its beneficial effects are not due to other effects of oxygen, namely, improvements in oxygen delivery to the tissues and dilation of the pulmonary vasculature. Another line of evidence concerning the effects of carotid body inhibition on dyspnea and respiratory control comes from studies on patients whose carotid bodies have been surgically resected.[122] In patients without severe lung disease, breathholding times are distinctly prolonged,[123] and the ventilatory response to exercise is slowed[124] (although the steady-state response is not attenuated).[125] In patients with severe obstruction, CO_2 retention at rest and exercise generally increases, with a consequent worsening of hypoxemia.[126] Such patients often report an improved exercise tolerance and a reduction in dyspnea. However, although no controlled trial has been performed, these patients appear to be at increased risk of ventilatory failure.[126] Whether a reversible (pharmacologic) blockade of carotid body function would obviate this important problem remains to be studied.

REFERENCES

1. von Euler C. Brain stem mechanisms for generation and control of breathing pattern. In: Cherniack NS, JG Widdicombe (eds). Handbook of Physiology. Vol 2. Part II. Section 3. Control of Breathing. Bethesda, MD: American Physiological Society, 1986, pp 1–67.
2. Long S, Duffin J. The neuronal determinants of respiratory rhythm. Prog Neurobiol 1986; 27:101–182.
3. Lipski J, Kubin L, Jodkowski J. Synaptic action of RB neurons on phrenic motoneurons studied with spike-triggered averaging. Brain Res 1983; 288:105–118.
4. Berger AJ, Mitchell RA, Severinghaus JW. Regulation of respiration. N Engl J Med 1977; 297:138–143.
5. Plum F, Alvord EC. Apneustic breathing in man. Arch Neurol 1964; 10:115–126.
6. Richter DW. Generation and maintenance of the respiratory rhythm. J Exp Biol 1982; 100:93–107.
7. Eyzaguirre C, Zapata P. Perspectives in carotid body research. J Appl Physiol 1984; 57:931–957.
8. McDonald DM. Peripheral Chemoreceptors. In: Hornbein TF (ed). Regulation of Breathing. Part I. New York: Marcel Dekker, Inc., 1981, pp 105–319.
9. Pallot DJ. The mammalian carotid body. Adv Anat Embryol Cell Biol 1987; 102:1–90.
10. Biscoe TJ, Purves MJ. Factors affecting the cat carotid chemoreceptor and cervical sympathetic activity with special reference to passive hind limb movements. J Physiol (Lond) 1967; 190:425–441.
11. Prabhakar NR, Mitra J, Lagercrantz H, et al. Substance P and hypoxic excitation of the carotid body. In: Henry J (ed). Substance P and Neurokinins. New York: Springer-Verlag, New York, Inc., 1987, pp 84–87.
12. Cherniack NS. Control of breathing in COPD. In: Cherniack NS (ed). Chronic Obstructive Pulmonary Disease. Philadelphia: W. B. Saunders Co., 1991, pp 117–126.

13. Bledsoe SW, Hornbein TF. Central chemoreceptors and the regulation of their chemical environment. In: Hornbein TF (ed). Regulation of Breathing. New York: Marcel Dekker, Inc., 1991, pp 347–406.
14. Mitchell RA, Loeschcke HH, Massion, WH, Severinghaus JW. Respiratory responses mediated through superficial chemosensitive areas on the medulla. J Appl Physiol 1963; 18:523–533.
15. Mitra J, Prabhakar NR, Pantaleo T, et al. Do structures in the region of the nucleus paragigantocellularis integrate and mediate ventilatory drive inputs? Soc Neurosci Abst 1986; 12:304.
16. Haxhiu MA, Mitra J, van Lunteren E, et al. Hypoglossal and phrenic responses to cholinergic agents applied to ventral medullary surface. Am J Physiol 1984; 247:R939–R944.
17. Haxhiu MA, Deal EC Jr, Trivedi RD, et al. Tracheal and phrenic responses to neurotensin applied to the ventral medulla. Am J Physiol 1988; 255:R780–786.
18. Loeschcke HH. Respiratory chemosensitivity in the medulla oblongata. Acta Neurobiol Exp (Warsz) 1973; 33:97–112.
19. Bruce EN, Cherniack NS. Central chemoreceptors. J Appl Physiol 1987; 62:389–402.
20. Miles R. Does low pH stimulate central chemoreceptors located near the ventral medullary surface? Brain Res. 1983; 271:349–353.
21. Widdicombe JG. The site of pulmonary stretch receptors in the cat. J Physiol (Lond) 1954; 125:336–351.
22. Sant'Ambrogio G. Information arising from the tracheobronchial tree of mammals. Physiol Rev 1982; 62:531–569.
23. Pack AI. Sensory inputs to the medulla. Annu Rev Physiol 1981; 43:73–90.
24. Berger AJ. Control of breathing. In: Murray JF, Nadel JA (eds). Textbook of Respiratory Medicine. Philadelphia: W. B. Saunders Co., 1988, pp 149–166.
25. Knowlton GC, Larrabee MG. A unitary analysis of pulmonary volume receptors. Am J Physiol 1946; 147:100–114.
26. Coleridge HM, Coleridge JCG. Reflexes evoked from the tracheobronchial tree and lungs. In: Cherniack NS, Widdicombe JG. (eds). Handbook of Physiology. Vol 2. Part II. Section 3. Control of Breathing. Bethesda, MD: American Physiological Society, 1986, pp 395–431.
27. Sampson SR, Vidruk EH. Properties of 'irritant' receptors in canine lung. Respir Physiol 1975; 25:9–22.
28. Widdicombe JG. Defensive mechanisms of the respiratory system. In: Widdicombe JG (ed). International Review of Physiology Respiratory Physiology II. Baltimore: University Park Press, 1977, pp 291–315.
29. Widdicombe JG. Nervous receptors in the respiratory tract and lungs. In: Hornbein TF (ed). Regulation of Breathing. Part I. New York: Marcel Dekker, Inc., 1981, pp 429–472.
30. Paintal AS. Vagal sensory receptors and their reflex effects. Physiol Rev 1973; 53:159–227.
31. Agostoni E, Chinnock JE, Daley MB, Burray JG. Functional and histological studies of the vagus nerve and its branches to the heart, lungs and abdominal viscera in the cat. J Physiol (Lond) 1957; 135: 182–205.
32. Coleridge JCG, Coleridge HMG. Afferent vagal C fibre innervation of the lungs and airways and its functional significance. Rev Physiol Biochem Pharmacol 1984; 99:1–110.
33. Duron B. Intercostal and diaphragmatic muscle endings and afferents. Hornbein TF (ed). In: Regulation of Breathing. Part I. New York, Marcel Dekker, Inc., 1981, pp 473–540.
34. Shannon R. Reflexes from respiratory muscles and costovertebral joints. In: Cherniack NS, Widdicombe JG (eds). Handbook of Physiology. Vol 2. Part I. Section 3. Control of Breathing. Bethesda, MD: American Physiological Society, 1986, pp 431–448.
35. Read DJC. A clinical method for assessing the ventilatory response to carbon dioxide. Aust Ann Med 1967; 16:20–32.
36. Kronenberg RS, Drage CW. Attenuation of the ventilatory and heart rate response to hypoxia and hypercapnia with aging in normal men. J Clin Invest 1973; 52:1812–1819.
37. Hirshman CA, McCullough RE, Weil JV. Normal values for hypoxic and hypercapnic ventilatory drives in man. J Appl Physiol 1975; 38:1095–1098.
38. Cummin RC, Saunders KB. The ventilatory response to inhaled CO_2. In: Whipp BJ (ed). The Control of Breathing in Man. Manchester: Manchester University Press, 1987, pp 45–67.
39. Whitelaw WA, Derenne JP, Milic-Emili J. Occlusion pressure as a measure of respiratory centre output in conscious man. Respir Physiol 1975; 23:181–199.
40. Cormack RS, Cunningham DJC, Gee JBL. The effect of carbon dioxide on the respiratory response to want of oxygen. Q J Exp Physiol 1957; 42:323–334.
41. Weil JV, Byrne-Quinn E, Sodal IE, et al. Hypoxic ventilatory drive in normal man. J Clin Invest 1970; 49:1061–1072.
42. Rebuck AS, Campbell EJM. A clinical method for assessing the ventilatory response to hypoxia. Am Rev Respir Dis 1974; 109:345–350.
43. Kety SS, Schmidt CF. The effects of altered arterial tensions of carbon dioxide and oxygen on cerebral blood flow and cerebral oxygen consumption of normal young men. J Clin Invest 1948; 27:484–495.
44. Ponten U, Siesjo BK. Gradients of CO_2 tension in the brain. Acta Physiol Scand 1966; 67:129–140.
45. Dejours P. Control of respiration by arterial chemoreceptors. Ann N Y Acad Sci 1963; 109:682–695.
46. Springer C, Cooper DM, Wasserman K. Evidence that maturation of the peripheral chemoreceptors is not complete in childhood. Respir Physiol 1988; 74:55–64.
47. Biscoe TJ, Purves MJ, Sampson SR. The frequency of nerve impulses in single carotid body chemoreceptor afferent fibres recorded in vivo with intact circulation. J Physiol (Lond) 1970; 208:121–131.
48. Robin ED, Whaley RD, Crump CH, et al. Acid-base relations between spinal fluid and arterial blood with special reference to control of ventilation. J Appl Physiol 1958; 13:385–392.
49. Fencl V, Vale JR, Broch JA. Respiration and cerebral blood flow in metabolic acidosis and alkalosis in humans. J Appl Physiol 1969; 27:67–76.
50. Collett PW, Roussos C, Macklem PT. Respiratory Mechanics. In: Murray JF, Nadel JA (eds). Textbook of Respiratory Medicine. Philadelphia: W.B. Saunders Co., 1988, pp 85–128.
51. Petersen ES. The control of breathing pattern. In: Whipp BJ (ed). The Control of Breathing in Man. Physiological Society Study Guides. Number 3. Manchester: Manchester University Press, 1987, pp 1–28.
52. Pengelly LD, Anderson AM, Milic-Emili J. Mechanics of the diaphragm. J Appl Physiol 1971; 30:797–805.
53. Newsom Davis J, Sears TA. The proprioceptive reflex control of the intercostal muscles during their voluntary activation. J Physiol (Lond) 1970; 209:711–738.
54. Cherniack NS, Altose MD. Respiratory responses to ventilatory loading. In: Hornbein TF (ed). Regulation of Breathing. Part II. New York: Marcel Dekker, Inc., 1981, pp 905–964.
55. Yamashiro SM, Daubenspeck JA, Lauritsen TN, Grodins FS. Total work of breathing optimization in CO_2 inhalation and exercise. J Appl Physiol 1975; 38:702–709.
56. Rochester DF, Arora NS, Braun NMT, Goldberg SK. The respiratory muscles in chronic obstructive pulmonary diseases. Bull Eur Physiopathol Respir 1979; 18:951–975.
57. Roussos CS, Macklem PT. Diaphragmatic fatigue in man. J Appl Physiol 1977; 43:189–197.
58. Roussos C. Moxham J. Respiratory muscle fatigue. In: Roussos C, Macklem PT (eds). Thorax. New York: Marcel Dekker, Inc., 1985, pp 829–870.
59. Wasserman K. Breathing during exercise. N Engl J Med 1978; 298:780–785.
60. Whipp BJ, Davis JA, Wasserman K. Ventilatory control of the 'isocapnic buffering' region in rapidly-incremental exercise. Respir Physiol 1989; 76:357–368.
61. Wasserman K, Whipp BJ, Casaburi R. Respiratory control during exercise. In: Cherniack NS, Widdicombe JG (eds). Handbook of Physiology. Vol 2. Part II. Chapter 17. Bethesda, MD: American Physiological Society, 1986, pp 595–619.
62. Dejours P. The regulation of breathing during muscular exercise in man: A neuro-humoral theory. In: Cummingham DJC, Lloyd BB (eds). The Regulation of Human Respiration. Oxford, England: Blackwell Scientific Publications, Inc., 1963, pp 535–547.
63. Wasserman K, Whipp BJ, Castagna J. Cardiodynamic hyper-

63. pnea: Hyperpnea secondary to cardiac output increase. J Appl Physiol 1974; 36:457–464.
64. Casaburi R. Analysis of the exercise hyperpnea using dynamic work rate forcings. In: Khoo MCK (ed). Modeling and Parameter Estimation in Respiratory Control. New York:Plenum Publishing Corp., 1989, pp 13–23.
65. Casaburi R, Barstow TJ, Robinson T, Wasserman K. Influence of work rate on ventilatory and gas exchange kinetics. J Appl Physiol 1989; 67:547–555.
66. West JB. Respiratory Physiology. Baltimore: Williams & Wilkins, 1979, pp 127–131.
67. Uchida Y. Tachypnea after stimulation of afferent cardiac sympathetic nerve fibers. Am J Physiol 1976; 230:1003–1007.
68. Kostreva DR, Hopp FA, Zuperku EJ, Kampine JP. Apnea, tachypnea and hypotension elicited by cardiac vagal afferents. J Appl Physiol 1979; 47:312–318.
69. Kan WO, Ledsome JR, Boulter CP. Pulmonary arterial distension and activity in phrenic nerve of anesthetized dogs. J Appl Physiol 1979; 46:625–631.
70. Jones PW, Huszczuk A, Wasserman K. Cardiac output as a controller of ventilation through changes in right ventricular load. J Appl Physiol 1982; 53:218–224.
71. Huszczuk A, Whipp BJ, Oren A, et al. Ventilatory responses to partial cardiopulmonary bypass at rest and exercise in dogs. J Appl Physiol 1986; 61:575–583.
72. Hollander AP, Bouman LN. Cardiac acceleration in man elicited by a muscle-heart reflex. J Appl Physiol 1975; 38:272–278.
73. Gelsema AJ, De Groot G, Bouman LN. Instantaneous cardiac acceleration in the cat elicited by peripheral nerve stimulation. J Appl Physiol 1983; 55:703–710.
74. Weissman ML, Wasserman K, Huntsman DJ, Whipp BJ. Ventilation and gas exchange during phasic hindlimb exercise in the dog. J Appl Physiol 1979; 46:878–884.
75. McCloskey DI, Mitchell JH. Reflex cardiovascular and respiratory responses originating in exercising muscle. J Physiol (Lond) 1972; 224:173–186
76. McAllen RM. Location of neurons with cardiovascular and respiratory function at the ventral surface of the cat's medulla. Neuroscience 1986; 18:43–49.
77. Grodins FS. Control theory and biological systems. New York: Columbia University Press, 1963.
78. Milhorn HT. The application of control theory to physiological systems. Philadelphia: W. B. Saunders Co., 1966.
79. Begin P, Grassino A. Inspiratory muscle dysfunction and chronic hypercapnia in chronic obstructive pulmonary disease. Am Rev Respir Dis 1991; 143:905–914.
80. Juan G, Calverley P, Talamo C. et al. Effect of carbon dioxide and acidemia on diaphragmatic function in human beings. N Engl J Med 1984; 310:874–879.
81. Wasserman K, Casaburi R, Sue, DY. Respiratory Acidosis. In: Glassock RG (ed). Current Therapy in Nephrology and Hypertension. 3rd ed. St. Louis: Mosby–Yearbook, Inc., 1992, pp 58–63.
82. Nocturnal Oxygen Therapy Trial Group. Continuous or nocturnal oxygen therapy in hypoxemic chronic obstructive pulmonary disease. Ann Intern Med 1980; 93:391–398.
83. Parot S, Saunier C, Gautier H, et al. Breathing pattern and hypercapnia in patients with obstructive pulmonary disease. Am Rev Respir Dis 1980; 121:985–991.
84. Parot S, Miara B, Milic-Emili J, Gautier H. Hypoxemia, hypercapnia, and breathing pattern in patients with chronic obstructive pulmonary disease. Am Rev Respir Dis 1982; 126:882–888.
85. Park SS. Factors responsible for carbon dioxide retention in chronic obstructive lung disease. Am Rev Respir Dis 1964; 92:245–254.
86. Gelb AF, Klein E, Schiffman P, et al. Ventilatory response and drive in acute and chronic obstructive pulmonary disease. Am Rev Respir Dis 1977; 116:9–16.
87. Bradley CA, Fleetham JA, Anthonisen NR. Ventilatory control in patients with hypoxemia due to obstructive lung disease. Am Rev Respir Dis 1979; 120:21–30.
88. Sorli J, Grassino A, Lorange G, Milic-Emili J. Control of breathing in patients with chronic obstructive lung disease. Clin Sci Mol Med 1978; 54:295–304.
89. Mountain R, Zwillich C, Weil J. Hypoventilation in obstructive lung disease. N Engl J Med 1978; 298:521–525.
90. Fleetham JA, Arnup ME, Anthonisen NR. Familial aspects of ventilatory control in patients with chronic obstructive pulmonary disease. Am Rev Respir Dis 1984; 129:3–7.
91. Casaburi R, Patessio A, Ioli F, et al. Reductions in exercise lactic acidosis and ventilation as a result of exercise training in patients with obstructive lung disease. Am Rev Respir Dis 1991; 143:9–18.
92. Cullen JH, Brum VC, Reidt WU. The respiratory effects of progesterone in severe pulmonary emphysema. Am J Med 1959; 27:551–557.
93. Tyler JM. The effect of progesterone on the respiration of patients with emphysema and hypercapnia. J Clin Invest 1960; 39:34–41.
94. Skatrud JB, Dempsey JA, Kaiser DG. Ventilatory response to medroxyprogesterone acetate in normal subjects: Time course and mechanism. J Appl Physiol 1978; 44:939–944.
95. Dolly FR, Block AJ. Medroxyprogesterone acetate and COPD: Effect on breathing and oxygenation in sleeping and awake patients. Chest 1983; 84:395–398.
96. Skatrud JB, Dempsey JA. Relative effectiveness of acetazolamide versus medroxyprogesterone acetate in correction of chronic carbon dioxide retention. Am Rev Respir Dis 1983; 127:405–412.
97. Melot C, Naeije R, Rothschild T, et al. Improvement in ventilation-perfusion matching by almitrine in COPD. Chest 1983; 83:528–533.
98. Gothe B, Cherniack NS, Bachand RT, et al. Long-term effects of almitrine bismesylate on oxygenation during wakefulness and sleep in chronic obstructive pulmonary disease. Am J Med 1988; 84:436–444.
99. Watanabe S, Kanner RE, Cutillo AG, et al. Long-term effect of almitrine bismesylate in patients with hypoxic chronic obstructive pulmonary disease. Am Rev Respir Dis 1989; 140:1269–1273.
100. Altose MD, Hudgel DW. The pharmacology of respiratory depressants and stimulants. Clin Chest Med 1986; 7:481–494.
101. Lugliani R, Whipp BJ, Wasserman K. Doxapram hydrochloride: A respiratory stimulant for patients with primary alveolar hypoventilation. Chest 1979; 76:414–419.
102. Haake RE, Saxon LA, Bander SJ, et al. Depressed central respiratory drive causing weaning failure: Its reversal with doxapram. Chest 1989; 95:695–697.
103. Eldridge FL, Millhorn DE, Waldrop TG, et al. Mechanism of respiratory effects of methylxanthines. Respir Physiol 1983; 53:239–261.
104. Murciano D, Aubier M, Lecocquic Y, et al. Effects of theophylline on diaphragmatic strength and fatigue in patients with chronic obstructive pulmonary disease. N Engl J Med 1984; 311:349–353.
105. Moxham J. Aminophylline and the respiratory muscles: An alternative view. Clin Chest Med 1988; 9:325–336.
106. Woodcock AA, Johnson MA, Geddes DM, Catecholamines and endogenous opiates at rest and exercise in athletes and patients with chronic airflow obstruction (abstract). Am Rev Respir Dis 1983; 122:264.
107. Santiago TV, Remolina C, Scoles V III, Edelman NH. Endorphins and the control of breathing. N Engl J Med 1981; 304:1190–1195.
108. Tabona MVZ, Ambrosino N, Barnes PJ. Endogenous opiates and the control of breathing in normal subjects and patients with chronic airflow obstruction. Thorax 1982; 38:834–839.
109. Tobin MJ, Jenouri G, Sackner MA. Effect of naloxone on breathing pattern in patients with chronic obstructive pulmonary disease with and without hypercapnia. Respiration 1983; 44:419–424.
110. Santiago TV, Sheft SA, Khan AU, Edelman NH. Effect of naloxone on the respiratory responses to hypoxia in chronic obstructive pulmonary disease. Am Rev Respir Dis 1984; 130:183–186.
111. Mitchell-Heggs P, Murphy K, Minty K, et al. Diazepam in the treatment of dyspnoea in the 'pink puffer' syndrome. QJ Med 1980; 41:9–20.
112. Woodcock AA, Gross ER, Geddes DM. Drug treatment of

113. Stark RD, Morton PB, Sharman P, et al. Effects of codeine on the respiratory responses to exercise in healthy subjects. Br J Clin Pharmacol 1983; 15:355–359.
114. Woodcock AA, Gross ER, Gellert A, et al. Effects of dihydrocodeine, alcohol and caffeine on breathlessness and exercise tolerance in patients with chronic obstructive lung disease and normal blood gases. N Eng J Med 1981; 305:1611–1616.
115. O'Neill PA, Morton PB, Stark RD. Chlorpromazine: A specific effect on breathlessness? Br J Clin Pharmacol 1985; 19:793–797.
116. Stark RD. Dyspnoea: Assessment and pharmacological manipulation. Eur Respir J 1988; 1:280–287.
117. O'Neill PA, Stretton TB, Stark RD, Ellis SH. The effect of indomethacin on breathlessness in patients with diffuse parenchymal disease of the lung. Br J Dis Chest 1986; 80:72–79.
118. Howard P, Cayton RM, Brennan SR, Anderson PR. Lignocaine aerosol and persistent cough. Br J Dis Chest 1977; 71:19–24.
119. Vyas MN, Banister EW, Morton JW, Grzybowski S. Response to exercise in patients with chronic airway obstruction. II. Effects of breathing 40 per cent oxygen. Am Rev Respir Dis 1971; 103:401–412.
120. Stein DA, Bradley BL, Miller WC. Mechanisms of oxygen effects on exercise in patients with chronic obstructive pulmonary disease. Chest 1982; 81:6–10.
121. Raimondi AC, Edwards RHT, Denison RM, et al. Exercise tolerance breathing a low-density gas mixture, 35% oxygen and air in patients with chronic obstructive bronchitis. Clin Sci 1970; 39:675–685.
122. Winter B. Bilateral carotid body resection for asthma and emphysema. Int Surg 1972; 57:445, 458–66.
123. Davidson JT, Whipp BJ, Wasserman K, et al. Role of the carotid bodies in breath-holding. N Engl J Med 1974; 290:819–822.
124. Wasserman K, Whipp BJ, Koyal SN, Cleary MG. Effect of carotid body resection on ventilatory and acid-base control during exercise. J Appl Physiol 1975; 39:354–358.
125. Lugliani R, Whipp BJ, Seard C, Wasserman K. Effects of bilateral carotid body resection on ventilatory control at rest and during exercise in man. N Engl J Med 1971; 285:1105–1105.
126. Stulbarg MS, Winn WR. Bilateral carotid body resection for the relief of dyspnea in severe chronic obstructive pulmonary disease: Physiologic and clinical observations in three patients. Chest 1989; 95:1123–1128.
127. Fenn WO, Craig AB. Effect of CO_2 on respiration using a new method of administering CO_2. J Appl Physiol 1963; 18:1023–1024.
128. Wasserman K, Hansen JE, Sue DY, Whipp BJ. Principles of Exercise Testing and Interpretation. Philadelphia: Lea & Febiger, 1987.

Chapter 6

Cardiovascular Consequences of Chronic Obstructive Pulmonary Disease

DOUGLASS A. MORRISON, M.D., F.A.C.C.
BRAM D. ZUCKERMAN, M.D.

Oxygen delivery is the life-sustaining function of the integrated cardiopulmonary and vascular systems. Both the heart and lungs require pulsatile perfusion of oxygenated blood to maintain their own functional integrity. For these and other reasons, the interactions of the heart and lungs are diverse. Nonetheless, and despite the advances in both cardiovascular medicine and pulmonary medicine, the dynamic interactions of the heart and lungs remain largely mysterious. With the advent of the separation of cardiology and pulmonary disease medicine (in contrast to the Belleview Chest Service of Andre Cournard, M.D., and Dickinson Richards, M.D.), chronic obstructive pulmonary disease (COPD) has been classified as a "pulmonary disease." The central theses of this chapter are as follows: (1) Like nearly every advanced cardiac or pulmonary entity, COPD does much of its "dirty work" by virtue of its effects on oxygen delivery; (2) oxygen delivery is a *cardiopulmonary* problem; (3) there are two sides and four chambers in the human heart; (4) cardiac function is impaired in COPD, but most of the direct impairment and the impairment that is of the greatest clinical significance accrues on the *right* side of the heart. Right ventricular and right atrial function have remained largely mysterious; and (5) much of the exercise intolerance and ultimate multisystem failure leading to death in the advanced COPD patient derive from the right cardiac consequences of his or her "pulmonary problem."

IS THERE A CARDIAC DYSFUNCTION IN CHRONIC OBSTRUCTIVE PULMONARY DISEASE?

Pathologic Evidence to Support a Cardiac Dysfunction in Chronic Obstructive Pulmonary Disease

Kountz, Alexander, and Prinzmetal reported on 17 autopsy cases of COPD in 1936.[1] They reported that 10 of the 17 cases had both right and left ventricular thickening (hypertrophy) and right ventricular dilatation. Scott and Garvin subsequently reported on 50 autopsy cases with emphysema and right ventricular hypertrophy.[2] These authors confirmed the association with left ventricular hypertrophy and also had clinical data on most of their patients that supported clinically significant failure of the right side of the heart.[2] The series of 52 cases of cor pulmonale reported by Zimmerman and Ryan also supported the clinically significant association of failure of the right side of the heart and left ventricular hypertrophy.[3] Michelson reported on 32 patients with chronic pulmonary disease, all of whom had biventricular hypertrophy at autopsy.[4] This study also included electrocardiographic data obtained ante mortem from most of the patients; right axis deviation, cor pulmonale, and regular sinus rhythm pattern were all noted frequently. Fluck and coworkers reported that 25% of 84 chronic bronchitic patients at autopsy had left ventricular hypertrophy greater than 17 mm.[5] More recently, Murphy and associates reported that 20 of 72 patients (28%) with chronic bronchitis and emphysema had post mortem left ventricular hypertrophy[6]; however, their data suggested that most of these patients had associated conditions, such as systemic hypertension or aortic stenosis, that might account for the left ventricular hypertrophy.

Taken together, these pathologic studies support the concept that right ventricular hypertrophy and dilatation frequently accompany chronic bronchitis and emphysema. Alternatively, left ventricular hypertrophy appears to be less common and often attributable to associated conditions.

Hemodynamic Evidence to Support Right Ventricular Dysfunction Secondary to Chronic Obstructive Pulmonary Disease

In 1946, Bloomfield and colleagues reported the right atrial and right ventricular pressures of 70 subjects (17 normal subjects and 53 patients with a variety of cardiopulmonary conditions).[7] They reported that right ventricular systolic and pulse pressures were elevated in most but not all patients with advanced pulmonary emphysema. Hickam and Cargill reported catheterization data from the right side of the heart during rest and exercise in a group of normal subjects and patients with emphysema and various cardiac pathologies.[8] They reported that the emphysema patients had pulmonary hypertension at rest and further elevations in blood pressure during mild supine exercise. Dexter and coworkers also provided reference pressures and flows against which those of COPD patients could be compared.[9] Harvey and coworkers[10] reported hemodynamic data on 48 patients with chronic pulmonary disease. Yu and associates reported data during resting from 18 patients with pulmonary emphysema.[11] They showed that pulmonary hypertension appeared to be related to the extent of anatomic emphysema, the severity of hypoxemia, and the severity of hypercapnia. Furthermore, they demonstrated that the pulmonary hypertension was "active" or "arteriolar," that is, the pulmonary wedge pressure was usually normal, and the pulmonary artery diastolic wedge pressure gradient was abnormally widened.

Williams and Behnke reported rest and supine exercise data from 53 patients with emphysema[12]; this series included 33 patients who had not had right ventricular failure and 20 patients who had been observed in failure but were clinically compensated at the time of study. This study suggested that resting cardiac output was normal or low and, especially in patients with a history of right ventricular failure, that the exercise increase in cardiac output was low relative to the exercise oxygen consumption seen in normal subjects.[12] Segal and Bishop looked specifically at the influence of blood viscosity and blood volume on pulmonary hypertension during rest and supine exercise in a group of 21 patients with chronic bronchitis and secondary polycythemia.[13] Although the resting cardiac outputs of most of these patients were considered normal, the majority of the patients had abnormally high pulmonary pressures and abnormally low cardiac output at exercise. It is interesting that venesection led to improvement in exercise hemodynamics in several of these patients, and the infusion of albumin, which led to an acute increase in blood volume, was accompanied by an increased cardiac output without an increase in pulmonary vascular resistance.[13]

Harris and coworkers examined the relationships between pressure and flow at rest and exercise in a group of normal subjects and patients with chronic bronchitis and mitral stenosis.[14] In contrast to the other two groups, bronchitics showed a curved relation between pressure and flow. Similarly, bronchitics had an inappropriately large increase in pulmonary pressure relative to flow during exercise.[14] Abraham and associates examined the effects of hypoxia and plasma volume expansion and noted that both mechanisms led to increased pulmonary artery pressures.[15]

Herles and colleagues noted elevations of pulmonary wedge pressure greater than 12 mm Hg in 20 of 121 patients with uncomplicated chronic bronchitis.[16] They inferred a postarteriolar component in the pulmonary hypertension noted in these patients. In a provocative study, Lockhart and coworkers examined this issue further.[17] They were unable to identify a simple relation among pulmonary functions, arterial blood gases, and the pulmonary wedge pressures of 87 patients with chronic bronchitis. Similarly, they measured esophageal pressures and concluded that high wedge pressures were not a simple function of increased intrathoracic pressures. This conclusion was also reached by Albert and associates based on a study of upright exercise in eight patients with COPD.[18]

Field and Cotes examined eight patients with bronchitis secondary to pneumonoconiosis.[19] They found that patients with chronic cough had an abnormal increase in pulmonary artery pressure when they exercised. They also found that this "load on the right ventricle" could be ameliorated by supplemental oxygen breathing. Lockhart and coworkers compared the hemodynamic effects of leg exercise and voluntary hyperventilation in a group of 12 patients with emphysema, bronchitis, or both.[20] They concluded that part of the elevation in pulmonary artery pressure and wedge pressure at exercise derived from intrathoracic pressure swings secondary to hyperventilation.

Weitzenblum and associates studied the hemodynamics of the right side of the heart during rest and exercise in 92 patients with stable chronic bronchitis.[21] They identified several subsets based upon the severity of pulmonary hypertension at rest and exercise but suggested that the cardiac output was nearly normal. Jezek and colleagues examined rest and exercise hemodynamics in 50 patients with COPD.[22] They also demonstrated that cardiac output versus oxygen consumption at exercise increased proportionally to the values that other researchers had obtained in older "normals." However, when right ventricular function was examined in terms of stroke volume versus right ventricular end-diastolic pressure, a significant abnormality was frequently found (19–40%). Romero-Colomer and Schrijen also concluded that exercise cardiac output increased normally in a group of 22 patients with COPD.[23]

Although primarily interested in repeat exercise tests (so as to also assess the reproducibility of measurements), Schrijen and Jezek obtained further rest and exercise hemodynamic data in 28 COPD patients.[24] They also documented nearly normal cardiac output responses; however, the data were not normal when compared with simultaneous right ventricular end-diastolic pressure.[24] Light and coworkers also compared the exercise oxygen consumption and cardiac output data obtained in their study of a group of 26 COPD patients with those of the normal subjects reported on by Granath and associates.[25, 26] They also concluded that exercise cardiac outputs were in the "normal range."[25]

Stewart and Lewis, however, reported low exercise outputs in 8 of the 20 COPD patients whom they studied.[27] Minh and associates and Mohsenifar and colleagues also concluded that cardiac output increase was a limiting factor in the exercise capacity of COPD patients.[28, 29] A critical point to remember in comparing the exercise cardiac output and oxygen consumption data of COPD patients with those of normal subjects is that normal subjects have normal arterial oxygen saturation, whereas most COPD patients are hypoxemic.[30] Accordingly, COPD patients might be expected to need higher cardiac outputs in order to maintain oxygen delivery.[30] In three separate studies of COPD patients, Morrison and coworkers demonstrated significant relationships between the function of the right side of the heart and rest or exercise cardiac output, and/or oxygen delivery.[31, 33] These data supported the concepts that part of these patients' exercise limitation is heart-related, and that the cardiac problem is associated primarily with the right ventricle.

A benchmark study by Burrows and associates supported an inverse relationship between the prognosis for 50 patients with COPD and their pulmonary vascular resistance.[34] Two studies by Weitzenblum and colleagues have supported the prognostic significance of the hemodynamics of the right side of the heart.[35, 36]

Together, the hemodynamic studies discussed support that (1) pulmonary hypertension is common in COPD, (2) pulmonary hypertension in COPD is probably caused by a series of factors that includes emphysema, hypoxemia, acidosis, passive elevation from left ventricular causes, and the effects of intrathoracic pressure variations, (3) whether exercise cardiac output is "normal" in most COPD patients is a moot point, (4) hypoxemia may mean cardiac output should be higher than "normal," and, finally, (5) right ventricular function, assessed in terms of either stroke volume to right ventricular end-diastolic pressure relations or right ventricular ejection fraction, is often abnormal in COPD. That is, there is a right ventricular dysfunction of COPD related in part to pulmonary hypertension, and this right ventricular dysfunction appears to be important in the exercise limitation and survival of these patients.[30]

Hemodynamic Evidence to Support a Clinically Relevant Left Ventricular Dysfunction in Chronic Obstructive Pulmonary Disease

Williams and coworkers tested left ventricular functional reserve by infusing methoxamine in 16 COPD patients.[37] Their results failed to support a significant left ventricular dysfunction. Rao and associates reported that four of eight patients with cor pulmonale showed evidence, including elevated pulmonary wedge pressure, to suggest left ventricular dysfunction.[38] All of the evidence cited, however, was nonspecific and would simply reflect generalized fluid retention from failure of the right side of the heart. In the previously cited study by Burrows and associates, only 1 of 50 patients appeared to have significant left ventricular dysfunction.[34] Similarly, Davies and Overy observed an elevation in left ventricular end-diastolic pressure in 12 patients with COPD.[39] In contrast, Baum and coworkers described abnormal left ventricular end-diastolic pressure, left ventricular function curves, or both, in 14 of 15 COPD patients.[40] In commenting on this and other studies, Fishman surmised that left ventricular hypertrophy and some degree of dysfunction might be attributable to severe blood gas abnormalities and polycythemia.[41] Kelly and colleagues used a dog model study to demonstrate that right ventricular pressure and volume loading were accompanied by some measurable left ventricular dysfunction.[42]

Khaja and Parker examined 20 patients with COPD.[43] They documented that right ventricular end-diastolic pressure increased abnormally with exercise, whereas left ventricular end-diastolic pressure remained normal.[43] Frank and associates performed extensive angiographic and metabolic studies on 11 patients with COPD; they concluded that left ventricular function was normal unless a second disease process was present.[44]

Steele and coworkers measured the left ventricular ejection fraction in 120 patients with COPD.[45] They observed no relationship between left ventricular ejection fraction and arterial blood gases and found evidence for concomitant coronary artery disease in most patients in whom the left ventricular ejection fraction was abnormal.[45] Unger and associates looked at 28 patients with COPD who were acutely dyspneic.[46] Although they found that it is was not possible clinically to predict the pulmonary wedge pressure in these patients and that some patients had an arbitrarily elevated pulmonary wedge pressure (greater than 12 mm Hg), most of their other data did not support a major left ventricular dysfunction attributable to uncomplicated COPD.[46] In commenting on Unger's study, Bahler reiterated that the wedge pressure (or left ventricular end-diastolic pressure) is influenced by intrathoracic pressure and that most studies had found normal ejection fractions in COPD patients unless these patients had concomitant left ventricular pathology.[47]

Matthay and colleagues, like Williams and associates, used provocative testing (dextran loading) to assess left ventricular function in a group of 26 patients with COPD.[48] Their data supported the concept that left ventricular function is normal in uncomplicated COPD.[48] Similarly, Kline and coworkers used both radionuclide and echocardiographic techniques in addition to direct hemodynamic measurements to study 27 COPD patients.[49] They also concluded that left ventricular function is usually normal in uncomplicated COPD.[49] Boushy and North performed catheterization of the right side of the heart in 136 COPD patients.[50] They found that the severity of emphysema did not correspond to the severity of hemodynamic abnormality. Both the Boushy and North study and a study by Schrijen and associates documented little change in hemodynamics over time.[50, 51]

Krayenbuehl and colleagues conducted an elegant angiographic study of 10 patients with severe pulmonary hypertension and compared the results with those of a normal control group at rest and during hand grip exercise.[52] They observed normal resting function but also an abnormal exercise response that appeared to involve a ventricular shape change related to ventricular interdependence. It should be noted that most of these patients had levels of pulmonary hypertension usually seen in primary pulmonary hypertension but not in COPD.

Kachel summarized much of this literature and concluded that when other causes of left ventricular dysfunction (such as systemic hypertension or coronary artery disease) had been excluded, few COPD patients had clinically significant left ventricular dysfunction.[53]

Christianson and coworkers also used cineangiography in the evaluation of 19 patients with COPD.[54] These investigators also found normal left ventricular systolic function in the absence of concomitant coronary artery disease. Gabinski examined the left ventricular hemodynamics and angiograms of 18 COPD patients.[55] He did find some subtle abnormalities of function.[55] Coronary angiography was not performed in these patients.

In summary, (1) subtle abnormalities of left ventricular function have been reported, usually in a minority of COPD patients. (2) The more carefully concomitant coronary artery disease, hypertensive disease, or valvular heart disease is excluded, the more infrequent and subtle the left ventricular dysfunction. (3) The most frequently reported abnormality is an elevation of filling pressures; this is clearly nonspecific and is influenced by ventricular compliance, ventricular interaction, and fluid status as well as by ventricular systolic function and intrathoracic pressure variations. (4) There are few data to support the contention that left ventricular dysfunction of COPD contributes in any clinically significant way to dyspnea in COPD patients.

CARDIAC FUNCTION AND THE TREATMENT OF CHRONIC OBSTRUCTIVE PULMONARY DISEASE

Hypoxia and Hypoxemia, and Their Effects on Cardiac Function

In honoring Dickinson W. Richards, Nobel laureate and pioneer in both circulatory and respiratory physiology, Heistad and Aboud summarized much of the systemic effects of hypoxia.[56] As they found in comparing the hemodynamics of the right and left sides of the heart in COPD, the primary action of hypoxemia appears to be in the pulmonary circuit.[57-59]

Von Euler and Liljestrand first described the effects of hypoxia on the pulmonary circulation in the cat.[57, 58] Motley and associates described the human development of pulmonary hypertension in response to short-term breathing of low oxygen mixtures.[59] Conversely, Kitchin and colleagues demonstrated in 20 COPD patients that pulmonary hypertension, particularly during exercise, could be ameliorated with supplemental oxygen breathing.[60] Levine and coworkers studied six patients with hypoxemia who were administered continuous oxygen for over 1 month.[61] Oxygen therapy was associated with improved clinical status, increased exercise tolerance, and declines in erythrocytosis and pulmonary resistance.

Cotes compared 16 patients with COPD with 10 healthy controls.[62] They documented reductions in pulmonary pressure and cardiac output in response to acute oxygen therapy. Abraham and associates studied six patients who were given oxygen over a 1- to 2-month period.[63] They documented that pulmonary pressure could be further reduced by chronically administering oxygen.[63] Horsfield and colleagues examined 17 COPD patients at rest and during exercise.[64] Abraham and associates followed eight patients serially after they recovered from acute respiratory failure.[65] The decrease in pulmonary pressure observed during recovery provided further support that hypoxic pulmonary vasoconstriction was a mechanism of pulmonary hypertension in these patients.

Neff and Petty reported on 33 patients with chronic airway obstruction who received from 7 to 41 months of continuous oxygen and who were believed to demonstrate a mortality benefit.[66] Ude and Howard studied acute oxygen use in 166 exacerbations of COPD among 40 patients and emphasized the need for controlled doses.[67] A study by Stark and coworkers further clarified dose response by showing that either 15 hours per day or 18 hours per day were associated with reductions in pulmonary resistance.[68] A subsequent study of five patients by Stark and coworkers showed associated reductions in pulmonary artery pressures and resistances as well as improved functional capacity.[69]

These observational studies set the stage for larger prospective randomized trials. The Nocturnal Oxygen Therapy Trial reported on 203 hypoxemic patients with chronic airflow obstruction randomly allocated to intermittent (12 h/day) or continuous (24 h/day) oxygen therapy.[70] Regardless of the level of pulmonary hypertension or the degree of exercise impairment, continuous oxygen therapy appeared to confer a survival benefit relative to the 12-hour therapy. The Medical Research Council Working Party randomly administered patients oxygen for at least 15 hours and compared them with patients who received no oxygen therapy.[71] This group demonstrated a mortality benefit as well. In a subsequent report from the Nocturnal Oxygen Therapy Trial group, Timms and associates demonstrated that the group receiving continuous oxygen also had improved pulmonary hemodynamics and cardiac function as shown by the right ventricular stroke work index.[72] The correlative data from this study suggested that most of the effect on right ventricular function accrued from a reduction in right ventricular afterload, but relief of myocardial ischemia was considered an alternative possibility. Flenley and Muir compared the patient selection for these two landmark trials and made at least two critical observations: (1) the relief of pulmonary hypertension seen in both was far more modest than was originally expected; and (2) although both of these trials limited their scope to patients with advanced COPD, in clinical practice many other patient groups might reasonably benefit from continuous oxygen therapy.[73]

The mechanisms by which oxygen confers clinical benefit have not been fully elucidated. MacNee and coworkers concluded from a hemodynamic and radionuclide angiographic study of COPD patients that right ventricular function was not improved by chronic oxygen therapy.[74] Two problems can be identified in their study: (1) the ejection fraction reflects loading conditions as well as contractile function, and (2) the calculation of end-diastolic and end-systolic volumes from a radionuclide ejection fraction and thermodilution stroke volume *assumes* no tricuspid regurgitation, a phenomenon almost certainly *not* encountered in pulmonary hypertensive patients during exercise.[74] In a subsequent review, Flenley and Muir cited much of the evidence for right ventricular hypertrophy, dilatation, and systolic dysfunction in pulmonary hypertensive COPD patients, especially in the subset of COPD patients with cor pulmonale.[75] They also reviewed the difficulties in showing cause and effect and, specifically, in separating afterload from contractility effects. They concluded that a combination of oxygen and other drugs might ultimately be synergistic in improving cardiac function in these patients.[75] In another state-of-the-art review, Fulmer and Snider reported the consensus views of the 1984 American College of Chest Physicians–National Heart, Lung, and Blood Institute National Conference on Oxygen Therapy.[76] This conference concluded that although the British Medical Research Council Study and the Nocturnal Oxygen Therapy Trial had been limited to COPD, careful evaluation could lead to the rational prescription of continuous oxygen therapy for stable hypoxemic patients with a number of other conditions. The conference also stated clearly that, "The reasons for either improved exercise capacity or endurance are unclear at this time." Similarly, Petty described the difficulties in "real-world" oxygen therapy prescription and appropriately emphasized the need for objective assessment of benefit after oxygen has been prescribed.[77]

A number of other observational studies have continued to address the issue of how chronic oxygen therapy leads to improved exercise capacity in stable hypoxemic pulmonary patients. Bradley and colleagues noted that the treadmill durations of 26 patients with COPD were better when they breathed supplemental oxygen as opposed to when they breathed compressed air, but they found no mechanistic explanation for these results when they studied the patients' blood gases.[78] Raffestin and coworkers had 20 COPD patients exercise on an ergometer while they monitored them using a catheter inserted in the right side of the heart.[79] As in the study of Minh and associates,[29] Raffestin and coworkers observed low mixed venous oxygen tensions during exercise (less than 30 mm Hg). Nevertheless, they separated their subjects into groups containing those with low and those with extremely low mixed venous tensions and concluded that an "unused oxygen reserve is still present at exhaustion in some patients." Given the inaccuracy implicit in using a simple number to reflect the adequacy of oxygen delivery to multiple organ systems, this conclusion is controversial.[30, 31] The conclusion that oxygen improved ventilatory mechanics and that this in turn contributed to improved exercise capacity is not supported by the data of Raffestin and coworkers. This conclusion was substantiated based on data on nine patients studied by Stein and associates.[80]

Although not an exercise study, we believe that the data reported by Degaute and colleagues on COPD patients in exacerbation is germane at this point.[81] Specifically, they demonstrated little response of pulmonary pressure to acute oxygen, but more important, the patients who showed their oxygen delivery to be improved by using supplemental oxygen were able to do so by having a higher cardiac output. These data are relevant to the chronic situation, where increased PaO_2 might be counterbalanced by a *decline* in hemoglobin, thus leaving arterial oxygen content unchanged.[31] MacNee and coworkers, although still finding the ejection fraction to be an incomplete means of assessing function, concluded from a study of 35 COPD patients and 30 normal subjects that right ventricular function, particularly during exercise, was improved by long-term oxygen administration.[82] Examining exercising COPD patients from the perspective of ventilatory rather than circulatory limitation, Light and colleagues could not find changes in ventilatory drive in patients who had responded to chronic oxygen administration with increased exercise capacity.[83]

In a study of acute oxygen administration (20 min), Morrison and associates demonstrated an improvement in right ventricular ejection fraction in patients who also had a decline in total pulmonary resistance.[84] In response to chronic oxygen administration, the same group found that improved right ventricular ejection fraction correlated with improved oxygen delivery.[31] More recently, a

4-year prospective exercise study has documented improved exercise capacity in association with the improved function of the right side of the heart expressed as exercise stroke volume to right ventricular end-diastolic pressure.[85] Like the earlier studies of the Edinburgh group, Morrison and associates did not observe improved right ventricular ejection fraction during exercise in the group with improved exercise capacity.

Further insights into both the mechanisms of the beneficial clincial effects of continuous oxygen therapy and of heart-lung interaction in COPD are derived from observations made during patient sleep. Catteral and colleagues documented that transient falls in oxygen saturation occurred commonly among COPD patients.[86] Both Fletcher and coworkers and Boysen and associates documented that nocturnal oxygen desaturation was associated with pulmonary hemodynamic abnormalities.[87, 88] This had in fact been the logic behind Stark's earlier studies of 12-hour versus 15-hour oxygen administration and the Nocturnal Oxygen Therapy Trial comparison of 12-hour versus 24-hour continuous oxygen therapy.[68, 70] Krieger and colleagues extended these observations by using multivariate analyses to show that both the daytime level of pulmonary function and nocturnal oxygen desaturation contributed to the development of pulmonary hypertension in COPD patients.[89] Fletcher and coworkers applied these results to their study and showed that supplemental oxygen could relieve both transient desaturation and transient elevations in pulmonary pressures and could lead to an increased cardiac output.[90]

Several other important studies of oxygen transport and of the effects of oxygen therapy in COPD are relevant to the more general question of cardiac function in this disease. As early as 1968, Filley and associates distinguished between COPD patients with or without normal cardiac output and oxygen transport.[91] Kawakami and colleagues observed that resting oxygen delivery as inferred from the mixed venous oxygen tension was predictive of survival, whereas pulmonary pressures and resistances were not.[93] Tenney and Mithoefer performed elegant mathematic analyses of oxygen delivery and subsequently applied them to patient studies.[94, 95] They believed mixed venous oxygen tension reflected the adequacy of whole-body oxygenation based on their analyses.

In summary, studies of oxygen therapy in COPD patients support that (1) hypoxemia is associated with pulmonary hypertension, impaired exercise capacity, and reduced survival; (2) oxygen therapy is associated with the relief of hypoxemia and pulmonary hypertension, improved exercise capacity, and enhanced survival; (3) pulmonary hypertension is not the whole explanation with regard to either exercise capacity or survival; (4) oxygen delivery to tissues and, specifically, the component of cardiac output appear to be quite important in both exercise limitation and survival; and finally (5) improved cardiac output appears to be related to improved right ventricular function in terms of stroke volume to end-diastolic pressure but not in terms of ejection fraction; this discrepancy likely accrues from changes in the amount of tricuspid regurgitation.[96]

Right ventricular function, which is linked to the abnormal pulmonary circuit, is likely of critical importance for oxygen delivery in the failing COPD patient during exercise or at rest. Accordingly, it is clinically relevant to both exercise capacity and survival. Left ventricular function is far less likely to be involved (other than by series and parallel links) unless there is additional disease (e.g., systemic hypertension, coronary artery disease).

PULMONARY VASCULAR IMPEDANCE AND HYPOXEMIA

In the preceding review of the clinical literature it has been frequently assumed that measurement of pulmonary vascular resistance can adequately describe right ventricular afterload. Variables such as compliance, elasticity, wave velocity, and wave reflections that are essential for describing the oscillatory component of the pulmonary pressure-flow relationship have not been available.[97] The oscillatory component may be important in determining how the normal right ventricle is coupled to the lung vasculature.[97-100] Increases in pulmonary artery stiffness or wave reflections, for example, can increase right ventricular systolic wall stress and thus diminish the stroke volume and power output of the right ventricle.[97-100] Changes in the pulsatile component of the pulmonary circulation may also affect the magnitude and manner in which oscillatory energy is dissipated in the lung vasculature. Because 30% of the total power expended by the right ventricle may be oscillatory, an increased focal dissipation of oscillatory energy in the precapillary area that is produced, for example, by an increase in proximal pulmonary artery stiffness may be an important stimulus for the structural, biochemical, and humoral responses noted in hypoxic pulmonary hypertension.[101] Main pulmonary artery impedance describes the summated effects of arterial wave reflections and elasticity in addition to pulmonary vascular resistance.[97] In other words, pulmonary vascular impedance may more fully describe right ventricular afterload than pulmonary vascular resistance. An appreciation of the physiologic significance of this approach can be obtained by reference to a simple physical model of pulmonary circulation.[97, 102]

In our model of pulmonary circulation, the pulmonary arterial tree is represented by a long elastic tube that is occluded at its end (Fig. 6–1, *left side, curve A*). Injection of a flow pulse at the origin of the tube produces a pressure wave that travels down the tube with a velocity that is proportional to the tube's stiffness. The pressure wave diminishes in amplitude owing to the viscous (frictional) dissipation of energy as it travels. When the incident wave reaches the end of the tube, it is completely reflected and travels back toward the origin. Figure 6–1 shows pressure waves generated at the origin of the tube when the reflecting site is moved closer to the tube's origin *(left side, curves B and D)*. With a more proximal reflecting site, the reflected wave merges

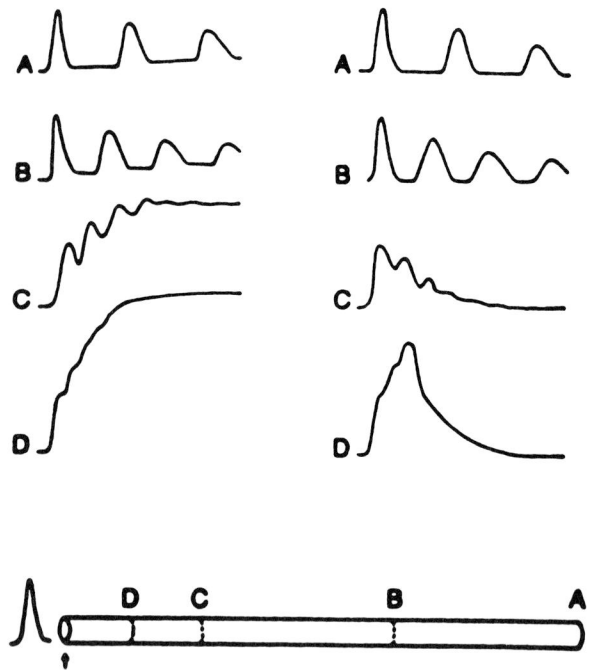

FIGURE 6-1. Curves A through D represent pressure waves measured at the origin of a distensible tube after a single injection of fluid (arrow) and when this tube was occluded closer and closer to the origin. The first wave results from injection, and the other waves occur as a result of wave reflections. Tracings on the *left side* result from complete occlusions; those on the *right side* result from incomplete occlusion. (Reprinted from O'Rourke MF, Yaginoma T. Wave reflections and the arterial pulse. Arch Intern Med 1984; 144:368. Copyright 1984, American Medical Association.)

with the incident wave, producing a "measured" pulmonary arterial pressure.

The site of major reflections in the pulmonary circulation is at the pulmonary arteriolar level.[97, 102, 103] A steady blood flow leaves the arterial system through these arterioles. Allowance can be made for this "runoff" from the arteriole system by only partially occluding the tube at points A through D (see Fig. 6-1, *right side*). Also, the pulmonary arterial tree consists of a "network of elastic tubes," with more peripheral arteries exhibiting increased stiffness.[97] The concept of forward and backward traveling pressure and of flow waves that summate to produce measured pressure and flow waves still applies, however.[97, 103–105] Finally, in our simple representation of pulmonary circulation we have modeled the heart as a pure "flow generator." Regardless of the timing of the returning reflected pressure pulses, the heart is able to produce the same flow input or stroke volume. In reality, however, returning reflected pressure waves that arrive during systole increase right ventricular wall stress and thus change the flow and power output of the right ventricle.[97–100]

Figure 6-2 illustrates representative micromanometric pressure and flow waveforms that were recorded in the main pulmonary artery of an open-chest calf during progressive hypoxia induced by inhalation of a 10% oxygen mixture. A steady rise in pressure and pulmonary vascular resistance occurred, so that at the time of the hypoxia #2, measurements of mean pulmonary artery pressure had almost doubled, pulmonary vascular resistance was tripled, and P_{O_2} had fallen from 375 mm Hg to 35 mm Hg. A No. 7F micromanometer with two pressure sensors 5 cm apart (SPC-770, Millar Instruments, Inc., Houston, TX) was used to measure pressure so that both proximal and distal pulmonary arterial pressures were obtained simultaneously. The transit time delay between the two pressure signals is a consequence of the fact that the pressure wave travels down the main pulmonary artery with a finite wave velocity.[97, 102]

In the control state, the pressure and flow waveforms are quite similar in shape during systole. Both pressure and flow demonstrate a rather flat and rounded peak. With progressive hypoxia, the proximal and distal pressures exhibit a late systolic rise in pressure even though there is an absence of any such rise in the flow waveform. Instead, the flow waveform shows a late systolic decrease in flow.

The observed changes in the pressure and flow recordings are largely produced by changes in the presence, timing, and magnitude of peripheral wave reflections. Reference to the corresponding frequency domain impedance spectra (Fig. 6-3), which were calculated from Fourier transforms of five consecutive pressure and flow pulses at each of the three reference states, emphasizes this point. With progressive hypoxia, the low-frequency values of the impedance modulus plot (0–8 Hz) are higher in value, and a rightward shift of both the impedance modulus and phase plots occurs. Less apparent is a small increase in the mean value of the moduli in the 8 to 28 Hz frequency range, which indicates that main pulmonary artery characteristic impedance (a term that describes main pulmonary elasticity and geometry) is increased.[97] Together, these changes indicate a large increase in the stiffness of the pulmonary arterial circulation. The increased arterial elasticity is probably the result of increased recruitment of arterial collagen fibers with increased pulmonary pressures as well as to the increased activation of smooth muscle in the large pulmonary arteries.[97, 101, 103] During hypoxia in the mid- to high-frequency range (8–28 Hz), a greater degree of oscillation of the impedance moduli around their average value or characteristic impedance is also observed. This spectral alteration implies that the magnitude of wave reflections produced at the arteriolar level increases substantially with hypoxia-induced increases in pulmonary vascular resistance.[97, 103]

Once the characteristic impedance value of the main pulmonary artery is determined, the effects of alterations in the presence, timing, and magnitude of wave reflections may also be observed in the time domain by utilizing the standard equations of the "arterial transmission line" theory.[104, 105] The results of this process are shown in Figure 6-4. The measured proximal pressure and flow waves illustrated in Figure 6-2 are shown decomposed into their forward and backward components. The measured pressure wave (PM) is equal to the sum of forward (PF) and backward (PB) pressure waves. An analogous equality applies to the measured flow wave (QM). During the baseline state, the back-

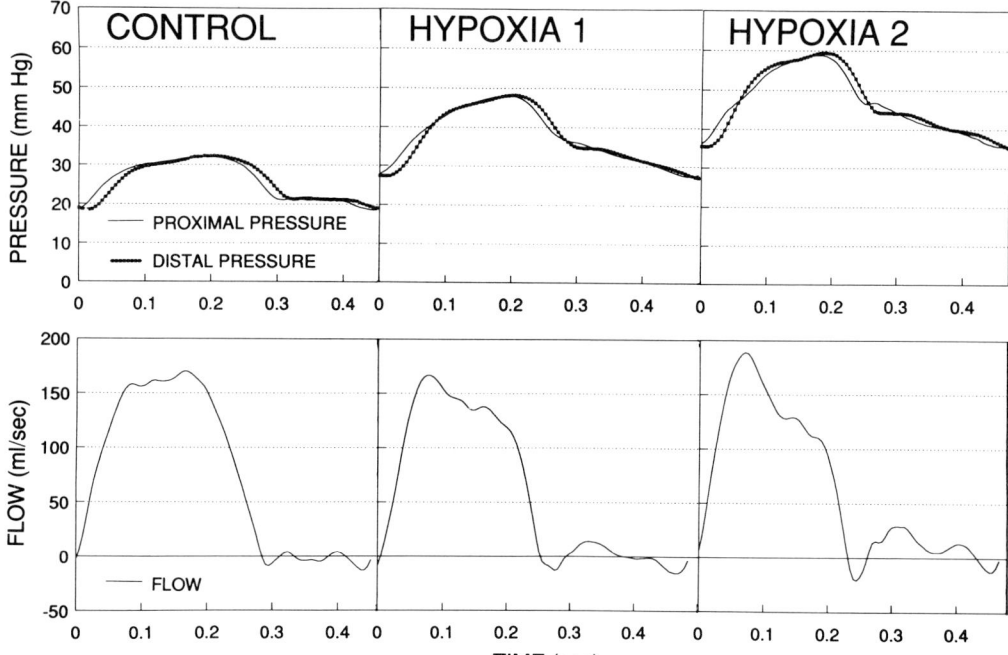

FIGURE 6–2. Typical pressure and flow tracings recorded under control, moderately hypoxic (HYPOXIA 1), and severely hypoxic (HYPOXIA 2) conditions.

ward pressure and flow waves demonstrate little oscillation, and the oscillation that does occur begins very late in systole. These observations imply that wave reflections are small, and they explain why the measured pressure wave is very similar in shape to the measured flow wave.[97, 104, 105] With increasing hypoxia, the backward pressure and flow waves appear earlier during the cardiac cycle and have a greater magnitude of oscillation. Thus, large increases in wave reflections and wave speed have occurred. These effects combine to produce a measured pressure wave that is augmented during systole and a measured flow wave that is reduced. In contrast to the simple tubular model shown in Figure 6–1, the hypoxia-induced increase in oscillatory afterload has combined with the increase in pulmonary vascular resistance to impair coupling between the right ventricle and pulmonary tree, and thus alter right ventricular performance.

Studies of the effects of oxygen on the oscillatory component of right ventricular afterload have also been studied in the dog and cat and have produced results similar to those shown for the calf.[103, 106, 107] Relatively little work has been performed on humans. The most important work on human subjects has been performed by Haneda and coworkers.[108] These investigators measured pulmonary impedance in a control group of human subjects and in patients with pulmonary venous hypertension, pulmonary arterial hypertension, and both pulmonary arterial hypertension and atrial septal defect. Impedance was determined both before and after the administration of oxygen. The two pulmonary arterial hypertension groups demonstrated significant shifts in

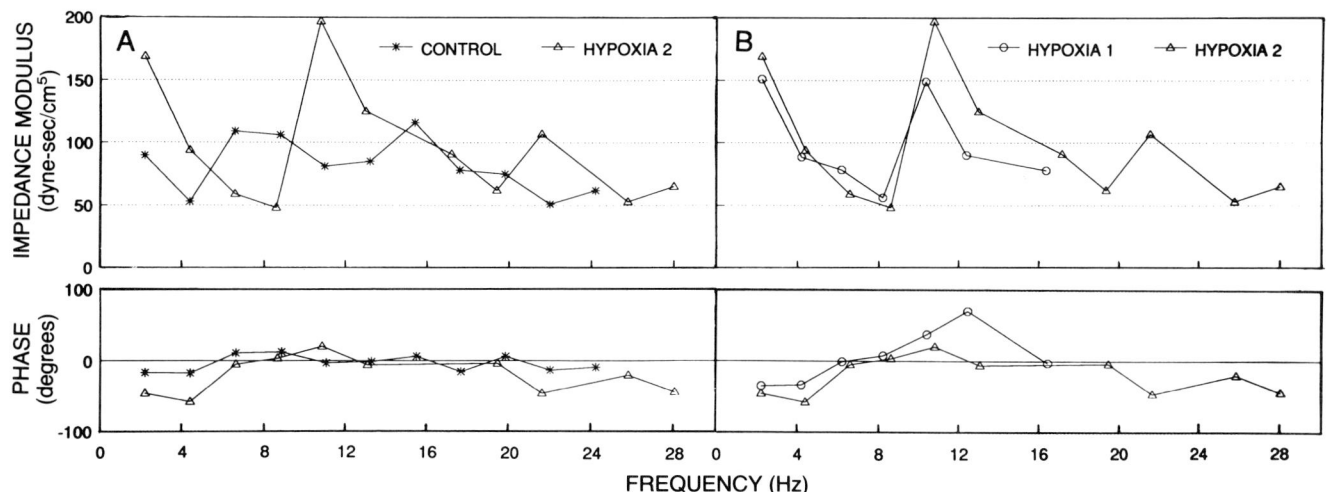

FIGURE 6–3. The corresponding impedance spectra for the data shown in Figure 6–2.

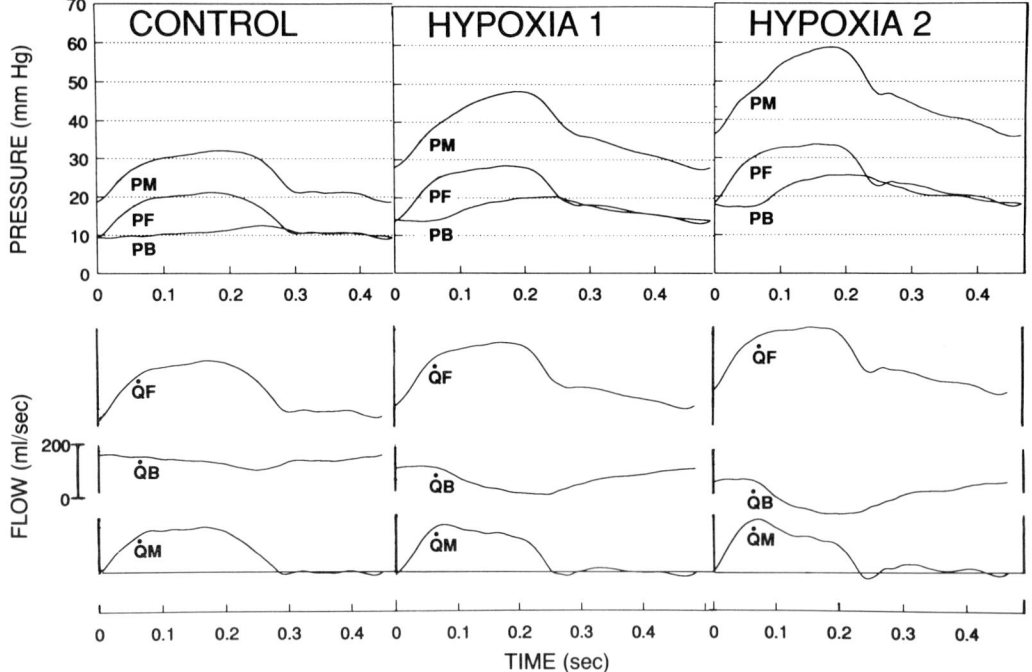

FIGURE 6–4. The measured proximal pressure and flow tracings (PM and Q̇M, respectively) are shown decomposed into forward and backward waves. The forward waves of pressure and flow (PE and Q̇F, respectively) have the same shape; the backward waves of pressure and flow waves (PB and Q̇B, respectively) also have the same shape, but the flow wave is inverted.

their impedance spectra during oxygen administration (Fig. 6–5). Because circulating norepinephrine levels decreased with the correction of hypoxemia in these groups, it was concluded that the decreased smooth muscle tone of large arteries as well as a drop in mean pressure were responsible for the impedance changes.

In both children and adults, other investigators have also shown increases in the hypertensive pulmonary impedance spectrum.[109–113] Studies by Yin and associates and Kussmaul and colleagues are of particular significance.[111, 112] Yin measured aortic and pulmonary input impedances simultaneously in a group of patients with pulmonary hypertension secondary to severe failure of the left side of the heart. Administration of the vasodilator nitroprusside appeared to have a greater effect on lowering pulmonary vascular impedance than systemic vascular impedance, suggesting that improvement of coupling between the right ventricle and pulmonary circulation is an important component of vasodilator action. Kussmaul determined pulmonary vascular impedance at rest and during exercise in a group of patients with ischemic heart disease and in a control group free of cardiac and pulmonary disease. Although no significant difference in impedance between the two groups at rest was found, and mean pulmonary pressure and characteristic impedance increased significantly only in the patients with ischemic heart disease when they exercised to their ischemic threshold. Interestingly, the increase in the oscillatory afterload component was not accompanied by any change in pulmonary vascular resistance. Further analysis of the exercise data, however, indicated that the oscillatory afterload change impaired the hydraulic efficiency of right ventricular and pulmonary artery coupling.

Additional human evidence for increased pulmonary impedance in pulmonary hypertension has probably been provided by noninvasive Doppler flow studies. Using a pulsed Doppler technique, several investigators have shown that with increased pulmonary pressures the flow wave changes from a round pattern to a more triangular one in a manner qualitatively similar to the transformation of the hypoxic calves' flow waveform shown in Figure 6–2.[114, 115] Additionally, the time to peak flow velocity has been negatively correlated with mean pulmonary artery pressure. These results suggest that altered timing and the intensity of reflected waves play an important role in the alteration of the human pulmonary hypertensive flow pulse. Further support for this argument, however, needs to be obtained by decomposing the human flow pulse into forward and backward components in a manner similar to that shown for the calf in Figure 6–4.

In conclusion, pulmonary vascular impedance can change markedly in pulmonary hypertension. More detailed work in this area should provide a clearer insight into how lung circulation and the right ventricle are altered in this disease, both before and after treatment.

SUMMARY

The literature reviewed in this chapter supports the concept that there is a right ventricular dysfunction in COPD patients that appears to be related to both abnormal pulmonary hemodynamics and hypoxemia. This right ventricular dysfunction seems to be clinically relevant to both exercise tolerance and survival. In contrast, clinically significant left ventricular dysfunction does not appear to develop from COPD that is uncomplicated by systemic hypertension or coronary artery disease.

The imperfect correlations between right ventricular

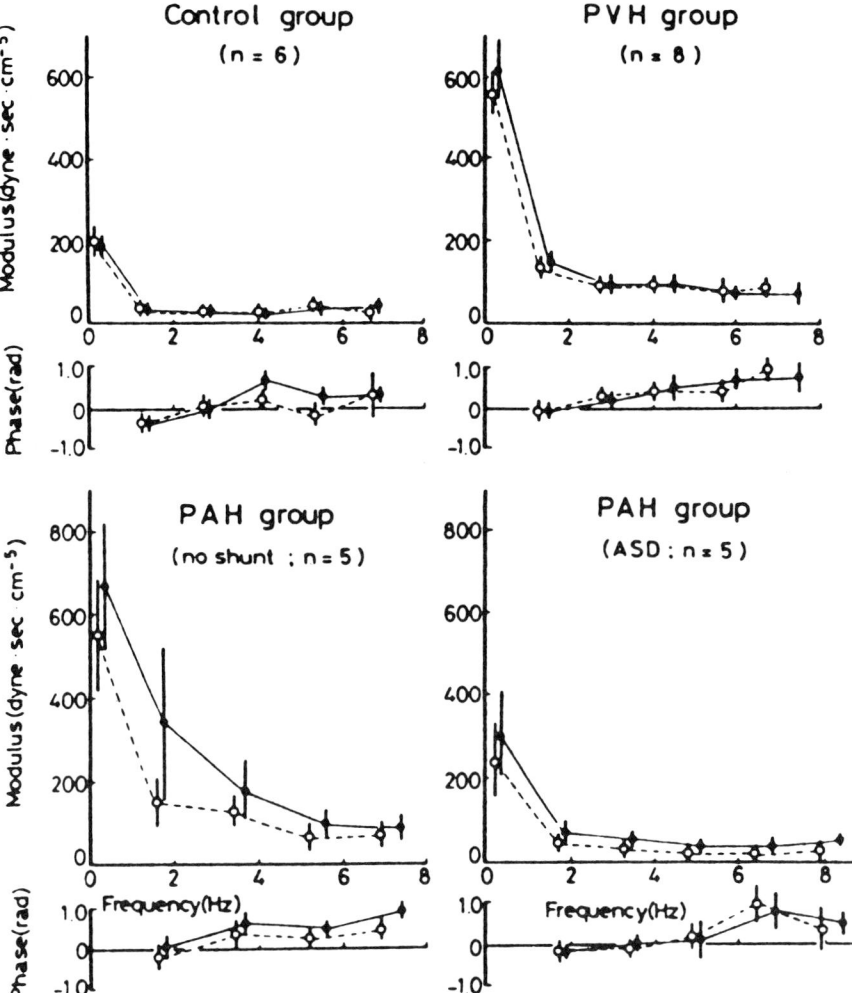

FIGURE 6-5. Average pulmonary arterial input impedance spectra in a group of normal subjects (control group) and in patients with pulmonary venous hypertension (PVH group), in patients with pulmonary arterial hypertension (PAH group), and in patients with pulmonary arterial hypertension and atrial septal defect (ASD). The *continuous lines* and *solid circles* were plotted while the subjects breathed oxygen. Pulmonary artery pressure and flow velocity were measured using catheter tip transducers. (Reprinted from Haneda R, Nakajima T, Shirato K, et al. Effects of oxygen breathing on pulmonary vascular input impedance in patients with pulmonary hypertension. Chest 1983; 83:523.)

ejection fraction and all conventional measures of pulmonary pressure and resistance have prompted us to consider more sophisticated measures of both the function of the right side of the heart and pulmonary hemodynamics. Specifically, the ejection fraction fails to account for tricuspid regurgitation, which is present with dilatation of the right side of the heart. In contrast, every study examining right ventricular stroke volume and filling pressures has demonstrated abnormal right ventricular function in COPD patients.

Similarly, a more complete description of the effect of the pulmonary circuit on the function of right side of the heart can be made by considering pulmonary impedance rather than pressure or resistance. The impedance spectrum takes into account both the oscillatory and steady-state components of afterload by describing the summated effects of arterial wave reflections and elasticity as well as pulmonary vascular resistance.

REFERENCES

1. Kountz WB, Alexander HL, Prinzmetal M. The heart in emphysema. Am Heart J 1936; 11:163–172.
2. Scott RW, Garvin CF. Cor pulmonale: Observations in 50 autopsy cases. Am Heart J 1941; 22:56–63.
3. Zimmerman HA, Ryan JM. Cor pulmonale. Dis Chest 1951; 20:286–289.
4. Michelson N. Bilateral ventricular hypertrophy due to chronic pulmonary disease. Dis Chest 1960; 38:435–446.
5. Fluck DC, Chandresekar RG, Gardner RV. Left ventricular hypertrophy in chronic bronchitis. Br Heart J 1966; 28:92–97.
6. Murphy ML, Adamson J, Hutcheson F. Left ventricular hypertrophy in patients with chronic bronchitis and emphysema. Ann Intern Med 1974; 81:307–313.
7. Bloomfield RA, Lawson HD, Cournand A, et al. Recording of right heart pressures in normal subjects and in patients with chronic pulmonary disease and various types of cardio-circulatory disease. J Clin Invest 1946; 25:639–664.
8. Hickam JB, Cargill WH. Effect of exercise on cardiac output and pulmonary arterial pressure in normal persons and in patients with cardiovascular disease and pulmonary emphysema. J Clin Invest 1948; 27:10–23.
9. Dexter L, Dow JW, Haynes FW, Whittenberger JL, et al. Studies of the pulmonary circulation in man at rest, normal variations and the interrelations between increased pulmonary blood flow, elevated pulmonary arterial pressure, and high pulmonary "capillary" pressures. J Appl Physiol 1951; 3:439–453.
10. Harvey RM, Ferrer I, Richards DW Jr, Cournand A. Influence of chronic pulmonary disease on the heart and circulation. Am J Med 1951; 10:719–738.
11. Yu PNG, Lovejoy FW, Joos HA, et al. Studies of pulmonary hypertension: I. Pulmonary circulatory dynamics in patients with pulmonary emphysema at rest. J Clin Invest 1953; 32:120–137.

12. Williams JF Jr, Behnke RH. The effect of pulmonary emphysema upon cardiopulmonary hemodynamics at rest and during exercise. Ann Intern Med 1964; 60:824–842.
13. Segel N, Bishop JM. The circulation in patients with chronic bronchitis and emphysema at rest and during exercise, with special reference to the influence of changes in blood viscosity and blood volume on the pulmonary circulation. J Clin Invest 1960; 45:1555–1568.
14. Harris P, Segel N, Bishop JM. The relation between pressure and flow in the pulmonary circulation in normal subjects and in patients with chronic bronchitis and mitral stenosis. Cardiovasc Res 1968; 2:73–83.
15. Abraham AS, Hedworth-Whitty RB, Bishop JM. Effects of acute hypoxia and hypervolaemia singly and together, upon the pulmonary circulation in patients with chronic bronchitis. Clin Sci 1967; 33:371–380.
16. Herles F, Jezek V, Daum S. Site of pulmonary resistance in cor pulmonale in chronic bronchitis. Br Heart J 1968; 30:654–660.
17. Lockhart A, Tzareva M, Nader F, et al. Elevated pulmonary artery wedge pressure at rest and during exercise in chronic bronchitis: Fact or fancy. Clin Sci 1969; 37:503–517.
18. Albert RK, Muramoto A, Caldwell J, et al. Increases in intrathoracic pressure do not explain the rise in left ventricular end-diastolic pressure that occurs during exercise in patients with chronic obstructive pulmonary disease. Am Rev Respir Dis 1985; 132:623–627.
19. Field GB, Cotes JE. Lability of pulmonary pressure/flow curves during exercise in clinically mild bronchitis: Evidence for a pulmonary vascular sluice in man. Clin Sci 1970; 38:461–477.
20. Lockhart A, Nader F, Tzareva M, Schrijen F. Comparative hyperventilation or pulmonary haemodynamics in chronic bronchitis and emphysema. Eur J Clin Invest 1970; 1:69–76.
21. Weitzenblum E, El Gharbi T, Vandevenne A, et al. Pulmonary haemodynamic changes during muscular exercise in "non-decompensated" chronic bronchitis. Bull Physiopathol Respir 1972; 8:49–71.
22. Jezek V, Schrijen F, Sadoul P. Right ventricular function and pulmonary hemodynamics during exercise in patients with chronic obstructive pulmonary disease. Cardiology 1973; 58:20–31.
23. Romero-Colomer P, Schrijen F. Pulmonary haemodynamics during exercise and maximum tolerated power in chronic broncho-pulmonary disease. Bull Physiopathol Respir 1974; 10:301–314.
24. Schrijen F, Jezek V. Haemodynamic variables during repeated exercise in chronic lung disease. Clin Sci Mol Med 1978; 55:485–490.
25. Light RW, Mintz HW, Linden GS, Brown SE. Hemodynamics of patients with severe chronic obstructive pulmonary disease during progressive upright exercise. Am Rev Respir Dis 1984; 130:391–395.
26. Granath A, Jonsson B, Strandell T. Circulation in healthy old men, studied by right heart catheterization at rest and during exercise in supine and sitting position. Acta Med Scand 1964; 176:425–446.
27. Stewart RI, Lewis CM. Cardiac output during exercise in patients with COPD. Chest 1986; 89:199–205.
28. Mohsenifar Z, Jasper AC, Koerner SK. Relationship between oxygen uptake and oxygen delivery in patients with pulmonary hypertension. Am Rev Respir Dis 1988; 138:69–73.
29. Minh VD, Lee HM, Vasquez P, et al. Relation of V_{O_2} max to cardiopulmonary function in patients with chronic obstructive lung disease. Bull Eur Physiopathol Respir 1979; 15:359–375.
30. Morrison DA. Editorial: Pulmonary hypertension in chronic obstructive pulmonary disease: The right ventricular hypothesis. Chest 1987; 92:387–389.
31. Morrison DA, Henry R, Goldman S. Preliminary study of the effects of low flow oxygen on oxygen delivery and right ventricular function in chronic lung disease. Am Rev Respir Dis 1986; 133:390–395.
32. Morrison DA, Collins CM, Stovall JR, Friefeld G. Reduced exercise capacity of chronic obstructive pulmonary disease patients exercising with noseclip mouthpiece. Am J Cardiol 1989; 64:1180–1184.
33. Morrison DA, Adcock K, Collins CM, et al. Right ventricular dysfunction and the exercise limitation of chronic obstructive pulmonary disease. J Am Coll Cardiol 1987; 9:1219–1229.
34. Burrows B, Ketel LJ, Niden AH, et al. Patterns of cardiovascular dysfunction in chronic obstructive lung disease. N Engl J Med 1972; 286:912–918.
35. Weitzenblum E, Hirth C, Ducolone A, et al. Prognostic value of pulmonary artery pressure in chronic obstructive pulmonary disease. Thorax 1981; 36:752–758.
36. Weitzenblum E, Sautegeau A, Ehrhart M, et al. Long-term course of pulmonary arterial pressure in chronic obstructive pulmonary disease. Am Rev Respir Dis 1984; 130:993–998.
37. Williams JF Jr, Childress RH, Boyd DL, et al. Left ventricular function in patients with chronic obstructive pulmonary disease. J Clin Invest 1968; 47:1143–1153.
38. Rao BS, Cohn KE, Eldridge FL, Hancock EW. Left ventricular failure secondary to chronic pulmonary disease. Am J Med 1968; 45:229–239.
39. Davies J, Overy HR. Left ventricular function in cor pulmonale. Chest 1970; 58:8–14.
40. Baum GL, Schwartz A, Llamas R, Castillo C. Left ventricular function in chronic obstructive pulmonary disease. N Engl J Med 1971; 285:361–365.
41. Fishman AP. Editorial: The left ventricle in chronic bronchitis and emphysema. N Engl J Med 1971; 285:361–365.
42. Kelly DT, Spotnitz HM, Beiser GD, et al. Effects of chronic right ventricular volume and pressure loading on left ventricular performance. Circulation 1971; 44:403–412.
43. Khaja F, Parker JO. Right and left ventricular performance in chronic obstructive lung disease. Am Heart J 1971; 82:319–327.
44. Frank MJ, Weisse AB, Moschos CB, Levinson GE. Left ventricular function, metabolism and blood flow in chronic cor pulmonale. Circulation 1973; 47:798–806.
45. Steele P, Ellis JH, Van Dyke D, et al. Left ventricular ejection fraction in severe chronic obstructive airways disease. Am J Med 1975; 59:21–28.
46. Unger K, Shaw D, Karliner JS, et al. Evaluation of left ventricular performance in acutely ill patients with chronic obstructive lung disease. Chest 1975; 68:135–142.
47. Bahler RC. Editorial: Assessment of left ventricular function in chronic obstructive pulmonary disease. Chest 1975; 68:132–133.
48. Matthay RA, Ellis JH, Steele PP. Effect of dextran loading on left ventricular performance in chronic obstructive pulmonary disease. Am Heart J 1976; 92:730–736.
49. Kline LE, Crawford MH, MacDonald WJ, et al. Noninvasive assessment of left ventricular performance in patients with chronic obstructive pulmonary disease. Chest 1977; 72:558–564.
50. Boushey SF, North LB. Hemodynamic changes in chronic obstructive pulmonary disease. Chest 1977; 72:565–570.
51. Schrijen F, Uffholtz H, Pohu JM, Poincelot F. Pulmonary and systemic hemodynamic evolution in chronic bronchitis. Am Rev Respir Dis 1978; 117:25–31.
52. Krayenbuehl HP, Turima J, Hess O. Left ventricular function in chronic pulmonary hypertension. Am J Cardiol 1978; 41:1150–1158.
53. Kachel RG. Left ventricular function in chronic obstructive pulmonary disease. Chest 1978; 74:286–290.
54. Christianson LC, Saah A, Fisher VJ. Quantitative left ventricular cineangiography in patients with chronic obstructive pulmonary disease. Am J Med 1979; 66:399–404.
55. Gabinski C. Left ventricular function in chronic obstructive pulmonary disease. Cor Vasa 1980; 22:238–244.
56. Heistad DD, Abboud F. Circulatory adjustments to hypoxia. Circulation 1980; 61:463–470.
57. von Euler US, Liljestrand G. Observations on the pulmonary arterial blood pressure in the cat. Acta Physiol Scand 1947; 12:301–320.
58. Fishman AP. Hypoxia on the pulmonary circulation: How and where it acts. Circ Res 1976; 38:221–231.
59. Motley HL, Cournand A, Werko L, et al. The influence of short periods of induced acute anoxia upon pulmonary artery pressure in man. Am J Physiol 1947; 150:315–320.
60. Kitchin AH, Louther CP, Matthews MB. The effects of exercise

and breathing oxygen-enriched air on the pulmonary circulation in emphysema. Clin Sci 1961; 21:93–106.
61. Levine BE, Bigelow DB, Hamstra RD, et al. The role of long-term continuous oxygen administration in patients with chronic airways obstruction with hypoxemia. Ann Intern Med 1967; 66:639–650.
62. Cotes JE, Pisa Z, Thomas AJ. Effect of breathing oxygen upon cardiac output, heart rate, ventilation, systemic and pulmonary blood pressure in patients with chronic lung disease. Clin Sci 1963; 25:305–321.
63. Abraham AS, Cole RB, Bishop JM. Reversal of pulmonary hypertension by prolonged oxygen administration to patients with chronic bronchitis. Circ Res 1968; 23:147–157.
64. Horsfield K, Segel N, Bishop JM. The pulmonary circulation in chronic bronchitis at rest and during exercise breathing air and 80% oxygen. Clin Sci 1968; 43:473–483.
65. Abraham AS, Cole RB, Green ID, et al. Factors contributing to the reversible pulmonary hypertension of patients with acute respiratory failure studied by serial observations during recovery. Circ Res 1969; 24:51–60.
66. Neff TA, Petty TL. Long-term continuous oxygen treatment in chronic oxygen airways obstruction. Ann Intern Med 1970; 72:621–626.
67. Ude AC, Howard P. Controlled oxygen therapy and pulmonary heart failure. Thorax 1971; 26:572–578.
68. Stark RD, Finnegan P, Bishop JM. Daily requirement of oxygen to reverse pulmonary hypertension in patients with chronic bronchitis. BMJ 1972; 3:724–728.
69. Stark RD, Finnegan P, Bishop JM. Long-term domiciliary oxygen in chronic bronchitis with pulmonary hypertension. BMJ 1973; 3:467–470.
70. Nocturnal Oxygen Therapy Trial Group. Continuous or nocturnal oxygen therapy in hypoxemic chronic obstructive lung disease. Ann Intern Med 1980; 93:391–8.
71. Medical Research Council Working Party. Long-term domiciliary oxygen therapy in chronic hypoxic cor pulmonale complicating chronic bronchitis and emphysema. Lancet 1981; 1:681–6.
72. Timms RM, Khaja F, Williams GW. NOTT Trial Group. Hemodynamic response to oxygen therapy in chronic obstructive pulmonary disease. Ann Intern Med 1985; 102:29–36.
73. Flenley DC. Long-term home oxygen therapy. Chest 1985; 87:99–103.
74. MacNee W, Wathen CG, Flenley DC, Muir AD. The effects of controlled oxygen therapy on ventricular function in patients with stable and decompensated cor pulmonale. Am Rev Respir Dis 1988; 137:425–434.
75. Flenley DC, Muir AL. Cardiovascular effects of oxygen therapy for pulmonary arterial hypertension. Clin Chest Med 1983; 4:297–308.
76. Fulmer JD, Snider GL. ACCP-NHLBI National Conference on Oxygen Therapy. Chest 1984; 86:234–247.
77. Petty TL. Who needs home oxygen? Am Rev Respir Dis 1985; 131:930–931.
78. Bradley BL, Garner AE, Billiu D, et al. Oxygen-assisted exercise in chronic obstructive lung disease. Am Rev Respir Dis 1978; 118:239–243.
79. Raffestin B, Escourrou P, Legrand A, et al. Circulatory transport of oxygen in patients with chronic airflow obstruction exercising maximally. Am Rev Respir Dis 1982; 125:426–431.
80. Stein DA, Bradley BL, Miller WC. Mechanism of oxygen effects on exercise in patients with chronic obstructive pulmonary disease. Chest 1982; 81:6–10.
81. Degaute JP, Domenighetti G, Naeije R, et al. Oxygen delivery in acute exacerbation of chronic obstructive pulmonary disease. Am Rev Respir Dis 1981; 124:26–30.
82. MacNee W, Morgan AD, Wathen CG, et al. Right ventricular performance during exercise in chronic obstructive pulmonary disease. The effects of oxygen. Respiration 1985; 48:206–215.
83. Light RW, Mahutte CK, Stansbury DW, et al. Relationship between improvement in exercise performance with supplemental oxygen and hypoxic ventilatory drive in patients with chronic airflow obstruction. Chest 1989; 95:751–756.
84. Morrison D, Caldwell J, Lakshminaryan S, et al. The acute effects of low flow oxygen and isosorbide dinitrate on left and right ventricular ejection fractions in chronic obstructive pulmonary disease. J Am Coll Cardiol 1983; 2:652–660.
85. Morrison DA, Stovall JR. Increased exercise capacity in hypoxemic patients after long-term oxygen therapy. Chest 1992; (in press).
86. Catterall JR, Douglas NJ, Calverley PMA, et al. Transient hypoxemia during sleep in chronic obstructive pulmonary disease is not a sleep apnea syndrome. Am Rev Respir Dis 1983; 128:24–29.
87. Krieger J, Sforza E, Apprill M, et al. Pulmonary hypertension, hypoxemia, and hypercapnea in obstructive sleep apnea patients. Chest 1989; 96:729–737.
88. Boysen PG, Block AJ, Wynne JW, et al. Nocturnal pulmonary hypertension in patients with chronic obstructive pulmonary disease. Chest 1979; 76:536–542.
89. Krieger J, Sforza E, Apprill M, et al. Pulmonary hypertension, hypoxemia, and hypercapnea in obstructive sleep apnea patients. Chest 1989; 96:729–737.
90. Fletcher EC, Levin DC. Cardiopulmonary hemodynamics during sleep in subjects with chronic obstructive pulmonary disease: The effect of short- and long-term oxygen. Chest 1984; 85:6–14.
91. Filley GF, Beckwitt HJ, Reeves JT, et al. Chronic obstructive bronchopulmonary disease: II. Oxygen transport in two clinical types. Am J Med 1968; 44:26–38.
92. Ashutosh K, Mead G, Dunsky M. Early effects of oxygen administration and prognosis in chronic obstructive pulmonary disease and cor pulmonale. Am Rev Respir Dis 1983; 127:399–404.
93. Kawakami Y, Kishi F, Yamamoto H, Miyamoto K. Relation of oxygen delivery, mixed venous oxygenation, and pulmonary hemodynamics to prognosis in chronic obstructive pulmonary disease. N Engl J Med 1983; 308:1045–1095.
94. Tenney SM, Mithoefer JC. The relationship of mixed venous oxygenation to oxygen transport with special reference to adaptations to high altitude and pulmonary disease. Am Rev Respir Dis 1982; 125:474–475.
95. Mithoefer JC, Holford FD, Keighley JFH. The effect of oxygen administration on mixed venous oxygenation in chronic obstructive pulmonary disease. Chest 1974; 66:122–132.
96. Morrison DA, Ovitt T, Hammermeister KE. Functional tricuspid regurgitation and right ventricular dysfunction in pulmonary hypertension. Am J Cardiol 1988; 62:108–112.
97. Milnor WR. Hemodynamics. Baltimore, MD: Williams & Wilkins, 1982.
98. Piene H, Sund T. Impedance matching between ventricle and load. Ann Biomed Eng 1984; 12:191–207.
99. Piene H, Sund T. Flow and power output of right ventricle facing load with variable input impedance. Am J Physiol 1979; 237:H125–H130.
100. Latson TW, Yin FCP, Hunter W. The effects of finite wave velocity and discrete reflections on ventricular loading. In: Yin FCP (ed). Ventricular/Vascular Coupling Clinical, Physiological and Engineering Aspects. New York: Springer-Verlag, New York, Inc. 1987; 334–394.
101. Hopkins RA. The pathophysiology of pulmonary vascular disease: In: Yin FCP (ed). Ventricular/Vascular Coupling Clinical, Physiological and Engineering Aspects, New York: Springer-Verlag, New York, Inc., 1987, 42–79.
102. O'Rourke MF, Yaginuma T. Wave reflections and the arterial pulse. Arch Intern Med 1984; 144:366–371.
103. Zuckerman B, Orton EC, Stenmark KR, et al. Alteration of the pulsatile load in the high altitude calf model of pulmonary hypertension. J Appl Physiol 1991; 70:859–868.
104. Van den Bos GC, Westerhof N, Randall OS. Pulse wave reflection: Can it explain the differences between systemic and pulmonary pressure and flow waves? A study in dogs. Circ Res 1982; 51:479–485.
105. Westerhof N, Spikema P, Van den Bos GC. Forward and backward waves in the arterial system. Cardiovasc Res 1972; 6:648–656.
106. Reuben SR, Swadling JP, Gersh BJ, de Lee G. Measurement of pulmonary artery distensibility in the dog. Cardiovasc Res 1970; 4:473–481.
107. Piene H. Some physical properties of the arterial bed deduced

from pulsatile arterial flow and pressure. Acta Physiol Scand 1976; 98:295–306.
108. Haneda R, Nakajima T, Shirato K, et al. Effects of oxygen breathing on pulmonary vascular input impedance in patients with pulmonary hypertension. Chest 1983; 83:520–527.
109. Milnor WR, Conti CR, Lewis KB, O'Rourke MF. Pulmonary arterial pulse wave velocity and impedance in man. Circ Res 1969; 25:637–649.
110. Reuben SR. Compliance of the human pulmonary arterial system in disease. Circ Res 1971; 29:40–50.
111. Yin FCP, Guzman P, Brin K, et al. Effect of nitroprusside on hydraulic vascular beds of the right and left ventricle in patients with heart failure. Circulation 1983; 67:1330–1339.
112. Kussmaul WG, Wieland J, Laskey W. Pressure-flow relations in the pulmonary artery during myocardial ischemia: Implications for right ventricular function in coronary disease. Cardiovasc Res 1988; 22:627–638.
113. Wilcox BR, Lucas C. Pulmonary input impedance in children with left-right shunt. J Surg Res 1980; 29:40–49.
114. Kitahatake A, Inove M, Asao M, et al. Noninvasive evaluation of pulmonary hypertension by a pulsed Doppler technique. Circulation 1983; 68:302–309.
115. Okamoto M, Miyatake K, Kinoshita N, et al. Analysis of blood flow in pulmonary hypertension with the pulsed Doppler flowmeter combined with cross sectional echocardiography. Br Heart J 1984; 51:407–415.

Chapter 7

Neurocognitive Aspects of Chronic Obstructive Pulmonary Disease

SEAN B. ROURKE, B.Sc., Hons. B.A.
IGOR GRANT, M.D.
ROBERT K. HEATON, Ph.D.

Both hypoxemia and hypercapnia can disturb cerebral functioning. For this reason, diseases such as chronic obstructive pulmonary disease (COPD) cannot be viewed as simply cardiopulmonary disorders. Recent evidence has shown that varying levels of both neuropsychologic impairment and psychiatric disturbances can occur in COPD. This chapter focuses on the neurocognitive aspects of COPD and reviews the current understanding regarding the causes and correlates of such complications.

This chapter begins with a description of how neuropsychology can contribute to the understanding of central nervous system functioning, and more specifically, to the delineation of brain and behavior relationships. Particular emphasis is placed on the types of questions that can be addressed from a neuropsychologic perspective to ascertain the causes and the extent of neurocognitive impairment in COPD patients at different stages of their disease. A summary of the results from high altitude studies follows; these results provide information regarding the acute effects of varying levels of hypoxemia on brain functioning and behavior. Next, an overview of the results from neuropsychologic studies in COPD is presented. This overview focuses mainly on two multicenter trials that attempted to delineate the chronic effects of hypoxemia on neurocognitive functioning. The effects of oxygen treatment on COPD patients are then described; this is followed by a review of the factors that may influence the effectiveness of oxygen therapy in the amelioration of neuropsychiatric symptoms. The influence of nocturnal oxygen desaturations on neuropsychologic functioning is discussed, followed by an outline of other potentially important variables and possible underlying mechanisms responsible for the neurobehavioral impairment that occurs in COPD. The chapter concludes by considering the clinical implications of the findings of studies in COPD.

NEUROPSYCHOLOGY: BRAIN AND BEHAVIOR RELATIONSHIPS

Several techniques can be employed to evaluate central nervous system functioning, including neurologic examinations, electrophysiologic and neuroradiologic studies, and neuropsychologic assessment. Of these various approaches, a neuropsychologic assessment is advantageous because it is a noninvasive technique that measures a key "product" of brain activity (cognition) and has considerable relevance to everyday functioning.[1–2]

The goal of a neuropsychologic assessment is to "produce a reliable and valid 'picture' of the relationships between brain and behavior."[3] Most often, a neuropsychologic assessment involves using a standardized battery of tests that has been designed to provide a relatively comprehensive sampling of general as well as specific indicators of cerebral functioning; the neuropsychologic tests in such a battery vary in their sensitivity and specificity for detecting various neurocognitive impairment,[4] since disease processes can affect different areas of the brain variably.

The numerous neuropsychologic batteries differ primarily in their theoretic origins.[5] Of these, the Halstead-Reitan Neuropsychological Battery (HRB) and related procedures have received the most extensive validation and application in a wide variety of neurologic and medical settings.[5, 6, 7] (See RM Reitan[6] for an extensive list of studies performed using the HRB on groups of subjects with and without brain damage or with many types of lesions and etiologies as well as with varying control or comparison groups.)

The HRB is a collection of tests that collectively sample intelligence, attention and concentration, language, abstracting ability, complex perceptual-motor integration (i.e., tests that require the subject to analyze perceptual information and then perform some specific action on the basis of his or her analysis, usually in the presence of a time constraint), sensation, motor ability, and memory. An advantage of the HRB is that it is able to produce normative data for all of its constituent tests; these data are corrected for age, education level, and sex.[8] A complete neuropsychologic evaluation using the Halstead-Reitan Neuropsychological Battery involves approximately 6 to 8 hours of testing. It is usually administered by trained psychometrists in a laboratory setting, and its results are interpreted by a neuropsychologist.

A standardized neuropsychologic battery, such as the Halstead-Reitan Neuropsychological Battery and related procedures, can be used to address the following questions about the neurobehavioral consequences of COPD: (1) Is there behavioral evidence to suggest impaired brain functioning with this disease and, if so, what is the nature of the abnormalities (i.e., which behaviors are affected and to what degree)? (2) What factors in the primary (lung) disease are related to the neurobehavioral abnormalities? (3) What is the natural history of the neurobehavioral impairments and can these impairments be ameliorated or reversed by effective treatment (e.g., by oxygen supplementation)? (4) What effects do the neurobehavioral abnormalities have on patients' everyday functioning and life quality, and to what degree do these effects improve with treatment? (5) Finally, what are the implications of the neuropsychologic findings for clinicians involved in the care of hypoxemia patients with COPD?

Since hypoxemia is a central derangement accompanying the progression of COPD, it is useful first to consider the current state of our knowledge regarding the acute effects of reduced PaO_2. Many insights have come from research of lung function at high altitudes.

ACUTE EFFECTS OF HYPOXEMIA ON NEUROCOGNITIVE FUNCTIONING: ALTITUDE STUDIES

Most altitude studies have examined only the effects of acute hypoxemia in medically healthy and relatively young persons. Therefore, we must be cautious when applying the data from such studies to the circumstances of older medically ill patients who experience chronic hypoxemia.

With increasing altitude and subsequent hypoxemia, subjects experience neurobehavioral impairment often similar to that seen in COPD. Certain neuropsychologic abilities are particularly susceptible to the effects of hypoxemia as a result of altitude. Sensory, motor, perceptual (especially visual), and complex perceptual-motor functions as well as abstraction, attention, and memory skills have been shown to be particularly sensitive.[9, 10] Most verbal functions, however, remain essentially intact. Several studies have indicated that these neurobehavioral deficits are transient,[11] whereas others have suggested mild but permanent impairment of motor speed and memory (particularly long-term visual memory).[10, 12] Methodologic differences may account for the differential results across altitude studies. Mood and affect changes (e.g., irritability and lability) have also been reported with hypoxemia occurring at high altitudes.[13]

There is considerable variability among individuals in their susceptibility to the effects of altitude. Hornbein and associates have suggested that this may be due to the variability in the hypoxic ventilatory response.[14] In the case of mountain climbers, other factors, such as extreme cold, illnesses secondary to travel in remote and primitive areas, injuries in falls, and sleep deprivation, also need to be considered during a psychologic evaluation. Nevertheless, Hornbein and associates have suggested that with prolonged and repeated exposure to hypoxemia at high altitudes, permanent impairment is likely, even without any obvious evidence of central nervous system dysfunction while individuals are at high altitude.[14]

RESULTS OF NEUROPSYCHOLOGIC STUDIES IN CHRONIC OBSTRUCTIVE PULMONARY DISEASE

In 1973, Krop and coworkers performed the first systematic neuropsychologic examination of COPD patients.[15] These authors were interested in whether continuous oxygen therapy could improve neuropsychologic functioning in hypoxemia patients with COPD. Twenty-two COPD patients participated in the study. The treatment group comprised 10 patients whose PaO_2 was 55 mm Hg or lower (mean age: 54 yr; mean level of education: 9.7 yr; mean PaO_2: 51 mm Hg; mean $PaCO_2$: 45.5 mm Hg; forced expiratory volume [FEV]: 0.77 L). The other 12 patients whose PaO_2 was 55 mm Hg or higher and who had similarly severe degrees of airway obstruction constituted the comparison group (mean age: 59 yr; mean level of education: 9.9 yr; mean PaO_2: 68 mm Hg; FEV: 0.76 L). A battery of neuropsychologic and personality tests was administered prior to and after 1 month of oxygen treatment. Only a few of the tests that normally appear in the Halstead-Reitan Neuropsychological Battery (described previously) were administered in this study.[15] Baseline testing without any supplemental oxygen was performed in both groups. However, it is important to note that follow-up testing was performed while the treatment group received oxygen therapy.

At baseline, hypoxemic patients were found to be impaired compared with the comparison group, particularly when they performed tests of perceptual-motor functions and of the speed of simple motor movement. No significant personality differences were observed between groups at baseline as measured by the Minnesota Multiphasic Personality Inventory (MMPI). Both groups scored higher on the hypochondriasis, depression, and hysteria scales with respect to published norms; this profile of MMPI scores was indicative of prominent distress, pessimism, and somatic preoccupation.

Continuous ambulatory oxygen therapy was administered to the treatment group for 1 month. No changes were observed in spirometric data (FEV and forced vital capacity [FVC]) or in the $PaCO_2$ in the treatment group. However, the mean PaO_2 improved from 51 mm Hg to 75 mm Hg. Neuropsychologically, treated patients improved significantly relative to the comparison group with respect to measures of intelligence, simple motor skills, perceptual-motor functions, and memory. Oxygen-treated patients also exhibited a significant improvement on the hypochondriasis, depression, hysteria, and social introversion scales of the MMPI. The results of the MMPI indicated that after oxygen therapy the treatment group became "more independent, less concerned with somatic problems, more outgoing, and in general, better able to deal with emotional stress."[15] According to the authors, the results of this first systematic neuropsychologic examination of COPD patients with hypoxemia were consistent with the expectation that oxygen deprivation can impair both cognitive and emotional functioning and that oxygen therapy can reverse deficits in these domains.

Despite the heuristic importance of this early study, some of its limitations must be recognized. First, the small number of subjects makes it difficult to determine whether the results are applicable to a larger population of COPD patients with varying levels of hypoxemia and other medical complications. Second, in the study, baseline cognitive and personality tests were performed while patients were not receiving oxygen, but the follow-up evaluations were conducted while the treatment group was administered supplemental oxygen. Therefore, it is difficult to determine whether the observed changes were associated with longer-lasting improvements in central nervous system function related to the 1 month of oxygen therapy or whether the effects were acute and transient. Third, it is unclear to what extent the clinical status of patients in both groups was stabilized at baseline before testing was performed. Conceivably, acute exacerbations in the more severely hypoxemic group at baseline would have been eased to some extent without the supplemental oxygen. Finally, it is likely that the comparison group also sustained some neurocognitive impairment, although to a lesser degree, due to mild levels of hypoxemia. However, because this study did not include a control group of matched subjects without COPD, this issue could not be addressed.

MULTICENTER INVESTIGATIONS

In the late 1970s and early 1980s two multicenter investigations conducted in the United States and in Canada examined clinical outcomes in large groups of patients at varying stages of disease—the Nocturnal Oxygen Therapy (NOT) Trial in 1980 and the Intermittent Positive-Pressure Breathing (IPPB) Trial in 1983.[16, 17] These two studies are particularly important because they have provided the most comprehensive neuropsychiatric evaluation and follow-up data to date about COPD patients with different degrees of hypoxemia.

Nocturnal Oxygen Therapy Trial

The main purpose of the NOT Trial was to investigate the differential effectiveness of continuous (at least 20 h/day) versus nocturnal (at least 12 h at night) oxygen treatment in the management of hypoxemic COPD.[16] In the neurobehavioral component, emphasis was placed on the qualitative nature of the neuropsychologic deficits exhibited in COPD patients as well as on the severity of these deficits.[18] The sample size and selection procedures made it possible to generalize the results more easily than was the case in the study by Krop and coworkers.[15] Patients were selected for the NOT Trial study if they were 35 years of age or older, had a resting PaO_2 of less than 60 mm Hg while they were clinically stable and breathing room air, displayed a ratio of FEV in 1 second to forced vital capacity (FEV_1/FVC) that was less than 70% after two inhalations of beta agonists from a metered-dose inhaler, and had a total lung capacity greater than 80% of the predicted norm. Patients were stabilized by medical therapy (bronchodilators, diuretics, and antibiotics, as clinically indicated) before baseline assessments were made to ensure that initial findings were not secondary to acute exacerbations of illness.[16]

The NOT Trial included a total of 203 hypoxemic patients with COPD. A representative subsample of these hypoxemic patients (N = 74) were matched to a comparison group of elderly subjects (N = 74) who had no history of COPD. Matching variables included age, sex, education, socioeconomic status, and place of residence. There were no significant demographic differences between the controls and the COPD patients. As a group, the ages of the representative hypoxemic patients with COPD were 64.4 ± 8.1 years, with a range of 43 to 84 years. The patients had received 9.8 ± 3.4 years of formal education, and they had the following pulmonary values: PaO_2: 51.2 mm Hg; $PaCO_2$: 43.7 mm Hg; pH: 7.41; hematocrit: 47.5 ml/dl; FEV_1: 0.74 ± 0.31 L; and FVC: 1.90 ± 0.67 L (refer to reference 16 for other physiologic data). Control subjects (mean age: 64.3 ± 10.5 yr; mean level of education: 10.1 ± 3.7 yr) in this study did not receive invasive tests but were shown to exhibit normal pulmonary function (FEV_1: 2.74 ± 0.83 L; FVC: 3.57 ± 1.0 L). Complete medical, neuropsychologic, and emotional and personality testing of COPD patients was performed at baseline prior to beginning oxygen therapy, and the major follow-up testing was done after 6 months of oxygen treatment. However, a smaller subsample was followed for 1 year (more on this later in this chapter). None of the subjects received supplemental oxygen during their follow-up evaluations.

Nocturnal Oxygen Therapy Trial: Neuropsychologic Findings

At baseline, hypoxemic patients performed significantly worse than controls on most neuropsychologic tests. Specifically, when compared with control subjects, the COPD patients demonstrated impairment "in their ability to acquire and retain new information, form new concepts and think flexibly, perform complex perceptual-motor maneuvers, engage in simple perceptual discriminations, and showed less motor dexterity, strength, and quickness."[18] When blind clinical ratings were performed on the neuropsychologic test results, 77% of COPD patients were classified as having clinically significant neuropsychologic deficits, with 42% exhibiting moderate to severe cerebral dysfunction (as compared with 14% of the control subjects).[18]

When neuropsychologic test results were grouped according to ability areas (e.g., global function, attention, verbal and language skills, abstraction, complex perceptual-motor skills, simple sensory and motor functions, and memory), hypoxemic patients were found to perform significantly worse than control subjects in all areas tested. However, it is interesting to note that the two groups displayed similar patterns of relative strengths and weaknesses. That is, attention, language, and simple sensory and memory functioning were the least affected in both groups, whereas abstraction, complex perceptual-motor integration, and simple motor abilities were relatively more impaired (Fig.7–1).

This suggests that the blind clinical raters did not compensate for normal variations of test performance caused by the advanced age and relatively low level of education of many of the subjects. Typical "population norms" for neuropsychologic tests tend to be most directly applicable to middle-age high school graduates,[8, 19] and the NOT Trial was conducted before demographically corrected normative data for the tests became available. Regardless, on the basis of the results

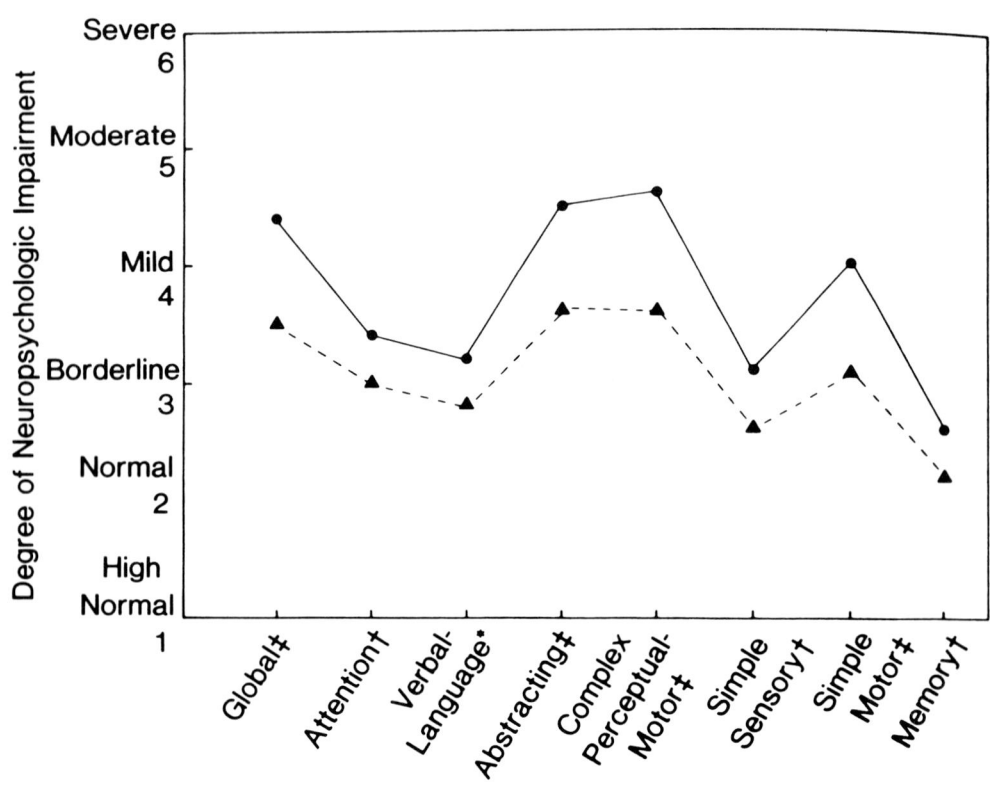

FIGURE 7–1. Group mean scores for patients with COPD (circles) and neighborhood controls (triangles) based on clinicians' ratings of neuropsychologic ability areas. The significance of differences between groups was based on the Mann-Whitney U test. (*: $P<.05$; †: $P<.01$; ‡: $P<.001$.) (From Grant I, Heaton RK, McSweeny AJ, et al. Neuropsychologic findings in hypoxemic chronic obstructive pulmonary disease. Arch Intern Med 1982; 142:1474. Copyright 1982, American Medical Association.)

presented, the investigators of the NOT Trial suggested that "COPD may not be related to any specific brain pathologic finding, but rather is aggravating neuropsychological decline that occurs as part of aging."[18]

In the search for medical predictors of neuropsychologic deficit, only weak relationships were found between neuropsychologic results and pulmonary function measures or hemodynamic indices. There was a slight tendency for patients with greater neuropsychologic deficits to be more hypoxemic, to have a lower level of oxygen transport, to be less polycythemic, and to have a lower exercise tolerance. A statistical procedure was carried out (stepwise forward multiple regression) that indicated that approximately 17% of the variance in the global neuropsychologic rating could be accounted for by the combination of resting arterial oxygen saturation (5%), education level (11%), and age (2%).[18] The low correlations between PaO_2 and impairment may have been the result of the restricted range of PaO_2 in this sample, that is, only more severely hypoxemic patients were studied in the NOT Trial.[16] This possibility was explored in the combined analyses of the NOT and the IPPB Trials (described later in this chapter).

Nocturnal Oxygen Therapy Trial: Life Quality Assessment Results

The life quality of hypoxemic patients with COPD was also addressed in the NOT Trial. Three self-report inventories were administered: the MMPI, the Profile of Mood Scale, and the Sickness Impact Profile. An additional inventory, the Katz Adjustment Scale, was administered to the spouse or another close relative of each patient. These instruments were used to evaluate (1) emotional functioning, including mood changes and other psychiatric symptoms; (2) social role functioning, including employment, home management, and social and family relationships; (3) activities of daily living, such as self-care skills and mobility; and (4) recreational pastimes and the ability to engage in pleasurable activities.[20]

The MMPI is a widely used objective test of personality and emotional disturbance. It consists of 566 true-false questions that measure 10 major dimensions of emotional status and psychopathology (hypochondriasis, depression, hysteria, psychopathic deviation, paranoia, psychasthenia, schizophrenia, mania, and social introversion). The Profile of Mood Scale consists of 65 adjectives that the patient rates on a five-point scale to describe recent mood. It provides a summary measure of total mood disturbance as well as individual scores relating to various affective dimensions. The Sickness Impact Profile is a questionnaire designed to measure sickness-related behavioral dysfunction. It yields summary scores for physical, psychosocial, and overall behavioral dysfunction as well as individual scores for 12 types of activities: ambulation, mobility, body care and movement, social interaction, communication, alertness behavior, emotional behavior, sleep and rest, eating, home management, recreation, and employment.

The results indicated that compared with control subjects, hypoxemic patients with COPD exhibited significant impairment in almost every area of life quality. Specifically, 42% of hypoxemic patients showed symptoms characteristic of reactive depression compared with only 9% of control subjects as indicated by their MMPI profiles (Fig. 7-2).

Furthermore, only 15% of the COPD patients were characterized as being free of emotional or personality disturbance based on clinical ratings of the MMPI, whereas 58% of control subjects were so described. The results obtained from the Profile of Mood Scale were generally consistent with those from the MMPI. That is, COPD patients described themselves as being "more tense, depressed, confused, fatigued, and sapped of vigor than do the controls."[20] The results from the Sickness Impact Profile indicated that COPD patients experienced moderate to severe impairment in almost all measured aspects of life quality (Fig. 7-3).

Finally, the relatives' views of life quality, as measured by the Katz Adjustment Scale, indicated that COPD patients were viewed as being "socially withdrawn and somewhat obstreperous."[20]

A moderate but statistically significant relationship was observed between life quality (i.e., overall Sickness Impact Profile score) and neuropsychologic functioning; patients with the most impaired life quality ratings exhibited the greatest neuropsychologic impairment. Owing to the relationship between emotional and neuropsychologic dysfunction, the authors suggested that "some of the emotional effects of hypoxemia may be the result of an inadequate supply of oxygen to the limbic system and other portions of the brain that mediate emotional behavior."[20] An alternative interpretation—that sickness-related emotional distress contributes directly to poor performance on neuropsychologic tests—was considered less likely because of inconsistent results from neuropsychologic studies using psychiatric patient groups.[21]

A statistical test (an exploratory multiple regression analysis) was carried out that indicated that age, socioeconomic status, and neuropsychologic functioning could account for 25% of the variance of life quality. It is striking that these three variables were more important with respect to life quality than was the pathophysiologic state of these patients.[20] Although this result must yet be reproduced, it implies that the severity of the pulmonary disease may not be the most important determinant of how well a patient copes with its effects. Rather, demographic and neurocognitive variables may be more salient.[20]

Intermittent Positive-Pressure Breathing Clinical Trial

The second multicenter investigation addressed the efficacy of IPPB for COPD patients. The IPPB Trial was also the first controlled clinical study to examine both the neuropsychologic functioning and the personality characteristics of mildly hypoxemic COPD patients (i.e., those with a $PaO_2 > 55$ mm Hg). COPD patients

84 CAUSES AND CONSEQUENCES OF CHRONIC PULMONARY DISEASE

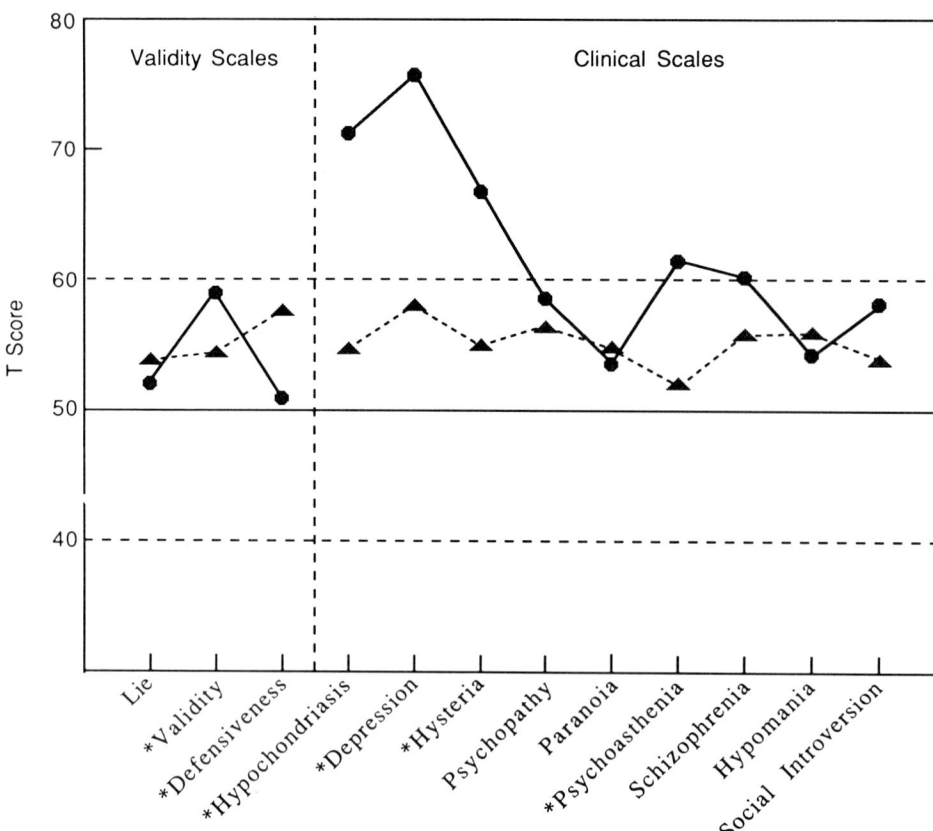

FIGURE 7–2. Mean Minnesota Multiphasic Personality Inventory profiles for patients with COPD and for control subjects. *Asterisks* indicate significant differences (*P* <.01) between patients with COPD and control subjects using paired tests (n = 52). A scaled male-female ratio was excluded because of the ambiguities of a mixed sex sample. (*solid line:* patients in the Nocturnal Oxygen Therapy Trial; *dotted line:* control subjects.) (From McSweeny AJ, Grant I, Heaton RK, et al. Life quality of patients with chronic obstructive pulmonary disease. Arch Intern Med 1982; 142:475. Copyright 1982, American Medical Association.)

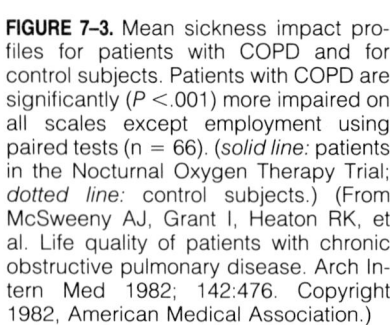

FIGURE 7–3. Mean sickness impact profiles for patients with COPD and for control subjects. Patients with COPD are significantly (*P* <.001) more impaired on all scales except employment using paired tests (n = 66). (*solid line:* patients in the Nocturnal Oxygen Therapy Trial; *dotted line:* control subjects.) (From McSweeny AJ, Grant I, Heaton RK, et al. Life quality of patients with chronic obstructive pulmonary disease. Arch Intern Med 1982; 142:476. Copyright 1982, American Medical Association.)

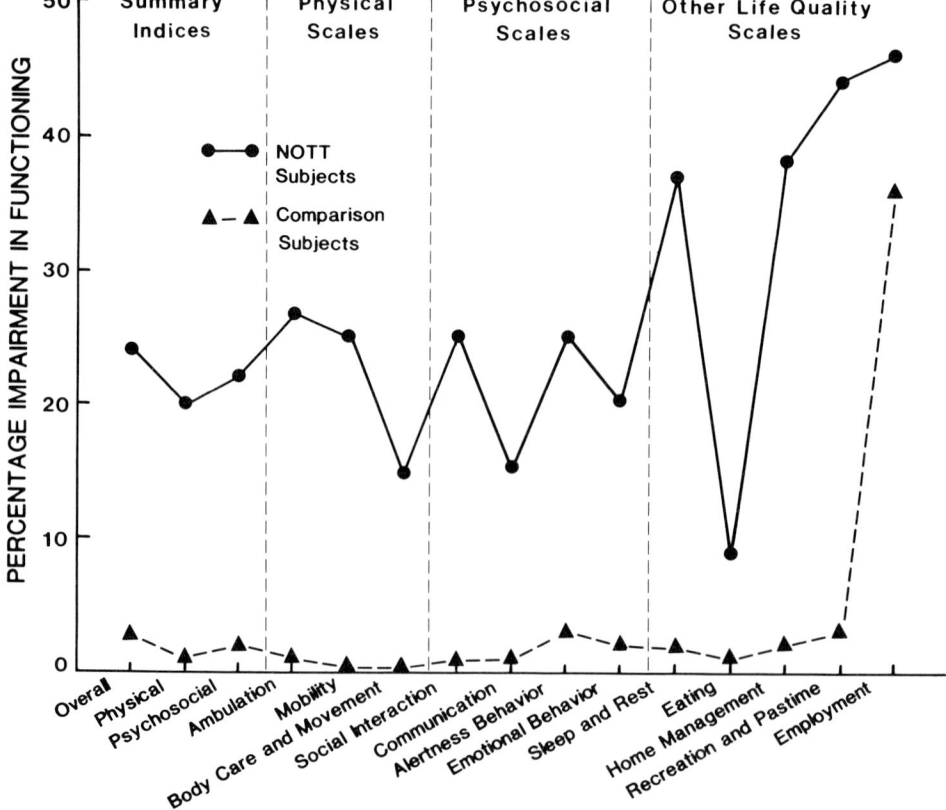

(N = 100) with a mean age of 61.5±7.4 years and a mean level of education of 9.9±3.1 years were compared with demographically matched controls (N = 25) with a mean age of 59.6±9.0 years and a mean education level of 10.5±3.3 years with respect to neuropsychologic and personality measures. The IPPB Trial employed matching procedures and testing instruments similar to those used in the NOT Trial; therefore, analyses could be carried out on the combined group at a later date. The patients chosen for the IPPB Trial were slightly younger but considerably less hypoxemic than those COPD patients in the NOT Trial (mean PaO_2 of 66.3 versus 51.2 mm Hg).[22, 23] They also manifested less severe abnormalities in other physiologic measures (e.g., mean PaO_2: 66.3±7.0 mm Hg; mean $PaCO_2$: 35.1±4.2 mm Hg; FEV_1: 1.10±0.4 L).

Intermittent Positive-Pressure Breathing Trial: Neuropsychologic Findings

All summary neuropsychologic measures were significantly worse for the mildly hypoxemic COPD group than the control group.[22] Moreover, as was the case in the NOT Trial, patients in the IPPB Trial were impaired in most ability areas relative to the control subjects. The cognitive skills affected included abstract reasoning, complex perceptual-motor integration, speed of performance, simple language function, and memory functions. As in the NOT Trial,[16] a modest but reliable relationship was observed between summary measures of neuropsychologic impairment and resting PaO_2.[18, 22]

Overall, IPPB patients performed better than those in the NOT Trial on the HRB. Comparison of scores across cognitive domains revealed some tests of the HRB were more sensitive to the effects of COPD than were others. For example, results of tests measuring abstraction ability and the ability to concentrate and attend to nonverbal stimuli were reliably worse in both the IPPB and the NOT Trial patients compared with those of control subjects. Furthermore, the two patient groups did not significantly differ with respect to these measures. In contrast, other tasks were differentially sensitive to the severity of disease, that is, the more severely hypoxemic COPD patients performed worse than the less hypoxemic patients on tests that measured the simple speed of motor activity, complex perceptual-motor ability, memory, and cognitive flexibility.[18, 22, 24]

Intermittent Positive-Pressure Breathing Trial: Life Quality Assessment Results

Results from the Sickness Impact Profile indicated that mildly hypoxemic COPD patients were significantly more impaired on almost all of the subscales (except those for eating, body care, and movement) than were the demographically matched controls. Although the degree of physical limitation was minimal in the mildly hypoxemic group, psychosocial limitation was nevertheless marked and included notable impairments in social interaction, recreation, and hobbies.[23]

Interestingly, when the mildly hypoxemic patients were compared with the severely hypoxemic patients from the NOT Trial group, the mildly hypoxemic patients had significantly less physical limitation (mean scores of 12% versus 20%, respectively, on the Sickness Impact Profile physical score) but comparable levels of psychosocial limitations (18% versus 22%, respectively). MMPI results were comparable with those obtained from the NOT Trial. These findings appear to suggest that the degree of physical limitation is related to the severity of pulmonary disease, whereas psychosocial impairment occurs earlier in the disease process.[23]

Combination NOT and IPPB Trial Data

The COPD patients in the NOT and IPPB trials differed in the degree of hypoxemia and other indices of disease severity.[16–18, 20, 22, 23] Because comparable psychosocial assessments were employed, the two populations could subsequently be combined to obtain a more representative sample of COPD patients and to make possible the relation of neuropsychologic performance to various levels of pulmonary function and other medical predictors.[24, 25] This pooling allowed stratification of patients into three hypoxemia "severity" groups: mild ($PaO_2 \geq 60$ mm Hg; N = 86), moderate (PaO_2 = 50 to 59 mm Hg; N = 155), and severe ($PaO_2 < 50$ mm Hg; N = 61). The three groups had the following mean values for PaO_2 and $PaCO_2$, respectively: mild group—67.8±6.3 mm Hg and 34.9±4.1 mm Hg; moderate group—54.4±2.7 mm Hg and 42.1±7.4 mm Hg; and severe group—44.4±4.1 mm Hg and 45.8±8.4 mm Hg.[25] (Refer to reference 25 for other pulmonary function and medical data.)

Despite comparable intelligence quotient values among COPD patients, those with the most severe hypoxemia tended to perform the most poorly on neuropsychologic tests. Control subjects had the best cognitive functioning as indicated by summary scores, such as the Average Impairment Rating; COPD patients with hypoxemia exhibited proportional increases (i.e., worse scores) based on their Average Impairment Rating. Both moderately and severely hypoxemic groups were indistinguishable with respect to their level of neuropsychologic impairment as measured by the Average Impairment Rating. Mild decrements in performance were observed on certain subtests as the level of hypoxemia increased. On the other hand, control subjects and mildly hypoxemic patients were observed to perform similarly on some measures.[25]

A factor analysis was used to reduce the large number of variables into the following factors: (1) verbal intelligence, (2) perceptual learning and problem-solving, (3) alertness and psychomotor speed, and (4) simple motor skills. When subtest scores were standardized so that they could be compared on the same scale, the overall pattern indicated that with increasing hypoxemia, patients scored progressively worse on all factors except verbal intelligence. Results were essentially unchanged after age was considered as a statistical factor (Fig. 7–4).[25]

A statistical procedure (stepwise linear regression with backward elimination) was performed to explore the contribution of various medical parameters as well as age and education to the prediction of neuropsychologic performance. Four variables accounted for a substantial proportion (40%) of the variability in neuropsychologic impairment: education (25%), age (5%), respiratory rate (5%), and PaO_2 (5%). Other regression analyses were performed using similar variables to predict performance on each of the factor-analytically derived composite scores. The results indicated that (1) education, as expected, contributed substantially to the verbal intelligence factor; (2) age and PaO_2 were the most important predictors of perceptual learning and problem-solving; (3) age, education, and respiratory rate were important in determining alertness and psychomotor speed; and (4) both demographic and medical variables influenced simple motor skills.[25] Overall, perceptual learning and problem-solving, which are tested by those areas of the HRB that are most sensitive to brain dysfunction, were best explained relative to the other three factors by a combination of aging and oxygen deprivation.[25]

The combination of the controlled NOT and IPPB Trials has provided extensive data on the neuropsychologic profile of a large group of COPD patients (N = 302) with varying levels of chronic hypoxemia and illness. Overall, 42% of the patients with COPD evidenced neuropsychologic deficits suggestive of impaired brain function.[25] Furthermore, when COPD patients were classified according to three hypoxemia levels, the mildly hypoxemic group (average PaO_2: 68 mm Hg) exhibited a 27% prevalence of impairment, the moderate group (average PaO_2: 54 mm Hg) had a 44% prevalence rate, and the severely hypoxemic group (average PaO_2: 44 mm Hg) had a prevalence rate of 61%.[25]

Effects of Oxygen Treatment

One hundred fifty of the COPD patients in the NOT Trial[16] were reevaluated after 6 months of oxygen therapy (78 patients received continuous oxygen therapy [COT] for 20 h/day, whereas 72 patients received nocturnal oxygen therapy [NOT] for 12 h/day). A subsample of those 150 patients (20 COT patients and 17 NOT patients) were examined at 1 year.[26] No selection bias was observed in the patients who underwent follow-up. During the first 6 months of oxygen therapy, no differences in the neuropsychologic outcomes of surviving NOT and COT patients were observed; however, survival rates indicated that COT was more effective after 12 months of oxygen treatment. In addition, those patients receiving COT exhibited significantly greater improvement on four of the five neuropsychologic summary measures during the second 6 months of treatment.[26] (Note: At follow-up all patients were tested while breathing room air.)

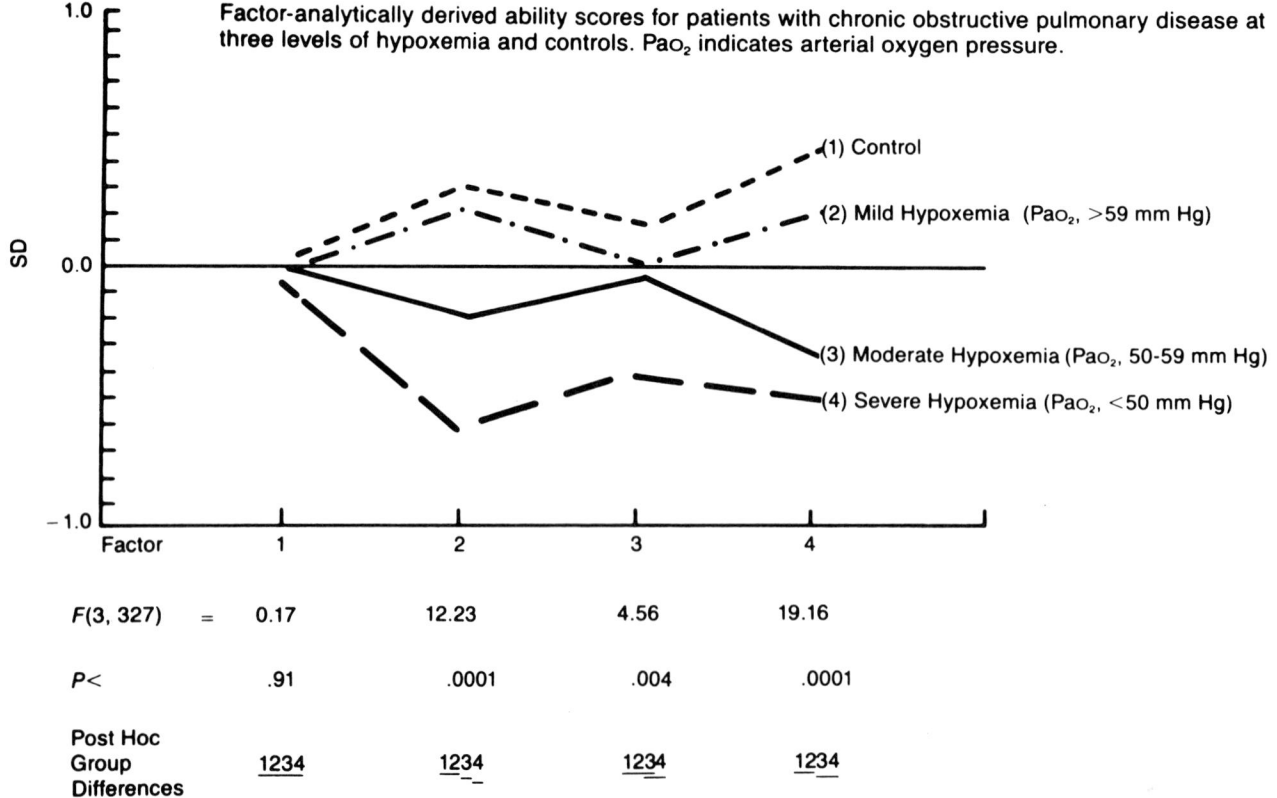

FIGURE 7–4. Factor-analytically derived ability scores for patients with COPD at three levels of hypoxemia and for control subjects. (From Grant I, Prigatano GP, Heaton RK, et al. Progressive neurophysiologic impairment and hypoxemia. Arch Gen Psychiatry 1987; 44:1003. Copyright 1987, American Medical Association.)

At 6 months, comparable rates of improvement were observed in both oxygen treatment programs, with 42% of COPD patients exhibiting modest neuropsychologic improvement. Most of these changes could not be explained by practice effects, since only 6% of nonpatient control subjects were rated as improved after 6 months on a clinical rating of global neuropsychologic functioning. Among patients, the cognitive areas in which improvement occurred included language function, abstraction and flexibility of thinking, simple sensory function, and simple motor abilities. However, the authors cautioned that these group differences were subtle and that neuropsychologic impairment was not entirely ameliorated by oxygen therapy.[26]

Whereas the neurocognitive improvement in the two treated groups (NOT versus COT) was similar at the 6-month assessment, the subgroup followed for 12 months showed a divergence, with those receiving COT apparently performing better than those on the nocturnal regimen.[26] The mean average impairment ratings for COT and NOT groups that completed neuropsychologic evaluations at baseline and after 6 and 12 months of oxygen treatment are shown in Figure 7–5.

However, contrary to the findings of Krop and co-workers,[15] no striking changes in the measures of life quality or emotional status were found at either the 6-month or 12-month assessment.[26] It is worth noting that "no change" in life quality may have indicated some benefit for COPD patients. That is, patients without treatment may have been expected to display some declines in their emotional and personality functioning over a 6- to 12-month study period.[26]

With respect to cardiopulmonary variables, no significant changes in the measures of pulmonary function, heart rate, or exercise tolerance were observed after 6 months of oxygen therapy in surviving COPD patients. As noted previously, however, there was a significant difference in the mortality rates between the two treated groups. That is, at 1 year the mortality rate was 21% in the NOT group but only 12% in the COT group. Those patients with the worst mood disturbances, neuropsychologic impairment, and physiologic measures of disease severity derived the greatest benefit from COT as indicated by their mortality rate.[26] After 2 years, the annual mortality rate rose to 41% in the NOT group and to 22% in the COT group. Similarly, in the British Medical Research Council Trial, which compared survival rates in hypoxemic COPD patients, 15 hours per day of oxygen therapy was associated with 5-year survival rate of 41%, whereas no oxygen treatment was associated with a 5-year survival rate of only 25%.[27]

The extent to which the levels of oxygen, carbon dioxide, and carbon monoxide affect neurocognitive performance, independently as well as interactively, is an area that requires further attention. Carbon dioxide was not significantly associated with cognitive impairment in the above studies; however, few of the patients studied had marked hypercapnia. Although factors other than PaO_2 probably contribute to cerebral disturbance in COPD, the fact that oxygen treatment is beneficial suggests that the correction of hypoxemia is one important variable. In the next section, possible mechanisms underlying this improvement are considered.

AMOUNT AND DURATION OF OXYGEN THERAPY IN RELATION TO NEUROCOGNITIVE FUNCTIONING

The administration of supplemental oxygen to patients with COPD and hypoxemia has been shown to improve neuropsychologic functioning, reduce pulmonary hypertension, and improve survival.[15, 25–29] It appears that oxygen therapy should be administered at least 19 hours per day, including during the hours of sleep, and in a dose sufficient to raise arterial PaO_2 to 65 to 80 mm Hg in those patients who have stable hypoxemia.[30] How-

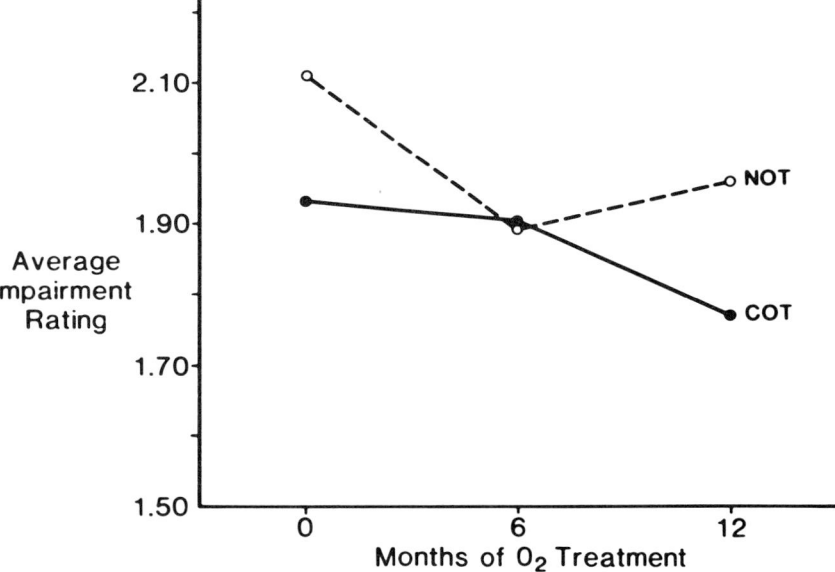

FIGURE 7–5. Mean average impairment ratings for continuous oxygen treatment *(solid line)* and nocturnal oxygen treatment *(dotted line)* groups that completed neuropsychologic evaluations at baseline and after 6 and 12 months of oxygen treatment. (From Heaton RK, Grant I, McSweeny AJ, et al. Psychologic effects of continuous oxygen therapy in hypoxemic chronic obstructive pulmonary disease. Arch Intern Med 1983; 143:1945. Copyright 1983, American Medical Association.)

ever, it is unclear how the changes in neuropsychologic functioning and survival may be related to the intensity and duration of oxygen therapy. Further inquiry is needed to determine the extent to which acute and long-term oxygen supplementation improves neurocognitive functioning.

Several investigators have propsed that two different mechanisms may be responsible for the neuropsychologic improvements that occur as a result of oxygen supplementation: (1) a short-term effect of oxygen on the activity and functioning of hypoxic neurons and (2) a long-term effect on the synthesis of macromolecules necessary for neurotransmitter synthesis or other metabolic requirements.[25, 26] Results from a study investigating the effects of acute oxygen therapy (lasting 6 h) on information processing by hypoxemic COPD patients with PaO_2 less than 55 mm Hg suggested that the first mechanism alone cannot improve cognitive functioning. Rather, Wilson and colleagues propose that activation of the second mechanism must occur before the first (acute) mechanism is activated in order for oxygen benefit to be optimum.[31] These researchers found no cognitive benefits from administering acute normobaric oxygen for 6 hours to COPD patients with hypoxemia. However, since the patients served as their own controls, it was not possible to determine the extent of the information processing deficits that would be expected in age-matched controls; therefore, it is diffcult to determine the amount of improvement that may have been expected as a result of acute oxygen supplementation.

A study involving short-term hyperbaric oxygen supplementation has been shown to improve cognitive functioning in a group of elderly patients with organic brain syndrome,[32] although other investigators have not been able to replicate these results.[33] On the other hand, earlier results from the work of Krop and coworkers[15] indicated the reversal of neuropsychologic deficits and emotional disturbances in patients after they received COT for 1 month. However, as was noted earlier, follow-up assessments were performed in the study by Krop and coworkers while the subjects were receiving supplemental oxygen. This was not the case in the NOT Trial[16, 18, 20, 25, 26]; in this study, more modest neuropsychologic improvements were recorded. Furthermore, the results of the NOT Trial[26] indicated that the administration of COT for 1 year had significant advantages for hypoxemic COPD patients (i.e., they displayed better neuropsychologic functioning and had a lower mortality rate) compared with NOT for the same period.

The severity of hypoxemia can fluctuate considerably during the day and night. Therefore, one possible mechanism of brain injury other than chronic hypoxemia might be the acute reduction in PaO_2 that occurs during sleep, especially in those COPD patients with sleep disordered breathing.

SLEEP FINDINGS

Normal subjects have been shown to experience nocturnal oxygen desaturations and subsequent hypoxemia, particularly during rapid eye movement sleep.[34-36] It has been suggested that males who snore heavily and who are asymptomatic for sleep apnea syndrome may have an increased risk of developing hypertension, angina, stroke, and neuropsychologic impairment due to nocturnal oxygen desaturations,[35, 37] and that these increased risks may not be reversible by NOT.[37, 38]

Other investigators have reported moderate neuropsychologic dysfunction in subjects with sleep apnea syndrome, normal arterial oxygen saturation levels during waking hours, and without COPD.[39] Patients with sleep apnea syndrome and associated hypoxemia have shown poorer cognitive functioning than such patients without hypoxemia.[40] Those patients with sleep apnea and hypoxemia exhibited impairments with respect to measures of attention, concentration, complex problem-solving, and the short-term recall of verbal and spatial information.

Although COPD patients may be chronically hypoxemic, some of them experience a significant worsening of hypoxemia during sleep due to nocturnal oxygen desaturations.[41, 45-47] For example, one study noted that 43% of COPD patients with a daytime PaO_2 of 60 to 70 mm Hg (excluding those with sleep apnea syndrome) were "nocturnal desaturators."[42] Similarly, it has been reported that 27% of COPD patients with a daytime PaO_2 greater than or equal to 60 mm Hg exhibited signs of nocturnal oxyhemoglobin desaturation related to rapid eye movement.[41] The risk was higher for patients with a daytime PaO_2 between 60 and 65 mm Hg (those who are on the steepest part of the oxyhemoglobin dissociation curve).

Most of the studies to date have related the degree of nocturnal hypoxemia in COPD to the degree of daytime hypoxemia[43]; however, a recent study indicates that daytime hypercapnia is also a risk factor for the development of nocturnal hypoxemia in patients who are normoxic while they are awake.[44] These nocturnal increases in hypoxemia most likely potentiate the physiologic and behavioral deficits observed in COPD patients.

Certain COPD patients (the so-called "blue bloaters") are particularly vulnerable to the experience of nocturnal desaturations and related hypoxemia.[48] These patients are often characterized by increased pulmonary artery pressure and polycythemia accompanied by symptoms of cor pulmonale.[45] Similarly, some COPD patients with cor pulmonale symptoms only exhibit slightly abnormal arterial blood gas characteristics while awake but show intermittent oxygen desaturations during sleep.[49] In contrast, other COPD patients (e.g., "pink puffers") exhibit normal regular respiratory patterns and show no evidence of oxygen desaturation during sleep.[50]

It is evident that the examination of sleep disordered breathing in COPD requires further attention; sleep disordered breathing may prove to be an important determinant of physiologic and behavioral parameters in COPD patients. It has also been proposed that males who snore heavily may potentially serve as a population in which the neurobehavioral effects of hypoxia might be modeled.[36]

OTHER POTENTIALLY IMPORTANT VARIABLES RESPONSIBLE FOR NEUROBEHAVIORAL IMPAIRMENT IN CHRONIC OBSTRUCTIVE PULMONARY DISEASE

Only a modest amount of variance in neuropsychologic performance in COPD patients can be attributed to PaO_2.[18, 22, 25] Measures of disease severity, such as pulmonary function tests, were not helpful in predicting neuropsychologic change (more on this point later in this chapter). These results suggest that other variables (e.g., age, level of education, desaturations during sleep, psychologic responses to chronic illness such as depression and anxiety, concurrent illnesses, increased susceptibility to diseases, increased fatigue, and sensory decrements) may be interacting both directly and indirectly to produce the neuropsychologic picture commonly seen in hypoxemic patients with COPD.

As part of the analysis of the combined NOT and IPPB Trials, a statistical procedure (stepwise logistic regression) was used to determine whether an equation could be developed to predict neuropsychologic deficit in COPD patients based on a combination of medical and sociodemographic variables. Four main predictors of neurobehavioral impairment in patients with COPD were obtained: age, level of education, PaO_2, and respiratory rate. FEV_1, FVC, $PaCO_2$, hematocrit, exercise capacity (measured using a bicycle ergometer), pH, hemoglobin levels, and systolic and diastolic blood pressures were not significantly associated with neuropsychologic performance.[25]

A heuristic model, such as the one that has been proposed by McSweeny and colleagues[20] to explain the variability in the life quality of patients with COPD, may be helpful in outlining the complexities with which neuropsychologic variables may potentially interact with other variables in COPD (Fig. 7–6). It is worth noting that age directly or indirectly influences every variable included.

It is well established that predictable neuroanatomic and neuropsychologic changes occur with age.[8, 19, 51] Performance on most neuropsychologic tests, including the Halstead-Reitan Neuropsychological Battery and other such tests, has been shown to be negatively correlated with age in both normal and patient populations. As a result, corrections need to be made for age as well as education, race, and sex before interpretations of neuropsychologic performance can be made; otherwise, normal subjects may easily be classified as brain-impaired.[8, 19, 51] Therefore, older people are more likely to have poorer neuropsychologic functioning than younger people regardless of whether they have COPD. Additionally, the elderly may lack compensatory reserve mechanisms[25] with which to cope with fluctuating hypoxemia during the day and particularly during sleep.

POSSIBLE MECHANISMS UNDERLYING HYPOXEMIA-INDUCED BRAIN DYSFUNCTION

Differing hypotheses have been proposed to explain how brain hypoxia may result in neuropsychologic impairment in COPD patients. Although cerebral hypoxia can impair the ability to generate energy (e.g., adenosine triphosphate production), the reduction in tissue PaO_2 necessary to impair oxidative metabolism must be profound (e.g., $PaO_2 < 20$ mm Hg). It is unlikely that such severe levels commonly occur in COPD; therefore, other mechanisms must be involved.[52]

More recent efforts have focused on the pathways responsible for the biosynthesis of various neurotransmitters. Acetylcholine has been implicated in the pathophysiology of hypoxic syndromes in that hypoxia might possibly lead to a reduction in acetylcholine synthesis.[9] However, cholinergic drug treatment only partially ameliorates hypoxia-induced behavioral deficits,[53] which suggests that other neurotransmitter systems may play a contributory role.[54]

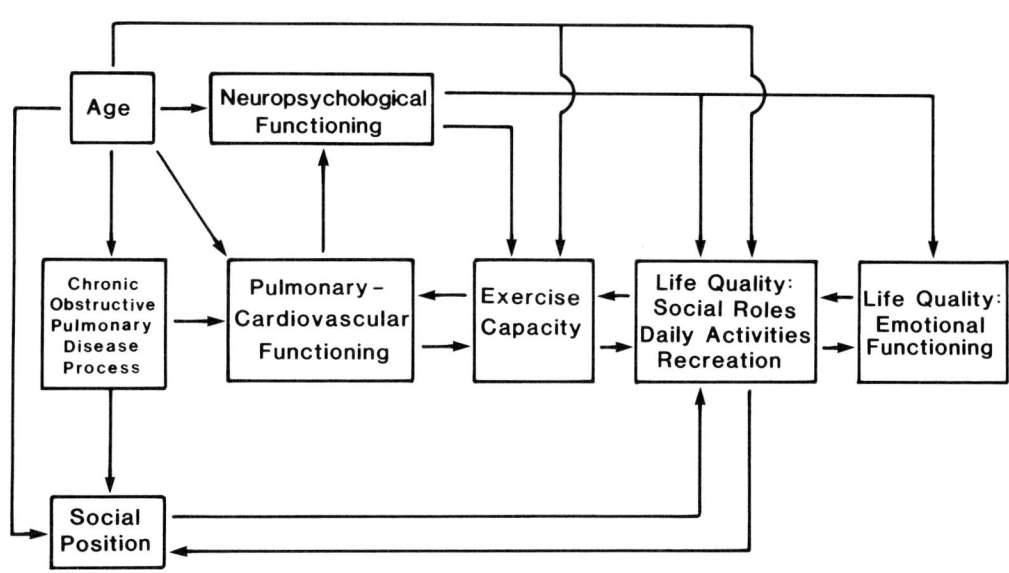

FIGURE 7–6. Heuristic model for the interrelation of COPD and other variables affecting life quality. (From McSweeny AJ, Grant I, Heaton RK, et al. Life quality of patients with chronic obstructive pulmonary disease. Arch Intern Med 1982; 142:477. Copyright 1982, American Medical Association.)

The interaction of aging, hypoxia, and acetylcholine release is an area that requires further attention.[56] Acetylcholine has been implicated in cognitive functions, particularly memory.[55] Results have also indicated that alterations in acetylcholine, dopamine, and glutamate metabolism accompany hypoxia, thiamine deficiency, and aging, which in turn affect motor performance and cognitive function.[56] Understanding the interactions among neurotransmitter mechanisms, hypoxia, and aging will "increase the possibility of developing better treatments for the multiple neurotransmitter deficiencies that accompany many metabolic, age-related, and chronic degenerative disorders."[56]

CLINICAL IMPLICATIONS OF NEUROPSYCHOLOGIC DEFICITS IN PATIENTS WITH CHRONIC OBSTRUCTIVE PULMONARY DISEASE

Patients with hypoxemic COPD display impairments in neurocognitive functioning and life quality in addition to their obvious cardiopulmonary abnormalities.[15-18, 20, 22-26] Many COPD patients display considerable neuropsychologic impairment in certain areas despite average verbal intellectual skills and the absence of any overt brain dysfunction.[24] As a result, referral for comprehensive neuropsychologic evaluation is recommended for COPD patients who (1) are elderly; (2) are experiencing difficulty with everyday functioning (e.g., vocational demands and interpersonal relationships); (3) are forgetful; (4) exhibit signs of psychomotor agitation; (5) display reduced PaO_2 levels; and (6) have concomitant medical disorders.

These neuropsychologic results are clinically important in that some patients may not be able to adhere accurately to rehabilitation programs (particularly to those programs that are complex or presented in an ambiguous fashion[18]) because of neuropsychologic deficits in abstraction and cognitive flexibility. Clinicians may experience increased compliance and success rates if they present treatment programs in a clear, straightforward, patient, and supportive manner.[18] Other relative weaknesses in the areas of complex perception and motor function integration and simple motor skills may manifest themselves in the form of psychomotor disturbance.

However, COPD patients do have some relative strengths that may help them cope with their illness. Memory and verbal skills, for example, appear to be relatively spared. The implications of these strengths are that COPD patients most likely are able to remember simple instructions concerning their treatment regimen and are able to communicate.[24] It can also be helpful for clinicians to explain the nature and severity of the neuropsychologic deficits to a patient's spouse and family members. This can help in their understanding the behavioral disturbances that are common in COPD patients and what compensatory and external support measures can be taken to maximize the patient's everyday functioning.[18] Finally, by taking into account each patient's unique expression of adaptive strengths and weaknesses, individually tailored rehabilitation regimens showing the greatest promise for success can be formulated and implemented.[57]

Further research is needed to investigate the underlying nature of the neurocognitive and life quality deficits in COPD patients and the relationship of these deficits to medical parameters. A delineation of the natural history of neuropsychologic functioning in COPD patients may help to explain the underlying mechanisms that may be involved and, subsequently, to indicate the most effective modes of intervention. Finally, oxygen supplementation, whether continuous or nocturnal, improves neurocognitive functioning. However, further study is needed to address the short-term and long-term effects of oxygen treatment on neuropsychologic functioning and the extent to which the neurocognitive improvements influence the life quality of COPD patients and their ability to comply with treatment regimens.

REFERENCES

1. Heaton RK, Pendleton MG. Use of neuropsychological tests to predict adult patients' everyday functioning. J Consult Clin Psychol 1981; 49:807–821.
2. McSweeny AJ, Grant I, Heaton RK, et al. Relationship of neuropsychological status to everyday functioning in healthy and chronically ill persons. J Clin Exp Neuropsychol 1985; 7:281–291.
3. Rourke BP, Bakker DJ, Fisk JL, Strang JD. Child Neuropsychology: An Introduction to Theory, Research, and Clinical Practice. New York: Guilford Press, 1983, p 112.
4. Lezak MD. Neuropsychological Assessment. 2nd ed. New York: Oxford University Press, Inc., 1983.
5. Grant I, Adams KM. Neuropsychological Assessment of Neuropsychiatric Disorders. New York: Oxford University Press, Inc., 1986, pp 3–86.
6. Reitan RM. Theoretical and methodological bases of the Halstead-Reitan Neuropsychological Test Battery. In: Grant I, Adams KM (eds). Neuropsychological Assessment of Neuropsychiatric Disorders. New York: Oxford University Press, Inc., 1986, pp 3–30.
7. Reitan RM, Wolfson D. The Halstead-Reitan Neuropsychological Test Battery: Theory and Clinical Interpretation. Tucson: Neuropsychology Press, 1985.
8. Heaton RK, Grant I, Matthews CG. Comprehensive Norms for an Expanded Halstead-Reitan Battery: Demographic Corrections, Research Findings, and Clinical Applications. Odessa, Florida: Psychological Assessment Resources, 1991.
9. Gibson GE, Pulsinelli W, Blass JP, Duffy TE. Brain dysfunction in mild to moderate hypoxia. Am J Med 1981; 70:1247–1253.
10. Townes BD, Hornbein TF, Schoene RB, et al. Human cerebral function at extreme altitude. In: West JB, Hahiri S (eds). High Altitude and Man. Bethesda, MD: American Physiological Society, 1984, pp 31–36.
11. Clark CF, Heaton RK, Wiens AN. Neuropsychological functioning after prolonged high-altitude exposure in mountaineering. Aviat Space Environ Med 1983; 54:202–207.
12. Cavaletti G, Garavaglia P, Arrigoni G, Tredici G. Persistent memory impairment after high altitude climbing. Int J Sports Med 1990; 11:176–178.
13. Flynn CF, Thompson TL. Effects of acute increases in altitude on mental status: Prevention and treatment. Psychosomatics 1990; 31:146–152.
14. Hornbein TF, Townes BD, Schoene RB, et al. The cost to the central nervous system of climbing to extremely high altitude. N Engl J Med 1989; 321:1714–1719.
15. Krop HD, Block AJ, Cohen E. Neuropsychologic effects of contin-

uous oxygen therapy in chronic obstructive pulmonary disease. Chest 1973; 64:317–322.
16. Nocturnal Oxygen Therapy Trial Group. Continuous or nocturnal oxygen therapy in hypoxemic chronic obstructive lung disease: A clinical trial. Ann Intern Med 1980; 93:391–398.
17. Intermittent Positive Pressure Breathing Trial Group. Intermittent positive pressure breathing therapy of chronic obstructive pulmonary disease: A clinical trial. Ann Intern Med 1983; 99:612–620.
18. Grant I, Heaton RK, McSweeny AJ, et al. Neuropsychologic findings in hypoxemic chronic obstructive pulmonary disease. Arch Intern Med 1982; 142:1470–1476.
19. Heaton RK, Grant I, Matthews CG. Differences in neuropsychological test performances associated with age, education, and sex. In: Grant I, Adams KM (eds). Neuropsychological Assessment of Neuropsychiatric Disorders. New York: Oxford University Press, Inc., 1986, pp 100–120.
20. McSweeny AJ, Grant I, Heaton RK, et al. Life quality of patients with chronic obstructive pulmonary disease. Arch Intern Med 1982; 142:473–478.
21. Heaton RK, Crowley TJ. Effects of psychiatric disorders and their somatic treatments on neuropsychological tests results. In: Filskov SB, Boll TJ (eds). Handbook of Clinical Neuropsychology. New York: John Wiley & Sons, Inc., 1981, pp 481–525.
22. Prigatano GP, Parsons O, Wright E, et al. Neuropsychological test performance in mildly hypoxemic patients with chronic obstructive pulmonary disease. J Consult Clin Psychol 1983; 51:108–116.
23. Prigatano GP, Wright EC, Levin D. Quality of life and its predictors in patients with mild hypoxemia and chronic obstructive pulmonary disease. Arch Intern Med 1984; 144:1613–1619.
24. Prigatano GP, Grant I. Neuropsychological correlates of COPD. In: McSweeny AJ, Grant I (eds). Chronic Obstructive Pulmonary Disease: A Behavioral Perspective. Vol 36. New York: Marcel Dekker, Inc., 1988, pp 39–57.
25. Grant I, Prigatano GP, Heaton RK, et al. Progressive neuropsychologic impairment and hypoxemia. Arch Gen Psychiatry 1987; 44:999–1006.
26. Heaton RK, Grant I, McSweeny AJ, et al. Psychologic effects of continuous and nocturnal oxygen therapy in hypoxemic chronic obstructive pulmonary disease. Arch Intern Med 1983; 143:1941–1947.
27. Report of the Medical Research Council Working Party. Long-term domiciliary oxygen therapy in chronic hypoxic cor pulmonale complicating chronic bronchitis and emphysema. Lancet 1981; 1:681–685.
28. Weitzenblum E, Sautegeau A, Ehrhart M, et al. Long-term oxygen therapy can reverse the progression of pulmonary hypertension in patients with chronic obstructive pulmonary disease. Am Rev Respir Dis 1985; 131:493–498.
29. Weitzenblum E, Oswald M, Mirhom R, et al. Evolution of pulmonary haemodynamics on COLD patients under long-term oxygen therapy. Eur Respir J 1989; 2:669S–673S.
30. Georgopoulos D, Anthonisen NR. Continuous oxygen therapy for the chronically hypoxemic patient. Ann Rev Med 1990; 41:223–230.
31. Wilson DK, Kaplan RM, Timms RM, Dawson A. Acute effects of oxygen treatment upon information processing in hypoxemic COPD patients. Chest 1985; 88:239–243.
32. Jacobs EA, Winter PM, Alvis HJ, Small SM. Hyperoxygenation effect on cognitive functioning in the aged. N Engl J Med 1969; 281:753–757.
33. Thompson LW, Davis GC, Obrist WD, Heyman A. Effects of hyperbaric oxygen on behavioral and physiological measures in elderly demented patients. J Gerontol 1976; 31:23–28.
34. Block AJ, Boysen PG, Wynne JW, Hunt LA. Sleep apnea, hypopnea, and oxygen desaturation in normal subjects: A strong male predominance. N Engl J Med 1979; 300:513–517.
35. Block AJ, Berry D, Webb W. Nocturnal hypoxemia and neuropsychological deficits in men who snore. Eur J Respir Dis 1986; 69:405S–408S.
36. Berry DTR, Webb WB, Block AJ, et al. Nocturnal hypoxia and neuropsychological variables. J Clin Exp Neuropsychol 1986; 8:229–238.
37. Block AJ, Hellard DW, Cicale MJ. Snoring, nocturnal hypoxemia, and the effect of oxygen inhalation. Chest 1987; 92:411–417.
38. Block AJ, Hellard DW, Switzer DA. Nocturnal oxygen therapy does not improve snorers' intelligence. Chest 1989; 95:274–278.
39. Greenberg GD, Watson RK, Deptula D. Neuropsychological dysfunction in sleep apnea. Sleep 1987; 10:254–262.
40. Findley LJ, Barth JT, Powers DC, et al. Cognitive impairment in patients with obstructive sleep apnea and associated hypoxemia. Chest 1986; 90:686–690.
41. Fletcher EC, Miller J, Divine GW, et al. Nocturnal oxyhemoglobin desaturation in COPD patients with arterial oxygen tensions above 60 mm Hg. Chest 1987; 92:604–608.
42. Levi-Valensi P, Aubry P, Rida Z. Nocturnal hypoxemia and long-term oxygen therapy in COPD patients with daytime Pao_2 60–70 mmHg. Lung 1990; 168 Suppl:770–775.
43. Stradling JR, Lane DJ. Nocturnal hypoxaemia in chronic obstructive pulmonary disease. Clin Sci 1983; 64:213–222.
44. Bradley TD, Mateika J, Li D, et al. Daytime hypercapnia in the development of nocturnal hypoxemia in COPD. Chest 1990; 97:308–312.
45. Tiep BL. Long-term home oxygen therapy. Clin Chest Med 1990; 11:505–521.
46. Flenley DC. Long-term home oxygen therapy. Chest 1985; 87:99–103.
47. Flenley DC. Sleep in chronic obstructive lung disease. Clin Chest Med 1985; 6:651–661.
48. Fletcher EC, Luckett RA, Miller T, et al. Pulmonary vascular hemodynamics in chronic lung disease patients with and without oxyhemoglobin desaturation during sleep. Chest 1989; 95:157–166.
49. Martin RJ. The sleep-related worsening of lower airways obstruction: Understanding and intervention. Med Clin North Am 1990; 74:701–714.
50. Douglas NJ, Calverley PMA, Leggett RJE, et al. Transient hypoxemia during sleep in chronic bronchitis and emphysema. Lancet 1979; 1:1–4.
51. Prigatano GP, Parsons OA. Relationship of age and education to Halstead Test performance in different patient populations. J Consult Clin Psychol 1976; 44:527–533.
52. Siesjo BK, Johannson H, Ljunggren B, Norberg K. Brain dysfunction in cerebral hypoxia and ischemia. In: Plum F (ed). Brain Dysfunction in Metabolic Disorders. New York: Raven Press, 1974, pp 75–112.
53. Gibson GE, Pelmas CJ, Petersen C. Cholinergic drugs and 4-aminopyridine alter hypoxic-induced behavioral deficits. Pharmacol Biochem Behav 1983; 18:909–916.
54. Freeman GB, Nielsen P, Gibson GE. Behavioral and neurochemical correlates of morphine and hypoxia interactions. Pharmacol Biochem Behav 1986; 24:1687–1693.
55. Bartus RT, Dean RL, Beer B, Lippa AS. The cholinergic hypothesis of geriatric memory dysfunction. Science 1982; 217:408–417.
56. Freeman GB, Gibson GE. Dopamine, acetylcholine, and glutamate interactions in aging. Ann N Y Acad Sci 1988; 515:191–202.
57. Greenberg GD, Ryan JJ, Bourlier PF. Psychological and neuropsychological aspects of COPD. Psychosomatics 1985; 26:29–33.

Chapter 8

Sleep Disordered Breathing

NEIL J. DOUGLAS, M.D., F.R.C.P.E.

Over 30 years ago, Robin reported that in seven patients with "emphysema and chronic hypercapnia," "alveolar" carbon dioxide tension increased by 10 mm Hg during sleep and that four of these patients exhibited Cheyne-Stokes respiration during sleep.[1, 2] Subsequent studies using an early ear oximeter[3] demonstrated that arterial oxygen saturation decreased in all the chronic obstructive pulmonary disease (COPD) patients studied during sleep. It was noted that the lowest saturations during sleep were recorded in those patients whose saturations were lowest when they were awake. These findings were confirmed and extended by the measurement of arterial blood gas tension in sleeping patients with COPD.[4] Later studies with electroencephalographic sleep staging demonstrated that the most severe hypoxemia and hypercapnia occurred during rapid eye movement (REM) sleep.[5-7]

The development of accurate oximeters has made possible the continuous measurement of overnight arterial oxygenation in patients with COPD. Douglas and colleagues[8] found that 23 of 28 episodes in which arterial oxygen saturation decreased by at least 10% occurred during REM sleep (Fig. 8–1); they also observed that during these episodes arterial oxygen tension dropped to as low as 26 mm Hg. These observations have subsequently been widely confirmed. They show that patients with COPD become hypoxemic during sleep and that the hypoxemia is most severe during REM sleep.[9-13] Hypoxemia during REM sleep in these patients is more severe during episodes when there are frequent eye movements (Fig. 8–2).[11, 14] During such hypoxemic episodes, arterial carbon dioxide tension increases, although the additional elevation in carbon dioxide tension is usually relatively small.[5, 6, 8, 15]

MECHANISMS OF HYPOXEMIA DURING SLEEP IN CHRONIC OBSTRUCTIVE PULMONARY DISEASE

The major factor causing REM hypoxemia in patients with COPD is hypoventilation, but a reduction in functional residual capacity and alterations in ventilation/perfusion matching also contribute to this phenomenon.

Hypoventilation

In normal subjects, ventilation during all sleep stages is reduced compared to that during wakefulness[16]; the same is true for patients with COPD.[13] The decrease in ventilation from wakefulness to non-REM sleep is relatively small, but during REM sleep intermittent marked hypoventilation occurs.[16] Such hypoventilation is most severe during periods of intense eye movements,[17-19] when tidal volume markedly decreases.

The typical desaturation occurring during REM sleep in patients with COPD (Fig. 8–3) is associated with hypoventilation and not with apneas.[11-14, 20] Although ventilation has not been accurately measured during sleep in COPD patients, surface measurements have shown that their breathing pattern during REM sleep is similar to that in normal subjects.[12] It has been estimated that alveolar ventilation during REM sleep in normal subjects is only about 60% of that during wakefulness.[16, 18] As patients with COPD have elevated physiologic dead spaces, the rapid shallow breathing that occurs during REM sleep produces an even greater

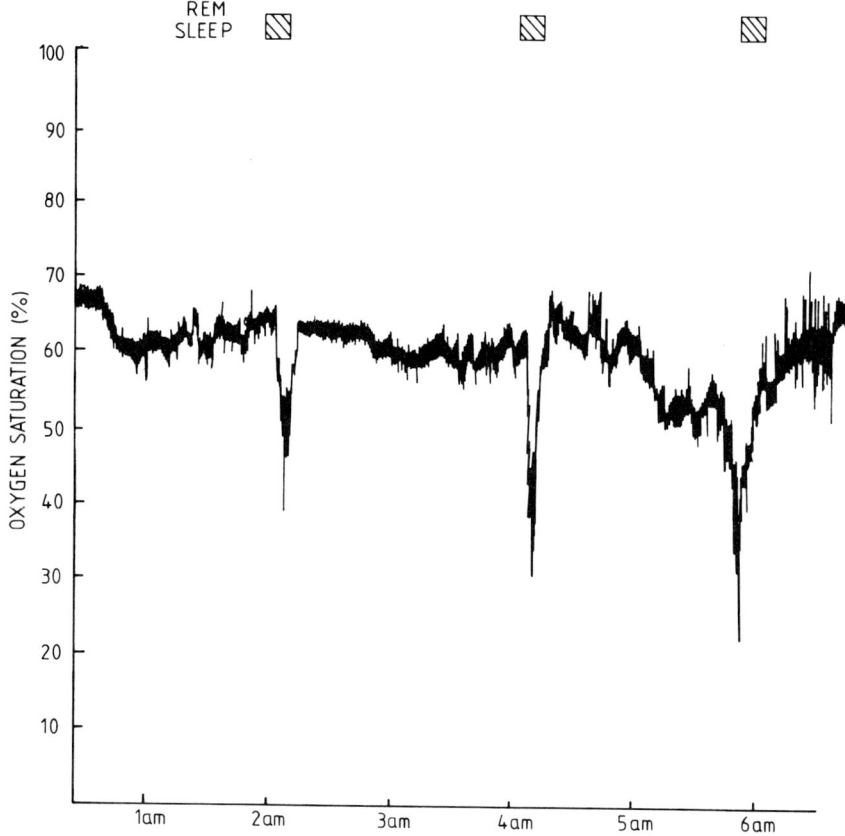

FIGURE 8–1. Oxygen saturation throughout the night in a patient with COPD. The *shaded areas* represent rapid eye movement (REM) sleep.

decrease in alveolar ventilation, which could account for all the hypoxemia observed in patients with COPD.[21]

Hypoventilation occurring during sleep has multiple causes. During non-REM sleep, ventilation in normal subjects decreases, despite an increase in occlusion pressure.[22, 23] This suggests that non-REM sleep hypoventilation may be partially caused by the increase in upper airways resistance that occurs during non-REM sleep.[24, 25] This effect is more pronounced as the ventilatory response to added resistance is impaired during non-REM sleep.[23, 26]

The increase in upper airways resistance is unlikely to

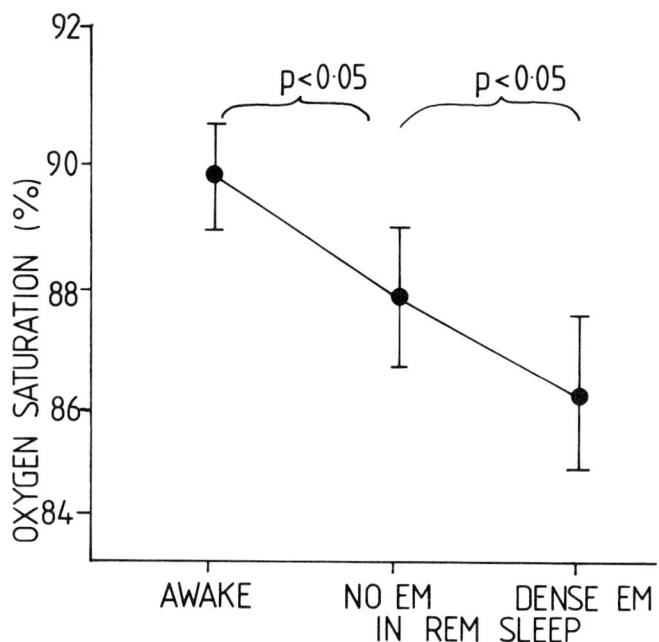

FIGURE 8–2. The effect of sleep stage on oxygen saturation in 18 patients with COPD. REM sleep is divided into periods with no eye movements (no EM) or periods with frequent eye movements (dense EM). (Data from George CF, West P, Kryger MH. Oxygenation and breathing pattern during phasic and tonic REM in patients with chronic obstructive pulmonary disease. Sleep 1987; 10:234–243.)

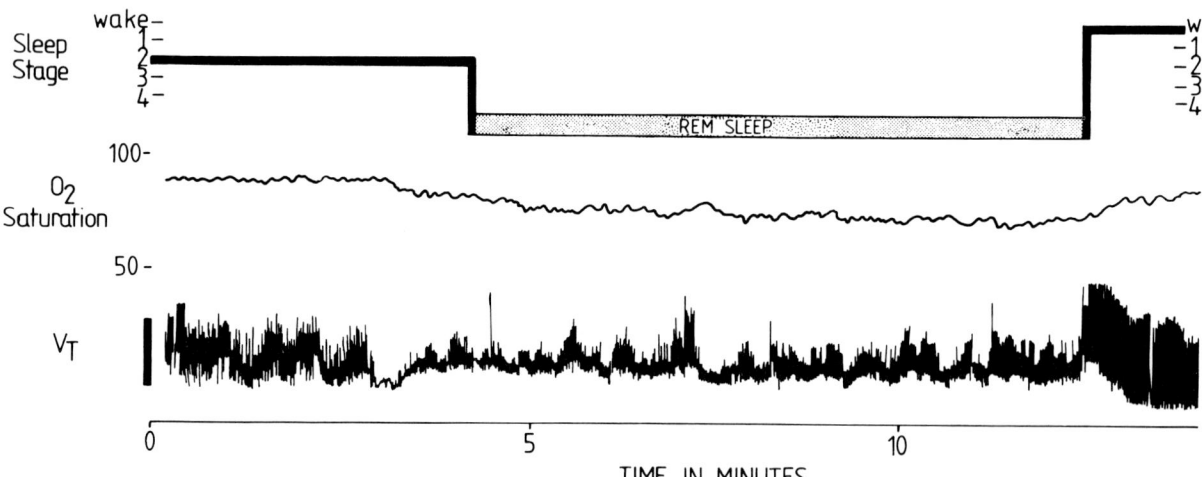

FIGURE 8–3. Changes in oxygen saturation and tidal volume (VT) in a patient with COPD during an episode of REM sleep. (Data from Fletcher EC, Gray BA, Levin DC. Non-apneic mechanisms of arterial oxygen desaturation during rapid-eye movement sleep. J Appl Physiol 1983; 54:632–639.)

be a major factor in the additional hypoventilation and hypoxemia of REM sleep because upper airways resistance is no greater in REM sleep than it is in non-REM sleep, at least in normal subjects.[25] Furthermore, although relatively few measurements have been made, the ventilatory response to added resistance appears to be similar in non-REM and REM sleep.[23, 26] During REM sleep, brain stem function in animals is altered by the phasic activity of respiratory neurons.[27] It seems likely that such diminution in respiratory output may be a major determinant of REM-related hypoventilation.

In addition, hypotonia of the intercostal muscles occurs during REM sleep[28]; this results in a reduction of the rib cage's contribution to ventilation.[19] In COPD patients with hyperinflation, this hypotonia has the further effect of "pulling in" the lower chest wall as the flattened diaphragm is contracted against a flaccid chest wall; this further decreases ventilation during REM sleep. This may explain why patients with COPD become relatively more hypoxemic during sleep than do patients with pulmonary fibrosis.[29] In addition, the "postural" hypotonia that occurs during REM sleep involves not only the intercostal muscles but also the accessory muscles of respiration,[30] which may be important in the maintenance of ventilation in patients with COPD.

A patient's normal defense mechanism in response to hypoxemia is to increase ventilation. However, during REM sleep, there is marked diminution of both the hypoxic[31, 32] and the hypercapnic[33, 34] ventilatory responses. This, therefore, permits REM hypoxemia to occur.

Decrease in Functional Residual Capacity

Functional residual capacity decreases during REM sleep in normal subjects.[25] Similar changes probably also occur in patients with COPD, although the only study of this that has been performed[13] used surface inductive plethysmography, which may not be quantitatively accurate when used during patient sleep.[35]

Ventilation/Perfusion Imbalance

Many investigators have claimed to show that ventilation/perfusion ($\dot{V}/\dot{Q}$) imbalance is a major cause of REM hypoxemia in patients with COPD.[5, 6, 20] However, the data on which this assumption is based depend largely on the existence of a steady state of gas transfer that does not occur during REM hypoxemia in COPD.[21] Nevertheless, the marked hypoventilation of REM sleep must be accompanied by an alteration in $\dot{V}/\dot{Q}$ matching; this is supported by the observation that cardiac output is maintained during episodes of hypoventilation, which in turn indicates changes in global $\dot{V}/\dot{Q}$ matching.[20, 21] However, current technology does not allow the relative importance of $\dot{V}/\dot{Q}$ matching changes to be assessed during this unsteady state.

Chronic Obstructive Pulmonary Disease Combined with the Sleep Apnea/Hypopnea Syndrome

Both COPD and the sleep apnea/hypopnea syndrome (SAHS) are relatively common conditions.[36–38] Thus, it is likely that the two conditions coexist in some patients by chance alone. The two conditions do coexist in some patients,[39–41] but studies performed in patients who were referred to respiratory clinics have not revealed any greater frequency of SAHS in patients with COPD than that which occurs in the normal population.[10–14]

Mechanisms of Hypoxemia During Sleep in Chronic Obstructive Pulmonary Disease: Conclusions

Hypoventilation is a major cause of hypoxemia during REM sleep in patients with COPD. In addition, the impairment of V̇/Q̇ matching and probably a reduction in functional residual capacity also contribute to this condition. In a small minority of patients with COPD, there may also be coexisting SAHS.

CONSEQUENCES OF HYPOXEMIA DURING SLEEP IN CHRONIC OBSTRUCTIVE PULMONARY DISEASE

REM hypoxemia produces a significant cardiovascular and neurophysiologic effect in patients with COPD and may also have hematologic effects. In addition, REM hypoxemia may contribute to nocturnal death.

Cardiac Dysrhythmias

Patients with COPD have an increased ventricular ectopic frequency during sleep.[42] However, in one study, no overall relationship between ventricular ectopic frequency and oxygen saturation was observed in 42 COPD patients, but ventricular ectopic frequency could be related to nocturnal oxygen saturation in 6 of the 20 patients in whom oxygen saturation decreased below 80%.[43] Flick and Block observed an insignificant tendency for nocturnal oxygen therapy to reduce ectopic frequency in their patients.[42] There is no evidence that such ventricular ectopic beats during sleep are of clinical importance.

Hemodynamics

Pulmonary arterial pressure increases during REM sleep as oxygenation decreases.[7, 8, 44] For example, Coccagna and Lugaresi[7] observed in 12 patients with COPD that mean pulmonary arterial pressure increased from 37 to 55 mm Hg during REM sleep, whereas the arterial oxygen tension decreased from 56 to 43 mm Hg. Boysen and colleagues[44] observed a close inverse correlation between oxygen saturation and mean pulmonary arterial pressure, and although the data were widely scattered, on average a 1% decrease in arterial oxygen saturation (SaO_2) resulted in a 1 mm Hg increase in pulmonary arterial pressure. During these REM hypoxemic episodes, cardiac output increases little if at all.[20, 21] The clinical significance of these episodes of pulmonary arterial pressure elevation is unknown. However, in rats, intermittent hypoxemia that was induced by breathing a 12% oxygen mixture for as little as 2 hours each day for 4 weeks significantly elevated right ventricular mass (Fig. 8–4).[45] It therefore seems possible that the intermittent REM hypoxemia observed in patients with COPD may have a similar effect on the human myocardium. Two studies have suggested that REM sleep hypoxemia in COPD may have effects similar to those of maximum exercise on the myocardium when it was assessed either in terms of myocardial oxygen consumption[46] or left ventricular ejection.[47]

A recent study compared pulmonary hemodynamics

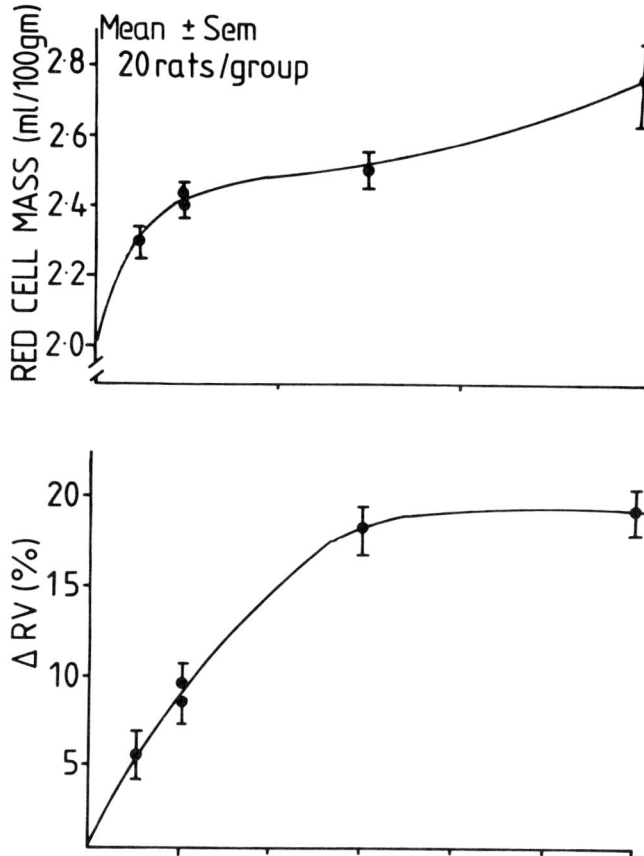

FIGURE 8–4. Percentage change in right ventricular mass (ΔRV%) and changes in red cell mass in rats spending the number of hours per day indicated over a 28-day period breathing a 12% oxygen mixture. The *two points* at the 4-hour time point represent results obtained in rats spending a single 4-hour period and rats spending eight 30-minute periods per day breathing a 12% oxygen mixture; the latter group of rats was used to simulate transient sleep hypoxemia. (Data from Moore-Gillon JC, Cameron IR. Right ventricular hypertrophy and polycythemia in rats after intermittent exposure to hypoxia. Clin Sci 1985; 69:595–599.)

in 36 patients with COPD who desaturated at night to at least 85% (with more than 5 min spent below 90%) in contrast to those in 30 patients who did not desaturate.[48] Those with such nocturnal desaturation had significantly higher daytime pulmonary arterial pressures and red blood cell masses than those who did not desaturate. Although the nocturnal hypoxemia may have produced these consequences, the nocturnal desaturators also had significantly lower daytime oxygenation levels, which could account for the hemodynamic and hematologic differences.

Polycythemia

Intermittent hypoxemia in rats results in the elevation of red blood cell mass (see Fig. 8–4).[45] Thus, the nocturnal desaturation that occurs in patients with COPD may also stimulate erythropoiesis. Morning erythropoietin levels have been found to be elevated in some patients with COPD.[49, 50] A recent preliminary report has suggested that patients whose oxygen saturation levels decrease below 60% at night may have progressive nocturnal increases in serum erythropoietin levels[51] but that more minor degrees of hypoxemia are not associated with a measurable elevation of erythropoietin concentrations.

Quality of Sleep

Both symptomatic inquiry[52] and objective assessment using polysomnography[12, 53–55] have shown that patients with COPD sleep poorly in comparison with normal subjects. Although arousal from sleep is common during episodes of desaturation,[54] the extent of sleep disruption appears to be at least as great in nondesaturating patients with COPD.[55] Despite the subjective and objective evidence of poor sleep quality, there is no evidence of objective daytime sleepiness in patients with COPD as assessed by the multiple sleep latency test.[56]

Death During Sleep in Chronic Obstructive Pulmonary Disease

Patients with COPD die more often at night than do age-matched controls, and death at night was found to be particularly common in COPD patients with hypoxemia and carbon dioxide retention.[57] In hypoxemic patients with COPD, nocturnal death is more common in those breathing air than in those receiving nocturnal oxygen therapy.[58] However, care must be taken not to equate nocturnal death with death during sleep.

Consequences of Chronic Obstructive Pulmonary Disease Combined with Sleep Apnea/Hypopnea Syndrome

Patients who have both COPD and SAHS are more likely to develop pulmonary hypertension,[59] failure of the right side of the heart,[40, 60] and carbon dioxide retention[61] than are patients with SAHS alone. This is probably because they have two causes for nocturnal hypoxemia, which together result in more severe nocturnal hypoxemia than would occur if they had only one of these conditions.

PREDICTION OF NOCTURNAL OXYGENATION

Trask and Cree[3] first observed in 1962 that the patients with COPD who were most hypoxemic when awake were those who became most hypoxemic during sleep. Since 1962 this has been widely confirmed by others.[12, 62, 63] Several equations have been derived to predict the extent of nocturnal hypoxemia. However, although all are statistically significant,[12, 62, 63] their clinical significance is limited because there is marked scatter around the regression lines,[63] especially in the most hypoxemic patients (Fig. 8–5). However, the derivation of such equations shows that the extent of nocturnal hypoxemia is related not only to daytime oxygenation but also to daytime arterial carbon dioxide tension[62, 63] and to the duration of REM sleep.[63]

There has been considerable attention devoted to so-called "nocturnal desaturators." Of 152 COPD patients with a daytime arterial oxygen tension of greater than 50 mm Hg, Fletcher and colleagues observed that 41 desaturated during sleep. They defined desaturation arbitrarily as the presence of oxygen saturation below 90% for at least 5 minutes and of a trough saturation of 85% or lower.[64] "Nocturnal desaturators" could not be distinguished from the nondesaturators by the results of respiratory function testing or by their symptoms. However, their mean arterial oxygen tension when awake was significantly lower (70 versus 76 mm Hg, respectively) and their arterial carbon dioxide tension was higher (41 versus 38 mm Hg, respectively) than those in patients who did not desaturate. Thus, this group of

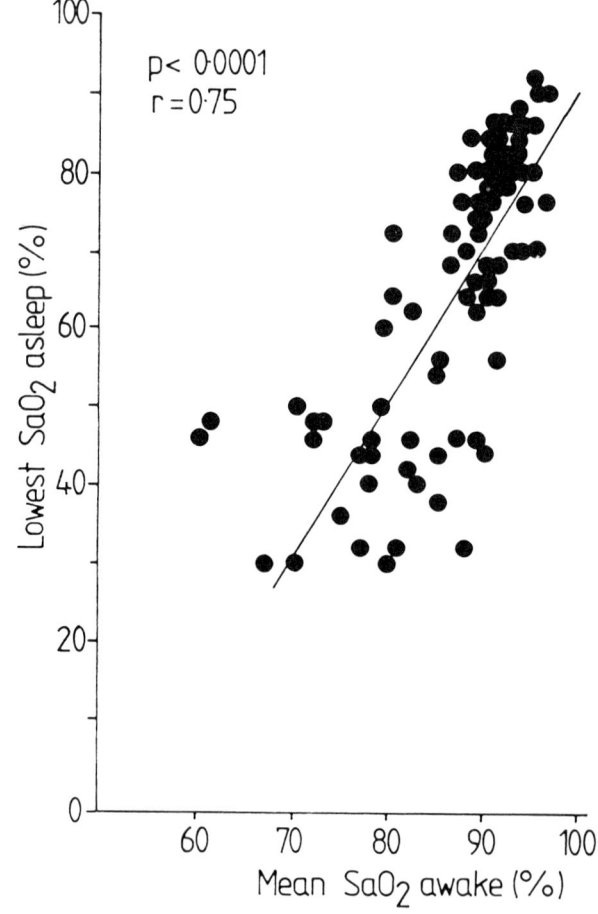

FIGURE 8–5. Relationship between mean oxygen saturation (SaO_2) during wakefulness and lowest nocturnal oxygenation during sleep in 97 patients with severe COPD. (Data from Connaughton JJ, Catterall JR, Elton RA, et al. Do sleep studies contribute to the management of patients with severe chronic obstructive pulmonary disease? Am Rev Respir Dis 1988; 138:341–345.)

patients would be expected to desaturate more readily than the remainder on the basis of the previously discussed regression relationships.[12, 62, 63] It remains to be proved whether this extent of nocturnal desaturation is of clinical importance, although one study showing no elevation of erythropoietin level in the presence of such minor desaturation casts doubt on its significance.[51]

CLINICAL VALUE OF STUDIES OF BREATHING AND OXYGENATION DURING SLEEP IN PATIENTS WITH CHRONIC OBSTRUCTIVE PULMONARY DISEASE

Performing polysomnography in patients with COPD could theoretically be of benefit as it might detect unsuspected SAHS by identifying clinically important excess hypoxemia during sleep in some patients or by guiding the selection of those patients who might benefit from nocturnal oxygen therapy. It might also be of use in determining what oxygen concentrations such patients should inspire at night. The latter two roles are discussed in the section on treatment.

Although no large population studies have been carried out, there is no evidence thus far to support that the prevalence of SAHS is greater in patients with COPD.[12] Current evidence suggests that when SAHS coexists with COPD, the typical symptoms of SAHS[65, 66] are present. It also suggests that sleep studies do not yield unsuspected cases of SAHS.[12, 63] Thus, the symptoms of SAHS should be sought in all patients with COPD, and, if major symptoms occur, clinical sleep studies should be performed.

Oxygenation during sleep can be predicted based on arterial blood gas tensions measured when patients are awake.[12, 63] However, such predictions produce considerable unexplained residual variance, the clinical significance of which is unclear. It has been claimed that measurements of nocturnal oxygenation in such patients can be a useful guide to treatment.[67] To establish the clinical importance of this variability among patients in the extent of sleep-related hypoxemia, Connaughton and colleagues[63] studied the relationship between nocturnal oxygen saturation and survival in 97 patients with COPD. Both mean nocturnal SaO_2 and the lowest SaO_2 during sleep were significantly related to survival, that is, the lower the level of nocturnal oxygenation, the worse the prognosis. However, neither nocturnal measure significantly improved the prediction of survival that could be obtained from the easier and cheaper measurements of oxygenation or vital capacity when patients are awake.[63]

These data were also analyzed to determine the significance of the scatter around the regression relationship between measurements of oxygen saturation and $PaCO_2$ taken when patients are awake with measures of oxygen saturation recorded during sleep. Those patients who had excess nocturnal hypoxemia—that is, those whose SaO_2 during sleep was lower than predicted from SaO_2 and $PaCO_2$ during wakefulness—had survival rates at a median of 70 months similar to those who became less hypoxemic at night relative to their oxygenation level and $PaCO_2$ when awake (Fig. 8–6). Therefore, there seems to be no clinical value in performing routine polysomnography in patients with COPD. It is this author's opinion that clinical sleep studies are currently indicated only in patients with COPD who are suspected of having SAHS based on suggestive symptoms or in those who have cor pulmonale or polycythemia and whose daytime arterial oxygen tension is greater than 60 mm Hg. In such patients, a complete polysomno-

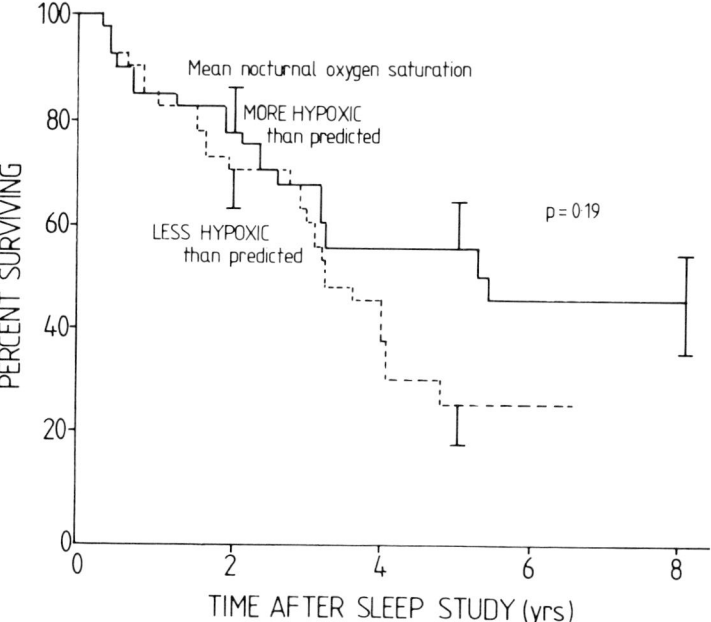

FIGURE 8–6. Effect of nocturnal oxygenation on survival in 66 patients with COPD. The survival of those who were less hypoxic than predicted and those more hypoxic than predicted is indicated from the regression equation between oxygen saturation during wakefulness and mean nocturnal oxygen saturation. (Reproduced from Connaughton JJ, Catterall JR, Elton RA, et al. Do sleep studies contribute to the management of patients with severe chronic obstructive pulmonary disease? Am Rev Respir Dis 1988; 138:341–345.)

graphic study is indicated because overnight oximetry alone can be very difficult to interpret in patients who are already hypoxemic when awake.

TREATMENT OF NOCTURNAL HYPOXEMIA IN CHRONIC OBSTRUCTIVE PULMONARY DISEASE

Oxygen Therapy

Nocturnal oxygen therapy improves oxygenation during sleep in patients with COPD,[8, 54, 68] although some degree of nocturnal desaturation still occurs, particularly during REM sleep. Occasionally, patients experience symptomatic carbon dioxide retention as a result of nocturnal oxygen therapy; this usually is manifested as morning headaches. Carbon dioxide retention may be a particular problem in patients with coexisting SAHS.[68]

The patients who become markedly hypoxemic at night are those who are already hypoxemic during the daytime.[63] Domiciliary oxygen therapy remains the only treatment that has been shown in controlled clinical trials to prolong life in such hypoxemic patients with COPD.[69, 70] As the period of oxygen administration always includes nighttime hours, it is tempting to assume that at least part of the benefit of oxygen therapy is due to a reduction in pulmonary arterial pressure elevation during REM sleep.[71]

In both the Nocturnal Oxygen Therapy Trial[69] and the British Medical Research Council[70] study, the choice of inspired oxygen concentration was entirely guided by daytime measures of oxygenation. There is no information available that can indicate the level of nocturnal oxygenation required to optimize survival. Thus, there is at present no routine place for studies of breathing and oxygenation during sleep in patients who are commencing oxygen therapy. Some researchers have suggested that such studies should be performed to ensure that a particular oxygen saturation is achieved throughout the night. However, this situation might need to be reviewed as further evidence becomes available. The only group in which this author believes polysomnography should be performed to evaluate oxygen therapy consists of those patients receiving oxygen who develop morning headaches, as this may indicate coexisting SAHS.[68]

Some[53, 68] but not all researchers[54, 72] have found that the correction of nocturnal hypoxemia improves sleep quality in patients with COPD. This disparity may have resulted from the differing severities of daytime hypoxemia and also from those studies[54, 68] that did not randomize the sequence of nights during which oxygen or air was administered and that did not employ a familiarization night. It seems likely that severely hypoxemic patients with COPD do sleep better when they are administered nocturnal oxygen therapy, although a carefully designed randomized study of a large number of patients is needed to test this hypothesis.

Almitrine

Almitrine is an investigational drug that raises arterial oxygen tension in patients with COPD. In a randomized double-blind study, a 2-week treatment course of almitrine administered in a dose of 50 mg twice daily improved oxygenation during sleep in patients with COPD but did not alter sleep quality.[73] Subsequent studies have confirmed that almitrine improves nocturnal oxygenation after 2 weeks[74] and also after 1 year.[75]

It was hoped that the combination of almitrine and nocturnal oxygen therapy might produce greater improvements in oxygenation and in the pressure of the right side of the heart than the use of either agent alone. However, this hope has not been fulfilled. No additional significant benefit in nocturnal oxygenation has been observed when the two treatments are combined. Similarly, there is no tendency for pulmonary arterial pressure to be higher when almitrine and oxygen therapy are combined than when oxygen alone is given.[76]

Further work is required before the role of almitrine can be established. Both the dosage used[77] and the importance of the peripheral neuropathy that can result from its use are yet to be defined.

Protriptyline

In an uncontrolled trial, Series and coworkers[78] recently reported that the administration of 20 mg of protriptyline daily improved nocturnal oxygenation in 11 patients with COPD. The observed improvement appeared to result from the suppression of REM sleep. However, all patients experienced mouth dryness, and 6 of the 11 had dysuria. A nonrandomized, nonblinded trial[79] suggests that protriptyline may improve daytime arterial oxygen and carbon dioxide tensions in patients with COPD, but side effects were again common and resulted in the discontinuation of therapy in 4 of the 14 patients within 10 weeks.

Medroxyprogesterone Acetate

Skatrud and associates[11] reported that medroxyprogesterone acetate improved arterial oxygen tension and reduced arterial carbon dioxide tension during both wakefulness and non-REM sleep in 5 of 17 hypercapnic patients with COPD. However, others found no significant change in the lowest oxygen saturation during sleep in 19 patients with COPD who were administered the drug in a double-blind placebo-controlled trial.[80] In addition, medroxyprogesterone acetate may cause troublesome side effects, including impotence in many male patients.

Acetazolamide

In five patients with hypercapnic COPD, acetazolamide improved both arterial oxygen tension during wakefulness and nocturnal oxygenation but did not alter arterial Pco_2 during sleep in two of the five patients.[81] However, the side effects of paresthesia, nephrolithiasis, and acidosis may limit the acceptability of acetazolamide.

Theophylline

The infusion of intravenous theophylline did not improve overnight oxygenation in 11 patients with COPD.[82]

Negative-Pressure Ventilation

Negative-pressure ventilation has been reported to reduce arterial carbon dioxide tension and to increase respiratory muscle strength in some patients with COPD.[83, 84] However, negative-pressure ventilation may result in the closure of the upper airways, as was observed in a study of five normal men in whom negative-pressure ventilation resulted in an increase in the number of apnea and in the impairment of sleep quality.[85] Thus, the value of using this technique in many patients with COPD is doubtful.

Intermittent Positive-Pressure Ventilation via Nasal Mask

Nocturnal intermittent positive-pressure ventilation via a nasal mask was originally developed for use in patients with kyphoscoliosis or neuromuscular disorders.[86–89] Some patients with COPD find this technique acceptable, and it has the added theoretical advantage over long-term oxygen therapy of reducing hypercapnia. However, there are relatively few data available on the use of nasal intermittent positive-pressure ventilation in patients with COPD. Carroll and Branthwaite[88] studied three patients with COPD who had rejected domiciliary oxygen therapy because of the limitation it imposed on their lifestyles as well as a fourth patient who had developed symptomatic hypercapnia when administered nocturnal oxygen therapy. These four patients tolerated nasal intermittent positive-pressure ventilation well in the medium term, but long-term data and data on the effect of nasal intermittent positive-pressure ventilation on survival in such patients are required before this promising technique can be widely advocated as a therapy of choice.

Hypnotics

Hypnotics are often used to treat sleep disturbance in patients with COPD. However, they should not be used in hypercapnic patients as they might further inhibit ventilatory responses and precipitate acute or chronic ventilatory failure. Benzodiazepines have been observed to increase sleep duration in some[90–92] but not all[93] studies

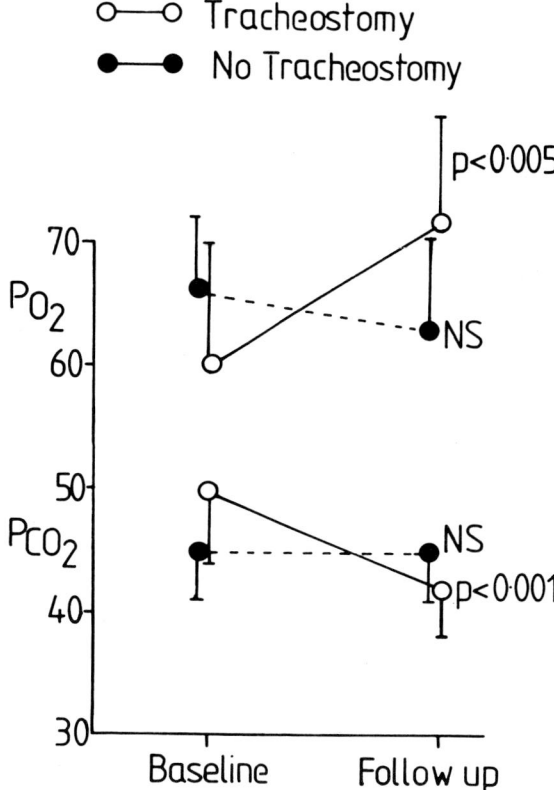

FIGURE 8–7. Arterial oxygen and carbon dioxide tensions during the daytime in two groups of patients who had both COPD and the sleep apnea/hypopnea syndrome. In those who accepted tracheostomy, arterial blood gas tensions improved at follow-up. However, there was no such change in those who declined tracheostomy (NS: not significant). (Data from Fletcher EC, Schaaf JW, Miller J, et al. Long-term cardiopulmonary sequelae in patients with sleep apnea and chronic lung disease. Am Rev Respir Dis 1987; 135:525–533.)

performed on normocapnic patients with COPD, but the frequency and severity of desaturation did increase in patients in one study.[90] Thus, even in normocapnic patients, hypnotics should only be used with great caution.

Alcohol

Alcohol ingestion before sleep may worsen nocturnal hypoxemia[94] and ventricular ectopic frequency[95] in COPD patients. Recent evidence suggests that heavy alcohol consumption by COPD patients may result in hypercapnic respiratory failure[96] and in failure of the right side of the heart[97] as well as lead to an increase in hypopneas and desaturation during sleep.[96] These data require further analysis; in particular, the interrelationship between excess alcohol consumption and body weight needs to be clarified. However, the two studies in combination do suggest that alcohol consumption should be discouraged in such patients. This may be particularly relevant to alcohol consumption in the evening, which has been clearly shown to contribute to the development of apneas and hypopneas during sleep.

Treatment of Chronic Obstructive Pulmonary Disease Combined with Sleep Apnea/Hypopnea Syndrome

There is little information concerning how to treat patients who have both COPD and SAHS. A nonrandomized study has shown that patients with both conditions improved their daytime arterial blood gas tensions (Fig. 8–7) and pulmonary arterial pressures only when SAHS was adequately treated (in this study by tracheostomy).[41] The patients who declined tracheostomy showed no such improvement, even though 9 of the 10 received domiciliary oxygen therapy. Thus, it is important to recognize coexisting SAHS in such patients and to treat it appropriately, usually by continuous positive airway pressure therapy with or without supplemental oxygen.

BREATHING DURING SLEEP IN CHRONIC OBSTRUCTIVE PULMONARY DISEASE: CONCLUSIONS

Patients with COPD become hypoxemic during sleep, particularly during REM sleep. The measurement of nocturnal hypoxemia and breathing patterns in individual patients does not provide prognostic information that might add significantly to more simple measurements of oxygenation and lung function that are made during wakefulness. A small minority of COPD patients may have concomitant SAHS, and any COPD patient with a history suggestive of SAHS should undergo a complete polysomnographic examination. Those found to have SAHS should be aggressively treated. Domiciliary oxygen therapy is the current treatment of choice in COPD patients who are hypoxemic during the day and night, although the roles of respiratory stimulants and of nasal intermittent positive-pressure ventilation may grow.

REFERENCES

1. Robin ED, Whaley RD, Crump CH, et al. The nature of the respiratory acidosis of sleep and of the respiratory alkalosis of hepatic comas (abstract). J Clin Invest 1957; 36:924.
2. Robin ED. Some interrelations between sleep and disease. Arch Intern Med 1958; 102:669–675.
3. Trask CH, Cree EM. Oximeter studies on patients with chronic obstructive emphysema, awake and during sleep. N Engl J Med 1962; 266:639–642.
4. Pierce AK, Jarrett CE, Werkle G, et al. Respiratory function during sleep in patients with chronic obstructive lung disease. J Clin Invest 1966; 45:631–636.
5. Koo KW, Sax DS, Snider GL. Arterial blood gases and pH during sleep in chronic obstructive pulmonary disease. Am J Med 1975; 58:663–670.
6. Leitch AG, Clancy LJ, Leggett RJE, et al. Arterial blood gas tensions, hydrogen ion, and electroencephalogram during sleep in patients with chronic ventilatory failure. Thorax 1976; 31:730–735.
7. Coccagna G, Lugaresi E. Arterial blood gases and pulmonary and systemic arterial pressure during sleep in chronic obstructive pulmonary disease. Sleep 1978; 1:117–124.
8. Douglas NJ, Calverley PMA, Leggett RJE, et al. Transient hypoxemia during sleep in chronic bronchitis and emphysema. Lancet 1979; 1:1–4.
9. Wynne JW, Block AJ, Hemenway J, et al. Disordered breathing and oxygen desaturation during sleep in patients with chronic obstructive lung disease (COLD). Am J Med 1979; 66:573–579.
10. Fleetham JA, Mezon B, West P, et al. Chemical control of ventilation and sleep arterial oxygen desaturation in patients with COPD. Am Rev Respir Dis 1980; 122:583–589.
11. Skatrud JB, Dempsey JA, Iber C, et al. Correction of CO_2 retention during sleep in patients with chronic obstructive pulmonary diseases. Am Rev Respir Dis 1981; 124:260–268.
12. Catterall JR, Douglas NJ, Calverley PMA, et al. Transient hypoxemia during sleep in chronic obstructive pulmonary disease is not a sleep apnea syndrome. Am Rev Respir Dis 1983; 128:24–29.
13. Hudgel DW, Martin RJ, Capehart M, et al. Contribution of hypoventilation to sleep oxygen desaturation in chronic obstructive pulmonary disease. J Appl Physiol 1983; 55:669–677.
14. George CF, West P, Kryger MH. Oxygenation and breathing pattern during phasic and tonic REM in patients with chronic obstructive pulmonary disease. Sleep 1987; 10:234–243.
15. Midgren B, Hansson L. Changes in transcutaneous PCO_2 with sleep in normal subjects and in patients with chronic respiratory diseases. Eur J Respir Dis 1987; 71:384–387.
16. Douglas NJ, White DP, Pickett CK, et al. Respiration during sleep in normal man. Thorax 1982; 840–844.
17. Aserinsky E. Periodic respiratory pattern occurring in conjunction with eye movements during sleep. Science 1965; 150:763–766.
18. Gould GA, Gugger M, Molloy J, et al. Breathing pattern and eye movement density during REM sleep in man. Am Rev Respir Dis 1988; 138:874–877.
19. Millman RP, Knight H, Kline LR, et al. Changes in compartmental ventilation in association with eye movements during REM sleep. J Appl Physiol 1988; 65:1196–1202.
20. Fletcher EC, Gray BA, Levin DC. Non-apneic mechanisms of arterial oxygen desaturation during rapid-eye movement sleep. J Appl Physiol 1983; 54:632–639.
21. Catterall JR, Calverley PMA, MacNee W, et al. Mechanism of transient nocturnal hypoxemia in hypoxic chronic bronchitis and emphysema. J Appl Physiol 1985; 59:1698–1703.
22. White DP. Occlusion pressure and ventilation during sleep in normal humans. J Appl Physiol 1986; 61:1279–1287.
23. Gugger M, Molloy J, Gould GA, et al. Ventilatory and arousal responses to added inspiratory resistance during sleep. Am Rev Respir Dis 1989; 140:1301–1307.
24. Lopes JM, Tabachnik E, Muller NL, et al. Total airway resistance and respiratory muscle activity during sleep. J Appl Physiol 1983; 54:773–777.
25. Hudgel DW, Martin RJ, Johnson B, et al. Mechanics of the respiratory system and breathing pattern during sleep in normal humans. J Appl Physiol 1984; 56:133–137.
26. Wiegand L, Zwillich CW, White DP. Sleep and the ventilatory response to resistive loading in normal men. J Appl Physiol 1988; 64:1186–1195.
27. Orem J. Medullary respiratory neuron activity: Relationship to tonic and phasic REM sleep. J Appl Physiol 1980; 48:54–65.
28. Tabachnik E, Muller NL, Bryan AC, et al. Changes in ventilation and chest wall mechanics during sleep in normal adolescents. J Appl Physiol 1981; 51:557–564.
29. Midgren B. Oxygen desaturation during sleep as a function of the underlying respiratory disease. Am Rev Respir Dis 1990; 141:43–46.
30. Johnson MW, Remmers JE. Accessory muscle activity during sleep in chronic obstructive pulmonary disease. J Appl Physiol 1984; 57:1011–1017.
31. Douglas NJ, White DP, Weil JV, et al. Hypoxic ventilatory response decreases during sleep in normal men. Am Rev Respir Dis 1982; 125:286–289.
32. Berthon-Jones M, Sullivan CE. Ventilatory and arousal responses to hypoxia in sleeping humans. Am Rev Respir Dis 1982; 125:632–639.
33. Douglas NJ, White DP, Weil JV, et al. Hypercapnic ventilatory response in sleeping adults. Am Rev Respir Dis 1982; 126:758–762.

34. Berthon-Jones M, Sullivan CE. Ventilation and arousal responses to hypercapnia in normal sleeping adults. J Appl Physiol 1984; 57:59–67.
35. Whyte KF, Gugger M, Gould GA, et al. Accuracy of the respiratory inductive plethysmograph in measuring tidal volume during sleep. J Appl Physiol 1991; 71:1866–1871.
36. Franceschi M, Zamproni P, Crippa D, et al. Excessive daytime sleepiness: A 1-year study in an unselected in-patient population. Sleep 1982; 5:239–247.
37. Lavie P. Incidence of sleep apnea in a presumably healthy, working population: A significant relationship with excessive daytime sleepiness. Sleep 1983; 6:312–318.
38. Stradling JR, Crosby JH. Predictors and prevalence of obstructive sleep apnoea and snoring in 1001 middle aged men. Thorax 1991; 46:85–90.
39. Guilleminault C, Cummiskey J, Motta J. Chronic obstructive airflow disease and sleep studies. Am Rev Respir Dis 1980; 122:397–406.
40. Bradley TD, Rutherford R, Grossman RF, et al. Role of daytime hypoxemia in the pathogenesis of right heart failure in the obstructive sleep apnea syndrome. Am Rev Respir Dis 1985; 131:835–839.
41. Fletcher EC, Schaaf JW, Miller J, et al. Long-term cardiopulmonary sequelae in patients with sleep apnea and chronic lung disease. Am Rev Respir Dis 1987; 135:525–533.
42. Flick MR, Block AJ. Nocturnal versus diurnal cardiac arrhythmias in patients with chronic obstructive pulmonary disease. Chest 1979; 75:8–11.
43. Shepard JW, Garrison MW, Grither DA, et al. Relationship of ventricular ectopy to nocturnal oxygen desaturation in patients with chronic obstructive pulmonary disease. Am J Med 1985; 78:28–34.
44. Boysen PG, Block AJ, Wynne JW, et al. Nocturnal pulmonary hypertension in patients with chronic obstructive pulmonary disease. Chest 1979; 76:536–542.
45. Moore-Gillon JC, Cameron IR. Right ventricular hypertrophy and polycythemia in rats after intermittent exposure to hypoxia. Clin Sci 1985; 69:595–599.
46. Shepard JW, Schweitzer PK, Keller CA, et al. Myocardial stress: Exercise versus sleep in patients with COPD. Chest 1984; 86:366–374.
47. Guilleminault C, Levy P, Romand PH, et al. Changes in left ventricular ejection fraction during arterial rapid eye movement sleep desaturation and exercise in chronic obstructive pulmonary disease and obstructive sleep apnea syndrome (abstract). Am Rev Respir Dis 1989; 139:A180.
48. Fletcher EC, Luckett RA, Miller T, et al. Pulmonary vascular hemodynamics in chronic lung disease patients with and without oxyhemoglobin desaturation during sleep. Chest 1989; 95:757–764.
49. Miller ME, Garcia JF, Cohen RA, et al. Diurnal levels of immunoreactive erythropoietin in normal subjects and subjects with chronic lung disease. Br J Haematol 1981; 49:189–200.
50. Wedzicha JA, Cotes PM, Empey DW. Serum immuno-reactive erythropoietin and hypoxic lung disease with and without polycythemia. Clin Sci 1985; 69:413–422.
51. Fitzpatrick MF, McMahon G, Whyte KF, et al. Does oxygen desaturation during sleep cause release of erythropoietin in patients with COPD? Am Rev Respir Dis 1990; 141:A375.
52. Cormick W, Olsen LG, Hensley MJ, et al. Nocturnal hypoxemia and quality of sleep in patients with chronic obstructive lung disease. Thorax 1986; 41:846–854.
53. Calverley PMA, Brezinova V, Douglas NJ, et al. The effect of oxygenation on sleep quality in chronic bronchitis and emphysema. Am Rev Respir Dis 1982; 126:206–210.
54. Fleetham J, West P, Mezon B, et al. Sleep, arousals and oxygen desaturation in chronic obstructive pulmonary disease. Am Rev Respir Dis 1982; 126:429–433.
55. Brezinova V, Catterall JR, Douglas NJ, et al. Night sleep of patients with chronic ventilatory failure and age-matched controls. Number and duration of ECG episodes of intervening wakefulness and drowsiness. Sleep 1982; 5:123–130.
56. Orr WC, Shamma-Othman Z, Levin D, et al. Persistent hypoxemia and excessive daytime sleepiness in chronic obstructive pulmonary disease. Chest 1990; 97:583–585.
57. McNicholas WT, Fitzgerald MX. Nocturnal deaths in patients with chronic bronchitis and emphysema. BMJ 1984; 289:878.
58. Douglas NJ. Breathing during sleep in patients with respiratory disease. In: Guilleminault C, Partinen M (eds). Obstructive Sleep Apnea Syndrome. New York: Raven Press, 1990, pp 37–48.
59. Weitzenblum E, Krieger J, Apprill M, et al. Daytime pulmonary hypertension in patients with obstructive sleep apnea syndrome. Am Rev Respir Dis 1988; 138:345–349.
60. Whyte KF, Douglas NJ. Peripheral edema in the sleep apnea/hypopnea syndrome. Sleep 1991; 14:354–356.
61. Bradley TD, Rutherford R, Lue F, et al. Role of diffuse airway obstruction in the hypercapnia of obstructive sleep apnea. Am Rev Respir Dis 1986; 134:920–924.
62. McKeon JL, Muree-Allan K, Saunders NA. Prediction of oxygenation during sleep in patients with chronic obstructive lung disease. Thorax 1988; 43:312–317.
63. Connaughton JJ, Catterall JR, Elton RA, et al. Do sleep studies contribute to the management of patients with severe chronic obstructive pulmonary disease? Am Rev Respir Dis 1988; 138:341–345.
64. Fletcher EC, Miller J, Devine GW, et al. Nocturnal oxyhemoglobin desaturation in COPD patients with arterial oxygen tensions above 60 mmHg. Chest 1987; 92:604–608.
65. Guilleminault C, van den Hoed J, Mitler MM. Clinical overview of the sleep apnea syndromes. In: Guilleminault C, Dement WC (eds). Sleep Apnea Syndromes. New York: Alan R. Liss, Inc., 1978, pp 1–12.
66. Whyte KF, Allen MB, Jeffrey AA, et al. Clinical features of the sleep apnoea/hypopnoea syndrome. Q J Med 1989; 72:659–666.
67. Phillipson EA, Remmers JE, (chairmen). Indications and standards for cardiopulmonary sleep studies. Am Rev Respir Dis 1989; 139:559–568.
68. Goldstein RS, Ramcharan V, Bowes G, et al. Effect of supplemental nocturnal oxygen on gas exchange in patients with severe obstructive lung disease. N Engl J Med 1984; 310:425–429.
69. Nocturnal Oxygen Therapy Trial Group. Continuous or nocturnal oxygen therapy in hypoxemic chronic obstructive lung disease: A clinical trial. Ann Intern Med 1980; 93:391–398.
70. Medical Research Council Working Party Report. Long-term domiciliary oxygen therapy in chronic hypoxic cor pulmonale complicating chronic bronchitis and emphysema. Lancet 1981; 1:681–686.
71. Fletcher EC, Levin DC. Cardiopulmonary hemodynamics during sleep in subjects with chronic obstructive pulmonary disease: The effect of short and long-term oxygen. Chest 1984; 85:6–14.
72. McKeon JL, Murree-Allen K, Saunders NA. Supplemental oxygen and quality of sleep in patients with chronic obstructive lung disease. Thorax 1989; 44:184–188.
73. Connaughton JJ, Douglas NJ, Morgan AD, et al. Almitrine improves oxygenation when both awake and asleep in patients with hypoxia and carbon dioxide retention caused by chronic bronchitis and emphysema. Am Rev Respir Dis 1985; 132:206–210.
74. Daskalopoulou E, Patakas D, Tsara V, et al. Comparison of almitrine bismesylate and medroxyprogesterone acetate on oxygenation during wakefulness and sleep in patients with chronic obstructive lung disease. Thorax 1990; 45:666–669.
75. Gothe B, Cherniack NS, Bachandrt RT, et al. Long-term effects of almitrine bismesylate on oxygenation during wakefulness and sleep in chronic obstructive pulmonary disease. Am J Med 1988; 84:436–443.
76. Rühle KH, Kempf P, Mössinger B, et al. Einfluss von Almitrin, einem Chemorezeptorenstimulator, auf die nächtliche Hyperkapnie und dem pulmonalarteriellen Druck unter O_2-Atmung bei chronisch obstruktiver Lungenerkrankung. Prax Clin Pneumol 1988; 42:411–414.
77. Howard P. Hypoxia, almitrine and peripheral neuropathy. Thorax 1989; 44:247–250.
78. Series F, Cormier Y, La Forge J. Changes in day and in night time oxygenation with protriptyline in patients with chronic obstructive lung disease. Thorax 1989; 44:275–279.
79. Series F, Cormier Y. Effects of protriptyline on diurnal and nocturnal oxygenation in patients with chronic obstructive pulmonary disease. Ann Int Med 1990; 113:507–511.
80. Dolly FR, Block AJ. Medroxyprogesterone acetate in COPD:

Effect on breathing and oxygenation in sleeping and awake patients. Chest 1983; 84:394–398.
81. Skatrud JB, Dempsey JA. Relative effectiveness of acetazolamide versus medroxyprogesterone acetate in correction of carbon dioxide retention. Am Rev Respir Dis 1983; 127:405–412.
82. Ebden P, Vathenen AS. Does aminophylline improve nocturnal hypoxia in patients with chronic airflow obstruction? Eur J Respir Dis 1987; 71:384–387.
83. Brown NMT, Marino WD. Effective daily intermittent rest of respiratory muscles in patients with severe chronic airflow limitation. Chest 1984; 85:59S–60S.
84. Crop AJ, Di Marco AF. Effects of intermittent negative pressure ventilation on respiratory muscle function in patients with severe chronic obstructive pulmonary disease. Am Rev Respir Dis 1987; 135:1056–1061.
85. Levy RD, Bradley TD, Newman SL, et al. Negative pressure ventilation: Effects on ventilation during sleep in normal subjects. Chest 1989; 95:95–99.
86. Ellis ER, Bye PTP, Bruderer JW, et al. Treatment of respiratory failure during sleep in patients with neuromuscular disease. Am Rev Respir Dis 1987; 135:148–152.
87. Kerby GR, Mayer LS, Pringleton SK. Nocturnal positive pressure ventilation via nasal mask. Am Rev Respir Dis 1987; 135:738–740.
88. Carroll N, Branthwaite MA. Control of nocturnal hypoventilation by nasal intermittent positive pressure ventilation. Thorax 1988; 43:349–353.
89. Ellis ER, Grunstin RR, Chan S, et al. Noninvasive ventilatory support during sleep improves respiratory failure in kyphoscoliosis. Chest 1988; 94:811–815.
90. Block AJ, Dolly FR, Slayton PC. Does flurazepam ingestion affect breathing and oxygenation during sleep in patients with chronic obstructive lung disease? Am Rev Respir Dis 1984; 129:230–233.
91. Wedzicha JA, Wallis PJW, Ingram DA, et al. Effect of diazepam on sleep in patients with chronic airflow obstruction. Thorax 1988; 43:729–730.
92. Midgren B, Hansson L, Skeidsvoll H, et al. The effects of nitrazepam and flunitrazepam on oxygen desaturation during sleep in stable hypoxemic non-hypercapnic COPD. Chest 1989; 95:765–768.
93. Cummiskey J, Guilleminault C, Rio GD, et al. The effects of flurazepam on sleep studies in patients with chronic obstructive pulmonary disease. Chest 1983; 84:143–147.
94. Easton PA, West P, Meatherall RC, et al. The effect of excessive ethanol ingestion on sleep in severe chronic obstructive pulmonary disease. Sleep 1987; 10:224–233.
95. Dolly FR, Block AJ. Increased ventricular ectopy and sleep apnea following ethanol ingestion in COPD patients. Chest 1983; 83:469–472.
96. Chan CS, Bye PTP, Woolcock AJ, et al. Eucapnia and hypercapnia in patients with chronic airflow limitation: The role of the upper airway. Am Rev Respir Dis 1990; 141:861–865.
97. Jalleh R, Fitzpatrick MF, Yildirim N, et al. Does alcohol consumption influence the development of cor pulmonale in patients with COPD? (abstract) Am Rev Respir Dis 1991; 143:A71.

Chapter 9

Dyspnea: Implications for Rehabilitation

KIERAN J. KILLIAN, M.D., F.R.C.P.C.

Physicians are faced with the task of alleviating dyspnea even though the fundamental basis of its origin remains poorly understood. A conscious sensation of discomfort accompanies breathing under various circumstances: respiratory loading (stiff lungs, obstructed airways), exercise, following hyperinflation, when the respiratory muscles are weak, and following the induction of fatigue. Formal attempts have been made to match these qualitative features to descriptive phrases,[1,2] but progress has not yet sufficiently advanced to promote a change in the current use of words. Throughout the 1965 "Breathlessness" symposium in Manchester, England, which was convened for the purpose of clarifying issues related to the perception of respiratory distress, the terms *dyspnea* and *breathlessness* were used interchangeably.[3] Hence, in the absence of a comprehensive knowledge of the sensory processes involved, a meaningful semantic definition is not possible. In the present state of understanding, dyspnea or breathlessness merely describes discomfort experienced and associated with the act of breathing unless differently stated in the context of its use.

HISTORICAL ASPECTS OF DYSPNEA

The first recorded references to dyspnea are difficult to pinpoint, but its early recognition was inescapable. The knowledge that the disease arises from natural causes and results in symptoms was recognized by Hippocrates (460–360 B.C.) and his followers.[4] Prior to Hippocrates's time, various gods and spirits were often invoked as causative agents, and such supernatural origins precluded human understanding. In these ancient times, symptoms and disease were considered synonymous. Until relatively recent times, disease was considered to be the result of an imbalance of the four basic humors—blood, black bile, yellow bile, and phlegm. Therapeutics was conceptually based on redressing the balance. Hence, the use of blood letting, emetics, laxatives, and the like was widespread. Morbid anatomy replaced imbalance as the cause of disease as anatomic dissection became widespread.[5] In the 18th and 19th centuries the presence of dyspnea in life was firmly matched to the associated morbid anatomy following death and thus became an integral component of language (e.g., "respiratory dyspnea," "cardiac dyspnea," and "renal dyspnea").

At the end of the 18th century, following the realization that combustion and respiration were synonymous, the study of physiology began to impact on the mechanism of dyspnea. The functional aspects of structure had little impact until this time. In the investigation of the physiology of respiration, the word *apnea* was widely used to describe the absence of contractile activity, whereas the word *dyspnea* was used to denote the intense contractile activity of the respiratory muscles.[6-9] Discomfort was assumed to accompany this activity. In time, the term lost its specific meaning and was used to describe discomfort in any circumstance. Hence, the factors controlling respiratory muscle activity were considered fundamental to the sensation of dyspnea.

Hypoxia and hypercapnia were believed to be the stimuli responsible for the control of respiratory muscle activity.[6,10,11] By the early 20th century, the role of hydrogen ions was included and considered the fundamental stimulus through which hypercapnia and hypoxia were mediated.[12,13] A relationship between the sensation of dyspnea and these stimuli was also tacitly assumed. In the early part of this century, Meakins[14] summarized the mechanisms of dyspnea as (1) a want of oxygen and (2) carbon dioxide retention (absolute or relative).

Evolution in the study of neural phenomena evolved somewhat independently but also impacted on the understanding of dyspnea. By the early 1800s, LeGallois[15] had established that breathing was dependent on neural activity in the medulla oblongata. He observed that the respiratory centers were excited by chemical stimulation (i.e., the presence of hydrogen ions, hypoxia, or hypercapnia) and that the activity in these centers provided a viable mechanism through which these stimuli could generate the conscious sensation of dyspnea. Intuitively, the activity in these neurons was considered to be fundamental in the genesis of dyspnea or perhaps even its source.

In the mid-18th century, Hering and Breuer[16] considered the control of respiration to be reflex and "self-steering" in nature. The belief that activity arising in the lung causes dyspnea was appealing in an era when morbid anatomy was the central focus of academic clinical activity.

Reflexes arising in the lung were considered important because they influenced the control of the respiratory centers and, in turn, respiratory muscle activity. As Hering and Breuer described:

"The lung, when it becomes more expanded by inspiration, or by inflation, exerts an inhibitory effect on inspiration and promotes expiration, and this effect is the greater the stronger the expansion. Every inspiration, therefore, in that it distends the lung brings about its own end by means of this distension, and thus initiates expiration."[16]

According to this view, when inspiration is hindered by mechanical loading, motor output is less inhibited and leads to a more prolonged forceful inspiration. At the extreme, inspiratory neurons would continue to act, exhaust themselves, and thus contribute to dyspnea. As Christie[17] summarized, "Though the conditions under which dyspnea occurs are various and manifold, giving rise to an impression of complexity, the fundamental causes are few and relatively simple. They consist of chemical and reflex disturbances." The later discovery of the peripheral chemoreceptor by J.F. Heyman, C. Heyman,[18] and Comroe[19] inevitably led to the idea that the peripheral chemoreceptor was important. Indeed, surgical excision of the carotid bodies was attempted, a practice later determined to be ineffective.

If any proposed mechanisms of dyspnea were to be considered valid, they had to be able to explain dyspnea in the context of disease. Means[20] noted that when ventilatory capacity declined as a consequence of disease, dyspnea became more intense. This provided sufficient explanation for the cause of dyspnea for clinical purposes. Disorders of ventilatory capacity were classified as obstructive and restrictive by Cournand and his colleagues.[21-23] Although initially expressed as an encroachment on ventilatory capacity, the ventilatory index (the ratio of expiratory ventilation to maximum voluntary ventilation and the ratio of expiratory ventilation to ventilatory capacity) owes its origin to these ideas. For practical purposes, an increased ventilatory index became regarded clinically as synonymous with dyspnea.

Mechanical stimuli fashioned by the forces generated by the respiratory muscles, the displacement achieved in the lungs and the chest wall, elastance, resistance, and the work of breathing provided a viable neurophysiologic source through which dyspnea might be centrally processed,[7-9,24-29] but no details about their contribution emerged. Mechanical stimuli were not the only stimuli considered. The oxygen cost of breathing increases in a positively accelerating manner as ventilation increases from 0.5 milliliters per liter of ventilation at low levels to greater than 2 milliliters per liter at high levels.[30-33] The oxygen cost of breathing was further increased in patients with pulmonary and cardiac diseases.[34]

McIlroy[35] suggested that the respiratory muscles incur an oxygen debt and that dyspnea is a consequence of this debt. The inadequate supply of oxygenated blood to the respiratory muscles in a manner similar to what occurs in claudication was forwarded by Harrison.[36] The belief that fatigue results from inadequate perfusion is a present day extension of this hypothesis.[37] Afferent neural activity arising in small myelinated and unmyelinated fibers lying in the interstitium of the respiratory muscles, which are stimulated as a direct or indirect consequence of tissue hypoxia, was the implied but unstated mechanism.

In summary, dyspnea was recognized, its prognostic significance understood, and its presence attributed to disease. At a physiologic level, the source of dyspnea was grafted to physiologic advances with no formal critical testing of any of the proposed mechanisms. Chemical, neural, metabolic, and mechanical stimuli competed for recognition as the primary stimulus. In the past, interest in the mechanism of the production of dyspnea was of little practical importance to the clinician because at a clinical level the mere recognition of "disease" ("respiratory dyspnea" or "cardiac dyspnea") was sufficient to provide what treatment was available. The net result was that dyspnea was never investigated in any formal sense.

MECHANISM OF DYSPNEA

The eyes, ears, nose, tongue, nasopharynx, and skin have receptors that have been found to respond to a range of physical stimuli, relay information to the central nervous system, and result in the generation of specific conscious sensations. With respect to this, dyspnea can be considered a conscious sensation mediated by specialized sense organs. The *kinesthetic sensory system* is one such system. Formal efforts to address the mechanism of dyspnea's generation from this kind of sensory perspective have been conspicuously absent. In fact, receptors stimulated during breathing were considered insentient. The belief that breathing is perceived only in the presence of dyspnea fostered the idea that some undefined sensory receptor mediated the sensation of dyspnea.

Peripheral and Central Chemoreceptor Stimulation. The idea that chemoreceptor stimulation or the central effects of chemoreceptors cause dyspnea has been inherent in the evolution of this subject over the past 200 years. However, experimental refutation or substantiation of their role in the generation of dyspnea has been difficult. When chemoreceptors are activated, motor output to the respiratory muscles, respiratory muscle activity, muscle and joint receptor activity, and pulmonary receptor activity all increase. Nonetheless, attempts have been made to investigate the sentient properties of chemoreceptors. Chemoreceptor activity increases with the cessation of breathing because $PaCO_2$ increases and PaO_2 declines. Discomfort increases as cessation is prolonged, and at the point of tolerance breathing is reestablished. Breathholding can be prolonged at tolerance by breathing a gas mixture that increases rather than decreases chemoreceptor activity.[38] This has been interpreted to mean that chemoreceptors themselves are insentient. In this view, the sensation of discomfort during breathholding is generated as a consequence of respiratory muscle contraction. Respiratory muscle activity is initially absent but then reappears and progressively increases as the breathholding is prolonged. In support of this interpretation, no discomfort is experienced with breathholding during total neuromuscular blockade.[39] These observations, correctly or incorrectly, led to the conclusion that chemoreceptors in isolation are insentient and that conscious sensation is generated as a secondary consequence of their stimulation.

Conflicting viewpoints have arisen as a consequence of experimental studies that have employed a variety of different approaches.[1, 2, 40–45] The distress experienced during breathing is greater with hypercapnic stimulation than with voluntarily induced ventilation of the same magnitude. The combined effect of chemoreceptor activity and other sources of afferent activity has been proposed as the explanation. However, the central motor output required to generate ventilation is dependent on the responsiveness of the alpha-motor neurons and on the responsiveness of the peripheral muscles, and neither have been excluded as a source of explanation. The addition of inspired CO_2 contributes to distress during total neuromuscular blockade. However, total neuromuscular blockade is essential, and acetylcholine produced under extreme circumstances may continue to gain access to the muscle. This also has not been excluded. Finally, breathing causes distress when it is too intense or too weak. The conscious awareness of appropriateness is difficult to conceive in the absence of chemoreceptor input. Increased chemoreceptor activity, whether central or peripheral, is associated with dyspnea, but whether dyspnea is a direct or an indirect consequence of this activity remains unresolved. The net result is that the nature of the sensation generated directly by chemoreceptor activity, if it exists at all, remains ill-defined.

Pulmonary Receptors (Stretch Receptors, Irritant Receptors, and C-Fibers). Pulmonary receptors are arguably the best-studied receptors associated with the act of breathing.[46] These receptors have the potential to influence respiratory sensation directly and indirectly. Direct probing of the intrapulmonary airway can be sensed and is similar to visceral sensation in the gastrointestinal tract. Stimulation of irritant receptors in the airway results in the substernal discomfort associated with tracheal inflammation. On the other hand, afferent sensory information from the lung parenchyma and vasculature and the airways (transmitted via stretch, irritant, and J-receptors and C-fibers) is well known to modify the control of breathing. By altering the control of breathing, the receptors indirectly influence the respiratory sensation generated by other receptors.

Because of the prominent role of stretch receptors in respiratory physiology, the question as to what role these receptors have in the conscious sensation of volume naturally arises. However, the nature of this role remains controversial.[47–53] Dyspnea during exercise clearly persists following heart and lung transplantation even though the lungs are no longer a source of afferent activity; thus, these receptors cannot be the sole mediators of dyspnea. Furthermore, the conscious appreciation of load is unchanged following vagal blockade.[54] Although not formally studied, the sensation of "tightness" associated with hyperinflation is often attributed to pulmonary receptors. However, it is equally plausible that sensory activity associated with inspiratory muscle activity under conditions of shortened muscle length and inefficient force generation could result in the same sensation. Although it is premature to exclude pulmonary receptors as factors contributing to conscious respiratory sensations, they are unlikely to be a central factor in the generation of dyspnea.

Muscular Receptors. Muscle spindles, tendon organs, free nerve endings lying within the muscles, and joint and skin receptors in the rib cage are all activated by the act of breathing. Golgi tendon organs are stimulated by tension in the muscle. Muscle spindles are stimulated by displacement or movement. Joint and skin receptors can also sense displacement. The conscious ability to perceive tension and displacement is central to both respiratory and peripheral skeletal muscles.[55–67] When the muscle is working at high intensity, over a long period of time, or both, pain is common. The stimulus for this is believed to be structural damage and the release of unspecified cellular products that stimulate free nerve endings.

Central Receptors. Sherrington[55] believed that muscular sensations were entirely caused by afferent feedback and not the "sense of innervation." However, the sensations of achieved tension and effort can be separated under conditions of fatigue or neuromuscular blockade by altering the length and velocity of contraction and by stimulating reflexes or by inhibiting alpha-motor neuron output.[59–61, 66, 68–71] Small interneurons located high in the central nervous system (corollary discharges from central motor neurons) transduce the intensity of the motor command and perform the role of a sensory receptor. Ventilatory effort is considered particularly important because these receptors are active when breathing is increased or loaded or when the respiratory muscles are weak, that is, in all of the circumstances in which dyspnea is experienced. Furthermore, when dyspneic patients are ventilated such that the respiratory muscles are inactive, the dyspnea is commonly relieved or even eliminated.

Upper Airway Receptors. The control of breathing is dependent on maintenance of the caliber of the upper airway, protection of the upper airway during eating, and the upper airway's role in speech.[72] Upper airway receptors clearly subserve these functions, and in so doing they must interact with the overall control mechanisms. A primary role for these receptors in the generation of dyspnea appears unlikely, but their activation during speech, swallowing, and coughing have indirect effects that result in dyspnea. Dyspnea is observed during eating and speech in patients with severe pulmonary impairment. Transient hypoventilation combined with subsequent hyperventilation may be the underlying cause of this phenomenon.

Role of Inappropriateness. The ability to consciously perceive various dimensions of respiratory sensation (e.g., effort, tension, and displacement) is now generally acknowledged. The interrelationships of these dimensions are also perceptible. The intensity of inspiratory muscle tension required for a given displacement in terms of volume and flow rate is the mechanism through which added loads are detected.[73, 74] In a similar fashion, the magnitude of ventilation for a given task is normally matched and consciously perceived. The respiratory muscle effort required for common tasks, such as walking and climbing stairs, and the magnitude of ventilation required for a given task all give rise to a sensation of "appropriateness." "Inappropriateness" is pervasive across sensory systems, is particularly sentient, and is readily recognized.[75] Respiration is usually not perceived, and conscious attention is seldom focused on the act of breathing. However, minor changes in the interrelationships of tension, length, velocity, and effort (i.e., inappropriateness) precipitate conscious attention in some individuals. On the other hand, total airway obstruction may fail to arouse some sleeping individuals.[76] The factors that facilitate the direction of attention have not been addressed. Anxiety arising as a consequence of inappropriateness is a source of discomfort, but inconsistent effects are difficult to study in that they require the identification of susceptible subjects. Psychologic factors have long been appreciated as elements that influence the perception of dyspnea even though the formal psychophysical study of these factors has been inadequate.

Fatigue. Dyspnea intensifies during prolonged exercise at both low and high power outputs, and it increases with the pressure generated by the inspiratory muscles, in response to their contractile behavior, and over the duration of respiratory muscle activity.[77, 78] The patient is aware that tension is declining and that effort is increasing when muscular fatigue occurs (so-called "failure of force development").[70] Effort is the most likely mechanism underlying the increase in respiratory distress during prolonged activity.

Quality of Respiratory Sensation. Discomfort is common to dyspnea in all conditions in which it occurs. However, the quality of the sensation during exercise, muscle weakness, loading, or bronchoconstriction varies. These differences arise as a consequence of multiple independent afferent inputs. Dyspnea may result from the summation of these multiple afferent inputs. However, it appears that dyspnea is closely related to effort that is independent of the input from other receptors and, hence, is somewhat independent of qualitative differences in the sensation. For example, high-velocity contractions cause distress as do high-tension contractions; both require excessive effort, but the afferent sensory information from the muscle in each form of contraction is widely different, as are the conscious qualitative sensory features of contraction.

In summary, the sensory receptors activated by breathing are the proximal source of afferent sensory information and are fundamental to the generation of respiratory sensations and dyspnea. There are a number of different receptor types. Each type responds to a different stimulus and each is associated with a unique quality, such as a sense of displacement or movement, a sense of tension, or a sense of effort. The quantity of sensation at any given receptor is a function of the intensity of its stimulation. The quality of respiratory sensation in general is a function of the various receptor types that are stimulated and of the intensity of stimulation. During breathing, many receptor types are stimulated simultaneously, and this makes possible a wide range of sensation qualities. The balance of evidence currently favors the notion that the intensity of dyspnea has its source in the motor nervous system, particularly in the mechanisms underlying the generation of the motor command.

PSYCHOPHYSICS

For any sensation, the linkages between the physical stimulus and perception consist of (1) the receptor that is activated by the stimulus, (2) the sensory nerves that transmit the stimulus to the central nervous system, (3) the processing of this afferent information in the central nervous system, which results in the formation of a sensory impression of peripheral receptor conditions, (4) interpretation of this sensory impression in light of previous experience and learning, and (5) the generation of conscious sensation. Psychophysics examines the quantitative relationship between the input parameters (the parameters of stimulation) and the output parameters (the evoked sensory response). Whereas the intervening unit processes cannot always be identified or measured because of technical difficulties, the relation between the conditions of stimulation and perception can be measured using psychophysical techniques.

Scaling studies are used to measure the magnitude of sensation. The operation performed consists of the matching of one continuum to another under preset

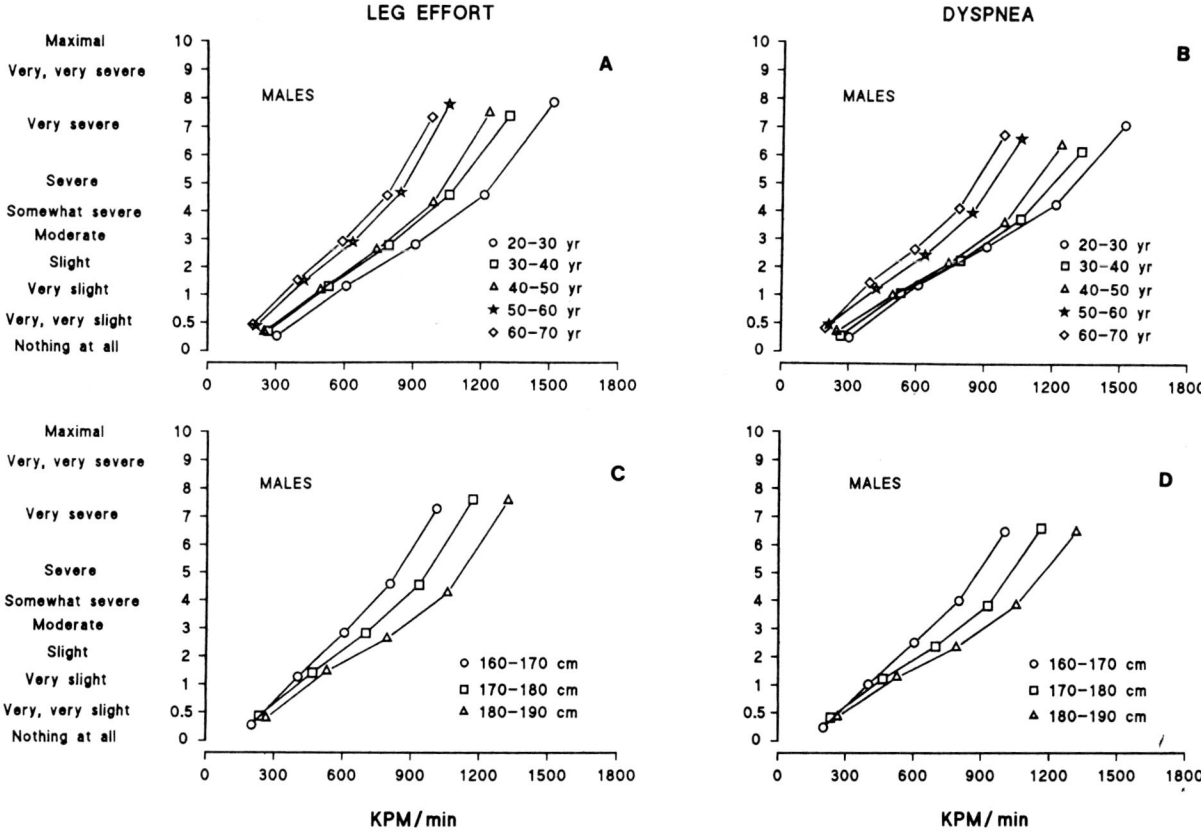

FIGURE 9–1. The mean intensity of leg effort (A and C) and dyspnea (B and D) experienced by normal male subjects stratified according to age and height during bicycle ergometry at various power outputs to maximum power output (n = 355). (Kpm: kilopound meters.)

rules (i.e., there exist nominal, ordinal, interval, and ratio scaling operations). Detailed information concerning the different types of operations is presented at length in the work of Stevens.[79, 80]

Sensory measurement was introduced by Fechner in the 1860s.[81] He determined sensory magnitude based on the summation of "just noticeable differences" from the absolute threshold of detection. However, just noticeable differences are not perceptually equal in magnitude as was originally postulated. The perceptual magnitude of each just noticeable difference increases systematically from the absolute threshold to the highest levels of stimulation.[82, 83]

Open magnitude scaling is a type of ratio scaling in which subjects select a number to represent the magnitude of a stimulus while maintaining proportionality in the sensory domain. For example, if one stimulus is perceived to be twice as intense as another, the number the subject selects to describe it is twice as great. The number range is freely selected by the subject such that the relevant measurement is the change in sensory magnitude combined with the change in stimulus intensity or in stimulation parameters. Open magnitude scaling is useful in defining the nature of the stimulus and the parameters of stimulation contributing to perceptual magnitude.[84] The effect of changing stimulus factors can be readily studied using this technique. Open magnitude scaling does not produce a direct measurement of absolute sensory intensity that can be transferred across individual subjects or across time in the same subjects.

Two scaling methods, open magnitude scaling and category scaling (Borg scaling and visual analog scaling), have been commonly used for the estimation of patient symptoms. Category scaling (interval scaling) is a method of scaling in which subjects rate perceptual magnitude by selecting from a range of numbers, lines of different lengths, or simple verbal expressions. These scales have fundamental problems because they do not preserve ratio relationships.[80, 85–89] However, they do have some distinct advantages. In particular, they (1) make possible a crude but very useful estimate of absolute magnitude, (2) permit comparison among individual subjects, and (3) are simple to use.

The direct measurement of symptoms is easy to perform when using visual analog scales and closed number scales. However, the doubling of a number or a line length by a subject does not indicate a doubling of perceptual magnitude.[85] The Borg scale was constructed to lessen this shortcoming.[90–95] The Borg scale provides a measurement related to absolute sensory magnitude, which is based on quantitative semantics (e.g., descriptors such as "slight," "moderate," or "severe"). Quantitative semantics are used in everyday life across all cultures and have crude but useful properties in the determination of absolute sensory magnitude. Furthermore, they have crude ratio properties relative to each other. Assigning numbers to these descriptors to reflect their ratio properties makes possible the quantitative measurement of absolute sensory magnitude using ratio properties. Thus, doubling a number implies doubling the perceived sensory magnitude. The Borg scale is therefore a means to combine the properties of open magnitude scaling with the properties of absolute magnitude scaling.

SYMPTOMS OCCURRING DURING EXERCISE IN NORMAL SUBJECTS

During exercise, the conditions at the various proximal receptors cannot be measured directly. However, the conditions of stimulation can be standardized for all subjects. A standardized incremental exercise test provides such conditions. In this test, the psychophysical relationship depends on the integrated interaction of all the unit processes outlined previously. Dyspnea and leg effort both increase during incremental exercise to capacity. At a given power output, the intensity is greater in women than in men, whereas it decreases as stature increases and increases with age in both sexes (Fig. 9–1). The magnitude is expressed by the following equations (height in cm, age in yr, men = 1, and women = 2).[96]

$$\text{Dyspnea} = 1.8 + 0.005 \text{ Kpm/min} + 0.02 \times \text{age} - 0.03 \times \text{height} + 0.72 \times \text{sex} \; (r = .71)$$

$$\text{Leg Effort} = 2.1 + 0.006 \text{ Kpm/min} + 0.03 \times \text{age} - 0.02 \times \text{height} + 0.64 \times \text{sex} \; (r = .75)$$

Symptom intensity is the same across sex, age, and stature when power output is expressed relative to capacity.[96] Normal standards and confidence limits for the symptoms of dyspnea and leg effort are expressed as percentile responses (Fig. 9–2).

In both normal subjects and patients, a point is reached at which exercise cannot continue and must be stopped. Discomfort attributed to breathing, the peripheral skeletal muscles, or both is cited as the most common form of distress.[96]

Dyspnea and peripheral muscular effort intensify during exercise (as described previously) and also as the duration of exercise is increased as illustrated in Figure 9–3 and as expressed by the following equations (MPO: maximum power output, K: constant):

$$\text{Dyspnea} = K \times \%\text{MPO}^{2.41} \times \text{time}^{0.47}$$

$$\text{Leg effort} = K \times \%\text{MPO}^{2.13} \times \text{time}^{0.39}$$

Doubling the intensity of activity results in a four- to five-fold increase in symptoms, whereas doubling the duration of activity results in only a 30 to 40% increase in symptoms.[77, 78] Reducing the intensity and increasing the duration of activity are extremely effective in the amelioration of symptoms.

The degree of limitation depends on the tolerance of the individual subject. Typically, subjects stop exercising when leg effort, dyspnea, or both become "very severe" (i.e., they exceed 7 on the Borg scale). Tolerance varies from "somewhat severe" (4) to "maximal" (10) (95% confidence limits) and is the same in health and disease.[96] In the presence of disease, limitation is experienced at lower work intensities because the pathophysiologic effects of disease contribute to excessive sensory receptor stimulation.[97] The combination of dyspnea and leg fatigue limits exercise in 42% of normal subjects, and leg fatigue alone limits exercise in 45%; 12% of subjects claimed dyspnea as the limiting factor when they were formally studied during incremental exercise testing.[96]

DYSPNEA AND LEG EFFORT IN CHRONIC AIRFLOW LIMITATION

Dyspnea and leg effort are both increased in the presence of airflow limitation. The intensity of dyspnea and of leg effort in patients with mild, moderate, and severe airflow limitation is illustrated in Figure 9–4.[97] Surprisingly, only 40% of these patients with stable chronic airflow limitation (forced expiratory volume in 1 second [FEV_1] < 40% of that predicted) were limited by dyspnea alone, 35% were limited by both dyspnea and leg fatigue, and 25% were limited by leg fatigue

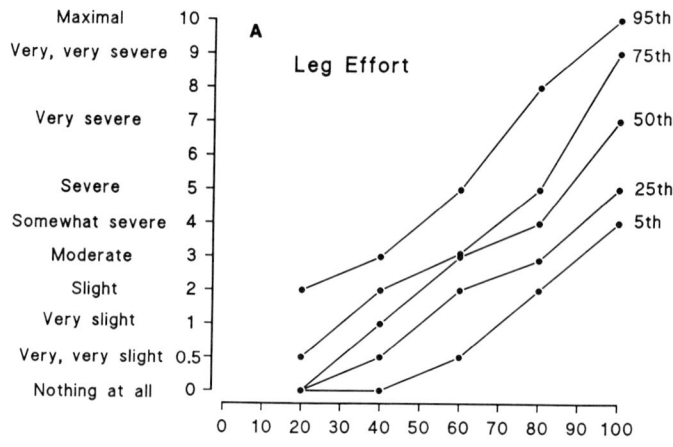

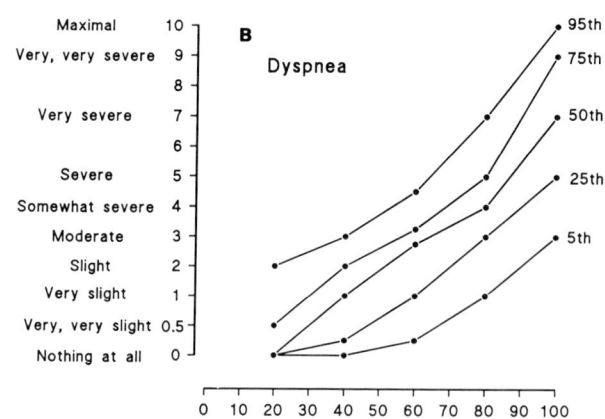

FIGURE 9–2. The intensity of leg effort (A) and dyspnea (B) expressed against power output (per cent of maximum) during incremental exercise on a bicycle ergometer to maximum capacity. Confidence limits are expressed as percentile responses.

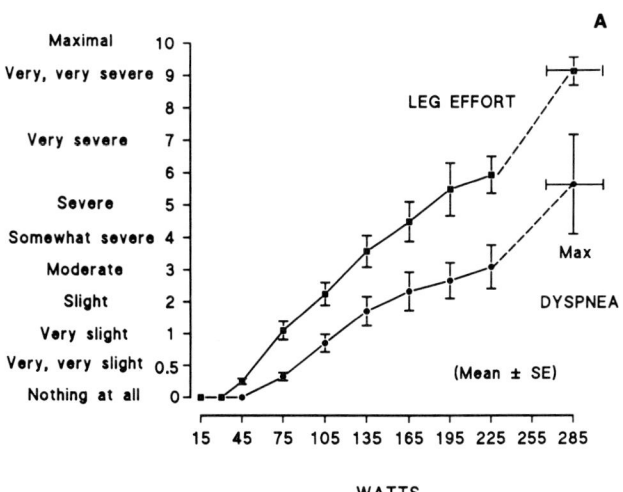
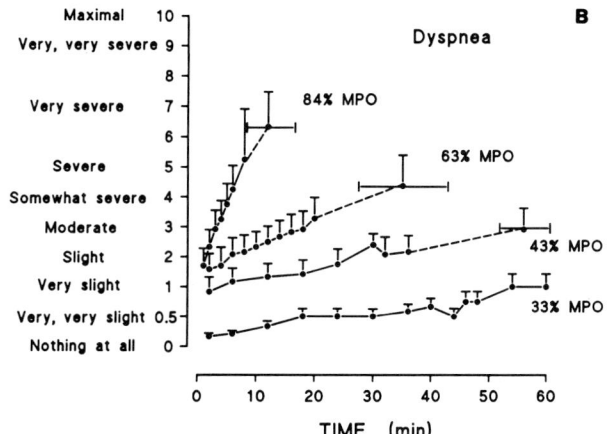
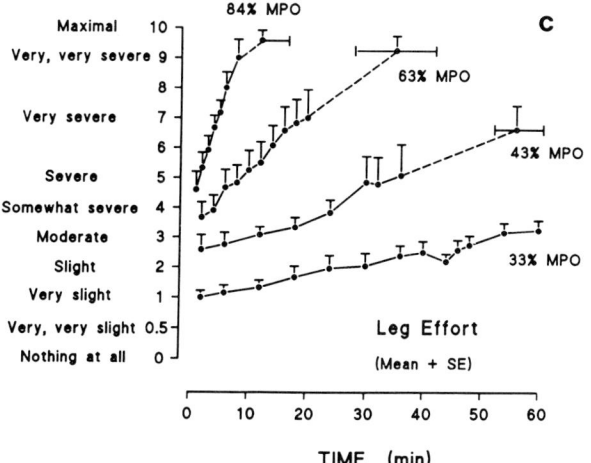

FIGURE 9–3. The intensity of dyspnea and leg effort experienced by normal subjects (n = 6) on a bicycle ergometer during incremental exercise (A) and during prolonged exercise (B and C) at four different but constant power outputs. (SE: standard error; MPO: maximum power output.)

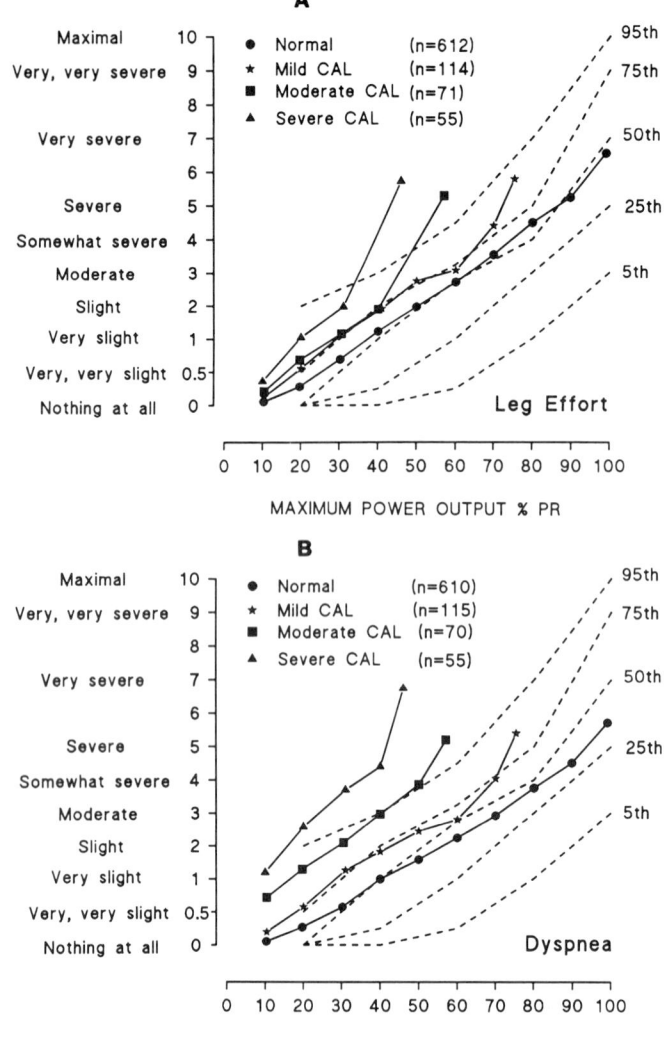

FIGURE 9-4. The mean intensity of leg effort (A) and dyspnea (B) experienced by patients with mild (FEV_1 60–80%), moderate (FEV_1 40–60%), and severe (FEV_1 <40%) chronic airflow limitation. Symptom intensity is superimposed on normal expected intensities; and confidence limits are expressed as percentile responses. (CAL: chronic airflow limitation; PR: predicted normal capacity.)

ventilation is increased, as occurs during exercise, voluntary hyperventilation, or reflexly driven hyperventilation; and (3) the action of the inspiratory muscles is impeded by the addition of resistive or elastic loads to breathing. In addition to airflow limitation, resistance, dynamic elastance, inspiratory pressures, and progressive hyperinflation all contribute to the perceived intensity of dyspnea. The strength of the inspiratory muscles also contributes to the intensity of dyspnea as expressed by the following equation (pred: predicted; MIP: maximum inspiratory pressure).[100]

$$\text{Dyspnea} = 1.80 + 0.05 \times \text{power \%pred} - 0.02 \times FEV_1 - 0.005 \times \text{MIP \%pred (SD 1.75; } r = .70)$$

During exercise, motor activation and sensory activation occur concomitantly in the respiratory and peripheral skeletal muscles. The motor and sensory activation for respiratory muscles is illustrated schematically in Figure 9–6. During exercise, the central receptors, muscle receptors, and pulmonary receptors are all stimulated to an extent determined by the strength of the respiratory muscles, the efficiency of force generation, the impedance opposing the action of the muscles, the efficiency of gas exchange, and the metabolic demand. The receptor that is overstimulated in all of these conditions is that for central motor output, and it is thus of particular importance. Although effort is a dominant contributor, intramuscular receptors, pulmonary receptors, and perhaps even chemoreceptors may under specific conditions be sentient and contribute to the quality of sensation known as dyspnea. Receptors that are stimulated are not unique to specific diseases and vary widely across and within disease processes.

Ventilatory, circulatory, and neuromuscular factors provide absolute limitations to exercise in both health and disease. These factors are well known and accepted, but there remains a wide variability in exercise performance in patients who have comparable levels of pulmonary impairment. This has always been somewhat of a concern from the simple perspective of discrete physiologic limiting factors. FEV_1 and carbon monoxide diffusing capacity (D_{LCO}) are values commonly used to quantify ventilatory and gas transfer capacity. Although there are obvious deficiencies with these simple measurements, collectively they account for 50% of the variability in maximum power output in patients with chronic airflow limitation in our experience (Fig. 9–7) and as expressed by the following multiple regression equation:

$$\text{MPO\%} = 13.6 + 0.57 \times FEV_1\% + 0.28 \times D_{LCO}\% \text{ (SD 17.6; } r = .71)$$

Arterial desaturation is seen in a minority of patients with stable chronic airflow limitation. Pulmonary hypertension restricts cardiac output and limits exercise in some patients. Muscle weakness also contributes to exercise intolerance. In essence, exercise is dependent on muscle fiber shortening, which is in turn under the volitional control of the central nervous system. The relationship between central motor output and muscular activity is complex but central to the sensation of effort.

alone.[98] The weakness of peripheral skeletal muscles contributes to exercise intolerance in these patients. When the static strength of major muscle groups was used to derive the categories of strength, working capacity was systematically greatest in those with the greatest overall strength (Fig. 9–5).[99]

The goals of rehabilitation are to enhance function, to minimize disability, and to ameliorate the limitation caused by dyspnea. Symptoms and the mechanisms of their generation play a prominent role in the achievement of these goals. Hence, an understanding of the symptoms and their mechanisms is essential. Both experimentally induced dyspnea and dyspnea that is a consequence of disease share common characteristics. The presence of dyspnea is confined to situations in which (1) the inspiratory muscles are weakened as a consequence of disease, hyperinflation, or fatigue; (2)

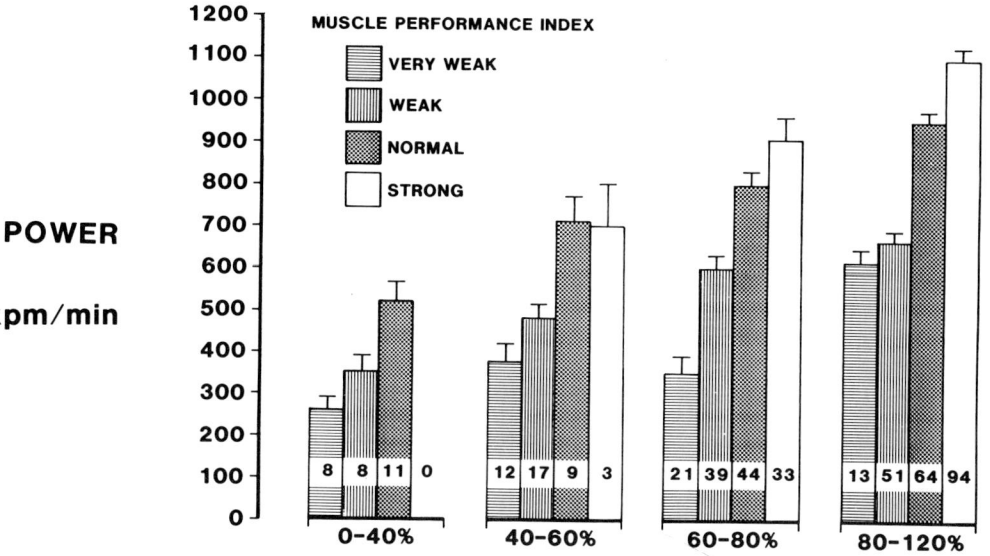

FIGURE 9–5. Maximum power output achieved by patients with mild, moderate, and severe airflow limitation. Each subgroup is divided into four categories based on measurements of quadriceps strength, handgrip, and inspiratory and expiratory muscle strength.

The responsiveness of the alpha-motor neurons can be facilitated by afferent feedback from muscle spindles or inhibited by tendon organs and small myelinated and unmyelinated intramuscular fibers. The responsiveness of a muscle to alpha-motor neuron activity depends on intramuscular homeostasis (particularly membrane charge), the amount of calcium released, and the availability of high-energy phosphates. To continue activity, adenosine triphosphate must be re-formed from creatine phosphate, the incomplete oxidation of glycogen to lactate, and the complete oxidation of carbohydrates and fats to CO_2 and water, which requires the delivery of oxygen by means of central cardiorespiratory and peripheral cardiovascular adaptations. It should not be forgotten that these factors contribute to limitation via the sensory system. In patients with chronic airflow limitation, exercise is limited by intolerable symptoms that include both dyspnea and peripheral muscle fatigue.

Interest in the mechanisms of symptom production has been of little practical importance because recognizing the presence of "disease" has been sufficient for management purposes. Dyspnea continues to be explained by physiologic advances without being subjected to formal critical testing, and chemical, neural, metabolic, and mechanical stimuli continue to compete as the primary initiators of dyspnea. In recent years, tech-

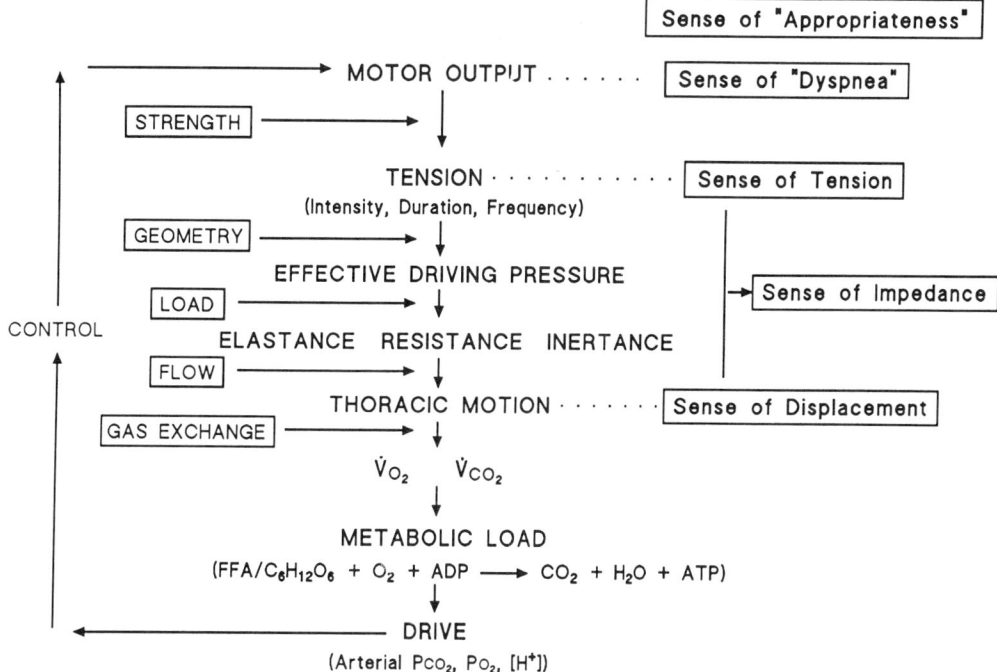

FIGURE 9–6. Schematic diagram illustrating the sequence of key unit physiologic processes that preserve respiratory homeostasis. The direct influence of these processes on muscular sensory receptors is illustrated on the right. On the left, some key factors that influence these processes are inserted. ($\dot{V}_{O_2}$: oxygen consumption per unit time; $\dot{V}_{CO_2}$: carbon dioxide consumption per unit time; FFA: free fatty acids; ADP: adenosine diphosphate; ATP: adenosine triphosphate.)

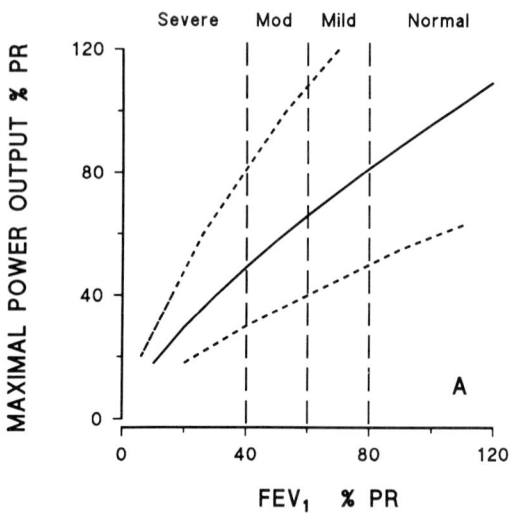 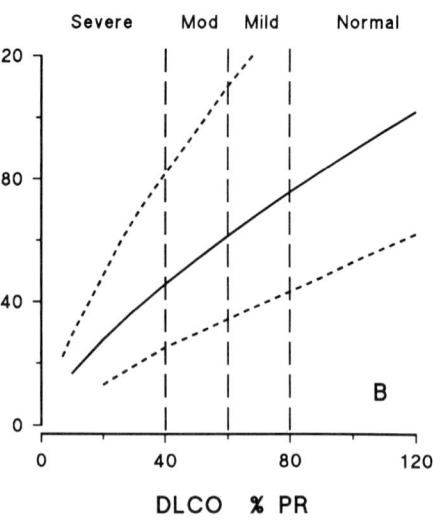

FIGURE 9–7. *A*, Maximum power output (per cent of predicted normal capacity) is expressed as a function of FEV_1 (per cent of predicted normal capacity). *B*, Diffusing capacity of the lungs for carbon monoxide (D_{LCO}, per cent of predicted normal capacity). ($MPO\% = 3.32 \times FEV_1\%^{0.73}$ [$r = 0.76$; $n = 898$]; $MPO\% = 3.09 \times D_{LCO}\%^{0.73}$ [$r = 0.58$; $n = 708$]; Mod: Moderate.)

niques for the measurement of the sensation of dyspnea in carefully controlled settings have made possible the experimental study of dyspnea. Although they have been the source for considerable progress in understanding the mechanisms of dyspnea, the practical contributions of these techniques to patient management remain to be established.

"No natural phenomenon can be adequately studied in itself alone, but to be understood must be considered as it stands connected with all of nature."—Sir Francis Bacon (1561–1626)

REFERENCES

1. Cockroft A, Adams L, Guz A. Assessment of breathlessness. Q J Med 1988; 1:669–676.
2. Simon PM, Schwartzstein RM, Weiss JW, et al. Distinguishable sensations of breathlessness induced in normal volunteers. Am Rev Respir Dis 1989; 140:1021–1027.
3. Howell JBL, Campbell EJM. Breathlessness. Oxford, England: Blackwell Scientific Publications, Inc., 1966.
4. Singer C. A Short History of Anatomy and Physiology from the Greeks to Harvey. New York: Dover Publications, Inc., 1957.
5. Morgagni G. The seats and causes of disease investigated by anatomy (De Sedibus et Causis Morborum per Anatomen Indagatis) In: Nuland SB (ed). Excerpts in Doctors: The Biography of Medicine. New York: Alfred A. Knopf, Inc., 1989, pp 145–170.
6. Pfluger E. On the causes of respiratory movement, and of dyspnea and apnea. (Über die Ursache der Atembewegungen, sowie der Dyspnoe und Apnoe.) Pflugers Arch Ges Physiol 1868; 1:61–106. Translation reprinted in West JB (ed). Translations in Respiratory Physiology. Stroudsburg, PA: Dowden, Hutchinson & Ross, Inc., 1975, pp 404–434.
7. Rohrer F. The correlation of respiratory forces and their dependence upon the state of expansion of the respiratory organs. (Der Zusammenhang der Atemkräfte und ihre Abhängigkeit vom Dehnungszustand der Atmungsorgane.) Pflugers Arch Ges Physiol 1916; 165:419–444. Translation reprinted in West JB (ed). Translations in Respiratory Physiology. Stroudsburg, PA: Dowden, Hutchinson & Ross, Inc., 1975, pp 67–88.
8. Rohrer F. The Physiology of Respiratory Movements (Physiologie der Atembewegung.) ATJ Bethe, et al (eds). Handbuch der Normalen und Pathologischen Physiologie. Berlin: Springer-Verlag, Inc., 1925, 70–127. Translation reprinted in West JB (ed). Translations in Respiratory Physiology. Stroudsburg, PA: Dowden, Hutchinson & Ross, Inc., 1975, pp 93–170.
9. Donders FC. Contribution to the mechanism of respiration and circulation in health and disease. (Beiträge zum Mechanismus der Respiration und Circulation im gesunden und kranken Zustande.) Z Rationel Med 1853; 3:287–319. Translation reprinted in West JB (ed). Translations in Respiratory Physiology. Stroudsburg, PA: Dowden, Hutchinson & Ross, Inc., 1975, pp 298–318.
10. Haldane SJ, Smith L. Carbon dioxide and regulation of breathing. In: Haldane JS, Priestly JG (eds). Respiration. Oxford, England: Clarendon Press, 1935.
11. Miescher-Rusch F. Bemerkungen zur Lehre von den Atembewegungen. Arch Anat Physiol (Leipzig) 1885; 355–380.
12. Winterstein H. The regulation of breathing by the blood. (Die Regulierung der Atmung durch das Blut.) Pflugers Arch Ges Physiol 1911; 138:167–184. Translation reprinted in West JB (ed). Translations in Respiratory Physiology. Stroudsburg, PA: Dowden, Hutchinson & Ross, Inc., 1975, pp 529–542.
13. Winterstein H. The reaction theory of respiratory regulation. (Die Reaktionstheorie der Atmungsregulation.) Pflugers Arch Ges Physiol 1921; 187:293–298. Translation reprinted in West JB (ed). Translations in Respiratory Physiology. Stroudsburg, PA: Dowden, Hutchinson & Ross, Inc., 1975, pp 543–548.
14. Meakins JM. The cause and treatment of dyspnea in cardiovascular disease. BMJ 1923; 1:1043–1055.
15. LeGallois CJJ. Experiments on the principle of life, and particularly on the principle of the notions of the heart, and on the seat of this principle (translation). In: Comroe JH Jr (ed). Pulmonary and Respiratory Physiology. Part II. Stroudsburg, PA: Dowden, Hutchinson & Ross, Inc., 1976, pp 12–16.
16. Breuer J, Hering E. Self-steering of respiration through the nervous vagus. Sitzber Math Naturw Cl 1868; 57:672–677. Reprinted in Comroe JH Jr (ed). Pulmonary and Respiratory Physiology. Part II. Stroudsburg, PA: Dowden, Hutchinson & Ross, Inc., 1976, pp 108–113.
17. Christie R. Dyspnea. Q J Med 1938; 7:421–454.
18. Heyman JF, Heyman C. Sur les modifications directes et sur la régulation réflèxe de l'activité du centre respiratoire de la tête isolée du chien. Arch Int Pharmacodyn Ther 1927; 33:273–191.
19. Comroe JH Jr. The location and function of the chemoreceptors of the aorta. Am J Physiol 1939; 127:176–191.
20. Means JH. Dyspnoea. Med Monograph 1924; 5:309–416.
21. Cournand A, Richards DW. Pulmonary insufficiency: I. Discussion of a physiological classification and presentation of clinical test. Am Rev Tuberc 1941; 44:26–41.
22. Cournand A, Richards DW. Pulmonary insufficiency: II. The effects of various types of collapse therapy upon cardiopulmonary function. Am Rev Tuberc 1941; 44:123–172.
23. Cournand A, Richards DW, Maier HC. Pulmonary insufficiency: III. Cases demonstrating advanced cardiopulmonary insufficiency following artificial pneumothorax and thoracoplasty. Am Rev Tuberc 1941; 44:272–287.
24. Wirz K. Changes in the pleural pressure during respiration, and

causes of its variability. (Das Verhalten des Druckes im Pleurarium bei der Atmung und die Ursachen seiner Veränderlichkeit.) Pflugers Arch Ges Physiol 1923; 199:1–56. Translation reprinted in West JB (ed). Translation in Respiratory Physiology. Stroudsburg, PA: Dowden, Hutchinson & Ross, Inc., 1975, pp 174–226.
25. Von Neergaard K, Wirz K. Method for measuring lung elasticity in living human subjects, especially in emphysema. (Über eine Methode zur Messung der Lungenelastizität am lebenden Menschen, insbesondere beim Emphysem.) 2 Klin Med 1927; 105:35–50. Translation reprinted in West JB (ed). Translations in Respiratory Physiology. Stroudsburg, PA: Dowden, Hutchinson & Ross Inc., 1975, pp 227–269.
26. Otis AB, Fenn WO, Rahn H. Mechanics of breathing in man. J Appl Physiol 1950; 2:592–607.
27. Marshall R, McIlroy MB, Christie RV. The work of breathing in mitral stenosis. Clin Sci 1954; 13:137–146.
28. Marshall R, Stone RW, Christie RV. Relationship of dyspnea to respiratory effort in normal subjects, mitral stenosis, and emphysema. Clin Sci 1954; 13:625–631.
29. Otis AB. The work of breathing. In: Fenn WO, Rahn H (eds). Handbook of Physiology. The Respiratory System. Vol 1. Part III. Bethesda, MD: American Physiological Society, 1964, pp 463–476.
30. Liljestrand G. Studies of the work of breathing. (Untersuchungen über die Atmungsarbeit. Scand Arch Physiol 35:199–293.). Translation reprinted in West JB (ed). Translations in Respiratory Physiology. Stroudsburg, PA: Dowden, Hutchinson, Ross, Inc., 1975, pp 438–513.
31. Cournand A, Richards DW, Bader RE, et al. The oxygen cost of breathing. Trans Assoc Am Physicians 1954; 67:162–173.
32. Bartlett RG, Brubach HF, Specht H. Oxygen cost of breathing. J Appl Physiol 1958; 12:413–424.
33. Campbell EJM, Westlake EK, Cherniack RM. The oxygen consumption and efficiency of the respiratory muscles of young male subjects. Clin Sci 1959; 18:55–64.
34. Fritis HW, Filler J, Fishman AP, et al. The efficiency of ventilation during voluntary hyperpnea: Studies in normal subjects and in dyspneic patients with either chronic pulmonary emphysema or obesity. J Clin Invest 1959; 38:1339–1348.
35. McIlroy MB. Dyspnea and the work of breathing in diseases of the heart and lungs. Prog Cardiovasc Dis 1958; 1:284–297.
36. Harrison TR. Shortness of breath. In: Beeson PB, Thorn GW, Resnik WH, et al. (eds). Principles of Internal Medicine. Philadelphia: Blakiston, 1950, pp 111–119.
37. Bellemare F, Grassino A. Effect of pressure and timing of contraction on human diaphragm fatigue. J Appl Physiol 1982; 53:1190–1195.
38. Fowler WS. Breaking point of breath-holding. J Appl Physiol 1954; 6:539–545.
39. Campbell EJM, Freedman S, Clark TJH, et al. The effect of muscular paralysis induced by tubocurarine on the duration and sensation of breath-holding. Clin Sci 1967; 32:425–432.
40. Adams L, Lane R, Shea SA, et al. Breathlessness during different forms of ventilatory stimulation: A study of mechanisms in normal subjects and respiratory patients. Clin Sci 1985; 69:663–672.
41. Chonan T, Mulholland MB, Cherniack NS, et al. Effects of voluntary constraining of thoracic displacement during hypercapnia. J Appl Physiol 1987; 63:1822–1828.
42. Schwartzstein RM, Simon PM, Weiss JW, et al. Breathlessness induced by dissociation between ventilation and chemical drive. Am Rev Respir Dis 1989; 139:1231–1237.
43. Chonan T, Mulholland MB, Altose MD, et al. Effects of changes in level and pattern of breathing on the sensation of dyspnea. J Appl Physiol 1990; 69:1290–1295.
44. Banzett RB, Lansing RW, Brown R, et al. 'Air hunger' from increased P_{CO_2} persists after complete neuromuscular block in humans. Respir Physiol 1990; 81:1–18.
45. Chonan T, Mulholland MB, Leitner J, et al. Sensation of dyspnea during hypercapnia, exercise, and voluntary hyperventilation. J Appl Physiol 1990; 68:2100–2106.
46. Coleridge HM, Coleridge JCG. Reflexes evoked from tracheobronchial tree and lungs. In: Geiger SR, Widdicombe JG, Cherniack NS, et al (eds). The Handbook of Physiology. Section 3. The Respiratory System. Bethesda, MD: American Physiological Society, 1986, pp 395–429.
47. Halttunen PK. The voluntary control in human breathing. Acta Physiol Scand Suppl 1974; 419:1–47.
48. Salamon M, Von Euler C, Franzen O. Perception of mechanical factors in breathing. Abstract presented at the National Symposium on Physical Work and Effort. Wenner-Gren Centre, Stockholm, 1975.
49. West DWM, Ellis CG, Campbell EJM. Ability of man to detect increases in his breathing. J Appl Physiol 1975; 39:372–376.
50. Katz-Salamon M. Perception of mechanical factors in breathing. In: Borg G (ed). Physical Work and Effort. Oxford, England: Pergamon Press, Inc., 1976, pp 101–113.
51. Stubbing DG, Killian KJ, Campbell EJM. The quantification of respiratory sensations by normal subjects. Respir Physiol 1981; 44:251–260.
52. Wolkove N, Altose MD, Kelsen SG, et al. Perception of lung volume and Weber's Law. J Appl Physiol 1982; 52:1679–1680.
53. DiMarco AF, Wolfson DA, Gottfried SB, et al. The sensation of inspired volume in normal subjects and quadriplegic patients. J Appl Physiol 1982; 53:1481–1486.
54. Guz A, Noble NIM, Widdicombe JG, et al. The role of vagal and glossopharyngeal afferent nerves in respiratory sensation, control of breathing and arterial pressure regulation in conscious man. Clin Sci 1966; 30:161–170.
55. Sherrington CS. The muscular sense. In: Shafer EA (ed). Textbook of Physiology. Vol 2. Edinburgh, Scotland: T.J. Pentland, 1900, pp 1002–1025.
56. Matthews PBC, Simmonds A. Sensations of finger movement elicited by pulling upon flexor tendons in man. J Physiol (Lond) 1974; 239:27P–28P.
57. McCloskey DI, Ebeling P, Goodwin GM. Estimation of weights and tensions and apparent involvement of a "sense of effort." Exp Neurol 1974; 42:220–232.
58. Gandevia SC, McCloskey DI. Joint sense, muscle sense, and their combination as position sense, measured at the distal interphalangeal joint of the middle finger. J Appl Physiol 1976; 260:387–407.
59. Gandevia SC, McCloskey DI. Sensation of heaviness. Brain 1977; 100:345–354.
60. Gandevia SC, McCloskey DI. Changes in motor commands, as shown by changes in perceived heaviness, during partial curarization and peripheral muscle anaesthesia in man. J Physiol (Lond) 1977; 272:673–689.
61. Roland PE, Ladegaard-Pederson H. A quantitative analysis of sensation of tension and kinaesthesia in man: Evidence for peripherally originating muscular sense and for a sense of effort. Brain 1977; 100:671–692.
62. McCloskey DI. Kinesthetic sensibility. Physiol Rev 1978; 58:763–820.
63. Gandevia SC, McCloskey DI. Interpretation of perceived motor commands by reference to afferent signals. J Physiol 1978; 283:493–499.
64. Matthews PBC. Evolving views on the internal operation and functional role of the muscle spindle. J Physiol 1981; 320:1–30.
65. Matthews PBC. Where does Sherrington's "muscular sense" originate? Muscles, joints, corollary discharges? Ann Rev Neurosci 1982; 5:189–218.
66. Gandevia SC. The perception of motor commands or effort during muscular paralysis. Brain 1982; 105:151–195.
67. Burgess PR, Wei JY, Clark FJ, et al. Signalling of kinesthetic information by peripheral sensory receptors. Ann Rev Neurosci 1982; 5:171–187.
68. Cafarelli E, Bigland-Ritchie B. Sensation of static force in muscles of different length. Exp Neurol 1979; 65:511–525.
69. Campbell EJM, Gandevia SC, Killian KJ, et al. Changes in the perception of inspiratory resistive loads during partial curarization. J Physiol 1980; 309:93–100.
70. Gandevia SC, Killian KJ, Campbell EJM. The effect of respiratory muscle fatigue on respiratory sensations. Clin Sci 1981; 60:463–466.
71. Cafarelli E. Peripheral contributions to the perception of effort. Med Sci Sports Exerc 1982; 14:382–389.
72. Widdicombe JG. Reflexes from the upper respiratory tract. In: Geiger SG, Widdicombe JG, Cherniack NS, et al (eds). Hand-

book of Physiology. Section 3. The Respiratory System. Vol 2. Part I. Bethesda, MD: American Physiological Society, 1986, pp 363–394.
73. Campbell EJM, Freedman S, Smith PS, et al. The ability of man to detect added elastic loads to breathing. Clin Sci 1961; 20:223–231.
74. Bennett ED, Jayson MIV, Rubenstein D, et al. The ability of man to detect added non-elastic loads to breathing. Clin Sci 1962; 23:155–162.
75. Campbell EJM, Howell JBL. The sensation of breathlessness. Br Med Bull 1963; 19:36–40.
76. McNicholas WT, Bowes G, Zamel N, et al. Impaired detection of added inspiratory resistance in patients with obstructive sleep apnea. Am Rev Respir Dis 1984; 129:45–48.
77. Kearon MC, Summers E, Jones NL, et al. Breathing during prolonged exercise in man. J Physiol 1991; 442:477–487.
78. Kearon MC, Summers E, Jones NL, et al. Effort and dyspnea during work of varying intensity and duration. Eur Respir J 1991; 4:917–925.
79. Stevens SS. On the theory of scales of measurement. Science 1946; 103:677–680.
80. Stevens SS. Psychophysics: Introduction to Its Perceptual, Neural, and Social Prospects. New York: John Wiley & Sons, Inc., 1975.
81. Fechner GT. Elemente der Psychophysik. Leipzig: Breitkopf und Hartel, 1860. English translation: Elements of Psychophysics. New York: Holt, Rinehart & Winston, Inc., 1966.
82. Stevens SS. On the psychophysical law. Psychol Rev 1957; 64:153–181.
83. Teghtsoonian R. On the exponents in Stevens' Law and the constant in Ekman's Law. Psychol Rev 1971; 78:71–80.
84. Marks LE. Sensory Processes: The New Psychophysics. New York: Academic Press, Inc., 1974.
85. Stevens SS, Galanter EH. Ratio scales and category scales for a dozen perceptual continua. J Exp Psychol 1957; 54:377–411.
86. Stevens SS. Problems and methods of psychophysics. Psychol Bull 1958; 55:177–196.
87. Stevens SS. Ratio scales, partition scales and confusion scales. In: Gulliksen H, Messick S (eds). Psychological Scaling: Theory and Applications. New York: John Wiley & Sons, Inc., 1960, pp 49–66.
88. Stevens SS. To honor Fechner and repeal his law. Science 1961; 133:80–86.
89. Stevens SS. Issues in psychophysical measurement. Psychol Rev 1971; 78:426–450.
90. Borg G. Interindividual scaling and perception of muscular force. K Fysiogr Sallsk Lund Forh 1961; 12:117–125.
91. Borg G. On quantitative semantics in connection with psychophysics. Educational and Psychological Research Bulletin, University of Umea 1964; 3.
92. Borg G, Hosman J. The metric properties of adverbs. Institute of Applied Psychology Report, University of Stockholm 1970; 7.
93. Borg G. A ratio scaling method for interindividual comparisons. Institute of Applied Psychology Report, University of Stockholm 1972; 27:1–12.
94. Borg G, Lindblad I. The determination of subjective intensities in verbal descriptions of symptoms. Institute of Applied Psychology Report, University of Stockholm 1976; 75.
95. Borg GA. A category scale with ratio properties for intermodal and interindividual comparisons. In: Geissler HG, Petzold P (eds). Psychophysical Judgment and the Process of Perception: Proceedings of the 22nd International Congress of Psychology. Amsterdam: North Holland Publishing Co., 1980, pp 25–34.
96. Killian KJ, Summers E, Jones NL, et al. Dyspnea and leg effort during incremental cycle ergometry. Am Rev Respir Dis (in press).
97. Jones NL, Kearon MC, Leblanc P, et al. Symptoms limiting activity in chronic airflow limitation (abstract). Am Rev Respir Dis 1989; 139:A319.
98. Killian KJ, Leblanc P, Martin DH, et al. Exercise capacity, ventilatory, circulatory, and symptom limitation in patients with chronic airflow limitation. Am Rev Respir Dis (in press).
99. Allard C, Jones NL, Killian KJ. Static peripheral skeletal muscle strength and exercise capacity in patients with chronic airflow limitation (abstract). Am Rev Respir Dis 1989; 139:A90.
100. Killian KJ, Summers E, Jones NL, et al. The contribution of pulmonary impairment to the perceived intensity of dyspnea during exercise (abstract). Am Rev Respir Dis 1990; 141:A553.

Chapter 10

Exercise Tolerance in the Pulmonary Patient

KARLMAN WASSERMAN, M.D., Ph.D.

During exercise, the cardiovascular and ventilatory systems must respond appropriately to achieve the increased cellular respiration required to generate the high-energy phosphate, adenosine triphosphate, that is needed for muscle contraction. Muscle respiration increases by a factor of 20 during brisk walking and by as much as a factor of 30 to 80 (depending on gender, age, and the level of fitness) at maximum exercise levels. The increase in external respiration must ultimately increase sufficiently to match the increase in cellular respiration (Fig. 10–1). Patients with lung diseases may have reduced exercise tolerance if (1) during exercise they cannot adequately rearterialize the venous blood (i.e., oxygenate the blood and eliminate CO_2) or (2) the cardiovascular response is inadequate to effect the transport of O_2 at the rate needed to support the increased cellular respiration required during exercise.

The symptoms limiting the exercise performance of the pulmonary patient are exertional dyspnea and fatigue. Both symptoms are almost always present, but usually dyspnea (breathlessness or shortness of breath) is the dominant symptom, particularly when hypoxemia, respiratory acidosis, or both develop during exercise. Because the patient's symptoms develop during exercise, it can be predicted that the patient's physiologic responses to exercise will reveal more information about his or her pathophysiology and symptoms than will resting measurements.

Perhaps surprisingly, the cardiac output increase that occurs in response to exercise is below that which is normal for the pulmonary patient,[1] and this factor may contribute to patient exercise limitation. The reduced cardiac output response to exercise may be a result of pathophysiologic mechanisms that (1) impede right-sided heart filling[2] and (2) restrict vasodilatation of the pulmonary circulation sufficiently to allow the right ventricle to drive blood through the lungs at a rate that is adequate to match the increase required by the left ventricle to support cell respiration.[3] Before these mechanisms can be discussed in greater detail, it is necessary to clarify what is meant by the term "pulmonary patient" and to describe his or her disease.

THE PULMONARY PATIENT

"Pulmonary patient" is an imprecise term because it conveys the idea that there is only one disease process that limits a patient's exercise capacity. In fact, a wide variety of diseases with different anatomic manifestations in the lungs may cause a reduction in exercise performance. The following pathophysiologic processes affect the exercise tolerance of the pulmonary patient:

1. Reduced expiratory airflow due to poor elastic recoil, such as that found in emphysema.
2. Increased airway resistance, such as that in patients with bronchitis and asthma.
3. Limitation in lung expansion caused by diffuse pulmonary fibrosis secondary to organic or inorganic dust exposure, gaseous injury to the lungs, chronic pulmonary infections, rheumatologic disorders, sarcoidosis, or idiopathic diseases (e.g., restrictive lung diseases).
4. Filling of small airways with cells or other material such as occurs in the presence of subacute inflam-

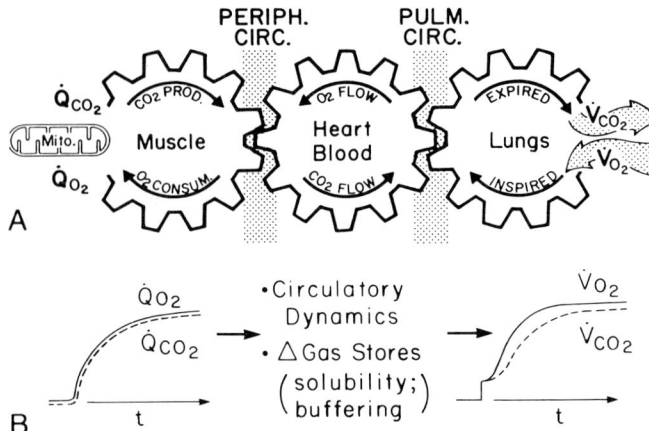

FIGURE 10-1. *A,* Physiologic requirements for the coupling of external respiration to cellular respiration during exercise. *B,* The dynamic responses of muscle O_2 consumption and CO_2 production to constant work rate exercise *(left),* and how this is modified at the airways *(right)* as a result of circulatory dynamics and changes in gas stores within the body. In true steady state, O_2 uptake at the lungs must equal O_2 consumption by the cells, and CO_2 output at the lungs must equal CO_2 production by the cells. (Modified from Wasserman K, Hansen JE, Sue DY, Whipp BJ. Principles of Exercise Testing and Interpretation. Philadelphia: Lea & Febiger, 1987, p 2.)

mation (caused by a reaction to inhaled dusts, infection, or a noninflammatory disease) or pulmonary alveolar proteinosis. The increased diffusion distance for O_2 results in a decrease in pulmonary capillary PO_2 because capillary residence time is decreased when exercise increases cardiac output.

5. Reduced pulmonary vascular bed and the bed's restricted ability to vasodilate during exercise as a result of pulmonary emboli, blood vessel scarring that accompanies chronic inflammatory processes of the lungs, or lung destruction caused by the release of proteolytic enzymes (as in emphysema).
6. Impaired cardiac output due to the effect of lung mechanics on cardiac filling.
7. Wasting of muscles of locomotion as a result of the inactivity precipitated by pulmonary disease.

RESTING VERSUS EXERCISE TESTS OF LUNG FUNCTION

Exercise intolerance is the usual complaint that prompts the patient with chronic pulmonary disease to consult with his or her physician. However, unless the resting pulmonary function measurements are severely disturbed, can the pulmonary physician truly understand the patient's exercise-induced symptoms? Respiratory function measurements recorded at rest provide information on the functional capacity of the patient's lungs, but they do not reveal the patient's ventilatory requirement during exercise. Patients with the same results from spirometric and arterial blood gas studies at rest may have markedly different ventilatory requirements. To determine the ventilatory requirement, exercise testing in which ventilation and gas exchange are measured is needed.

TABLE 10-1. BASIS OF DIFFERENT VENTILATORY REQUIREMENTS FOR A GIVEN LEVEL OF EXERCISE

1. Arterial CO_2 set-point
2. Physiologic V_{DS}/V_T
3. Arterial hypoxemia
4. State of cardiovascular and muscular fitness
5. Pulmonary vascular disease
6. Increased carboxyhemoglobin concentration

The primary factors that lead to these differences in ventilatory requirement are listed in Table 10-1, and the mechanisms for each is as follows:

I. Arterial CO_2 set-point: Patients who regulate arterial P_{CO_2} at widely different set-points have widely different alveolar ventilation requirements. A patient who regulates arterial P_{CO_2} at 30 mm Hg requires 67% more alveolar ventilation than a patient with the same forced expiratory volume in 1 second (FEV_1) but who regulates arterial P_{CO_2} at 50 mm Hg. The regulatory mechanism appears to be "tighter" in the former patient than in the latter, since the former patient seems to tolerate less variation in Pa_{CO_2} and in pH than does the latter. Thus, the patient with the lower arterial P_{CO_2} set-point is likely to experience a greater degree of breathlessness at any metabolic rate compared with the patient with the higher arterial P_{CO_2} set-point.

II. Ventilation/perfusion ($\dot{V}_A/\dot{Q}$) mismatching with a dominance of high $\dot{V}_A/\dot{Q}$ lung units: Patients with lung units in which ventilation relative to perfusion is high have a high fraction of tidal volume (V_T) that is physiologic dead space (DS). Thus, the calculated ratio of physiologic dead space to tidal volume (V_{DS}/V_T) is increased. This increases the ventilatory requirement for a given level of exercise.

III. Arterial hypoxemia with an increased difference between alveolar and arterial O_2 pressures ($P_{A{O_2}} - Pa_{O_2}$): Arterial hypoxemia and increased $P_{A{O_2}} - Pa_{O_2}$ may result from any of four pathophysiologic states (Table 10-2):
  1. Low $\dot{V}_A/\dot{Q}$ lung units: Underventilation of perfused lung units results in regional reductions in alveolar O_2 tension. Thus, the blood that passes through these lung units remains incompletely saturated. At rest, significant hypoxemia does not result from this mechanism unless $\dot{V}_A/\dot{Q}$ is less than 0.5; however, hypoxemia does occur during exercise even when $\dot{V}_A/\dot{Q}$ is greater than 0.5 because mixed venous O_2 content decreases. This is the most common mechanism

TABLE 10-2. MECHANISMS OF ARTERIAL HYPOXEMIA AND OF AN INCREASED DIFFERENCE IN ALVEOLAR AND ARTERIAL P_{O_2} IN PATIENTS WITH LUNG DISEASES

1. Low $\dot{V}_A/\dot{Q}$
2. Diffusion block for O_2
3. Reduced red blood cell residence time in pulmonary capillaries
4. Right-to-left shunt through a patent foramen ovale

leading to hypoxemia in patients with obstructive lung diseases.

2. Diffusion block: When the alveoli are filled with fluid, cells, or the products of cell degeneration, the distance between the lung gas containing O_2 and the blood in the capillary is increased. This can result in a decreased O_2 tension in the red blood cells passing through the capillaries. Thus, this blood is only partially saturated with O_2 during its transit through this diseased lung region. The degree of arterial O_2 unsaturation increases with exercise. Examples of diseases that characterize this pathophysiology are those that are manifested by subacute inflammation (such as "walking" pneumonias) and pulmonary alveolar proteinosis.

3. Shortened red blood cell residence time: Certain disorders are associated with a reduced capillary bed. As a consequence of capillary bed reduction, the increased cardiac output, which must be compatible with the subject's increased O_2 requirement, results in an increased red blood cell velocity through the bed. Thus, the red blood cell residence time in the capillary can become critically short (<0.3 sec),[4] particularly during exercise, so that there is incomplete oxygenation of the blood during the period that the red blood cells are exposed to gas in the gas exchange blood vessels. An example of this pathophysiology occurs in pulmonary vascular occlusive diseases, such as recurrent pulmonary emboli.

4. Right-to-left shunt through a patent foramen ovale: Arterial hypoxemia may result from the opening of an incompletely sealed foramen ovale when the increase in venous return causes right atrial pressure to exceed left atrial pressure during exercise. In such cases, larger decreases in arterial P_{O_2} than those for the other mechanisms of hypoxemia result.[6] Since approximately 25% of all people have an unsealed foramen ovale, 25% of patients with chronic pulmonary disease are candidates to develop hypoxemia from this mechanism during exercise.

IV. State of cardiovascular and muscular fitness: The ventilatory response to exercise might be quite different among patients, depending on their state of cardiovascular fitness or muscular conditioning. Since the less cardiovascularly fit or deconditioned patient develops a greater lactic acidosis in response to exercise, he or she would have more ventilatory drive owing to increased fixed acid production than a more fit subject. The hydrogen ions produced by the formation of lactic acidosis stimulate the carotid bodies to increase ventilatory drive.[7] The increased lactic acidosis resulting from inadequate O_2 transport to metabolically active cells not only increases ventilatory drive but also reduces aerobic adenosine triphosphate regeneration. Thus, two patients with the same degree of mechanical impairment during breathing, the same CO_2 set-point, and the same V_D/V_T might have considerably different ventilatory requirements because of differences in cardiovascular fitness.

V. Increased pulmonary vascular resistance: The systemic circulation is unable to deliver adequate O_2 to the cells of the body when the supply of blood from the right to the left side of the heart is impeded by increased pulmonary vascular resistance. Because the left ventricular output does not fulfill the O_2 requirement of the muscle cells at low work rates in this condition, lactic acidosis develops. This in turn stimulates ventilatory drive.

VI. Increased carboxyhemoglobin levels (e.g., in the cigarette smoker): An increase in carboxyhemoglobin level reduces hemoglobin sites that are most readily available to provide O_2 to the cells. The mechanism for the increased ventilatory drive in this clinical state appears to be the increased lactic acidosis resulting from an imbalance between O_2 supply and O_2 requirement. This condition is associated with an increased ventilatory drive during exercise at work rates above the subject's lactic acidosis threshold.[8]

In summary, it would be impossible to classify the degree of a patient's exercise limitation based on resting pulmonary function measurements alone. Obviously, patients with very poor resting pulmonary function can be recognized as being incapable of a significant amount of exercise. However, there are levels of impairment of resting pulmonary function for which symptoms can vary widely because there are widely different pathophysiologic states that can affect the exercise ventilatory requirement (see Table 10–1). Thus, exercise tests are needed to determine the extent of exercise impairment in these patients.

PATHOPHYSIOLOGIC MECHANISMS LIMITING EXERCISE IN PATIENTS WITH A CHRONIC OBSTRUCTIVE PULMONARY DISEASE

It should be emphasized that the term COPD does not describe one disease but rather the state in which airway obstruction is the predominant functional abnormality. It encompasses a number of diseases, including emphysema, bronchitis, and asthma. To illustrate some of the physiologic disturbances that occur during exercise in COPD, the metabolic cost, ventilatory requirement, and lactic acidosis that developed in response to exercise were compared in two groups of patients with different degrees of airway obstruction caused by emphysema[5,9] and in normal adult subjects (Table 10–3). The physiologic responses were determined for an O_2 uptake ($\dot{V}O_2$) of approximately 1.0 liter per minute, the O_2 consumption normally required for walking at a moderate pace on a zero grade. It should be noted that the work rate that could be performed by the COPD patients was reduced as compared with the norm for the same $\dot{V}O_2$. This might be accounted for in part by the increased work of breathing of the COPD patient and

TABLE 10-3. EFFECT OF AIRWAY OBSTRUCTION DUE TO EMPHYSEMA ON AVERAGE BLOOD LACTATE CONCENTRATION, MINUTE VENTILATION, AND WORK RATE AT AN O_2 CONSUMPTION OF APPROXIMATELY 1.0 LITER PER MINUTE

FEV_1 (L)	$\dot{V}O_2$ (L/min STPD)	WR (Watts)	$\dot{V}E$ (L/min BTPS)	$\dot{V}E/\dot{V}O_2$	La (mM/L)	$La/\dot{V}O_2$
1.02	0.90	35	35	39	3.03	3.37*
1.80	1.05	34	36	34	2.95	2.80†
Normal	≈1.00	50	25	25	<1.00	<1.00‡

*All data in row from Cooper CB, Daly JA, Burns MR et al. Lactic acidosis contributes to the production of dyspnea in chronic obstructive pulmonary disease. Am Rev Respir Dis 1991; 143:A80.
†All data in row from Casaburi R, Patessio A, Ioli F, et al. Reductions in exercise lactic acidosis and ventilation as a result of exercise training in obstructive lung disease. Am Rev Respir Dis 1991; 143:9–18.
‡All data in row from Wasserman K, Hansen JE, Sue DY, Whipp BJ. Principles of Exercise Testing and Interpretation. Philadelphia: Lea & Febiger, 1987, Chapters 1, 3, and 4.
Key: FEV_1: forced expiratory volume in 1 second; WR: work rate; $\dot{V}E$: expiratory volume; La: blood lactate concentration; STPD: standard temperature and pressure, dry; BTPS: body temperature, ambient pressure, saturated.

in part by the effect of the increased blood lactate level on metabolic rate.[10] Minute ventilation ($\dot{V}E$) is increased relative to $\dot{V}O_2$ ($\dot{V}E/\dot{V}O_2$) by 36% in the moderately obstructed patient and 55% in the severely obstructed patient; this reflects the increase in V_{DS}/V_T caused by $\dot{V}A/\dot{Q}$ mismatching. Blood lactate concentration is significantly elevated at a $\dot{V}O_2$ of 1.0 liter per minute. The lactate level increase is more marked in the more obstructed patient, but it is considerably elevated for obstructed patients in both groups above that level expected for normal, moderately sedentary subjects. This suggests that these patients are significantly detrained. Supporting this conclusion are the findings of Casaburi and coworkers,[5] which demonstrate a reduction in lactate concentration and exercise ventilation and improved exercise tolerance following exercise training. Alternatively, the lactic acidosis that these patients develop at low work rates may be due to impaired cardiovascular function.

A number of mechanisms that affect ventilation interact to reduce exercise tolerance and increase breathlessness during exercise in the COPD patient (Fig. 10–2). COPD patients may have an increased ventilatory drive (Fig. 10–2, *left side*) owing to four mechanisms:

1. Inefficiency of gas exchange created by $\dot{V}A/\dot{Q}$ mismatching. The increase in V_{DS}/V_T caused by $\dot{V}A/\dot{Q}$ mismatching requires that $\dot{V}E$ be increased so that the lungs are able to eliminate a given amount of metabolic CO_2 at a given $PaCO_2$ set-point.
2. Arterial hypoxemia. Arterial hypoxemia caused by the increased perfusion of poorly ventilated lungs (low $\dot{V}A/\dot{Q}$ ratio lung units) stimulates the carotid bodies to increase ventilatory drive.
3. The development of lactic acidosis at exceptionally low work rates. The hydrogen ions produced when lactate accumulates serve not only to reduce the bicarbonate concentration (which increases the hydrogen ion stimulus to breathe) but also to increase CO_2 production that results from the bicarbonate buffering of lactic acid.
4. Metabolic cost of work. The O_2 requirement to perform a given amount of work is increased in COPD patients, possibly owing to the increased metabolic cost of breathing. This may be the reason for the reduced rate of external work performed for the same metabolic rate as shown in Table 10–3.

Confounding the increased ventilatory requirement in COPD patients is a reduced ability to breathe caused by increased airway resistance and reduced elastic recoil (Fig. 10–2, *right side*).

The high expiratory resistance resulting from the reduced elastic recoil pressure in emphysema patients becomes more prominent as tachypnea develops (the equal pressure point moves upstream in the airway). The breathing rate increases because of the need to increase minute ventilation so that gas exchange at the lungs matches the gas exchange requirements of the cells. As a result of the reduced expiratory time and the need to increase expiratory flow, the emphysema patient

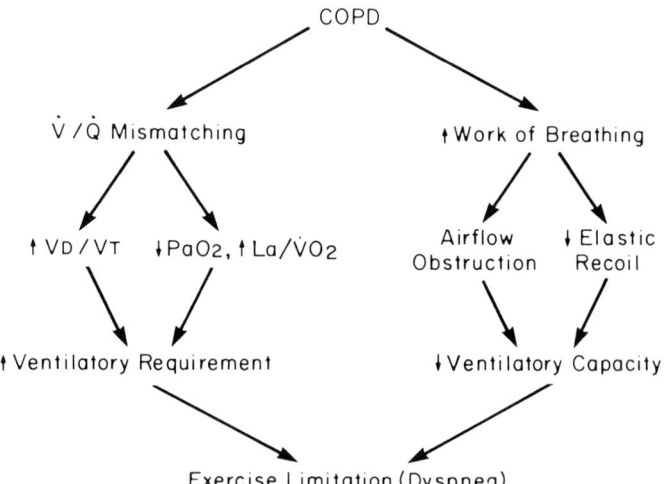

FIGURE 10–2. Factors that play a role in the onset of exercise limitation and dyspnea in patients with COPD. COPD patients have both an increase in ventilatory requirement to perform exercise and a reduction in ventilatory capacity. See text for a detailed discussion of each of the factors shown. ($\dot{V}/\dot{Q}$: ventilation-perfusion ratio; V_{DS}/V_T: dead space-tidal volume ratio; $La/\dot{V}O_2$: ratio of lactate to oxygen consumption.) (Modified from Wasserman K, Hansen JE, Sue DY, Whipp BJ. Principles of Exercise Testing and Interpretation. Philadelphia: Lea & Febiger, 1987, p 52.)

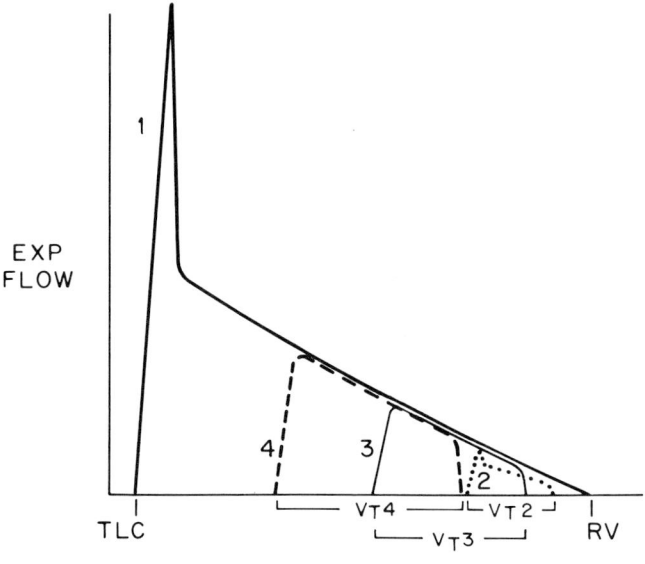

FIGURE 10–3. Curve 1 shows the maximum expiratory (EXP) flow curve from total lung capacity (TLC) to residual volume (RV). Curve 2 shows the expiratory flow over the volume change for tidal breathing at rest. Curve 3 demonstrates the increase in expiratory flow and end tidal volume during exercise, illustrating the increase in FRC resulting from air trapping. Curve 4 is the flow-volume curve for a higher exercise work rate in which expiratory flow must increase with the increase in tidal volume. As with curve 3, the maximum expiratory flow reaches the outer limits of the forced expiratory flow-volume curve (curve 1), and FRC increases owing to increasing work rate and air trapping.

is forced to breathe at a higher lung volume because he or she reaches the limits of maximum flow at lower lung volumes (Fig. 10–3). Thus, his or her FRC increases as work rate increases (Fig. 10–3). This hyperinflated state likely adds to the sensation of breathlessness because receptors in the intercostal muscles, which are sensitive to muscle shortening and tension, are stimulated.[11]

CHARACTERISTIC ABNORMAL RESPONSES TO EXERCISE IN OBSTRUCTIVE LUNG DISEASE

Table 10–4 summarizes the abnormal responses to exercise that are characteristically observed in patients with obstructive lung diseases. Generally, these patients can increase their ventilation in response to exercise to a level that is approximately equal to their maximum voluntary ventilation.[3] The breathing reserve, which is defined as the difference between the maximum voluntary ventilation and the maximum exercise ventilation, is usually less than 10 liters per minute in these patients. Exercise study reports from representative cases are provided in reference 12.

As a result of $\dot{V}_A/\dot{Q}$ mismatching, the physiologic dead space and the V_{DS}/V_T of patients with COPD are increased. This results in a reduced fraction of the breath that is effective alveolar ventilation and in a reduced ventilatory efficiency. Consequently, to eliminate the CO_2 produced and to replace the O_2 in the blood that was consumed due to increased exercise metabolism, patients with COPD usually have a high ventilatory requirement relative to their metabolic rate. This is manifested as an increased ventilatory equivalent for O_2 or CO_2—measurements that are easily made noninvasively during exercise testing. This increased ventilatory equivalent might be offset by a high Pa_{CO_2} set-point. But even a high set-point is rarely sufficiently high in the ambulatory patient to normalize the value of the ventilatory equivalent.

In COPD patients with poor ventilatory reserve, ventilatory compensation for the exercise metabolic acidosis (reduction in Pa_{CO_2} in response to metabolic acidosis) usually does not develop. Therefore, the steepening of ventilation as the work rate approaches its maximum and the increase in ventilatory equivalent for CO_2 at the maximum exercise level observed in normal subjects or in patients with cardiovascular defects are not observed in these patients. Therefore, a respiratory acidosis is generally evident at the maximum exercise level.[13] However, this is not a consistent finding, since patients with milder airway obstruction hyperventilate in response to the exercise metabolic acidosis.

Arterial hypoxemia commonly develops in COPD patients as the result of low $\dot{V}_A/\dot{Q}$ lung units, right-to-left shunt through a patent foramen ovale, or both (pathophysiologic mechanisms 1 and 4 of Table 10–2).

The heart rate reserve (predicted maximum heart rate minus maximum exercise heart rate) is generally high in patients with severe obstructive lung disease. As a result of ventilatory limitation, these patients are unable to increase their work rate to a level sufficiently high to fully stress their cardiovascular system. However, the magnitude of the heart rate reserve is not precisely reflected in the degree of airway obstruction because of variability in cardiovascular fitness.

The O_2 uptake per heart beat ($\dot{V}_{O_2}/HR$) or O_2-pulse is characteristically low in patients with COPD and heart disease.[13] The O_2-pulse is equal to the product of stroke volume and the difference between arterial and venous O_2. Thus, any factor causing stroke volume to be reduced causes the O_2-pulse to be reduced as well. Consequently, it might be predicted that the stroke volume

TABLE 10–4. CHARACTERISTIC ABNORMAL RESPONSES TO EXERCISE IN OBSTRUCTIVE LUNG DISEASE

1. Reduced breathing reserve
2. Increased V_{DS}/V_T
3. Increased ventilatory equivalent for CO_2 and O_2 ($\dot{V}_E/\dot{V}_{CO_2}$, $\dot{V}_E/\dot{V}_{O_2}$)
4. Increased difference between arterial and end tidal CO_2 pressures (Pa_{CO_2} − $P_{ET CO_2}$)
5. Increased difference between alveolar and arterial O_2 pressures ($P_{A O_2}$ − Pa_{O_2}) and between end tidal and arterial O_2 pressures ($P_{ET O_2}$ − Pa_{O_2})
6. No increase in ventilatory equivalent for CO_2 at maximum exercise
7. Respiratory acidosis
8. Hypoxemia depending on the presence of low $\dot{V}_A/\dot{Q}$ lung units
9. High heart rate reserve
10. Low O_2-pulse
11. Exercise metabolic (lactic) acidosis

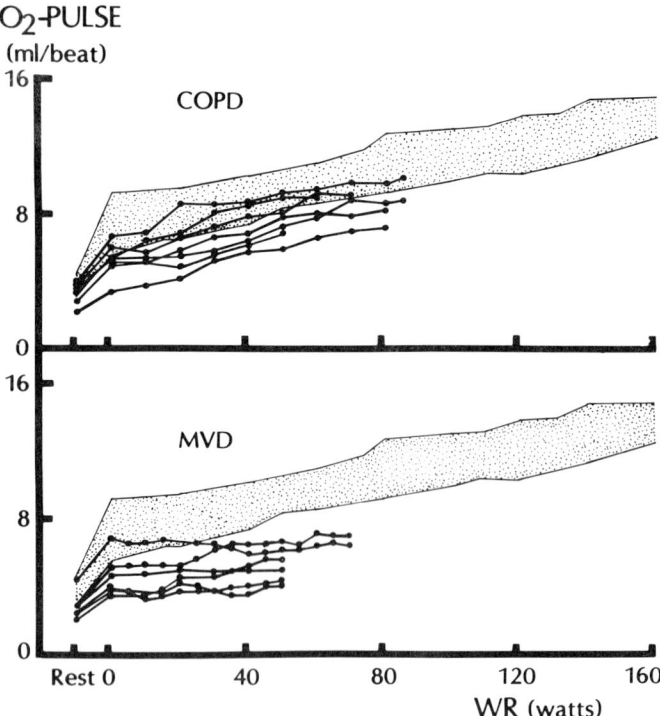

FIGURE 10–4. Oxygen pulse versus work rate (WR) in normal subjects (stippled area), in patients with COPD (solid lines and points, upper panel) and in patients with mitral valve disease (MVD, lower panel). (From Nery LE, Wasserman K, French W, et al. Contrasting cardiovascular and respiratory responses to exercise in mitral valve and chronic obstructive pulmonary diseases. Chest 1983; 83:446–453.)

and O_2-pulse are reduced both in patients with primary heart disease and in those with COPD but for different reasons. Because patients with cardiac disease generally tend to reach their maximum arteriovenous O_2 differences at a relatively low work rate, they may not increase their O_2-pulses beyond that achieved at their lowest work rates (Fig. 10–4).[13] Also, the values at their maximum work rates are low because of their reduced stroke volumes. In contrast, as a result of less primary cardiac limitation, the COPD patients apparently do not reach their maximum arteriovenous O_2 differences at maximum exercise despite their low resting and exercise stroke volumes. Thus, although they are reduced, their O_2-pulses continue to increase during exercise (see Fig. 10–4).

The physiologic basis for the reduction in stroke volume in obstructive lung disease patients is likely limited cardiac filling imposed by the high intrathoracic pressure that occupies most of the respiratory cycle in addition to increased pulmonary vascular resistance. The former mechanism should be more marked during exercise in patients with emphysema as breathing rate increases.

Also limiting the size of the stroke volume and causing the reduction in O_2-pulse in COPD patients is the failure of the right ventricular wall to thicken adequately to overcome the increased pulmonary vascular resistance. This restricts the ability of the blood to readily flow from the right ventricle to the left atrium in these patients. This hypothesis is reflected in the reduced right ventricular ejection fraction and increased left ventricular ejection fraction that occur in response to exercise in these patients.[14]

Finally, the lactic acidosis that develops in these patients at relatively low metabolic rates (see Table 10–4) undoubtedly contributes to their exercise limitation. This low work rate–related lactic acidosis is likely to be a result of the relatively sedentary behavior of the COPD patients. Since the hydrogen ions produced with lactate stimulate respiratory chemoreceptors (particularly the carotid bodies[8]), the low work rate–related lactic acidosis must contribute to patient exercise limitation. Casaburi and coworkers[5] supported this by demonstrating that exercise training in moderately obstructed COPD patients can result in a reduction in lactic acidosis and ventilation during exercise as well as in improved exercise tolerance.

The mechanisms limiting exercise tolerance in patients with obstructive lung diseases are summarized in Table 10–5. Three major factors—increased work of breathing, increased ventilatory drive, and impaired cardiac output—contribute to the exercise intolerance. The mechanisms underlying these disturbances were discussed earlier.

PATHOPHYSIOLOGIC MECHANISMS LIMITING EXERCISE IN PATIENTS WITH INTERSTITIAL PULMONARY FIBROSIS

Pulmonary fibrosis occurs as a consequence of a number of chronic inflammatory disorders, including those caused by inhaled inorganic and organic dusts, infections (such as those due to *Mycobacterium tuberculosis*), sarcoid reactions, and vasculitides, and those disorders that are idiopathic. Patients with interstitial pulmonary fibrosis characteristically experience exertional dyspnea, which limits exercise performance. Interestingly, exercise testing reveals that mechanisms that are not predictable from the pathology likely contribute to this symptom. Physiologic measurements made during exercise testing suggest that a reduced functional pulmonary capillary bed and increased pulmonary vascular resistance are usually dominant factors.

Four mechanisms might contribute to the symptom of

TABLE 10–5. MECHANISMS LIMITING EXERCISE TOLERANCE IN OBSTRUCTIVE LUNG DISEASES

1. Increased work of breathing
2. Increased ventilatory drive
    a. Decreased PaO_2
    b. Increased V_{DS}/V_T
    c. Decreased pH
    d. Increased metabolic requirement
3. Impaired cardiac output increase
    a. Decreased cardiac filling due to increased intrathoracic pressure during exhalation
    b. Increased pulmonary vascular resistance during exhalation due to increased alveolar pressure and the loss of functional pulmonary vessels because of underlying lung disease

TABLE 10–6. PATHOPHYSIOLOGIC RESPONSES TO EXERCISE IN RESTRICTIVE LUNG DISEASES

1. Reduced peak $\dot{V}O_2$
2. Reduced anaerobic threshold
3. Reduced ratio of the change in oxygen consumption to the change in work rate ($\Delta\dot{V}O_2/\Delta WR$)
4. Increased V_{DS}/V_T
5. Increased ventilatory equivalent for O_2 and CO_2
6. Hypoxemia that is usually progressive
7. Ratio of tidal volume to inspiratory capacity (V_T/IC) ≈ 1 at low levels of work

---

exertional dyspnea in patients with pulmonary fibrosis: (1) an increase in arterial hypoxemia, (2) increased hydrogen ion level as a result of the lactic acidosis resulting from the lower than normal cardiac output response to exercise, (3) an increased physiologic V_{DS}/V_T, and (4) the increased inspiratory work owing to decreased lung compliance.

Abnormal physiologic responses to exercise that are characteristic of restrictive lung disease patients are listed in Table 10–6. Anatomically, pulmonary fibrosis generally appears to obliterate the small blood vessels. The peak $\dot{V}O_2$ that occurs in response to maximum-effort exercise is reduced. This is usually accompanied by a reduced anaerobic threshold, which is apparently caused by increased pulmonary vascular resistance that in turn leads to a reduction in the cardiac output response to exercise.

The reduced capillary bed observed in this disorder likely results in a shortened red blood cell residence time. Thus, there is less time for the establishment of a P_{O_2} diffusion equilibrium between pulmonary capillary red blood cells and alveolar gas. This is likely to be the major mechanism for the progressive hypoxemia that is observed as work rate increases.

However, the difficulty in increasing cardiac output in response to the work rate increase that occurs in pulmonary fibrosis creates an imbalance in O_2 supply and O_2 requirement in the actively contracting muscles. Thus, lactic acidosis develops at low work rates. The hydrogen ions from the lactic acid are undoubtedly an additional stimulus for ventilatory chemoreceptors. An abnormally small rise in $\dot{V}O_2$ for the work rate increase also occurs. This suggests that the regeneration of high-energy phosphate by aerobic mechanisms is impaired. Inadequate aerobic high-energy phosphate resynthesis likely leads to fatigue or the inability to maintain muscular contraction during exercise.

$\dot{V}_A/\dot{Q}$ mismatching is also characteristic of patients with pulmonary fibrosis. Owing to the loss of blood vessels associated with this disease, $\dot{V}_A/\dot{Q}$ mismatching is principally of the high-$\dot{V}_A/\dot{Q}$ type. Thus, the physiologic V_{DS}/V_T and ventilatory equivalent for O_2 and CO_2 are abnormally high. In contrast to what occurs in COPD, arterial hypoxemia resulting from a low $\dot{V}_A/\dot{Q}$ is probably not an important cause of exercise hypoxemia in this type of disorder.

At rest, there may be very little hypoxemia and increased alveoloarterial P_{O_2} difference in patients with pulmonary fibrosis. During exercise, the hypoxemia becomes more marked and progressively increases as work rate is increased.[12] Because the magnitude of the hypoxemia cannot be predicted from resting pulmonary function measurements, it is imperative to measure the arterial O_2 tension during exercise. This is especially important when evaluating how much O_2 is needed during exercise in the treatment of patients with pulmonary fibrosis.

In patients with pulmonary fibrosis, V_T usually increases until it reaches the inspiratory capacity. It is then fixed at that level, and further increases in $\dot{V}_E$ are achieved by increasing breathing frequency. Thus, these patients breathe unusually rapidly in response to exercise, even more so than do obstructive lung disease patients.[12] The ratio of tidal volume to the inspiratory capacity usually approaches one and remains fixed at that level as work rate increases.

ALVEOLAR FILLING DISORDERS

There are pulmonary disorders in which inflammatory cells or other material fills perfused alveoli and increases the distance between alveolus and capillary. In these cases, neither airflow limitation nor reduced lung compliance impairs function significantly. Increasing the diffusion distance between alveolar gas and red blood cells requires that red blood cell residence time in capillaries be increased to achieve diffusion equilibrium for O_2. However, this is not possible because cardiac output, and therefore pulmonary blood flow, must be maintained to support the metabolic rate. Consequently, this alveolocapillary pathology results in hypoxemia that is worsened by exercise.

PULMONARY VASCULAR OCCLUSIVE DISEASE

Patients with a reduced pulmonary capillary bed and an inability to expand it during exercise can experience several types of pathophysiologic limitation. As a result of the increased pulmonary blood flow that occurs with exercise, the red blood cell residence time in the restricted pulmonary capillary bed may decrease to critically short periods. This causes a disequilibrium between the O_2 in the alveolar gas and in pulmonary capillary blood as it enters the pulmonary vein.[4] This O_2 disequilibrium becomes more marked, and arterial hypoxemia worsens as pulmonary blood flow increases during exercise.

Hypoxemia may also result from a right-to-left shunt in patients with pulmonary vascular disease, since 25% of people have a potentially patent foramen ovale. Thus, when right atrial pressure increases because of these patients' inability to develop pulmonary vasodilatation in response to the increased venous return induced by exercise, a right-to-left shunt that worsens with increasing exercise level can develop.

Other physiologic abnormalities found in patients with pulmonary vascular occlusive disease include factors 1 to 6 listed in Table 10–6. Thus, the physiologic changes that occur during exercise are similar to those found in patients with restrictive lung diseases with the exception that the evidence for mechanical limitation for lung expansion is absent.

NONCARDIOPULMONARY FACTORS THAT CONTRIBUTE TO EXERCISE INTOLERANCE IN PATIENTS WITH LUNG DISEASE

A number of conditions amplify the symptom of exertional dyspnea and reduce exercise tolerance in patients with either lung or heart disease (Table 10–7). These conditions are worth mentioning because they explain why a patient's symptoms may be more marked than those predicted based on evaluations of the lungs or the heart at rest. Furthermore, these conditions may be modified by treatment when they are recognized.

An important nonpulmonary and noncardiac factor is the increase in carboxyhemoglobin level that accompanies cigarette smoking. The hemoglobin bound by carbon monoxide is usually that which unloads O_2 most readily. Increased carboxyhemoglobin levels that result from smoking reduce both the maximum O_2 consumption and the anaerobic threshold by approximately the same per cent as the per cent increase in carboxyhemoglobin level.[15] Since the anaerobic threshold occurs in the work rate range usually performed by the patient during normal daily activity, its reduction is of functional importance. The increased carboxyhemoglobin concentration raises the level of lactate at any work level above the anaerobic threshold of the subject and lowers the anaerobic threshold.

By reducing the blood's O_2 carrying capacity, anemia can further reduce exercise performance. Like an increase in carboxyhemoglobin concentration, anemia limits O_2 delivery to the cells, which induces low work rate–related lactic acidosis. The latter provides an additional stimulus to breathe and contributes to a patient's exertional dyspnea.

Obesity is an extremely important cause of exercise limitation because of its prevalence in the population of the United States. Obesity forces the metabolic requirement to increase for any given work rate. The increased O_2 cost of cycling work that is a result of obesity is substantial.[16] However, the magnitude of the increase in $\dot{V}O_2$ due to excessive body weight is even greater for ambulatory activities than for cycling work. Not only is the metabolic rate increased so that a given amount of external work can be performed by obese patients, but ventilatory mechanics are also altered by obesity because it reduces the FRC[17] and promotes atelectasis. The latter causes resting hypoxemia that may disappear with exercise.

Obesity might also reduce cardiac reserve, since a higher than normal cardiac output response is required to perform any given amount of external work. Because of the relatively high cardiac output required at rest (and to a greater degree during exercise), blood pressure is usually increased at rest and more markedly during exercise. This systemic hypertension increases left ventricular afterload. If cardiac function is already compromised, the exercise-induced hypertension may cause heart failure. Thus, obesity, in combination with the underlying defect in lung function, might limit the patient beyond the degree expected based on data from pulmonary function tests performed at rest.

Metabolic disturbances, such as chronic metabolic acidosis secondary to uremia, diabetes, or acetazolamide treatment for glaucoma, might result in a low arterial P_{CO_2} set-point and require that ventilation be increased relative to the metabolic rate. When a patient has a limited ability to increase his or her ventilation, lowering the arterial P_{CO_2} set-point might significantly worsen dyspnea.

SUMMARY

Pulmonary patients are not limited solely by abnormal pulmonary function. Their limitation must be studied during exercise because the degree of exercise $\dot{V}A/\dot{Q}$ mismatching and hypoxemia cannot be predicted from measurements taken at rest. The effect of the accompanying pulmonary vascular disease is best quantified during exercise. Also, the amount of ventilation required for exercise, which is quite predictable in the normal subject, is unpredictable in the patient with lung disease. However, the ventilatory requirement is almost always greater than normal. Breathing disorders might also affect the cardiac output response to exercise, even in patients who do not have underlying cardiac disease, and cause lactic acidosis at an unusually low work rate. Finally, other factors, such as obesity, cigarette smoking, anemia, and other illnesses unrelated to the lung, can cause metabolic disturbances and stimulate the ventilatory requirement to increase to a level higher than that for normal subjects. In the presence of these factors, the pulmonary patient is more symptomatic than would be expected based on pulmonary function measurements taken at rest.

REFERENCES

1. Degre S, Sergysels R, Messin R, et al. Hemodynamic responses to physical training in patients with chronic lung disease. Am Rev Respir Dis 1974; 110:395–402.
2. Butler J, Schrigen F, Henriquez A, Cause of the raised wedge pressure on exercise in chronic obstructive lung disease. Am Rev Respir Dis 1988; 138:350–354.
3. Wasserman K, Hansen JE, Sue DY, Whipp BJ. Principles of Exercise Testing and Interpretation. Philadelphia: Lea & Febiger, 1987, Chapters 1, 3, and 4.

TABLE 10–7. NONCARDIOPULMONARY FACTORS CONTRIBUTING TO EXERCISE INTOLERANCE IN PATIENTS WITH LUNG DISEASE

1. Carboxyhemoglobinemia
2. Anemia
3. Obesity
4. Chronic metabolic acidosis

4. Comroe JH Jr, Forster RE, DuBois AB, et al. The Lung: Clinical Physiology and Pulmonary Function Tests. 2nd ed. Chicago: Year Book Medical Publishers, Inc., 1962, pp 126–127.
5. Casaburi R, Patessio A, Ioli F, et al. Reductions in exercise lactic acidosis and ventilation as a result of exercise training in obstructive lung disease. Am Rev Respir Dis 1991; 143:9–18.
6. Sietsema KE, Simon JI, Wasserman K. Pulmonary hypertension presenting as a panic disorder. Chest 1987; 91:910–912.
7. Wasserman K, Whipp BJ, Koyal SN, Clearly M. Effect of carotid body resection on ventilatory and acid-base control during exercise. J Appl Physiol 1975; 39:354–358.
8. Koike A, Wasserman K, Armon Y, Weiler-Ravell D. The work-rate-dependent effect of carbon monoxide on ventilatory control during exercise. Respir Physiol 1991; 85:169–183.
9. Cooper CB, Daly JA, Burns MR, et al. Lactic acidosis contributes to the production of dyspnea in chronic obstructive pulmonary disease. Am Rev Resp Dis 1991; 143:A80.
10. Roston WL, Whipp BJ, Davis JA, et al. Oxygen uptake and lactate kinetics during exercise in man. Am Rev Respir Dis 1987; 135:1080–1084.
11. Campbell EJM, Agostoni E, Newsom-Davis J. The Respiratory Muscles: Mechanics and Neurocontrol. Philadelphia: W.B. Saunders Co., 1970.
12. Wasserman K, Hansen JE, Sue DY, Whipp BJ. Exercise Testing and Interpretation. Philadelphia: Lea & Febiger, 1987.
13. Nery LE, Wasserman K, French W, et al. Contrasting cardiovascular and respiratory responses to exercise in mitral valve and chronic obstructive pulmonary diseases. Chest 1983; 83:446–453.
14. Matthay RA, Burger HJ, Davies R, et al. Right and left ventricular exercise performance in chronic obstructive pulmonary disease: Radionuclide assessment. Ann Intern Med 1980; 93:234–239.
15. Koike A, Weiler-Ravell D, McKenzie DK, et al. Evidence that the metabolic acidosis threshold is the anaerobic threshold. J Appl Physiol 1990; 68:2521–2526.
16. Wasserman K, Whipp BJ. Exercise physiology in health and disease (state of the art). Am Rev Respir Dis 1975; 112:219–249.
17. Ray CS, Sue DY, Bray G, et al. Effect of obesity on respiratory function. Am Rev Respir Dis 1983; 128:501–506.

Chapter 11

Acute and Chronic Respiratory Failure

THOMAS K. ALDRICH, M.D.

Respiratory failure, a common cause of disability and death in a wide variety of primary respiratory and nonrespiratory illnesses, is defined as a major abnormality of pulmonary gas exchange. Criteria for its diagnosis are arbitrary, but most authorities agree that an arterial P_{O_2} less than 50 mm Hg (recorded while the subject is breathing room air) or an arterial P_{CO_2} greater than 50 mm Hg usually indicates the presence of respiratory failure. Two major types of respiratory failure are distinguished: oxygenation failure and ventilatory pump failure.[1] In each type, the onset of the condition, which may be acute or chronic, has important implications for the resulting functional impairment.

OXYGENATION FAILURE

Oxygenation failure is manifested by hypoxemia and is usually accompanied by low or normal P_{CO_2}. Acute oxygenation failure typically results from cardiogenic or noncardiogenic pulmonary edema, extensive pneumonia, lobar atelectasis, or pulmonary embolism, whereas chronic oxygenation failure may be a consequence of congenital heart disease combined with right-to-left shunt, interstitial pneumonitis, or chronic bronchitis.

The origins of hypoxemia are usually attributed to one or more of five physiologic mechanisms: inadequate partial pressure of inspired oxygen, global hypoventilation, right-to-left shunting, ventilation/perfusion ($\dot{V}/\dot{Q}$) mismatching, or incomplete diffusion equilibrium (Table 11–1).[2] In most cases of oxygenation failure, right-to-left shunting, $\dot{V}/\dot{Q}$ mismatching, or both are the major causes of hypoxemia. Diffusion disequilibrium probably contributes to hypoxemia in conditions characterized by a combination of widened alveolocapillary distance and shortened pulmonary capillary transit times, such as extensive destruction and fibrosis of pulmonary parenchyma, especially when the cardiac output is high (as during exercise). The recent observation by Light that excessive intrapulmonary oxygen consumption can account for some of the hypoxemia of dogs with experimental lobar pneumonia[3] suggests that this mechanism may contribute to hypoxemia in some cases of extensive pulmonary inflammation.

VENTILATORY PUMP FAILURE

Failure of the ventilatory pump results in the retention of carbon dioxide due to alveolar hypoventilation, which in turn can be caused by global hypoventilation, $\dot{V}/\dot{Q}$ mismatching, or a combination of the two.[4] Global hypoventilation directly lowers alveolar ventilation. $\dot{V}/\dot{Q}$ mismatching increases physiologic dead space; this requires an increase in minute ventilation to achieve an unchanged alveolar ventilation. If minute ventilation cannot be increased, alveolar ventilation decreases and P_{CO_2} rises.

In ventilatory pump failure, hypercapnia is often accompanied by hypoxemia, which is usually readily reversible with improved ventilation or with small amounts of supplemental oxygen. Acidemia is pronounced in acute ventilatory pump failure, whereas the metabolic compensation for chronic hypercarbia (bicar-

TABLE 11-1. MECHANISMS OF HYPOXEMIA

Mechanism	Measured F_{IO_2}* and P_b†	Measured P_{aCO_2}	Improvement on Oxygen	Change on Exercise	Discrepancy Among $\dot{V}_{O_2}$‡ Measurements
Inadequate P_{IO_2}§	Low F_{IO_2} or Pb	Normal or low	Good	Worsens	Slight
Hypoventilation	Normal	High	Good	N.A.‖	Slight
Shunt	Normal	Variable	*Slight*	Worsens	Slight
$\dot{V}/\dot{Q}$¶ mismatch	Normal	Variable	Good	*Often improves*	Slight
Diffusion disequilibrium	Normal	Normal or low	Good	Worsens	Slight
Intrapulmonary oxygen consumption**	Normal	Variable	Good	N.A.‖	*Higher by gas collection than by the Fick method*

The distinguishing characteristics of hypoxemia are shown in italics.
*Fraction of inspired oxygen.
†Barometric pressure.
‡Oxygen consumption.
§Pressure of inspired oxygen.
‖Not applicable (i.e., exercise tests would not be performed).
¶Ventilation/perfusion.
**Never occurs without coexisting shunts, $\dot{V}/\dot{Q}$ mismatch, or both.

bonate retention) ameliorates the acidemia in chronic ventilatory pump failure[5] (Fig. 11–1).

Chronic ventilatory failure can result from one or more of three abnormalities: inadequate ventilatory drive, excessive respiratory load, or inadequate inspiratory muscle endurance (Fig. 11–2).

Inadequate Ventilatory Drive

Suppression of the normal ventilatory drive leads to reduced alveolar ventilation and to CO_2 retention. Although this is the least common of the three major causes of ventilatory failure, it can contribute to exacerbations of ventilatory failure resulting from other causes. Acute failure of ventilatory drive most often results from overdoses of sedative, narcotic, or hypnotic drugs. In patients with other types of ventilatory failure, metabolic alkalosis or administration of excessive oxygen can contribute to reductions in minute ventilation and exacerbate CO_2 retention.

Most metabolic encephalopathies, such as hepatic or uremic encephalopathy, are associated with increased (rather than decreased) ventilatory drive and with hypocapnia (rather than with hypercapnia). An exception is myxedema, which often impairs ventilatory drive. Similarly, although most structural injuries of the brain are associated with hypocapnia rather than with hypercapnia, occasionally bilateral brain stem injuries result in profound depressions of ventilatory drive. Although anatomic lesions of the brain stem have not been consistently found, the primary hypoventilation syndrome probably represents an example of a primary defect of brain stem function that results in alveolar hypoventilation.

Finally, central respiratory drive can be influenced by peripheral events in the tracheobronchial tree and in the respiratory muscles. Increasing evidence suggests that animals and humans subjected to excessive respiratory loads reduce their ventilatory drive in order to reduce their required level of effort and to prevent peripheral inspiratory muscle fatigue, which is potentially more damaging.[6] The mechanism responsible for the "central fatigue" is unknown, but it may involve an endogenous opioid-mediated stress response,[7] reflex inhibition of interneurons or respiratory motor neurons,[8] or fatigue of the motor neurons themselves.[9] Although further CO_2 retention occurs when ventilatory drive is reduced in this way, reduced ventilatory drive has the benefit of reducing the respiratory load, approximately in proportion to the reduction in minute ventilation. Excessive central fatigue may well be an immediate

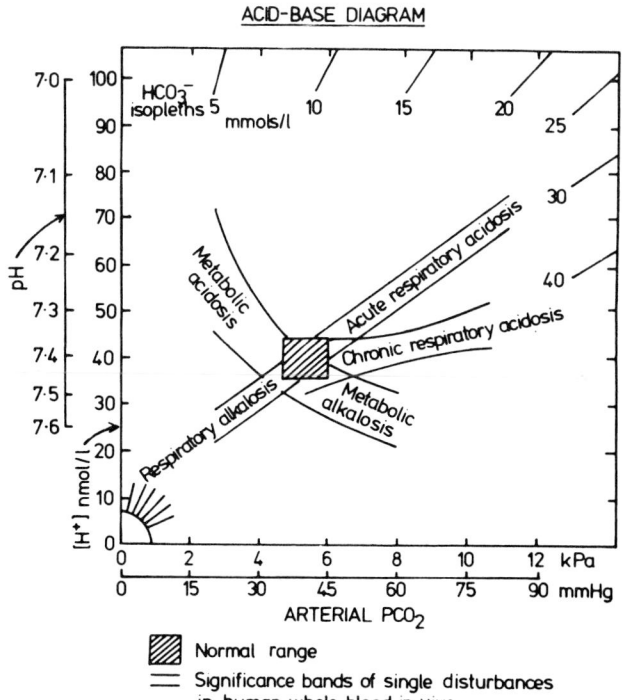

FIGURE 11–1. Diagnosis of acid-base derangements. Arterial pH, P_{CO_2}, and bicarbonate concentration are displayed. Ninety-five per cent confidence limits for isolated respiratory or metabolic acidosis or alkalosis are shown. If the values from a clinical sample fall outside the confidence intervals, a mixed acid-base disorder is likely. (From Flenley DC. Another non-logarithmic acid-base diagram? Lancet 1971; 1:961–965.)

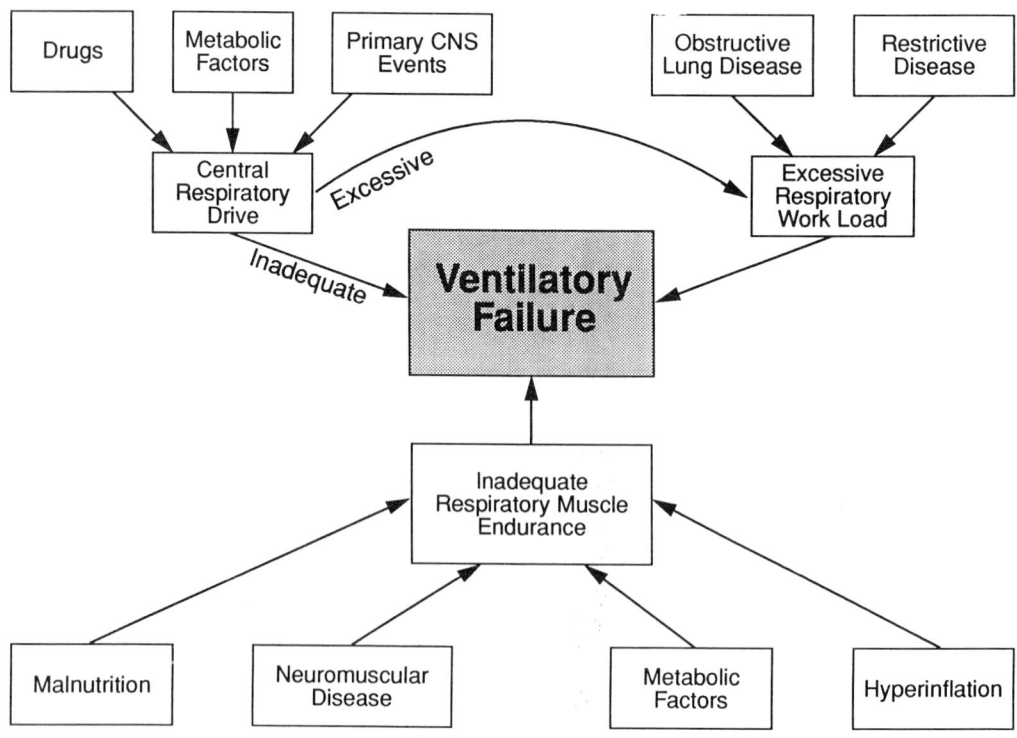

FIGURE 11-2. Factors that can contribute to ventilatory failure. (CNS: central nervous system.) (Adapted from Karpel JP, Aldrich TK. Respiratory failure and mechanical ventilation: Pathophysiology and the methods of promoting weaning. Lung 1986; 164:309–324.)

precipitant of respiratory arrest in many patients with progressive ventilatory failure.[10]

Excessive Respiratory Load

Most of the respiratory workload is inspiratory; the energy required for expiratory airflow is expended during the inspiratory phase and stored as elastic recoil pressure of the lungs for release during the expiratory phase.[11] Even in chronic obstructive pulmonary disease (COPD) or asthma, recoil provides enough driving pressure for expiratory airflow, and the majority of the respiratory work continues to be carried out by the inspiratory muscles. The expiratory muscles, especially the abdominal muscles, are particularly necessary to provide the driving pressure for an effective cough. They also perform inspiratory work in some patients by contracting during the expiratory phase and in turn forcing the diaphragm cephalad, which provides negative (inspiratory) diaphragmatic recoil during the subsequent inspiration.[12]

Three types of inspiratory loads are customarily recognized: resistive, elastic, and inertial (Table 11–2).[11] Resistive loads are caused by the frictional resistance encountered by gases flowing through narrowed bronchi; the severity of the load depends on the geometry of the bronchi, the density of the gas, and the flow rate. Upper airway obstruction and appliances such as endotracheal tubes produce the most severe inspiratory resistive loads. In COPD, although expiratory resistances are extraordinarily high, inspiratory resistances are only moderately elevated.[13]

Excessive elastic loads are due to decreased compliance of the lungs or chest wall; the severity of this load increases with the increasing stiffness of the tissues that are expanded and with increasing tidal volumes. Kyphoscoliosis produces the most severe elastic loads owing to

TABLE 11-2. FACTORS THAT CAN CONTRIBUTE TO EXCESSIVE RESPIRATORY WORKLOAD

Resistive Loads
  Anatomic upper airway obstruction
  Mucus
  Bronchial wall edema
  Bronchospasm
  Turbulent flow

Elastic Loads
  Chest wall distortion
  Obesity
  Pleural fibrosis or effusion
  Pulmonary resection
  Pulmonary fibrosis
  Pulmonary edema
  Hyperinflation

Inertial Loads
  Mass loading (obesity)

Threshold Loads
  Dynamic hyperinflation (intrinsic PEEP)

Increased Minute Ventilation
  Increased CO_2 production
    (exercise, fever, shivering, increased respiratory quotient)
  Increased dead space
  Metabolic acidosis
  Anxiety, dyspnea

Ventilatory Muscle Inefficiency

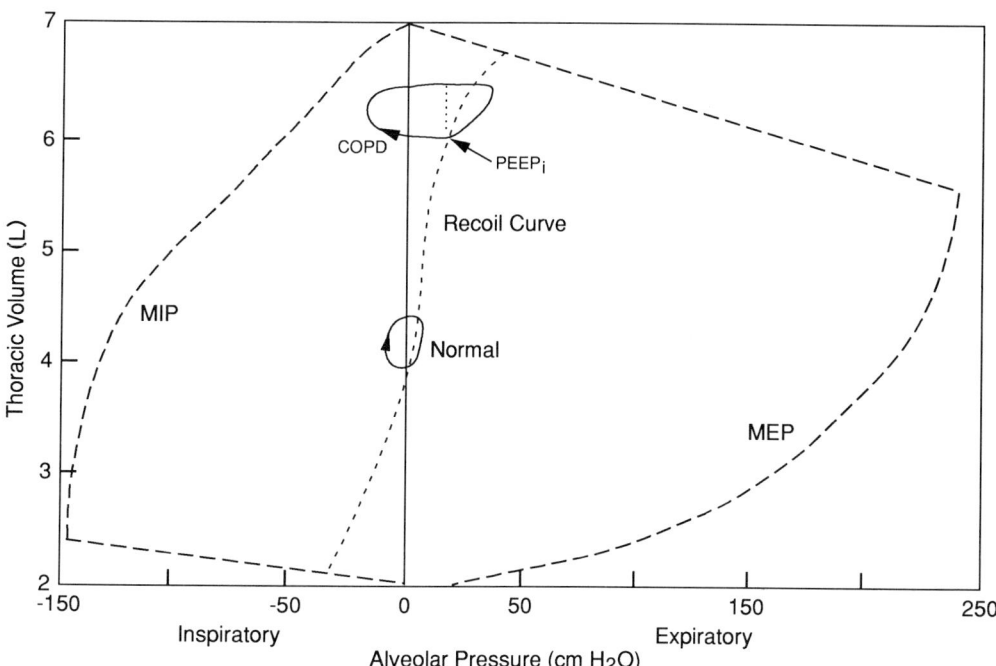

FIGURE 11–3. Effect of dynamic hyperinflation on the pressure-volume relationships of the respiratory system. The *inner dashed line* represents the respiratory system recoil pressure, that is, the pressure that must be opposed by respiratory muscle effort to maintain any particular lung volume with the glottis open. The *outer dashed lines* identify the limits of alveolar pressures during maximum static efforts. The *loops* trace typical tidal breaths for a normal subject and for a patient with an acute exacerbation of COPD. For the COPD patient, at end-expiration substantial positive alveolar pressure is still present, and must be opposed by inspiratory muscle effort before inspiratory airflow can occur. The majority of the work of breathing is required to overcome this threshold load. (MIP: Maximum static inspiratory pressure; MEP: maximum static expiratory pressure; PEEP$_i$: intrinsic positive end-expiratory pressure. Adapted from Rahn H, Otis AB, Chadwick LE, Fenn WO. The pressure-volume diagram of the thorax and lung. Am J Physiol 1946; 146:161–178.)

the loss of thoracic volume and ankylosis of the costovertebral joints; CO_2 retention is not uncommon in kyphoscoliosis. Pleural effusion, pulmonary fibrosis, atelectasis, and pulmonary edema are other common causes of increased elastic loads. These conditions contribute to the respiratory workload, but it is unusual for one of these conditions to be the sole cause of ventilatory failure. When CO_2 retention occurs in a patient with one of these conditions, a careful search often reveals one or more additional major contributing conditions.

In asthma and especially in emphysema, both of which are characterized by hyperinflation (particularly during acute exacerbations), pulmonary compliance is typically higher than normal. Significant elastic loads may be present, however, if the hyperinflation is severe enough that the tidal volume occurs near total lung capacity, where the pressure-volume curve is relatively flat.

Inertial loads are the forces that oppose acceleration or deceleration of the gases and tissues put into motion by respiratory efforts. They are proportional to the mass of the tissues and gases and are thought to be negligible except in morbid obesity.[14]

A fourth type of load, the *threshold load*, has recently been shown to be common among patients with obstructive pulmonary disease.[15] During acute exacerbations of COPD, when expiratory airflow is severely limited, the related dyspnea often prompts a patient to make inspiratory efforts before the respiratory system returns to its normal resting point at which recoil pressure is absent (i.e., functional residual capacity [FRC]). The consequent dynamic hyperinflation dictates that substantial positive (expiratory) respiratory system recoil pressure (termed *auto-positive end-expiratory pressure* [*auto-PEEP*] or *intrinsic PEEP*) is present at end-expiration (Fig. 11–3). Furthermore, substantial effort must be made by the inspiratory muscles to bring the alveolar pressure down below atmospheric pressure before any inspiratory airflow can occur. The result is an inspiratory threshold load that differs from resistive loads in that it is independent of inspiratory flow rate. Also, it differs from elastic loads in that it is independent of tidal volume. This threshold load accounts for a major proportion of the respiratory workload, not only in mechanically ventilated patients but also in many ambulatory patients with COPD, especially but not only in those with CO_2 retention.[16]

Any condition that increases minute ventilation requirements increases respiratory workload approximately in proportion. In patients with marginal tolerance of resting minute ventilation, the increased load resulting from the increased minute ventilation during exercise is the immediate cause of their exercise intolerance. Other conditions that commonly increase minute ventilation requirements include increased physiologic dead space, metabolic acidosis, septicemia, anxiety, and, occasionally, an abrupt increase in carbohydrate intake with a resultant increase in CO_2 production.[17] Thus, although it cannot be the sole cause of ventilatory failure, excessive ventilatory drive can precipitate ventilatory failure in an otherwise marginally compensated patient.

Finally, much of the energy expenditure of the inspiratory muscles is not reflected by pressure-volume work.[18] For example, in a patient with phrenic nerve palsy, the remaining nonparalyzed inspiratory muscles must compensate for the flail motion of the paralyzed hemidiaphragm, which consumes oxygen and energy substrates and performs mechanical work that is not readily measurable as a pressure-volume or a pressure-time product. Less dramatic inefficiencies of inspiratory

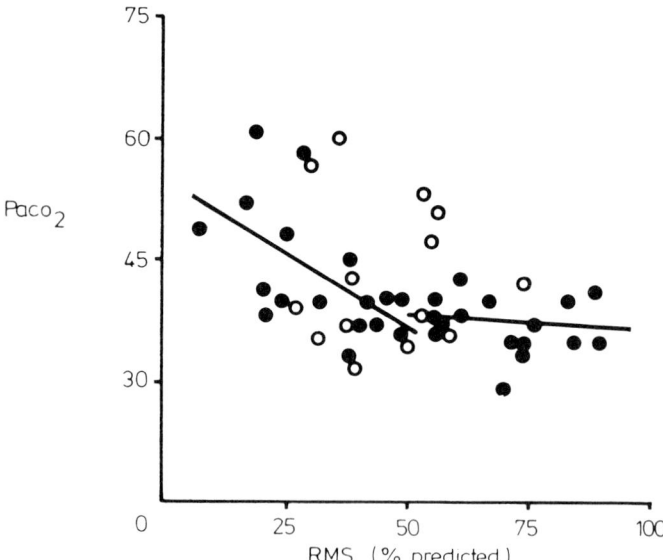

FIGURE 11-4. The influence of respiratory muscle strength (RMS) on $Paco_2$. RMS is calculated as the average of the maximum static inspiratory and expiratory mouth pressures and is expressed as per cent predicted. The *closed circles* represent patients with proximal myopathies without interstitial lung disease, whereas the *open circles* identify patients with both myopathy and interstitial pneumonitis. (From Braun NMT, Arora NS, Rochester DF. Respiratory muscle and pulmonary function in polymyositis and other proximal myopathies. Thorax 1983; 38:616–623.)

muscle action contribute to the inspiratory muscles' burden and are thought to be particularly important in obesity[14] and in COPD.[19]

Inadequate Inspiratory Muscle Endurance

Like all striated muscles, the inspiratory muscles are susceptible to weakening by neuromuscular diseases.[20] Respiratory complications, due in part to inspiratory muscle weakness, are the most common causes of death in Duchenne type muscular dystrophy and other serious muscle diseases and cause some of the most serious complications of Guillain-Barré syndrome and myasthenia gravis. Among patients without intrinsic pulmonary or chest wall disease, ventilatory failure, as manifested by carbon dioxide retention, usually begins to occur when the respiratory muscle strength falls below about 50% of that predicted (Fig. 11–4).[21] When pulmonary conditions such as kyphoscoliosis, aspiration pneumonia, microatelectasis, or interstitial pneumonitis are present, the threshold for ventilatory failure is closer to normal.

Even in the absence of neuromuscular disease, a number of conditions that commonly occur in chronically or acutely ill patients can impair inspiratory muscle endurance and increase the risk of ventilatory failure (Table 11–3). Muscle wasting is a prominent feature of malnutrition and does not spare the inspiratory muscles.[22] Surprisingly, in most cases of malnutrition, the muscle fibers that are most susceptible to atrophy are the strong but fatigable fast-twitch fibers[23]; the relatively weaker but fatigue-resistant slow-twitch fibers are less affected. Consequently, although malnutrition causes marked weakness of the inspiratory muscles, their endurance, which is particularly important for the repetitive efforts required for breathing, is better preserved.

A number of metabolic factors can also reduce the strength and endurance of otherwise normal inspiratory muscles. Examples include conditions that impair oxygen and substrate delivery to contracting muscles, such as hypoxemia, anemia, and reduced cardiac output[24]; electrolyte imbalances, such as hypophosphatemia,[25] hypomagnesemia,[26] and hypocalcemia[27]; respiratory or metabolic acidosis[28]; and the cachexia-producing effects of cancer or acute or chronic infections.[29–31] A wide variety of drugs, usually in overdose but occasionally at doses generally considered safe, can also interfere with normal muscle function.[32] Examples include adrenocorticosteroids, which can promote atrophy of respiratory and nonrespiratory muscles, and aminoglycoside antibiotics or calcium channel blockers, which can impair neuromuscular transmission.

Two intrinsic properties of muscles, the length-tension relationship and the force-velocity relationship, are relevant to their strength during normal tidal volume contractions. Like all striated muscles, the inspiratory muscles are weaker if they contract at shorter than normal fiber length.[33] Thus, as shown in Figure 11–3, maximum static inspiratory pressure decreases as lung volume approaches total lung capacity. In a patient with emphysema, in whom functional residual capacity is chronically far above normal, or in a patient with asthma and acute hyperinflation, the inspiratory muscles are

TABLE 11-3. CAUSES OF INADEQUATE INSPIRATORY MUSCLE STRENGTH AND ENDURANCE

Neuromuscular Disease

Malnutrition

Reduced Oxygen Delivery
  Anemia
  Hypoxemia
  Reduced cardiac output

Acidosis

Electrolyte Disorder
  Hypophosphatemia
  Hypomagnesemia
  Hypocalcemia
  Hypokalemia
  Hyperkalemia

Cachexia
  Acute (infection-related)
  Chronic (in cancer, chronic infections, and other wasting illnesses)

Drugs
  Adrenocorticosteroids (atrophy)
  Aminoglycoside antibiotics (neuromuscular blockade)
  Calcium channel blockers (neuromuscular blockade)

Intrinsic Properties
  Length-tension relationship
  Force-velocity relationship

Disuse and Detraining

Fatigue

weaker and more fatigable than normal simply because of their length-tension relationships. The force-velocity relationship indicates that when muscles contract rapidly, they are capable of less force generation than when they contract more slowly.[34] Consequently, the maximum respiratory pressures achievable during maximum static efforts (MIP, see Fig. 11–3) overestimate the pressure reserve available to inspiratory muscles. In patients with obstructive airways disease, the prolonged expiratory phase reduces the time available for the inspiratory phase and requires the inspiratory muscles to contract at relatively high velocity; therefore, the extent that the maximum static inspiratory pressure overestimates pressure reserve is even more pronounced in COPD patients than in normal subjects.

Finally, like other striated muscles, the inspiratory muscles are at least theoretically susceptible to detraining or atrophy from disuse or to transient weakness (fatigue) from overuse. Changes of disuse atrophy in limb skeletal muscles occur within 2 to 4 days of the onset of disuse[35]; if the same is true of inspiratory muscles, a brief period of controlled mechanical ventilation may result in clinically important inspiratory muscle atrophy, which could contribute to the perpetuation of ventilatory failure. It has been clearly established that inspiratory muscles can be fatigued by experimental overuse, but it is not yet clear whether patients with chronic lung or neuromuscular disease allow their inspiratory muscles to be overused to the point of fatigue or whether they unconsciously reduce their level of respiratory effort to avoid fatigue.[36]

The Balance Between Load and Endurance

Patients with chronic ventilatory failure usually have both an increased respiratory workload and reduced inspiratory muscle endurance due to a variety of the primary and secondary conditions described above (Fig. 11–5). Optimal management of respiratory failure requires consideration of all possible contributing factors and the treatment of all correctable problems. In many cases, even when the primary problem leading to respiratory failure cannot be corrected, this approach can tip the balance away from ventilatory failure.

CLINICAL CHARACTERISTICS OF RESPIRATORY FAILURE

Symptoms

The major symptom of acute respiratory failure is usually dyspnea. Although the severity of dyspnea is generally in proportion to the severity of the pulmonary functional impairment, there is a wide range of sensitivities to the sensation among individual patients. Paradoxically, the sensation of dyspnea does not always occur in proportion to the severity of CO_2 retention because dyspnea often provokes tachypnea and hyperventilation. Furthermore, the additional respiratory

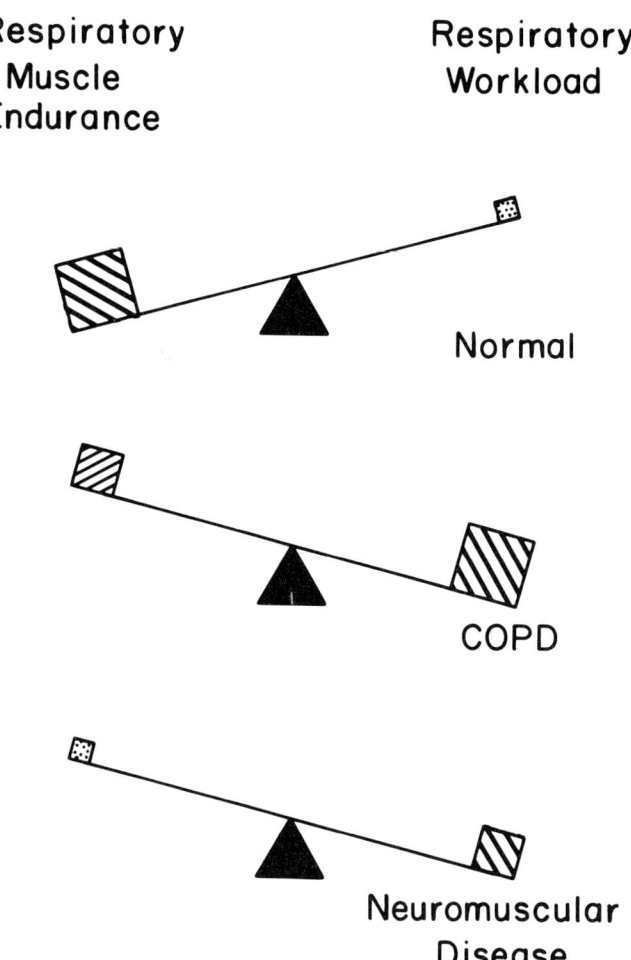

FIGURE 11–5. A schematic representation of the balance between inspiratory muscle endurance and respiratory workload. In healthy individuals, the balance strongly favors endurance, that is, no ordinary activity requires more than a small fraction of the available endurance. In contrast, patients with COPD must contend with large increases in the workload, and their endurance is also limited. Similarly, patients with neuromuscular disease have decreased endurance, but they are also faced with increases in their respiratory workload. In both cases, the result frequently is inadequate endurance relative to the workload.

workload that accompanies hyperventilation may add to a patient's dyspnea and help perpetuate a vicious circle. By the same argument, a patient who accepts a degree of CO_2 retention may suffer less dyspnea than a patient with identically severe pulmonary function who requires an unremittingly high level of respiratory effort to maintain a normal arterial P_{CO_2}.[37]

In chronic ventilatory failure, the severity of dyspnea is much more variable. Thus, in neuromuscular diseases characterized by slowly progressive ventilatory failure, such as amyotrophic lateral sclerosis or Duchenne type muscular dystrophy, dyspnea may be absent most of the time. In such cases, the occurrence of dyspnea often signals the onset of an acute complication such as pneumonia.

A number of adaptive mechanisms contribute to the reduced importance of dyspnea in chronic ventilatory failure. One mechanism is the retention of bicarbonate, which reduces acidosis. This in turn reduces ventilatory drive and workload while at the same time perhaps prevents further acidosis-related impairments in inspiratory muscle function. Another adaptive response to ventilatory failure may be the elaboration of endogenous opioids in response to the stress of loaded breathing, which reduces drive at the expense of further CO_2 retention.[38] Dyspnea is discussed in more detail in Chapter 9.

Other major symptoms of ventilatory failure depend upon its etiology. In patients with COPD, cough, sputum production, and wheezing are prominent symptoms. When these complaints are episodic, especially when they are associated with identifiable allergic or irritant precipitating factors, an asthmatic component may be present; this is important to recognize because of asthma's often excellent response to adrenocorticosteroids, bronchodilators, or both. For patients with heart failure, orthopnea may be severe, peripheral edema may be present, and palpitations or angina may accompany the shortness of breath that occurs during exercise. Although cough is not uncommon in heart failure, it is usually not the productive cough that is typical of COPD.

Regardless of the pathogenesis of ventilatory failure, its severity is almost always increased at night or during sleep. Paroxysmal nocturnal dyspnea, therefore, is by no means diagnostic of congestive heart failure. Furthermore, since patients may be unaware of the occurrence or severity of sleep disturbances, either daytime somnolence due to chronic sleep deprivation or morning headaches due to nocturnal hypoxia may be the major symptom of developing ventilatory failure.

Intellectual and perceptual dysfunctions are additional complications of the hypoxemia and, to a lesser extent, of the hypercapnia of ventilatory failure.[39] Their manifestations depend on the severity and rate of onset of hypoxia. Agitation or a subtle impairment of memory or judgment is characteristic of mild hypoxia, whereas stupor or coma occurs in severe hypoxia. Although acclimatization to hypoxia ameliorates the symptoms to some extent,[40] the demonstrated beneficial effects of supplemental oxygen on intellectual function[41] show that intellectual dysfunction persists during chronic hypoxia.

Signs of Ventilatory Failure

Most of the signs of respiratory failure are nonspecific and related more to the underlying disease that resulted in respiratory failure than to the respiratory failure itself. In many cases, clinical signs of respiratory failure are subtle or absent, and the diagnosis is made only after blood gas analysis. For example, anemic patients often are not cyanotic, even during severe hypoxemia, because cyanosis is present only when more than approximately 5 g/dl desaturated hemoglobin are present in the arterial circulation.

Abnormalities of respiratory pattern are among the most useful signs for alerting the clinician to the presence of respiratory failure and, in some cases, for providing clues regarding its etiology.[42] Rapid shallow breathing, the most common pattern observed in patients with respiratory failure, is entirely nonspecific. Nevertheless, it is often the first indicator of the presence of respiratory failure, and its recognition leads to further investigation and therapy. Bradypnea (respiratory rate less than 10 breaths per minute) is unusual; when present, it may suggest bilateral brain stem lesions, brain stem compression at the level of the lower pons, or, most commonly, overdose of narcotic drugs. Central neurogenic hyperventilation, ataxic respirations, or the Cheyne-Stokes pattern may indicate the presence of medullary, cerebellar, or metabolic defects, but these conditions do not usually result in respiratory failure.

Other useful clues to the presence and type of respiratory failure include visible contractions of respiratory muscles. Most patients with respiratory failure and dyspnea have evident contractions of the accessory muscles of respiration or of the alae nasi. Many patients also have visible contractions of the abdominal muscles during the expiratory phase; these contractions assist expiratory flow and, more important, displace the diaphragm into a longer, more favorable position on its length-tension curve.[12] A few patients have paradoxical inward inspiratory motion of the abdomen in the absence of abdominal muscle contraction, a sign of diaphragmatic paresis or possibly of impending diaphragmatic fatigue.[43]

Depending on the origin of respiratory failure, various abnormalities of percussion and auscultation of the lung fields may be present. Expiratory wheezes are characteristic of obstructive pulmonary disease, whereas inspiratory stridor suggests the presence of upper airway obstruction. The timing of auscultatory crackles often suggests their origin—early inspiratory crackles are characteristic of bronchitis, whereas end-inspiratory crackles suggest congestive heart failure or interstitial pneumonitis.[44] Dullness to percussion over a portion of the lung fields suggests pulmonary consolidation when bronchial breath sounds are present in the same region or indicates pleural effusion when breath sounds are absent.

Finally, a few nonpulmonary findings may be helpful in identifying and classifying respiratory failure. For example, clubbing of the fingers may suggest congenital heart disease as a cause of oxygenation failure or bronchiectasis in ventilatory pump failure. Another example is the onset of peripheral edema, which may suggest congestive heart failure as the primary or a contributing cause of respiratory failure, or, more commonly, the onset of cor pulmonale (failure of an otherwise normal right ventricle) caused by the excessive afterload imposed by hypoxia-related pulmonary hypertension. In some patients with relatively normal daytime blood gas parameters, signs of cor pulmonale provide the first clue to the occurrence of respiratory failure during sleep.

Laboratory Findings

As noted above, arterial blood gas measurements establish the diagnosis of respiratory failure. These measurements are also crucial for following the progress of disease and its treatment. The recent widespread adoption of pulse oximetry for noninvasive measurements of arterial oxygen saturation has markedly improved the precision and the safety of monitoring patients with hypoxemic respiratory failure. Unfortunately, there has not been similar progress in noninvasive monitoring of respiratory acidosis in ventilatory failure. In stable patients without tachypnea, end tidal carbon dioxide measurements correlate well with arterial P_{CO_2}, but among patients with acute respiratory illnesses, in whom accurate noninvasive measurements of Pa_{CO_2} would be most desirable, the lack of a stable end-expiratory CO_2 concentration makes end tidal airway CO_2 concentration unreliable as an index of Pa_{CO_2}. Also, although transcutaneous P_{CO_2} measurements show promise for the future, procedures for their calibration and lengthy equilibration times make currently available instruments too cumbersome for routine use.

Aside from the study of blood gases, the laboratory examination in respiratory failure is relatively nonspecific. Polycythemia may suggest chronic hypoxia, but it may also occur in smokers and patients with renovascular disease and in primary polycythemia. High venous bicarbonate levels, which may suggest chronic hypoventilation, are also present in metabolic alkalosis. Characteristic abnormalities of other routine blood test findings occur in infections, malnutrition, collagen-vascular and metabolic diseases, and other conditions, but they are not specific for any particular cause of respiratory failure. As an illustration of a nonspecific laboratory finding, thyroid hormone levels are often abnormally low in patients with respiratory failure, even in the absence of clinical myxedema, because of reductions in the concentrations of binding proteins and because of the reduced metabolism of triiodothyronine to thyroxine in euthyroid sick syndrome.[45]

Both chest radiography and electrocardiography are indispensable for the diagnosis and management of respiratory failure. Occasionally, as in pneumothorax or acute myocardial infarction, these tests provide the definitive diagnosis. More commonly, as in pulmonary edema or pneumonia, they complement other examinations. In some cases, as in pulmonary embolism, chest films and electrocardiograms are most helpful in ruling out other possible diagnoses.

The examination of expectorated or suctioned sputum is also particularly helpful. The amount and character of the sputum demonstrate to what extent it may be contributing to the respiratory workload. Furthermore, a brief microscopic examination of unstained sputum often provides helpful clues to its origin; thus, a predominance of granulocytes indicates probable infection, whereas a predominance of eosinophils (readily distinguishable from granulocytes even without staining) strongly suggests asthma or asthmatic bronchitis.[46] Finally, in patients with purulent sputum, findings from Gram's staining usually allow the selection of an appropriate, relatively narrow-spectrum antibiotic.

Pulmonary function testing is often useful for the diagnosis of respiratory failure and especially for following its progress. Simple spirometry, now readily available for bedside use, can usually differentiate obstructive from restrictive conditions and can provide evidence for or against upper airway obstruction. The spirometric measurements—vital capacity and forced expiratory volume in one second—are maximal at expiratory muscle efforts that are well below the maximum; above a threshold value, the results are independent of driving pressure. Thus, although patient cooperation is required, as long as a reasonable effort is made, these measurements are reliable. In the Guillain-Barré syndrome or myasthenia gravis—conditions often associated with the rapid worsening of ventilatory function—regular monitoring of vital capacity identifies patients with impending respiratory arrest and allows elective (rather than emergent) intubation for mechanical ventilatory support.

The maximum inspiratory pressure test is also a useful bedside test for detecting and especially for ruling out inspiratory muscle weakness. The subject makes a strong inspiratory effort against an occluded airway, and the resulting negative airway pressure is noted. Because there is no airflow during the test, the pressure change at the airway opening is identical to the pressure change in the thorax, regardless of airways resistance. Unfortunately, unlike the spirometric measurements, the maximum static inspiratory pressure is entirely effort-dependent. The inability of many chronically ill patients to give a maximum effort on command decreases the specificity of the maximum static inspiratory pressure for detecting inspiratory muscle weakness.[47]

In some cases of respiratory failure, measurements of lung volumes, compliance, resistance, or diffusing capacity, or any combination of these measurements are necessary to elucidate the cause or to follow progress. Occasionally, tests of heart rate, ventilation, arterial oxygen saturation, and oxygen consumption during exercise are necessary to differentiate cardiac from pulmonary causes of chronic respiratory insufficiency. When diaphragmatic paralysis is suspected, fluoroscopy of the diaphragm during a rapid inspiratory effort ("sniff" test) can help to confirm or rule out the diagnosis.

MANAGEMENT OF RESPIRATORY FAILURE

The cornerstone of the management of respiratory failure is treatment of the underlying disease. In many cases, however, respiratory failure persists despite optimal treatment of the underlying disease, and specific or nonspecific supportive measures must be used. Careful attention to secondary or complicating conditions often controls symptoms and partially relieves functional disabilities, even when no progress can be made in reversing the primary disease. Thus, for treatment of respiratory failure, all possible contributing factors should be identified, and those that are amenable to treatment should be optimally treated.

Oxygenation Failure

Supportive treatment for oxygenation failure consists primarily of the administration of supplemental oxygen. Techniques for oxygen administration are discussed in Chapter 15. Drugs to improve the matching of ventilation and perfusion, such as almitrine bismesylate, may prove to be useful in the management of chronic hypoxemia if problems with side effects can be overcome.[48]

When adequate oxygenation cannot be achieved by less invasive means, mechanical ventilation is indicated, often with positive end-expiratory pressure. Mechanical ventilation can improve hypoxemia more effectively than supplemental oxygen alone because it allows more homogeneous inflation of the lungs, thus improving the matching of ventilation to perfusion, and because it helps to open regions of microatelectasis. Extracorporeal membrane oxygenation is effective treatment for severe hypoxemia, but its side effects, especially in adults, as well as its expense make it impractical for all but a few severely hypoxemic patients who require temporary support for reversible disease or those who are awaiting lung transplantation.[49]

Reductions in Load

For asthma and chronic airways obstruction, reductions in load constitute the mainstay of treatment. Bronchodilators, antibiotics for excessive purulent sputum production due to bronchitis, and mucolytics are examples of drugs designed primarily to reduce the work of breathing. These drugs may be effective even in the absence of diagnosed obstructive airways disease. Diuretics and inotropic agents can result in improved pulmonary compliance and reduced work of breathing in congestive heart failure, and adrenocorticosteroids can often reduce resistive loads in asthma and elastic loads in certain cases of interstitial pneumonitis.

In patients with large pleural effusions, thoracentesis can substantially, but usually temporarily, reduce elastic workload. The improvement varies with the amount of fluid removed and with the ability of the underlying lung to re-expand.[50] Patients who derive substantial benefit from thoracentesis but in whom the fluid rapidly reaccumulates may require pleurodesis or pleuroperitoneal shunting.

To the extent that microatelectasis contributes to elastic loading in neuromuscular disease or other conditions associated with shallow breathing, incentive spirometry, which encourages regular sighing, can re-expand regions of microatelectasis and prevent the development of lobar atelectasis.[51] In some patients who are unable to voluntarily generate adequate-volume sighs, the regular administration of several sequential large-volume breaths by Ambu bag or positive-pressure ventilator (as in intermittent positive-pressure breathing) may serve the same function.[52]

Position changes can also affect respiratory workload. In the upright position, the diaphragm's inspiratory excursions are assisted by the effects of gravity. Although the resultant shortening of the diaphragm can worsen its length-tension relationships, the increase in chest wall compliance, particularly in obese patients, results in a better balance between load and endurance. Furthermore, the increase in functional residual capacity in the upright posture often improves oxygenation and decreases the risk of progressive atelectasis in patients with rapid shallow breathing.

Any treatment that reduces minute ventilation requirements also reduces the respiratory workload. An example is sodium bicarbonate administration for patients with metabolic acidosis who can tolerate the sodium load, especially those with renal tubular acidosis. A change in diet, with a reduction in carbohydrate intake and an increase in fat intake, results in a decrease in respiratory quotient, which in turn results in a decrease in the carbon dioxide production for any given oxygen consumption and a corresponding reduction in minute ventilation requirement.[53] The encouragement of pursed-lip breathing is another way of reducing minute ventilation requirements in patients with COPD. Pursed-lip breathing works primarily by slowing the respiratory rate, which allows an increase in tidal volume, reduces the ratio of dead space to tidal volume, and thus reduces total minute ventilation.[54]

A promising new treatment for ventilatory failure is the transtracheal administration of air or oxygen. Implanted transtracheal catheters, which were developed as a more efficient and less obtrusive method than nasal cannulas to deliver low-flow oxygen,[55] appear to have two additional advantages, especially when they deliver relatively high flows (up to 10 or 15 L/min) of air or air supplemented with oxygen.[56, 57] First, the continuous flow washes out CO_2 from the upper airway; this decreases the amount of effective dead space and thus reduces minute ventilation requirements. Second, to the extent that the upper airway offers resistance to the backflow of the tracheal gases, positive airway pressure is produced; this helps to maintain airway patency and relieves some of the inspiratory work of breathing in a manner analogous to that of continuous positive airway pressure.

Several important benefits of exercise training also stem from reductions in minute volume requirements.[58] First, exercise training often causes a degree of desensitization to sensations of dyspnea; this results in a reduced minute ventilation for any given activity. Second, training usually promotes improved exercise efficiency, which means that higher exercise levels can be tolerated for any given oxygen consumption. Third, in patients who are able to exercise to anaerobic threshold, a peripheral muscle training effect occurs; this effect increases the anaerobic threshold and decreases lactic acid production during exercise. The decreased severity of metabolic acidosis and the lower respiratory quotient both reduce minute ventilation requirements. Exercise training is discussed in more detail in Chapter 16.

Improvements in Inspiratory Muscle Function

When inspiratory muscle weakness is caused by identifiable neuromuscular disease, specific treatment is the most appropriate approach. Unfortunately, specific treatment is only available for a small minority of patients with neuromuscular disease, such as those with myasthenia gravis, some cases of collagen-vascular disease, and electrolyte or nutritional deficiencies.

For all patients with respiratory failure, however, adequate oxygenation and correction of any electrolyte or acid-base abnormalities minimize the contribution of those abnormalities to the imbalance between workload and endurance. For patients in circulatory shock, cardiac inotropic agents may restore adequate delivery of oxygen and energy substrates to the contracting inspiratory muscles, while at the same time improving washout of metabolites.[24]

For patients with hyperinflation, measures to reduce functional lung volumes improve inspiratory muscle strength by placing the muscles at a more advantageous point on their length-tension curve.[33] Such measures include bronchodilation and any treatment, such as pursed-lip breathing, that reduces the respiratory rate or, to a lesser extent, the tidal volume.

Nutritional support is a two-edged sword in patients with ventilatory failure. On the one hand, it increases carbon dioxide production (as compared to the fasting state), even when carried out with high-fat, low-carbohydrate formulas.[17] On the other hand, nutritional support prevents the glycogen depletion that may occur in hard-working inspiratory muscles,[59, 60] and it can prevent the malnutrition-associated inspiratory muscle atrophy that is apparent after days to weeks of partial or total starvation.[61] Furthermore, the prevention of malnutrition-associated defects in immune function[62] and in the pulmonary clearance of microorganisms[63] would improve both workload and endurance. Most authorities believe that the benefits of nutritional support outweigh its harmful effects.[64–66] In malnourished COPD patients, a balanced[64] or fat-weighted[65] diet is recommended; such a diet should yield enough calories to provide approximately 1.7 times the measured resting energy expenditure,[64, 66] which equals about 1.9 to 2 times the value calculated using the Harris-Benedict equations.[67] Nutritional support is discussed more thoroughly in Chapter 25.

Pharmacologic treatment to improve inspiratory muscle function nonspecifically has been sought for many years. The methylxanthines, caffeine, and theophylline have been clearly shown to improve the isolated diaphragm's response to low-frequency stimulation in the range of 1 to 20 Hz.[68–70] Methylxanthines do not improve maximum inspiratory pressures[71] because they do not improve the diaphragm's response to high-frequency stimulation.[68, 69, 72] Since tidal breathing efforts are the result of low-frequency phrenic nerve impulses,[73] isolated enhancements of the low-frequency response might be expected to improve the balance between workload and endurance. However, it is not clear whether patients with acute or chronic illness experience the same improvements in low-frequency response or whether those improvements are substantial enough to reduce symptoms or disability.[74, 75]

Studies have reported acute improvements in inspiratory muscle function following the administration of a number of other drugs, including beta$_2$ sympathetic agonists,[76–79] cardiac inotropic agents,[79, 80] and the acetylcholine esterase inhibitor neostigmine.[76] In most cases, the reports have remained unconfirmed or have been refuted by other investigators.[81, 82] Longer-term therapy with anabolic steroids[83, 84] or with growth hormone[85] has been suggested to strengthen inspiratory muscle, but this approach as yet remains unproved.

Finally, inspiratory muscle endurance training has been advocated for patients with chronic ventilatory failure. If training could improve these patients' inspiratory muscle endurance, their tolerance of a chronic irreversible respiratory load would be improved. Training usually consists of one to three daily 15- to 30-minute periods of isocapnic hyperventilation,[86] inspiratory flow-resistance loading,[87] or inspiratory threshold loading.[88] Such training has been carried out in ambulatory patients with chronic airways obstruction,[86–88] kyphoscoliosis,[89] neuromuscular diseases,[90, 91] and even in patients receiving mechanical ventilation.[92] Because endurance training is best accomplished by frequent periods of acutely fatiguing exertion,[93] the results of this technique are critically dependent on the patient's motivation. Generally, threshold loading has had the most success. Inspiratory muscle training is discussed in more detail in Chapter 17.

Adjustments of Drive

As noted above, inadequate ventilatory drive is an uncommon cause of ventilatory failure, except in cases of drug overdose. Patients with drug overdoses are treated supportively and with the expectation that ventilatory drive will recover. Since the recovery of ventilatory drive sometimes lags behind the level of consciousness in cases of benzodiazepine overdose, intensive monitoring should continue for up to 1 day after the resolution of coma induced by benzodiazepines.[94]

In the occasional case of ventilatory failure associated with myxedema, treatment with thyroid hormones is indicated. In patients with metabolic alkalosis and the resultant carbon dioxide retention, chloride repletion with saline and potassium chloride is usually effective. Occasionally, more aggressive treatment is indicated, such as either the administration of the carbonic-anhydrase–inhibiting diuretic acetazolamide or cautious infusions of dilute hydrochloric acid.

In cases in which no etiology can be established, trials of drug treatment to enhance drive are indicated,[95] since any such treatment also increases respiratory workload. Even in the absence of metabolic alkalosis, acetazolamide can enhance drive in some patients by inducing mild metabolic acidosis. Progesterone and doxapram are two centrally acting drugs that can occasionally improve ventilatory drive in the primary hypoventilation syndrome. In patients who do not respond to drug treatment, phrenic nerve pacing may be indicated.[96]

As discussed above, many patients with ventilatory

failure suffer from excessive rather than inadequate drive and would benefit from treatments to inhibit ventilatory drive in order to reduce respiratory load and dyspnea. Major tranquilizers,[97, 98] benzodiazepines,[98] and narcotics[99–101] have been used in carefully selected cases of intolerable load-associated dyspnea or of intractable exercise intolerance. Narcotics have proved to be the most successful and have the advantage that their effects can be relatively easily reversed with narcotic antagonists. Several studies have demonstrated reductions in dyspnea and improvements in exercise tolerance after the administration of narcotics.[99–101] The sedating and drive-suppressing effects of narcotics are difficult to control, however, and their use can lead to serious risks of apnea and death. Nevertheless, such treatments are occasionally justified in a carefully monitored setting for competent patients with particularly severe disabling dyspnea.

Mechanical Ventilation

When ventilatory failure cannot be controlled by less invasive means because of impending or actual respiratory arrest or intolerable dyspnea, mechanical ventilation is indicated. Although considerable inspiratory muscle activity persists in many patients receiving mechanical ventilation, the ventilator eliminates the risk that insufficient power will be available for adequate alveolar ventilation. In most acute cases, the goal of mechanical ventilation is temporary support until the underlying disease or the exacerbation of disease that resulted in acute respiratory failure can be controlled.

In chronic ventilatory failure, the goal of treatment depends on the severity of disease. In patients who are completely ventilator-dependent, the goal is simply life support. In patients who can tolerate spontaneous breathing for various lengths of time, the goal may be to prevent or reverse inspiratory muscle fatigue. In many of these patients, ventilatory support is provided only at night to ensure a period of rest for the ventilatory muscles, to prevent sleep deprivation caused by sleep-disordered breathing, and to prevent cor pulmonale by ensuring adequate oxygenation for at least several hours per day.

Mechanical ventilation is usually accomplished in the assist/control mode by a volume ventilator that provides positive-pressure breaths via an endotracheal tube or tracheostomy (i.e., intermittent positive-pressure breathing). Alternate modes of positive-pressure mechanical ventilation include intermittent mandatory ventilation, in which assisted or controlled mechanical breaths are interspersed with spontaneous patient-initiated breaths; continuous positive airway pressure, in which airway pressure remains higher than atmospheric pressure throughout the respiratory cycle, thus providing a small inspiratory assist and eliminating the excess work of breathing imposed by intrinsic positive end-expiratory pressure; and pressure-support ventilation, which provides a more consistent inspiratory assist by means of a computer-controlled constant level of positive inspiratory airway pressure throughout the inspiratory effort. Alternative delivery methods, suitable mainly for patients with chronic ventilatory failure who do not require full-time ventilatory support, include negative-pressure ventilation by cuirass or body ventilator and nasal or face-mask ventilation with intermittent positive-pressure breathing or continuous positive airway pressure. These techniques have been particularly successful in patients with neuromuscular causes of respiratory failure.[102, 103] Each mode of ventilation has advantages and disadvantages under various clinical circumstances; the appropriate mode is usually the one that provides the most patient comfort. Mechanical ventilation is discussed in more detail in Chapters 20 and 36.

Recent developments that have resulted in improved quality of life for patients receiving chronic mechanical ventilation include an increasing focus on providing care at home, simplified methods to allow speech despite positive-pressure ventilation through a tracheostomy, and reductions in the size, weight, and noise level of mechanical ventilators.[104] In spite of these advances, many patients with chronic respiratory or neuromuscular illnesses, their family members, and many physicians regard chronic mechanical ventilation as unacceptable and decide or recommend against its consideration, even to preserve life. Although there are no data describing the preferences of competent patients, many patients faced with an immediate choice between mechanical ventilation or death choose mechanical ventilation, regardless of their previous attitudes.[104] For competent, motivated patients with supportive families or other care providers, therefore, chronic mechanical ventilation is increasingly becoming an acceptable treatment.

CONCLUSION

Respiratory failure may be acute or chronic and may be characterized by inadequate oxygenation, inadequate ventilation, or both. Chronic respiratory failure is usually caused by failure of the ventilatory pump, which in turn usually results from a combination of increased respiratory workload and inadequate inspiratory muscle endurance. Although weakness is the major contributor to ventilatory failure in neuromuscular diseases, the workload is often increased by kyphoscoliosis, recurrent aspiration, microatelectasis, upper airway obstruction, or any of these factors in combination. In chronic lung disease, in which excessive workload is the major problem, inspiratory muscle function is often impaired by malnutrition, electrolyte imbalances, an unfavorable position on the length-tension curve as a result of hyperinflation, inspiratory muscle detraining, or any combination of these. In both cases, the result is often an unfavorable imbalance between load and endurance, both components of which must be addressed for satisfactory resolution of the symptoms and disabilities of ventilatory failure.

REFERENCES

1. Roussos C, Macklem PT. The respiratory muscles. N Engl J Med 1982; 307:786–797.
2. West JB. Pulmonary Pathophysiology: The Essentials. Baltimore: Williams & Wilkins, 1982.
3. Light RB. Intrapulmonary oxygen consumption in experimental pneumococcal pneumonia. J Appl Physiol 1988; 64:2490–2495.
4. West JB. Assessing pulmonary gas exchange. N Engl J Med 1987; 316:1336–1338.
5. Flenley DC. Another non-logarithmic acid-base diagram? Lancet 1971; 1:961–965.
6. Aldrich, TK. Central fatigue of the rabbit diaphragm. Lung 1988; 166:233–242.
7. Scardella AT, Parisi RA, Phair DK, et al. The role of endogenous opioids in the ventilatory response to acute flow-resistive loads. Am Rev Respir Dis 1986; 133:26–31.
8. Road J, Vahi R, Del Rio P, Grassino A. In vivo contractile properties of fatigued diaphragm. J Appl Physiol 1987; 63:471–478.
9. Kernell D, Monster AW. Motoneurone properties and motor fatigue. Exp Brain Res 1982; 46:197–204.
10. Yanos J, Keaney MF III, Leisk L, et al. The mechanism of respiratory arrest in inspiratory loading and hypoxemia. Am Rev Respir Dis 1990; 141:933–937.
11. Cherniack NS, Milic-Emili J. Mechanical aspects of loaded breathing. In: Roussos C, Macklem PT; The Thorax. Lung Biology in Health and Disease. Vol 29. New York: Marcel Dekker, Inc., 1985, pp 751–786.
12. Martin JG, DeTroyer A. The behaviour of the abdominal muscles during inspiratory mechanical loading. Respir Physiol 1982; 50:63–73.
13. Aldrich TK, Shapiro SM, Sherman MS, Prezant DJ. Alveolar pressure and airways resistance during maximal and submaximal respiratory efforts. Am Rev Respir Dis 1989; 140:899–906.
14. Sharp JT. The chest wall and respiratory muscles in obesity, pregnancy, and ascites. In: Roussos C, Macklem PT. The Thorax. Lung Biology in Health and Disease. Vol 29. New York: Marcel Dekker, Inc., 1985, pp 999–1021.
15. Pepe PE, Marini JJ. Occult positive end-expiratory pressure in mechanically ventilated patients with airflow obstruction: The auto-PEEP effect. Am Rev Respir Dis 1982; 126:166–170.
16. Haluszka J, Chartrand DA, Grassino AE, Milic-Emili J. Intrinsic PEEP and arterial P_{CO_2} in stable patients with chronic obstructive pulmonary disease. Am Rev Respir Dis 1990; 141:1194–1197.
17. Fraser IM. Effects of refeeding on respiration and skeletal muscle function. Clin Chest Med 1986; 7:131–139.
18. Roussos C. Energetics. In: Roussos C, Macklem PT. The Thorax. Lung Biology in Health and Disease. Vol 29. New York: Marcel Dekker, Inc., 1985, pp 437–492.
19. Tobin MJ. Respiratory muscle involvement in chronic obstructive pulmonary disease and asthma. Probl Respir Care 1990; 3:375–395.
20. Aldrich TK, Aldrich MS. Primary muscle disorders. In: Kamholz SL (ed). Pulmonary Aspects of Neurological Diseases. New York: PMA Publishing, 1987, pp 85–100.
21. Braun NMT, Arora NS, Rochester DF. Respiratory muscle and pulmonary function in polymyositis and other proximal myopathies. Thorax 1983; 38:616–623.
22. Arora NS, Rochester DF. Effect of body weight and muscularity on human diaphragm muscle mass, thickness, and area. J Appl Physiol 1982; 52:64–70.
23. Sieck GC, Lewis MI, Blanco CE. Effects of undernutrition on diaphragm fiber size, SDH activity, and fatigue resistance. J Appl Physiol 1989; 66:2196–2205.
24. Aubier M, Viires N, Syllie G, et al. Respiratory muscle contribution to lactic acidosis in low cardiac output. Am Rev Respir Dis 1982; 126:648–652.
25. Planus RF, McBrayer RH, Koen PA. Effect of hypophosphatemia on pulmonary muscle performance. Adv Exp Med Biol 1982; 151:283–290.
26. Malloy DW, Dhingra S, Solven FS. Hypomagnesemia and respiratory muscle power. Am Rev Respir Dis 1984; 129:497–498.
27. Aubier M, Viires N, Piquet J, et al. Effects of hypocalcemia on diaphragmatic strength generation. J Appl Physiol 1985; 58:2054–2061.
28. Juan G, Calverley P, Talamo C, et al. Effect of carbon dioxide on diaphragmatic function in human beings. N Engl J Med 1984; 310:874, 879.
29. Tracey KJ, Vlassara H, Cerani A. Cachectin/tumor necrosis factor. Lancet 1989; 1:1122–1126.
30. Meir-Jedrzejowicz A, Brophy C, Green M. Respiratory muscle weakness during upper respiratory tract infections. Am Rev Respir Dis 1988; 138:5–7.
31. Drew JS, Farkas GA, Pearson RD, Rochester DF. Effects of a chronic wasting infection on skeletal muscle size and contractile properties. J Appl Physiol 1988; 64:460–465.
32. Aldrich TK, Prezant DJ. Adverse effects of drugs on the respiratory muscles. Clin Chest Med 1990; 11:177–189.
33. Braun NMT, Arora NS, Rochester DF. Force-length relationship of the normal human diaphragm. J Appl Physiol 1982; 53:405–412.
34. Luff AR. The force-velocity relationship of respiratory muscles. In: Sieck GC, Gandevia SC, Cameron WE (eds). Respiratory Muscles and Their Neuromotor Control. Neurology & Neurobiology. Vol 26. New York: Alan R. Liss, 1987, pp 403–413.
35. Witzmann FA, Kim DH, Fitts RH. Hindlimb immobilization: Length-tension and contractile properties of skeletal muscle. J Appl Physiol 1982; 53:335–345.
36. Aldrich TK. Respiratory muscle fatigue. Probl Respir Care 1990; 3:329–342.
37. Rochester DF, Arora NS, Braun NMT, Goldberg SK. The respiratory muscles in chronic obstructive pulmonary disease. Bull Eur Physiopathol Respir 1979; 15:117–123.
38. Santiago TV, Remolina C, Scoles V, Edelman NH. Endorphins and the control of breathing: Ability of naloxone to restore flow-resistive load compensation in chronic obstructive pulmonary disease. N Engl J Med 1981; 304:1190–1195.
39. Gibson ME, Pulsinelli W, Blass JP, Duffy TE. Brain dysfunction in mild to moderate hypoxia. Am J Med 1981; 70:1247–1254.
40. Robin ED. Of men and mitochondria: Coping with dysoxic hypoxia. Am Rev Respir Dis 1980; 122:517–531.
41. Nocturnal Oxygen Therapy Trial Group. Continuous or nocturnal oxygen therapy in hypoxemic chronic obstructive lung disease. Ann Intern Med 1980; 93:391–398.
42. Plum F, Posner JB. The Diagnosis of Stupor and Coma. Philadelphia: F.A. Davis Co., 1980.
43. Cohen CA, Zagelbaum G, Gross D, et al. Clinical manifestations of inspiratory muscle fatigue. Am J Med 1982; 73:308–316.
44. Nath AR, Capel LH. Inspiratory crackles: Early and late. Thorax 1982; 29:223–227.
45. Wartofsky L, Burman KD. Alterations in thyroid function in patients with systemic illness: The euthyroid sick syndrome. Endocr Rev 1982; 3:164–217.
46. Epstein RL. Constituents of sputum: A simple method. Ann Intern Med 1972; 77:259–265.
47. Multz AS, Aldrich TK, Prezant DJ, et al. Maximal inspiratory pressure is not a reliable test of inspiratory muscle strength in mechanically ventilated patients. Am Rev Respir Dis 1990; 142:579–582.
48. Watanabe S, Kanner RE, Cutillo AG, et al. Long-term effect of almitrine bismesylate in patients with hypoxemic chronic obstructive pulmonary disease. Am Rev Respir Dis 1989; 140:1269–1273.
49. Egan TM, Duffin J, Glynn MF, et al. Ten-year experience with extracorporeal membrane oxygenation for severe respiratory failure. Chest 1988; 94:681–687.
50. Light RW, Stansbury DW, Brown SE. Changes in pulmonary function following therapeutic thoracentesis. Changes in pul-

monary function following therapeutic thoracentesis. Chest 1981; 80:374–380.
51. Bartlett RH, Gazzaniga AB, Geraghty TR. Respiratory maneuvers to prevent postoperative pulmonary complications. JAMA 1973; 224:1017–1021.
52. Sinha R, Bergofsky EH. Prolonged alteration of lung mechanics in kyphoscoliosis by positive pressure hyperinflation. Am Rev Respir Dis 1972; 106:47–57.
53. Goldstein S, Askanazi J, Weissman C, et al. Energy expenditure in patients with chronic obstructive pulmonary disease. Chest 1987; 91:222–224.
54. Tiep BL, Burns M, Kao D, et al. Pursed lips breathing training using ear oximetry. Chest 1986; 90:218–221.
55. Walsh DA, Govan JR. Long-term continuous domiciliary oxygen therapy by transtracheal catheter. Thorax 1990; 45:478–481.
56. Wesmiller SW, Hoffman LA, Soiurba FC, et al. Exercise tolerance during nasal cannula and transtracheal oxygen delivery. Am Rev Respir Dis 1990; 141:789–791.
57. Bergofsky EH, Hurewitz AN. Airway insufflation: Physiologic effects on acute and chronic gas exchange in humans. Am Rev Respir Dis 1989; 140:885–890.
58. Casaburi R, Storer TW, Wasserman K. Mediation of reduced ventilatory response to exercise after endurance training. J Appl Physiol 1987; 63:1533–1538.
59. Gaesser GA, Brooks GA. Glycogen repletion following continuous and intermittent exercise to exhaustion. J Appl Physiol 1980; 49:722–728.
60. Ferguson GT, Irvin CG, Cherniack RM. Relationship of diaphragm glycogen, lactate, and function to respiratory failure. Am Rev Respir Dis 1990; 141:926–932.
61. Sieck GC, Lewis MI, Blanco CE. Effects of undernutrition on diaphragm fiber size, SDH activity and fatigue resistance. J Appl Physiol 1989; 66:2196–2205.
62. Good RA. Nutrition and immunity. J Clin Immunol 1981; 1:3–11.
63. Niederman MS, Merrill WW, Ferranti RD, et al. Nutritional status and bacterial binding in the lower respiratory tract in patients with chronic tracheostomy. Ann Intern Med 1984; 100:795–800.
64. Donahoe M, Rogers RM. Nutritional assessment and support in chronic obstructive pulmonary disease. Clin Chest Med 1990; 11:487–504.
65. Angelillo VA, Sukhdarshan B, Durfee D, et al. Effects of low and high carbohydrate feedings in ambulatory patients with chronic obstructive pulmonary disease and chronic hypercapnia. Ann Intern Med 1985; 103:883–885.
66. Efthimiou J, Fleming J, Gomes C, et al. The effect of supplemental oral nutrition in poorly nourished patients with chronic obstructive pulmonary disease. Am Rev Respir Dis 1988; 137:1075–1082.
67. Harris JA, Benedict FG. A biometric study of basal metabolism in man. Carnegie Institute of Washington. Publication 270, 1919.
68. Jones DA, Howell S, Roussos C, et al. Low-frequency fatigue in isolated skeletal muscles and the effects of methylxanthines. Clin Sci 1982; 63:161–167.
69. Esau SA. Effect of theophylline on membrane potential and contractile force in hamster diaphragm muscle in vitro. J Clin Invest 1986; 77:638–640.
70. Supinski GS, Deal EC, Kelsen SG. Comparative effects of theophylline and adenosine on respiratory, skeletal, and smooth muscle. Am Rev Respir Dis 1986; 133:809–813.
71. Foxworth JW, Reisz GR, Knudson SM, et al. Theophylline and diaphragmatic contractility: Investigation of a dose-response relationship. Am Rev Respir Dis 1988; 138:1532–1534.
72. Reid MR, Miller MJ. Theophylline does not increase maximal tetanic force or diaphragm endurance in vitro. J Appl Physiol 1989; 67:1655–1661.
73. Iscoe S, Dankoff R, Migicousky R, et al. Recruitment and discharge frequency of phrenic motoneurones during inspiration. Respir Physiol 1978; 26:113–128.
74. Murciano D, Aubier M, Lecocguic Y, et al. Effects of theophylline on diaphragmatic strength and fatigue in patients with chronic obstructive pulmonary disease. N Engl J Med 1984; 311:349–353.
75. Moxham J. Aminophylline and the respiratory muscles: An alternative view. Clin Chest Med 1988; 9:325–336.
76. Howell S, Fitzgerald RS, Roussos C. Effects of neostigmine and salbutamol on diaphragmatic function. Respir Physiol 1985; 62:15–29.
77. Aubier MA, Viires N, Murciano D, et al. Effects and mechanism of action of terbutaline on diaphragmatic contractility and fatigue. J Appl Physiol 1984; 56:922–929.
78. Suzuki S, Numata H, Sano F, et al. Effects and mechanism of fenoterol on fatigued canine diaphragm. Am Rev Respir Dis 1988; 137:1048–1054.
79. Aubier M, Murciano D, Menu Y, et al. Dopamine effects on diaphragmatic strength during acute respiratory failure in chronic obstructive pulmonary disease. Ann Intern Med 1989; 110:17–23.
80. Aubier M, Viires N, Murciano D, et al. Effects of digoxin on diaphragmatic strength generation. J Appl Physiol 1985; 58:2054–2061.
81. Javaheri S, Smith JT, Thomas JP, et al. Albuterol has no effect on diaphragmatic fatigue in humans. Am Rev Respir Dis 1988; 137:197–201.
82. Sherman MS, Aldrich TK, Chaudhry I, Nagashima H. The effect of digoxin on contractility and fatigue of isolated rat and guinea pig hemidiaphragms. Am Rev Respir Dis 1988; 138:1180–1184.
83. de Boisblanc BP, Jawda A, Svec F, et al. Effect of anabolic steroids on diaphragmatic tension generation in a rat model of cystic fibrosis (abstract). Am Rev Respir Dis 1990; 141:A548.
84. Prezant DJ, Gentry EI, Valentine DE. Diaphragm contractility and fatigue after combined treatment with dexamethasone and testosterone (abstract). Am Rev Respir Dis 1991; 143:A567.
85. Suchner U, Rothkopf MM, Stanislaus G, et al. Growth hormone and pulmonary disease: Metabolic effect in patients receiving parenteral nutrition. Arch Intern Med 1990; 150:1225–1230.
86. Belman MJ, Mittman C. Ventilatory muscle training improves exercise capacity in chronic obstructive pulmonary disease patients. Am Rev Respir Dis 1980; 121:273–280.
87. Pardy RL, Rivington RN, Despas PJ, Macklem PT. The effects of respiratory muscle training on exercise performance in chronic airflow limitation. Am Rev Respir Dis 1981; 123:426–433.
88. Larson JL, Kim MJ, Sharp JT, Larson DA. Inspiratory muscle training with a pressure threshold breathing device in patients with chronic obstructive pulmonary disease. Am Rev Respir Dis 1988; 138:689–696.
89. Hornstein S, Inman S, Ledsone JR. Ventilatory muscle training in kyphoscoliosis. Spine 1987; 12:859–863.
90. Gross D, Ladd HW, Riley EJ, et al. The effect of training on strength and endurance of the diaphragm in quadriplegia. Am J Med 1980; 68:27–35.
91. DiMarco AF, Kelling JS, DiMarco MS, et al. The effect of inspiratory resistive training on respiratory muscle function in patients with muscular dystrophy. Muscle Nerve 1985; 8:284–290.
92. Aldrich TK, Karpel JP, Uhrlass RM, et al. Weaning from mechanical ventilation: Adjunctive use of inspiratory muscle resistive training. Crit Care Med 1989; 17:143–147.
93. Delateur BJ, Lehmann JF, Giaconi R. Mechanical work and fatigue: Their roles in the development of muscle work capacity. Arch Phys Med Rehabil 1975; 57:319–324.
94. Jedeikin R, Menutti D, Bruderman I, Hoffman S. Prolonged respiratory center depression after alcohol and benzodiazepines. Chest 1985; 87:262–264.
95. Altose MD, Hudgel DW. The pharmacology of respiratory depressants and stimulants. Clin Chest Med 1986; 7:481–494.
96. Glenn WWL, Hokomb WG, Gee JBL, et al. Central hypoventilation: Long-term ventilatory assistance by radiofrequency electrophrenic respiration. Ann Surg 1970; 172:755–773.
97. Stark RD, Gambes SA, Lewis JA. Methods to assess breathlessness in healthy subjects: A critical evaluation and application to analyze the acute effects of promethazine on breathlessness induced by exercise or by exposure to raised levels of carbon dioxide. Clin Sci 1981; 61:429–439.
98. Woodcock AA, Gross ER, Gellert A, et al. Drug treatment of breathlessness: Contrasting effects of diazepam and promethazine in pink puffers. BMJ 1981; 283:343–346.

99. Johnson MA, Woodcock AA, Geddes DM. Dihydrocodeine for breathlessness in "pink puffers". BMJ 1983; 286:675–677.
100. Light RW, Muro JR, Sato RI, et al. Effects of oral morphine on breathlessness and exercise tolerance in patients with chronic obstructive pulmonary disease. Am Rev Respir Dis 1989; 139:126–133.
101. Santiago TV, Johnson J, Riley DJ, Edelman NH. Effects of morphine on ventilatory response to exercise. J Appl Physiol 1979; 47:112–118.
102. Bach JR, Alba AS. Noninvasive options for ventilatory support of the traumatic high level quadriplegic patients. Chest 1990; 98:613–619.
103. Bach JR, Alba AS. Management of chronic alveolar hypoventilation by nasal ventilation. Chest 1990; 97:52–57.
104. Life-sustaining technologies and the elderly. Washington, DC: US Congress, Office of Technology Assessment; July 1987. US Library of Congress publication OTA-BA-306, Catalog No. 87-619835.

Chapter 12

Course and Prognosis in Patients with Chronic Airflow Obstruction: Possible Implications for Therapy

DIRKJE S. POSTMA, M.D.
GERARD H. KOËTER, M.D.
PETER J. WIJKSTRA, M.D.

Chronic airflow obstruction (CAO) is, as its name implies, a disease in which airflow obstruction is persistently present, despite therapy. It largely occurs in older persons and is strongly related to smoking, although not all smokers are affected, suggesting that endogenous factors do influence this disease process.[1] One of the main features observed in CAO patients is a decline in forced expiratory volume in 1 second (FEV_1) that is far more rapid than that in healthy individuals. In normal individuals, the FEV_1 decreases by 20 to 30 ml per year. In patients with CAO the FEV_1 decreases by 40 to 100 ml per year, but even higher values up to 200 ml per year have been reported.[2]

Understanding the mechanisms responsible for the increased fall in lung function over time in patients with CAO is very important because this may lead to adequate intervention measures that may result in less morbidity or even fewer deaths. Studies conducted in the late 1980s reported an increase in CAO-related mortality that has been observed in many countries.[3-6] This disease is not only a nuisance for the patient but also constitutes a significant economic and social burden for society.

In this chapter, the course of patients with established CAO characterized by mild to moderate or severe airflow obstruction is described with regard to prognostic factors and these factors' possible meaning for therapeutic intervention.

PROBLEMS OF DIAGNOSIS

Recent cross-sectional and longitudinal reports on the increase in mortality as a result of CAO have shown that the disease's increased incidence rate is quite real.[6,7] However, it is not certain whether the individuals in these studies who are characterized as having CAO recognize their disease and seek medical advice to prevent the further deterioration of their lung function. CAO is generally a disease diagnosed at middle age, and it is just at this time that a deterioration of overall physical condition presents itself. Some insidiously occurring symptoms, such as some daily coughing and some breathlessness experienced when climbing several flights of stairs, are often attributed to the aging process. At a more advanced age, physical fitness is of lesser importance because of the more sedentary life style of the elderly. A recent Australian epidemiologic study showed that individuals poorly perceive their deteriorating lung function (Fig. 12–1).[1] The investigators established an FEV_1 less than 60% of predicted as the

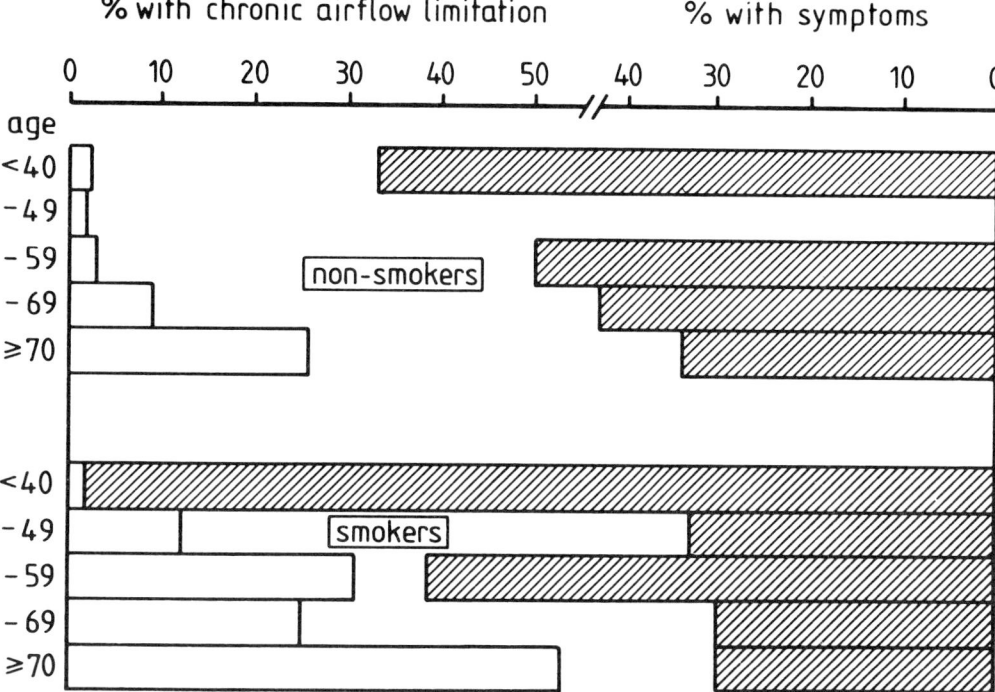

FIGURE 12-1. Prevalence of individuals with airflow obstruction (white bars) in an Australian population stratified for age (yr), and the percentage of those individuals (striped bars) with chest symptoms. (From Peat JK, Woolcock AJ, Cullen K. Decline of lung function and development of chronic airflow limitation: A longitudinal study of nonsmokers and smokers in Busseltons, Western Australia. Thorax 1990; 45:32–37.)

cut-off level for abnormality and observed an increasing incidence of abnormal lung function with increasing age. Two per cent of the nonsmokers under the age of 40 years and 26% of the individuals over the age of 70 years had abnormal lung function. Percentages were, as could be expected, considerably higher in smokers of all ages, although the trend was the same. However, 67% of the younger, nonsmoking group with abnormal lung function and 34% of the older group were reported to have symptoms. CAO may thus go unrecognized until severe and irreversible loss of FEV_1 has occurred. Because CAO is a common cause of disability and a risk factor for other serious illnesses, early identification of CAO patients is an unsolved but essential health care issue. Studies are under way to investigate whether specific therapy (apart from smoking cessation), including the inhalation of corticosteroids, may change the course of disease. There are reasons to assume that this is possible. Therefore, awareness of the possible presence of CAO, especially in smokers, is one of the major goals for every clinician in the future.

PREDICTORS OF THE COURSE OF DISEASE: MORTALITY

Table 12–1 summarizes the results of some studies on the predictors of survival in patients with CAO. Their different results are addressed in this section.

Age and FEV_1

Mortality is higher in patients with CAO than in an age-matched and gender-matched healthy population. All clinical and population-based studies show that mortality is higher with increasing baseline age and decreasing baseline degree of airways obstruction as measured by FEV_1 (Fig. 12–2). These two parameters are the most important determinants of mortality. Compared with age and level of FEV_1, all other influences are relatively minor.

Smoking

Smoking is strongly associated with the development of CAO. The positive relationship of smoking cessation to longer survival has been addressed in only one study (Fig. 12–3).[2] This may be largely the result of the study's long duration of follow-up compared with the periods of other studies, as the influence of smoking cessation on survival became apparent only after approximately 6 years of follow-up.

Allergy

Most investigations studying survival in CAO have excluded subjects with "asthmatic" features. Burrows and coworkers[17] investigated individuals in a random population. One hundred twenty subjects 40 to 75 years of age were selected from 207 individuals whose first spirometric examination showed their FEV_1 to be less than 65% of that predicted. They all consulted with a physician for asthma, chronic bronchitis, emphysema, or "bronchial trouble." In addition, the ratio of FEV_1 to forced vital capacity (FVC) had to be less than 75% if the subjects were to be included. Twelve patients under age 40 years were excluded because of clear asthmatic features, and 37 subjects were not considered

TABLE 12-1. PREDICTORS OF MORTALITY

Reference	No. of Patients	Follow-up (yr)	Baseline			Rev	Predictors
			FEV_1 in L (SD)	FEV_1 % Pred (SD)	Age in Yr (SD)		
IPPB Trial Group[8, 9]	985	3	1.03	36 (11)	61 (7)	BM	Age FEV_1 pb TLC Maximum work Heart rate
Boushy et al.[10]	663	2–7	—	—	—	ND	FEV_1 Age D_{LCO} Pa_{CO_2} N_2 washout
Burrows et al.[11]	200	3–7	1.0 (0.4)	34 (12)	59 (8)	BM	FEV_1 Heart rate Decline in FEV_1
Traver et al.[12]	200	15	1.0 (0.4)	34 (12)	59 (8)	BM	Age FEV_1 pb Cor pulmonale (< 65 years)
Kanner et al.[13]	84	7–13	—	—	—	BM	FEV_1*/FVC FEV_1* Pa_{O_2}* Pa_{CO_2}* Smoking* Decline in FEV_1* Reversibility* D_{LCO}*
Postma et al.[14] Smit et al.[15]	129	6–10	0.6 (0.1)	25 (9)	54 (9)	AC	Reversibility P pulmonale RV%TLC
Postma et al.[16]	129	14–18	0.6 (0.1)	25 (9)	54 (9)	AC	Reversibility FEV_1%FIV_1 Smoking

*Unadjusted data (i.e., not corrected for confounders).
Key: FEV_1%Pred: FEV_1, per cent predicted; Rev: reversibility resulting from bronchodilator therapy; BM: beta mimetic; pb: postbronchodilator; TLC: total lung capacity; ND: not done; D_{LCO}: carbon monoxide diffusing capacity; AC: anticholinergic; SD: standard deviation.

because of their age (over 75 years). Burrows and coworkers identified patients as having CAO if they reported never to have had asthma, did not have allergies, and had smoked previously. A group comprising chronic asthmatic bronchitic patients who had a diagnosis of asthma, were nonsmokers, or did not have allergies was identified. The patients in this group were mostly women and had a lower mortality rate than those in the CAO group with comparable FEV_1 levels. However, the "asthmatic" group had smoked less (18 pack years [number of packs of cigarettes smoked per day multiplied by the number of years of smoking]) than the CAO group (51 pack years). Smoking was associated with mortality, but it was not accounted for in the analysis. There has been only one study of patients with advanced airflow obstruction (FEV_1 < 1.25 L) that showed that the number of reactive skin test results was not related to survival.[14]

Further studies are necessary to determine whether allergic individuals with smoking-related airflow obstruction have a better survival rate.

Airway Hyperresponsiveness

After the presence of airflow obstruction, airway hyperresponsiveness is one of the most important find-

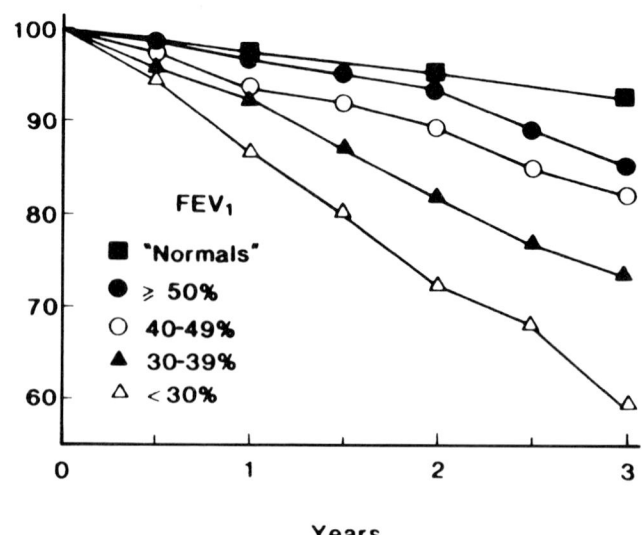

FIGURE 12-2. Survival curves stratified for the level of airflow obstruction. (FEV_1: forced expiratory volume in 1 second). (From Anthonisen NR, Wright EC, Hodgkin JE. Prognosis in chronic obstructive pulmonary disease. Am Rev Respir Dis 1986; 133: 14–22.)

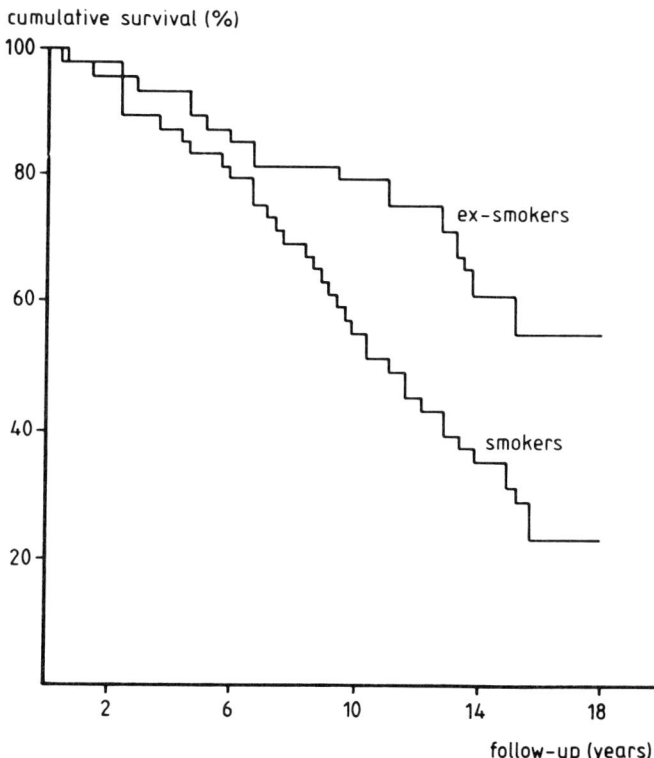

FIGURE 12–3. Survival curves with respect to smoking habits. (From Postma DS, Sluiter HJ. Prognosis of chronic obstructive pulmonary disease: The Dutch experience. Am Rev Respir Dis 1989; 14:S100–S105.)

ings in subjects with CAO. Airway hyperresponsiveness is defined as an exaggerated bronchoconstrictor response to various physical, chemical, or pharmacologic stimuli. It is experienced as an increase in dyspnea or even wheezing during exposure to irritants such as cold weather, air pollution, fog, smoke, and perfume. There have been several population-based reports relating airway hyperresponsiveness to the presence of pulmonary symptoms[18–20] and to the development of CAO.[21, 22]

Cross-sectional studies[23–29] have documented the occurrence of airway hyperresponsiveness to histamine and methacholine in the majority of patients with CAO. There are some caveats in these studies; most of them may have had a selection bias owing to the hospital recruitment of patients, and only two of the studies had healthy control groups.[24, 27] Moreover, none of these studies compared the results in healthy subjects and in patients after adjustment for the level of FEV_1. This is an important issue, as the degree of airway hyperresponsiveness is inversely associated with the level of pulmonary function both in population-based studies[18, 20] and in patients with CAO.[30, 31] Some studies suggest that baseline airway caliber is not the only factor determining the degree of airway hyperresponsiveness. Patients with chronic bronchitis, which is defined as the presence of chronic sputum and cough, may have airway hyperresponsiveness without airflow obstruction. Moreover, Yan and associates[32] showed that a significant decrease in airway hyperresponsiveness occurred after fenoterol pretreatment in 11 subjects with CAO; however, no increase in FEV_1 was observed. Thus, it seems likely that the presence of airway hyperresponsiveness in subjects with CAO is partially determined by airflow obstruction, but airflow obstruction is not the only factor.

The only study to investigate the relationship of histamine responsiveness and survival examined 129 patients with advanced CAO (mean FEV_1 = 0.61 L and 25% of predicted). The mean provocation concentration of histamine that caused a decrease of 20% in FEV_1 from baseline FEV_1 was 4 mg/ml (normal values > 32 mg/ml) in these patients.[33] All patients reacted. Histamine responsiveness did not show a significant relationship with mortality when FEV_1 and reversibility were taken into account. However, results may be different in patients with less advanced stages of disease.

Several studies of CAO patients have used bronchodilator response rather than bronchoconstrictor response as a measure of responsiveness. However, the two measures are not interchangeable. In patients with fixed airflow obstruction in whom no reversibility occurs during bronchodilator administration, bronchoconstriction in response to histamine or methacholine may still be experienced. Moreover, studies of hospital-selected patients report only a moderate correlation between the bronchodilator and bronchoconstrictor responses.[34]

Reversibility of Airflow Obstruction

Several investigations of patients with CAO have indicated that a higher degree of improvement (reversibility) in FEV_1 after administration of a bronchodilator is associated with longer survival (after adjustment for the initial level of FEV_1). Beta agonists[9, 11, 12] and anticholinergics[14] have the same result. Two studies showed that reversibility was not related to longer survival when the postbronchodilator FEV_1 was taken into account.[9, 11] Based on these studies, it appears that fixed obstruction determines survival, at least in patients treated with bronchodilators.

Kanner and colleagues[13] presented different results, stating that greater degrees of bronchodilator response were associated with reduced 12-year survival rates. This may reflect population differences, as these investigators included pure chronic bronchitis patients and asthmatic patients, whereas the other studies did not. Furthermore, adjustment for the level of FEV_1 was not carried out.

Some of the other studies that have been mentioned also excluded patients with asthmatic features, possibly resulting in a lower level and narrower range of bronchodilator response. Recent epidemiologic investigations by Burrows and coworkers[17] have shown that patients termed "chronic asthmatic bronchitics" (mostly female, atopic individuals with positive skin test results, elevated immunoglobulin E levels, or eosinophilia) had a better survival rate than patients with CAO (as identified by a respiratory disease questionnaire and FEV_1). In addition, the Intermittent Positive-Pressure Breathing (IPPB) trial,[35] in which asthmatic individuals were excluded, reported that postbronchodilator FEV_1 was greater than 50% of predicted and that those patients who complained the most of wheezing had a less rapid decline in FEV_1 at follow-up. These results support the findings that patients with more "asthmatic" features, such as reversibility, have a better prognosis.

Exercise Tolerance

One study has investigated exercise tolerance and exercise heart rate as variables for survival.[9] It was reported that these variables are the next in importance for survival after age and FEV_1. The influence of these parameters on survival was, however, minor. It is not yet clear whether improvement of exercise tolerance results in longer survival.

Other Parameters

Hogg and associates[36] showed that the level of FEV_1 in smokers does not reflect the degree of emphysematous involvement in pathologic and anatomic substrates. In patients with established airflow obstruction it is thus still possible that more emphysematous destruction of lung tissue is important with respect to prognosis. Indeed, the IPPB trial[8,9] showed that measurements thought to reflect emphysema (carbon monoxide diffusing capacity, functional residual capacity, and total lung capacity, although only in patients with FEV_1 between 30 and 39% of that predicted) were only minimally related to survival. This is in accordance with other studies that showed that a greater abnormality in lung function parameters reflecting emphysema, such as diffusing capacity,[10-12] total lung capacity, residual volume as a per cent of total lung capacity (RV%TLC), and specific compliance,[16] as well as the ratio of FIV_1 to forced inspiratory volume in 1 second (FIV_1)[16] are related to a greater decline in lung function and a lower survival rate.

PREDICTION OF THE COURSE OF DISEASE: DECLINE IN LUNG FUNCTION

Table 12–2 summarizes the results of studies on the decline in FEV_1 in patients with CAO. Several factors are related to the decline in FEV_1. However, in some cases, two studies showed that a given factor correlated in an opposite direction to the decline in FEV_1.

Age and FEV_1

One of the most extensive and comprehensive studies on the course of CAO has been published by Anthonisen and colleagues.[9] The results are of the IPPB trial,[8] which studied 985 subjects between the ages of 30 and 74 years and with established CAO without asthmatic features. As a result of the selection criteria, the mean FEV_1 of the subjects was 36% (SD: 11%) of that predicted, and postbronchodilator FEV_1 was only 5% better. Although the follow-up period was rather short (3 years), the results are of importance because of the large number of patients who were available for analysis. Mean FEV_1 decline was 48 ml per year (SD: 99 ml/yr) in those patients who were observed for at least 2 years. Patients with low FEV_1 exhibited a slow decline and little variability in FEV_1, a phenomenon the authors attribute to a survivor effect. Patients with low baseline FEV_1 only generated FEV_1 follow-up data when the decline was small, since many of those with a substantial decrease in FEV_1 died.

Other studies[2,34] did not show a significant relationship between initial FEV_1 and a decrease in FEV_1 during follow-up. This may, however, be accounted for by the relatively small range in baseline FEV_1 values.

Smoking

The IPPB trial[8,9] was unable to show that smoking influenced the decline in FEV_1. This does not imply that

TABLE 12–2. STUDIES RELATING AIRWAY HYPERRESPONSIVENESS AND REVERSIBILITY TO DECLINE IN FEV_1

Study	No. of Patients	Follow-up (yr)	FEV_1%Pred (%Pred)	Age (yr)	Test	Factors*
Barter et al.[23]	34	5	—	56 (6)	Mch BM	FEV_1/FVC Smoking Airway hyperresponsiveness Reversibility
Kanner et al.[37]	84	≥2	—	±50	BM	Reversibility
Campbell et al.[34]	66	4–6	84 (15)	53 (6)	BM	Residence Smoking Reversibility Age Occupational exposure
Anthonisen et al.[9]	985	3	36 (11)	61 (7)	BM	Reversibility Wheezing Psychologic disturbances
Postma et al.[2,38]	81	12–20	63 (12)	48 (9)	HIST AC	Smoking Airway hyperresponsiveness Reversibility

*Factors significantly related to decline in FEV_1.
Key: Mch: methacholine; BM: beta mimetic; HIST: histamine; AC: anticholinergic.

smoking cessation does not influence the rate of FEV_1 decline, since smoking cessation is not a random event. The incidence of smoking decreased in the IPPB study as baseline FEV_1 decreased. Thus, patients may have only stopped smoking because they had relatively large annual decreases in FEV_1. Another study in patients with a mean FEV_1 of 63% of predicted showed a positive correlation between the increase in the annual decline in FEV_1 and the number of pack years of smoking.[38]

Allergy

Allergy as defined by skin test reactivity was not related to the rate of FEV_1 decline in two studies.[34, 14] There are no other data available with regard to allergy and its relationship to the decline of FEV_1 in CAO.

Airway Hyperresponsiveness

Barter and Campbell[23, 34] were the first to investigate methacholine response and bronchodilator response as they related to the annual rate of decline of FEV_1 in patients with mild airflow obstruction. Bronchodilator response and methacholine response were related to each other and positively related to the decline in FEV_1. Methacholine responsiveness was, however, measured at the end of the study. As mentioned previously, a higher degree of airway hyperresponsiveness is associated with a lower baseline FEV_1. It is therefore not surprising that the subjects with the largest fall in FEV_1 over 4 to 6 years of follow-up demonstrated the highest level of airway hyperresponsiveness at the end of the study. The increased responsiveness may be simply be the result of decreased function. Bronchodilator response at the beginning of follow-up was positively related to the annual decrease in FEV_1. One third of the patients initially selected were lost at follow-up. Some caution must therefore be taken with the interpretation of the results.

One other study investigated 81 patients with mild to moderate airflow obstruction at a university chest clinic for 12 to 20 years. The study showed that the level of airway hyperresponsiveness that was assessed at the beginning of the investigation was related to an accelerated decline in FEV_1 that was independent of initial FEV_1 and reversibility.[38]

Reversibility of Airflow Obstruction

The IPPB trial included patients with severe to moderate airflow obstruction (FEV_1 36% of predicted) with only mild or hardly any bronchodilator response (postbronchodilator FEV_1 41% of predicted). It showed that, independent of initial FEV_1 level, the bronchodilator response was related to the decline in FEV_1 in that the higher the reversibility, the slower the decline—a finding that was particularly striking in the patients with the greatest bronchodilator response (Fig. 12–4). The results

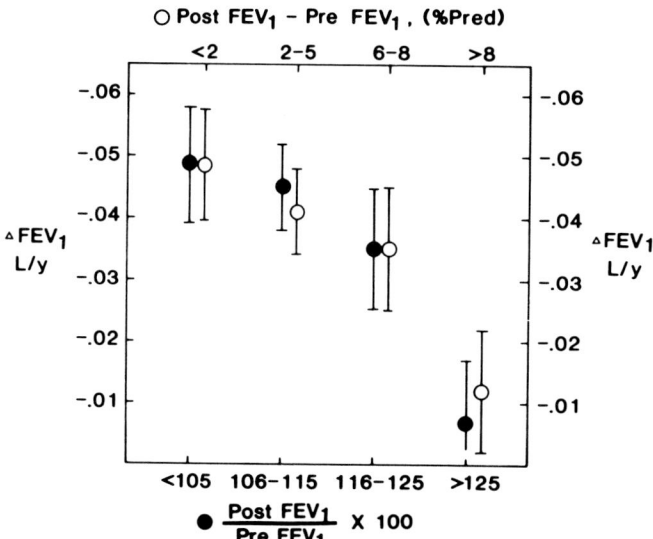

FIGURE 12–4. Relationship between bronchodilator response (abscissa) and the annual decline in FEV_1 (Δ FEV_1, L/y, ordinate). Bronchodilator response is expressed as the per cent increase in FEV_1 above baseline and is relative to predicted FEV_1. (From Anthonisen NR. Prognosis in chronic obstructive pulmonary disease: Results from multicenter clinical trials. Am Rev Respir Dis 1989; 140:S95–S99.)

were the same when bronchodilation was expressed as a percentage above baseline or as a percentage predicted. This is in contrast to a retrospective study of patients with severe airflow obstruction (FEV_1 25% of predicted and postbronchodilator FEV_1 38% of predicted) in which the bronchodilator response expressed as a percentage above baseline was no longer significantly related to survival after approximately 20 years.[16]

Nevertheless, both studies show that reversibility is positively related to survival when it is expressed as percentage predicted. This is important because this reversibility parameter has been shown to be independent of the baseline FEV_1 level.[39] This is not the case with the increase in FEV_1 expressed as a percentage above baseline. In this situation, it is obvious that reversibility increases with lower baseline FEV_1.[14]

The results discussed contradict those of a number of other studies.[13, 23, 34] These studies have reported that in smokers with well-preserved FEV_1 at baseline, the rate of FEV_1 decline is directly related to bronchodilator response. Apart from previously mentioned caveats in these studies, one of the differences between them and the Anthonisen[9] and Postma[2, 38] studies is that the patients reported by Barter and Campbell[23] were not systematically treated with bronchodilators. It may be possible that untreated patients with bronchodilator response show a relatively rapid rate of FEV_1 decline that is reversed by bronchodilator therapy. Another explanation may be that the mechanism of airflow obstruction is different in those with and in those without large bronchodilator response. Further studies, like the Lung Health Study sponsored by the National Institutes of Health,[40] have yet to show whether bronchodilator therapy influences the rate of decline of FEV_1 in patients with moderate or severe airflow obstruction.

Conclusions

Based on the available data on the relationship between patient characteristics and prognosis, whether expressed as a survival rate or as a decline in FEV_1, some conclusions may be drawn. Age and level of FEV_1 are the most important predictors of prognosis in patients with CAO. After these factors, smoking, the reversibility of airflow obstruction during bronchodilator use, and the level of airway hyperresponsiveness may be of importance. Some studies show that the presence of emphysematous features has a negative effect on prognosis and that in advanced disease the presence of hypoxemia and hypercapnia is a negative sign.[10-13] These findings may have implications for the institution of therapy, as it is worthwhile to learn whether the improvement of those factors that are related to prognosis may also alter the course of disease. One promising finding in this respect is the observation that the institution of oxygen therapy in hypoxemic patients improves prognosis.[41, 42] If hypoxemia is treated with continuous oxygen therapy, the outlook for the patient appears to be no different from that for the patient with a similar level of airflow obstruction but without baseline hypoxemia (Fig. 12–5).[9]

Predictors of Prognosis, and Drug Therapy

The major symptoms of patients with CAO can be broadly divided into those associated with airway narrowing (e.g., dyspnea and wheezing) and those associated with chronic expectoration and the increased tendency for bronchopulmonary infections. In attempting to modify the insidious course of chronic airway obstruction by treatment, one generally tries to achieve the following goals:

- A sustained improvement of symptoms in the stable state, resulting from either the improvement of pulmonary function or the decrease in expectoration and cough.
- A reduction in the frequency or length of exacerbations of symptoms.
- A slowing of the progressive decline in FEV_1 after the start of treatment.
- An improvement of the quality of life.

Clearly, the third goal necessitates a long-term follow-up period to prove the effect, particularly since an absence of response for the first two goals for improvement does not necessarily preclude a long-term beneficial effect.

Improvement of Symptoms and FEV_1: Smoking

Smoking cessation reduces chronic cough and expectoration and the frequency of bronchopulmonary infections. In younger smokers there is usually some early improvement of airway function, but this improvement is smaller or absent in older smokers. Even in smokers with established CAO and severe airflow obstruction, it is worthwhile to encourage them to quit smoking, since quitting reduces (but does not stop) the decline of FEV_1. Physicians must be careful in explaining to patients what the benefits of smoking cessation are: probably not an immediate improvement of FEV_1, but a slower decline to a rate that is only slightly greater than in those who have never smoked as well as an improved survival rate after about 6 years (see earlier). The influence of smoking cessation on airway hyperresponsiveness is yet not known. Definite information must come from the Lung Health Study sponsored by the National Institutes of Health.[40] Preliminary results in a few patients[43] did not show attenuation of airway hyperresponsiveness after

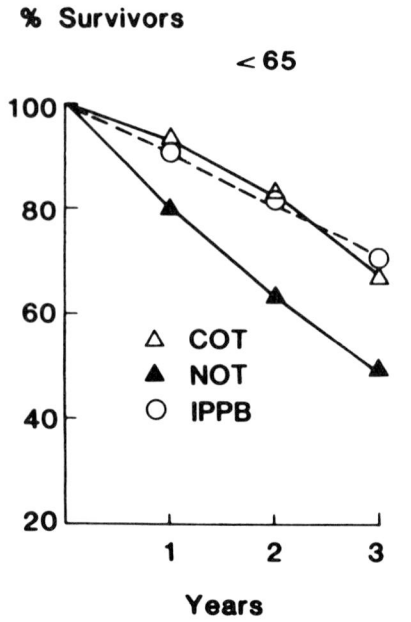
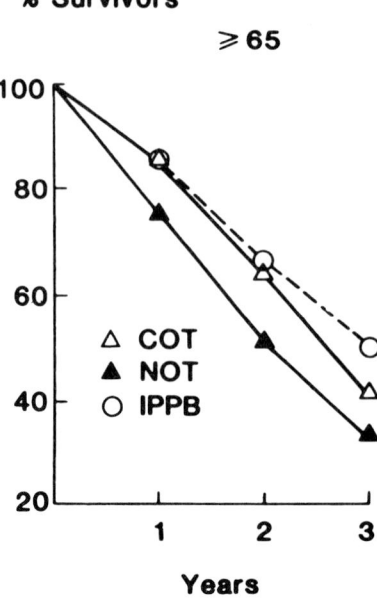

FIGURE 12–5. Comparison of survival rates in intermittent positive-pressure breathing and nocturnal oxygen therapy trials. All baseline FEV_1s below 30% of predicted. (NOT: nocturnal oxygen therapy; IPPB: intermittent positive-pressure breathing; COT: continuous oxygen therapy). (From Anthonisen NR. Prognosis in chronic obstructive pulmonary disease: Results from multicenter clinical trials. Am Rev Respir Dis 1989; 140:S95–S99.)

smoking cessation. Nevertheless, the beneficial effect of smoking cessation in patients with CAO is now generally accepted.

Improvement of Symptoms: Exacerbations

Patients with CAO frequently suffer from exacerbations of their symptoms, especially as a result of bacterial bronchopulmonary infections. This is an important factor that affects both quality of life and working capacity.

Three multicenter studies have examined the effects of treatment with oral N-acetylcysteine on the number and duration of exacerbations of symptoms (Table 12–3).[44–46] The number of self-reported exacerbations varied considerably among individuals in all trials, and, obviously, patients with the highest number had the best chance for improvement during therapy. There were great differences between the three trials with respect to the rates of exacerbation; these differences were most likely the result of differences in patient selection. Nevertheless, there was a tendency for a lower number of exacerbations in the active treatment groups. In the study conducted by the British Thoracic Society,[46] differences could not be attributed to variations in baseline exacerbation rates between the group administered N-acetylcysteine and that receiving a placebo. Differences between the effects of a placebo and N-acetylcysteine use did not reach statistical significance as a result of high standard deviations. Moreover, it is not clear how reproducible self-reported exacerbation rates are.

One double-blind multicenter study[47] conducted in 1990 showed that adjunct therapy with iodinated glycerol improved symptoms and shortened exacerbation duration significantly in the whole group studied, although only to a small extent in chronic bronchitis patients. Whether objective pulmonary function measurements and survival time were also improved is not known from this study; nevertheless, the patients' well-being did improve, a fact of great importance.

Improvement of FEV_1: Bronchodilators

Whether intermittent bronchodilator therapy, bronchodilator administration three to four times per day, or bronchodilator therapy only for symptomatic relief is the best policy in the treatment of airflow obstruction is still a matter of debate. However, symptomatic relief of a patient's dyspnea is an important issue and it is quite clear that this comfort should not be withheld from a patient. It seems appropriate to test which bronchodilators have the best effect, both subjectively and objectively. Some patients show hardly any increase in FEV_1 when using a beta mimetic agent but have a substantial increase when receiving an anticholinergic drug. In other patients, the bronchodilator effect may be very small; however, patients do have a relief of symptoms and may even show improvement in their 12-minute walking distances.

It must be remembered, however, that the prescription rate a physician gives to a patient is probably not similar to the actual intake rate. Based on the results of the 3-year prospective IPPB trial,[8,9] it has become clear that only one half of the patients who were studied followed their treatment program as prescribed. Younger patients with less obstruction and smokers tended to be noncompliant. In this study, there was little difference in mortality when it was analyzed with respect to compliance. Results regarding the influence of compliance on the decline of FEV_1 are not available. One study[2] showed that when patients were asked to describe their use of medication in a blinded trial, those patients who reported that they forgot to take their medication 2 to 3 days per week or more had a more rapid decline in FEV_1 (108 ± 33 ml/yr) than that of the patients who reported taking their medication at most once per week (58 ± 26 ml/yr). These results could not be explained by smoking habits, as a comparable number of patients smoked in both groups. Since 89% of the patients used anticholinergics, 12% used beta adrenergics, and only 0.5% inhaled corticosteroids, it was not possible to draw conclusions about the influence of the type of drug on the decline of FEV_1. The results of this questionnaire suggest that daily bronchodilator therapy may be of importance in preventing FEV_1 decline, at least in those patients with moderate to severe airflow obstruction (i.e., those with a mean FEV_1 of 1.9 L [64% of predicted]).

These last results are at variance with those of a prospective bronchodilator trial examining 223 patients with moderate airflow obstruction (inclusion criterion: $FEV_1 > 50\%$ of that predicted).[48] One hundred sixty patients completed the 2-year study using *single-bronchodilator* therapy in those who were only treated symptomatically. The annual FEV_1 decline in continuously treated patients was higher (72 ml/yr) than those who were only treated symptomatically (20 ml/yr). This study did include asthmatic patients, and decline in FEV_1 appeared to be similar in asthmatic and chronic bronchitic individuals, a finding that is not generally observed. This does not imply that all bronchodilator therapy is bad. FEV_1 was rather high in the patients under study (mean: 79% of that predicted). Thus, these

TABLE 12–3. EXACERBATION OF INFECTION RATE IN ORAL N-ACETYLCYSTEINE TREATMENT

References	No. of Patients	Age (yr)	FEV_1 %Pred	Mean Exacerbations (per Winter)	
				Placebo	N-Acetylcysteine
Multicenter study group[44]	495	—	>40%	2.0	0.8
Boman et al.[45]	203	52	mean 80%	1.7	1.2
British Thoracic Society[46]	181	63	mean 30%	2.6	2.1

patients may use their bronchodilators for relief of their symptoms of dyspnea only incidentally. However, in advanced disease, in which FEV_1 is very low, it may well be that patients use their bronchodilators more often per day to suppress dyspneic sensations; this results in continous use. It is still questionable whether bronchodilator therapy improves prognosis in these patients. Another striking observation of the previously cited bronchodilator study is that the treatment regimen did not influence symptoms, experienced health, or exacerbations. Thus, patients did not perceive their deteriorating lung function. It is important that physicians explain to their patients that deterioration of their lung function may occur even when they do not perceive it themselves. Regular lung function measurements seem to be appropriate to alert physicians to impending worsening prognosis.

Improvement of FEV_1: Corticosteroids

Corticosteroids have been used in the treatment of asthma and CAO since 1950, when the first preparations of biosynthetically derived analogs of the adrenal cortical hormones became available. Today, approximately 40 years later, their role in the management of CAO is still a controversial issue, whereas their role in the treatment of asthma is firmly established. Oral and inhaled corticosteroids exert a beneficial effect on the degree of airway hyperresponsiveness and airflow obstruction in asthma, both after short-term and longer treatment periods.[49-51] It is generally believed that this attenuation takes place via the dampening of airway inflammation underlying the increased airway responsiveness in these patients.[52]

The finding of a deleterious influence of airway hyperresponsiveness on the development of airflow obstruction and on the progressive loss of lung function in patients with CAO, especially in smokers, has led to greater interest in this phenomenon in CAO. Can anti-inflammatory therapy attenuate airway hyperresponsiveness in patients with CAO, and, if airway hyperresponsiveness occurs, does its attenuation result in a slowing of FEV_1 decline? At this time it is clear from many studies of asthmatic patients that inhaled corticosteroids may moderately reduce the severity of airway hyperresponsiveness. A study conducted in 1990 showed that in mild asthmatics airway hyperresponsiveness improves even after a 1-year follow-up treatment program including the daily administration of 800 μg inhaled budesonide. A few patients even reached a level of airway hyperresponsiveness in the normal range.[51]

The few results pertaining to CAO are not promising. Results of *oral* corticosteroids use in 25 smokers (mean FEV_1 of 62% of that predicted) and 32 ex-smokers (mean FEV_1 of 62% predicted) with CAO are summarized in Table 12-4.[53] These results show that *short-term* oral corticosteroids use does not attenuate airway hyperresponsiveness in CAO. It could even lead to the worsening of airway hyperresponsiveness in smokers, possibly as a result of the continuation of the deleterious effect of smoking on airway inflammation, whereas the corticosteroids dampen the defense. Other *short-term* studies show conflicting results (Table 12-5), largely because of patient selection differences.[54]

There appears to be both a dose effect and a time effect relationship between oral corticosteroid use and the level of FEV_1.[55] Given these effects, it is clear that "responders" and "nonresponders" to therapy seem to have a broad spectrum of FEV_1 values. Factors other than baseline FEV_1 must therefore predict the individual corticosteroid response. However, all variables mentioned in the literature seem to give rise to conflicts concerning the number of eosinophils in peripheral blood or sputum and the reversibility of airflow obstruction. Studies that show that there is an excess of eosinophils in peripheral blood[56-60] report a higher proportion of responders (with a mean of 28% responders) to corticosteroids than do studies of patients with low eosinophil counts (i.e., with a mean of 5% responders).[56, 62] Further studies with larger numbers of patients and sufficient variation in FEV_1 may have to elucidate whether eosinophils, neutrophils, or the degree of reversibility, or any combination of these factors determine corticosteroid response.

Two studies have shown the beneficial effect of the *long-term* use of oral corticosteroids on the course of FEV_1 in patients with moderate and severe airflow obstruction. In the first study,[64] patients with positive skin test results were not excluded, which raised the possibility that more "asthma-like" patients were included even if they had an FEV_1 below 1 L (mean of 25% of that predicted). In the second study of 138 patients[65] with moderately severe airflow obstruction (FEV_1 of 63% of predicted and FEV_1/FVC of 48%), patients with allergies were excluded. Both studies showed a close correlation between the pattern of change in FEV_1 and the intake and dosage of prednisolone. Below a dosage of 10 mg prednisolone per day (i.e., 7.5 or 5 mg), FEV_1 declined continuously. When 10 mg prednisolone or more was given, FEV_1 remained

TABLE 12-4. AIRWAY HYPERRESPONSIVENESS AFTER PREDNISOLONE ADMINISTRATION*

		Before		After	
	No. of Patients	$PC_{20}HIST$†	FEV_1%Pred	$PC_{20}HIST$	FEV_1%Pred
Smokers	25	4.72	61.5	3.78	59.6
Ex-smokers	32	5.69	62.4	6.52	61.4

*After eight daily doses of 40 mg each.
†Provocation concentration of histamine (mg/ml) causing a decrease of 20% in FEV_1 from baseline FEV_1.

stable or even improved. Both studies were retrospective in nature and had a long period of follow-up (14–20 yr), but any interpretation of the data should be carried out carefully. Nevertheless, 53 patients could be regarded as their own controls since corticosteroids were instituted or withheld during follow-up in these patients. The same results were observed in these patients as in those mentioned earlier: improvement of FEV_1 after institution of corticosteroid therapy and deterioration after its termination. It took, however, between 6 months and 2 years before the effects of corticosteroids on FEV_1 could be observed. Regardless, the study indicated that the results of therapy in patients with CAO are quite different from the effects observed in patients with asthma.

Only some investigations of the *short-term* use of inhaled corticosteroids by patients with CAO have been conducted.[66-69] One recent study showed that 12 of 34 patients with CAO responded with a 10% or greater increase in either FEV_1, FVC or peak expiratory flow rate after the daily administration of 1500 μg of beclomethasone dipropionate.[65] According to the immunoglobulin E and skin test data provided, this study did include some allergic individuals. Hence individuals chosen because they were definitely nonasthmatic did not show any attenuation of airway hyperresponsiveness or improvement of FEV_1, even with therapy durations and inhaled corticosteroid doses that have a clear effect in asthmatics. However, smoking cessation, which presumably also has anti-inflammatory effects, does not result in a similar improvement in FEV_1 in the short term but is highly effective in the attenuation of the decline in FEV_1. There is one abstract reporting on 59 patients with CAO with moderate airflow obstruction who were prospectively studied for 2 years with respect to the use of inhaled budesonide (1600 μg per day), inhaled budesonide and prednisolone (1600 μg and 5 mg per day, respectively) or a placebo.[70] Results suggest that patients taking inhaled corticosteroids had a slower decline in FEV_1 and fewer symptoms after 2 years of follow-up. Moreover, their symptom exacerbations tended to be of a shorter duration. There were some patients who derived greater benefit from inhaled corticosteroids, but the authors could not identify which characteristics predicted this tendency.

REHABILITATION OF PATIENTS WITH CHRONIC AIRFLOW OBSTRUCTION

Patients with advanced chronic airflow obstruction who have had optimal medical treatment including bronchodilators and corticosteroids but who are nevertheless still limited in their daily activities are good candidates to enter a rehabilitation program. In 1974, the American College of Chest Physicians accepted the following definition of pulmonary rehabilitation:

"Pulmonary rehabilitation may be defined as an art of medical practice wherein an individually tailored, multidisciplinary program is formulated which through accurate diagnosis, therapy, emotional support and education stabilizes or reverses both the physio- and psychopathology of pulmonary diseases

TABLE 12–5. BASELINE DATA AND CORTICOSTEROID RESPONSES IN SELECTED STUDIES

	Study*									
	1	2	3	4	5	6	7	8	9	10
No. of patients	16	10	16	46	43	10	24	13	31	57
Dose of steroids (mg/day)	40	5	40	32	40	30	30	32	35	40
Duration (days)	14	7	14	14	14	14	7	14	14	8
Responders (%)	12	0	43	17	35	30	33	8	13	7
(number)	2	0	7	8	15	3	8	1	4	4
Age (yr)	60	62	63	74	60	61	—	63	63	56
Male (%)	100	100	96	85	76	100	83	92	64	100
History of allergy†	No	No	No	Yes	Yes	—	No	No	No	No
Eosinophil excess	Yes	Yes	Yes	Yes	Yes	—	Yes	No	—	No
FEV_1 (L)	1.24	1.11	0.85	1.03	1.02	0.81	0.74	1.16	0.84	1.98
FEV_1 %pred	35	—	33	37	37	—	7	—	—	63
FVC (L)	2.74	2.28	1.92	—	2.22	2.56	—	2.43	2.15	—
FEV_1/FVC (%)	45	49	45	—	44	—	—	48	—	45
FEV_1 increase‡ (ml)	120	90	85	156	160	162	177	70	—	200
FEV_1 increase (%)	12	13	10	15	15	21	27	6	—	12
Sputum production (%)	100	100	61	—	82	80	100	—	—	63
	Effect Prednisolone Above Placebo									
FEV_1 (ml)	112	−3	12	110	150	34	15	100	82	−50
FVC (ml)	27	−2	22	—	200	159	—	0	119	—
PEFR (L/min)	—	—	44	—	23	—	—	—	9	—
Complaints	No	—	Yes	—	Yes	Yes	Yes	4	—	Yes
12 MD§	—	—	47	—	52	38	—	—	—	—

*1: Eliasson et al.[55]; 2: Evans et al.[56]; 3: Lam et al.[57]; 4: Mendella et al.[58]; 5: Mitchell et al.[59]; 6: O'Reilly et al.[61]; 7: Shim et al.[60]; 8: Strain et al.[62]; 9: Stokes et al.[63]; 10: Renkema[70].
†Personal or family history at atopy.
‡Increase in FEV_1 after inhalation of a beta agonist.
§Walking distance at 12 minutes.

and attempts to return the patient to the highest possible functional capacity allowed by his pulmonary handicap and overall life situation."[71]

In this definition, it is clear that a rehabilitation program has to be carried out by a multidisciplinary team of health care professionals. The main aim of this team is to improve the disease state of chronic obstructive pulmonary disease (COPD) patients so that they are able to function independently of others.[72] Rehabilitation programs have mostly been carried out in a clinical setting. In this setting, all members of the team are accessible and, thus, multidisciplinary treatment is feasible. On the other hand, outpatient programs are more convenient for the patient, and such training programs can be supervised by a physiotherapist.

Although most pulmonary rehabilitation programs are developed for patients with COPD, patients with other lung diseases can also participate.[73]

Quality of Life

It is known that a difference sometimes exists between the outcome of disease (with regard to lung function tests) and the quality of life of COPD patients.[74] Therefore, it is important that when all effects of a pulmonary rehabilitation program are to be measured, changes in quality of life are also considered. Several investigators have developed and validated a technique that measures quality of life. Jones and colleagues[75] investigated the correlation between the results of the Sickness Impact Profile and some physiologic parameters and showed the Sickness Impact Profile to be a valid measure of general health in patients with chronic airflow limitation.

Because of the weak relationship among pulmonary function, exercise capacity, and quality of life, Guyatt and coworkers.[76] developed a chronic respiratory disease questionnaire to determine the effect of treatment on quality of life in clinical trials. They followed 31 patients who participated in inpatient pulmonary rehabilitation programs for 6 months. After 6 months, 24 patients demonstrated substantial improvement in quality of life based on their answers to the questionnaire. After another 6 months, improved quality of life was sustained in 11 patients and declined in 20 patients. In the study of Bebout and associates,[77] in which 75 patients with COPD participated in a rehabilitation program, 43 patients were followed over 92 months. During this period, more than 50% of the patients reported improvement in dyspnea classification, the ability to go outside, the frequency of difficult breathing episodes, and self-assurance.

Available data suggest that pulmonary rehabilitation of patients with COPD has a positive effect on quality of life, but further research on this aspect of rehabilitation has to be done.

Level of Function

Most patients show an improved ability to carry out daily life activities after a rehabilitation program. Some of these patients are even able to continue or return to their employment. For instance Haas and Cardon[78] found that 25% of 252 patients with COPD who took part in a pulmonary rehabilitation program were able to work full-time for 5 years after the program. This was true for only 3% of 50 patients in the control group. Cox[79] also observed a significant increase in daily physical activities in a rehabilitation group compared with the control group.

In another study, Petty and coworkers[80] found that 32% of a group of 182 patients who participated in a pulmonary rehabilitation program were at least working part-time when they entered the rehabilitation program. When the patients were compared with the nonworking patients, these investigators did not find a difference in lung function test results; the only differences observed were in exercise capacity and age. These observations make it clear that variables other than the degree of pulmonary impairment are more important in determining how the patient functions during his or her daily activities. Schrier and associates[81] therefore recommend that the health care of patients with CAO should focus both on somatic problems and on psychosocial problems.

Survival

Studies that have examined the survival rates of COPD patients during pulmonary rehabilitation show variable results.[82] There have been no prospective studies of pulmonary rehabilitation programs with regard to mortality. Haas and Cardon[78] compared 252 patients who participated in a rehabilitation program with 50 control subjects and found that the survival rate in the rehabilitation group was 22%, whereas it was 42% in the control group. However, Anthonisen and colleagues[83] reported an improvement in survival rate over 3 years of follow-up for the rehabilitation group. One of the main reasons for the absence of data on survival rates in the literature is that most pulmonary rehabilitation studies did not have follow-up periods sufficiently long to evaluate survival, whereas others did not include a control group.

CONCLUSION

The overall results of findings in the literature do not provide sufficient grounds for the institution of long-term vigorous therapy for CAO. However, circumstantial data do lead one to suspect that treatment directed at the improvement of airflow obstruction may alter the course of disease. One study shows that anti-inflammatory therapy over 2 years of follow-up attenuates the decline of lung function. However, some patients gain more from this therapy than others. Future studies must reveal which patients should receive bronchodilators and anti-inflammatory therapy. Long-term, prospective studies are as warranted because the observations of short-term studies, in contrast to those made in studies of asthmatic patients, do not provide data on certain effects. In addition to objective measurements (e.g., FEV_1 and airway hyperresponsiveness), subjective data and information on a patient's quality of life and his or her symptom exacerbations should be included for final evaluation. In this respect, prospective long-term trials investigating rehabilitation programs both in clinical and home settings are of great importance.

REFERENCES

1. Peat JK, Woolcock AJ, Cullen K. Decline of lung function and development of chronic airflow limitation: A longitudinal study of non-smokers and smokers in Busseltons, Western Australia. Thorax 1990; 45:32–37.
2. Postma DS, Sluiter HJ. Prognosis of chronic obstructive pulmonary disease: The Dutch experience. Am Rev Respir Dis 1989; 14:S100–S105.
3. Thom TJ. International comparisons in COPD mortality. Am Rev Respir Dis 1989; 140:S27–S34.
4. Manfreda J, Mao Y, Litven W. Morbidity and mortality from chronic obstructive pulmonary disease. Am Rev Respir Dis 1989; 14:S19–S26.
5. Feinleib M, Rosenberg HM, Collins JG, et al. Trends in COPD morbidity and mortality in the United States. Am Rev Respir Dis 1989; 140:S9–S18.
6. Lebowitz MD. The trends in airway obstructive disease morbidity in the Tucson epidemiological study. Am Rev Respir Dis 1989; 140:S35–S41.
7. Higgins MW, Keller JB. Trends in COPD morbidity and mortality in Tecumseh, Michigan. Am Rev Respir Dis 1989; 140:S42–S48.
8. IPPB Trial Group. Intermittent positive pressure breathing therapy of chronic obstructive pulmonary disease. Ann Intern Med 1983; 99:612–620.
9. Anthonisen NR, Wright EC, Hodgkin JE. Prognosis in chronic obstructive pulmonary disease. Am Rev Respir Dis 1986; 133:14–22.
10. Boushy SF, Thompson HK, North LB, et al. Prognosis in COPD. Am Rev Respir Dis 1973; 108:1373–1382.
11. Burrows B, Earl RH. Course and prognosis of chronic obstructive lung disease. N Engl J Med 1969; 280:397–404.
12. Traver GA, Cline MG, Burrows B. Predictors of mortality in COPD. Am Rev Respir Dis 1979; 119:895–902.
13. Kanner RI, Renzetti AP, Stanish WM, et al. Predictors of survival in subjects with chronic airflow obstruction. Am J Med 1983; 74:249–255.
14. Postma DS, Burema J, Gimeno F, et al. Prognosis in severe chronic obstructive pulmonary disease. Am Rev Respir Dis 1979; 119:357–367.
15. Smit JM, Burema J, May JF, et al. Prognosis in severe chronic airflow obstructive pulmonary disease with regard to the electrocardiogram. J Electrocardiol 1983; 76:77–81.
16. Postma DS, Gimeno F, Van der Weele LTH, Sluiter HJ. Assessment of ventilatory variables in survival prediction of patients with chronic airflow obstruction: The importance of reversibility. Eur J Respir Dis 1985; 67:360–368.
17. Burrows B, Bloom JW, Traver GA, Cline MG. The course and prognosis of different forms of chronic airways obstruction in a sample from the general population. N Engl J Med 1987; 317:1309–1314.
18. Rijcken B, Schouten JP, Weiss ST, et al. The relationship between airway responsiveness to histamine and pulmonary function level in a random population sample. Am Rev Respir Dis 1988; 137:826–832.
19. Welty C, Weiss ST, Tager IB, et al. The relationship of airway responsiveness to cold air, cigarette smoking and atopy to respiratory symptoms and pulmonary function in adults. Am Rev Respir Dis 1984; 130:198–203.
20. Sparrow D, O'Connor G, Colton T, et al. The relationship of nonspecific bronchial responsiveness to the occurrence of respiratory symptoms and decreased levels of pulmonary function: The Normative Aging Study. Am Rev Respir Dis 1987; 135:1255–1260.
21. Pham QT, Mur JM, Chau N, et al. Prognostic value of acetylcholine challenge test: A prospective study. Br J Ind Med 1984; 41:267–271.
22. Parker DR, O'Connor GT, Sparrow D, et al. The relationship of nonspecific airway responsiveness and atopy to the rate of decline of lung function. Am Rev Respir Dis 1990; 141:589–594.
23. Barter CE, Campbell AH. Relationship of constitutional factors and cigarette smoking to decrease in 1-second forced expiratory volume. Am Rev Respir Dis 1976; 113:305–314.
24. Klein RC, Salvaggio FE. Nonspecificity to the bronchoconstriction effect of histamine and acetylmethylcholine in patients with obstructive airway disease. J Allergy 1966; 37:158–168.
25. Parker CD, Bilbo RE, Reed CE, et al. Methacholine aerosol as test for bronchial asthma. Arch Intern Med 1965; 115:452–458.
26. Laitinen LAI. Histamine and methacholine challenge in the testing of bronchial reactivity. Scand J Respir Dis (Suppl) 1974; 86:9–48.
27. Muitari A. The value of the methacholine test as a diagnostic method in bronchospastic disorders. Ann Med Int Fenn 1968; 57:197–203.
28. Ramsdell JW, Nachtwey FJ, Moser KM. Bronchial hyperreactivity in chronic obstructive bronchitis. Am Rev Respir Dis 1982; 126:829–832.
29. Bahous J, Cartier A, Ouimet G, et al. Nonallergic bronchial hyperexcitability in chronic bronchitis. Am Rev Respir Dis 1988; 137:281–285.
30. Ramsdale EH, Morris MM, Roberts RS, Hargreave FE. Bronchial responsiveness to methacholine in chronic bronchitis: Relationship to airflow obstruction and cold air responsiveness. Thorax 1984; 39:912–918.
31. Dutoit JI, Woolcock AJ, Salme CM, et al. Characteristics of bronchial hyperresponsiveness in smokers with chronic airflow limitation. Am Rev Respir Dis 1986; 134:498–501.
32. Yan K, Salome CM, Woolcock J. Prevalence and nature of bronchial hyperresponsiveness in subjects with chronic obstructive pulmonary disease. Am Rev Respir Dis 1985; 132:25–29.
33. Postma DS, Steenhuis GJ, Sluiter HJ. Prognosis in adult patients with airflow obstruction. In: Sluiter HJ, Van der Lende R, Gerritsen J, Postma DS (eds): Bronchitis IV: Fourth International Symposium. Assen, The Netherlands: VanGorcum, 1989, pp 350–367.
34. Campbell AH, Barter CE, O'Connel JM, Huggins R. Factors affecting the decline of ventilatory function in chronic bronchitis. Thorax 1985; 40:741–748.
35. Anthonisen NR. Prognosis in chronic obstructive pulmonary disease: results from multicenter clinical trials. Am Rev Respir Dis 1989; 140:S95–S99.
36. Hogg JC, Pare PD, Wright JL. The relationship between airway pathology and airway obstruction. In: Sluiter HJ, Van der Lende R, Gerritsen J, Postma DS (eds). Bronchitis IV: Fourth International Symposium. Assen, The Netherlands: VanGorcum, 1989, pp 123–134.
37. Kanner RE, Renzetti AD, Klauber ME, et al. Variables associated with changes in spirometry in patients with obstructive lung disease. Am J Med 1979; 67:44–49.
38. Postma DS, de Vries K, Koeter GH, Sluiter HJ. Independent influence of reversibility of air-flow obstruction and nonspecific hyperreactivity on the long-term course of lung function in chronic air-flow obstruction. Am Rev Respir Dis 1986; 134:276–280.
39. Brand PLP. Value of physiological and psychological variables in determining respiratory symptoms and quality of life in adult patients with an obstructive airways disease (abstract). Am Rev Respir Dis 1990; 141:A760.
40. Anthonisen NR. Lung health study. Am Rev Respir Dis 1989; 140:871–872.
41. Medical Research Council Working Party. Long term domiciliary oxygen therapy in chronic cor pulmonale complicating chronic bronchitis and emphysema. Lancet 1981; i:681–686.
42. Nocturnal Oxygen Therapy Trial Group. Continuous or nocturnal oxygen therapy in hypoxemic chronic obstructive pulmonary disease: A clinical trial. Ann Intern Med 1980; 93:391–398.
43. Pride NB. Epidemiology of obstruction, exacerbation and hyperreactivity. Effects of glucocorticosteroids and other anti-inflammatory treatment. Agents Actions 1990; 30:S59–S72.
44. Multicenter study group. Long term oral acetylcysteine in chronic

45. Boman G, Backer U, Larsson S, et al. Oral acetylcysteine reduces exacerbation rate in chronic bronchitis: Report of a trial organized by the Swedish Society for Pulmonary Diseases. Eur J Respir Dis 1983; 64:405–415.
46. British Thoracic Society Research Committee. Oral N-acetylcysteine and exacerbation rates in patients with chronic bronchitis and severe airways obstruction. Thorax 1985; 40:832–835.
47. Petty TL. The national mucolytic study. Results of a randomized, double-blind, placebo-controlled study of Iodinated glycerol in chronic obstructive bronchitis. Chest 1990; 84:75–83.
48. Van Schayck CP, Dompeling E, Van Herwaarden CLA, et al. Bronchodilator treatment in moderate asthma or chronic bronchitis: Continuous or on demand? BMJ 1991; 303:1426–1431.
49. Kraan J, Koëter GH, van der Mark THW, et al. Changes in bronchial hyperreactivity induced by 4 weeks of treatment with antiasthmatic drugs in patients with allergic asthma: A comparison between budesonide and terbutaline. J Allergy Clin Immunol 1985; 76:628–639.
50. Kerrebijn KF, Van Essen-Zandvliet EEM, Neijens HJ. Effect of long-term treatment with inhaled corticosteroids and beta-agonists on the bronchial responsiveness in children with asthma. J Allergy Clin Immunol 1987; 79:653–659.
51. Juniper EF, Kline PA, Van Zieleghem MA, et al. Effect of long-term treatment with an inhaled corticosteroid (budesonide) on airway hyperresponsiveness and clinical asthma in nonsteroid-dependent asthmatics. Am Rev Respir Dis 1990; 142:832–836.
52. Barnes PJ. New concept in the pathogenesis of bronchial hyperresponsiveness and asthma. J Allergy Clin Immunol 1989; 83:1013–1026.
53. Renkema TEJ, Postma DS, Sluiter HJ. Modulation of airway hyperreactivity by prednisolone in patients with emphysema (abstract). Am Rev Respir Dis 1988; 137:242.
54. Postma DS, Renkema TEJ, Koëter GH. Effects of corticosteroids in "chronic bronchitis" and "chronic obstructive airway disease." Agents Actions 1990; 30:41–57.
55. Eliasson O, Hoffman J, Trueb D, et al. Corticosteroids in COPD. A clinical trial and reassessment of the literature. Chest 1986; 89:484–490.
56. Evans JA, Morrison IM, Saunders KB. A controlled trial of prednisone, in low dosage, in patients with chronic airways obstruction. Thorax 1974; 29:401–406.
57. Lam WK, So SY, Yu DYC. Response to oral corticosteroids in chronic airflow obstruction. Br J Dis Chest 1983; 77:189–198.
58. Mendella LA, Manfreda J, Warren CPW, Anthonisen NR. Steroid response in stable chronic obstructive pulmonary disease. Ann Intern Med 1982; 96:17–21.
59. Mitchell DM, Gildeh P, Rehahn M, et al. Effects of prednisolone in chronic airflow limitation. Lancet 1984; ii:193–195.
60. Shim C, Stover DE, Williams MH Jr. Response to corticosteroids in chronic bronchitis. J Allergy Clin Immunol 1978; 62:363–367.
61. O'Reilly JF, Shaylor JM, Fromings KM, Harrison BDW. The use of the 12 minute walking test in assessing the effect of oral steroid therapy in patients with chronic airways obstruction. Br J Dis Chest 1982; 76:374–382.
62. Strain DS, Kinasewitz GT, Franco DP, George RB. Effect of steroid therapy on exercise performance in patients with irreversible chronic obstructive pulmonary disease. Chest 1985; 88:718–721.
63. Stokes TC, O'Reilly JF, Shaylor JM, Harrison BDW. Assessment of steroid responsiveness in patients with chronic airflow obstruction. Lancet 1982; ii:345–348.
64. Postma DS, Steenhuis EF, van der Weele LTH, Sluiter HJ. Severe chronic airflow obstruction: Can corticosteroids slow down progression? Eur J Respir Dis 1985; 67:56–64.
65. Postma DS, Peters I, Steenhuis EJ, Sluiter HJ. Moderately severe chronic airflow obstruction. Can corticosteroids slow down progression? Eur Respir J 1988; 1:22–26.
66. Engel T, Heining JH, Madsen O, et al. A trial of inhaled budesonide on airway responsiveness in smokers with chronic bronchitis. Eur Respir J 1989; 2:935–939.
67. Auffarth B, Postma DS, De Monchy JGR, et al. Effects of inhaled budesonide on spirometry, reversibility, airway responsiveness and cough threshold in smokers with COPD. Thorax 1991; 46:372–378.
68. Pride NB, Taylor RG, Lim H, et al. Bronchial hyperresponsiveness as a risk factor for progressive airflow obstruction in smokers. Bull Eur Physiopathol Respir 1987; 23:369–375.
69. Weir DC, Gove RI, Robertson AJ, Burge PS. Corticosteroid trials in non-asthmatic chronic airflow obstruction. Thorax 1990; 45:112–117.
70. Renkema TEJ. A two-year prospective study on the effect of inhaled and inhaled plus oral corticosteroids in chronic airflow obstruction (abstract). Am Rev Respir Dis 1990; 141:A468.
71. American Thoracic Society: Pulmonary rehabilitation. Am Rev Respir Dis 1981; 124:663–666.
72. Lertzmann MM, Cherniack RM. Rehabilitation of patients with chronic obstructive pulmonary disease. Am Rev Respir Dis 1976; 114:1145–1165.
73. Foster S, Thomas HM. Pulmonary rehabilitation in lung disease other than Chronic Obstructive Pulmonary Disease. Am Rev Respir Dis 1990; 141:601–604.
74. Guyatt GH, Berman LB, Townsend M, et al. A measure of quality of life for clinical trials in chronic lung disease. Thorax 1987; 42:773–778.
75. Jones PW, Baveystock CM, Littlejohns P. Relationship between general health measured with the sickness impact profile and respiratory symptoms, physiological measures, and mood in patients with chronic airflow limitation. Am Rev Respir Dis 1989; 140:1538–1543.
76. Guyatt GH, Berman LB, Townsend M. Longterm outcome after respiratory rehabilitation. Can Med Assoc J 1987; 137:1089–1095.
77. Bebout DE, Hodgkin JE, Zorn EG, et al. Clinical and physiological outcomes of a university-hospital pulmonary rehabilitation program. Respir Care 1983; 28:1468–1473.
78. Haas A, Cardon H. Rehabilitation in chronic obstructive pulmonary disease: A 5-year study of 252 patients. Med Clin North Am 1969; 53:593–606.
79. Cox NJM. Effects of a pulmonary rehabilitation programme in patients with obstructive lung disease. Nijmegen, The Netherlands: University of Nijmegen; 1990. Thesis.
80. Petty TL, MacIlroy ER, Swigert MA, Brink GA. Chronic airway obstruction, respiratory insufficiency and gainful employment. Arch Environ Health 1970; 21:71–78.
81. Schrier AC, Dekker FW, Kaptein AA, Dijkman JH. Quality of life in elderly patients with chronic nonspecific lung disease seen in family practice. Chest 1990; 98:894–899.
82. Hodgkin JE. Pulmonary rehabilitation. In: Hodgkin JE, Petty TL (eds). Chronic Obstructive Pulmonary Disease: Current Concepts. Philadelphia: W.B. Saunders Co., 1987; pp 154–171.
83. Anthonisen NR, Wright EC, Hodgkin JE. Prognosis in chronic obstructive pulmonary disease. Am Rev Respir Dis 1986; 133:14–20.

2

Therapeutic Modalities in Pulmonary Rehabilitation

Chapter 13

Pharmacologic Therapy

MICHAEL W. OWENS, M.D.
WILLIAM M. ANDERSON, M.D.
RONALD B. GEORGE, M.D.

The therapeutic agents discussed in this chapter are primarily those used in the management of chronic obstructive pulmonary disease (COPD), which is the most common cause of pulmonary disability.[1] The treatments of restrictive lung disease, asthma, and cystic fibrosis are not discussed here, as they are the subjects of subsequent chapters. Likewise, nutrition, psychotherapeutic drugs, agents designed to reduce the sensation of dyspnea, and techniques used to aid in smoking cessation are the subjects of other chapters. This discussion addresses agents used in the management of airways obstruction (such as anti-inflammatory agents), drugs used in the control of airways secretions, antimicrobial agents, drugs for the prevention of respiratory infections, and agents that affect the respiratory muscles and the control of respiration. We present an outline of recommended strategies for managing patients with COPD, including those who experience acute exacerbations of symptoms.

Since COPD is defined as a disorder in which airflow obstruction does not change markedly over time,[2] patients should not expect rapid responses or cures, and therapy must often be continued over long periods. It is important that the clinician select agents whose toxicity is limited or can be controlled and that are relatively inexpensive. The benefits or lack of benefit derived from drug use should be monitored objectively by serial determination of airflow and the maintenance of flow sheets that are easy to read and readily available. The treatment regimen must be designed to be as simple as possible to ensure patient compliance when only limited benefits from therapy can be foreseen.

BRONCHODILATORS

Sympathomimetic Agents

These drugs are widely considered as first-line treatment for COPD. Beta-adrenergic agonists increase cyclic adenosine monophosphate (cAMP) formation, which in turn results in a change in intracellular calcium ion concentrations.[3] The stimulation of beta receptors results in multiple effects on the respiratory and cardiovascular systems. Beta$_1$ receptor stimulation primarily causes positive chronotrophy and inotrophy of the heart, whereas beta$_2$ receptor stimulation primarily causes respiratory system changes, such as the relaxation of bronchial smooth muscle, the prevention of smooth muscle contraction by various stimuli in a dose-related response, increased mucus clearance, pulmonary artery dilation, and the decreased release of mediators from basophils and mast cells. Beta-adrenergic agonists may reduce bronchial microvascular hyperpermeability. The stimulation of beta$_2$ receptors also causes skeletal muscle tremors and probably results in some direct cardiac stimulation.[4]

There are four classes of beta-adrenergic agonists: catecholamines, resorcinols, saligenins, and pro-drugs. The catecholamines have mixed alpha-adrenergic, beta$_1$-adrenergic and beta$_2$-adrenergic effects. Epinephrine, isoproterenol (a synthetic derivative of epinephrine), and isoetharine are members of this group. The catecholamines' duration of action is only 1 to 2 hours because these drugs are rapidly methylated in the lung by catechol-O-methyltransferase.[5] The disadvantages of drugs in this group include their short half-lives and lack of beta$_2$-adrenergic specificity as well as the development of tolerance in some patients.[6] Metaproterenol, terbutaline, and fenoterol are members of the resorcinol group. These more selective beta$_2$-adrenergic drugs are not methylated, and their duration of action is much longer than that of catecholamines (about 4–6 hr).[7,8] The members of the saligenin group, which are relatively beta$_2$-selective and have longer half-lives than isoproterenol, include albuterol and pirbuterol. Pirbuterol differs from albuterol only in its substitution of a nitrogen atom for a carbon atom in the benzene ring. Bitolterol, an example of a pro-drug, is inactive until it is cleaved in the lung by esterase to produce its active form, colterol. Esterase levels are higher in the lung than in the heart; this means that fewer cardiac side effects occur when pro-drugs as opposed to other types of medication are used.

The side effects of beta-adrenergic drugs involve several organ systems. Muscle tremor is present in varying degrees in all patients taking beta$_2$-specific agents. Peripheral vasodilation results in a mild reflex increase in pulse rate. Catecholamines can cause hyperglycemia, hypokalemia, hypophosphatemia, hypocalcemia, hypomagnesemia, and increased levels of lactate, pyruvate, and ketones.

Reversible airflow obstruction is often present in patients with COPD. Reversibility may be difficult to detect at a given time; hence, multiple tests may need to be performed.[9] A significant bronchodilator response can be found in approximately 40% of patients with COPD.[10] Even patients without an objective improvement in airflow may have improvement in dyspnea and functional status over time if they undergo aggressive bronchodilator therapy.[11,12]

When inhaled, beta-adrenergic agents are quite effective and cause minimal side effects. Other advantages of these agents include ease of application, portability, and the rapid onset of action. Aerosols may be produced by hand-held pressure nebulizers, by metered-dose inhalers (MDIs) using freon or other compressed propellants, or by using the pressure of rapid inhalation and a mixing chamber to suspend an agent in powder form (e.g., by using a product such as Rotohaler). MDIs are the most commonly recommended dispensers because of their portability and effectiveness. The direct application of the adrenergic agent to the airway mucosa produces relief of bronchospasm and makes possible the use of much lower doses than those required for systemic therapy. Side effects of the new beta$_2$-adrenergic aerosols are minimal when they are administered at recommended doses. A small number of patients develop muscle tremor and tachycardia; however, these symptoms gradually diminish as the aerosols are used.

There are two significant problems with the otherwise ideal inhaled beta$_2$-adrenergic agents: they have a relatively short duration of action (3–6 hours for the newer drugs), and they require an adequate inhalation technique in order to reach their site of action. With careful instruction, the majority of patients can use their inhalers properly; however, physicians should question and reinstruct patients in MDI use at each visit if necessary.[13]

TABLE 13–1. RECOMMENDED PROCEDURES FOR THE OPTIMUM USE OF METERED-DOSE INHALERS*

1. Shake the inhaler
2. Breathe out to end-expiration (the end of a normal breath)
3. Open the mouth wide and hold canister in the upright position 2 to 4 cm from mouth
4. While breathing in deeply and slowly (inspiration time approximately 5 seconds), depress the top of the canister
6. Repeat as often as prescribed by physician, allowing at least 1 to 2 minutes between actuations

*From Guidry GG, George RB. ACCP Pulmonary and Critical Care Update. 1990, Vol 6, Lesson 1.

Many clinicians refer to the package insert recommendations, which suggest that the patient keep his or her mouth closed while using the mouthpiece. Dolovich and coworkers showed that this method results in greater deposition of aerosols in the mouth and throat rather than in the lung parenchyma; therefore, the technique outlined in Table 13–1 is recommended.[14] Spacers and reservoir devices are useful for some patients (e.g., for children, elderly patients, and neurologic patients) to decrease the proximal deposition of large particles.[15] Spacers allow for large particle deposition outside the mouth, whereas aerosol reservoirs make it possible to avoid the need for coordinating inhaler activation and inspiration by providing an aerosol chamber.[16] Powder generators that deliver aerosol agents in powder form as the patient inspires are also effective.

Hand-held nebulizers are often used for aerosol delivery in hospitals and clinics, especially when pulmonary patients experience acute attacks. However, these nebulizers are bulky, expensive, and subject to bacterial contamination. They require more medication (up to 10 times the MDI dose) to achieve an equivalent effect because the majority of the agent-suspending aerosol is lost in the equipment and surrounding atmosphere. Properly used MDIs have been shown to be equally as effective as hand-held nebulizers both in chronic stable COPD and during acute exacerbations.[17,18] Nevertheless, hand-held nebulizers are popular with patients and allow busy hospital personnel to deliver adequate dose levels without constant supervision.

The administration of beta-adrenergic agents by either oral or parenteral methods is less satisfactory because of its higher dose requirements and significant side effects.[19] Sustained-release oral preparations of beta$_2$-adrenergic drugs are available. Their major advantage is a longer duration of action compared with that of inhaled forms. They may be an alternative to sustained-release theophylline in patients with nocturnal symptoms. Parenteral beta-adrenergic agents are used primarily in younger patients, who appear to tolerate their side effects better.[20]

Anticholinergic Bronchodilators

Anticholinergic drugs are among the first agents ever used for the treatment of airflow obstruction. Parasympathetic mechanisms control the airway caliber.[21] Normally, there is a basal level of bronchomotor tone caused by tonic parasympathetic stimulation. Anticholinergic agents antagonize the action of acetylcholine at parasympathetic postganglionic effector cell junctions by competing with acetylcholine for receptors. Acetylcholine stimulates the enzyme guanyl cyclase to produce increased levels of guanosine 3',5'-cyclic monophosphate (cGMP). Elevated cGMP levels can cause both bronchial smooth muscle contraction and mast cell degranulation. The goal of anticholinergic therapy is to decrease the level of intracellular cGMP. Anticholinergic agents also block reflex bronchoconstriction that is caused by inhaled irritants, and they attenuate the release of mediators from mast cells after parasympathetic stimulation. Anticholinergic drugs reach their peak effect 30 to 60 minutes after inhalation.

Atropine sulfate, a tertiary ammonium compound of atropine, is well absorbed from the gastrointestinal tract into the bloodstream. It travels to the brain, where it crosses the blood-brain barrier. It is also rapidly absorbed from the lungs following aerosol inhalation, meaning that it can result in toxicity when it is inhaled at usual bronchodilating doses. Common, dose-dependent side effects include dry mouth, tachycardia, blurred vision, and problems with urination. Patients with narrow-angle glaucoma or prostatic hypertrophy should not be given atropine sulfate.

Ipratropium bromide (a quaternary derivative of atropine sulfate) results in fewer side effects than atropine sulfate because it is poorly absorbed from the bronchial mucosa. Other inhaled anticholinergic agents, such as glycopyrrolate, have been effective, but in general the preferred anticholinergic agent for the treatment of COPD is inhaled ipratropium bromide.[22]

Anticholinergics are as effective as sympathomimetic agents in patients with COPD.[23-26] Marini and Lakshminarayan found that 11 of 15 patients with COPD who initially demonstrated a less than 15% increase in forced expiratory volume in 1 second (FEV_1) after the inhalation of isoproterenol subsequently increased their FEV_1 by greater than 15% after the inhalation of atropine.[27] Another study showed that inhaled atropine significantly increased the FEV_1 in patients with irreversible (after the inhalation of metaproterenol) COPD.[28] The bronchodilation caused by ipratropium bromide appears to be at least equivalent to that caused by beta-adrenergic drugs.[29]

Anticholinergics may be more effective when used on a long-term basis than beta-adrenergic drugs. Taskin and colleagues found that ipratropium bromidecaused significantly more bronchodilation than metaproterenol and that the resultant bronchodilation was more prolonged.[30] This effect was observed over 3 months of therapy (Fig. 13–1). Ipratropium bromide use has not been associated with tachyphylaxis when taken for as long as 5 years.[31] Two studies have suggested that ipratropium bromide has a steroid-sparing effect.[32, 33]

The bronchodilating effects of beta-adrenergic and anticholinergic agents are independent. Sympathomimetic drugs primarily affect the smaller distal airways, whereas anticholinergics primarily affect the larger central airways. Atropine decreases cGMP, and beta-adrenergics increase cAMP; both of these processes result in bronchodilation. The combination of anticholinergics and beta-adrenergic agents usually produces greater increases in airflow than the use of either agent alone.[34-36] Douglas and coworkers administered subjects inhaled salbutamol (albuterol) until their respiratory flow rates had reached a plateau. Next, they administered inhaled ipratropium bromide (80 µg), which resulted in a further improvement in flow rates.[37] However, Rebuck and associates found that ipratropium bromide did not act synergistically with sympathomimetics and methylxanthines in the treatment of acute exacerbations of COPD, but they did find it to be an equally effective alternative to the sympathomimetics (Fig. 13–2).[38]

Methylxanthines

Methylxanthines (e.g., caffeine, theophylline, and theobromine) have been used in the treatment of COPD

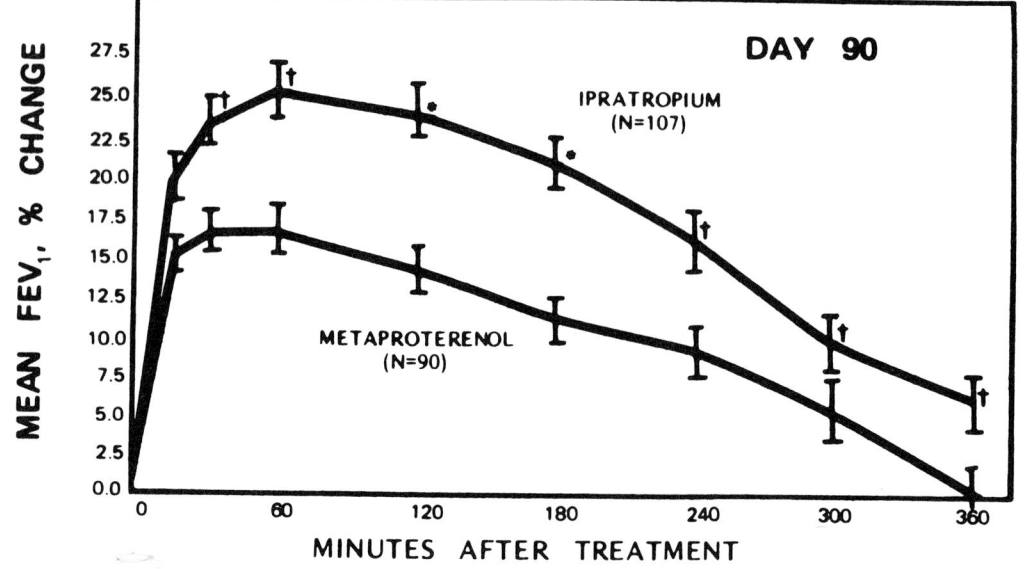

FIGURE 13–1. Mean per cent changes in FEV_1 at serial times after inhalation of ipratropium (40 µg) or metaproterenol (1500 µg) after a 90-day trial period of daily use (*P<.01, comparison of adjusted group means from an analysis of covariance; †P<.05, comparison of adjusted group means from an analysis of covariance). (Reprinted from Tashkin DP, Ashutosh K, Blecker ER, et al. Comparison of the anticholinergic bronchodilator ipratropium bromide with metaproterenol in chronic obstructive pulmonary disease: A 90-day multi-center study. Am J Med 1986; 81:81–90.)

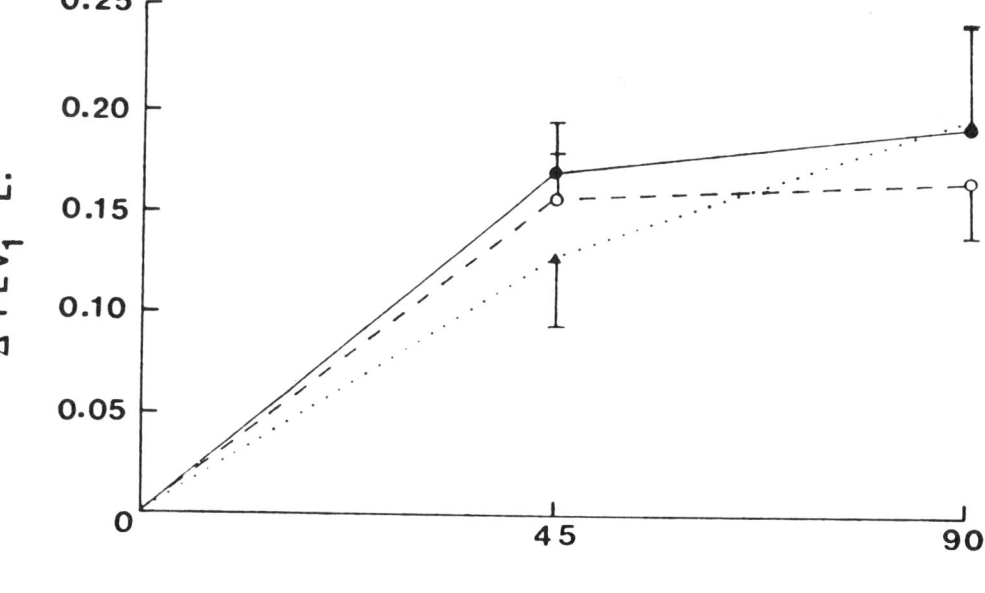

FIGURE 13-2. Mean increases in FEV₁ above baseline after inhalation of ipratropium bromide *(triangles)*, fentoterol *(open circles)*, or their combination *(solid circles)* in 51 patients with COPD. (Reprinted from Rebuck AS, Chapman KR, Abboud P. Nebulized anticholinergic and sympathomimetic treatment of asthma and chronic airway disease in the emergency room. Am J Med 1987; 82:59–64.)

for many years. Theophylline has been available for over 40 years, yet its mechanism of action remains unclear. It relaxes bronchial smooth muscle (especially if it is constricted), increases diaphragm contractility, and reduces diaphragm susceptibility to fatigue.[39] Theophylline increases mucociliary clearance in some patients and reduces mediator release from mast cells.[40] Theophylline also inhibits phosphodiesterase (the enzyme that inactivates cAMP), which results in an increase in the level of cAMP within the cells. However, this effect occurs only minimally at therapeutic serum concentrations.[41] The mechanism of action has also been attributed to the antagonism of adenosine, but this is unlikely to occur at concentrations within the usual therapeutic range.[42]

Bronchodilation secondary to theophylline is directly proportional to the log of the serum concentration in the range of 3 to 25 μg/ml.[43] Serum levels less than 10 μg/ml minimally improve lung function, and levels greater than 20 μg/ml are associated with significant side effects; therefore, recommended therapeutic levels in the past have been in the range of 10 to 20 μg/ml.[43] Since theophylline has a narrow range in which it is both therapeutic and nontoxic, we prefer the use of lower serum levels in adults, that is, in the range of 8 to 12 μg/ml. Theophylline should not be used if its level in the blood cannot be reliably determined. Theophylline plasma half-lives vary among patients (Table 13–2). Those who rapidly metabolize the drug require larger and more frequent doses. Theophylline half-life is decreased in children, smokers, and marijuana users, in those on high-carbohydrate/low-protein diets, and in patients taking drugs that induce the formation of hepatic enzymes (e.g., phenobarbital and phenytoin). Theophylline's half-life is increased in neonates and elderly patients, in those with acute and chronic hepatic dysfunction, congestive heart failure, or febrile illness, and in those taking other drugs (e.g., macrolide and quinolone antibiotics, allopurinol, cimetidine, troleandomycin, and propranolol). Acute viral illnesses and influenza vaccine are associated with an increased half-life of theophylline.[44, 45] Changes in body position during sleep may decrease theophylline absorption rate in some patients.[46]

The intravenous administration of aminophylline (which consists of 85% theophylline) is often used together with beta-adrenergic agents and corticosteroids in the management of acute exacerbations of COPD. Its efficacy in this situation is uncertain. A recent study found that the addition of aminophylline to inhaled metaproterenol, oral antibiotics, and intravenous methylprednisolone during acute exacerbations of COPD did not improve bronchodilation, arterial blood gas parameters, or dyspnea, but it did cause more frequent side effects than the administration of these drugs alone.[47] If aminophylline is to be used, a loading dose of 6 to 8

TABLE 13-2. SOME FACTORS THAT ALTER THE HALF-LIFE OF THEOPHYLLINE

Decrease in Half-Life
  Age (e.g., in children)
  Smoking
  Marijuana use
  High-carbohydrate/low-protein diet
  Drugs (phenobarbital and phenytoin)

Increase in Half-Life
  Age (e.g., in neonates and in the elderly)
  Liver disease
  Congestive heart failure
  Drugs (erythromycin, quinolone antibiotics, allopurinol, cimetidine, troleandromycin, and propranolol)
  Influenza vaccine
  Acute viral illness
  Fever
  Obesity

mg/kg may be given over 20 to 30 minutes if the patient has not been taking theophylline orally. The loading dose should be based on the ideal body weight in order to avoid overdose in obese patients. A loading dose should not be given if the patient has been taking theophylline orally or if a serum theophylline level is unavailable. A starting maintenance dose of 0.5 mg/kg per hour for adults should be adjusted based on serum levels obtained 12 and 24 hours after starting the infusion. Adjustments are made based on linear kinetics. For instance, if the level is 6 µg/ml, then doubling the infusion rate increases the level to approximately 12 µg/ml after four to five half-lives (24–30 hours). If toxic symptoms appear (e.g., tachycardia, ectopic beats, nausea, vomiting, anxiety, and headache), the infusion should be stopped, and the level should be checked both immediately and again in 6 to 8 hours. The level should have decreased to one half of the original level. Additional side effects of theophylline include diarrhea, abdominal pain, anorexia, and the relaxation of the lower esophageal sphincter, which leads to gastroesophageal reflux. A small percentage of patients cannot tolerate even minimal doses of theophylline. The risk of seizures and cardiac arrhythmias increases at levels greater than or equal to 30 µg/ml. Another potential manifestation of theophylline toxicity is the development of multifocal atrial tachycardia.[48] Such serious complications are associated with a significant increase in mortality during acute exacerbations of COPD.

Theophylline use has decreased in recent years because it requires systemic administration and causes significant side effects. Furthermore, safer, more effective agents are available. However, sustained-release preparations of oral theophylline may be a useful adjunct for patients with COPD. Stable blood levels can be achieved over a 24-hour period using sustained-release agents; thus, theophylline administered in this way might be useful for patients with nocturnal symptoms. Since sustained-release theophylline reaches peak serum levels after 4 to 8 hours in most patients, the vulnerable period that may occur 3 to 4 hours after inhaled agents are given is avoided. We know of no indication for the use of oral short-acting theophylline in adults with COPD.

Recent studies of patients with COPD have shown that the FEV_1 and forced vital capacity (FVC) increase only slightly in most patients at serum levels between 10 and 20 µg/ml.[49] Theophylline does not result in an increase in the 12-minute walking distance or change the results of progressive cycle ergometry when its action is compared to that of a placebo.[50] Although flow rates improved modestly, most patients did not show improvement in their symptoms of wheezing, breathlessness, or cough, nor in their sense of well-being. However, some studies suggest that theophylline improves functional status and dyspnea even without improving airflow.[11, 51, 52] Better functional status and lessened dyspnea may relate to improvements of respiratory muscle function.[52]

Disagreement concerning findings that indicate the benefits or lack of benefits of theophylline use in patients with COPD is probably explained by differences among the populations studied. Ideally, aminophylline should be used only in patients who are likely to benefit from it. The presence of improvement of the FEV_1 after the inhalation of isoproterenol predicts with good sensitivity (75%) and specificity (96%) which patients with COPD will respond to oral methylxanthines.[53] An improvement of more than 25% after the inhalation of isoproterenol suggests that a patient will likely respond to theophylline.

Glucocorticoid Agents

Although the usefulness of glucocorticoids in the treatment of asthma is well established, their effectiveness in the management of patients with COPD is less clear. The mechanism of glucocorticoid action is unknown, but it probably involves a variety of factors, such as a decrease in the number, activity, and directed migration of inflammatory cells,[54] a decrease in arachidonic acid metabolites,[55] an increase in beta$_2$-adrenergic responsiveness,[56] prevention of increases in vascular permeability,[57] and a decrease in airway hypersensitivity.[58, 59] These effects are not immediate and take at least 6 or 12 hours to appear.[60] Steroids can be administered orally, parenterally, or by inhalation.

The prolonged administration of systemic steroids is associated with significant side effects, including adrenal suppression, hypertension, diabetes, Cushing's syndrome, and impairment of the host's immune defense mechanisms. If oral therapy is necessary, it should proceed on an alternate-day regimen if possible, and should include the lowest possible dose of a medium-duration preparation (such as prednisone). Prednisone is metabolized in the liver to its active form prednisolone; therefore, patients with liver disease may respond more rapidly to methylprednisolone, which does not undergo hepatic conversion.[60]

Inhaled steroids have minimal systemic absorption and essentially do not cause systemic side effects. They are not associated with signs of hyperadrenocorticism, and daily doses of up to 800 µg cause only minimal pituitary and adrenal suppression.[61] About 10% of patients develop candidiasis, dysphonia (secondary to local deposition of the drug in the mouth and pharynx), or both. Rinsing and gargling with water after the use of inhaled steroids helps to prevent oral side effects; if oropharyngeal candidiasis does occur, it can be treated with topical therapy. The usual daily dose of inhaled steroids is approximately equivalent to 10 to 15 mg/day of prednisone. There is a dose-related response with inhaled doses up to 1600 µg/day. Beclomethasone is available in the United States at a concentration of 42 µg per single inhalation. Flunisolide is available at a concentration of 250 µg per inhalation, and triamcinolone is available at a concentration of 100 µg per inhalation. Inhalation of a beta$_2$-adrenergic agonist prior to steroid inhalation aids in preventing the airway irritation that some patients develop with steroid use. The addition of inhaled steroids may make possible a decrease of the dose of chronically administered oral steroids and should be attempted in all patients who require long-term systemic corticosteroid therapy.

Corticosteroids are frequently used in the treatment of COPD, despite the fact that they are effective in only a minority of patients. Albert and coworkers have shown that intravenous steroids improve airflow during acute exacerbations of COPD.[62] The duration of respiratory failure was reduced in patients who received methylprednisolone 0.5 mg/kg every 6 hours compared with those who received a placebo. At any point after the first 12 hours after administration, a significant improvement in airflow was observed in the treated group compared with the placebo group. In another study, the use of steroids in this setting did not improve airflow during the first 4 hours after administration or decrease hospital admissions.[63]

The indications for steroids in patients with stable COPD are less clear. Only 15 to 30% of patients with stable COPD benefit from steroid therapy.[64-66] However, an individual patient may respond much better than the group as a whole and may benefit from the addition of steroids to his or her regimen. Mendella and associates have demonstrated that the response to inhaled isoproterenol is a good predictor of the response to oral steroids.[64] Almost all steroid responders showed a 15% or greater increase in FEV_1 after the inhalation of isoproterenol, whereas patients who exhibited a less than 10% increase in FEV_1 were less likely to respond. Shim and colleagues have suggested that eosinophils detected in sputum using Wright's staining are an indicator of response to steroids,[66] but this finding was not substantiated in a later report.[67] The absence of a response to steroids in a clinically stable patient does not preclude a response during acute exacerbations.

Patients with irreversible COPD (i.e., those who do not have an increase in respiratory flow rates after conventional therapy) may have a subjective improvement in symptoms after treatment with corticosteroids. It has been hypothesized that this subjective improvement might be secondary to an increase in exercise tolerance that is independent of any measurable improvement in airway mechanics. This hypothesis was not substantiated in the study by Strain and coworkers, who performed maximum exercise testing in patients after placebo and after steroid. They found that patients with stable COPD did not show improved exercise tolerance after steroid therapy.[68]

A trial course of steroids is indicated in patients with moderate to severe COPD who are not controlled with the other measures outlined earlier. An objective improvement in pulmonary function should be documented. If there is improvement, the lowest dose that maintains the improvement should be used. If daily doses of 15 mg or less of oral prednisone can be used, it is advisable to substitute an inhaled steroid for prednisone. Patients receiving higher doses of prednisone should be maintained on alternate-day regimens, if possible.

ANTITUSSIVES, EXPECTORANTS, AND MUCOLYTICS

Many disease processes are associated with symptoms of cough and expectoration, and chronic coughing (greater than 3 wk in duration) is a common symptom in patients seeking medical attention.[69] Coughing may be a sign of a serious underlying disease (e.g., cancer or COPD) or may be in response to minor acute irritation. The cause of a chronic cough can be identified in most patients.[70] Specific therapy should be provided to treat the specific cause once it is identified. If it is not identified, chronic cough can be treated nonspecifically (e.g., using antitussives and expectorants) if it is a nuisance or if it causes other medical problems.

A recent review analyzed the clinical efficacy of drugs that are available as antitussives, mucolytics, and expectorants.[71] The authors classified nonspecific antitussive drugs according to their primary mode of action. Ipratropium bromide, iodinated glycerol, and guaimesal are effective antitussive drugs in patients with chronic bronchitis.[72-74] These agents work by altering mucociliary factors that irritate cough receptors. Although local and intravenous lidocaine is effective at decreasing cough in patients undergoing bronchoscopy, no controlled studies have demonstrated its usefulness in patients with chronic cough. Morphine, codeine, dextromethorphan, diphenhydramine, caramiphen, viminol-p-hydroxybenzoate, and levodropropizine are effective antitussive agents that increase the threshold or latency of the cough center.[71] In addition to altering mucociliary factors, ipratropium bromide may work as an antitussive by increasing the threshold or latency of the efferent limb of the vagus nerve.[72]

For patients with chronic bronchitis, only a hypertonic saline aerosol has been shown to improve cough clearance; however, no associated improvements in pulmonary function or symptoms have been found.[75]

MANAGEMENT AND PREVENTION OF RESPIRATORY INFECTIONS

Extensive clinical literature produced over the past 25 years has documented the role of infectious agents in the production of both chronic bronchitis and recurrent episodes of acute exacerbations of bronchitis.[76-78] It has been estimated that about one half of the acute episodes are accounted for by infectious causes. These acute exacerbations are characterized by an increase in cough and dyspnea and by changes in the type and amount of sputum produced; fever, leukocytosis, and new infiltrates are often absent on chest radiographs. Bacteria, including *Streptococcus pneumoniae* and *Haemophilus influenzae*, are present in the sputum of about one half of all patients, whereas other infectious agents, including the influenza and parainfluenza viruses, rhinovirus, coronavirus, and *Mycoplasma pneumoniae*, are other pathogens that are recognized during acute exacerbations.[79]

Of the wide variety of bacteria and viruses that pass through the oral cavity and pharynx of the normal person, only a small minority are able to persist and become established as "normal flora." Certain bacteria and viruses as well as mycoplasma adhere to the epithelial cells of the respiratory mucous membranes by means of adhesive molecules on their surfaces that are recognized by specific receptor molecules on the epithelial cells. In normal subjects, pharyngeal contents are frequently aspirated in small amounts into the trachea; despite these inoculations, the trachea remains sterile in most normal persons. Patients with chronic bronchitis, however, do not have sterile tracheas even when no clinical evidence of infection is present.[80] Microbes that make up the normal flora of the pharynx become attached to the epithelium of the trachea and large bronchi of patients with chronic bronchitis. These organisms are often associated with acute exacerbations of bronchitis. Antibiotic therapy for acute exacerbations is designed to treat the bacterial components of lower respiratory tract infections.

Antibiotic Therapy

The effectiveness of antibiotic therapy in the treatment of acute exacerbations of chronic bronchitis has been the subject of debate.[79–81] The most comprehensive study reported to date was that of Anthonisen and associates; they treated 362 exacerbations of chronic bronchitis in 173 patients over a 3-year period.[81] One hundred eighty of the episodes were treated with a placebo and 182 episodes were managed with a 10-day course of an oral broad-spectrum antibiotic. The patients were followed closely for a period of 3 weeks after entry into the study. The antibiotics used were trimethoprim-sulfamethoxazole (one tablet twice per day), amoxicillin (250 mg four times per day), or doxycycline (in an initial dose of 200 mg followed by doses of 100 mg per day). The results of this study are summarized in Table 13–3. The investigators found that the three antibiotic regimens did not differ in their efficacy and that patients who received antibiotics had less deterioration of their symptoms and a higher success rate. They also found that when peak respiratory flow rate was measured on day 6 of the trial, it was significantly more improved in those patients who received antibiotics. The incidence of side effects was similar both in patients treated with antibiotics and in those treated with a placebo. Anthonisen and associates concluded that there is a significant benefit associated with the use of antibiotics to treat acute exacerbations of COPD.

The choice of antibiotic is also a subject of controversy. In the report of Anthonisen and associates, patients with COPD had an average of one exacerbation every 8.5 months, or an average frequency of 1.3 exacerbations per year.[81] Thus, courses of antibiotic therapy are often prescribed several times for the same patient. For this reason, most authors agree that the antibiotic should be orally administered, nontoxic, and relatively inexpensive.

The selection of antibiotics for the treatment of the acute exacerbation of chronic bronchitis is based on the appearance of the sputum after Gram's staining and on the known incidence of bacteria that are associated with acute exacerbations.[82] The sputum, if it is carefully collected and stained, is useful in guiding therapy. The presence of neutrophils and mixed bacterial flora is the most common finding in chronic bronchitis and indicates a mixed bacterial infection. Recommended antibiotics include ampicillin, amoxicillin, a tetracycline, or co-trimoxazole. These antibiotics are likely to control the most common organisms, including *Haemophilus influenzae* and pneumococci. The absence of neutrophils suggests a noninfectious cause of the exacerbation, such as inhaled toxins or allergens, whereas the presence of neutrophils in the absence of bacteria suggests a viral infection, *Mycoplasma pneumoniae*, a *Legionella* organism, or previous antibiotic therapy. The Gram-negative diplococcus *Moraxella (Branhamella) catarrhalis*, which was formerly considered a saprophyte, is now thought to be an important respiratory pathogen in patients with COPD.[83] The significance of this fact is that this organism often produces beta-lactamase and is thus resistant to ampicillin and amoxicillin; therefore, treatment with co-trimoxazole, erythromycin, or a tetracycline is indicated. If small gram-negative coccobacilli predominate, *H. influenzae* infection is likely. Although ampicillin and amoxicillin are usually effective against this organism, some strains collected from patients with COPD have been found to be beta-lactamase producers. If the infection is severe or does not respond to initial antibiotic therapy, a beta-lactamase–resistant antibiotic, such as the combination of amoxicillin and clavulanic acid (Augmentin) or an oral cephalosporin, such as cefaclor, may be indicated.[84]

An antibiotic therapy duration of 7 to 10 days has been recommended by several authors.[80, 81, 84] We prefer to treat patients for at least 10 days, since bronchial clearance mechanisms are abnormal in patients with COPD. Because of altered mucociliary clearance, mucous gland hypertrophy, and the distortion of the architecture of the bronchial walls, mucus clearance is relatively ineffective, and thus the pooling of secretions within the airways occurs where antibiotic penetrance is inadequate. Measures to improve mucus clearance are an important part of the management of these patients. In the study by Anthonisen and associates,[81] respiratory flow rates continued to improve during the 2-week period following the initiation of antibiotic therapy; this suggests that prolonged treatment is important following acute exacerbations of COPD.

Management of Severe Infections

The management program outlined above is indicated for the treatment of acute bronchitis in patients who do

TABLE 13–3. OUTCOME OF THERAPY IN EXACERBATIONS OF CHRONIC BRONCHITIS: ANTIBIOTICS COMPARED WITH PLACEBO*

Outcome	Antibiotics†	Placebo
Deterioration	18 (10%)‡	34 (19%)
Success	124 (68%)‡	99 (55%)
No change	34 (19%)	42 (23%)
Other	6 (3%)	5 (3%)
Total	182 (100%)	180 (100%)

*Data from Anthonisen NR, Manfreda J, Warren MD, et al. Antibiotic therapy in exacerbations of chronic obstructive pulmonary disease. Ann Intern Med 1978; 106:200.
†Amoxicillin, doxycycline, or trimethoprim-sulfamethoxazole.
‡$P<.05$ between study groups.

not have fever or new infiltrates as determined from a chest radiograph. Indications for hospitalization in this population differ from those in otherwise normal patients, since these patients are already chronically ill and may have defective immune systems. Hospitalization is indicated if the acute exacerbation does not respond as expected to the therapeutic measures outlined, if acute respiratory failure occurs, if there is evidence for left-sided heart failure or cor pulmonale, if other significant diseases such as cardiac or renal disease become more severe as a result of the exacerbation, or if complications such as atelectasis or pneumothorax occur.[2]

Patients with pneumonia (as indicated by the detection of new infiltrates on a chest radiograph, purulent sputum, fever, and an elevated white blood cell count) should be hospitalized for a period of intensive therapy and observation. Although the oral antibiotics discussed earlier may be effective, an initial period of intravenous antibiotic administration combined with fluid administration is often helpful. A recent study conducted in Spain indicated that in older patients with severe community-acquired pneumonia the overall mortality was 21%.[85] The average age of the patients in this study was 57 years, and 46% of the patients (71% of those who died) had a concurrent chronic debilitating disease. Although 38% of the patients had pneumococcal infections, Gram-negative bacilli were responsible for these infections in 25% of the cases. Thus, it was concluded that in such a population of severely ill adults with underlying chronic disease, the use of broad-spectrum antibiotic treatment in combination with erythromycin and a third-generation cephalosporin drug is indicated for initial empirical therapy.[85] An alternative program would include a cephalosporin combined with an aminoglycoside.

Although sputum culture is usually not indicated during acute exacerbations of COPD, patients with severe pneumonia who require hospitalization and those who do not respond to initial empiric therapy are candidates for sputum culturing and sensitivity testing. Changes in antibiotic therapy should be made cautiously and based on objective data, such as that provided by Gram's staining and the culture of respiratory secretions, since response is much slower in this population than in previously healthy adults. Methods to obtain uncontaminated sputum for culture, including transtracheal aspiration and fiberoptic bronchoscopy using a protected brush catheter for specimen collection, are rarely indicated in such patients who have community-acquired pneumonias.[86, 87]

Prophylaxis for Respiratory Infections

The prevention of acute exacerbations of COPD incorporates such general health measures as adequate nutrition and fluid intake, the avoidance of cigarette smoke, and methods to improve mucus clearance. Specific measures designed to improve immunologic host defenses against infectious agents consist of vaccination against common viral and bacterial pathogens and the administration of amantadine, an oral antiviral agent. Future preventive therapy will likely include measures to prevent the adherence of pathogenic organisms to the respiratory epithelial cells and measures to alter immune response.

Influenza vaccine has proved to be of great value in reducing both morbidity and mortality during epidemics of influenza.[2] The protection rate associated with the administration of influenza vaccine is 60 to 80%. The vaccine itself is relatively innocuous, having only a 2% rate of mild febrile reactions and muscle aching that may persist for a few hours. Hypersensitivity reactions are limited to patients who are allergic to egg protein. The severe reactions that occurred following swine influenza vaccination in 1976 have not been noted with the use of current vaccines against types A and B influenza virus. Annual vaccination is recommended for all patients with COPD unless a specific contraindication is present, such as allergy to egg protein. The vaccine is altered each year based on the known incidence of virus types in the environment and is generally available in the early fall. Patients with COPD should be immunized as soon as possible after the vaccine becomes available each year.

The mortality rate for pneumococcal pneumonia has remained stable over the past 30 years in spite of advances in antibiotic therapy. There are approximately 500,000 cases of pneumococcal pneumonia in the United States each year, and it has been estimated that 5% of these patients die.[88] For this reason, attempts have been made to control pneumococcal infections with vaccines, which at first contained 14 pneumococcal serotypes but later contained 23 serotypes. These vaccines contain purified capsular polysaccharide extracted from the pneumococcus and have proved effective in preventing pneumococcal pneumonia and bacteremia in young men at high risk, such as military recruits.[89] Unfortunately, the efficacy of the vaccine in preventing pneumococcal pneumonia in patients with COPD has not been established. A large cooperative study begun by the Veterans Administration in 1981 tested the effects of the 14-valent pneumococcal vaccine in a total of 2295 high-risk patients, 539 of whom had chronic pulmonary disease. They were unable to demonstrate any efficacy of the vaccine in preventing pneumonia or acute exacerbations of bronchitis in this population, nor did they find the vaccine effective in any subgroup. Patients were affected equally by those serotypes contained in the vaccine as well as by other serotypes. They concluded that chronically ill patients (who are the most susceptible to pneumococcal infection) may have an impaired immune response to the vaccine. Nevertheless, the United States Public Health Service recommends the use of the current 23-serotype vaccine in all persons over 50 years of age and in those with chronic pulmonary disease. A single dose is thought to be sufficient because the duration of protection has not been determined. Future recommendations may indicate the need for revaccination after a period of several years.[2]

Purified polysaccharide vaccines against *H. influenzae* have been developed.[90] Although one such vaccine alone was not effective when tested in young children, a protein-conjugated form of the vaccine has been shown to be efficacious.[91-93] Anti-*Pseudomonas* vaccines have been developed and tested in patients with cystic fibrosis, and vaccines against other Gram-negative rods are currently being investigated for use in patients with severe pneumonia. These vaccines are of little potential use for the usual patient with COPD, since Gram-negative bacteria are unlikely to be responsible for the usual infectious exacerbations. Furthermore, most older patients with COPD have antibodies against a wide variety of organisms as a result of previous exposure. The vaccines may be available in the future, however, for the treatment of more severe infections in hospitalized patients.

Amantadine hydrochloride is a tricyclic amine that inhibits an early stage of replication of the influenza A virus. In several studies it has been shown to be both therapeutic and protective with respect to influenza A viral infections.[2, 94] Amantadine is not effective against other viral infections, such as influenza B. Thus, it should only be considered for use when influenza A epidemics are likely, such as during the winter and early spring in the United States. Estimates of the efficacy of amantadine in preventing influenza range from 50 to 90%.[2] For therapy of viral infections, it must be administered within 48 hours of the onset of illness. For preventive purposes, the antiviral agent is given to high-risk individuals during an epidemic along with the vaccine and continued for 2 weeks (until the vaccine becomes effective). The recommended adult dose of amantadine is 100 mg twice daily for patients under the age of 65 years; for those over 65 years of age an initial loading dose of 200 mg is followed by 100 mg daily. Side effects, especially in the elderly, include mental changes, ataxia, tremor, and convulsions. Confusion has been reported in 3 to 7% of treated patients.

PHARMACOTHERAPY OF THE RESPIRATORY MUSCLES

The preceding sections have addressed therapy for diseases of the gas-exchanging organ, the lungs. In this section, we consider therapy of the other major "organ" of the respiratory system—the respiratory muscles. The diaphragm is the major muscle of resting inspiration. Like the heart, the diaphragm must intermittently and continuously contract to maintain life. Unfortunately, unlike the heart, pharmacotherapy of this vital organ is in its infancy. Over the past 10 years, multiple studies have reported the beneficial effects of drugs such as the methylxanthines, beta-adrenergic agonists, dopamine, and various respiratory stimulants. In this section, the controversies concerning these studies are addressed, and then an overview of adverse drug effects on the respiratory muscles is presented.

Methlyxanthines

The methylxanthines include caffeine (1,3,7-trimethylxanthine) and theophylline (1,3-dimethylxanthine), which have specific effects on the diaphragm. Caffeine has been shown to increase the release and inhibit the reuptake of Ca^{2+} in intact cells and in the sarcoplasmic reticulum store of Ca^{2+} in skeletal muscle.[95, 96] Theophylline's primary effect on the diaphragm may be to increase Ca^{2+} movement across cell membranes. Other effects of the methylxanthines include augmentation of neurotransmitter release at the neuromuscular junction, an increase in miniature action potentials at muscle endplates, and the increase of end-plate potential in response to the electrical stimulation of motor nerves.

In 1981, Aubier and colleagues reported the effects of aminophylline on respiratory muscle function in humans.[39] When infused at therapeutic doses in volunteers, the drug resulted in a 15% increase in transdiaphragmatic pressure (a measure of muscle strength), while maintaining the electromyographic activity of the diaphragm at a constant level. This study further demonstrated that theophylline infusion prior to the induction of fatigue by resistive loaded breathing resulted in the rapid recovery of contractile tension. When theophylline was administered following fatigue, the resulting transdiaphragmatic pressure exceeded the baseline levels for any given level of phrenic nerve stimulation. More recently, Aubier and colleagues have shown that a 2-month treatment regimen of sustained-release theophylline in patients with obstructive pulmonary disease (FEV_1 of 35.5% of that predicted) could improve respiratory muscle performance by 29%.[52] Multiple human and animal studies have reported similar results and have confirmed that chronic therapy can improve diaphragmatic contractility.[95, 97]

In spite of these encouraging results, contrary opinions exist.[79] Moxham has suggested that the techniques used in Aubier's early work are difficult to perform, thus making it difficult for other investigators to confirm his results.[98] Furthermore, the significant improvement in pulmonary function and little change in pulmonary resistance noted by Murciano and coworkers[99] have been cited as evidence against a beneficial effect of theophylline on the diaphragm. In addition, we have been unable to demonstrate an improvement in exercise performance following aminophylline therapy in a small group of patients with irreversible airway obstruction.[100] Regardless of the negative reports, theophylline should be considered for individualized therapy for the patient with COPD whose respiratory muscle weakness or fatigue is a major problem (e.g., for the patient with impending respiratory failure during acute exacerbations).

There has been insufficient study of caffeine's effects on human diaphragm function. One study has shown that caffeine can increase the tension in skeletal muscle when administered at therapeutic doses; another has shown that a 40% increase in diaphragmatic contractility occurs when caffeine is administered.[95] Whether the consumption of caffeinated beverages can improve respiratory muscle function is unknown.

Sympathomimetic Agents

In view of the abundance of beta-adrenergic receptors in the diaphragm, it would seem that beta-adrenergic agonist drugs would have a significant effect on muscle function. In a dog model, this is true for the nonspecific beta-adrenergic agonist isoproterenol. Howell and co-workers have shown a small (11–12%) improvement in diaphragmatic contractility when isoproterenol was administered during fatigue; they also observed a minimal improvement in diaphragmatic contractility during hypercapnia when the drug was used.[101, 102]

Animal studies investigating the beta$_2$-specific adrenergic agonist terbutaline have revealed that this agent has variable effects on the rested diaphragm; however, contractility was increased significantly in fatigued diaphragms after the drug's use.[103, 104] The rate of decline in tension could be decreased during fatigue in these studies. The beneficial effects of terbutaline could be blocked by propranolol, a fact which confirms its mode of action. There are few studies of the effects of beta$_2$-adrenergic agonists on human respiratory muscle function. However, one report of the effect of albuterol in five normal subjects with diaphragmatic fatigue induced by breathing in the presence of inspiratory resistance suggests that there is no beneficial effect of this drug.[105] More clinical trials are needed to determine whether the beneficial effects of terbutaline and albuterol (as reported in animal studies) can be observed in humans, whose diaphragms have a muscle fiber composition of a different metabolic type than that of laboratory animals.

Inotropic Agents

Unlike other skeletal muscles, the diaphragm depends on extracellular Ca^{2+} for activation.[106] This dependence appears to be similar to that of cardiac muscle, in which Ca^{2+} ions cross the muscle cell membrane and induce Ca^{2+} release from the sarcoplasmic reticulum. Digitalis can enhance the levels of intracellular Ca^{2+} and augment myocardial contraction through the inhibition of Na^+–K^+ exchange, which inhibits the outward extrusion of cellular Ca^{2+} via Na^+–Ca^{2+} exchange. In patients with COPD, Aubier and colleagues have shown that there is a 20% increase in diaphragmatic strength without a change in cardiac output when digoxin is administered.[107] A more pronounced improvement in diaphragmatic strength has been noted in similar patients following an infusion of dopamine (10 μg/kg/min); this improvement is accompanied by a 40% improvement in cardiac output.[99] Further studies are needed to evaluate whether chronic administration of these agents can improve diaphragmatic function directly or by increasing cardiac output and oxygen delivery.

Respiratory Stimulants

Several agents that stimulate ventilation at the central or peripheral level have been developed. They have been used to treat acute respiratory failure and to delay or avoid mechanical ventilation while treatment of the acute disorder is carried out. In addition, stimulant therapy of COPD has been undertaken to improve hypoxemia and possibly avoid long-term oxygen therapy.[108, 109] Stimulant use has also become an alternative therapy in obstructive sleep apnea when nasal continuous positive airway pressure cannot be used.[110–112]

Doxapram is a central respiratory stimulant that may delay the need for mechanical ventilation when administered to patients with COPD in acute respiratory failure. In a double-blind cooperative study, doxapram decreased the oxygen-associated elevation in Pa_{CO_2} and decline in pH.[108] In another study, this agent was shown to improve spontaneous ventilation, leading to successful weaning from mechanical ventilation.[109] Side effects, including restlessness, seizures, and cardiac irritability, have limited doxapram's usefulness.

Progesterone and derivative acetate compounds have been shown to improve arterial hypoxemia, reduce hypercapnia, and increase pH during wakefulness in patients with COPD.[113] These drugs have also been shown to improve arterial hypoxemia during sleep in these patients; however, other parameters of sleep disordered breathing or measures of the severity of obstructive sleep apnea may not be significantly improved. Other studies have found that patients with obstructive sleep apnea derive no benefit from these agents.[110] Poor patient compliance with the use of these medications due to sexual dysfunction, breast tenderness, and hirsutism as well as thromboembolic phenomena has limited their use. Whether other progestational agents with more respiratory stimulatory effect, such as chlormadinone acetate, improve ventilation during wakefulness and sleep is unknown.[111]

The respiratory stimulant acetazolamide, which causes metabolic acidosis by inhibiting carbonic anhydrase, has been shown to result in a 69% reduction in the frequency of centrally mediated sleep apnea.[112] The drug may be useful in the patient with this disorder who cannot tolerate nasal continuous positive airway pressure. Bicarbonate wasting combined with electrolyte abnormalities may be a problem with prolonged use of the drug.

Buspirone is a centrally acting stimulatory drug that is marketed as an anxiolytic agent. It has a unique dose-dependent stimulatory effect on respiration, which is primarily the result of an increase of tidal volume; it also increases respiratory rate.[114] Unlike the benzodiazepines, which have depressant neural effects mediated by the receptors for gamma-aminobutyric acid, buspirone is believed to have agonist actions on serotonin $5-HT_{1A}$ receptors. Thus, buspirone may prove to be useful in patients with anxiety and respiratory disease without causing undesirable respiratory depression.

In contrast to the centrally stimulating agents discussed earlier, almitrine bismesylate may act on peripheral chemoreceptors and enhance hypoxic pulmonary vasoconstriction.[115, 116] Minute ventilation is increased with increased PaO_2, predominately as a result of an improvement in ventilation/perfusion mismatching. The drug causes increased pulmonary artery pressure as well as systemic hypertension, unexplained weight loss, and peripheral neuropathies. At the present time, the drug is available in Europe but not in the United States, and a recent multicenter trial conducted in the United States to test the drug was cancelled.

Adverse Effects of Pharmacotherapy

Many therapeutic agents have been shown to have depressant effects on the respiratory muscles (Table 13–4). Narcotics, hypnotics, and sedatives are in common use, and their central hypoventilatory effects may have detrimental effects on any rehabilitation program.[117] Alcohol may blunt the ventilatory response to hypoxia and hypercapnia and exacerbate obstructive sleep apnea. Alcoholism is a cause of cardiomyopathy, and a recent study in patients with cardiomyopathy revealed that 42% had significantly decreased skeletal muscle strength and that 46% had histologic evidence of a skeletal myopathy. The estimated total intake of alcohol correlated directly with muscle strength and cardiac output, whereas an inverse relationship of alcohol intake to cardiac ejection fraction was shown.[118]

Motor neuropathies and neuromuscular blockade may occur when agents such as antibiotics, antiarrhythmics, and chemotherapeutic drugs are used. Aminoglycosides may produce significant neuromuscular blockade and the potential for diaphragm weakness. Therapy with neostigmine (to a maximum dose of 0.07 mg/kg), calcium gluconate (to a maximum dose of 25 mg/kg), or both may be conducted if appropriate cardiopulmonary monitoring is used.[117, 119] Corticosteroids, which are fre-

TABLE 13–4. DRUGS THAT CAN IMPAIR RESPIRATORY MUSCLE FUNCTION*

Type of Drug	Type of Impairment			
	Central Hypoventilation	**Motor Neuropathies**	**Neuromuscular Blockade**	**Myopathies**
CNS agents	Narcotics† Sedatives† Alcohol†	Tricyclics Ergot compounds Phenytoin† Methaqualone	Benzodiazepines Lithium Phenytoin	Narcotics General anesthetics Antipsychotics Lithium Diazepam Levodopa MAO inhibitors
Muscle relaxant	Baclofen		Neuromuscular blockers† Dantrolene	Suxamethonium
Antimicrobial		Sulfonamides Isoniazid† Other anti-TB drugs Dapsone Colistin Metronidazole Nitrofurantoin	Aminoglycosides† Macrolides† Polymyxin B† Colistin Tetracyclines	Amphotericin B Isoniazid Emetine Penicillins
Antirheumatic		Gold† Indomethacin Colchicine Phenylbutazone D-Penicillamine	D-Penicillamine† Chloroquine	D-Penicillamine Gold Chloroquine
Cardiovascular	Clonidine Lidocaine Loop diuretics	Perhexiline† Amiodarone† Captopril† Hydralazine Disopyramide Clofibrate	β-blocker Ca^{2+} blockers† Quinidine Procainamide Lidocaine Trimethaphan	Diuretics† β-blockers Clofibrate† Procainamide† EACA† Amiodarone Nifedipine Hydralazine
Hormone		Danazol	ACTH Corticosteroids Thyroid hormones Contraceptives	Corticosteroids† Thyroid hormone Danazol Vasopressin
Antineoplastic		Vincristine† Procarbazine Cytarabine Chlorambucil		Vincristine
Other	Antihistamines Cimetidine $NaHCO_3$	Vaccines† Cimetidine Chlorpropamide Tolbutamide	Nicotine $MgSO_4$	β-agonists Cimetidine Phenformin Amphetamines

*From Aldrich TK, Prezant DJ. Adverse effects of drugs on the respiratory muscles. Clin Chest Med 1990; 11:177–189.
†Common or severe.
Key: CNS: central nervous system; MAO: monoamine oxidase; TB: tuberculosis; EACA: ε-aminocaproic acid; ACTH: adrenocorticotropic hormone.

TABLE 13–5. THERAPEUTIC AGENTS USED IN THE MANAGEMENT OF PATIENTS WITH CHRONIC OBSTRUCTIVE PULMONARY DISEASE

Maintenance Therapy
Bronchodilators
    Beta-adrenergic agonists
    Anticholinergics
    Methylxanthines
    Others
Mucolytics, expectorants, and antitussives
Other therapeutic agents

Prevention of Acute Exacerbations
Anti-inflammatory agents
    Corticosteroids
    Others
Vaccines
Antiviral agents

Management of Acute Exacerbations
Oxygen
Bronchodilators
Antibiotics
Other therapeutic agents

quently used in patients in pulmonary rehabilitation programs, may inhibit neuromuscular transmission at the postsynaptic level.[117] Furthermore, these agents may induce muscle atrophy specific to the respiratory muscles, an effect that may not be predicted from an evaluation of peripheral skeletal muscles.[117, 120]

Based on the preceding discussion, it is apparent that the evaluation of specific therapy for the enhancement of respiratory muscle function is still in its initial stages. However, considerable information is available concerning adverse drug effects and drug interactions that may delay progress in an otherwise effective rehabilitation program.

MANAGEMENT STRATEGIES FOR CHRONIC OBSTRUCTIVE PULMONARY DISEASE

This chapter has attempted to summarize the available data addressing the pharmacologic therapy of patients with chronic airways obstruction. The therapeutic agents discussed are designed to be used in a comprehensive treatment program with careful subjective and objective monitoring. The therapeutic agents commonly used in the management of COPD are listed in Table 13–5. Their use should be designed to maintain optimum levels of pulmonary function, a minimum of side effects, and a low cost as well as to prevent acute exacerbations and to manage these exacerbations when they occur. Optimum therapy also includes the avoidance of agents that worsen the disease (Table 13–6).

Improving Patient Compliance with Therapeutic Regimens

Recent studies show that patients with COPD poorly adhere to prescribed medication regimens. Dolce and associates followed 78 patients with COPD treated in a medicine clinic and closely observed their adherence patterns.[121] They found that prescribed drug regimens were relatively complex and included an average of six medications per patient. Approximately one half of the patients overused their medications, whereas the remainder underused their medications. Adherence was best for relatively short-term regimens, such as those including steroids and antibiotics, and was worse for long-term therapy, such as that requiring the use of bronchodilators. Approximately one in three patients demonstrated a faulty technique in the use of his or her MDI. Poor patient compliance with the medical regimens (41%) was attributed to patients' claims that they felt good.

Therapeutic regimens for patients with COPD tend to be complicated in that they include both oral medications and inhaled agents. It has been demonstrated that considerable time must be spent to educate patients on the importance of their therapy. Careful instruction in the use of an MDI requires about 20 minutes.[122] These educational sessions must be repeated periodically if optimum adherence is to be expected.[122]

In order to optimize compliance, the regimen should be made as simple as possible. This may itself cause problems, since longer-acting drugs may be more expensive. If possible, maintenance drugs should be administered no more than twice daily (with the addition of inhaled bronchodilators when symptoms occur). It is clear that when regimens involve administration more often than twice daily, patient compliance decreases dramatically.[122]

Agents to Avoid in the Treatment of Patients with Chronic Obstructive Pulmonary Disease

Some therapeutic agents that may increase bronchospasm are listed in Table 13–6. If possible, these agents should be avoided, especially during acute exacerbations of COPD. The beta-adrenergic blocking drugs are among the most widely used therapeutic agents, especially in older patients who may also have hypertension or coronary artery disease. Two beta-blocking agents, atenolol and metoprolol, are relatively cardioselective and are preferred if beta-adrenergic blockade is absolutely necessary. Their cardioselective qualities are relative and disappear when higher doses are necessary. The combined alpha-adrenergic and beta-adrenergic blocking agent labetalol has been shown to be relatively safe for use in patients with COPD; however, bronchial obstruction occurs when this agent is used in high doses.[123]

Captopril was the first angiotensin converting enzyme

TABLE 13–6. SOME AGENTS TO AVOID IN PATIENTS WITH CHRONIC OBSTRUCTIVE PULMONARY DISEASE

Beta-adrenergic blocking agents
Angiotensin converting enzyme inhibitors
Inhaled agents
    Acetylcysteine
    Cigarette smoke
    Toxic fumes (e.g., insecticides and room deodorizers)

(ACE) inhibitor commercially available in the United States, and soon after its appearance it was reported to cause the so-called "cough syndrome."[124] This syndrome has subsequently been reported with the use of all ACE inhibitors and is thought to be an effect of ACE inhibition itself rather than an idiosyncratic side effect. The cough syndrome is associated with increased sensitivity to nonspecific inhalation challenge; it is now believed to occur in 10 to 12% of all patients receiving ACE-inhibitor therapy.[125]

Several inhaled substances are likely to cause bronchospasm in patients with COPD, especially during acute exacerbations of their illness when the degree of bronchospasm becomes more severe. Among the agents that may cause or worsen bronchospasm is the mucolytic drug acetylcysteine, which may induce an allergic reaction. Passive exposure to cigarette smoke has been shown to produce COPD and is a common cause of exacerbations of chronic illness.[126] Other toxic fumes, such as insecticide sprays, aerosol deodorizers, and cleaning fluids, may also induce acute attacks.

REFERENCES

1. The health consequences of smoking: Chronic obstructive lung disease. A report of the Surgeon General, 1984. Bethesda, MD, 1984. US Department of Health and Human Services Publication 84-50205.
2. American Thoracic Society. Standards for the diagnosis and care of patients with chronic obstructive pulmonary disease (COPD) and asthma. Am Rev Respir Dis 1987; 136:225–244.
3. Robertson C, Levison H. Bronchodilators in asthma. Chest 1985; 87(Suppl):64–68.
4. Tattersfield AE, Britton JR. Beta-adrenoceptor agonists. In: Barnes PJ, Rodger IW, Thomson NC (eds). Asthma: Basic Mechanisms and Clinical Management. 2nd ed. London: Academic Press, Inc., 1989, pp 563–590.
5. Freedman BJ, Hill GB. Comparative study of duration of action and cardiovascular effects of bronchodilator aerosols. Thorax 1971; 26:46.
6. Miller J, Kessler F, Weisinger P. Double-blind one-year clinical study of fenoterol metered-dose inhaler: Preliminary results of a cooperative study. Ann Allergy 1977; 39:418.
7. Paterson JW, Woolcock AJ, Shenfield GM. Bronchodilator drugs. Am Rev Respir Dis 1979; 120:1149–1188.
8. Miller WC, Rice DL. A comparison of oral terbutaline and fenoterol in asthma. Ann Allergy 1980; 44:15–18.
9. Anthonisen NR, Wright EC. The IPPB Trial Group: Response to inhaled bronchodilators in COPD. Chest 1987; 91:36S–39S.
10. Berger R, Smith D. Acute postbronchodilator changes in pulmonary function parameters in patients with chronic airways obstruction. Chest 1988; 93:541–546.
11. Guyatt GH, Townsend M, Pugsley SO, et al. Bronchodilators in chronic airflow limitation: Effects on airway function, exercise capacity, and quality of life. Am Rev Respir Dis 1987; 135:1969–1974.
12. Berger R, Smith D. Effects of inhaled metaproterenol and exercise performance in patients with stable "fixed" airway obstruction. Am Rev Respir Dis 1988; 138:624–629.
13. Shim C, Williams MH Jr. The adequacy of inhalation of aerosol from canister nebulizer. Am J Med 1980; 69:891–894.
14. Dolovich M, Ruffin RE, Roberts R, et al. Optimal delivery of aerosols from metered-dose inhalers. Chest 1981; 80(Suppl):911–915.
15. Sackner MA, Kim CS. Auxiliary MDI aerosol delivery systems. Chest 1985; 88(Suppl 2):161–170.
16. Tobin MJ, Jenouri G, Danta I, et al. Response to bronchodilator drug administration by a new reservoir aerosol delivery system and a review of other auxiliary delivery systems. Am Rev Respir Dis 1982; 126:670–675.
17. Turner JR, Corkery KJ, Echman D, et al. Equivalence of continuous flow nebulizer and metered dose inhaler with resevoir bag for treatment of acute air flow obstruction. Chest 1988; 93:476–481.
18. Jasper AC, Mohsenifar A, Kahan S, et al. Cost-benefit comparison of aerosol bronchodilator delivery methods in hospitalized patients. Chest 1986; 91:614–618.
19. Popa VT. Clinical pharmacology of adrenergic drugs. J Asthma 1984; 21:183–207.
20. Pany WH, Martorano F, Cotton EK. Management of life threatening asthma with intravenous isoproterenol infusions. Am J Dis Child 1976; 130:39–42.
21. Gross N. Role of ipratropium bromide in chronic obstructive pulmonary disease. Am Rev Respir Dis 1984; 129:856–870.
22. Johnson BE, Suratt PM, Gal TJ, et al. Effect of inhaled glycopyrrolate and atropine in asthma. Chest 1984; 85:325–328.
23. Altounyan REC. Variation of drug action on airway obstruction in man. Thorax 1964; 19:406–415.
24. Astin TW. Reversibility of airways obstruction in chronic bronchitis. Clin Sci 1972; 42:726–733.
25. Klock LE, Miller TD, Morris AH, et al. A comparative study of atropine sulfate and isoproterenol hydrochloride in chronic bronchitis. Am Rev Respir Dis 1975; 112:371–376.
26. Barber PV, Chatterjee SS, Scott R. A comparison of ipratropium bromide, deptropine citrate and placebo in asthma and chronic bronchitis. Br J Dis Chest 1977; 71:101–104.
27. Marini JJ, Lakshminarayan S. The effect of atropine inhalation in "irreversible" chronic bronchitis. Chest 1980; 77:591–596.
28. Passamonte PM, Martinez AJ. Effect of inhaled atropine or metaproterenol in patients with chronic airway obstruction and therapeutic serum theophylline levels. Chest 1984; 85:610–615.
29. Hughes JA, Tobin MJ, Bellamy D, Hutchinson DCS. Effects of ipratropium bromide and fenoterol aerosols in pulmonary emphysema. Thorax 1982; 37:667–670.
30. Taskin DP, Ashutosh K, Bleecker ER, et al. Comparison of the anticholinergic bronchodilator ipratropium bromide with metaproterenol in chronic obstructive pulmonary disease: A 90-day multi-center study. Am J Med 1986; 81(Suppl 5A):81–90.
31. Minette A. The effects of long-term treatment with SCH 1000 MDI. Postgrad Med J 1975; 51(Suppl):153–154.
32. Ajewski Z, Popiak B. The relation between permanent administration of atrovent and the dose of steroids in chronic bronchitis (abstract). Scand J Respir Dis 1979; 103(Suppl):205.
33. Jilg J. Long-term treatment with SCH 1000 MDI in out-patients with chronic bronchitis (abstract). Postgrad Med J 1975; 51(Suppl):7–13.
34. Lightbody IM, Ingram CG, Legge JS, Johnston RN. Ipratropium bromide, salbutamol and prednisolone in bronchial asthma and chronic bronchitis. Br J Dis Chest 1978; 72:181–186.
35. Wilson RHL, Battaglia PJ, Wilson NL. Crossover study with nebulized bronchodilators and atropine. Chest 1978; 73(Suppl):998–1000.
36. Petrie GR, Palmer KNV. Comparison of aerosol ipratropium bromide and salbutamol in chronic bronchitis and asthma. BMJ 1975; 1:430–432.
37. Douglas NJ, Davidson I, Sudlow MF, Flenley DC. Bronchodilation and the site of airway resistance in severe chronic bronchitis. Thorax 1979; 34:51–56.
38. Rebuck AS, Chapman KR, Abboud P. Nebulized anticholinergic and sympathomimetic treatment of asthma and chronic airway disease in the emergency room. Am J Med 1987; 82:59–64.
39. Aubier M, DeTroyer A, Sampson M, et al. Aminophylline improves diaphragmatic contractility. N Engl J Med 1981; 305:249–252.
40. Persson CGA. Some pharmacological aspects of xanthines in asthma. Eur J Respir Dis 1980; 61(Suppl):7–16.
41. Polson JB, Krzanowski JJ, Goldman AL, et al. Inhibition of human pulmonary phosphodiesterase activity by therapeutic levels of theophylline. Clin Exp Pharmacol Physiol 1978; 5:536–539.
42. Fredholm BB. Theophylline actions of adenosine receptors. Eur J Respir Dis 1980; 109(Suppl):29–36.

43. Mitenko PA, Ogilvie RE. Rational intravenous dose of theophylline. N Engl J Med 1973; 289:600–603.
44. Chang KC, Lauer BA, Bell TD, Chai H. Altered theophylline pharmacokinetics during acute respiratory viral illness. Lancet 1978; 1:1132–1133.
45. Renton KW, Gray JD, Hall RI. Decreased elimination of theophylline after influenza vaccination. Can Med Assoc J 1980; 123:288–290.
46. Reed CE, Li JTC. Nocturnal asthma: Approach to the patient. Am J Med 1988; 85(Suppl):14–16.
47. Rice KL, Leatherman JW, Duane PG, et al. Aminophylline for acute exacerbations of chronic obstructive pulmonary disease: A controlled trial. Ann Intern Med 1987; 107:305–309.
48. Levine JH, Michael JR, Guarnieri T. Multifocal atrial tachycardia: a toxic effect of theophylline. Lancet 1985; 1:12–14.
49. Eaton ML, Green BA, Church TR, et al. Efficacy of theophylline in "irreversible" airflow obstruction. Ann Intern Med 1980; 92:758–761.
50. Eaton ML, McDonald FM, Church TR, et al. Effects of theophylline on breathlessness and exercise tolerance in patients with chronic airflow obstruction. Chest 1982; 82:538–542.
51. Mahler D, Matthay RA, Synder PE, et al. Sustained-release theophylline reduces dyspnea in nonreversible obstructive airway disease. Am Rev Respir Dis 1985; 131:22–25.
52. Murciano P, Audair MH, Pariente R, Aubier M. A randomized, controlled trial of theophylline in patients with severe chronic obstructive pulmonary disease. N Engl J Med 1989; 320:1521–1525.
53. Dull WL, Alexander MR, Sadoul P, Woolson RF. The efficacy of isoproterenol inhalation for predicting the response to orally administered theophylline in chronic obstructive pulmonary disease. Am Rev Respir Dis 1982; 126:656–659.
54. Pauwell R. Mode of action of corticosteroids in asthma and rhinitis. Clin Allergy 1986; 16:281–288.
55. Blackwell GJ, Carnuccio R, Rosa M, et al. Macrocortin: A polypeptide causing the anti-phospholipase effect of corticosteroids. Nature 1980; 287:147–149.
56. Townley RG, Reeb R, Fitzgibbons T, et al. The effect of corticosteroids on the beta-adrenergic receptors in bronchial smooth muscle. J Allergy 1970; 45:118–121.
57. Bork J, Goldschmidt T, Smedegard G, et al. Methylprednisolone acts at the endothelial cell level reducing inflammatory responses. Acta Physiol Scand 1985; 123:221–224.
58. Easton JG. Effect of an inhaled corticosteroid on methacholine airway reactivity. J Allergy Clin Immunol 1981; 67:388–390.
59. Ryan G, Latimer KM, Juniper EF, et al. Effect of beclomethasone dipropionate on bronchial responsiveness to histamine in controlled nonsteroid-dependent asthma. J Allergy Clin Immunol 1985; 75:25–30.
60. Powell LW, Axelsen E. Corticosteroids in liver disease: Studies on the biological conversion of prednisone to prednisolone and plasma protein binding. Gut 1972; 13:690–696.
61. Davies G, Thomas P, Broder I, et al. Steroid-dependent asthma treated with inhaled beclomethasone dipropionate: A long-term study. Ann Intern Med 1977; 86:549–553.
62. Albert RK, Martin TR, Lewis SW. Controlled clinical trial of methylprednisolone in patients with chronic bronchitis and acute respiratory insufficiency. Ann Intern Med 1980; 92:753–758.
63. Emerman CL, Connors AF, Lukens TW, et al. A randomized control trial of methylprednisolone in the emergency treatment of acute exacerbations of COPD. Chest 1989; 95:563–567.
64. Mendella LA, Manfreda J, Warren CPW, Anthonisen NR. Steroid response in stable chronic obstructive pulmonary disease. Ann Intern Med 1982; 96:17–21.
65. Harding SM, Freedman S. A comparison of oral and inhaled steroids in patients with chronic airways obstruction: Features determining response. Thorax 1978; 33:214–218.
66. Shim C, Stover DE, Williams MH Jr. Response to corticosteroids in chronic bronchitis. J Allergy Clin Immunol 1978; 62:363–367.
67. Stokes TC, Shaylor JM, O'Reilly JF, Harrison BDW. Assessment of steroid responsiveness in patients with chronic airflow obstruction. Lancet 1982; 2:345–348.
68. Strain DS, Kinasewitz GT, Franco DP, George RB. Effect of steroid therapy on exercise performance in patients with irreversible chronic obstructive pulmonary disease. Chest 1986; 88:718–721.
69. Office Visits to Internists: The National Ambulatory Medical Care Survey. United States, 1975. Hyattsville, MD: National Center for Health Statistics, Vital and Health Statistics; 1978. US Department of Health, Education, and Welfare publication (PHS) 79-1787, pp 4–29.
70. Irwin RS, Curley FJ, French CL. Chronic cough: The spectrum and frequency of causes, key components of the diagnostic evaluation, and outcome of specific therapy. Am Rev Respir Dis 1990; 141:640–647.
71. Irwin RS, Curley FJ: The treatment of cough. A comprehensive review. Chest 1991; 99:1477–1484.
72. Chafouri MA, Patil KD, Kass I. Sputum changes associated with the use of ipratropium bromide. Chest 1987; 86:387–393.
73. Petty TL. The National Mucolytic Study: Results of a randomized double-blind, placebo-controlled study of iodinated glycerol in chronic obstructive bronchitis. Chest 1990; 97:75–83.
74. Jager EGH. Double-blind, placebo-controlled clinical evaluation of Guaimesol in outpatients. Clin Ther 1989; 11:341–362.
75. Clark SW, Lopez-Vidriero MT, Pavia D, Thomson ML. The effect of sodium 2-mercaptoethane sulphonate and hypertonic saline aerosols on bronchial clearance in chronic bronchitis. Br J Clin Pharmacol 1979; 7:39–44.
76. Lambert HF, Stern H. Infective factors in exacerbations of bronchitis and asthma. BMJ 1972; 3:323–327.
77. Tager I, Speizer FE. Role of infection in chronic bronchitis. N Engl J Med 1975; 292:563–571.
78. Gump DW, Phillips CA, Forsyth BR, et al. Role of infection in chronic bronchitis. Am Rev Respir Dis 1976; 113:465–474.
79. Bates JH. The role of infection during exacerbations of chronic bronchitis. Ann Intern Med 1982; 97:130–131.
80. Nicotra MB, Rivera M, Awe RI. Antibiotic therapy of acute exacerbations of chronic bronchitis. Ann Intern Med 1982; 97:18–21.
81. Anthonisen NR, Manfreda J, Warren MD, et al. Antibiotic therapy in exacerbations of chronic obstructive pulmonary disease. Ann Intern Med 1978; 106:196–204.
82. Penn RL, George RB. Antibiotics in COPD: If chronic disease becomes acute. J Respir Dis 1986; 7:13–16.
83. Irwin RS, Corao WM, Erikson AD, et al. Characterization by transtracheal aspiration of the tracheobronchial microflora during acute exacerbations of chronic bronchitis (abstract). Am Rev Respir Dis 1980; 121:150.
84. Brown RB. Managing exacerbations of chronic bronchitis. J Respir Dis 1990; 11:353–364.
85. Pachow J, Prados MD, Capote F, et al. Severe community-acquired pneumonia. Etiology, prognosis and treatment. Am Rev Respir Dis 1990; 142:369–373.
86. Thorsteinsson SB, Musher DM, Fagan T. The diagnostic value of sputum culture in acute pneumonia. JAMA 1975; 233:894–895.
87. Simberkoff MS, Cross AP, Al-Ibram M, et al. Efficacy of pneumococcal vaccine in high-risk patients: Results of a Veterans Administration cooperative study. N Engl J Med 1987; 315:1318–1327.
88. Recommendations of the Immunization Practices Advisory Committee: Update: Pneumococcal polysaccharide vaccine usage, United States. MMWR 1984; 33:273–281.
89. MacLeod CM, Hodges RG, Heidelberger M. Prevention of pneumococcal pneumonia by immunization with specific capsular polysaccharides. J Exp Med 1945; 82:445–465.
90. Peltola H, Käyhty H, Virtanen M, Mäkelä PH. Prevention of Hemophilus influenzae type b bacteremic infections with the capsular polysaccharide vaccine. N Engl J Med 1984; 310:1561–1566.
91. Anderson P, Pichishero ME, Insel RA. Immunization of 2-month-old infants with protein-coupled oligosaccharides derived from the capsule of Hemophilus influenzae type b. J Pediatr 1985; 107:346–351.
92. Gilleland HE Jr, Gilleland LB, Matthews-Greer JM. Outer membrane protein F preparation of Pseudomonas aeruginosa as a vaccine against chronic pulmonary infection with heterologous immunotype strains in a rat model. Infect Immun 1988; 56:1017–1022.

93. Woods DE, Bryan LE. Studies on the ability of alginate to act as a protective immunogen against infection with *Pseudomonas aeruginosa* in animals. J Infect Dis 1985; 151:581–588.
94. Van Voris LP, Betts RF, Hayden FG, et al. Successful treatment of naturally occurring influenza A/USSR/77 H1N1. JAMA 1981; 245:1128–1131.
95. Aubier M. Pharmacotherapy of respiratory muscles. Clin Chest Med 1988; 9:311–324.
96. Anderson WMcD, Zavecz JH, Levine SN. Sarcoplasmic reticulum and diaphragmatic fatigue. J Appl Physiol (in press).
97. Kuci JH, Sieck GC. Chronic aminophylline administration: Effect on diaphragm contractility and fatigue resistance in vitro. Am Rev Respir Dis 1991; 144:121–125.
98. Moxham J. Aminophylline and the respiratory muscles: An alternative view. Clin Chest Med 1988; 9:325–336.
99. Murciano D, Pamela F, Mal H, et al. Effects of dopamine on diaphragmatic strength generation in patients with chronic obstructive pulmonary disease during acute respiratory failure. Am Rev Respir Dis 1988; 137:A319.
100. Vereen LE, Kinasewitz GT, George RB. Effect of aminophylline on exercise performance in patients with irreversible airway obstruction. Arch Intern Med 1986; 146:1349–1351.
101. Howell S, Roussos C. Isoproterenol and aminophylline improve contractility of fatigued canine diaphragm. Am Rev Respir Dis 1984; 129:118–124.
102. Howell S, Fitzgerald RS, Roussos C. Effects of aminophylline, isoproterenol, and neostigmine on hypercapnic depression of diaphragmatic contractility. Am Rev Respir Dis 1985; 132:241–247.
103. Aubier M, Viires N, Murciano D, et al. Effects and mechanisms of action of terbutaline on diaphragmatic contractility and fatigue. J Appl Physiol 1984; 56:922–929.
104. Zavecz JH. Fatigue of the guinea-pig diaphragm in vitro: Effect of terbutaline and caffeine. Res Comm Subst Abuse 1984; 5:303–312.
105. Javaheri S, Smith JT, Thomas JP, et al. Albuterol has no effect on diaphragmatic fatigue in humans. Am Rev Respir Dis 1988; 137:197–201.
106. Zavecz JH, Anderson W, Adams B. Effect of amiloride on diaphragmatic contractility: Evidence of a role for Na^+-Ca^{2+} exchange. J Appl Physiol 1991; 70:1309–1314.
107. Aubier M, Murciano D, Viires N, et al. Effects of digoxin on diaphragmatic strength generation in patients with chronic obstructive pulmonary disease during acute respiratory failure. Am Rev Respir Dis 1987; 135:544–548.
108. Moser KM, Luchsinger PC, Adamson JS, et al. Respiratory stimulation with intravenous doxapram in respiratory failure. N Engl J Med 1973; 288:427–431.
109. Haake RE, Saxon LA, Bander SJ, et al. Depressed central respiratory drive causing weaning failure: Its reversal with doxapram. Chest 1989; 95:695–697.
110. Cook W, Benich JJ, Wooten SA. Indices of severity of obstructive sleep apnea syndrome do not change during medroxyprogesterone acetate therapy. Chest 1989; 96:262–266.
111. Kimura H, Tatsumi K, Kunitomo F, et al. Progesterone therapy for sleep apnea syndrome evaluated by occlusion pressure responses to exogenous loading. Am Rev Respir Dis 1989; 139:1198–1206.
112. White DP, Zwillch DW, Pickett CK, et al. Central sleep apnea: Improvement with acetazolamide therapy. Arch Intern Med 1982; 142:1816–1819.
113. Dolly FR, Block AJ. Medroxyprogesterone acetate and COPD. Chest 1983; 84:394–398.
114. Garner SJ, Eldridge FL, Wagoner PG, et al. Buspirone, an anxiolytic drug that stimulates respiration. Am Rev Respir Dis 1989; 139:946–950.
115. Watanabe S, Kanner RE, Cutillo AG, et al. Long-term effect of almitrine bismesylate in patients with hypoxic chronic obstructive pulmonary disease. Am Rev Respir Dis 1989; 140:1269–1273.
116. Herve P, Musset D, Simonneau G, et al. Almitrine decreases the distensibility of the large pulmonary arteries in man. Chest 1989; 96:572–577.
117. Aldrich TK, Prezant DJ. Adverse effects of drugs on the respiratory muscles. Clin Chest Med 1990; 11:177–189.
118. Urbano-Marquez A, Estruch R, Navarro-Lopez F, et al. The effects of alcoholism on skeletal and cardiac muscle. N Engl J Med 1989; 320:409–415.
119. Sokoll MD, Ferfis SD. Antibiotics and neuromuscular function. Anesthesiology 1981; 55:148–159.
120. Ferguson GT, Irvin CG, Cherniack RM. Effect of corticosteroids on respiratory muscle histopathology. Am Rev Respir Dis 1990; 142:1047–1052.
121. Dolce JJ, Crisp C, Monzella B, et al. Medication adherence patterns in chronic obstructive pulmonary disease. Chest 1991; 99:837–841.
122. Guidry GG, George RB. Compliance with drug therapy. In: ACCP Pulmonary and Critical Care Update. Vol 6. Lesson 1. 1990; pp 1–5.
123. George RB, Manocha K, Burford, JG, et al. Effects of labetalol in hypertensive patients with chronic obstructive pulmonary disease. Chest 1983; 83:457–460.
124. Coulter DM, Edwards IR. Cough associated with captopril and enalapril. BMJ 1987; 294:1521–1523.
125. George RB. Management of hypertension in patients with obstructive airway disease. Chest 1985; 88(Suppl):190–193.
126. The health consequences of involuntary smoking: A report of the Surgeon General. Rockville, MD: Office on Smoking and Health; 1986. US Department of Health and Human Services publication 87-8398.

Chapter 14

Controlled Breathing Techniques and Chest Physical Therapy in Chronic Obstructive Pulmonary Disease and Allied Conditions

L. JACK FALING, M.D.

Controlled breathing techniques (breathing training) and chest physical therapy are two major components of the multidisciplinary approach to the rehabilitation of patients with chronic obstructive pulmonary disease (COPD) and the related disorders of bronchiectasis, cystic fibrosis, and chronic asthma. Although only smoking cessation and long-term oxygen therapy are known to prolong life in patients with COPD, it is likely that chest physical therapy, especially postural drainage, does the same for persons with cystic fibrosis and widespread bronchiectasis. Although it does not prolong life, breathing training does help to restore patients to their highest possible functional capacity and to improve their quality of life.

The first part of this chapter addresses the controlled breathing techniques of pursed-lip breathing (PLB), the bending forward posture, and diaphragmatic breathing exercises. These techniques are employed to diminish dyspnea and increase the efficiency of the respiratory muscles. The second part describes the chest physical therapy modalities that enhance the clearance of airway secretions; these modalities include postural drainage, chest percussion, vibration, directed cough, and the forced expiratory technique. With few exceptions, these methods have remained largely unchanged since they were first described in the late 1800s and the first half of the 20th century. However, new investigational methodologies, such as modern respiratory mechanics, electrophysiologic muscle testing, and lung radioaerosol clearance studies, now provide an improved understanding as to how these modalities work, what physical therapy techniques are most beneficial to patients, and what types of lung disease can be treated with their use.

It must be emphasized that most patients require detailed and repeated instruction in most breathing exercises and chest physical therapy modalities before they are able to carry out these techniques routinely. Such instruction is best performed by experts in these methods, such as pulmonary nurse specialists and respiratory and physical therapists. The core of an instruction program should be conducted in an ambulatory outpatient setting, although inpatient hospital instruction is frequently provided at the outset for acutely ill, more severely debilitated patients. Involvement of other family members is strongly encouraged and is often essential to perform techniques such as chest percussion. Each patient should be evaluated separately and prescribed only those treatment modalities that are likely to be of benefit. For example, it makes no sense to prescribe postural drainage and chest percussion if a patient does not hypersecrete mucus. In addition, patients may need to temporarily alter their physical modality regimen during an acute exacerbation of their lung disease. The benefits of these programs are not usually apparent from the results of pulmonary function testing and are judged mainly by the presence of reduced dyspnea, increased exercise tolerance, and diminished anxiety and panic attacks.

CONTROLLED BREATHING TECHNIQUES (BREATHING TRAINING)

Controlled breathing techniques (or breathing training) were first promoted in the United States over 30 years ago by Alvan Barach and William F. Miller, who recognized that chronic obstructive lung disease patients could lessen their dyspnea by consciously altering their breathing patterns.[1,2] These physicians described and employed the three major breathing training techniques that are used today: PLB, the bending forward posture, and controlled abdominal breathing. However, we are only now beginning to understand how these breathing techniques relieve dyspnea and improve respiratory function. These methods are employed primarily in the long-term management of ambulatory patients with severe chronic obstructive lung disorders, although they might also prove helpful to such patients during acute exacerbations of their disease. Although most of these patients have conventional COPD with emphysema and chronic bronchitis, the controlled breathing techniques can also benefit patients with other disorders of airway obstruction, such as cystic fibrosis, bronchiectasis, and chronic asthma.

The goals of controlled breathing techniques are (1) to restore the diaphragm to a more normal position and function, (2) to decrease the respiratory rate by employing a breathing pattern that diminishes air trapping and improves the respiratory duty cycle, (3) to diminish the work of breathing, and (4) to reduce dyspnea and allay patient anxiety.

Pursed-Lip Breathing

PLB is usually the easiest breathing technique for patients with chronic airflow obstruction to learn and is often used instinctively by those who find it helpful. Patients inhale through their nose for several seconds with their mouths closed; they then exhale slowly for 4 to 6 seconds through pursed lips held in a whistling or kissing position. This is done with or without contraction of their abdominal muscles during exhalation. During PLB, no expiratory airflow occurs through the nose because of the involuntary elevation of the soft palate, which totally occludes the entrance to the nasopharynx.[3] PLB should be utilized during and following exercise and with any activity that causes a patient to experience tachypnea leading to progressive air trapping. Barach, who had pulmonary emphysema and employed PLB himself, noted that dyspnea was relieved almost immediately after PLB was begun.[4]

Although a number of studies have investigated the physiologic responses to PLB, we cannot yet fully explain why some patients intuitively employ this breathing technique or why it may lessen dyspnea. Thoman and coworkers,[5] Mueller and associates,[6] and Roa and colleagues[7] all observed that an important response to PLB is a substantial increase in tidal volume (V_T) along with a reduced respiratory rate and minute ventilation (V_E). Mueller and associates noted that the COPD patients who experienced the greatest relief of dyspnea following PLB demonstrated the largest increases in V_T as well as the most marked decreases in respiratory rate.[6] This benefit was noted when patients exercised and when they were at rest. It is possible that dyspnea is lessened with PLB because patients shift their breathing pattern from a rapid respiratory rate, which is under involuntary brain stem respiratory center control, to a slower, more controlled pattern that is governed by voluntary cortical function.

Both Thoman and coworkers[5] and Mueller and associates[6] showed that PLB during rest reduced $PaCO_2$; Mueller and associates also showed that this technique significantly improved PaO_2 in their resting patients. More recently, Tiep and coworkers showed that PLB significantly improved arterial oxygen saturation (SaO_2) measured by ear oximetry in 12 stable resting COPD patients compared with when PLB was not used by these patients.[8] Only Mueller and associates evaluated arterial blood gases in their COPD patients who used PLB during exercise, and they noted no change in these parameters.[6]

It is also important that both Thoman and coworkers[5] and Ingram and Schilder[9] showed that functional residual capacity decreases insignificantly following PLB. This failure to diminish end-expiratory lung volume makes it unlikely that improved dyspnea with PLB is the result of restoring the diaphragm to a more cranial position within the thorax, where it would be stationed on a more advantageous portion of its length-tension curve.

Another recognized benefit of PLB, and an alternative explanation for why PLB relieves dyspnea, is this technique's capacity to increase expiratory airway pressure, thus inhibiting dynamic expiratory airway collapse. Dynamic compression of airways with airway collapse during exhalation often occurs in COPD patients during exercise as well as at rest because the loss of lung elastic recoil forces (as occurs in emphysema) and diffuse airways narrowing require these patients to actively employ their expiratory muscles. The positive pleural pressure generated by a forced exhalation is transmitted to the intrathoracic airways, which are more collapsible in COPD patients than in normal persons; this causes premature airway closure and expiratory flow limitation. Ingram and Schilder demonstrated the benefit of PLB on lung mechanics in a subgroup of COPD patients employing an apparatus that included a rubber stopper with a small 4-mm orifice to mimic the pursed-lip technique.[9] Inspiratory and expiratory nonelastic airway resistance was measured with the stopper in place or not in place in 15 older men with COPD. The eight men who experienced spontaneous relief of dyspnea when they employed self-generated PLB were found to have a significantly greater diminution in nonelastic (airway) expiratory resistance when they used the artificial stopper system than did the seven patients who claimed no benefit from true PLB. Because these eight men also had substantially greater differences between their nonobstructive expiratory resistance (stopper not in place) and inspiratory resistance, Ingram and Schilder concluded that these eight patients had collapsible large airways, but that PLB considerably lessened their dynamic airways collapse and the expected increase in expiratory airways resistance. PLB achieved this by shifting a large portion of the expiratory pressure drop from the airways to the airway opening.

Somewhat surprisingly, no group of investigators has shown that PLB diminishes the work of breathing, as might be expected in view of the lessened dyspnea that PLB often produces. This was the case in the study by Mueller and associates, who found that PLB failed to decrease patient oxygen consumption ($\dot{V}_{O_2}$), even though the patients in the study reduced their $\dot{V}_E$.[6] They concluded that the expected decrease in respiratory muscle oxygen consumption caused by a decreased $\dot{V}_E$ must have been offset by an increased amount of work performed per breath that was a result of the greater V_T exhibited by all their patients as well as by the added expiratory resistance produced by the pursed lips. Similarly, Ingram and Schilder calculated that PLB incorporating the artificial PLB system actually increased total respiratory work in their patients because of the need for greater pressure during exhalation to generate flow and volume changes.[9] More recently, Roa and coworkers also showed that PLB substantially increased the inspiratory work of breathing in 12 patients with chronic airways obstruction.[7] Although Tiep and coworkers did not objectively measure work of breathing, they observed that COPD patients who employed properly taught but imposed PLB appeared to work harder and did not assume PLB naturally or for more than brief periods.[8]

In a recent abstract, Roa and coworkers examined the specific effects of PLB on respiratory muscle function for the first time.[7] They studied the effects of PLB on ventilatory muscle recruitment by continuously measuring pleural, gastric, and transdiaphragmatic pressures (Ppl, Pg, and Pdi, respectively) using transnasally placed esophageal and gastric balloons. In resting COPD patients, PLB clearly shifted a major portion of the inspiratory work of breathing from the diaphragm to the rib cage muscles. This was manifested by a decrease in positive Pg and by a more negative Ppl during inspiration while PLB was employed during exhalation. This is illustrated in Figure 14–1, which shows the Pg–Ppl plots before and during PLB in their 12 patients. The more positive Δ Pg/Δ Ppl slope suggests that active recruitment of the accessory rib cage muscles has taken place and that the diaphragm may be resting during PLB. It is possible that a temporary reduction in diaphragmatic (but not overall respiratory muscle) work during PLB may help explain the reduction in dyspnea experienced by many COPD patients who employ this technique.

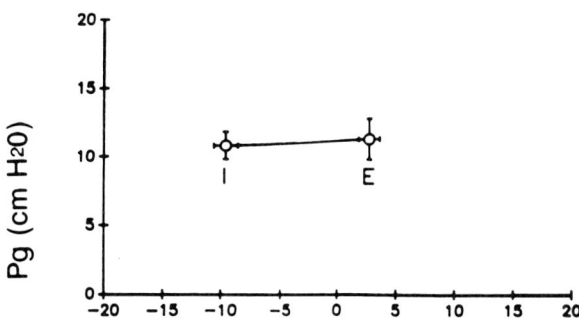

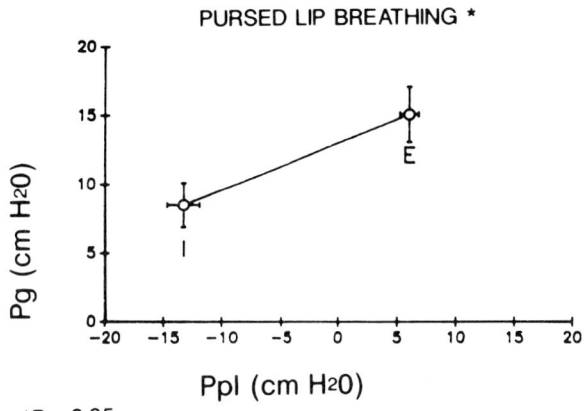

*P <0.05

FIGURE 14–1. The plot of gastric (Pg) and pleural (Ppl) pressures during inspiration (I) and expiration (E) in 12 COPD patients during normal tidal breathing *(upper panel)* and during pursed-lip breathing (PLB, *lower panel*). During PLB, gastric pressures are less positive and pleural pressures are more negative during inspiration (I) than with tidal breathing. The more positive Δ Pg/Δ Ppl slope during PLB suggests that active recruitment of accessory rib cage muscles has occurred and that the diaphragm may be resting. Data are expressed as mean ± SD, and P signifies difference in slope between tidal breathing and PLB. (From Roa J, Epstein S, Breslin E, et al. Work of breathing and ventilatory muscle recruitment during pursed lip breathing in patients with chronic airway obstruction. Am Rev Respir Dis 1991; 143:A77.)

Head Down and Bending Forward Postures

The supine position and, to an even greater extent, the head down (Trendelenburg) and leaning forward postures frequently relieve dyspnea in COPD patients. These techniques have often been used alone but may be combined with abdominal breathing exercises and PLB to manage dyspnea. Over 30 years ago, Barach and Beck observed that the head down position appeared to alleviate dyspnea by reducing respiratory effort and that it was accompanied by a prompt decline in accessory respiratory muscle use.[10] They postulated that elevating a depressed, flattened diaphragm through the upward cranial shift of the abdominal contents improved its contractile performance. Fluoroscopy has confirmed that these positional changes displace the diaphragm toward the head, and shifts greater than 3 cm have been observed in COPD patients.[11] However, these positions have produced less dramatic changes in total diaphragmatic excursions. Barach and Beck recorded only about a 2-cm increase in diaphragmatic excursion during quiet respiration in COPD subjects with their heads tilted downward by 12 to 18 degrees,[10] whereas Gayrard and associates, who also employed the head down position with or without abdominal weights in similar patients, observed only negligible improvement in diaphragmatic excursions during tidal breathing or during the performance of forced respiratory maneuvers compared with the improvement they noted in excursions when patients were in the supine position.[11]

The head down position, used infrequently today, is accomplished using a slant board (identical to that employed for postural drainage) or an equivalent aid, such as foot blocks, to elevate the foot of the bed or cot. Patients are most comfortable when placed in a 10- to 20-degree head down position. With the more commonly used leaning forward position, patients assume a posture in which the trunk is bent forward 20 to 45 degrees from the vertical axis. This posture can be assumed while the patient is seated or walking. In the seated position, patients can support themselves by bracing their elbows or hands on their knees or on a table. During walking, patients can be instructed or assisted in using this position by employing a walker or by using canes in both hands.

Improved mechanical efficiency of the diaphragm appears responsible for the relief of dyspnea and for the physiologic benefit seen with the head down and leaning forward positions. Other physiologic gains have been minimal, with the exception of a 20% reduction in $\dot{V}_E$ and stable arterial blood gas parameters noted in two studies that employed the head down position.[10, 12] In addition, bracing the arms while seated or walking in the leaning forward position may help to optimize the function of several of the accessory muscles of inspiration, such as the latissimus dorsi and the pectoralis major and minor.[13] In addition to insertion points on the rib cage, these muscles have an extrathoracic, shoulder girdle anchoring point. Such bracing, which fixes these muscles on their extrathoracic anchoring point, permits them to lengthen and exert a greater pulling force on the ribs.

Sharp and colleagues have identified the physiologic basis as to why these postures allow the diaphragm to function more effectively in some COPD patients and why they aid in reducing dyspnea.[14] They recognized that a subgroup of COPD patients with paradoxical (inward) inspiratory motion of their upper anterior abdominal wall (caused by the passive ascent of the diaphragm in the standing and upright seated positions) experienced major relief of their dyspnea while leaning forward. About one half of these patients also had relief of dyspnea while in the supine position. In many cases, simply observing a patient's breathing pattern made possible the detection of this inspiratory paradox. The patients in this subgroup had hyperinflated lungs with much greater total lung capacity, functional residual capacity, and residual volume; these factors resulted in the greater depression of their diaphragms in comparison with that of the COPD subjects without paradoxical abdominal motion and with no postural relief of dyspnea. Electromyographic recordings of respiratory muscle activity, Pdi, and magnetometrically determined thoracoabdominal diameters showed that the hyperinflated COPD subjects switched to a normal outward abdominal motion during inspiration when in the supine position or when leaning forward while seated. Their inspiratory Pdis were higher when they were in these positions as opposed to when they were standing or seated in an erect position; this is because their inspiratory Pg became more positive or less negative, indicating a partial return of diaphragmatic function. At the same time, the electromyographic activity of their sternocleidomastoid and scalene muscles significantly diminished, indicating that reduced work was being performed by the accessory inspiratory muscles. Those COPD patients with no decrease in their dyspnea during these postural changes failed to show these physiologic changes or demonstrated them to a lesser extent.

Druz and Sharp have further clarified the effects of various postures on respiratory muscle function in their studies of the electrical and mechanical activity of the diaphragm in eight normal persons and in six COPD patients with markedly hyperinflated lungs and low, flat diaphragms as indicated by their chest radiographs.[15] In contrast to the normal subjects, the four COPD subjects who experienced postural relief of dyspnea while in the supine or leaning forward positions experienced a substantial reduction in their ΔPdi (the inspiratory phasic change in transdiaphragmatic pressure) while they were standing or seated erect; this finding indicated reduced diaphragmatic function (Fig. 14–2). Like the normal subjects, the COPD patients displayed a marked increase in their ΔEdi, (the phasic inspiratory amplitude of their diaphragmatic electromyogram and an index of phrenic nerve activity) while in these positions. Therefore, the diminished mechanical output of their diaphragms in the standing and seated erect postures was not caused by reduced phrenic nerve activity but rather stemmed from a further unfavorable change in diaphragmatic configuration and muscle fiber length. However, when in the supine or leaning forward positions, these four COPD postural responders displayed both a substantial decrease in their Edi and an increase in their ΔPdi (see Fig. 14–2). Because of this, their neuromuscular efficiency index (ΔPdi/ΔEdi) increased significantly owing to improved diaphragmatic contraction together with reduced diaphragmatic excitation; in contrast, this index was reduced when they stood or were seated upright. The improved length-tension status of their diaphragms while in the supine or leaning forward postures permitted their diaphragms to generate greater pressure for a reduced neurogenic input; in other words, the improved status increased the diaphragm's efficiency in transducing electrical activity into pressure. These changes as well as the previously noted decline in accessory respiratory muscle activity probably account for the reduced dyspnea these patients experienced. For

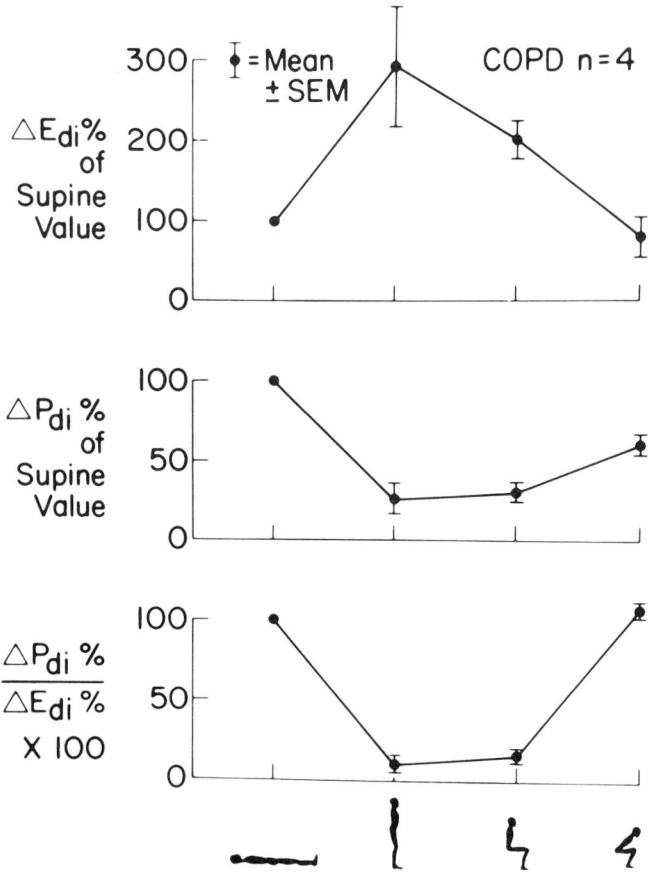

FIGURE 14-2. Data on four COPD patients in supine, standing, erect sitting, and forward leaning positions (Δ Edi: inspiratory phasic change in the moving average integral of the diaphragmatic electromyelogram; Δ Pdi: inspiratory phasic change in the transdiaphragmatic pressure). The ratio of Δ Pdi% to Δ Edi% is an index of the efficiency of the diaphragm. (From Druz WS, Sharp JT. Electrical and mechanical activity of the diaphragm accompanying body position in severe chronic obstructive pulmonary disease. Am Rev Respir Dis 1982; 125:275–280.)

paucity of data assessing its use. On the other hand, mechanically induced elevation of the diaphragm by abdominal strapping in severely hyperinflated COPD patients actually reduced exercise endurance during leg cycling.[17] This was the case even though abdominal strapping increased Pdi during exercise by 40%, and no evidence of inspiratory muscle fatigue was apparent just before exercise ended. Abdominal strapping must have created other unfavorable effects, such as the forcing of the inspiratory rib cage and accessory respiratory muscles to function over a less effective portion of their length-tension curves. Strapping also probably prevented rapid relaxation of the abdominal muscles at end-expiration; this impedes passive diaphragmatic descent during inspiration, which serves as an adjunct to diaphragmatic contraction in generating an adequate $\dot{V}_E$ during exercise.[17]

Diaphragmatic Breathing Exercises and Allied Maneuvers

Early investigators emphasized the importance of diaphragmatic breathing exercises in managing patients with obstructive lung disorders.[1] Possible benefits from such exercises include improved lung mechanics, increased ventilatory efficiency, and the more even distribution of inspired gas. Although some patients claim clinical improvement and reduced dyspnea with diaphragmatic breathing, physiologic studies have been inconclusive and conflicting as to its effectiveness. For this reason, prescription of this technique should be accompanied by close clinical monitoring to ascertain its efficacy. If patients fail to show clinical improvement (less dyspnea and increased exercise tolerance) after a reasonable trial of properly performed diaphragmatic breathing, this treatment should be discontinued. Diaphragmatic breathing training that attempts to enhance diaphragmatic function through improved positioning of the diaphragm is believed to differ from ventilatory muscle training, which uses isocapnic hyperventilation or inspiratory resistance breathing in the hope of improving respiratory muscle strength and endurance. However, it is likely that the benefits of these two basically different rehabilitation modalities overlap to some extent, and studies combining both of these techniques in a single training program remain to be performed.

Although all patients with chronic airways obstruction can be taught breathing exercises, these exercises are considered to be most helpful for patients with hyperinflated lungs and depressed diaphragms who have pulmonary emphysema as a major component of their lung disease. Inspecting a patient's breathing pattern and palpating his or her lower thorax and upper abdomen usually suffice to assess if he or she is using the respiratory muscles properly and effectively. Accessory neck muscle use, predominantly upper chest wall expansion along with inward movement of the lower ribs, and failure of the abdomen to expand on inspiration (or paradoxically move inward) all signify diaphragmatic

unclear reasons, the two COPD subjects who noted no postural relief of dyspnea experienced little improvement of their ΔPdi/ΔEdi when they were in the supine or bent forward positions because of an actual increase of their ΔEdi and only a slight increase in their ΔPdi. Further studies are needed to elucidate why diaphragmatic function failed to improve with the supine or leaning forward postures in this COPD subgroup, and similar studies remain to be performed in less severely compromised and less hyperinflated COPD patients.

Justification for employing the leaning forward position during exercise is supported by the recent findings of Delgado and coworkers that dyspnea was diminished and exercise tolerance was improved during walking in the leaning forward posture (at a 45-degree angle) in COPD patients who had developed paradoxical diaphragmatic motion during exercise in the upright position.[16] This improvement was accompanied by the return of normal chest wall–abdominal motion during breathing in one patient and by a shift to only partial inspiratory paradox in a second. However, such posturing during exercise requires further study because of the dysfunction. Patients with such features should benefit the most from diaphragmatic breathing instruction. This technique requires conscious patient effort and has never been documented to become an automatic function. Breathing training should be instructed by a specialist in the method. The technique is easily taught to most patients but can be difficult for those with the poorest diaphragm function. Specific instructions for diaphragmatic breathing are shown in Table 14–1. After mastering the technique, patients should practice these exercises for at least one-half hour two to three times per day, initially in the supine or head down position and while sitting, and later while standing or walking or during daily living activities. Diaphragmatic breathing is frequently combined with PLB and the leaning forward position to achieve maximum relief of dyspnea.

Table 14–2 presents the results of six studies that evaluated the effects of breathing exercises in patients with chronic airways obstruction.[2, 18–22] All patients received supervised breathing training, although the specific exercises differed somewhat among study groups. Patients exercised several times per day in most studies, although Miller's patients trained four to six times per day.[23] Clinical or physiologic re-evaluation (or both) was conducted from about 2 weeks to 1 year following the onset of the exercise program. Most programs lasted 1 to 3 months. Evaluation consisted of clinical assessment in one study,[18] physiologic testing in three studies,[2, 20, 22] and both clinical and physiologic evaluation in two studies.[19, 21] A wide range of physiologic parameters were analyzed.

Although the studies utilizing clinical evaluation showed substantial clinical benefit in most patients, only Miller's patients achieved statistically significant improvement of multiple pulmonary function indices.[2] They showed significant improvement in forced expiratory flow, lung volumes, ventilatory parameters, and arterial blood gas indices. The remaining investigators concluded that extended diaphragmatic breathing training failed to significantly improve pulmonary function in their patients.[19–22] Becklake and associates commented that "benefit claimed by the subject was more likely to be the result of his mental attitude than of true physical improvement."[19] It is difficult to explain why only Miller's patients achieved significant pulmonary function improvement, but this may stem from his more comprehensive training program and his requirement that patients "practice prodigiously" (at least 4–6 times per day).[23] In addition, breathing training was begun only after optimal improvement had been attained using intensive conventional methods including smoking cessation, secretion management, and bronchodilator administration. Although their overall results were disappointing, most of the other investigators noted that a few of their subjects improved considerably. Sinclair had five such patients,[21] McNeill and McKenzie had three,[20] and Becklake and associates had one.[19] It is apparent that some patients' pulmonary function is helped by breathing training, but at present we are unable to predict in advance which patients respond to this rehabilitation modality.

Only Miller and coworkers studied the long-term effects of breathing training on a number of physiologic parameters following exercise, but they limited exercise to 1 minute of one-step climbing.[2] In comparison with postexercise studies prior to training, they observed a significant rise in patients' arterial oxygen saturation and oxygen removal per liter of ventilation and a significant decline in their $Paco_2$, which indicated improved alveolar ventilation and alveolar gas exchange. Only patients with a maximum breathing capacity greater than 40% of that predicted (which indicates less severe disease) achieved a decrease in their exercise $\dot{V}_E$, demonstrating a reduced ventilatory requirement. However, all but one patient noted a reduced duration of dyspnea after exercise following training.

The early effects of diaphragmatic breathing training have been studied with respect to its influence on ventilatory parameters, the distribution of inspiratory gas, and chest wall mechanics. Campbell and Friend (Table 14–2) noted that the early benefits of diaphragmatic-type breathing included a major decrease in respiratory rate and in $\dot{V}_E$ as well as an increase in V_T and "a lowering of the end respiratory level" (reduced functional residual capacity).[22] Willeput and colleagues had similar findings.[24] The changes these investigators observed were the same as those seen when patients performed PLB. Several other groups have also noted reductions in respiratory rate and increases in V_T but no changes in $\dot{V}_E$ or functional residual capacity.[25, 26]

Theoretically, diaphragmatic breathing should create regional changes in the configuration of the chest wall and cause larger Ppl swings at the lung bases than at the apices. This change from a constant Ppl gradient

TABLE 14–1. TECHNIQUE OF DIAPHRAGMATIC BREATHING*

1. Diaphragmatic exercises should be preceded by the inhalation of a bronchodilator if a patient has reversible airway obstruction and by postural drainage or controlled cough, or both, if airway secretions are a major problem. Patients should use O_2 if they receive home O_2 therapy.
2. The patient lies supine or tilted 15 to 25 degrees in the head down position.
3. The patient places his or her dominant hand on the upper midabdomen and the nondominant hand on the upper anterior chest. This permits monitoring of an inspiratory outward motion of the abdomen while minimizing chest excursions. The patient relaxes the chest wall and accessory respiratory muscles.
4. The patient breathes more slowly and deeply, inspiring through the nose and expiring slowly with pursed lips. A conscious effort is made to employ only the diaphragm during inspiration and to maximize abdominal protrusion. The anterior abdominal wall muscles are consciously contracted during inspiration to facilitate diaphragmatic movement and to improve lower rib cage expansion.
5. The patient can employ abdominal wall muscle contraction during expiration to displace the diaphragm more cephalad. An 8- to 10-lb abdominal weight placed on or strapped to the lower abdomen can also be used to assist this activity.
6. Once they are mastered lying down, the same exercises should be repeated while sitting and later while standing in a forward leaning posture.

*From Faling LJ. Pulmonary rehabilitation: Physical modalities. Clin Chest Med 1986; 7:599–618.

TABLE 14-2. RESULTS OF STUDIES EVALUATING BREATHING EXERCISES IN PATIENTS WITH CHRONIC AIRWAYS OBSTRUCTION*

Reference	Patient Population	No. of Patients	Breathing Technique	Duration Technique Employed	Measurement(s) Performed	Improvement
Livingstone et al.[18] (1935)	Asthma	75	Emphasize lung expiration to elevate diaphragm for 10 min 2–3 times/day.†	1 yr	Clinical assessment	52/75 had excellent, very good, or much improved status.
Becklake et al.[19] (1954)	Emphysema with or without bronchitis or asthma	10	Prolong expiration, improve diaphragmatic movement, general relaxation 2 times/day.	Mean of 24 days (range 13–46 days)	Subjective improvement, VC, TLC, FRC, RV, MBC, and Sao_2	8/10 had moderate to marked subjective improvement. Only one patient showed improvement of multiple physiologic tests. Average per cent change of all tests considered insignificant.
Miller[2] (1954)	Obstructive bronchitis, asthmatic bronchitis, bronchiectasis	24	Diaphragmatic training as per Asthma Research Council† and Miller[2] 4–6 times/day.	From 6 wk to 2 mo	Maximum diaphragmatic excursion, RR, V_T, $\dot{V}_E$, FVC, FEV_3, MBC, IC, ERV, MEP, Sao_2, $Paco_2$, pHa, and Hct (all at rest)	Significant increases in maximum diaphragmatic excursion, V_T, IC, FVC, FEV_3, MBC, MEP, Sao_2, and pHa. Significant decreases in RR, $Paco_2$, and Hct.
McNeill et al.[20] (1955)	Asthma, bronchitis	33 (17 of whom completed exercises)	Asthma Research Council technique† 2 times/day.	1–3	EFR_{40}	Improvement in 11 patients, worsening in 6; mean improvement for group was 4% (not significant).
Sinclair[21] (1955)	Emphysema with or without asthma or bronchitis	22	‡Emphasize abdominal-diaphragmatic breathing. Taught on a daily or weekly basis.	Mean of 8.1 wk (3–14 wk)	Clinical assessment, maximum diaphragmatic excursion, VC, TLC, FRC, RV, MBC, $\dot{V}_E$, alveolar N_2%, and Sao_2 (all tests not performed in all subjects)	Slight increases in VC, MBC, $\dot{V}_E$, Sao_2, and maximum diaphragmatic excursion (no indicator significant for entire group). Slight decrease in RV, TLC, and alveolar N_2% (no indicator significant for entire group). Five patients had appreciable improvement of PFTs. Seven claimed marked clinical improvement. Seven claimed moderate improvement, and eight were unchanged.
Campbell et al.[22] (1955)	Emphysema	12	‡Emphasize abdominal-diaphragmatic breathing. Taught 3 times/wk for 4–6 weeks.	Acute effects after instruction, and long-term effects after 3 mo	*Acute effects:* V_T, RR, $\dot{V}_E$, He mixing efficiency, $\dot{V}O_2$, and slow space/FRC *Long-term effects:* Lung volumes, MBC, and He mixing efficiency	*Acute effects:* Increase in V_T, decrease in RR and $\dot{V}_E$. $\dot{V}O_2$, He mixing efficiency, and slow space/FRC were unchanged. *Long-term effects:* No change in lung volumes, He mixing efficiency, or MBC.

*From Faling LJ. Pulmonary rehabilitation: Physical modalities. Clin Chest Med 1986; 7:599–618.
†Asthma Research Council. Physical Exercises for Asthma. 8th ed. London: Asthma Research Council, 1949.
‡Reed JMW. In: Marshall G, Perry KMA (eds). Diseases of the Chest. 1st ed. London: Butterworth's, 1952.
Key: VC: vital capacity; TLC: total lung capacity; FRC: functional residual capacity; RV: residual volume; MBC: maximum breathing capacity; RR: respiratory rate; FVC: forced vital capacity; FEV_3: forced expiratory volume in 3 seconds; IC: inspiratory capacity; ERV: expiratory reserve volume; MEP: maximum expiratory pressure; pHa: arterial pH; Hct: hematocrit; EFR_{40}: forced expiratory flow at 0.25 seconds of a FVC × 40; alveolar N_2%: intrapulmonary gas-mixing efficiency expressed as alveolar nitrogen per cent after 7 min of O_2 breathing; He: helium; slow space/FRC: poorly ventilated space/functional residual capacity (in per cent and determined based on He breathing); PFTs: pulmonary function tests.

down the lung should preferentially deliver inhaled gas to the more compliant lung bases, thus improving ventilation/perfusion relationships. However, three studies of COPD patients that evaluated this possibility using nitrogen washout curves or inhaled or intravenous xenon 133 were unable to demonstrate any redistribution of ventilation in a comparison of diaphragmatic and conventional breathing.[25-27] This was the case even though Sackner and coworkers, employing strain gauges, recorded larger abdominal excursions during diaphragmatic breathing,[26] and Grimby and associates, using magnetometers, showed that the abdomen's contribution to ventilation increased from 40 to 67% when this breathing method is employed.[25]

Another possible benefit of diaphragmatic breathing in COPD patients is that it might improve the mechanical efficiency of breathing. This possibility was addressed by Sackner and coworkers[28] and Willeput and colleagues[24] by studying the effects of diaphragmatic breathing on thoracoabdominal motion in COPD subjects. Sackner and coworkers monitored the separate rib cage and abdominal movement of patients in the supine and upright positions by employing respiratory inductive plethysmography, whereas Willeput and colleagues assessed these movements in seated subjects using magnetometers. Both groups noted that diaphragmatic breathing resulted in increased asynchronous* and paradoxical† motion of the rib cage and abdomen. Willeput and colleagues found such changes limited to the rib cage, with paradoxical outward chest wall movement during exhalation in 9 of their 11 patients.[24] Sackner and coworkers calculated inspiratory and expiratory indices of asynchrony to quantitate discoordination between the rib cage and abdomen and observed that both were abnormally increased in COPD patients in the supine position during abdominal (diaphragmatic) breathing as compared with during their usual, natural breathing pattern. Paradoxical rib cage motion during inspiration and expiration was also increased, but it resolved when patients returned to an upright position.[28] Both Willeput and colleagues and Sackner and his coworkers concluded that these chest wall effects of diaphragmatic breathing would distort the rib cage and abdominal compartments away from their normal relaxation characteristics, thus increasing patients' work of breathing. For these reasons, diaphragmatic breathing is probably less mechanically efficient than natural breathing in COPD patients.

In conclusion, the long-term and short-term benefits of diaphragmatic breathing exercises remain unclear, and the occasional clinical benefit that has been noted might represent a placebo effect. Since only a few investigators have documented improved physiologic parameters using this technique, further investigation is needed to fully justify diaphragmatic breathing as an effective modality for managing COPD patients and to explain why some COPD patients show clinical benefit with its use.

CHEST PHYSICAL THERAPY

Normal and Abnormal Mucociliary Clearance in Chronic Obstructive Pulmonary Disease

Normal Respiratory Mucus and Mucus Clearance

The mucociliary system is responsible for normal airway mucus transport and consists of ciliated epithelial cells covered by a thin layer of mucus. This system protects the airway by trapping and eliminating a wide range of inhaled materials, including allergens, dusts, noxious gases, and microorganisms.

Abnormal Mucociliary Clearance and Cough in Chronic Obstructive Pulmonary Disease and Related Conditions

Many factors and conditions adversely affect mucociliary transport in COPD and cause the retention and stasis of airway secretions. These effects come about as a result of increases in the production of mucus, by alterations in its physical properties, impairment of ciliary function, the loss of ciliated epithelial cells, as well as various combinations of these disturbances. Disabling the mucociliary system causes airway mucus impaction and impaired gas exchange. Obstructive atelectasis, bronchopulmonary infection, and acute respiratory insufficiency often occur in this setting.

Goals of Chest Physical Therapy

The goal of chest physical therapy in COPD patients is to facilitate the removal of excess or retained airway secretions, thus reducing resistance to airflow and the work of breathing, improving pulmonary gas exchange, and decreasing the incidence of bronchial infection. In addition, atelectasis caused by mucus impaction within airways may be prevented; if it is already present, it may be corrected. Chest physical therapy is employed in hospitalized COPD patients experiencing acute exacerbations of their disease as well as postoperatively to reduce respiratory complications. In ambulatory patients with airways obstruction, it is prescribed mainly for patients with chronic bronchitis who produce large amounts of mucus and for patients with cystic fibrosis and bronchiectasis.

Techniques of chest physical therapy include postural drainage, chest percussion, vibration, directed cough, and the forced expiratory technique. In many instances, conclusions regarding the possible benefits of these methods in COPD patients with chronic bronchitis and emphysema were derived from observations made in patients with cystic fibrosis and bronchiectasis. Although such comparison is justified for COPD patients who are mucus hypersecretors, the overall advantages of chest

---

*A difference in the rate of change of rib cage and abdominal compartmental excursions during tidal breathing.
†Opposite movement of one compartment (rib cage or abdomen) during tidal breathing.

physical therapy in COPD are less conclusive than the long-acknowledged value of these therapeutic approaches in cystic fibrosis and bronchiectasis.

Definition of Techniques

Postural drainage employs gravity to help drain mucus from the airways of individual lung lobes and segments. The Trendelenburg posture with varying degrees of rotation is usually employed with an angle of drainage between 10 and 45 degrees (except when the upper lobes are drained, which is accomplished when the patients are upright or lying flat). Although large drainage angles are frequently poorly tolerated by many persons with severe airways obstruction, COPD patients were recently found to have negligible alterations in lung volumes and no decrease in arterial oxygen saturation when they were studied in the head down position up to a 25-degree head down tilt.[29] In patients who have predominantly unilateral lung disease, positioning the "good" lung in the downward position usually improves arterial blood oxygenation, but care must be taken to ensure that drainage from the uppermost part of the diseased lung does not spill into and compromise the dependent "good" lung.

Patients can create various postural drainage positions by employing a tilt board (such as an ironing board) or by tilting a bed or cot. Patients can also use pillows on a bed or a couch or on the floor to create more comfortable postural drainage positions and angles. An inhaled bronchodilator can be used 10 to 20 minutes prior to postural drainage to facilitate secretion movement. Generous daily fluid intake (1–2 L) seems advisable based on findings of the adverse effects of dehydration on tracheal clearance in dogs and of its reversal by rehydration.[30] However, the benefits of vigorous hydration in humans on the viscoelastic properties of airway mucus and on the ease of sputum expectoration are less certain, and no improvement in sputum production has been observed in patients with chronic bronchitis.[31] Also, inhaled moisture from a nebulizer or humidifier is mainly beneficial to patients with a tracheostomy who have lost the "air-conditioning" function of the upper respiratory tract. Postural drainage should be carried out two to three times per day, with each complete treatment lasting 30 to 45 minutes. Each postural drainage position may be sustained for 5 to 10 minutes or longer if secretion clearance remains incomplete. Because of enhanced airway secretion retention during sleep, postural drainage is especially helpful after awakening in the morning and should be performed frequently during periods of increased sputum production. To avoid gastroesophageal reflux as well as nausea and emesis, it is prudent to delay head down drainage for 1 to 2 hours after meals; this may be of even greater importance for patients who are fed using a nasogastric tube, since such a tube encourages esophageal reflux by compromising lower esophageal sphincter function. Following a period of postural drainage, controlled cough or the forced expiratory technique is essential to clear bronchial secretions directed to the large airways by postural drainage.[32] Determination of the lung zones that require drainage is based on a knowledge of a patient's underlying lung disorder, on careful auscultation of the patient's thorax for rhonchi, wheezes, or diminished breath sounds due to mucus airway plugging, and on the examination of chest radiographs for signs of focal or diffuse disease. Ambulatory patients quickly learn to use the drainage positions that provide the greatest benefit.

Percussion, vibration, and shaking are frequently used during postural drainage to loosen airway secretions. Percussion is applied throughout the entire respiratory cycle by striking the thoracic cage with cupped hands or by employing a mechanical percussor. The technique is thought to transmit energy from the chest wall to the airways, thus loosening airway secretions from bronchial walls. Percussion is administered by trained personnel or family members and is delivered at a frequency of about 5 Hz for 1 to 5 minutes over the zone of the chest that is draining. However, the optimal force and duration of percussion are unknown, and percussion for periods longer than 5 minutes is justified if secretions are believed to persist in the percussed lung zone. A thin towel or other suitable wrap is draped over the percussed zone in patients with sensitive skin and should probably be routinely employed in older patients whose skin is fragile. Extreme caution is needed when treating patients with severe osteoporosis or other fragile bone disorder, and percussion should not be delivered to the spine, sternum, or soft tissues overlying the kidneys or other vital organs.

Vibration is administered by exerting a downward pressure over a draining zone at a frequency of 10 to 15 Hz employing hands crossed in a manner similar to that used in cardiopulmonary resuscitation. When applied manually, it is most beneficial during exhalation. Mechanical vibrators can also be used, but they should be continuously applied throughout the respiratory cycle at a frequency of about 13 Hz.[33] Chest shaking (at 2 Hz) has also been employed to help loosen airway secretions, but such low-frequency movements probably do not provide additional benefit.[33]

Cough—either voluntarily or as a reflex—can be an effective means to expel excess mucus from the larger airways. Following a rapid inspiration that exceeds normal V_T, transient glottic closure together with expiratory muscle contraction generate pleural and abdominal pressures between 50 and 100 mm Hg. The sudden release of such pressures creates high but transient air velocities; in normal persons, these velocities approach 200 to 250 m/sec in central airways, which are compressed and narrowed by the large extraluminal Ppl.[34] These high airflows generate large shear forces by coupling the expired air with the mucus adhering to airway walls; such shearing causes airway secretions to be expelled.

Although only large airways (up to the sixth or seventh generation of branching) are cleared by cough at high lung volumes, airway collapse extends upstream to smaller airways during cough at lower lung volumes; it is probable that cough under these circumstances also propels mucus from small bronchi to the larger, central bronchi.³² In a mechanical model of the trachea, the clearance of mucus simulants by artificial cough increased linearly with increasing mucus depth.³⁵ This supports the clinical observation that cough is an ineffective means for clearing mucus from the airways of both normal persons and of patients with lung disease who do not produce excess mucus³⁶; it is apparent that a critical depth of airway mucus is necessary before cough becomes helpful. Cough is most effective in the upright or seated positions, since higher cough pressures and flow rates can be generated in these positions as compared with other body positions.³⁷

Since the "cleansing" action of cough in large airways takes place mainly during the first one or two coughs of a cough sequence,³⁸ and because frequent uncontrolled cough may induce fatigue, chest wall pain, and dyspnea as well as worsen bronchospasm, controlled cough and the forced expiratory technique (huffing) have been advocated as preferred alternatives.³⁹ During controlled cough, patients are instructed to inspire deeply, hold their breath for several seconds, and then cough two or three times with their mouth open and without taking another breath. Patients can then take another slow deep inhalation, and then repeat the cough procedure. After undertaking this two or three times, patients should rest and breathe normally for several minutes before repeating their controlled coughing.

The forced expiratory technique (huffing) consists of one or two forced exhalations (but without glottic closure as in cough) starting at midlung volume and continuing to a low lung volume. This is followed by expectoration or a controlled cough at high lung volume to clear mucus from the central airways and then by a period of relaxed, preferably diaphragmatic breathing. The rationale for the forced expiratory technique is that it creates less fatigue, is less likely to provoke bronchospasm, and produces less dynamic airway collapse because transpulmonary pressures are reduced. The forced expiratory technique functions in part by creating two-phase air-liquid flow, that is, the simultaneous flow of gas and liquid in the airways.⁴⁰ With the forced expiratory technique, airflow rates may be high enough to permit airflow through airways totally plugged by mucus, thus propelling the mucus toward the mouth. Although most published reports on the forced expiratory technique relate to patients with cystic fibrosis and bronchiectasis, this approach should also prove beneficial for COPD patients with mucus hypersecretion.

Another adjunct to cough is positive expiratory pressure physiotherapy.⁴¹ Theoretically, this technique represents another method to limit dynamic expiratory airway closure while also increasing lung volume and directing air distal to and behind airway secretions so that these secretions can be more easily expelled. Positive expiratory pressure is performed while the patient is seated and can be carried out in the home setting without assistance. The positive expiratory pressure apparatus consists of either a face mask or a mouthpiece (including a nose clip) with a one-way valve to which variable expiratory resistance is applied.⁴¹ The system and a pressure manometer to display actual positive expiratory pressure levels are commercially available. A resistance that provides a positive expiratory pressure level of 10 to 20 cm H_2O in midexhalation is selected. The technique is employed for 5 to 15 breaths and is followed by the forced expiratory technique and spontaneous cough as needed. The treatment protocol may be repeated over a 10 to 30 minute period.

Chest Physical Therapy in Specific Lung Disorders

Whereas the various components of chest physical therapy have been critically evaluated in bronchiectasis and cystic fibrosis and make possible a logical treatment approach, a similar assessment has not yet been carried out for all lung diseases for which chest physical therapy might provide benefit. In these conditions, chest physical therapy is described in general terms and includes postural drainage, percussion, and vibration, even though a clear understanding of which of these components of chest physiotherapy is most beneficial in a specific setting is lacking.

Chest Physical Therapy in Chronic Obstructive Pulmonary Disease Patients

Stable Disease

Chest physical therapy in stable COPD patients causes immediate increases in sputum expectoration. The greatest benefit is derived by patients who produce the largest daily sputum volumes. Four of five studies that recorded changes in sputum volume or weight[42–45] reported increased sputum production during or immediately following chest physical therapy; Mohsenifar and coworkers, however, noted no sputum increase (all but one patient expectorated less than 5 ml of sputum during chest physical therapy) in their 20 patients who had moderate daily sputum production (< 30 ml/24 h).[46] Similarly, chest physical therapy in stable COPD patients accelerates mucus clearance from central and, to a lesser extent, peripheral lung zones based on radiotracer studies,[42, 43] and it seems that both postural drainage and cough are needed to maximize this effect.[42, 43]

Chest physical therapy in stable COPD patients provides little benefit to short-term pulmonary function. Of five studies measuring pulmonary function changes,[44–48] only Feldman and associates[48] recorded significant improvement following a regimen of postural drainage, percussion, vibration, and cough; however, this benefit was limited to flows at low lung volume, indicating that there is some improvement of small airways function but none of forced expiratory volume in 1 second (FEV_1) and a transient reduction in peak expiratory flow rate (PEFR). The other studies found no significant change in a wide range of parameters, including those for arterial blood gases, spirometric indices (forced vital capacity and FEV_1) and flows at high (PEFR and forced expiratory flow between 200 and 1200 mL of forced vital capacity [$FEF_{200-1200}$]) and low ($FEF_{50\%}$, $FEF_{75\%}$, and $FEV_{25-75\%}$) lung volumes. This lack of improvement may reflect the poor correlation of airway function (especially large airway function) with the amount of expectorated sputum as well as a requirement for longer-term physiotherapy, since pulmonary function changes may lag substantially behind changes in sputum expectoration and bronchial clearance, perhaps because of difficulty or delay in the clearing of secretions in small airways.

Acute Disease

The value of chest physical therapy in acute COPD exacerbations is even more uncertain. In six studies,[49–54] chest physical therapy produced little if any improvement of the parameters that were monitored. The exacerbations were all of acute bronchitis with the exception of a few cases of pneumonia. Anthonisen and colleagues[50] as well as Newton and coworkers[53] compared the hospital courses of acutely ill COPD patients treated with conventional therapy alone (oxygen, antibiotics, bronchodilators, and diuretics) with that of patients who received conventional therapy and chest physical therapy (Newton and coworkers also employed intermittent positive-pressure breathing). Length of hospital stay[53] and temperature curves[50] were the same in both groups. There were also no significant differences in the course of arterial blood gas parameters,[50, 53] spirometric indices,[53] or daily sputum volumes,[50, 53] except for in a small subgroup of men with initial mild hypoxemia ($PaO_2 > 60$ mm Hg) who produced more sputum when therapy included chest physical therapy and intermittent positive-pressure breathing.[53] Both groups concluded that chest physical therapy failed to improve upon the conventional management of their patients.

Three studies have assessed the immediate impact of chest physical therapy on lung mechanics[51, 52] and arterial blood gas indices[52, 54] during an acute COPD exacerbation. Although Newton and Stephenson observed no improvement in vital capacity, FEV_1, specific conductance, or arterial blood gas parameters following a regimen of postural drainage, vibration, and chest percussion,[52] and Buscaglia and St. Marie recorded a stable oxygen saturation after vigorous chest physical therapy,[54] Campbell and colleagues actually noted a decline in FEV_1 in similarly treated patients.[51] This did not happen if chest percussion and vibration were omitted from the chest physical therapy regimen; this lead Newton and coworkers to speculate that this decline may have been due to bronchoconstriction triggered by these maneuvers.

Is chest physical therapy ever beneficial in COPD patients with an acute bronchitic exacerbation? This remains uncertain, but patients producing large quantities of sputum may have an immediate benefit based on the observation of Campbell and colleagues of an increased FEV_1 in one patient during an exacerbation of bronchitis,[51] and the discovery of Wollmer and coworkers of greater radioaerosol clearance in two patients with very high sputum yields when both percussion and postural drainage were employed.[49]

Bronchiectasis

Chest physical therapy remains the cornerstone of therapy for bronchiectasis except in patients with "dry" bronchiectasis who fail to produce sputum. Ideally, treatment consists of self-administered postural drainage and the forced expiratory technique.[39] The addition of percussion or vibration further enhances sputum expectoration but does not improve tracheobronchial clearance as assessed by radioaerosol studies using inhaled particles tagged with a gamma-emitting radionuclide like technetium 99m.[55] However, the inhalation of a beta-adrenergic agonist just prior to initiating postural drainage and the forced expiratory technique substantially increases both sputum production and lung radioaerosol clearance.[56] Family members can usually be instructed to assist in chest physical therapy if necessary, especially during acute exacerbations. Such therapy has been demonstrated to quickly ameliorate airflow obstruction in one study[57] but not in another.[58] Also, no short-term improvement in oxygen saturation occurred in the second study.[58] Although the extended effects of chest physical therapy on pulmonary function in bronchiectasis remain to be evaluated, long-term clinical experience attests to its value in maintaining patients' functional capacity and in reducing infectious exacerbations. It is probable that many of the newer approaches to managing airway secretions in cystic fibrosis are also applicable to patients with bronchiectasis.

Cystic Fibrosis

Chest physical therapy is essential in managing cystic fibrosis and should be administered for the lifetime of cystic fibrosis patients. Such therapy is partly responsible for the increasing life expectancy of children and young adults with the disease. It delays the development of severe airways obstruction, the worsening of bronchiectasis, and destructive lower respiratory infections caused by *Staphylococcus aureus*, *Pseudomonas aeruginosa* (including mucoid strains), and by other bacterial pathogens. Besides enhancing airway mucus clearance, chest physical therapy in cystic fibrosis improves large[48, 59] and small airways function.[48] Failure to administer chest physical therapy for several weeks promotes the worsening of pulmonary function, which may be reversed by reinitiating therapy.[60] Although conventional chest physical therapy, which emphasizes postural drainage, is the mainstay for managing infants and young children with cystic fibrosis, alternative, self-administered methods warrant a trial in older children and adults. Vigorous self-directed cough[61, 62] and the forced expiratory technique[39] are both effective for expectorating pulmonary secretions in stable patients and are equally efficacious in therapist-administered chest physical therapy. Sleeping in the head down position (20-degree tilt) further improves sputum production in patients with copious secretions and may obviate the need for daytime postural drainage if combined with the forced expiratory technique.[63] The frequency of treatments must be individualized depending on the severity of cystic fibrosis, but at a minimum should be carried out at least after awakening in the morning and before sleep at night, even if the patient feels well and has minimal or no sputum production. Supervised, directed coughing in combination with the forced expiratory technique is equally beneficial in conventional physical therapy for managing acute exacerbations in cystic fibrosis,[64] but it seems prudent to provide traditional chest physical therapy to acutely ill patients, since postural drainage can augment the clearance benefit of the forced expiratory technique in cystic fibrosis.[39]

Mechanical chest percussors have also been used in cystic fibrosis patients[65, 66] but probably do not supplement the benefits of the forced expiratory technique combined with postural drainage.[67] Mask positive expiratory pressure can also enhance mucus clearance in cystic fibrosis[68, 69]; however, this technique can diminish the effectiveness of postural drainage and the forced expiratory technique when combined with them.[41] Because these physical therapy adjuncts are easy to administer, may shorten treatment sessions, and allow independent therapy, their value in cystic fibrosis warrants further study. All but the most disabled patients should be encouraged to engage in daily physical exercise, especially in running and swimming. These activities can be as effective as chest physical therapy in clearing airway secretions in children.[70] In adult cystic fibrosis patients, exercise using a bicycle ergometer aids sputum expectoration but is less beneficial than chest physiotherapy in this regard.[71]

Asthma

There is no evidence to support the use of chest physical therapy in managing asthma.[72] Pharmacologic treatment with bronchodilators and corticosteroids remains the cornerstone of therapy even in acute asthma and status asthmaticus. Nevertheless, impaction of large and especially small airways with thick, tenacious mucus is probably universally present in status asthmaticus, and patients often have serious difficulty expectorating these mucus plugs. Gentle chest physical therapy can be attempted in such patients, although there is no consensus as to which physical therapy techniques are most effective in asthma and are least likely to worsen bronchospasm. Treatment sessions with postural drainage, percussion, and vibration should be short, and their efficacy should be judged based on alterations in dyspnea, arterial blood gas parameters, and the quantity of expectorated sputum. An anecdotal report notes that vigorous chest physical therapy in mechanically ventilated patients with status asthmaticus can mobilize large amounts of sputum (30–40 ml per treatment), significantly decrease peak inspiratory ventilator pressures, and reduce the chest radiographic findings of hyperinflation caused by the trapping of air behind airway obstructions.[73]

Pneumonia

Chest physical therapy including postural drainage, percussion, and vibration has not been shown to hasten the clinical or roentgenographic resolution of primary pneumonia in otherwise well patients without endobronchial lesions, underlying chronic obstructive lung disease, respiratory muscle weakness, or the need for mechanical ventilatory support.[74, 75] However, chest physical therapy is clearly indicated in pneumonia patients who have underlying COPD, bronchiectasis, or another lung disorder and who cannot clear their own airway secretions. The chest physical therapy regimen selected in this setting should be the one that most benefits a patient's underlying obstructive lung disorder.

Preoperative and Postoperative Respiratory Care

Atelectasis is a common postoperative pulmonary complication in patients with underlying obstructive lung disorders and occurs most often following upper abdominal and cardiothoracic surgery. Additional risk factors include advanced age (> 60 yr), obesity, and ongoing cigarette use. The causes of postoperative atelectasis are many and include impaired tracheobronchial mucus transport following general anesthesia,[76] poorly understood diaphragmatic dysfunction,[77] pain-induced impairment of cough and sigh maneuvers, excessive analgesia, and immobility. Intraoperative lung contusion and phrenic nerve injury caused by cryocardioplegia are additional mechanisms unique to cardiothoracic surgery.[78] However, general anesthesia does not seem to adversely alter the viscoelastic and transport properties of normal human respiratory tract mucus; it is therefore probable that a reduced postoperative mucus transport rate is caused by ciliary depression by anesthetic gases.[79]

Preventive measures are the cornerstone of appropriate preoperative and postoperative respiratory care. The most important of these measures are deep breathing techniques that induce maximum inspiratory volumes. The ability of these modalities to significantly reduce postoperative pulmonary complications is well documented. Such methods include intermittent positive-pressure breathing, incentive spirometry, and deep breathing exercises.[80] Continuous positive airway pressure by mask using a pressure of 7.5 to 15 cm H_2O can also prevent postsurgical atelectasis and quickly restore functional residual capacity to close to preoperative levels.[81, 82] Because intermittent positive-pressure breathing is expensive and causes more side effects than other methods,[80] we prefer the other expansion modalities, especially incentive spirometry.

Patients should receive instruction in the techniques discussed prior to surgery and undergo treatment postoperatively for 15 minutes every 2 to 3 hours while awake during the first 3 to 5 days after surgery. These methods should be prescribed primarily for obstructive lung disease patients undergoing upper abdominal and cardiothoracic surgery but may also be worthwhile following less serious operations if patients have severe pulmonary function impairment. The routine addition of chest physical therapy to lung expansion manuevers in all COPD patients is probably not helpful and may increase patient discomfort.[32] The use of chest physical therapy in combination with deep breathing techniques should be limited to patients who produce a large amount of sputum (> 30 ml/day). This approach, together with general prophylactic measures—including smoking cessation before elective operations, late-morning surgery for patients with excessive early-morning sputum production, frequent side-to-side turning postoperatively, the judicious use of analgesics, and early ambulation—can substantially reduce the incidence of postsurgical pulmonary complications.

Obstructive Atelectasis Due to Retained Airway Secretions

In contrast to its lesser role in preventing atelectasis, chest physical therapy should be routinely employed in COPD patients who develop obstructive atelectasis as a result of mucus impaction in the airways. This problem is frequently encountered postoperatively in patients who have undergone abdominal or thoracic surgery as well as in seriously ill COPD patients (who are often in an intensive care setting) with a wide range of superimposed disorders, including drug overdose, trauma, paralysis, or other major illness. Along with intensified bronchodilator therapy, breathing exercises, and directed cough, such patients should receive generous chest physical therapy combined with postural drainage and percussion directed to the involved lung zone or zones. Chest physical therapy with percussion and vibration can even by employed in trauma patients with rib fractures or a flail chest as long as such treatment is not given directly over the trauma site and the therapist monitors for accidental rib displacement during the treatment. This approach is usually successful in quickly resolving atelectasis resulting from the plugging of large airways; one publication noted complete resolution of atelectasis in three of eight patients following a single treatment and the restoration of 50% of lung volume in three others.[83] Most of the volume loss in this group was restored in 24 hours. On the other hand, atelectasis caused by retained secretions within small airways resolves more slowly; only about 60% of normal lung volume is restored following 48 hours of aggressive therapy.[83] Atelectasis of this type is often identified by the presence of air bronchograms within the atelectatic lung as observed on plain chest radiographs; this indicates the patency of the large central bronchi.

Fiberoptic bronchoscopy with lavage and suctioning of obstructed airways is no better than conventional chest physical therapy in resolving atelectasis caused by the plugging of either large or small airways with mucus.[83] This procedure should be reserved for patients whose atelectasis is unresponsive to chest physical therapy. This conservative approach is also justified before instituting other techniques to treat atelectasis, such as maximum-volume intermittent positive-pressure breathing[84] and lung expansion employing a fiberoptic bronchoscope with a balloon cuff.[85] However, continuous positive-pressure breathing using expiratory pressures between 5 and 15 cm H_2O administered as positive end-expiratory pressure using a ventilator[86] or as continuous positive airway pressure using a nasal[87] or facial mask[88] may provide more rapid resolution of atelectasis that is unassociated with large airway obstruction. Further investigation is needed to compare the efficacy of chest physical therapy and continuous positive-pressure breathing in resolving atelectasis of this type. It should also be noted that studies evaluating the benefits of intermittent positive-pressure breathing and continuous positive-pressure breathing in treating atelectasis were carried out in patients without COPD. Since these techniques can promote further air trapping and carry a risk of hyperinflation and pneumothorax, they should be utilized cautiously in COPD patients.

Metabolic Effects and Complications of Chest Physical Therapy

Chest physical therapy can substantially increase patients' metabolic rate, and with physical therapy oxygen consumption and carbon dioxide production average close to 40% above those levels found during sleep.[89] These parameters may remain above resting values for up to 45 minutes after chest physical therapy is completed. Since major increases in heart rate and the product of heart rate and systolic blood pressure (an indicator of myocardial oxygen demand) also occur, chest physical therapy is believed to constitute a major metabolic and hemodynamic stress and might be hazardous to COPD patients who also have serious underlying cardiovascular disorders.[89] It seems prudent to institute electrocardiographic and hemodynamic monitoring in such patients, and higher concentrations of inspired oxygen should probably be employed during and for 30 minutes to 1 hour after chest physical therapy is completed.

Serious complications are infrequent during chest physical therapy. Only a few deaths have been reported,[90] and they have usually been caused by massive pulmonary hemorrhage from a lung abscess or bronchopulmonary fistula.

Other adverse side effects of chest physical therapy, such as those due to the mechanical effects of changes in body position (e.g., displacement of intravascular lines and endotracheal tubes, or fractures and dislocations), are more common[91] but can often be anticipated and minimized. The most important adverse occurrence is hypoxemia. An average decrease in PaO_2 of 19 mm Hg was observed in one group of 17 patients following postural drainage and chest percussion[92]; similarly, significant falls in SaO_2 from above 90 to 85% or below were found in 5 to 9 patients with cystic fibrosis.[93] However, hypoxemia does not always occur with chest physical therapy,[94] and PaO_2 may actually improve.[95] Hypoxemia with chest physical therapy occurs in patients with minimal or no airways secretions[94] as well as in patients who produce copious sputum.[93] Of importance, PaO_2 appears to decrease less as baseline hypoxemia becomes more pronounced, so that chest physical therapy need not be withheld from patients with low baseline PaO_2 values.[96] However, the number of patients with obstructive lung disease in this study is not specified. Chest physical therapy–related hypoxemia may be worsened by chest percussion,[94] by placing the diseased lung in the dependent position,[92] and by endotracheal suctioning.[97] Supplemental oxygen (administered at 3 L/min via nasal cannula) did not prevent chest physical therapy–related hypoxemia in cystic fibrosis patients but did promote a quicker return of SaO_2 to baseline levels after the completion of therapy.[93] However, thoracic expansion exercises together with pauses for relaxation and controlled breathing prevented decreases in SaO_2 in another group of patients with cystic fibrosis.[98] Although the mechanism of hypoxemia after chest physical therapy is not certain, it may be the result of a shifting of mucus from the peripheral to the central airways, which causes blockage at this level and ventilation/perfusion mismatch. The widespread availability of ear oximetry now permits continuous monitoring of SaO_2 during chest physical therapy and, if needed, supplemental oxygen supply can be easily adjusted to maintain SaO_2 at a safe level of 90% or greater.

Chest physical therapy does not appear to have a major effect on lung mechanics, although one study did note a modest but transient fall in FEV_1 immediately after chest percussion in 40% of patients treated during an acute exacerbation of chronic bronchitis.[51] Since most of these patients had evidence of hyperreactive airways, chest percussion should probably be preceded by the use of an aerosolized bronchodilator, and special caution is warranted when this technique is administered to asthmatics who are experiencing an acute asthma attack or who are in status asthmaticus. Neither postural drainage alone nor directed cough seems to cause a similar decline in FEV_1.

SUMMARY

Chest physical therapy in stable COPD patients is responsible for an immediate increase in sputum expectoration, with the greatest sputum increases occurring in those who cough up the largest daily amounts of sputum. Also, chest physical therapy in this group enhances mucus clearance from central and, to a lesser extent, peripheral lung zones; postural drainage and cough are both required to maximize this effect. There is little or no early positive effect of chest physical therapy on pulmonary function in stable COPD patients, except for a modest improvement in small airways function. With respect to acute COPD exacerbations, only patients producing the largest quantities of sputum are likely to be aided by the addition of chest physical therapy to their treatment regimens.

Chest physical therapy remains an essential component in the therapy of bronchiectasis and cystic fibrosis. The frequency of treatments must be individualized based on the severity of disease and the quantity of airway secretions that must be cleared. Standard chest physical therapy with postural drainage, cough, and the forced expiratory technique is the cornerstone of such treatment regimens. Newer modalities, such as mechanical chest percussion and mask positive expiratory pressure, warrant further clinical trials before they can be routinely used in these disorders.

Chest physical therapy should be used sparingly in patients with stable and acute asthma. In pneumonia, it is clearly indicated in only those patients who have underlying obstructive airways disease and who cannot clear their own airway secretions. Similarly, the addition of routine chest physical therapy to lung expansion manuevers is mostly unhelpful in preoperative and postoperative respiratory care and should be employed only in those patients who are major sputum producers (> 30 ml/day). However, chest physical therapy is essential for the management of obstructive atelectasis resulting from the plugging of both large and small airways by mucus in postoperative COPD patients or COPD patients seriously ill with a wide range of superimposed disorders.

REFERENCES

1. Barach AL. Breathing exercises in pulmonary emphysema and allied chronic respiratory disease. Arch Phys Med Rehab 1955; 36:379–390.
2. Miller WF. A physiologic evaluation of the effects of diaphragmatic breathing training in patients with chronic pulmonary emphysema. Am J Med 1954; 17:471–477.
3. Rodenstein DO, Stanescu DC. Absence of nasal air flow during pursed lips breathing. Am Rev Respir Dis 1983; 128:716–718.
4. Barach AL. Physiologic advantages of grunting, groaning and pursed-lip breathing: Adaptive symptoms related to the development of continuous positive pressure breathing. Bull N Y Acad Med 1973; 49:666–673.
5. Thoman RL, Stoker GL, Ross JC. The efficacy of pursed-lips breathing in patients with chronic obstructive pulmonary disease. Am Rev Respir Dis 1966; 93:100–105.
6. Mueller RE, Petty TL, Filley GF. Ventilation and arterial blood gas changes induced by pursed lips breathing. J Appl Physiol 1970; 28:784–789.
7. Roa J, Epstein S, Breslin E, et al. Work of breathing and ventilatory muscle recruitment during pursed lip breathing in patients with chronic airway obstruction. Am Rev Respir Dis 1991; 143:A77.
8. Tiep BL, Burns M, Kao D, et al. Pursed lips breathing training using ear oximetry. Chest 1986; 90:218–221.
9. Ingram RH Jr, Schilder DP. Effect of pursed lips expiration on the pulmonary pressure-flow relationship in obstructive lung disease. Am Rev Respir Dis 1967; 96:381–387.
10. Barach AL, Beck GJ. The ventilatory effects of the head-down position in pulmonary emphysema. Am J Med 1954; 16:55–60.
11. Gayrard P, Becker M, Bergofsky EH. The effects of abdominal weights on diaphragmatic position and excursion in man. Clin Sci 1968; 35:589–601.
12. Erwin WS, Zolov D, Bickerman HA. The effect of posture on respiratory function in patients with obstructive pulmonary emphysema. Am Rev Respir Dis 1966; 94:865–872.
13. Celli BR. Importance of the respiratory muscles in rehabilitation. Probl Respir Care 1990; 3:459–482.
14. Sharp JT, Drutz WS, Moisan T, et al. Postural relief of dyspnea in severe chronic obstructive pulmonary disease. Am Rev Respir Dis 1980; 122:201–211.
15. Druz WS, Sharp JT. Electrical and mechanical activity of the diaphragm accompanying body position in severe chronic obstructive pulmonary disease. Am Rev Respir Dis 1982; 125:275–280.
16. Delgado HR, Braun SR, Skatrud JB, et al. Chest wall and abdominal motion during exercise in patients with chronic obstructive pulmonary disease. Am Rev Respir Dis 1982; 126:200–205.
17. Dodd DS, Brancatisano TP, Engel LA. Effect of abdominal strapping on chest wall mechanics during exercise in patients

with severe chronic air-flow obstruction. Am Rev Respir Dis 1985; 131:816–821.
18. Livingstone JL, Gillespie M. The value of breathing exercises in asthma. Lancet 1935; 2:705–708.
19. Becklake MR, McGregor M. Goldman HI, Braudo JL. A study of the effects of physiotherapy in chronic hypertrophic emphysema using lung function tests. Dis Chest 1954; 26:180–191.
20. McNeill RS, McKenzie JM. An assessment of the value of breathing exercises in chronic bronchitis and asthma. Thorax 1955; 10:250–252.
21. Sinclair JD. The effect of breathing exercises in pulmonary emphysema. Thorax 1955; 10:246–249.
22. Campbell EJM, Friend J. Action of breathing exercises in pulmonary emphysema. Lancet 1955; 1:325–329.
23. Miller WF. Physical therapeutic measures in the treatment of chronic bronchopulmonary disorders: Methods for breathing training. Am J Med 1958; 24:929–940.
24. Willeput R, Vachaudez JP, Lenders D, et al. Thoracoabdominal motion during chest physiotherapy in patients affected by chronic obstructive lung disease. Respiration 1983; 44:204–214.
25. Grimby G, Oxhoj H, Bake B. Effects of abdominal breathing on distribution of ventilation in obstructive lung disease. Clin Sci Mol Med 1975; 48:193–199.
26. Sackner MA, Silva G, Banks JM, et al. Distribution of ventilation during diaphragmatic breathing in obstructive lung disease. Am Rev Respir Dis 1974; 109:331–337.
27. Brach BB, Chao RP, Sgroi VL, et al. Xenon washout patterns during diaphragmatic breathing. Studies in normal persons and patients with chronic obstructive pulmonary disease. Chest 1977; 71:735–739.
28. Sackner MA, Gonzalez HF, Jenouri G, Rodriguez M. Effects of abdominal and thoracic breathing on breathing pattern components in normal subjects and in patients with chronic obstructive pulmonary diesase. Am Rev Respir Dis 1984; 130:584–587.
29. Marini JJ, Tyler ML, Hudson LD, et al. Influence of head-dependent positions on lung volume and oxygen saturation in chronic air-flow obstruction. Am Rev Respir Dis 1984; 129:101–105.
30. Chopra SK, Taplin GV, Simmons DH, et al. Effects of hydration and physical therapy on tracheal transport velocity. Am Rev Respir Dis 1977; 115:1009–1014.
31. Shim C, King M, Williams MH Jr. Lack of effect of hydration on sputum production in chronic bronchitis. Chest 1987; 92:679–682.
32. Sutton PP, Pavia D, Bateman JRM, Clarke SW. Chest physiotherapy: A review. Eur J Respir Dis 1982; 63:188–201.
33. King M, Phillips DM, Gross D, et al. Enhanced tracheal mucus clearance with high frequency chest wall compression. Am Rev Respir Dis 1983; 128:511–515.
34. Evans JN, Jaeger MJ. Mechanical aspects of coughing. Pneumonologie 1975; 152:253–257.
35. King M, Brock G, Lundell C. Clearance of mucus by simulated cough. J Appl Physiol 1985; 58:1776–1782.
36. Camner P, Mossberg B, Philipson K, Strandberg K. Elimination of test particles from the human tracheobronchial tract by voluntary coughing. Scand J Respir Dis 1979; 60:56–62.
37. Burford JG, George RB. Respiratory physical therapy in the treatment of chronic bronchitis. Semin Respir Infect 1988; 3:55–60.
38. Harris RS, Lawson TV. The relative mechanical effectiveness and efficiency of successive voluntary coughs in healthy young adults. Clin Sci 1968; 34:569–577.
39. Sutton PP, Parker RA, Webber BA, et al. Assessment of the forced expiration technique, postural drainage and directed coughing in chest physiotherapy. Eur J Respir Dis 1983; 64:62–68.
40. Clarke SW. Rationale of airway clearance. Eur Respir J 1989; 2(Suppl 7):599S–604S.
41. Hofmeyr JL, Webber BA, Hodson ME. Evaluation of positive expiratory pressure as an adjunct to chest physiotherapy in the treatment of cystic fibrosis. Thorax 1986; 41:951–954.
42. Bateman JRM, Newman SP, Daunt KM, et al. Regional lung clearance of excessive bronchial secretions during chest physiotherapy in patients with stable chronic airways obstruction. Lancet 1979; 1:294–297.
43. Bateman JRM, Newman SP, Daunt KM, et al. Is cough as effective as chest physiotherapy in the removal of excessive tracheobronchial secretions? Thorax 1981; 36:683–687.
44. March H. Appraisal of postural drainage for chronic obstructive pulmonary disease. Arch Phys Med Rehabil 1971; 52:528–530.
45. May DB, Munt PW. Physiologic effects of chest percussion and postural drainage in patients with stable chronic bronchitis. Chest 1979; 75:29–32.
46. Mohsenifar Z, Rosenberg N, Goldberg HS, Koerner SK. Mechanical vibration and conventional chest physiotherapy in outpatients with stable chronic obstructive lung disease. Chest 1985; 87:483–485.
47. Oldenburg FA Jr, Dolovich MB, Montgomery JM, Newhouse MT. Effects of postural drainage, exercise, and cough on mucus clearance in chronic bronchitis. Am Rev Respir Dis 1979; 120:739–745.
48. Feldman J, Traver GA, Taussig LM. Maximal expiratory flows after postural drainage. Am Rev Respir Dis 1979; 119:239–245.
49. Wollmer P, Ursing K, Midgren B, Eriksson L. Inefficiency of chest percussion in the physical therapy of chronic bronchitis. Eur J Respir Dis 1985; 66:233–239.
50. Anthonisen P, Riis P, Sogaard-Anderson T. The value of lung physiotherapy in the treatment of acute exacerbations in chronic bronchitis. Acta Med Scand 1964; 175:715–719.
51. Campbell AH, O'Connell JM, Wilson F. The effect of chest physiotherapy upon the FEV_1 in chronic bronchitis. Med J Aust 1975; 1:33–35.
52. Newton DAG, Stephenson A. Effect of physiotherapy on pulmonary function. Lancet 1978; 2:228–229.
53. Newton DAG, Bevans HG. Physiotherapy and intermittent postive-pressure ventilation of chronic bronchitis. Br Med J 1978; 2:1525–1528.
54. Buscaglia AJ, St. Marie MS. Oxygen saturation during chest physiotherapy for acute exacerbation of severe chronic obstructive pulmonary disease. Respir Care 1983; 28:1009–1013.
55. Sutton PP, Lopez-Vidriero MT, Pavia D, et al. Assessment of percussion, vibratory-shaking and breathing exercises in chest physiotherapy. Eur J Respir Dis 1985; 66:147–152.
56. Sutton PP, Gemmell HG, Innes N, et al. Use of nebulised saline and nebulised terbutaline as an adjunct to chest physiotherapy. Thorax 1988; 43:57–60.
57. Cochrane GM, Webber BA, Clarke SW. Effects of sputum on pulmonary function. Br Med J 1977; 2:1181–1183.
58. Mazzocco MC, Owens GR, Kiriloff LH, Rogers RM. Chest percussion and postural drainage in patients with bronchiectasis. Chest 1985; 88:360–363.
59. Tecklin JS, Holsclaw DS. Evaluation of bronchial drainage in patients with cystic fibrosis. Phys Ther 1975; 55:1081–1084.
60. Desmond KJ, Swhwenk WF, Thomas E, et al. Immediate and long-term effects of chest physiotherapy in patients with cystic fibrosis. J Pediatr 1983; 103:538–542.
61. Rossman CM, Waldes R, Sampson D, Newhouse MT. Effect of chest physiotherapy on the removal of mucus in patients with cystic fibrosis. Am Rev Respir Dis 1982; 126:131–135.
62. de Boeck C, Zinman R. Cough versus chest physiotherapy: A comparison of the acute effects on pulmonary function in patients with cystic fibrosis. Am Rev Respir Dis 1984; 129:182–184.
63. Verboon JML, Bakker W, Sterk PJ. The value of the forced expiration technique with and without postural drainage in adults with cystic fibrosis. Eur J Respir Dis 1986; 69:169–174.
64. Bain J, Bishop J, Olinsky A. Evaluation of directed coughing in cystic fibrosis. Br J Dis Chest 1988; 82:138–148.
65. Maxwell M, Redmond A. Comparative trial of manual and mechanical percussion technique with gravity-assisted bronchial drainage in patients with cystic fibrosis. Arch Dis Child 1979; 54:542–544.
66. Flower KA, Eden RI, Lomax L, et al. New mechanical aid to physiotherapy in cystic fibrosis. BMJ 1979; 2:630–631.
67. Murphy MB, Concannon D, FitzGerald MX. Chest percussion: Help or hindrance to postural drainage? Ir Med J 1983; 76:189–190.
68. Falk M, Kelstrup M, Andersen JB, et al. Improving the ketchup bottle method with positive expiratory pressure, PEP, in cystic fibrosis. Eur J Respir Dis 1984; 65:423–432.
69. Van Asperen PP, Jackson L, Hennessy P, Brown J. Comparison

of a positive expiratory pressure (PEP) mask with postural drainage in patients with cystic fibrosis. Aust Paediatr J 1987; 23:283–284.
70. Zack M, Oberwaldner B, Hansler F. Cystic fibrosis: Physical exercise versus chest physiotherapy. Arch Dis Child 1982; 57:587–589.
71. Sahl W, Bilton D, Dodd M, Webb AK. Effect of exercise and physiotherapy in aiding sputum expectoration in adults with cystic fibrosis. Thorax 1989; 44:1006–1008.
72. Kirilloff LH, Owens GR, Rogers RM, Mazzocco MC. Does chest physical therapy work? Chest 1985; 88:436–444.
73. Kigin CM. Breathing exercises in chest physical therapy. Chest 1987; 92:190.
74. Graham WGB, Bradley DA. Efficacy of chest physiotherapy and intermittent positive-pressure breathing in the resolution of pneumonia. N Engl J Med 1978; 299:624–627.
75. Britton S, Bejstedt M, Vedin L. Chest physiotherapy in primary pneumonia. BMJ 1985; 290:1703–1704.
76. Gamsu G, Singer MM, Vincent HH, et al. Postoperative impairment of mucous transport in the lung. Am Rev Respir Dis 1976; 114:673–679.
77. Dureuil B, Vires N, Cantineau J-P, et al. Diphragmatic contractility after upper abdominal surgery. J Appl Physiol 1986; 61:1775–1780.
78. Pearce W, Baile EM, Hards J, et al. Phrenic nerve function and its relationship to atelectasis after coronary artery bypass surgery. Chest 1988; 93:693–698.
79. Rubin BK, Finegan B, Ramirez O, King M. General anesthesia does not alter the viscoelastic or transport properties of human respiratory mucus. Chest 1990; 98:101–104.
80. Celli BR, Rodriguez KS, Snider GL. A controlled trial of intermittent positive pressure breathing, incentive spirometry, and deep breathing exercises in preventing pulmonary complications after abdominal surgery. Am Rev Respir Dis 1984; 130:12–15.
81. Stock MC, Downs JB, Gauer PK, et al. Prevention of postoperative pulmonary complications with CPAP, incentive spirometry, and conservative therapy. Chest 1985; 87:151–157.
82. Paul WL, Downs JB. Postoperative atelectasis: Intermittent positive pressure breathing, incentive spirometry, and facemask positive end-expiratory pressure. Arch Surg 1981; 116:861–863.
83. Marini JJ, Pierson DJ, Hudson LD. Acute lobar atelectasis: A prospective comparison of fiberoptic bronchoscopy and respiratory therapy. Am Rev Respir Dis 1979; 119:971–978.
84. O'Donohue WJ Jr. Maximum volume IPPB for the management of pulmonary atelectasis. Chest 1979; 76:683–687.
85. Harada K, Mutsuda T, Saoyama N, et al. Re-expansion of refractory atelectasis using a bronchofiberscope with a balloon cuff. Chest 1983; 84:725–728.
86. Fowler AA, Scoggins WG, O'Donohue WJ Jr. Positive end-expiratory pressure in the management of lobar atelectasis. Chest 1978; 74:497–500.
87. Duncan SR, Negrin RS, Mihm FG, et al. Nasal continuous positive airway pressure in atelectasis. Chest 1987; 92:621–624.
88. Williamson DC III, Modell JH. Intermittent continuous positive airway pressure by mask. Arch Surg 1982; 117:970–972.
89. Weissman C, Kemper M, Damask MC, et al. Effect of routine intensive care interactions on metabolic rate. Chest 1984; 86:815–818.
90. Tyler ML. Complications of positioning and chest physiotherapy. Respir Care 1982; 27:458–466.
91. Mackenzie CF, Ciesla N, Imle PC, Klemic N. Chest physiotherapy in the intensive care unit. Baltimore: Williams & Wilkins, 1981.
92. Huseby J, Hudson L, Stark K, Tyler M. Oxygenation during chest physiotherapy (abstract). Chest 1976; 70:430.
93. McDonnell T, McNicholas WT, FitzGerald MX. Hypoxaemia during chest physiotherapy in patients with cystic fibrosis, Ir J Med Sci 1986; 155:345–348.
94. Connors AF Jr, Hammon WE, Martin RJ, Rogers RM. Chest physical therapy: The immediate effect of oxygenation in acutely ill patients. Chest 1980; 78:559–564.
95. Holody B, Goldberg HS. The effect of mechanical vibration physiotherapy on arterial oxygenation in acutely ill patients with atelectasis or pneumonia. Am Rev Respir Dis 1981; 124:372–375.
96. Tyler ML, Hudson LD, Grose BL, Huseby JS. Prediction of oxygenation during chest physiotherapy in critically ill patients. Am Rev Respir Dis 1980; 121 (Part 2):218.
97. Gormezano J, Branthwaite MA. Effects of physiotherapy during intermittent positive pressure ventilation. Anaesthesia 1972; 27:258–264.
98. Pryor JA, Webber BA, Hodson ME. Effect of chest physiotherapy on oxygen saturation in patients with cystic fibrosis. Thorax 1990; 45:77.

Chapter 15

Long-term Oxygen Therapy

CHRISTOPHER B. COOPER, M.D.

"There is some use of air, which we do not yet so well understand, that makes it so continuously needful to the life of animals." Boyle, 1670.

Several hundred years have now elapsed since scientists first appreciated that there was some constituent of the atmosphere that was fundamental to human existence. Elemental oxygen was jointly discovered in the 1770s by the Swedish pharmacist Carl Wilhelm Scheel and the English cleric Joseph Priestley. Priestley wrote in 1774 that he had extracted air that burned with a remarkably vigorous flame. Scheel probably discovered oxygen somewhere between 1770 and 1773, and similarly called it "fire air." Both Priestley and Scheel realized that oxygen could be not only beneficial but also dangerous. In 1777, Lavoisier coined the term "oxygine," which is derived from the Greek for "acid producer." Hence, around the time of its discovery, the essential nature of oxygen was appreciated, and its potential for harmful effects was realized.

HISTORY OF OXYGEN THERAPY

Origins of Oxygen Therapy

In 1775, Priestley first suggested the therapeutic use of oxygen, claiming it was "salutory to the lungs in morbid cases." In 1779, Ingen-Housz recommended breathing 16,000 to 20,000 cm^3 daily for therapeutic purposes. The first clearly documented medical application of oxygen was recorded by Beddoes and Watt[1] in *Considerations on the Medicinal Use of Factitious Airs*. In 1798, Beddoes established a pneumatic institute in Clifton, England, and began the therapeutic administration of oxygen. Nonetheless, oxygen therapy was not widely accepted at this time. The therapeutic use of oxygen enjoyed a brief resurgence during the 1832 cholera epidemic, and in the 1840s oxygen began to be used in anesthesia. Probably the first use of oxygen in the United States was documented in 1887 by George Holzapple, who treated a case of pneumococcal pneumonia with oxygen generated from the heating of potassium chloride and manganese oxide in test tubes. Oxygen therapy became established as a respected therapeutic modality at the time of World War I, when Haldane[2] described its use in the treatment of chlorine gas poisoning. In 1921, Leonard Hill described the first oxygen tent for the treatment of "edema and chronic ulcer of the lung." Also in the United States, in 1922, Alvin Barach described the systemic use of oxygen for lobar pneumonia. Barach was undoubtedly the pioneer of modern oxygen therapy and pulmonary rehabilitation. He also devised the first truly portable devices for giving oxygen to patients with emphysema. In the 1950s, he described the relief of dyspnea using oxygen contained in small transfilling bottles. Cotes and Gilson[3] also used portable compressed gas cylinders and were the first to document an increase in patient exercise capacity with oxygen therapy.

The Modern Era of Oxygen Therapy

In the latter half of the 1960s, a number of investigators in Denver, Colorado, began the systematic examination of the beneficial effects of oxygen therapy in patients with chronic hypoxemia. These investigations laid the foundations for modern oxygen therapy and stimulated the expansion of clinical research in this field. Levine and coworkers[4] demonstrated in a small group of patients that oxygen therapy could correct pulmonary hypertension induced by chronic hypoxemia as well as reduce red blood cell mass and increase exercise tolerance. Similar findings were reported by Abraham associates.[5] Petty and Finigan[6] demonstrated clinical benefits from prolonged ambulatory oxygen therapy in 20 patients. Soon afterward, improved survival was reported in patients with cor pulmonale.[7] In the United Kingdom, Stark and colleagues[8, 9] were exploring the daily duration of oxygen therapy required to reduce pulmonary hypertension. These early studies led to the design of two multicenter trials, one in the United States[10] and the other in the United Kingdom.[11] The Nocturnal Oxygen Therapy (NOT) trial compared continuous oxygen therapy (COT; in practice, 17.7 hr/day) with oxygen therapy given overnight (12 hr/day). The Medical Research Council (MRC) study tested whether oxygen therapy given for 15 hours per day improved survival compared with no oxygen therapy at all. There were some important differences among the patient groups studied. Those in the NOT trial were somewhat older and did not have carbon dioxide retention. The severity of hypoxemia in both groups was similar, and both groups had modest pulmonary hypertension at entry into the studies. The results suggested that 18% of the MRC patients who received no oxygen would have been alive after 5 years according to a calculated annual percentage risk factor of 30%. This observation corresponds with the results of earlier studies. The survival rate was significantly better for patients who received oxygen for 15 hours, but it was better still for those from the NOT trial who received oxygen for about 18 hours. The combined results (Fig. 15–1) indicated that long-term oxygen therapy (LTOT) could be advantageous if given for as long as possible during every 24-hour period. In the NOT trial, pulmonary hemodynamics were compared at the onset and after 6 months of LTOT.[12] A reduction in pulmonary artery pressure (P_{PA}) was seen at rest in the group receiving COT and in both groups during exercise. Similar changes in pulmonary vascular resistance were observed; these differences were greater during exercise. In the same report, Timms and coworkers[12] showed that survival up to 8 years was related to the decrease in mean P_{PA} during the first 6 months of treatment. Ashutosh and associates[13] reported that a decrease in P_{PA} greater than 5 mm Hg was associated with improved survival in patients receiving LTOT. Following these important studies, it has been widely concluded that improved survival results primarily from the reversal of pulmonary hemodynamic disturbances by oxygen therapy. Alternative explanations are conceivable. It is possible that the correlation of mortality with pulmonary hypertension is an epiphenomenon accompanying important pathophysiologic events elsewhere in the body. Recent analyses have demonstrated a relentless decline in airway function despite LTOT[14] and have shown a persistently strong association between the severity of airflow obstruction and survival.[15] Careful analysis of the combined results of the NOT trial and the MRC study reveals an important difference in survival prospects. In the NOT group, those patients who were prescribed COT received on average 17.7 hours per day as compared with the patients of the two other treatment groups who received oxygen between 12 and 15 hours per day. The difference in the duration of oxygen therapy between these groups was not considerable, yet

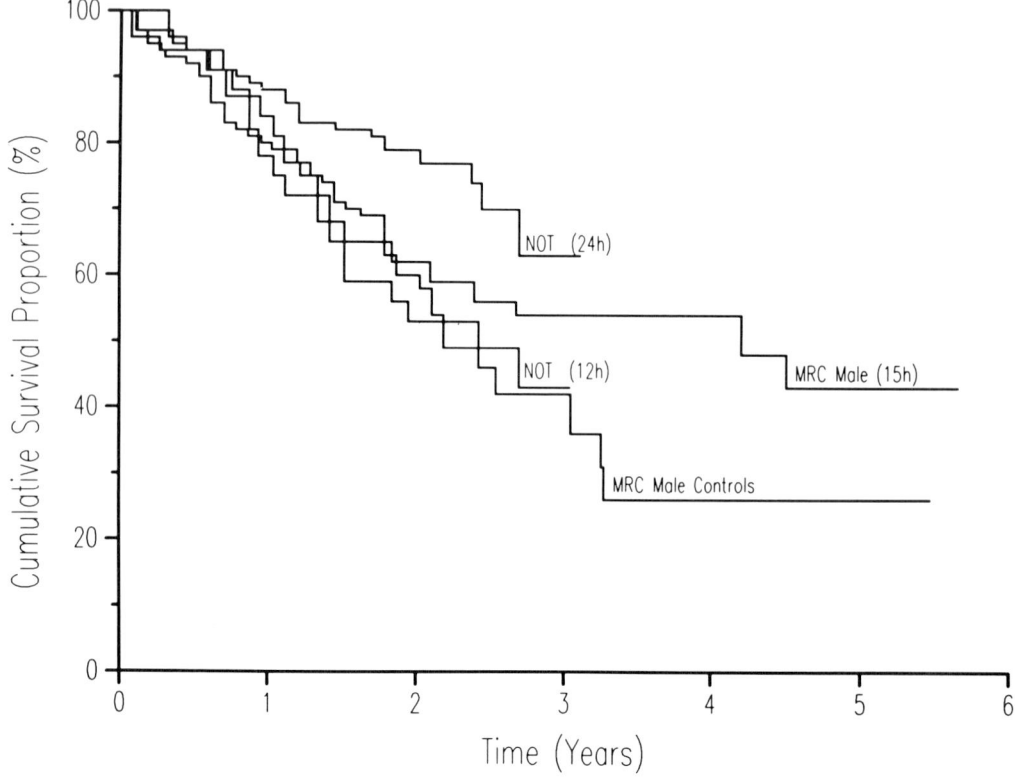

FIGURE 15–1. Combined data from the Nocturnal Oxygen Therapy (NOT) Trial of the National Institutes of Health (NIH) and the Medical Research Council (MRC) Study showing the improvement in survival proportional to the duration of oxygen therapy (h) each day. MRC controls received no oxygen. Note that the NOT (24 h) group also had access to ambulatory oxygen therapy. (Data from Nocturnal Oxygen Therapy Trial Group. Continuous or nocturnal oxygen therapy in hypoxemic chronic obstructive lung disease. Ann Intern Med 1980; 93:391–398 *and* Medical Research Council Working Party. Long-term domiciliary oxygen therapy in chronic hypoxic cor pulmonale complicating chronic bronchitis and emphysema. Lancet 1981; i:681–686.)

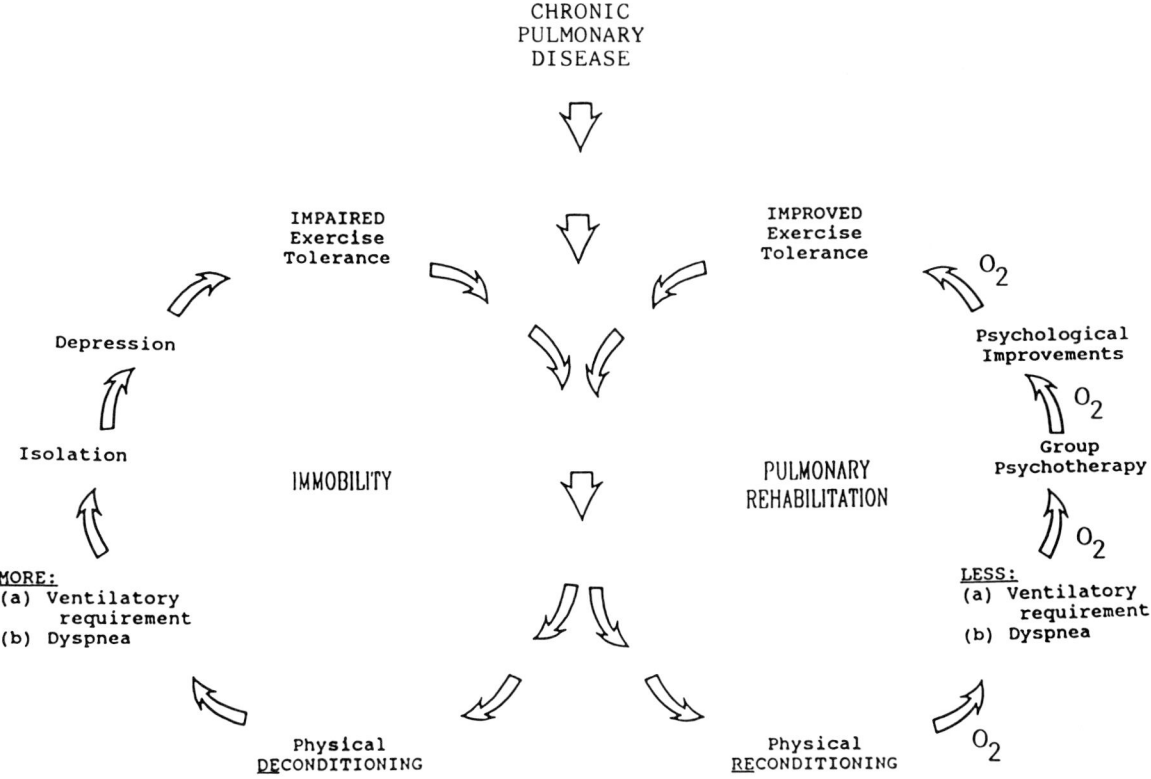

FIGURE 15-2. Diagram to show the "vicious cycle of chronic pulmonary disease" (*left side*), whereby immobility leads to physical deconditioning, worsening symptoms, social isolation, and further impairment of exercise tolerance. Conversely, the "favorable cycle of pulmonary rehabilitation" (*right side*) leads to physical reconditioning, improvement of symptoms, psychologic benefits, and progressive improvement in exercise tolerance.

the greater survival rate of the COT group was striking. This observation raises the possibility that the additional benefit observed in the COT group was a result of the provision of portable or ambulatory oxygen therapy. The importance of ambulatory capability in LTOT has always been recognized in the United States.[16] This is not to say that stationary oxygen sources are not beneficial, but they do not by themselves produce the most desirable outcome in the rehabilitation of chronically hypoxemic patients. LTOT should be considered in the overall context of comprehensive care programs for chronic hypoxemic lung disease patients. In other words, it should be regarded as an integral component of pulmonary rehabilitation. Figure 15-2 shows the vicious circle of immobility and physical deconditioning in chronic lung disease. Although fixed oxygen sources correct hypoxemia, they do not necessarily break this vicious circle because they encourage immobility and prevent physical reconditioning.

PHYSIOLOGIC MECHANISMS OF OXYGEN THERAPY

The rationale for oxygen therapy is based on our understanding of the pathophysiology of hypoxia and hypoxemia. Correction of hypoxia preserves vital organ functions. PaO_2 is determined primarily by three factors: (1) the fractional concentration of inspired oxygen (FIO_2), (2) alveolar ventilation ($\dot{V}A$), and (3) ventilation/perfusion ($\dot{V}/\dot{Q}$) relationships. Hypoxemia therefore occurs at high altitude when FIO_2 is reduced, in the presence of alveolar hypoventilation, and with abnormalities of $\dot{V}/\dot{Q}$ distribution that are associated with various pulmonary and cardiac diseases. Oxygen therapy effectively raises FIO_2. However, the increase in PaO_2 that occurs is highly dependent on the degree of ventilation/perfusion inequality; for example, it is maximum when venous admixture is least and becomes negligible when shunt or venous admixture approaches 50% of the cardiac output. Several factors may lessen the increase in PaO_2 that can be anticipated from oxygen therapy. These factors include absorption atelectasis and the reversal of hypoxic pulmonary vasoconstriction, both of which might worsen $\dot{V}/\dot{Q}$ imbalance and also a decrease in ventilation. PaO_2 is one of the important determinants of tissue oxygen delivery, but oxygen transport to metabolizing tissues necessitates the integrated actions of the respiratory, cardiovascular, and hematologic systems. Oxygen delivery to tissues is therefore also dependent on cardiac output and individual organ perfusion or capillarity. The oxygen-carrying capacity of the blood is determined by the hemoglobin concentration and hemoglobin affinity for oxygen, which in turn is influenced by pH, PCO_2, and erythrocyte levels of 2,3-diphosphoglycerate. Oxygen-carrying capacity is reduced in the presence of elevated levels of carboxyhemoglobin.

In considering the physiologic effects of oxygen therapy, it is necessary to examine each component of this integrated system. Most studies have been performed using subjects with COPD because they constitute the majority of patients with chronic hypoxemia. Many of the responses to oxygen therapy that COPD patients demonstrate can be assumed to apply to patients with other chronic pulmonary diseases. The physiologic effects of oxygen therapy are subdivided into alterations of ventilation, respiratory system mechanics, hemodynamics, tissue oxygenation, neuropsychiatric function, prognosis, and survival. Effects of oxygen on respiratory sensation are considered later in this chapter.

Ventilation

Generally, investigators have found that oxygen has no effect on resting ventilation in patients with COPD.[17-21] During exercise, ventilation was found to be reduced at submaximum work rates. Cotes and associates[18] showed a ventilation reduction of 26% when patients breathed 66% oxygen, whereas Pierce and colleagues[22] found a reduction of 25% when their subjects breathed 40% oxygen. In the study by Pierce and colleagues,[22] this reduction in ventilation was associated with hypercapnia during exercise. A reduction in submaximum ventilation has also been demonstrated in patients with restrictive lung disease who breathed 60% oxygen.[23] Reductions in ventilation are usually associated with a decrease in respiratory rate.[24, 25] Pierce and colleagues[22] showed a decrease in respiratory rate of 23%. Certain studies have suggested that the reduction in ventilation and respiratory rate is caused by diminished ventilatory drive.[20, 26] Grassino and coworkers[26] showed a reduction in airway occlusion pressure ($P_{0.1}$) and mean inspiratory flow rate (V_T/T_I) but not in respiratory rate and breathing cycle pattern. Scano and associates[20] also showed a reduction in $P_{0.1}$ and V_T/T_I.

Mechanics of the Respiratory System

Oxygen therapy is associated with a reduction in airways resistance.[27] In the study of Scano and associates,[22] minute ventilation ($\dot{V}_E$) and mean inspiratory flow rate were related to $P_{0.1}$ (as an index of ventilatory drive). Both were reduced for a given value of $P_{0.1}$, suggesting improvement in the impedance of the respiratory system. Several studies have demonstrated an increase in the ratio of dead space to tidal volume (V_{DS}/V_T).[21, 28, 29] Lee and Read[28] suggested that this change was caused by the reversal of hypoxic pulmonary vasoconstriction, which results in abnormally low $\dot{V}/\dot{Q}$ areas. However, these investigators used 100% oxygen and, therefore, their findings could also be explained by atelectasis. Rebuck and Vandenberg[29] correlated the decrease in V_{DS}/V_T with a decrease in P_{PA}. Several investigators have attempted to correlate the improvement in exercise tolerance observed when patients breathe oxygen with reduced mechanical demands on the respiratory muscles.[22, 30-33] In normal subjects, Bye and colleagues[30] demonstrated that breathing 40% oxygen reduced ventilation and electromyographic signs of diaphragm fatigue. These changes were accompanied by a reduction in ratings of perceived exertion. In eight patients with COPD, oxygen therapy was also shown to postpone electromyographic signs of diaphragm fatigue and paradoxical abdominal movements.[25]

Hemodynamic Effects

When oxygen is administered to normal subjects, a decrease in heart rate is observed. Cotes and associates[18] demonstrated similar changes in subjects with COPD. Selinger and coworkers[34] showed an increase in heart rate when LTOT was discontinued in a similar group of COPD patients. The decrease in heart rate is associated with a reduction in cardiac output.[18, 35] The effects of oxygen on left ventricular ejection fraction are uncertain. Some investigators could not demonstrate changes in this parameter.[21, 36] However, Ashutosh and associates[13] showed that left ventricular ejection fraction increased in some COPD patients who demonstrated a decrease in P_{PA} greater than 5 mm Hg when breathing 28% oxygen. Morrison and colleagues[37] showed improvement in right ventricular ejection fraction in 12 COPD subjects after these subjects breathed oxygen via nasal cannulas for 3 weeks.

The acute administration of oxygen is well known to cause a decrease in P_{PA}.[5] Abraham and coworkers[38] demonstrated this decrease in their subjects after 24 hours of 28% oxygen therapy and after 20 minutes of 100% oxygen therapy. Conversely, terminating oxygen therapy for COPD patients caused an increase in mean P_{PA} from 30 to 35 mm Hg.[34] P_{PA} decreases with acute administration of oxygen,[4, 5, 39, 40] presumably as a result of the elimination of pulmonary vasoconstriction.[38] Weitzenblum and associates[41] demonstrated that the progressive increase in P_{PA} in COPD is reversed by LTOT. They studied 16 patients using repeated pulmonary artery catheterization. The first measurements were recorded on average 47 months before LTOT, the second measurements were taken just prior to the commencement of LTOT, and the third measurements were recorded after an average of 31 months of treatment. A sustained decrease in P_{PA} has also been reported by other investigators.[5, 9, 11, 40, 42] Fletcher and Levin[43] demonstrated that oxygen therapy also eliminated nocturnal decreases in arterial oxygen saturation (SaO_2), resulting in lower overnight P_{PA}. The absence of pulmonary vasodilatation in response to increased FIO_2 has been associated with worse prognosis in COPD,[36] whereas Ashutosh and associates[13] demonstrated that a decrease in P_{PA} greater than 5 mm Hg was associated with better prognosis in COPD.

Tissue Oxygenation

In normal subjects who exercise at a given work rate, hypoxia is associated with higher $\dot{V}_E$ and blood lactate levels.[44] Stein and colleagues[31] compared arterial lactate levels in patients with COPD who breathed room air and oxygen. Oxygen therapy reduced arterial lactate level, carbon dioxide output, and $\dot{V}E$. Similar reductions in blood lactate level have been shown in patients with restrictive lung disease.[23] Reduction in metabolic acidosis associated with exercise might reflect improved oxygen delivery to tissues. Oxygen therapy increased oxygen delivery in two studies.[37, 45] This was shown to be due to an increase in arterial oxygen content. In the study by Degaute and coworkers,[45] some subjects did not demonstrate improved oxygen delivery because of a concomitant decrease in cardiac output. This was also demonstrated in the study of Corriveau and associates.[35] Selinger and coworkers[34] showed that withdrawal from LTOT led to a reduction in oxygen delivery and a decrease in mixed venous oxygen tension ($P\bar{v}O_2$).

Neuropsychiatric Function

Many hypoxemic COPD patients have impairment in cerebral function in addition to their pulmonary and cardiovascular abnormalities. Early in the 1970s, the findings of two short-term studies demonstrated improved neuropsychologic functioning in COPD patients when they were breathing oxygen as compared with baseline observations made when they were breathing air.[46, 47] It is not clear from these reports whether the changes represented a temporary effect or a more stable improvement in brain function. As part of the NOT trial, 150 hypoxemic patients with COPD were given detailed neuropsychologic and life quality examinations before and after 6 months of supplemental oxygen treatment. Assessments before and after the treatment period were conducted while the patients were breathing air. Forty-two per cent of patients showed some neuropsychiatric improvement after 6 months of therapy, although they reported little change in their emotional status or quality of life.[48] These findings suggest that correction of tissue hypoxia may be important in producing selective psychologic benefits, particularly in the area of cognitive functioning in patients with hypoxemic COPD.

Hematologic Effects

Several studies have demonstrated the reversal of secondary polycythemia by LTOT.[4, 6, 10, 11, 44, 47] One study of COPD patients demonstrated improved platelet survival time with oxygen therapy.[50]

OXYGEN THERAPY IN PULMONARY REHABILITATION

The systematic investigation of oxygen therapy in pulmonary rehabilitation began in the 1950s.[3, 51] Cotes and Gilson[3] reported lower levels of ventilation in patients with chronic ventilatory insufficiency and advocated portable and domiciliary oxygen prescription. Barach, in one of his many studies,[51] was the first to report improvement of dyspnea with the use of a lightweight oxygen cylinder. Woolf and Suero[52] reported the successful use of oxygen to enable patients to participate in a program of pulmonary rehabilitation (patients were unable to enter the program if they breathed room air alone). Despite the potential for combined benefits from oxygen and physical exercise, only one study has attempted systematically to investigate oxygen in this context.[53] The investigators of this study compared the effects of portable liquid oxygen with those of liquid air during a 5-week program of physical training. Their patients had previously participated in a longer program of pulmonary rehabilitation. When exercise testing was performed while patients breathed room air, PaO_2 and heart rate at rest were lower in the group that had trained with oxygen. However, no benefits were demonstrated in terms of ventilation and dyspnea or of subjective assessments of activity. Patients reported improvements whether they used compressed air or oxygen, providing one of the earlier demonstrations of a placebo effect. In this section, the role of oxygen therapy in pulmonary rehabilitation is considered with regard to (1) its potential for improving exercise tolerance and (2) its effects on symptoms of disability.

Exercise Tolerance

Numerous studies have demonstrated improvements in exercise tolerance in hypoxemic patients when they breathe oxygen at various concentrations compared to when they breathe room air. Improvements have also been demonstrated in normoxic patients who show desaturation during exercise. Several studies have demonstrated increased exercise endurance times in COPD patients breathing oxygen.[3, 31, 32, 47, 54–57] Other studies have demonstrated improved exercise tolerance in patients with restrictive lung disease[23] and cystic fibrosis.[58] Generally, these studies have demonstrated a reduction in submaximum exercise ventilation. The effect of oxygen on maximum exercise capacity is unclear. Some investigators have reported increases in maximum work rate or maximum oxygen uptake ($\dot{V}O_2$max),[31, 32, 59] whereas others have reported no change.[23, 54, 55, 58] Leggett and Flenley[60] reported that the additional work of carrying portable oxygen equipment offset the benefit of the oxygen therapy. The study by Davidson and colleagues[57] compared portable oxygen therapy with compressed air use (both in portable cylinders) and showed that there was benefit from oxygen therapy despite the additional load of carrying the apparatus. The same study showed that this benefit increased with an increase in oxygen flows. Other investigators have shown that lower concentrations of inspired oxygen were equally effective. Cotes and Gilson[3] showed that 30% oxygen was equally effective as 50% or 100% oxygen. In contrast, Longo and coworkers[61] found no improvement in exercise tolerance with oxygen therapy at 2 or 4 L/min in 27 COPD patients with mild hypoxemia.

One of the challenges of oxygen therapy with exercise is the identification of those patients who will benefit. Davidson and colleagues[57] showed that the benefits of oxygen therapy were not related to spirometric measures or to initial exercise capacity. However, the increase in exercise endurance was inversely correlated with the gas transfer coefficient (D_{LCO}/V_A). Other investigators have attempted to link the improvements associated with oxygen therapy to the elimination of exercise-related desaturation.[23, 55, 60–62] In COPD patients, no such correlation has been found. However, in patients with restrictive lung disease, the increased exercise endurance time they obtained when breathing oxygen correlated with the decrease in SaO_2 produced by exercising while breathing room air.[23] Further studies of the physiologic effects of oxygen and exercise in combination are required to answer these questions.

Symptomatic Improvements

Oxygen therapy is likely to have an important physiologic effect on peripheral chemoreceptor drive. Reduced carotid body activation, resulting from an increase in PaO_2, is suggested as an important mechanism in reducing dyspnea both in normal subjects[63, 64] and in patients with COPD.[65] Conversely, almitrine bismesylate, a carotid body stimulant, increases ventilation and dyspnea and usually improves PaO_2 owing to more homogeneous $\dot{V}/\dot{Q}$ matching.[66] Several studies have examined the effects of oxygen therapy on dyspnea. Barach[51] showed that there is reduced dyspnea with the use of lightweight oxygen cylinders. Woodcock and coworkers[62] demonstrated reduced dyspnea in emphysematous patients who used portable oxygen equipment. Similar effects were shown in patients with restrictive lung disease.[23] Swinburn and associates[56] showed that there was less dyspnea at a given work rate in five patients breathing oxygen who had demonstrated desaturation during exercise.

The study of Lilker and colleagues[53] did not demonstrate a change in dyspnea or subjective improvements that could be related to oxygen. Conversely, patients felt better whether they used either portable compressed air or oxygen, demonstrating an important placebo effect. The placebo effect of oxygen may account for about 50% of its apparent benefits.[67] Figure 15–3 shows reductions in dyspnea reported by Davidson and colleagues[57]; they demonstrated that higher oxygen flows resulted in greater reductions in dyspnea early in exercise.

Whenever oxygen is prescribed for the alleviation of dyspnea, then benefit should first be demonstrated using objective physiologic measurements. Other symptomatic benefits are less easy to quantitate. Improvements in perceived exertion might relate to the neuropsychiatric benefits already described. The contribution of better oxygenation to increased motivation, a greater willingness to exercise, and the alleviation of depression are factors that are not yet fully elucidated.

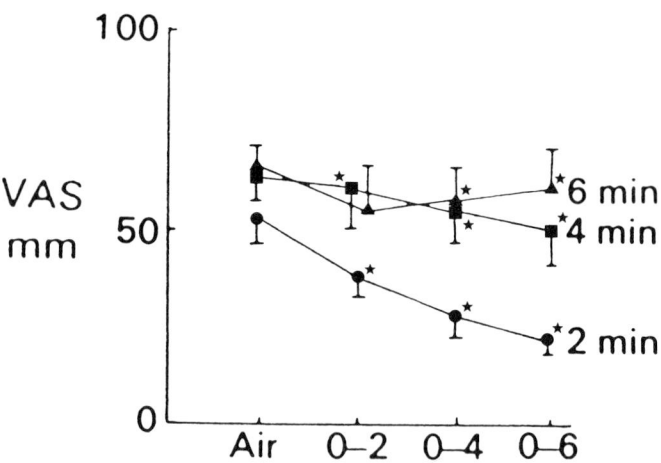

FIGURE 15–3. Visual analog scores (VAS) for breathlessness in 17 COPD subjects after 2, 4, and 6 minutes of constant load exercise on a bicycle ergometer while breathing either air or supplemental oxygen at flows of 2 (0–2), 4 (0–4), or 6 (0–6) L/min. The reductions in breathlessness were greatest after 2 minutes and with increasing oxygen flows (*star*: $P<.05$ compared with air). (Modified from Davidson AC, Leach R, George RJD, et al. Supplemental oxygen and exercise ability in chronic obstructive airways disease. Thorax 1988; 43:965–971.)

CLINICAL INDICATIONS FOR OXYGEN PRESCRIPTION

LTOT is expensive, and therefore prescription should be based on sound clinical justification. Various countries, including the United States, have developed guidelines for the prescription of LTOT. However, the scientific basis for such treatment is not yet complete. Since there are different modes of oxygen supply and delivery, criteria should allow the physician sufficient latitude to choose an appropriate system for the individual patient. Adequate data for the efficacy of LTOT currently exist only for COPD patients, but most investigators believe that these data also apply to chronically hypoxemic patients with other lung diseases such as cystic fibrosis, pulmonary fibrosis secondary to interstitial pneumonitis or chronic granulomatous disease, and severe restrictive lung disease (e.g., kyphoscoliosis).

Prescription of LTOT is based primarily on the patient's demonstration of chronic hypoxemia while he or she breathes room air at sea level. Arterial blood gas analysis is desirable, but criteria based on pulse oximetry have also been utilized. PaO_2 is often unstable because it depends not only on the clinical state of the patient but also on the degree of hyperventilation, which influences PaO_2 by its effects on alveolar PCO_2.

Expected Prevalence of Chronic Hypoxemia

A community survey performed in 1985 in Sheffield, England, predicted that 0.3% of the population had chronic hypoxemia sufficient to justify the prescription of LTOT based on existing criteria in the United Kingdom.[68] This estimate means that 60,000 patients require

LTOT in England and Wales and 750,000 require such treatment in the United States. If these estimates are accurate and the selection criteria on which they are based are accepted as appropriate, then these figures suggest that LTOT is considerably underprescribed in the United Kingdom, whereas in the United States the majority of suitable patients are being treated.

Prescription Criteria

Strict criteria for the prescription of LTOT have now been published in several countries. In the United States, LTOT prescription is largely based on recommendations from two conferences on home oxygen therapy held in Denver, Colorado, in 1986 and 1988.[16, 69] The criteria have been reviewed, and those currently applicable are shown in Table 15–1. Prescription of LTOT requires the physician to complete a Certificate of Medical Necessity that demonstrates appropriate levels of PaO_2 or SaO_2. Consideration is given to the fact that some patients with PaO_2 above 55 mm Hg may have evidence of hypoxic organ dysfunction; therefore, patients with PaO_2 up to 59 mm Hg and with certain clinical features (shown in Table 15–1) are also eligible for LTOT. Prescribing practices for LTOT are strongly influenced by political and economic factors. Current mechanisms of reimbursement are based on oxygen flow requirements and therefore discourage the prescription of oxygen-conserving devices. Also, no provision is made for the treatment of patients with unstable hypoxemia. A third Oxygen Consensus Conference held in Washington D.C. in March 1990[70] has recommended modifications to the existing Health Care Financing Administration regulations that would address these particular problems.

In the United Kingdom, LTOT is prescribed entirely under the jurisdiction of the National Health Service. The prescription criteria include spirometric values and the need to demonstrate clinical stability. There is provision for the prescription of palliative oxygen therapy to patients in special circumstances; these patients might not necessarily be hypoxemic.[71] Current arrangements for the provision of LTOT in the United Kingdom encourage the use of oxygen concentrators and overlook the importance of ambulatory oxygen therapy. There has been an attempt to unify European guidelines for the prescription of LTOT.[72] The criteria were not well defined but are essentially similar to those that apply in the United States. In Sweden, 33% of LTOT patients have pulmonary diseases other than COPD.[73]

The Thoracic Society of Australia has also issued guidelines for LTOT.[74] They include provision for the prescription of oxygen to patients who demonstrate desaturation during exercise and also to patients with refractory dyspnea associated with cardiac failure. A survey in New South Wales reported that 76% of patients receiving LTOT had COPD.[75] These investigators also demonstrated that cost reductions of the LTOT service could be achieved by rationalization and central administration.

Clinical Stability

Ever since the recruitment of patients for the NOT trial,[10] it has been appreciated that many patients show spontaneous improvement in PaO_2 regardless of oxygen prescription. Timms and coworkers[76] reported that 45% of patients initially screened for the NOT trial were no longer eligible to be included after 4 weeks because of an increase in their PaO_2 to greater than 55 mm Hg. Other investigators have made similar observations.[77, 78] In the study of Levi-Valensi and associates,[77] 30% of stable hypoxemic patients judged to be suitable for LTOT demonstrated an increase in PaO_2 to above 59 mm Hg after 3 months of prospective study without oxygen use. It was not possible to predict which patients would demonstrate this improvement. Appreciation of spontaneous improvement in PaO_2 is important, but the implications for the prescription of LTOT have yet to be clearly defined. O'Donohue[78] reported an improvement in PaO_2 during transtracheal oxygen therapy and suggested that this might be a beneficial effect of the oxygen therapy rather than a spontaneous alteration of the underlying clinical state. Variation in PaO_2 is important in the context of prescribing LTOT, and specific mechanisms to explain the observed increases in PaO_2 need further investigation.

Efficacy

When LTOT is prescribed, it is essential to confirm an adequate increase in PaO_2. Figure 15–4 shows the

---

TABLE 15–1. PRESCRIBING CRITERIA FOR LONG-TERM OXYGEN THERAPY

United States: CMN Form HCFA-484
1. $PaO_2 \leq 55$ mm Hg or
   $SaO_2 \leq 88\%$ (breathing room air)
2. $PaO_2 \leq 59$ mm Hg and evidence of at least one of the following: pulmonary hypertension (P wave > 3 mm in leads II, III, or aVF), cor pulmonale (dependent edema), or erythrocytosis (Hct >56%)

Annual update of CMN required for patients meeting criteria of 1. Revised CMN required after 3 months for patients meeting criteria of 2.

United Kingdom: DHSS Drug Tariff, 1986[71]
1. Absolute indications: COPD ($FEV_1 < 1.5$ L, FVC < 2.0 L); hypoxemia ($PaO_2 < 55$ mm Hg); hypercapnia ($PaCO_2 > 45$ mm Hg); and edema. Stability demonstrated over 3 wk
2. As in 1., but without edema or $PaCO_2 > 45$ mm Hg
3. Palliative therapy may be prescribed

Europe: Report of a SEP Task Group, 1989[72]
1. $PaO_2 < 55$ mm Hg; "steady-state COPD"
2. PaO_2 55–65 mm Hg with additional features as on United States CMN Form HCFA-484
3. Restrictive disease with $PaO_2 < 55$ mm Hg

Australia: Thoracic Society of Australia, 1985[74]
1. $PaO_2 < 56$ mm Hg, COPD, RVH, polycythemia, and edema
2. Desaturation < 90% on exercise
3. Refractory dyspnea associated with cardiac failure

Key: CMN: Certificate of Medical Necessity; RVH: right ventricular hypertrophy; Hct: hematocrit; DHSS: Department of Health and Social Security; FVC: forced vital capacity; SEP: European Society of Pneumology.

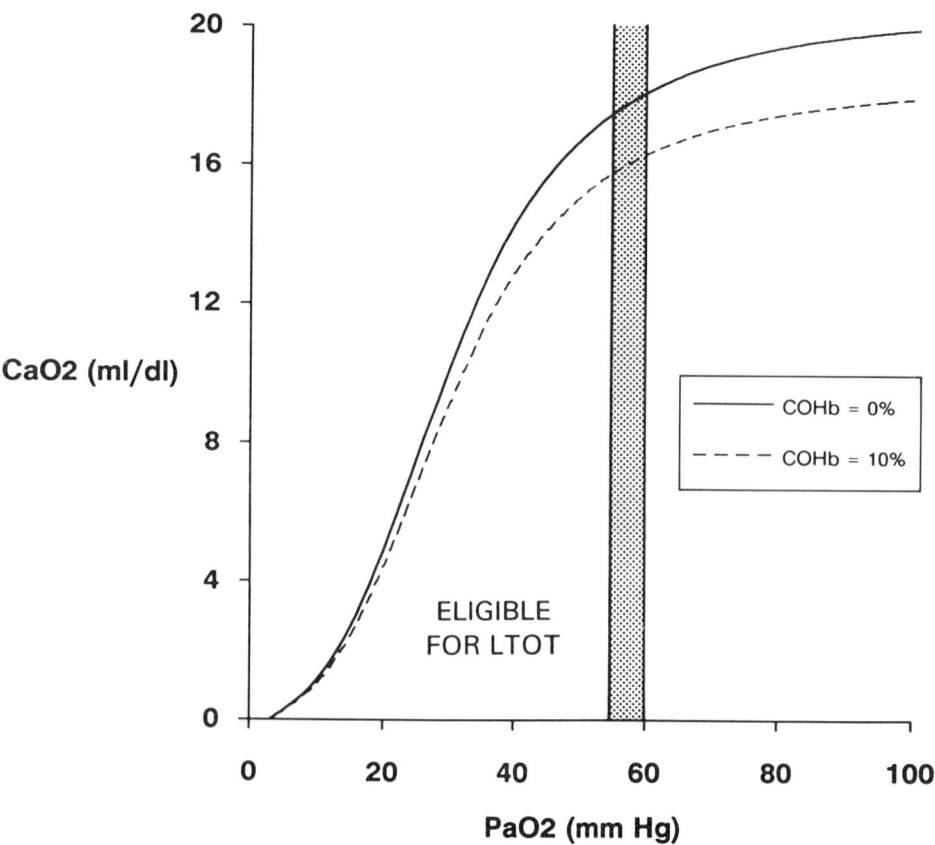

FIGURE 15–4. Relationship between arterial oxygen content (CaO_2) and PaO_2 assuming normal adult hemoglobin at a concentration of 15 g/dl, $PaCO_2$ at 40 mm Hg, and HCO_3 at 25 mEq/L. According to current prescribing criteria in the United States, subjects falling to the left of the *shaded area* are eligible for long-term oxygen therapy (LTOT). Those within the *shaded area* are eligible if they meet the additional clinical criteria shown in Table 15–1. CaO_2 is reduced by the presence of carboxyhemoglobin (COHb).

relationship between arterial oxygen content and PaO_2. Owing to the sigmoidal shape of this relationship, it is apparent that oxyhemoglobin saturation is almost complete when PaO_2 is greater than 80 mm Hg. In the treatment of chronically hypoxemic patients, an adequate arterial oxygen content is generally achieved above this level of PaO_2, assuming that the patient does not have anemia or an unduly high carboxyhemoglobin level. Usually, the amount of oxygen therapy can be adjusted to suit individual needs and to obtain a PaO_2 greater than 80 mm Hg. It is also important to demonstrate that oxygen therapy does not provoke excessive hypercapnia.[79] Adequate oxygenation is usually achieved with flows of 1 to 3 L/min through nasal cannulas.[76]

Tobacco Smoking

Patients receiving LTOT are usually discouraged from continuing smoking. Yet, studies have shown that 8 to 10% of these patients continue to smoke.[73, 80]

Oxygen Therapy in Special Situations

Current prescribing criteria in the United States also make provision for patients with hypoxemia during exercise or sleep. Normally, it is necessary to increase oxygen flow by 1 L/min during exercise or during sleep when worsening hypoxemia has been demonstrated to occur. A portable oxygen system is recommended if PaO_2 falls below 55 mm Hg during exercise.[16] Hypoxemia during sleep is now recognized in patients with COPD,[81, 82] kyphoscoliosis,[83] cystic fibrosis,[84] and interstitial lung disease.[30] Nocturnal decreases in SaO_2 are associated with increased PPA,[43, 85] leading some investigators to speculate that these hemodynamic disturbances might contribute to cor pulmonale.[86] Patients who are demonstrated to have nocturnal desaturation show abnormal hemodynamic responses to exercise.[87] Nocturnal oxygen therapy improves overnight PaO_2 without causing an adverse or unacceptable increase in $PaCO_2$.[88] Furthermore, nocturnal oxygen supplementation eliminates nocturnal desaturation and normalizes PPA.[43, 85]

Special considerations are required for hypoxemic patients who travel by air. Although usual cruising altitudes of commercial aircraft are higher than 30,000 feet, most domestic aircraft cabins are pressurized to be equivalent to an altitude of only about 8000 feet. Normal subjects and patients can expect a fall in PaO_2 between 16 and 32 mm Hg at this altitude. Patients with chronic hypoxemia who are already receiving LTOT or those with borderline hypoxemia need careful evaluation before traveling by air. One approach is use of the Hypoxia-Altitude Simulation Test.[89] COPD patients with a resting PaO_2 less than 72 mm Hg while breathing room air are likely to have a decrease in PaO_2 to less than 50 mm Hg while breathing 15% oxygen, which simulates an altitude of 8000 feet.[89] Patients with PaO_2 values below these thresholds should be recommended for supplemental oxygen during their flight. Airline travel is certainly inadvisable for any chronically hypoxemic patient whose clinical condition is unstable.

Adherence to Guidelines

Several studies in the United Kingdom have examined the appropriateness of oxygen therapy prescribing practices in relation to the published guidelines. The results were generally disappointing. They showed that only 43 to 54% of patients fulfilled the criteria.[90, 91] Between 26 and 44% of patients were not monitored by a pulmonary specialist.[90-92] Furthermore, patients were often elderly and severely disabled, and many died soon after the initiation of LTOT.[80, 92] Closer adherence to guidelines is likely in the United States because of reimbursement regulations. Nonetheless, further investigation is required to challenge the effectiveness and appropriateness of current prescribing patterns.

EQUIPMENT FOR THE SUPPLY AND DELIVERY OF OXYGEN

Oxygen Supply

Many different types of apparatuses are available for the supply of oxygen in the domiciliary setting. One important principle should not be overlooked: if patients are to become mobile, oxygen therapy must be nonrestricting, and thus the equipment for oxygen supply must allow the patient to be ambulatory at least part of the time. Essentially, there are four sources of supply of domiciliary oxygen: compressed gas cylinders, liquid oxygen, molecular sieve oxygen concentrators, and newer membrane separators. Each is discussed in turn.

Compressed Gas Cylinders. Compressed gas cylinders have been the traditional source of oxygen supply. They are relatively inexpensive and release 100% oxygen up to high flow rates. Compressed gas cylinders store oxygen under high pressure (2000–3000 psi). The pressurized gas is regulated to about 50 psi before reaching the flow meter. Portable (i.e., small) compressed gas cylinders are generally heavier than portable liquid systems. Furthermore, portable oxygen cylinders have a very limited duration of supply and need frequent filling. Transfilling of high-pressure oxygen cylinders is discouraged in the home, and thus frequent deliveries may be required from the oxygen vendor. An H-size cylinder, weighing about 850 lb, serves as a useful stationary supply; it has a capacity of 6840 L and provides approximately 57 hours of oxygen therapy at a flow rate of 2 L/min. E-size and smaller cylinders are suitable for portable oxygen supply, particularly if they are made of aluminum. E-size cylinders weigh between 13 and 17 lb, contain 625 L of oxygen, and provide 5 hours of oxygen therapy at a flow rate of 2 L/min. The smallest available cylinders (C-size) contain only about 240 L of oxygen and provide a short duration of oxygen (about 2 hr) at 2 L/min (Table 15–2).

Liquid Oxygen Supply. The principal advantage of liquid oxygen systems is that they require smaller storage volume than pressurized gas (one liter of oxygen in liquid form is equivalent to about 860 L in the gas phase). A further advantage is that these systems are low-pressure systems. Liquid oxygen supply offers the best opportunities for portability and pulmonary rehabilitation to date. Portable units are generally lightweight (see Table 15–2) and are easily transfilled from larger stationary sources. Liquid oxygen, like compressed gas, provides 100% oxygen concentration at all flow rates. Liquid systems require periodic venting to atmosphere to prevent pressure build-up (an evaporative loss of about 1 lb of oxygen per day can be expected). The range of flows available with liquid systems is limited by the warming capacity of a unit and by its ability to evaporate gas from a liquid tank. Several systems that weigh about 9.5 to 11 lb and provide 8 to 9 hours of oxygen at a flow rate of 2 L/min are available. The smallest available unit weighs 6.5 lb and provides about 4 hours of oxygen at 2 L/min. Generally, liquid oxygen is more expensive than pressurized gas, but the additional costs are reasoned to be justified if the patients are capable and determined to make more than three trips out of the home each week.[93]

Molecular Sieve Oxygen Concentrators. Oxygen concentrators are currently the least expensive means of providing oxygen therapy. Their major disadvantage is that they are fixed units, that is, they depend on an electricity supply. Therefore, an alternative back-up system for the provision of oxygen is usually necessary. Molecular sieves usually incorporate two sieve beds containing zeolight (synthetic aluminum silicate), which is a compound capable of entrapping gas molecules according to their size and polarity. In general, these devices work by alternately using the sieve beds in a synchronized absorption/desorption fashion; separated oxygen is then stored in a separate accumulation tank. Molecular sieves concentrate oxygen to about 96%. Argon is also concentrated and comprises about 4% of the outflow. Clinical experience has now defined certain characteristics of molecular sieves that are worthy of comment. First, they are complex apparatuses with many moving parts that clearly require frequent maintenance to ensure proper functioning. Several groups of investigators have demonstrated a decrease in oxygen concentration when higher flow rates are used.[94-96] Currently, the only way to avoid this problem is to increase the size of the sieve beds. Several manufacturers now make molecular sieve concentrators that produce about 93% oxygen at a flow rate of 5 L/min. These devices generally weigh about 50 lb. There is an additional range of devices capable of producing 90 to 93% oxygen up to flow rates of about 3 L/min; these devices are somewhat lighter in weight because they have smaller sieve beds. Evidently, there is a limit to which the molecular sieves can be reduced in size without impairing the efficiency of the apparatus. Another concern is the significant decrease in outflow oxygen concentration with the increasing duration of service of the equipment.[97, 98] A French study[98] surveyed 2414 operational oxygen concentrators during 1 month in 1988.

TABLE 15–2. EQUIPMENT FOR OXYGEN SUPPLY

Apparatus	Weight (lb)	Capacity (L)	Performance
Cylinders			
H-size	150.0	6840	57.0 h at 2 L/min
G-size		3600	
F-size		1360	
E-size	17.0	680	5.0 h at 2 L/min
E-size (aluminum)	13.0	680	5.0 h at 2 L/min
E-size (Oxymatic)		680	40.0 h at 2 L/min
D-size		420	3.5 h at 2 L/min
D-size (Oxymatic)		420	3.5 h at 2 L/min
C-size		240	2.0 h at 2 L/min
C-size (aluminum)	10.0	240	2.0 h at 2 L/min
C-size (Oxymatic)		240	14.0 h at 2 L/min
Mini (Oxylite)	4.0		9.5 h at 2 L/min
Liquid			
Walker (Linde)	6.5		4.0 h at 2 L/min
C-1000 (Puritan Bennett)	7.5		8.5 h at 2 L/min
C-T (Puritan Bennett)	8.4		
OMS I (Pulsair)	7.5	400	10.0 h at 2 L/min
OMS II (Pulsair)	10.3	824	23.0 h at 2 L/min

Apparatus	Weight (lb)	Performance
Molecular sieves		
PVO2D (DeVilbiss)	46	93% O_2 at 3 L/min
MC44D (DeVilbiss)	48	90% O_2 at 5 L/min
H-300 (Healthdyne)	40	90% O_2 at 3 L/min
BX-5000 (Healthdyne)	53	90% O_2 at 5 L/min
DC-100* (Roman)	29	93% O_2 at 2 L/min
AC-300* (Roman)	34	93% O_2 at 3 L/min
Emperor (Roman)	49	93% O_2 at 5 L/min
Mobilaire III (Invacare)	51	94% O_2 at 3 L/min
Mobilaire V (Invacare)	54	94% O_2 at 5 L/min
Spirit (Kee-Ox)	46	93% O_2 at 3 L/min
Elite (Kee-Ox)	56	90% O_2 at 5 L/min
429a (Puritan Bennett)		92% O_2 at 4 L/min
590 (Puritan Bennett)		90% O_2 at 5 L/min
Membrane separators		
Oxycare	35	45% O_2 at 10 L/min
OE Plus (Gulfstream)	68	40% O_2 at 6 L/min

(Values of % O_2 are ± 3%.)
*Samsonite suitcase.

Their average oxygen output concentration was 92%, but a significant decrease was noted with increasing duration of service, even when the apparatuses were subjected to regular maintenance. Certain investigators[96, 97] have revealed serious malfunctions in a small proportion of cases. Clearly, molecular sieve oxygen concentrators require systematic technical checks in order to ensure good working order. One study implied that built-in flow devices may not be particularly accurate.[94] Newer models are now incorporating an oxygen concentration indicator that alerts the patient to decreasing oxygen concentration. Molecular sieves do not concentrate water vapor, and therefore humidification is usually necessary when high flows are required. The possibility of concentrating toxic gases, particularly in heavily polluted areas, also has to be considered; furthermore, industrial pollution is thought to contribute to premature exhaustion of the sieve beds.[97] Despite certain shortcomings, these oxygen concentrators have an obvious advantage in that no refilling is required. The greatest disadvantage of the oxygen concentrators at present is that they are fixed installations that limit a patients' physical activities. Therefore, oxygen concentrators are appropriate if patients are housebound and can only ambulate to a limited extent about the home. For patients for whom both ambulation and economy are concerns, the concentrator can be supplemented by a portable system such as an E-size cylinder with an oxygen conservation device.

Membrane Separator Oxygen Enrichers. An alternative system for concentrating oxygen from air uses a polyethylene membrane and a compressor to effect a differential separation of gases. Such membranes usually are permeable both to oxygen and water vapor, and therefore the outflow gas is adequately humidified. At present, this apparatus is capable of producing an oxygen concentration of about 45%. Nevertheless, a satisfactory increase in oxygen saturation (to over 91%) can be achieved in patients, taking account of the fact that the flow rate must be about three times greater than that used with a molecular sieve concentrator.[95] Membrane separators have certain technical advantages over molecular sieve concentrators. First, they have few moving parts (the only necessary servicing is replacement of the inlet filter). These devices are therefore ideal for rural areas, where back-up services are not easily provided. Also, there are economic advantages in low maintenance costs. Although membrane separators produce a lower oxygen concentration, their performance is consistent over a wide range of flow rates. The absence of the need for humidification offers another economic advantage and renders these systems ideal for transtracheal oxygen therapy in which mucosal drying is a particular problem. Membrane separators may therefore be ideal for this form of oxygen delivery. Membrane separators are much safer than molecular sieves from the point of view of fire hazard. Furthermore, they serve as bacterial filters, since the polyethylene membranes are an absolute barrier to foreign materials larger than individual molecules.

General Considerations Regarding the Installation of Equipment for Oxygen Therapy. Providers of durable medical equipment for domiciliary use should have trained staff who are capable of instructing patients in the proper use of their oxygen equipment. Continuing patient education is also important because chronic hypoxemia impairs memory and may lead to difficulties in operating the equipment. An ideal service would provide regular follow-up visits and a 24-hour emergency contact. It is also desirable that the vendor of oxygen equipment bill the third party payer for the equipment, thus relieving the patient of this responsibility.

Oxygen Delivery

Systems for the delivery of oxygen to the patient can generally be divided into those providing low flow and those providing high flow. With low-flow systems, the gas flow is less than the patient's inspiratory demand, and therefore a proportion of the inspirate is room air. High-flow systems exceed the patient's inspiratory demand, either because of the gas flow itself or through the entrainment of room air due to gas viscosity. In general, the provision of steady-flow oxygen is wasteful, since the major benefit of oxygen delivery is derived at the beginning of inspiration. A variety of devices are available for oxygen delivery. Traditional face masks and nasal cannulas are the most frequently encountered, but transtracheal oxygen therapy (TTOT) is increasing in popularity, and various oxygen-conserving devices may be used to improve efficiency. Each of these systems is considered in turn.

Face Masks. Using a tightly fitting face mask is one of the most effective means of oxygen delivery; however, it is far less well tolerated than are nasal cannulas.[99] Fixed-performance masks utilize a high oxygen flow that generally exceeds the peak inspiratory flow rate. These masks provide a constant, predetermined oxygen concentration but may be less reliable in breathless patients with abnormal patterns of breathing. Variable performance masks generally use lower flows and cannot provide a predictable oxygen concentration. Masks contain a reservoir of about 100 to 200 ml of gas, and with lower flows partial rebreathing is possible. Decreasing $\dot{V}E$ usually increases FIO_2 when variable performance masks are used. Variations in breathing pattern (i.e., in inspiratory flow rate) have also been shown to produce large variations in FIO_2.[100] Masks make eating, expectorating, and talking awkward. They operate best at higher flows and therefore are not especially reliable when an FIO_2 less than 35% is required.

Nasal Cannulas. Nasal cannulas are undoubtedly the most commonly used means of oxygen delivery. They are inexpensive and relatively comfortable and allow the patient to eat, sleep, talk, and expectorate. Surprisingly, the FIO_2 is independent of whether a patient breathes through his or her nose or mouth.[101] The elevation of FIO_2 above that of room air is modest even at higher flow rates via nasal cannulas (Table 15–3).[102–104] Nasal cannulas may produce dermatitis and mucosal drying; to some extent, these problems can be prevented by adequate humidification. Unlike with the use of face masks, carbon dioxide rebreathing does not occur. However, nasal cannulas are generally less efficient than face masks.

Transtracheal Oxygen Therapy. The direct introduction of oxygen flow into the trachea was first described by Heimlich.[105] The technique has gradually gained popularity over recent years, and several large groups of investigators have now reported their experience with its use.[106–108] TTOT has obvious cosmetic advantages in that it enhances a patient's personal image and thus helps him or her to avoid social isolation (Fig. 15–5). Furthermore, patients are more likely to be compliant with this therapy. Oxygen flow requirements are reduced, equipment is lighter, and mobility may be improved. The patient also has a better sense of taste and experiences better oxygenation. High patient acceptance overrides many of the potential problems with this mode of oxygen delivery. Christopher and colleagues[109] demonstrated that TTOT may be effective in hypoxemia, which is refractory to oxygen therapy via nasal cannulas or face masks. The same group of investigators[107] reported their experience in 100 patients treated over a 2-

TABLE 15–3. TRACHEAL FRACTION OF OXYGEN WITH NASAL CANNULAS

Flow (L/min)	Estimated FIO_2 (%)	Tracheal FO_2* (%)
1	24	22.7
2	28	24.3
3	32	25.0
4	36	26.3
5	40	
6	44	

*Data from Schacter EN, Littner MR, Luddy P, et al. Monitoring of oxygen delivery systems in clinical practice. Crit Care Med 1980; 8:405–409.

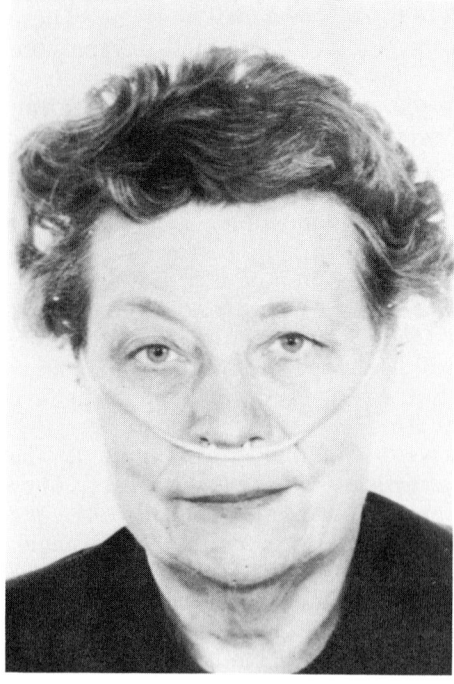 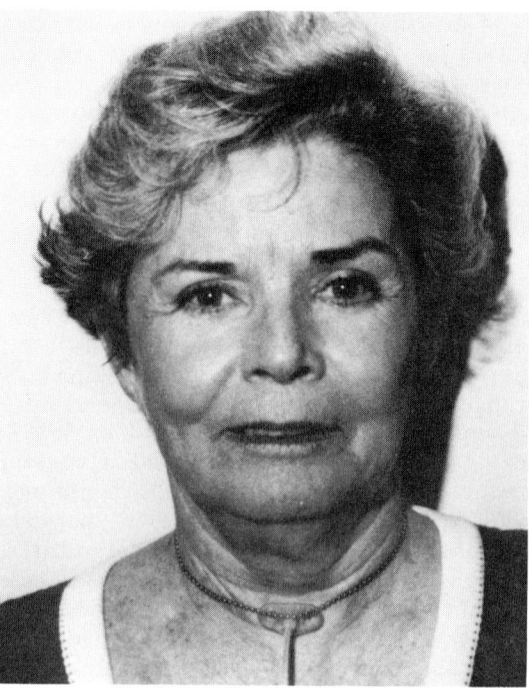

FIGURE 15–5. Photographs to illustrate the cosmetic advantage of transtracheal oxygen delivery (*right*) compared with the appearance of a patient using traditional nasal cannulas (*left*). Better patient acceptance is likely to be associated with improved compliance and greater physiologic benefits.

year period in Denver, Colorado. Overall patient acceptance was 96%. This group advocates a stenting technique that allows the minitracheostomy tract to become established. TTOT is delayed to reduce the incidence of subcutaneous emphysema. During the first 6 to 8 weeks, patients are taught to clean their transtracheal oxygen catheters in place using saline and special cleaning rods. Thereafter, the tracheostomy tract should be epithelialized, and patients can change their catheter twice daily without the need for guidewires. Another group[110] reported their experience with the Heimlich technique using 16-gauge angiocatheters. The formation of mucus balls was less likely with these narrower-gauge catheters, but a higher incidence of catheter failure was reported. Generally, TTOT reduces oxygen flow requirements by 25 to 55% compared with those of continuous flow therapy via nasal cannulas.[106–108, 110] Flow savings were observed in 97% of all patients. The trachea clearly acts as an anatomic reservoir that stores oxygen during the last part of exhalation. Flow requirements have also been demonstrated to be reduced during exercise.[107] Several investigators have reported an increased exercise tolerance in TTOT patients.[111–113] Reduction in dyspnea has also been reported.[106, 110, 111, 114, 115]

TTOT improves patient compliance[106] and is associated with symptomatic improvement[112] and improved quality of life.[109, 110] The study of Couser and Make[115] demonstrated that increasing TTOT flows caused a reduction of inspired volume at the mouth; this was largely due to a reduction in V_T. These investigators proposed that the bulk flow of oxygen into the trachea reduced the inspiratory volume and possibly reduced inspiratory muscle work as a result. Since the upper respiratory tract is bypassed in TTOT, humidification is required, especially at higher flow rates. In this setting, membrane separator oxygen concentrators may be particularly useful. One group[114] has described the use of tunneled tubing to form a totally implanted system for TTOT. The principal indications, disadvantages, and complications of TTOT are shown in Table 15–4. Larger series have shown overall complication rates between 8 and 12%.[106–108] TTOT is ideal for highly motivated and responsible patients who are capable of appropriate maintenance of the transtracheal catheter. A knowledgeable team of health care professionals is essential to provide patient training and follow-up care. Smaller series have reported greater problems[111] and difficulties

TABLE 15–4. INDICATIONS AND COMPLICATIONS OF TRANSTRACHEAL OXYGEN THERAPY

Complications of Therapy	Incidence (%)
Mucus balls (symptomatic)	25
Cough	5–15
Superficial infection	3–7
Subcutaneous emphysema	4–10
Catheter blockage	6.5
Catheter failure	3–4*
Catheter dislodgment	12–22
Reinsertion failure	3.5–7
Keloid	7
Hypercapnia	6
Late hemoptysis	2
Contact dermatitis	2
Bleeding	1–2
Bronchospasm	1–2
Cephalad catheter displacement	1–2
Pneumonia	1
Pneumomediastinum	1
Abscess	1
Cardiac dysrhythmia	1

*Incidence of catheter fracture requiring bronchoscopic extraction: 1–2%.

in establishing a new program.[116] The most common complication of TTOT is the formation of mucus balls, which is caused by the drying effects of oxygen, an increased amount of secretions, and poor patient adherence to catheter cleaning schedules. These problems are often transient, but serious airflow obstruction has been reported in three studies.[108, 116, 117] Hoarseness is a rare complication unless the cricothyroid membrane is punctured. At night, patients often inadvertently dislodge their catheters, and the minitracheostomy tract may close within 1 to 2 hours. The incidence of such lost tracts is reported to be from 7 to 33%.[107, 108, 116] Walsh and Govan[118] demonstrated a small increase in $Paco_2$ with TTOT, but this did not appear to have adverse clinical consequences. Overall, the complication rates from TTOT are low, although certain studies have shown that a high proportion of patients discontinue therapy.[118] Mortality rates were high in several reported studies,[108, 118] although deaths are usually reported to be related to underlying lung disease and are not a direct consequence of the TTOT. Clearly, the influence of TTOT is difficult to determine without painstaking, randomized controlled trials, and further investigation in this area is clearly warranted.

Reservoir Oxygen-Conserving Devices. Recognizing that the continuous flow of oxygen is inefficient, several conserving systems have been devised to maximize the delivery of oxygen at the beginning of inspiration. These systems include reservoir devices and demand or pulsed oxygen delivery. They have the potential for reducing the cost of domiciliary oxygen therapy by reducing oxygen flow requirements; this in turn reduces the size and weight of oxygen equipment. Two types of reservoirs are available for use with nasal cannulas. The mustache nasal cannula is a storage device with an internal diaphragm and a reservoir of about 20 ml in volume. The reservoir is filled with oxygen during the expiratory phase. On inspiration, the diaphragm collapses, providing a volume of oxygen at the beginning of the breath. During the remainder of inspiration, the diaphragm remains collapsed, and the reservoir functions as a conventional nasal cannula. This system was first described by Tiep and coworkers.[119] Using a similar device, Moore-Gillon and associates[120] measured transcutaneous Po_2 and Pco_2 and demonstrated an efficiency of 2:1 compared with that of standard nasal cannulas. Soffer and colleagues[121] showed oxygen flow savings of 75% at rest and of 50% during exercise. Carter and coworkers[122] demonstrated 3:1 savings during treadmill exercise. Clearly, the effectiveness of the mustache reservoir varies among individual patients, and this may reflect different degrees of mouth breathing.[95] The long-term efficacy of these devices has been questioned. Evans and associates[123] found some reduction in the improvement of Pao_2 after 1 hour of use. Disadvantages include an unsightly appearance that discourages patients from wearing the device in public or for prolonged periods. Claiborne and colleagues[124] showed that 43% of patients discontinued use of the device after only 1 month. The safe life span of this equipment is not yet established. The membrane must be replaced fairly frequently, and this has obvious cost implications.

Respiratory Phased Demand or Pulse Delivery. These systems deliver a fixed or variable volume of oxygen at the end of exhalation and during early inspiration (at a time when the inspired gas contributes most to blood oxygen saturation). This approach is increasing in popularity, and 11 manufacturers currently market this type of equipment. Only the first 25 to 50% of inspiratory time is devoted to alveolar filling, whereas the last one third of the inspired volume tends to enter dead space. Therefore, oxygen flow during the latter part of inspiration and throughout expiration is wasted (i.e., 60–70% of the cycle). The principle of pulsed oxygen delivery was first described by Cotes and Gilson.[3] The device that they first devised utilized an inhalation pressure detector. Then, in 1963, Cotes[125] described a "palm breathing device," which was triggered by the thumb. Pflug and coworkers[126] described an inspiratory system electrically actuated by chest wall motion that provided a 50% reduction in oxygen flow requirement. Modern systems are generally operated by thermistor detectors or pressure sensors. Electromechanical reliability must be carefully examined, and, ideally, a system should provide a fail-safe mechanism to deliver oxygen if the sensor fails. One obvious problem is that rapid, shallow breathing may cause near-continuous activation of the valve without oxygen conservation.[95] In general, pulsed oxygen delivery produces savings in oxygen flow requirements varying between 3:1 and 7:1.[127] Oxygen delivery needs to be increased during exercise,[127] but the efficiency of the system is still maintained.[128] Winter and associates[129] reported that lower flow requirements produced a similar Pao_2 in chronically hypoxemic patients.

Several devices that provide either variable pulse cycles or variable pulse volumes are commercially available. These devices generally operate at 20 to 50 psi. Some are suitable for attachment to hospital wall outputs, and others may be combined with portable systems that use compressed gas cylinders or liquid oxygen. The potential for oxygen flow savings increases the useful duration of portable oxygen systems to the point where patients may now enjoy adequate oxygen supply and delivery throughout the day, thus enabling them to revert toward normal physical activities. Pulsing devices represent a small additional weight to portable systems. Their long-term performance needs further investigation.[130] Attention also needs to be devoted to safety features. Adjustment of sensitivity settings is often inadequate; this leads to difficulties during sleep or activity. Internal batteries hold a limited charge and thus need frequent replacement. Humidification is usually not necessary with oxygen-pulsing devices because of the reduction in flow of dry oxygen gas. Furthermore, oxygen flow savings have obvious cost implications.

Innovative Combinations for the Supply and Delivery of Oxygen

In assessment of the currently available methods for the supply and delivery of oxygen, it appears that transtracheal oxygen administration is the least obtrusive and offers good patient compliance, but it is also the most invasive technique. In contrast, reservoir devices are the least expensive, simple, and reliable, but they are also the most obtrusive. Pulsing or demand oxygen flow is most efficacious but is often subject to mechanical failure.

Certain innovative combinations that offer a wider range of portability and durations of adequate oxygen flow are now emerging. Portable oxygen concentrators may soon become reality as a result of interesting developments in the area of membrane separators. Reduction in the size and weight of oxygen concentrators may also be facilitated by the addition of oxygen-conserving devices that improve the efficiency of oxygen delivery. Effective combinations of pulsed delivery devices and lightweight portable cylinders are now commercially available. One such system weighs only 5 lb and is claimed to be capable of delivering oxygen for 14 hours at a flow rate of 2 L/min. Pulsed TTOT has now been reported.[131, 132] Using this combination of techniques, flow savings are between 2:1 and 3:1, that is, they are similar to those described for other devices.

ASSESSMENT OF OXYGENATION

Detection of Hypoxemia

Hypoxemia is often difficult to detect based on clinical criteria because its manifestations are nonspecific and frequently difficult to distinguish from symptoms or signs of the underlying disease. Hemodynamic disturbances are generally mediated through adrenergic mechanisms that can be invoked in a variety of clinical circumstances. Neuropsychiatric features of hypoxemia range from mild confusion to coma. With lesser degrees of hypoxemia, the neurologic manifestations can be expected to be subtle. Cyanosis is not an especially reliable physical sign, especially when there is skin pigmentation. Nevertheless, cyanosis may be detected when concentrations of reduced hemoglobin reach about 1.5 g/dl. Cyanosis is absent in anemia and may be present in polycythemia even when there is normal SaO_2. An important distinction must be drawn between central cyanosis associated with pulmonary or cardiovascular pathology and peripheral cyanosis, which might be evident whenever peripheral circulation is sluggish or inadequate, for example in peripheral vascular disease or in hyperviscosity syndromes. Because physical examination is insufficient for confident assessment of oxygenation, it is necessary to rely on other forms of measurement.

Monitoring Oxygen Therapy

Tissue oxygenation is determined not only by PaO_2 but also by tissue perfusion and oxygen consumption. The goal of oxygen therapy is to improve tissue oxygenation by raising PaO_2. Effective oxygen therapy should restore normal tissue oxygenation without requiring an excessively high inspired oxygen concentration (i.e., FIO_2). Since PaO_2 is a vital factor in the assessment of tissue oxygenation, several methods are available for its measurement.

Arterial Blood Gas Analysis. Arterial blood can be sampled intermittently by arterial puncture or from an indwelling arterial catheter. In vitro blood gas analysis is the gold standard for the measurement of PaO_2. Laboratory technical errors can generally be reduced by proficiency testing in blood gas laboratories.[133] Complications of arterial puncture are uncommon, although pain and bruising occur in about 33% of patients, especially when needles larger than 23 gauge are used.

Methods of continuous intra-arterial PaO_2 measurement have been described.[134] These include polarographic oxygen cathodes, semipermeable membrane tips coupled to a mass spectrometer, and fiberoptic catheters that are sturdy and fast-responding. The future should witness further development and refinement of these methodologies. Prior to radial artery puncture, an Allen test should be performed to assess the adequacy of ulnar artery perfusion to the hand.

Ear or Finger Oximetry. Continuous measurement of SaO_2 can be achieved using pulse oximetry, which employs the principle that light transmission through an adequately perfused ear lobe or through finger pulp is directly proportional to the oxygen saturation of perfusing blood. Modern instruments use two wavelengths. Pulse oximeters are generally reliable for values of SaO_2 between 50 and 100%, provided that significant quantities of carboxyhemoglobin or bilirubin are not present.[135] Measurements are artificially low in the presence of jaundice and are artificially high if carboxyhemoglobin levels are greater than about 3%. Performance of these instruments is influenced by skin pigmentation, skin thickness, low tissue perfusion, and probe motion. Generally, they are accurate to within 2% of SaO_2, and their response time is adequate for most clinical purposes.[136] The obvious disadvantage of SaO_2 measurements is that PaO_2 must decrease to less than 60 mm Hg before appreciable decreases in SaO_2 occur, and therefore changes in PaO_2 above this threshold may be missed. Cutaneous oximetry also does not take account of pH or $PaCO_2$.

Transcutaneous Oxygen Tension. It is possible to measure transcutaneous PO_2 using heated polarographic electrodes maintained at 43 to 45°C. These electrodes contain an electrolyte solution that is in contact with the skin, which is covered by a Teflon membrane. The raised temperature is necessary to promote local hyperemia, but it also affects transcutaneous PO_2 by shifting the oxyhemoglobin saturation curve to the right. Also, it is necessary to change the site of a transcutaneous electrode about every 4 hours to avoid skin injury caused by the temperature of the electrode. Transcutaneous PO_2 reflects a balance between oxygen delivery to the skin and cutaneous oxygen consumption.[137] Transcutaneous PO_2 approximates the PO_2 of arterialized capillary blood and is on average 20 mm Hg lower than PaO_2.[138] This discrepancy is predictable and can be corrected. However, in certain clinical situations, there is a dissociation between transcutaneous Po_2 and Pao_2. These situations include critical hypotension[139] and peripheral vascular disease.[140, 141]

Several studies have attested to the accuracy and usefulness of transcutaneous Po_2 measurements in neonatal intensive care. However, technical problems and calibration difficulties may limit the usefulness of this technique for the routine clinical monitoring of adults. Errors occur with thicker skin and when veins encroach upon the field of the electrode. Further clinical experience in adults is needed to determine whether transcutaneous monitors will obviate the need for arterial blood gas analysis.

Tissue Oxygenation

Measurement of tissue or cellular Po_2 is technically feasible using microelectrode techniques. However, such measurement is unlikely to have clinical importance, since an individual tissue does not necessarily typify the body as a whole. Two approaches can be used to assess the overall adequacy of tissue oxygenation.

Mixed Venous Oxygen Tension. Several investigators have proposed the use of $P\bar{v}o_2$ to indicate mean tissue Po_2. The oxygen tension of a pulmonary artery blood sample provides an integrative value depending on Sao_2, hemoglobin, and cardiac output in relation to $\dot{V}o_2$. This is probably a reasonable assumption, but $P\bar{v}o_2$ is influenced by the contribution of blood leaving organs that have widely different oxygen consumptions. Low $P\bar{v}o_2$ indicates an overall problem with tissue oxygenation that is a result, for example, of increased tissue oxygen consumption during exercise or, alternatively, of reduced oxygen delivery. However, a normal $P\bar{v}o_2$ cannot be understood to mean normal tissue Po_2. There is no consensus as to what absolute value of $P\bar{v}o_2$ equates to an adequate tissue oxygenation. Certain organs may be critically hypoxic even though $P\bar{v}o_2$ gives an impression of adequate overall oxygenation.

Lactic Acidosis. An alternative approach to assess the adequacy of tissue oxygenation is to examine organ function and metabolic acid-base status. Both are reliable indicators of tissue hypoxia. The presence of lactic acidosis is evidence that tissue oxygen requirement exceeds oxygen delivery; this invokes anaerobic metabolic pathways. Bye and coworkers[23] have shown that the administration of oxygen reduces the lactic acidosis resulting from exercise, at least in patients with interstitial lung disease.

Summary

Various methods are available for the assessment of oxygenation. In clinical practice, pulse oximetry is readily available and reasonably reliable. In vitro arterial blood gas analysis remains the gold standard until other techniques prove themselves to be technically reliable and easily applicable in the clinical setting.

COMPLIANCE WITH OXYGEN THERAPY

The effectiveness of LTOT is crucially dependent on patient compliance. There are several factors that can potentially reduce patient compliance with oxygen therapy. Some patients do not perceive symptomatic improvement and are thus not convinced of the benefit of their oxygen treatment. Others are self-conscious about their appearance while carrying oxygen equipment or wearing an oxygen delivery device on the face. Others have unrealistic fears of danger from their equipment. Some patients are dissuaded from using adequate oxygen therapy because of its cost, and others are deterred because of the stigma of disability. The physician thus has an important role. Patient compliance can be improved with careful education that stresses the rehabilitative role of oxygen therapy in improving longevity and quality of life. Several studies conducted in Europe have evaluated patient compliance with LTOT. Carefully educated patients in the United Kingdom who were monitored in the hospital and in their own homes were found to be using their domiciliary oxygen for 14 to 15 hours per day.[97, 142] One study in France[143] showed that only 38% of patients followed their prescription and used their oxygen for more than 15 hours per day. Patients with worse hypoxia were generally more compliant. Another French study[144] demonstrated that patients invariably overestimate the daily duration of oxygen therapy that they have undergone. Patient compliance tends to improve with careful home monitoring.[90, 97, 144] Some studies have shown that significant numbers of patients (8–10%) continue to smoke while receiving LTOT.[73, 80]

Patient education dispels fears of danger from use of the equipment and lessens the stigma of disability. Improvements in apparatuses for oxygen delivery will lead to better cosmetic appearances and greater patient acceptance. Earlier prescription of LTOT will discourage the impression that oxygen is reserved for those with terminal illness. Close patient monitoring is essential either during hospital visits or during visits to the patients' homes.

ECONOMIC CONSIDERATIONS

About 800,000 patients currently receive LTOT in the United States. Comparing this figure with the estimated prevalence of chronic hypoxemia in the community, it would seem that appropriate numbers of patients are receiving LTOT based on the existing guidelines.[68] LTOT raises complex cost-benefit considerations. The study of Cooper and associates[15] demonstrated that life expectancy can be doubled by LTOT, but this finding implies that the earlier introduction of LTOT leads to greater benefit in terms of extra years of life. Each added life-year costs approximately the equivalent of 1 year's prescription of LTOT. Thus, the cost of an additional year of life is probably low when compared with that for the treatment of other severely debilitating diseases such as end-stage renal disease and severe hypertension. Duration of survival is important, but it is not the only aspect to be considered in the cost-benefit analysis of LTOT. Equally important is a patient's quality of life in terms of his or her ability to perform usual daily activities with satisfactory neuropsychiatric function. LTOT certainly leads to improvement in neuropsychiatric status.[48] Improvement in the ability to perform activities of daily living is probably only achieved when portable oxygen therapy is prescribed and when patients enjoy the combined benefits of oxygen and physical exercise. Occasionally, patients are able to return to work if they have sedentary occupations, but human productivity is a relatively minor component in this economic analysis.

The average costs of oxygen therapy vary considerably in different regions of the United States. Also, they vary according to the type of apparatus prescribed. At the present time, average costs for the rental of an oxygen concentrator range from $280 to $350 per month. The rental cost of liquid oxygen apparatuses for both stationary and portable supply ranges from $120 to $150 per month, but the actual cost of liquid oxygen is an additional $450 per month (assuming the patient consumes 2 L/min for 15 hr/day). The costs of oxygen supplied in compressed gas cylinders probably range from $500 to $1000 per month. The relative costs of refilling compressed gas cylinders are greater for the smaller portable apparatuses. Overall, these figures indicate that portable oxygen systems are generally more expensive, but their additional value in terms of physiologic benefits and of the reduction of other health care costs (e.g., hospitalization) has yet to be properly evaluated. The approximate cost comparisons indicate that one arterial blood gas analysis is equivalent to 1 to 2 days of oxygen therapy and that 1 day in the hospital is equivalent to about 1 month of oxygen therapy.

Reimbursement Issues

The economics of LTOT are largely influenced by legislation relating to reimbursement. In the United States, home oxygen therapy constitutes 45% of all costs of durable medical equipment. Usually, 80% of these costs are covered by insurance such as Medicare. In many other countries, systems of socialized medicine bear the full cost of the domiciliary oxygen service. Frequently, prescribing restrictions intended to contain costs seriously limit the development of an appropriate clinical service; as a result, deserving patients are denied the optimum benefits of oxygen therapy. United States legislation of 1987 (commonly called the "Six-Point Plan") provides less reimbursement for lower oxygen flow requirements and thus does not encourage the prescription of oxygen-conserving devices. Furthermore, reimbursement is not available for more than one oxygen supply system within the home; therefore, if a fixed installation such as an oxygen concentrator is covered, an additional back-up or portable system is not paid for. The cost of servicing oxygen concentrators is generally not covered, nor is the cost of electricity.

Generally, the cost of the oxygen itself represents only a small contribution to the overall costs of LTOT. It is hoped that future developments in the technology for oxygen supply and delivery together with more widespread use of oxygen-conserving techniques will lead to more economical LTOT service. Anomalies in reimbursement mechanisms must be addressed to facilitate more widespread prescription of oxygen-conserving devices and portable oxygen therapy. Portable oxygen therapy might eventually be proved to provide the greatest cost benefit. Also, the characteristics of those patients for whom the cost-benefit relationship is most favorable have yet to be identified.

COMPLICATIONS AND TOXICITY OF OXYGEN THERAPY

Scheel and Priestley both appreciated the potential toxic effects of oxygen at the time of its discovery. In 1785, Lavoissier noted congestion in the lungs of guinea pigs at autopsy after they had received oxygen therapy. The concept of oxygen toxicity was firmly established by Paul Bert in 1878. Hazards of modern oxygen therapy can be broadly divided into nonmedical (or physical) risks and medical (or clinical) complications.

Nonmedical Hazards

Despite the complexity of some oxygen equipment, patients generally adjust to using oxygen therapy in the home within a very short period of time.[145] However, the danger of burns must be considered. Although oxygen itself is neither explosive nor combustible, it does support combustion, and the higher the concentration of oxygen, the greater the burning speed and the temperature of the flame. Patients are at obvious risk of igniting plastic tubing and facial hair when they smoke cigarettes during oxygen therapy. Fire hazards are considerably reduced when lower concentrations of oxygen are used. West and Primeau[146] demonstrated that when plastic cannulas conduct 100% oxygen flowing at 2 L/min, they could ignite within 1 second and burn with a flame greater than 3000°C. In contrast, with 40% oxygen flowing at 2 L/min, cannulas were only scorched, and with higher flows the flame was self-extinguished. Leakage from high-pressure cylinders or evaporation from liquid reservoirs enhances the flammability of nearby combustible materials. When high-pressure cylinders (2400 psi) are stored close to sources of extreme heat, a pressure increase within the cylinders occurs. Safe storage is therefore essential. Also, oil and grease should not be allowed to contaminate valves, regulators, or connectors, since this increases the risk of combustion. Cylinders should be properly secured so that they can not tip over; they should also be transfilled with caution. Generally, patients do not transfill high-pressure cylinders within the home.

Liquid oxygen is safer in certain respects than pressurized gas, and with liquid oxygen systems fire hazards are negligible. Evaporation does not elevate room F_{IO_2} sufficiently to create a measurable change.[147] The boiling point of oxygen is $-297°$ F. Therefore, a risk of frostbite or cold burns from patient contact with metal tubing or connectors does exist. Liquid oxygen is stored in relatively low-pressure systems, and rupture usually leads to rapid decompression without risk of explosion.

Molecular sieve oxygen concentrators are generally quite safe, although the need for frequent preventive maintenance must be emphasized. Concentrators include various electrical components that are in close proximity to oxygen tanks and polyvinyl chloride tubing. Therefore, there is a small but potential fire hazard from such apparatuses. Membrane separators that produce lower oxygen concentrations are considerably safer. Furthermore, they produce a constant gas flow and contain no electrical relays, valves, or oxygen storage tanks; these factors minimize any fire risk.

Pulmonary Oxygen Toxicity

Inhalation of high concentrations of oxygen causes a variety of clinical problems. These include acute tracheobronchitis, bronchopulmonary dysplasia, and pathophysiologic changes that are most consistent with the adult respiratory distress syndrome. When normal subjects breathe 100% oxygen for a few hours, they typically develop substernal burning and impaired mucociliary clearance. These symptoms rapidly resolve when room air is breathed. Bronchopulmonary dysplasia is usually encountered in neonates; however, an adult equivalent characterized by fibroblastic and epithelial cell proliferation has been described.

Of greatest concern in prolonged oxygen therapy is the possibility of parenchymal injury in the lung. A precise safety threshold to prevent such injury has not been established. Normal subjects who breathe 100% oxygen produce symptoms at 24 hours, whereas if they breathe 50% oxygen or less for up to 7 days they do not seem to develop clinically significant lung impairment. Parenchymal pulmonary oxygen toxicity is possible with LTOT.[148] Fifty per cent of COPD patients receiving LTOT for between 7 and 61 months had histologic changes consistent with pulmonary oxygen toxicity. Nevertheless, the survival advantages of this therapy should outweigh these risks. The pathophysiologic mechanisms involved in pulmonary oxygen toxicity are not clearly defined, but the popular hypothesis invokes a role for the oxidant-antioxidant balance in the cellular milieu of the lung. Hyperoxia probably leads to increased production of free radicals such as O_2^-, H_2O_2, and $OH\cdot$ by endoplasmic reticulum and mitochondria. These potentially damaging substances cause structural and metabolic changes that ultimately lead to cell death. Type I alveolar endothelial cells are particularly susceptible, and their injury leads to the proliferation of type II cells. The histopathology of pulmonary oxygen toxicity is nonspecific.[149,150] Diffuse alveolar damage is described with capillary proliferation, hemosiderosis, interstitial fibrosis, and epithelial dysplasia. It is probable that antioxidant defense mechanisms play an important role in preventing pulmonary oxygen toxicity. Animal studies suggest that high levels of superoxide dismutase and peroxidase might increase tolerance to elevated F_{IO_2}.[151] The role of antitoxin, vitamin E, and other free radical scavengers is not yet established in this situation.

Unfortunately, as of yet, no reliable index of pulmonary oxygen toxicity exists. Clinical guidelines therefore encourage the use of the minimum F_{IO_2} needed to achieve adequate tissue oxygenation. The toxic effects of oxygen are determined by its pressure rather than its concentration (with the exception of absorption atelectasis, discussed later). For example, Morgan and colleagues[152] showed that astronauts could breathe 100% oxygen for prolonged periods if its pressure was considerably less than 1 atmosphere. In the clinical setting, an optimum P_{O_2} is 90 to 110 mm Hg. Further increases in pressure have an insignificant effect on hemoglobin oxygen saturation and arterial oxygen content (see Fig. 15-4).

Hypercapnia

Oxygen may potentially worsen ventilatory failure because it (1) removes the hypoxic stimulus to ventilation and (2) reverses hypoxic vasoconstriction. Both mechanisms predictably lead to hypercapnia. Campbell[153] recognized the importance of hypoxic drive when PaO_2 was less than 65 mm Hg. He introduced the concept of using controlled oxygen therapy to reduce the risk of hypercapnia when hypoxic drive was eliminated in patients who had lost carbon dioxide responsiveness. Barach[154] argued that limited hypercapnia was an adaptive response that enabled greater carbon dioxide elimination at a given level of $\dot{V}_E$. Nevertheless, the potential for hypercapnia with serious clinical consequences does exist, although this probably rarely occurs with LTOT because the average F_{IO_2} usually does not exceed 40%. Several groups of investigators have stressed that the small increase in $PaCO_2$ that occurs with oxygen therapy is not detrimental to the patient.[91, 143, 155–157] Neff and Petty[7] demonstrated that moderate hypercapnia is well tolerated in the long term.

Absorption Atelectasis

This complication of oxygen therapy is dependent on the fractional concentration of oxygen in the alveolar gas rather than on oxygen pressure. Oxygen breathing leads to progressive washout of nitrogen from alveolar spaces and therefore increases the potential for alveolar collapse. Alveolar collapse is normally prevented by nitrogen, a gas that is nonabsorbable at normal atmospheric pressures. Evidence of absorption atelectasis can be seen as an increase in a patient's alveolar-arterial oxygen gradient after he or she has breathed pure oxygen for more than 1 hour.

Miscellaneous Complications

Hyperbaric oxygen is known to cause retrolental fibrodysplasia. Neonates are particularly susceptible to this complication. Oxygen is also well known for its effects of pulmonary vasodilatation; however, it also has the capability of causing systemic vasoconstriction, which might tend to offset the potential improvement in tissue oxygen delivery. In its various forms, oxygen therapy has definite psychologic effects, including dependency. The placebo effect of oxygen therapy has already been discussed.

FUTURE DIRECTIONS FOR OXYGEN THERAPY

Oxygen therapy, with its numerous physiologic benefits and its potential for improved survival in patients with chronic hypoxemia, plays an important role as an integral component of pulmonary rehabilitation. When compared with other medications for chronic diseases, it is relatively inexpensive. There are several clinical and technologic challenges ahead. There is a need for more clinical studies to define the contribution of ambulatory oxygen therapy to improving survival and quality of life and also to reducing overall health care costs. Physiologic studies are needed to define the combined effects of exercise training and oxygen therapy. The technologic challenges mainly concern the development of safe, portable, and unobtrusive apparatuses for the provision of ambulatory oxygen therapy. Oxygen itself is inexpensive, and it is hoped that technologic progress will lead to less expensive equipment for its supply and delivery. One exciting area of study in this respect is transtracheal oxygen therapy, which is readily accepted by patients and clearly more efficient in producing physiologic benefits. Efforts are also under way to develop a portable oxygen concentrator. However, there is a limit to which molecular sieves can be reduced in size before their efficiency is compromised. Perhaps this difficulty can be overcome using membrane separators, which are potentially more compact and reliable at higher flows. Progress has already been made in the development of lightweight cylinders and liquid oxygen tanks incorporating demand delivery devices that extend their ambulatory capability. There will always be challenges to improving the aesthetics, cost, and convenience of these apparatuses. Technologic advances are also likely in the area of the monitoring of oxygenation, including in the techniques of pulse oximetry and transcutaneous oxygen electrodes.

Finally, there remain challenges in defining which patient groups stand to derive the greatest benefit from oxygen therapy. Further studies of the role of oxygen therapy in reducing dyspnea are also indicated. Currently, LTOT is prescribed for many terminally ill patients who have limited prospects for improved survival or for a return to normal physical activities. Earlier prescription of LTOT needs further investigation. The combination of oxygen therapy with exercise training might prove to be a more important objective than simply the extension of the daily duration of oxygen therapy.

REFERENCES

1. Beddoes T, Watt J. Considerations of the medicinal use of factitious airs: and on the manner of obtaining them in large quantities. Bristol: Johnson, 1794.
2. Haldane JS. The therapeutic administration of oxygen. BMJ 1917; 1:181–183.
3. Cotes JE, Gilson JC. Effect of oxygen on exercise ability in chronic respiratory insufficiency: Use of portable apparatus. Lancet 1956; 2:872–876.
4. Levine BE, Bigelow DV, Hamstra RD, et al. The role of long-term continuous oxygen administration in patients with chronic airway obstruction with hypoxemia. Ann Intern Med 1967; 66:639–650.
5. Abraham AS, Hedworth-Whitty RB, Bishop JM. Effects of acute hypoxia and hypervolemia singly and together, upon the pulmonary circulation in patients with chronic bronchitis. Clin Sci 1967; 33:371–380.
6. Petty TL, Finigan MM. The clinical evaluation of prolonged ambulatory oxygen therapy in patients with chronic airway obstruction. Am J Med 1968; 45:242–252.
7. Neff TA, Petty TL. Long-term continuous oxygen therapy in chronic airway obstruction: Mortality in relationship to cor pulmonale, hypoxia and hypercapnia. Ann Intern Med 1970; 72:621–626.
8. Stark RD, Finnegan P, Bishop JM. Daily requirement of oxygen to reverse pulmonary hypertension in patients with chronic bronchitis. BMJ 1972; 3:724–728.
9. Stark RD, Finnegan P, Bishop JM. Long-term domiciliary oxygen in chronic bronchitis with pulmonary hypertension. BMJ 1973; 3:467–470.
10. Nocturnal Oxygen Therapy Trial Group. Continuous or nocturnal oxygen therapy in hypoxemic chronic obstructive lung disease. Ann Intern Med 1980; 93:391–398.
11. Medical Research Council Working Party. Long term domiciliary oxygen therapy in chronic hypoxic cor pulmonale complicating chronic bronchitis and emphysema. Lancet 1981; i:681–686.
12. Timms RM, Khaja FU, Williams GW, et al. Hemodynamic response to oxygen therapy in chronic obstructive pulmonary disease. Ann Intern Med 1985; 102:29–36.
13. Ashutosh K, Mead G, Dunksy M. Early effects of oxygen administration and prognosis in chronic obstructive pulmonary disease and cor pulmonale. Am Rev Respir Dis 1983; 127:399–404.
14. Cooper CB, Howard P. An analysis of sequential physiologic changes in hypoxic cor pulmonale during long term oxygen therapy. Chest 1991; 100:76–80.
15. Cooper CB, Waterhouse J, Howard P. Twelve year clinical study of patients with hypoxic cor pulmonale given long term domiciliary oxygen therapy. Thorax 1987; 42:105–110.
16. Conference Report: Problems in prescribing and supplying oxygen for Medicare patients. Am Rev Respir Dis 1986; 134:340–341.
17. Kitchin AH, Lowther CP, Matthews MB. The effects of exercise and of breathing oxygen-enriched air on the pulmonary circulation in emphysema. Clin Sci 1961; 21:93–106.
18. Cotes JE, Pisa Z, Thomas AJ. Effect of breathing oxygen upon cardiac output, heart rate, ventilation, systemic and pulmonary blood pressure in patients with chronic lung disease. Clin Sci 1963; 25:305–321.
19. Holt JH, Branscomb BV. Hemodynamic responses to controlled 100% oxygen breathing in emphysema. J Appl Physiol 1965; 20:215–220.
20. Scano G, Van Meerhaeghe A, Willeput R, et al. Effect of oxygen on breathing during exercise in patients with chronic lung disease. Eur J Respir Dis 1982; 63:23–30.
21. Hunt JM, Copeland J, McDonald CF, et al. Cardiopulmonary response to oxygen therapy in hypoxaemic chronic airflow obstruction. Thorax 1989; 44:930–936.

22. Pierce AK, Paez PN, Miller WF. Exercise training with the aid of a portable oxygen supply in patients with emphysema. Am Rev Respir Dis 1965; 91:653–659.
23. Bye PTP, Anderson ASD, Woolcock AJ, et al. Bicycle endurance performance of patients with interstitial lung disease breathing air and oxygen. Am Rev Respir Dis 1982; 126:1005–1012.
24. Wasserman K, Whipp BJ, Casaburi R, et al. Ventilatory control during exercise in man. Bull Eur Physiopathol Respir 1979; 15:27–51.
25. Bye PTP, Esau SA, Levy RD, et al. Ventilatory muscle function during exercise in air and oxygen in patients with chronic airflow limitation. Am Rev Respir Dis 1985; 132:236–240.
26. Grassino A, Sorli J, Lorange F, et al. Respiratory drive and timing in chronic obstructive pulmonary disease. Chest 1978; 73(Suppl):290–293.
27. Austin TW, Penman WB. Airway obstruction due to hypoxemia in patients with chronic lung disease. Am Rev Respir Dis 1967; 95:567–575.
28. Lee J, Read J. Effect of oxygen breathing on distribution of pulmonary blood flow in chronic obstructive lung disease. Am Rev Respir Dis 1967; 96:1173–1180.
29. Rebuck AS, Vandenberg RA. The relationship between pulmonary arterial pressure and physiologic dead space in patients with obstructive lung disease. Am Rev Respir Dis 1973; 107:423–428.
30. Bye PTP, Esau SA, Walley KR, et al. Ventilatory muscles during exercise in air and oxygen in normal men. J Appl Physiol 1984; 56:464–471.
31. Stein DA, Bradley BL, Miller WC. Mechanisms of oxygen effects on exercise in patients with chronic obstructive pulmonary disease. Chest 1982; 81:6–10.
32. Vyas MN, Banister EW, Morton JW, et al. Response to exercise in patients with chronic airway obstruction: II. Effects of breathing 40 per cent oxygen. Am Rev Respir Dis 1971; 103:401–412.
33. Criner GJ, Celli BR. Ventilatory muscle recruitment in exercise with O_2 in obstructed patients with mild hypoxemia. J Appl Physiol 1987; 63:195–200.
34. Selinger SR, Kennedy TP, Buescher P, et al. Effects of removing oxygen from patients with chronic obstructive pulmonary disease. Am Rev Respir Dis 1987; 136:85–91.
35. Corriveau ML, Rosen BJ, Dolan GF. Oxygen transport and oxygen consumption during supplemental oxygen administration in patients with chronic obstructive pulmonary disease. Am J Med 1989; 87:633–637.
36. Keller R, Ragaz A, Borer P. Predictors for early mortality in patients with long-term oxygen home therapy. Respiration 1985; 48:216–221.
37. Morrison DA, Henry R, Goldman S. Preliminary study of effects of low flow oxygen on oxygen delivery and right ventricular function in chronic lung disease. Am Rev Respir Dis 1986; 133:390–395.
38. Abraham AS, Cole RB, Green ID, et al. Factors contributing to the reversible pulmonary hypertension of patients with acute respiratory failure studied by serial observations during recovery. Circ Res 1969; 24:51–60.
39. Burrows B, Kettel LJ, Niden AH, et al. Patterns of cardiovascular dysfunction in chronic obstructive lung disease. N Engl J Med 1972; 286:912–918.
40. Petty TL, Neff TA, Creagh E, et al. Outpatient oxygen therapy in chronic obstructive pulmonary disease. A review of 13 years' experience and an evaluation of modes of therapy. Arch Intern Med 1979; 139:28–32.
41. Weitzenblum E, Sautegeau A, Ehrhart M, et al. Long-term oxygen therapy can reverse the progression of pulmonary hypertension in patients with chronic obstructive pulmonary disease. Am Rev Respir Dis 1985; 131:493–498.
42. Leggett RJ, Cooke NJ, Clancy L, et al. Long-term domiciliary oxygen therapy in cor pulmonale complicating chronic bronchitis and emphysema. Thorax 1976; 31:414–418.
43. Fletcher EC, Levin DC. Cardiopulmonary hemodynamics during sleep in subjects with chronic obstructive pulmonary disease. The effect of short- and long-term oxygen. Chest 1984; 85:6–14.
44. Adams RP, Welch HG. Oxygen uptake, acid-base status, and performance with varied inspired oxygen fractions. J Appl Physiol 1980; 49:863–868.
45. Degaute J-P, Domenighetti G, Naeije R, et al. Oxygen delivery in acute exacerbation of chronic obstructive pulmonary disease. Effects of controlled oxygen therapy. Am Rev Respir Dis 1981; 124:26–30.
46. Krop HD, Block AJ, Cohen E. Neuropsychologic effects of continuous oxygen therapy in chronic obstructive pulmonary disease. Chest 1973; 64:317–322.
47. Block AJ, Castle JR, Keitt AS. Chronic oxygen therapy. Treatment of chronic obstructive pulmonary disease at sea level. Chest 1974; 65:279–288.
48. Heaton RK, Grant I, McSweeney AJ, et al. Psychologic effects of continuous and nocturnal oxygen therapy in hypoxemic chronic obstructive pulmonary disease. Arch Intern Med 1983; 143:1941–1947.
49. Chamberlain DA, Millard FJC. The treatment of polycythemia secondary to hypoxic lung disease by continuous oxygen administration. Q J Med 1963; 128:341–350.
50. Johnson TS, Ellis JH Jr, Steel PP. Improvement in platelet survival time with oxygen in patients with chronic obstructive airway disease. Am Rev Respir Dis 1978; 117:255–257.
51. Barach AL. Ambulatory oxygen therapy: Oxygen inhalation at home and out-of-doors. Dis Chest 1959; 35:229–241.
52. Woolf CR, Suero JT. Alterations in lung mechanics and gas exchange following training in chronic obstructive lung disease. Dis Chest 1969; 55:37–44.
53. Lilker ES, Karnick A, Lerner L. Portable oxygen in chronic obstructive lung disease with hypoxemia and cor pulmonale. A controlled double-blind crossover study. Chest 1975; 68:236–241.
54. Raimondi AC, Edwards RHT, Denison DM, et al. Exercise tolerance breathing a low density gas mixture, 35% oxygen and air in patients with chronic obstructive bronchitis. Clin Sci 1970; 39:675–685.
55. Bradley BL, Garner AE, Billiu D, et al. Oxygen-assisted exercise in chronic obstructive lung disease. Am Rev Respir Dis 1978; 118:239–243.
56. Swinburn CR, Wakefield JM, Jones PW. Relationship between ventilation and breathlessness during exercise in chronic obstructive airways disease is not altered by prevention of hypoxemia. Clin Sci 1984; 67:515–519.
57. Davidson AC, Leach R, George RJD, et al. Supplemental oxygen and exercise ability in chronic obstructive airways disease. Thorax 1988; 43:965–971.
58. Nixon PA, Orenstein DN, Curtis SE, et al. Oxygen supplementation during exercise in cystic fibrosis. Am Rev Respir Dis 1990; 142:807–811.
59. Wilson BA, Welch HG, Liles JN. Effects of hyperoxic gas mixtures on energy metabolism during prolonged work. J Appl Physiol 1975; 39:267–271.
60. Leggett RJE, Flenley DC. Portable oxygen and exercise tolerance in patients with chronic hypoxic cor pulmonale. BMJ 1977; 2:84–86.
61. Longo AM, Moser KM, Luchsinger PC. The role of oxygen therapy in the rehabilitation of patients with chronic obstructive pulmonary disease. Am Rev Respir Dis 1971; 103:690–697.
62. Woodcock AA, Gross ER, Geddes DM. Oxygen relieves breathlessness in "pink puffers." Lancet 1981; i:907–909.
63. Chronos N, Adams L, Guz A. Effect of hyperoxia and hypoxia on exercise-induced breathlessness in normal subjects. Clin Sci 1988; 64:531–537.
64. Ward SA, Whipp BJ. Effects of peripheral and central chemoreflex activation on the isopnoeic rating of breathing in exercising humans. J Physiol 1989; 411:27–43.
65. Lane R, Cockcroft A, Adams L, et al. Arterial oxygen saturation and breathlessness in patients with chronic obstructive airways disease. Clin Sci 1987; 72:693–698.
66. Tweney J. Almitrine bismesylate: Current status. Bull Eur Physiopathol Respir 1987; 23:153S–165S.
67. Waterhouse JC, Howard P. Breathlessness and portable oxygen in chronic obstructive airways disease. Thorax 1983; 38:302–306.
68. Williams BT, Nicholl JP. Prevalence of hypoxaemic chronic

obstructive lung disease with reference to long-term oxygen therapy. Lancet 1985; ii:369–372.
69. Conference Report. Further recommendations for prescribing and supplying long-term oxygen therapy. Am Rev Respir Dis 1988; 138:745–747.
70. Conference report: New problems in supply, reimbursement, and certification of medical necessity for long-term therapy. Am Rev Respir Dis 1990; 142:721–724.
71. The Drug Tariff. Introduction of oxygen concentrators to the domiciliary oxygen therapy service. London, 1986. Department of Health and Social Security publication No. FPN 398.
72. Report of a SEP Task Group: Recommendations for long term oxygen therapy (LTOT). Eur Respir J 1989; 2:160–164.
73. Strom K, Boe J. A national register for long-term oxygen therapy in chronic hypoxia: Preliminary results. Eur Respir J 1988; 1:952–958.
74. Breslin ABX, Colebatch HJH, Engel L, et al. Domiciliary oxygen treatment. Med J Aust 1985; 142:508–510.
75. McKeon JL, Saunders NA, Murree-Allen K. Domiciliary oxygen: Rationalization of supply in the Hunter region from 1982–1986. Med J Aust 1987; 146:73–78.
76. Timms RM, Kvale PA, Anthonisen NR, et al. Selection of patients with chronic obstructive pulmonary disease for long-term oxygen therapy. JAMA 1981; 245:2514–2516.
77. Levi-Valensi P, Weitzenblum E, Pedinielli J-L, et al. Three-month follow-up of arterial blood gas determinations in candidates for long-term oxygen therapy: A multicentric study. Am Rev Respir Dis 1986; 133:547–551.
78. O'Donohue WJ Jr. Effect of oxygen therapy on increasing arterial oxygen tension in hypoxemic patients with stable chronic obstructive pulmonary disease while breathing ambient air. Chest 1991; 100:968–972.
79. Stretton TB. Provision of long term oxygen therapy. Thorax 1985; 40:801–805.
80. McCallion J, Pearce SJ. Oxygen concentrators: Which patients are being treated and are the DHSS guidelines being followed? (abstract) Thorax 1988; 44:859P.
81. Douglas NJ, Calverley PMA, Leggett RJE, et al. Transient hypoxaemia during sleep in chronic bronchitis and emphysema. Lancet 1979; i:1–4.
82. Tirlapur VG, Mir MA. Nocturnal hypoxemia and associated electrocardiographic changes in patients with chronic obstructive airways disease. N Engl J Med 1982; 306:125–130.
83. Mezon BL, West P, Israels J, et al. Sleep breathing abnormalities in kyphoscoliosis. Am Rev Respir Dis 1980; 122:617–621.
84. Francis PWJ, Muller NL, Guiwitz D, et al. Hemoglobin desaturation: Its occurrence during sleep in patients with cystic fibrosis. Am J Dis Child 1980; 134:734–740.
85. Boysen PG, Block AJ, Wynne JW, et al. Nocturnal pulmonary hypertension in patients with chronic obstructive pulmonary disease. Chest 1979; 76:536–542.
86. DeMarco FJ, Wynne JW, Block AJ, et al. Oxygen desaturation during sleep as a determinant of the "blue and bloated" syndrome. Chest 1981; 79:621–625.
87. Fletcher EC, Luckett RA, Miller T, et al. Exercise hemodynamics and gas exchange in patients with chronic obstruction pulmonary disease, sleep desaturation, and a daytime PaO$_2$ above 60 mm Hg. Am Rev Respir Dis 1989; 140:1237–1245.
88. Goldstein RS, Rancharan V, Bowes G, et al. Effect of supplemental nocturnal oxygen on gas exchange in patients with severe obstructive lung disease. N Engl J Med 1984; 310:425–429.
89. Gong H, Tashkin DP, Lee EY, et al. Hypoxia-altitude simulation test. Evaluation of patients with chronic airway obstruction. Am Rev Respir Dis 1984; 130:980–986.
90. Walshaw MJ, Lim R, Evans CC, et al. Prescription of oxygen concentrators for long-term oxygen treatment: Reassessment in one district. BMJ 1988; 297:1030–1032.
91. Baudouin SV, Waterhouse JC, Tahtamouni T, et al. Long term domiciliary oxygen treatment for chronic respiratory failure reviewed. Thorax 1990; 45:195–198.
92. Dilworth JP, Higgs CMB, Jones PA, et al. Prescription of oxygen concentrators: Adherence to published guidelines. Thorax 1989; 44:576–578.
93. McDonald GJ. Long-term oxygen therapy delivery systems. Respiratory Care 1983; 28:898–905.
94. Johns DP, Rochford PD, Streeton JA. Evaluation of six oxygen concentrators. Thorax 1985; 40:806–810.
95. Gould GA, Scott W, Hayhurst MD, et al. Technical and clinical assessment of oxygen concentrators. Thorax 1985; 40:811–816.
96. Bongard JP, Pahud C, De Haller R. Insufficient oxygen concentration obtained at domiciliary controls of eighteen concentrators. Eur Respir J 1989; 2:280–282.
97. Evans TW, Waterhouse J, Howard P. Clinical experience with the oxygen concentrator. BMJ 1983; 287:459–461.
98. Sous-Commission Technique ANTADIR. Home controls of a sample of 2,414 oxygen concentrators. Eur Respir J 1991; 4:227–231.
99. Green ID. Choice of method for administration of oxygen. BMJ 1967; 3:593–596.
100. Leigh JM. Variation in performance of oxygen therapy devices. Anesthesia 1970; 25:210–222.
101. Gould GA, Forsyth IS, Flenley DC. Comparison of two oxygen conserving nasal prong systems and the effects of nose and mouth breathing. Thorax 1986; 41:808–809.
102. Robertson GS. Cricothyroid puncture in the assessment of equipment for postoperative oxygen therapy. Lancet 1969; i:801–803.
103. Gibson RL, Comer PB, Beckham RW, et al. Actual tracheal concentrations with commonly used oxygen equipment. Anesthesiology 1976; 44:71–73.
104. Schacter EN, Littner MR, Luddy P, et al. Monitoring of oxygen delivery systems in clinical practice. Crit Care Med 1980; 8:405–409.
105. Heimlich HJ. Respiratory rehabilitation with transtracheal oxygen system. Ann Otol Rhinol Laryngol 1982; 91:643–647.
106. Heimlich HG, Carr GC. Transtracheal catheter technique for pulmonary rehabilitation. Ann Otol Rhinol Laryngol 1985; 94:502–504.
107. Christopher KL, Spofford BT, Petrun MD, et al. A program for transtracheal oxygen delivery: Assessment of safety and efficacy. Ann Int Med 1987; 107:802–808.
108. Hoffman LA, Johnson JT, Wesmiller SW, et al. Transtracheal delivery of oxygen: Efficacy and safety for long-term continuous therapy. Ann Otol Rhinol Laryngol 1991; 100:108–115.
109. Christopher KL, Spofford BT, Brannin PK, et al. Transtracheal oxygen therapy for refractory hypoxemia. JAMA 1986; 256:494–497.
110. Banner NR, Govan JR. Long term transtracheal oxygen delivery through microcatheter in patients with hypoxaemia due to chronic obstructive airways disease. BMJ 1986; 293:111–114.
111. Hoffman LA, Dauber JH, Ferson PF, et al. Patient response to transtracheal oxygen delivery. Am Rev Respir Dis 1987; 135:153–156.
112. Bloom BS, Daniel JM, Wiseman M, et al. Transtracheal oxygen delivery and patients with chronic obstructive pulmonary disease. Respir Med 1989; 83:281–288.
113. Wesmiller SW, Hoffman LA, Sciurba FC, et al. Exercise tolerance during nasal cannula and transtracheal oxygen delivery. Am Rev Respir Dis 1990; 141:789–791.
114. Johnson LP, Cary JM. The implanted intratracheal oxygen catheter. Surg Gynecol Obstet 1987; 165:75–76.
115. Couser JI Jr, Make BJ. Transtracheal oxygen decreases inspired minute ventilation. Am Rev Respir Dis 1989; 139:627–631.
116. Adamo JP, Mehta AC, Stelmach K, et al. The Cleveland Clinic's initial experience with transtracheal oxygen therapy. Respir Care 1990; 35:153–160.
117. Fletcher EC, Nickeson D, Costarangos-Galarza C. Endotracheal mass resulting from a transtracheal oxygen catheter. Chest 1988; 93:438–439.
118. Walsh DA, Govan JR. Long term continuous domiciliary oxygen therapy by transtracheal catheter. Thorax 1990; 45:478–481.
119. Tiep BL, Nicotra NB, Carter PR, et al. Low-concentration oxygen therapy via a demand oxygen delivery system. Chest 1985; 87:636–638.
120. Moore-Gillon JC, George RJD, Geddes DM. An oxygen conserving nasal cannula. Thorax 1985; 40:817–819.
121. Soffer M, Tashkin DP, Shapiro BJ, et al. Conservation of oxygen

122. Carter R, Williams JS, Berry J, et al. Evaluation of the pendant oxygen-conserving nasal cannula during exercise. Chest 1986; 89:806–810.
123. Evans TW, Waterhouse JC, Suggett AJ, Howard P. A conservation device for oxygen therapy in COPD. Eur Respir J 1988; 1:959–961.
124. Claiborne RA, Paynter DE, Dutt AK, et al. Evaluation of the use of an oxygen conservation device in long-term oxygen therapy. Am Rev Respir Dis 1987; 136:1095–1098.
125. Cotes JE. Continuous versus intermittent administration of oxygen during exercise to patients with chronic lung disease. Lancet 1963; i:1075–1077.
126. Pflug AE, Cheney FW Jr, Butler J. Evaluation of an intermittent oxygen flow system. Am Rev Respir Dis 1972; 105:449–452.
127. Tiep BL, Lewis Y, Branum N, et al. Respiratory management at home. Phys Med Rehabil 1988; 2:385–403.
128. Tiep BL, Carter R, Nicotra B, et al. Demand oxygen delivery during exercise. Chest 1987; 91:15–20.
129. Winter RJD, George RJD, Moore-Gillon JC, et al. Inspiration-phased oxygen delivery. Lancet 1984; i:1371–1372.
130. Block AJ. Intermittent flow oxygen devices: Technically feasible, but rarely used. Chest 1984; 86:657–658.
131. Leger P, Gerard M, Robert D. Simultaneous use of a pulsed dose demand valve (PDV) with a transtracheal catheter (TTC): An optimal O_2 saving for long term O_2 therapy (abstract). Am Rev Respir Dis 1986; 133:350.
132. Tiep BL, Christopher KL, Spofford BT, et al. Pulsed nasal and transtracheal oxygen delivery. Chest 1990; 97:364–368.
133. Hansen JE. Participant responses to blood gas proficiency testing reports. Chest 1992; 101:1240–1244.
134. Bromberg PA, Lewis BF. Monitoring oxygen therapy. Am Rev Respir Dis 1980; 122:55–59.
135. Chaudhary BA, Burki NK. Ear oximetry in clinical practice. Am Rev Respir Dis 1978; 177:173–175.
136. Saunders NA, Powles ACP, Rebuck AS. Ear oximetry: Accuracy and practicability in the assessment of arterial oxygenation. Am Rev Respir Dis 1976; 113:745–749.
137. Wyss CR, Matsen FA, King RV, et al. Dependence of transcutaneous oxygen tension on local arterial-venous pressure gradient in normal subjects. Clin Sci 1981; 60:499–506.
138. Gothgen I, Jacobsen E. Transcutaneous oxygen tension measurement: I. Age variation and reproducibility. Acta Anaesthesiol Scand Suppl 1978; 67:66–70.
139. Peabody JL, Willis MM, Gregory GA, et al. Clinical limitations and advantages of transcutaneous oxygen electrodes. Acta Anaesthesiol Scand Suppl 1978; 68:76–82.
140. Dowd GSE, Linge K, Bentley G. Transcutaneous PO_2 measurement in skin ischemia. Lancet 1982; i:48.
141. Wyss CR, Matsen FA, Simmons CW, et al. Transcutaneous oxygen tension measurements on limbs of diabetic and nondiabetic patients with peripheral vascular disease. Surgery 1984; 95:339–346.
142. Pilot development of domiciliary oxygen concentrators. Manchester, 1983. North Western Regional Health Authority report No. 4/9/176.
143. Vergeret G, Tunon de Lara M, Douvier JJ, et al. Compliance of COPD patients with long term oxygen therapy. Eur J Respir Dis 1986; 69(Suppl 146):421–425.
144. Prignot J. Home monitoring of patients on long-term oxygen therapy. Bull Int Union Tuberc Lung Dis 1987; 62:33–34.
145. Heiny LW. High pressure medical oxygen equipment in the home. Respir Care 1974; 19:521–526.
146. West GA, Primeau P. Nonmedical hazards of long-term oxygen therapy. Respir Care 1983; 28:906–912.
147. Petty TL. The success and safety of home oxygen (editorial). Respir Care 1974; 19:496–498.
148. Petty TL, Stanford RE, Neff TA. Continuous oxygen therapy in chronic airway obstruction: Observations on possible oxygen toxicity and survival. Ann Intern Med 1971; 75:361–367.
149. Pratt PC. The reaction of the human lung to enriched oxygen atmosphere. Ann N Y Acad Sci 1965; 121:809–822.
150. Pratt PC. Pathology of pulmonary oxygen toxicity. Am Rev Respir Dis 1974; 110:51–57.
151. White CW, Avraham KB, Stanely PF, et al. Transgenic mice with expression of elevated copper-zinc superoxide dismutase in the lungs are resistant to pulmonary oxygen toxicity. J Clin Invest 1991; 87:2162–2168.
152. Morgan TE Jr, Cutler RG, Shaw EG, et al. Physiologic effect of exposure to increased oxygen tension at 5 psi. Aerospace Med 1963; 34:720–726.
153. Campbell EJM. A method of controlled oxygen administration which reduces the risk of carbon-dioxide retention. Lancet 1960; ii:12–14.
154. Barach AL. Hypercapnia in chronic obstructive lung disease: An adaptive response to low-flow oxygen therapy. Chest 1974; 66:112–113.
155. Morse JO, Kettel LJ, Diener CF, et al. Effect of long-term, continuous oxygen therapy in patients with severe chronic hypercapnia. Am Rev Respir Dis 1973; 107:1064–1066.
156. Stewart BN, Hood CI, Block AJ. Long-term results of continuous oxygen therapy at sea level. Chest 1975; 68:486–492.
157. Lertzman MM, Cherniack RM. Rehabilitation of patients with chronic obstructive pulmonary disease. Am Rev Respir Dis 1976; 114:1145–1165.

Chapter 16

Exercise Training in Chronic Obstructive Lung Disease

RICHARD CASABURI, Ph.D., M.D.

Patients with lung disease suffer from a progressive reduction in their level of physical activity. Since lung disease makes exertion unpleasant, these patients become sedentary. The resultant chronic inactivity deconditions the muscles of locomotion. This in turn makes physical activity even more unpleasant and thus reinforces the sedentary lifestyle. This process of progressive disability can be depicted as a downward spiral (Fig. 16–1).

A major goal of pulmonary rehabilitation is to interrupt this downward spiral by enabling patients to tolerate a higher level of activity. Undoubtedly, much of the benefit of pulmonary rehabilitation is psychologic. Patients become convinced that the shortness of breath they experience is not harmful. They may, in fact, become *desensitized* to the sensation of dyspnea. (Chapter 18 provides an excellent overview of the budding science of dyspnea modulation.) One important way to achieve the psychologic benefit of rehabilitation is through a program of progressive supervised exercise. If the only goal of rehabilitation is to achieve this psychologic benefit, then the mode or pattern of exercise is probably not of crucial importance. However, if the goal is to improve the patient's *physiologic* ability to perform exercise, then the design of the exercise program is much more important.

If we are to consider the physiologic requirements of exercise, it is necessary to appreciate that the body depends on the integrated responses of a number of organ systems to transport oxygen from the atmosphere to exercising muscle and to expel carbon dioxide from the body. Oxygen must be carried by pulmonary ventilation from the environment to the alveolocapillary interface. The relation of ventilation to perfusion and the diffusion characteristics of this interface determine oxygen transport from the alveoli to the blood. Appropriate vasodilation and the recruitment of pulmonary circulation are key features of the exercise response because they accommodate the greatly increased cardiac output without inordinately increasing pressures in the right side of the heart. A reduction in afterload of the left side of the heart is also required, and the vasculature of the exercising muscles must dilate greatly to accomplish this. The blood flow that reaches the capillaries of muscles must carry an adequate oxygen supply; anemia, carbon monoxide, and a lack of full hemoglobin oxygen saturation decrease oxygen delivery. Finally, oxygen must diffuse from muscle capillaries to the mitochondria to participate in oxidative phosphorylation and in consequent adenosine triphosphate production.

The physiologic disadvantages that the patient with obstructive lung disease faces when he or she attempts to meet the greatly increased demand for oxygen supply imposed by exercise are worth considering. In particular, the work of breathing is increased by both high airways resistance and hyperinflation; as a result, the respiratory muscles are placed at a mechanical disadvantage. Thus, the increase in ventilation demanded by exercise comes at a high metabolic cost. Worse yet, the amount of ventilation required is extraordinarily large because the lung of the pulmonary disease patient exchanges gas poorly. Gas that ventilates unperfused airspaces (alveolar dead space) is wasted in terms of oxygen and carbon dioxide transport. Mismatching of ventilation to perfu-

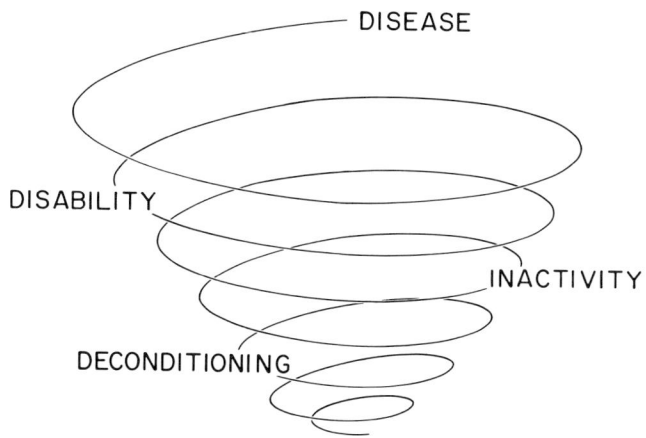

FIGURE 16–1. Symbolic representation of the downward spiral that progressively restricts the level of activity tolerated by patients with lung disease.

sion yields arterial hypoxemia. The cardiovascular system is also impacted by obstructive lung disease. Even when overt cor pulmonale is not present, pulmonary vascular reserve is diminished. Pulmonary artery pressure rises abnormally, and cardiac output may be limited, thus compromising oxygen delivery to the muscles.

Many patients with obstructive lung disease are limited by the amount of ventilation they can achieve, that is, they are "ventilatorily limited" (Fig. 16–2). As their level of activity increases, so does their ventilatory requirement. When this requirement exceeds the amount of ventilation that can be sustained, exercise cannot continue. It is important to realize that it is essentially meaningless to ask which of the physiologic abnormalities associated with a patient's disease is the principal factor limiting his or her exercise tolerance. Each abnormality directly or indirectly adds to the ventilatory requirement for exercise and thus contributes to the ventilatory limitation. Amelioration of any contributing abnormality has the potential to improve exercise tolerance in the ventilatorily limited patient.

Unfortunately, few therapeutic modalities have been demonstrated to reduce the ventilatory requirement or relieve the ventilatory limitation. Bronchodilator or antiinflammatory therapy may reduce the work of breathing and sometimes (but not always) lessens ventilation/perfusion imbalance; however, the reversibility of airflow obstruction typically is modest. Supplemental oxygen therapy has three potentially beneficial effects: (1) the attenuation of carotid chemoreceptor drive, (2) improvement in oxygen delivery (through an increase in the oxygen content of the blood), and (3) hemodynamic improvement (as a result of pulmonary vasodilation). As is detailed in Chapter 17, respiratory muscle training or rest therapy is designed to lessen the ventilatory limitation; whether either of these approaches constitutes practical therapy has yet to be firmly established. Studies of pharmacologic or dietary means to reduce ventilatory requirement during exercise have been less than encouraging.[1-4] Lung or heart-lung transplantation is likely an effective method to increase exercise tolerance[5] (see Chapter 35) but is not an option for most patients.

It is against this background that the potential physiologic benefits of exercise training for the patient with obstructive lung disease can be considered. Although there is a growing body of knowledge regarding the responses of lung disease patients to exercise training, it is dwarfed by the extensive literature concerning exercise training in healthy subjects. Review of this literature provides a framework for considering training strategies for the patient with lung disease.

EXERCISE TRAINING IN HEALTHY INDIVIDUALS

Structural and Physiologic Changes that Result from Training

The changes that result from training can be divided into those structural changes that occur in muscle and in other organ systems and those changes in physiologic responses that accompany the stress of exercise.[6] Sports scientists make a strong distinction between two kinds of training strategies.[7] "Aerobic" (or "endurance") training seeks to improve an athlete's ability to perform sustained tasks; long distance runners and swimmers, for example, perform this kind of training. On the other hand, "strength" training seeks to improve an athlete's ability to perform explosive tasks, such as weight lifting or sprinting. Since the major focus of pulmonary rehabilitation is to increase a patient's ability to sustain tasks, discussion of endurance training seems more relevant.

Structural Adaptations. Human skeletal muscles are composed of two major kinds of fibers.[8] One type

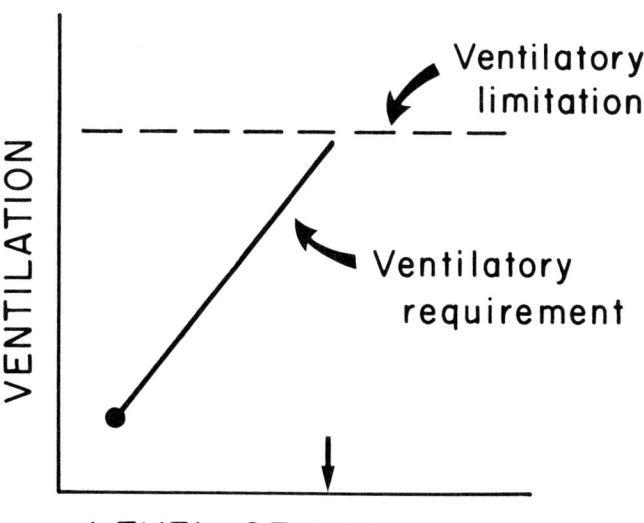

FIGURE 16–2. Schematic illustration of the factors limiting exercise tolerance in the ventilatorily limited patient. The ventilatory requirement rises as the level of activity increases. When the ventilatory requirement exceeds the sustainable ventilation, exercise cannot continue. Measures that decrease the ventilatory requirement at a given level of activity or that ameliorate the ventilatory limitation predictably increase exercise tolerance.

contracts slowly but has a high capacity for prolonged repetitive contraction (termed type I, slow-twitch, or oxidative muscle fibers). The other fiber type contracts quickly but has a limited capacity for sustained contraction (termed type II, fast-twitch, or glycolytic muscle fibers). The distribution of these two fiber types within a given muscle is determined by heredity[9] and is thus not subject to modification by training.[10] However, endurance training produces profound changes within fiber types. As a result of training, subpopulations of type II fibers undergo change. Specifically, type IIb fibers, which have a low oxidative potential, transform into type IIa fibers, which have a higher capacity for oxidative metabolism.[11] Likewise, type I fibers undergo dramatic structural and biochemical changes.[8] These fibers hypertrophy and the number and size of their mitochondria increase. Furthermore, in these fibers both the concentration of enzymes that facilitate the Krebs cycle and the concentration of mitochondrial enzymes that facilitate oxidative phosphorylation increase.[12] In this way, the capacity to oxidatively metabolize pyruvate (the end product of glycolysis), fatty acids, and ketone bodies[8] is increased. These changes would be of no benefit, however, if the ability to deliver oxygen to the site of oxidative metabolism was not improved. Myoglobin levels within trained muscle are higher; this contributes to the transport of oxygen from muscle capillaries to the site of metabolism.[13] However, the key change seems to be the proliferation of muscle capillaries.[14] As a result of training, the increase in the number of muscle capillaries exceeds the increase in muscle fiber size, so that more capillaries surround a given fiber. Thus, a given capillary supplies a smaller area of muscle fibers. Diffusion distance from the oxygen source (hemoglobin in muscle capillaries) to the oxygen sink (the mitochondria) decreases.

It is important to point out that these structural changes in skeletal muscle that are brought about by endurance training are seen only in the muscle groups involved in the training regimen[15] (i.e., training is specific to the muscle groups involved[6]). For example, walking or running does not induce changes in the arm muscles. Improvements in the performance of stationary bicycle exercise may not carry over fully to running, since a somewhat different group of muscles is involved. However, some of the structural changes that result from endurance training are of general benefit; these are principally changes that occur in the cardiovascular system.[6, 16, 17] The heart hypertrophies and undergoes a demonstrable increase in wall thickness and chamber size. Blood volume increases due to both increases in plasma volume and in total hemoglobin level. Cardiac output at the maximum exercise level is higher after training, although cardiac output at rest and at a given level of exercise is not much changed. However, stroke volume is higher after training both at rest and during exercise. Thus, heart rate at rest and at a given level of exercise is distinctly lower. Both systolic and diastolic blood pressures are somewhat lower during exercise, especially in previously hypertensive subjects. Finally, oxygen extraction by the trained muscle is more complete and is manifested by a higher arteriovenous oxygen content difference at a given level of exercise.

Body composition changes are usually seen as a result of a program of endurance training.[18, 19] Body weight decreases as lean body mass (measured, for example, by underwater weighing) increases. The quantity of body fat usually decreases.

Physiologic Responses to Exercise. Athletes who exercise at increasing work rates reach a point at which both oxygen transport to muscle and whole-body oxygen uptake ($\dot{V}O_2$) fail to increase further. Exhaustion is reached soon afterward. Endurance training increases maximum $\dot{V}O_2$ by increasing the arteriovenous oxygen content difference and the maximum cardiac output.[18] As a result, maximum exercise tolerance also increases. It is perhaps more important that the ability to tolerate submaximum exercise improves.[20] This seems to be related to the fact that the increased capacity for aerobic exercise produced by endurance training forestalls the onset of anaerobic metabolism (i.e., the anaerobic threshold is higher).[21-25] Anaerobic metabolism is inefficient in terms of substrate utilization,[26] and lactic acid, the by-product of anaerobic metabolism, has a number of undesirable effects. For example, oxygen requirements for a given level of work are increased; the reasons for this are not totally understood.[25, 27] Furthermore, carbon dioxide output is increased because the buffering of lactic acid by sodium bicarbonate generates this gas.[26] Ventilation is stimulated in order to clear the added carbon dioxide load and because metabolic acidosis directly stimulates the carotid bodies.[28]

Because endurance training increases oxygen delivery to the exercising muscles, a higher level of exercise can be tolerated without lactic acidosis. In other words, the anaerobic threshold (the $\dot{V}O_2$ above which sustained increases in blood lactate levels are seen) rises. Consequently, at a given heavy work rate, the level of blood lactate is lower after a program of endurance training (Fig. 16–3). Because blood lactate level is lower, a number of physiologic responses are altered. Both $\dot{V}O_2$ and carbon dioxide output are reduced[25, 30, 31] (Fig. 16–4). The reduction in ventilation is easily demonstrated and is roughly 7 L/min lower for every 1 mEq/L that blood lactate level decreases as a result of training[29] (Fig. 16–5). Despite the lower ventilation, both arterial pH and $PaCO_2$ (see Fig. 16–4) are higher. It is important to stress that the alterations that are produced by training are only observed at work rates above the anaerobic threshold. For work rates below the anaerobic threshold, the changes in $\dot{V}O_2$, carbon dioxide output, and ventilation are negligible or nonexistent.

There are changes in the response to exercise that are seemingly unrelated to lactate production and that occur as a result of endurance training. Blood catecholamine levels (e.g., epinephrine and norepinephrine levels) are often substantially reduced,[32] sometimes by as much as 90% at heavy work rates[25] (see Fig. 16–3); other hormonal responses are reduced as well.[32, 33] The increase in body temperature that occurs with exercise is ameliorated (see Fig. 16–3).[25, 34] Finally, subjective ratings of perceived exertion for a given work rate are lower.[35]

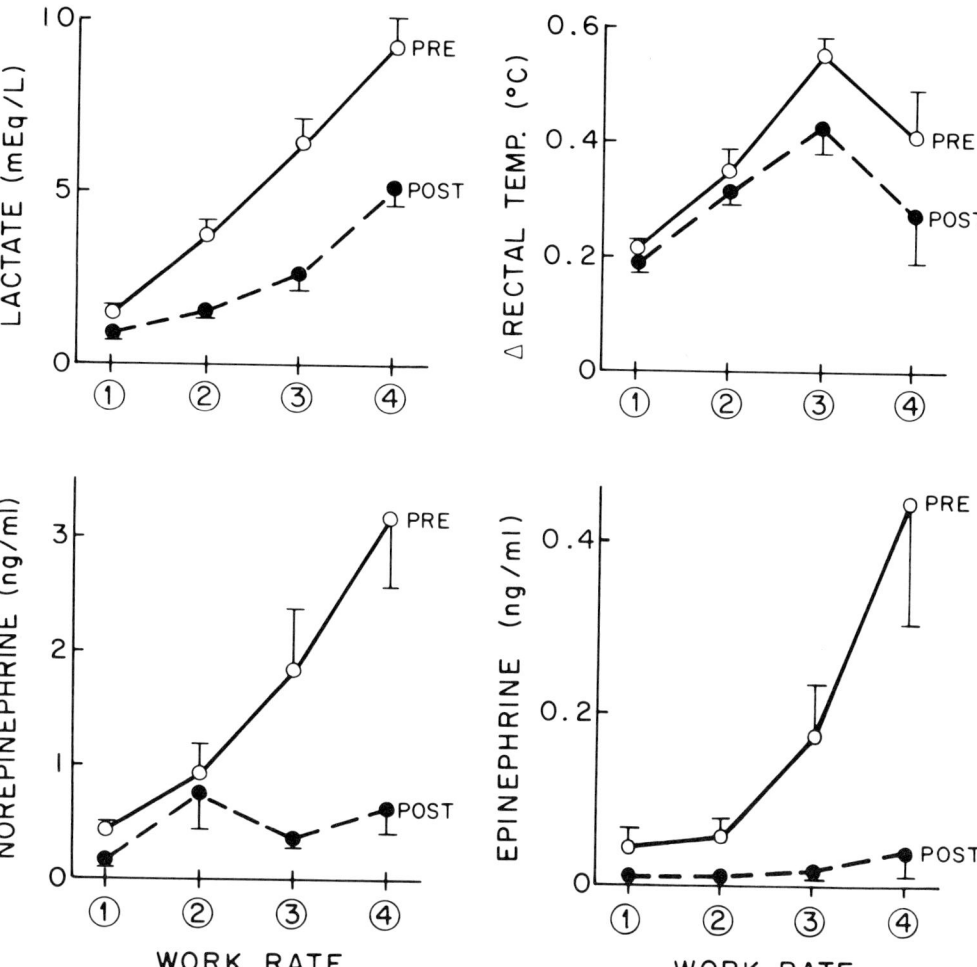

FIGURE 16–3. Effect of endurance training on physiologic responses to exercise (end-exercise blood lactate, norepinephrine, and epinephrine levels, and the difference between resting and end-exercise rectal temperature). Shown are the average (± 1SE) of 10 healthy subjects' responses to 15 minutes of constant work rate exercise before (*open circles*) and after (*closed circles*) a program of endurance exercise training (8 weeks for 45 minutes per day, 5 days per week at above anaerobic threshold work rates). Each performed four work rates, which were calculated from pretraining determinations as 90% AT (1), AT + 25%Δ (2), AT + 50%Δ (3), and AT + 75%Δ (4), where AT is the anaerobic threshold and Δ is the difference between work rates corresponding to the AT and maximum oxygen consumption ($\dot{V}O_2max$). (From Casaburi R, Storer TW, Wasserman K. Mediation of reduced ventilatory response to exercise after endurance training. J Appl Physiol 1987; 63:1533–1538.)

Characteristics of an Effective Training Program

Two factors substantially inhibit our ability to specify how best to induce a physiologic training effect from a program of endurance training. The first likely comes as a surprise to those unfamiliar with this line of research: we have only the slightest clue as to what effective stimulus induces the structural changes in skeletal muscle. (See Saltin and Gollnick[8] for some interesting speculations.) Although one might reasonably suppose that some sort of trophic substance is elaborated by the exercising muscle, none has been implicated. Furthermore, there is no strong evidence that any particular change in the intramuscular environment (e.g., hypoxia or acidosis) is linked to the training stimulus. Thus, this is an area that is in need of intensive investigation. The second problem we have in determining how best to induce a training effect is that studies designed to isolate critical determinants are difficult to perform. Because a training response requires weeks to develop, a prolonged observation period is also needed. Intersubject differences usually necessitate the study of rather large groups of subjects. Assessing any performance-based endpoint (e.g., the endurance of a task) is very difficult because motivational factors are involved; at the very least, a control group is required for such assessment.

Despite these difficulties, substantial progress has been made in defining the parameters of an effective training program. Acknowledged determinants include the intensity of the exercise, the duration of the exercise session, the frequency of exercise sessions, the duration of the training program, the mode of exercise, and the initial fitness level and age of the participants.[18, 36] It is known that most of these determinants are interactive[37]; a fairly wide range of parameters can be combined to yield an effective program of endurance training.

Exercise Intensity. The prescription of exercise intensity has two major tenets. First, it is widely believed that there is a threshold intensity under which no training effect is achieved, no matter how great the frequency of exercise sessions and the duration of the exercise program.[36] Second, it is believed that if the rate of work is above the intensity threshold, the total amount of work per session is the principal determinant of the training response (i.e., a short session of high-intensity exercise may be as effective as a longer session of moderate-intensity exercise).[18, 36] However, these tenets are not beyond questioning and should be closely examined.

A major stumbling block in exercise prescription is deciding which physiologic variable to use to define

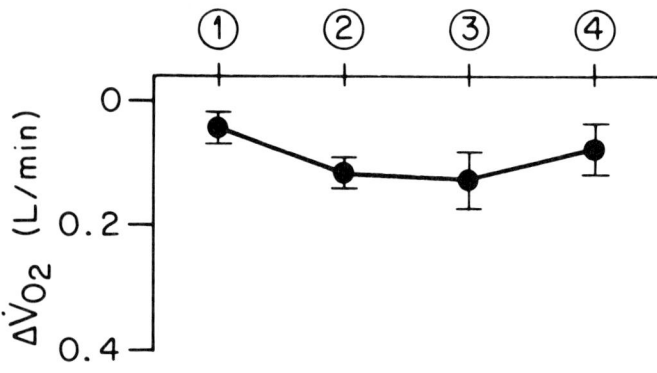
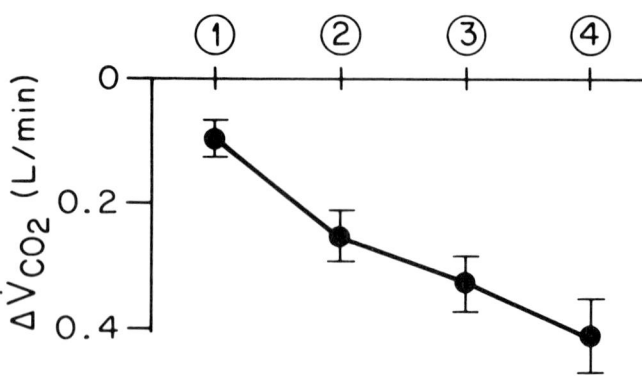
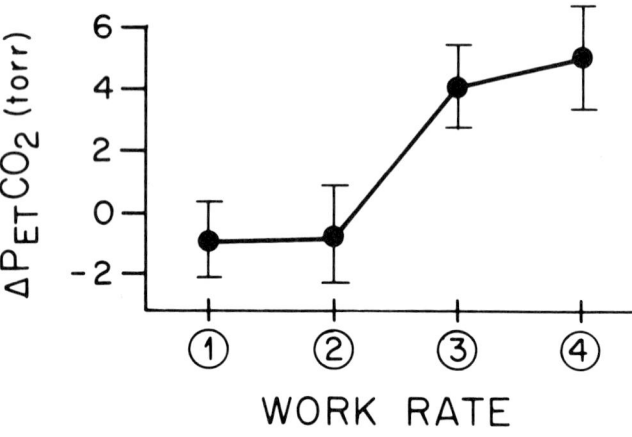

FIGURE 16–4. Endurance training produces decreases in $\dot{V}O_2$ and carbon dioxide output ($\dot{V}CO_2$) for work rates above the AT. Furthermore, owing to the decreased hydrogen ion stimulation of ventilation, arterial PCO_2 (approximated by end tidal PCO_2 [$P_{ET}CO_2$]) is higher after training. The *points* are the average ($\pm$ 1 SE) difference between the pretraining and post-training responses of 10 healthy subjects. See Figure 16–3 for definitions of the work rates studied. (From Casaburi R, Storer TW, Wasserman K. Mediation of reduced ventilatory response to exercise after endurance training. J Appl Physiol 1987; 63:1533–1538.)

variables have been investigated: heart rate, oxygen uptake, and blood lactate level.

Using heart rate as a descriptor of exercise intensity is advantageous in that it is easy to measure. Furthermore, as training proceeds, a given heart rate becomes associated with a higher rate of work[6]; this provides a continuing stimulus. However, heart rate has only a remote relation to conditions in the exercising muscle; therefore, the theoretical basis for using heart rate to define the critical training intensity is necessarily weak. The intensity threshold has been asserted to be roughly 60% of the maximum heart rate, or 50% of the heart rate reserve (i.e., the per cent difference between maximum heart rate and resting heart rate).[36] Because predicted maximum heart rate is strongly dependent on age, the critical training heart rate decreases with age (e.g., it is roughly 140 beats/min at age 20 yr and 105 beats/min at age 65 yr).[6] However, the exercise intensity corresponding to a given heart rate varies widely among subjects.[38] Also, some studies have shown that programs featuring long exercise sessions may achieve a measurable training effect even if heart rate is below traditional measures of the critical heart rate.[39, 40]

The most-cited critical intensity in terms of oxygen uptake is 50% of maximum oxygen consumption ($\dot{V}O_2$max). Unless training is to take place on a calibrated ergometer (e.g., a calibrated bicycle ergometer), the heart rate that yields the selected per cent of $\dot{V}O_2$max is determined empirically, and then this heart

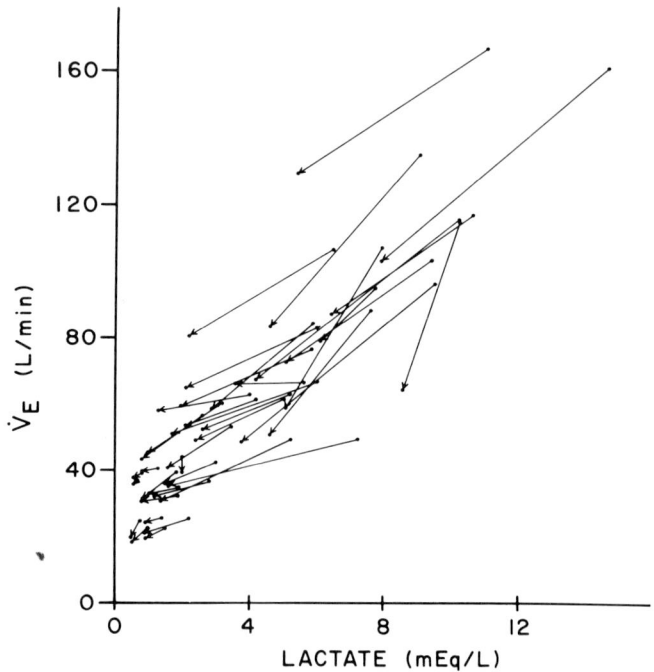

FIGURE 16–5. Relationship between the reduction in end-exercise ventilation ($\dot{V}E$) and end-exercise blood lactate level produced by endurance training in healthy subjects. Lines connect before and after training responses to identical exercise tests. See Figure 16–3 for descriptions of the subjects and the work rates studied. The reduction in ventilation is highly correlated with the reduction in blood lactate level. (From Casaburi R, Storer TW, Wasserman K. Mediation of reduced ventilatory response to exercise after endurance training. J Appl Physiol 1987; 63:1533–1538.)

exercise intensity. As was mentioned earlier, since we do not know the effective stimulus for the training response, we have no guide to help in the selection of the most relevant marker of training intensity. Three rate is used as the target for training sessions. Although earlier studies seemed to indicate that no measurable physiologic training effect was obtained at work rates below 50% $\dot{V}O_2$max, some recent studies specifically designed to address this issue have found distinct physiologic training effects at work rates lower than the traditional threshold.[39, 41, 42]

Using blood lactate levels to select work rates for exercise training has been suggested by several authors.[43–45] This method has the intuitive attraction that work rates above the lactate threshold place more stress on the body in terms of substrate utilization, local hypoxemia, and acidosis. Furthermore, the anaerobic threshold occurs in the range of 50% $\dot{V}O_2$[46] (or at 50% of heart rate reserve) in many healthy subjects. Although earlier studies suggested that this concept might be valid,[22, 47] more recent studies have shown that work rates not associated with elevated blood lactate levels can yield an appreciable training effect.[39, 48] In our own laboratory,[39] three groups of healthy subjects were assigned to train at a work rate equal to 80% of the anaerobic threshold, at a work rate mildly above the anaerobic threshold, or at a work rate appreciably above the anaerobic threshold. The length of the daily session was adjusted so that subjects performed the same amount of work per session regardless of group assignment. After a 5-week training program, the three groups were indistinguishable in terms of blood lactate level reductions, ventilation, oxygen uptake, and heart rate at a given level of heavy exercise; that is, the group training below the anaerobic threshold manifested no less a training effect than those training above the anaerobic threshold.

The existence of less than firm guidelines for designing an adequate training intensity for healthy subjects suggests that applying these guidelines to patient groups may be difficult.

Session Duration. Although no clear duration threshold has been demonstrated, it has been shown for moderate training intensities that sessions 10 to 15 minutes in duration yield an appreciably lower training effect than do sessions 30 to 60 minutes in duration.[18, 49] Since very high-intensity training predisposes subjects to injury and poor compliance, high-intensity, short-duration sessions are usually not recommended. It seems reasonable to conclude that training sessions of continuous exercise should last at least 20 minutes (and preferably 30–60 min) to be effective.

Does dividing the training session into two or three shorter sessions per day influence the results of the overall training program? Although little information exists on this point, it seems likely that divided sessions are satisfactory.

Session Frequency. There is a consensus that it is advisable to train 3 to 5 days per week.[18, 36, 37] It is possible to achieve increased aerobic fitness from as little as 2 days per week of training, but fewer benefits have usually been derived from such a regimen. There is little evidence that increasing the number of training sessions from five per week to seven per week is of benefit,[18] and daily training sessions are rarely practical.

Duration of the Program. Individuals who enter a training program are advised to continue training for life. It is also true that by progressively increasing the training work rate, it may be possible to achieve progressive increases in aerobic fitness over a period of many months. The time course of changes in a number of physiologic variables has been measured following the onset of an exercise training program of constant intensity. If the training work rate is kept constant, then these variables approach a new steady state exponentially. The half time of this exponential response differs somewhat among variables but is roughly 10 days.[50, 51] Thus, after about 3 to 4 weeks, no further increases in $\dot{V}O_2$max nor decreases in heart rate, blood lactate level, or epinephrine level are seen in response to a steady work rate.[48, 50, 51] Since most training programs do not maintain a constant intensity (training work rate is advanced as greater exercise intensities are tolerated), a training period longer than 3 weeks is required. Most investigators have used program durations in the 5- to 10-week range if their objectives were to achieve a substantial physiologic training effect.

Mode of Exercise. A variety of exercise modes have been shown to induce a training effect. If the activity causes a substantial increase in metabolic rate, and if the frequency, duration, and intensity of the exercise are sufficient (see earlier), an improvement in the aerobic performance of the muscle groups involved will be achieved.[18] Activities in this category include running, rapid walking, bicycling, swimming, and arm cranking.[36] It is important to remember that performance will be improved only in the muscle groups that are trained. Pollock and coworkers specifically demonstrated that subjects who were randomly included in training programs featuring running, walking, or bicycling that elicited heart rates of roughly 175 beats per minute achieved the same increases in $\dot{V}O_2$max.[52]

Initial Level of Fitness. The potential improvement in measures of aerobic fitness (when calculated as a per cent increase) is highest in previously sedentary subjects and is lowest in subjects who are already very fit.[18, 37, 53] This factor often makes comparison of published studies with different selection criteria difficult.

Age of the Participants. It has been well demonstrated that aerobic fitness can be improved even in geriatric subjects.[54–56] Since predicted maximum heart rate and oxygen uptake are lower in the elderly, training work rates are also lower. The anaerobic threshold is a higher fraction of $\dot{V}O_2$max in older subjects than in younger subjects. It therefore seems advisable to set a somewhat higher target training intensity if that target is to be specified in terms of a per cent of $\dot{V}O_2$max.

Maintaining Fitness. Experimental studies in which training programs are followed by the abrupt resumption of sedentary behavior show that the structural and physiologic changes that accompany training regress almost as fast as they were achieved. A substantial loss of fitness is seen within 2 weeks, and a return to pretraining status occurs after 10 weeks to 8 months of detraining.[18, 36, 57, 58] Thus, the effects of training programs are transitory unless exercise continues. However, based on available evidence, it seems likely that once a given level of aerobic fitness has been achieved, a less vigorous program suffices to maintain that fitness level. Modest decreases in session frequency and session duration can be accommodated without significant reductions in $\dot{V}O_2$max.[59, 60] However, a reduction in training intensity is associated with a decrease in aerobic fitness.[61]

BENEFITS OF EXERCISE PROGRAMS IN PULMONARY REHABILITATION*

"... an exercise program was instituted with subsequent marked improvement of capacity to exercise ... The progressive improvement in ability to walk without dyspnea suggested that a physiologic response similar to a training program in athletes may have been produced ..."

Alvan Barach and associates, 1952[62]

Virtually every program of pulmonary rehabilitation includes exercise. This has come about as a result of the pioneering work not only of Alvan Barach but, somewhat later, of William Miller and Thomas Petty as well. The result of their work was a change of opinion in the pulmonary medicine community. Instead of stressing rest and the avoidance of dyspnea, the community recognized that dyspnea was not itself harmful to the patient with obstructive lung disease. On the contrary, it became clear that these lung disease patients seemed to benefit from an increased level of activity.

Over the past 30 years, a number of investigators have attempted to formally document the benefits of exercise in the context of pulmonary rehabilitation programs. Their studies are reviewed later in this chapter; however, in fairness to these investigators, a distinction should be made. It is probably not appropriate to refer to the exercise that patients perform in most of this literature as exercise training. It might be useful to define a program of exercise training as one that has been specifically designed to elicit physiologic changes in the exercising muscles and in other organ systems. With a very few exceptions, exercise programs for chronic obstructive pulmonary disease (COPD) patients have not been designed as training programs in this sense.

Table 16–1 is a summary of 37 reports in the scientific literature that address exercise programs for COPD patients. Although an attempt has been made to comprehensively review this literature and to correctly characterize authors' findings, the goal of a complete summary of the work in this area has probably not been achieved.

---

*Most of this discussion is focused on the results of exercise programs for obstructive lung disease patients. Specific information regarding the training of patients with restrictive lung disease can be found in Chapter 32. Chapter 31 presents the results of training in asthmatic subjects.

Characteristics of Patients and Exercise Programs

Patient Characteristics. A total of 933 patients were observed in the 37 studies presented in Table 16–1. The average age of these patients was 61 years; thus, this population not only had lung disease but was also largely geriatric. It should be noted, however, that several reports have documented that the physiologic principles of exercise training apply to older as well as to younger individuals.[54–56] At present, men comprise the majority of all COPD patients; as a result, women were somewhat underrepresented in this group of 933 patients, constituting only 19% of the population. Thus, the overall conclusions that can be drawn from this literature can only be applied with certainty to men with COPD.

The average forced expiratory volume in 1 second (FEV_1) of the patients studied was approximately 1.1 L. This means that most of the patients studied were classified as having moderately severe or severe deficits in lung mechanics. Indeed, this reflects the practice of American pulmonary rehabilitation programs to enroll patients who are in an advanced stage of their disease. Twenty of these 37 studies reported arterial blood gas parameters that were measured at rest and prior to program initiation. The average mean PaO_2 reported in these studies was 69 ± 9 mm Hg. Thus, most patients who were studied were moderately hypoxemic. In only two studies—those of Pierce and colleagues[64] and Petty and coworkers[69]—was the average PaO_2 less than 60 mm Hg. Average $PaCO_2$ in these twenty studies was 42 ± 4 mm Hg; in other words, the majority of patients did not manifest carbon dioxide retention. In only three studies—those of Miller and associates,[63] Pierce and colleagues,[64] and Brundin and coworkers[75, 76]—was the average $PaCO_2$ greater than 45 mm Hg (the first two studies contained only four patients each). It might be noted that obstructed patients (even those with only mild obstruction) who demonstrate normal $PaCO_2$ regulation at rest generally retain carbon dioxide during exercise or at least fail to decrease $PaCO_2$ in response to lactic acidosis of exercise.[101]

In summary, the typical patients in these studies were men between 60 and 70 years of age with moderately severe airways obstruction and moderate hypoxemia but without carbon dioxide retention.

Exercise Programs. There is considerable variability among the exercise regimens that these 933 patients were asked to undergo as part of their rehabilitation programs. This may well reflect the wide range of exercise modalities available in the clinical practice of pulmonary rehabilitation. The duration of the exercise programs ranged from 12 days[97] to 1 year or more.[69, 75, 76, 81, 82] Table 16–2 summarizes the distribution of exercise program durations. The most common duration was 6 weeks (11 studies). Ten studies were of 4 months' duration or longer. On the other hand, five studies were less than 5 weeks in duration. In the context of physiologic responses to exercise training, it is worth mentioning that, although the biochemical signs of a training response can be seen as early as 1 week after the start of a vigorous program, it is generally believed that at least 5 weeks of progressive intensification of the program are necessary to yield a substantial training response. Thus, in the majority of patients who were included in the exercise studies reported, the program durations were sufficient to elicit a physiologic training response.

The frequency of sessions in these studies' programs also varied. In 14 programs, patients exercised several times per day; unfortunately, in several of these 14 studies, the investigators neglected to state how many times *per week* exercise sessions occurred. In other programs, sessions took place once per day several times per week. In 13 studies, exercise sessions were conducted daily or 5 times per week, and in 7 programs, sessions were held 3 or 4 times per week. Only one exercise program featured two or fewer sessions per week.[75, 76] Thus, based on what is known regarding the training responses of healthy subjects, sessions conducted 3 days per week or more produce a physiologic training effect when they are part of an otherwise adequate exercise program.

The amount of time patients spent exercising per day also varied widely among the studies. Several programs divided a day's exercise regimen into several sessions. As studies of healthy subjects have failed to discern appreciable differences among the effects of a single exercise session and those of divided sessions, whose individual durations sum to the same total exercise time as the single session (interval training),[18] it is probably reasonable to consider the total time spent exercising as the relevant variable. Table 16–3 shows the distribution of session durations among the 37 studies. Most studies of healthy subjects have shown that sessions of 30 to 45 minutes in duration are effective in inducing physiologic changes. Sessions shorter than 20 minutes in duration are considerably less effective. Based on this criterion, a substantial minority of the exercise programs in Table 16–1 feature sessions that are probably not sufficiently long to elicit a physiologic training effect.

It is most difficult to evaluate the adequacy of exercise intensity in most of these 37 studies. A substantial majority of the studies used subjective measures of exercise intensity (e.g., exercise intensity was "advanced as tolerated"). As discussed earlier, the concept of the existence (and appropriate measure) of a critical training intensity in healthy subjects is quite controversial. However, it is generally agreed that gauging exercise intensity by a physiologic yardstick (e.g., heart rate, $\dot{V}O_2$, or blood lactate level) is desirable. It is important to note that some researchers have asserted that many, if not most, patients with COPD are unable to exercise at a work rate that is sufficiently intense to stress the exercising muscles appreciably.[88, 102, 103] This assertion has intuitive appeal, since the exercise tolerance of many patients is limited by shortness of breath rather than by discomfort in the exercising muscles. Recent work that has focused on the design of adequate training intensities for COPD patients is explored later in this chapter. Furthermore, an important point has been made by Ries and Archibald.[95] Target training intensities based on heart rate or $\dot{V}O_2$ criteria that are adequate for healthy subjects may well be inappropriately low for COPD patients. It seems probable that work rates that approach the ventilatory limits of the patient may be well tolerated and effective.

Mode of Exercise. In the context of studying the capacity of exercise programs to increase exercise tolerance, it is important that the exercise testing modality induce the utilization of the same muscles that are trained during the exercise program. Although it may be argued that, for instance, bicycle ergometer testing of the benefits of a program of treadmill walking is suboptimal, there may be extenuating factors that encourage its use. For several reasons, the bicycle ergometer is a efficacious testing instrument when the physiologic responses to exercise are studied. The quantitation of the work performed is relatively straightforward. In contrast, the metabolic cost of treadmill, stepping, or walking exercise is difficult to predict and is very much a function of body weight. Exercise efficiency (measured by indirect calorimetry as the $\dot{V}O_2$ required for a given amount of external work performed) varies only over a narrow range in bicycle ergometer exercise[104] but varies appreciably with walking or stepping exercise. If the patient uses a wise pacing strategy or holds on to the handrails of the treadmill or stepping machine, his or her $\dot{V}O_2$ for a given speed or grade can be altered.[80, 103] Thus, a "learning effect" can be mistaken for a physiologic training effect. These considerations make the bicycle ergometer the preferable testing instrument, except for the rare patient who is unfamiliar with pedaling and in those programs in which the exercise does not involve the legs (e.g., arm training, which is discussed later in this chapter).

With respect to the preferred mode of exercise for rehabilitative purposes, studies of healthy subjects have shown that there is not a great difference among, for example, cycling, treadmill, walking, and stair climbing exercises as long as the metabolic cost of each is roughly equal.[18] Walking or treadmill exercise has a slight advantage over bicycle ergometer (or bicycle) exercise in that it involves a somewhat larger muscle mass. However, the metabolic cost of bicycle ergometer exercise is much easier to predict and makes possible easier exercise prescription.

Oxygen Supplementation. There is little question that patients with arterial PO_2 less than 55 mm Hg require chronic supplemental oxygen therapy.[105, 106] Exercise-induced hypoxemia is variably seen in patients with COPD. Its presence cannot be reliably predicted on the basis of resting spirometry or carbon monoxide diffusing capacity.[107, 108] A preliminary exercise test that features blood gas measurements (or at least pulse oximeter measurements) is advisable.

For those patients without substantial desaturation, the need for supplemental oxygen therapy is less clear. Certainly, oxygen therapy is expensive and should not be administered if no benefit is conferred. Yet, in 6 of the 37 studies cited in Table 16–1, oxygen was supplied routinely to patients undergoing rehabilitative exercise. This practice might be defended in that supplemental

Text continued on page 216

TABLE 16–1. SUMMARY OF STUDIES INVESTIGATING RESPONSES

Reference	Total No. of Subjects / Males (%) / Average Age	Average FEV$_1$ / Pao$_2$ (or Sao$_2$) and Paco$_2$	Program Duration / Session Frequency / Daily Duration	Exercise Intensity	Mode of Exercise During Program/During Testing
Miller and Taylor[63] (1962)	4 / 100 / 59 yr	0.8 L / — / —	3–6 wk / 1–2 per day / —	"maximum tolerated"	treadmill/treadmill
Pierce et al.[64] (1964)	9 / 100 / 55 yr	0.9 L / Pao$_2$ = 67 mm Hg / Paco$_2$ = 47 mm Hg	8 wk / 5–10 per day / 10–25 min/day	"lower than maximal speed"	treadmill/treadmill
Pierce et al.[65] (1965)	4 / 100 / 59 yr	0.9 L / Pao$_2$ = 52 mm Hg / Paco$_2$ = 51 mm Hg	10 wk / 5–10 per day / 25–100 min/day	"1/2–3/4 maximum attainable speed"	treadmill/treadmill
Paez et al.[66] (1967)	8 / 100 / 58 yr	26% pred / Sao$_2$ = 86% / Paco$_2$ = 45 mm Hg	3 wk / 5 per day / —	"to tolerance"	treadmill/cycle
Christie[67] (1968)	10 / 100 / 60 yr	0.7 L / — / —	8 wk / 1 per day / 15 min plus ½–1 mile walk per day	"adjusted to patient's condition"	stepping and walking/stepping
Woolf and Suero[68] (1969)	14 / 93 / 59 yr	21% pred / Pao$_2$ = 63 mm Hg / Paco$_2$ = 45 mm Hg	4–8 wk / 5 days/wk / 60 min/day	"as tolerated"	treadmill/treadmill
Petty et al.[69] (1969)	138 / 87 / 61 yr	1.0 L / Pao$_2$ = 58 mm Hg / Paco$_2$ = 38 mm Hg	Evaluations at 3, 6, and 12 mo / 1 per day / 60 min/day	"as tolerated"	walking/treadmill
Nicholas et al.[70] (1970)	8 / 93 / 61 yr	0.9 L / Pao$_2$ = 75 mm Hg / Paco$_2$ = 42 mm Hg	6 mo / 3 per wk / 30 min/day	"as tolerated"	walking/treadmill
Bass et al.[71] (1970)	11 / 91 / 61 yr	— / — / —	18 wk / 3 per day / —	"as tolerated"	cycle/cycle
Vyas et al.[72, 73] (1971)	11 / — / 61 yr	0.9 L / Pao$_2$ = 72 mm Hg / Paco$_2$ = 39 mm Hg	10 wk / 1–2 per day / 20–30 min/day	"as tolerated"	cycle/cycle
Holten[74] (1972)	15 / 80 / 56 yr	MVV = 39 L/min / Pao$_2$ = 67 mm Hg / Paco$_2$ = 45 mm Hg	4 wk / 2 per day / 12 min/day	"increased as tolerated"	cycle/cycle
Brundin[75, 76] (1974)	24 / 100 / 61 yr	0.8 L / Pao$_2$ = 60 mm Hg / Paco$_2$ = 48 mm Hg	6–18 mo / ½–2 per wk / 16 min/day	"increased as tolerated"	cycle/cycle
Degre et al.[77] (1974)	11 / 100 / 50 yr	42% pred / Pao$_2$ = 76 mm Hg / Paco$_2$ = 38 mm Hg	6 wk / 3 per wk / 25 min/day	75% of maximum work rate	cycle/cycle
Alpert et al.[78] (1974)	5 / 100 / 65 yr	26% pred / Pao$_2$ = 61 mm Hg / —	18 wk / 3 per day / 60 min/day	"increased as tolerated"	cycle/cycle
McGavin et al.[79] (1977)	12 / 100 / 61 yr	1.0 L / — / —	12 wk / 5 per wk / 5–10 min/day	"suit the individual's ability"	stairs/walking and cycle
Chester et al.[80] (1977)	21 / 100 / 51 yr	1.3 L / Pao$_2$ = 66 mm Hg / Paco$_2$ = 36 mm Hg	4 wk / 1 per day / 15 min/day	70% of maximum HR	treadmill/cycle and treadmill
Mertens et al.[81] (1978)	13 / 100 / 53 yr	1.6 L / Pao$_2$ = 88 mm Hg / Paco$_2$ = 36 mm Hg	1 yr / daily / —	"graded"	walking or jogging/cycle
Sinclair and Ingram[82] (1980)	17 / — / 66 yr	1.1 L / — / —	1 yr / daily / 15 min	"according to ability"	walking and stair climbing/walking
Moser et al.[83] (1980)	42 / 52 / 67 yr	0.9 L / Pao$_2$ = 78 mm Hg / —	6 wk / 3 per day / 30 min/day	"highest level tolerated"	treadmill or walking/treadmill

OF PATIENTS WITH COPD TO EXERCISE PROGRAMS

Routine O_2 Supplementation	Control Group	Inpatient or Outpatient Program Supervised Exercise	Improved Spirometry	Increased Exercise Endurance	Increased $\dot{V}O_2$ max	Change in Response to Identical Work Rate
yes	no	inpatient yes	—	yes	—	—
no	no	inpatient yes	no	yes	yes	decreases in HR (24%), $\dot{V}_E$ (40%), and $\dot{V}O_2$ (23%)
yes	no	inpatient yes	FEV_1 increased 13%	yes	—	decreases in $\dot{V}_E$ (29%) and $\dot{V}O_2$ (24%)
one half of subjects with O_2, one half without	no	inpatient yes	no	yes	—	no change in $\dot{V}_E$
no	no	inpatient yes	no	yes	yes	decrease in $\dot{V}_E$; no change in $\dot{V}O_2$
no	no	inpatient yes	no	yes	—	1.7 mEq/L decrease in La
no	no	outpatient only first 10 sessions	no	yes	—	decrease in $\dot{V}O_2$ (15%) at 6 mo
no	no	outpatient yes	no	yes	yes	—
no	no	outpatient no	no	yes	—	no change in $\dot{V}_{EQ}O_2$
no	no	inpatient and outpatient yes	no	yes	yes	decrease in $\dot{V}_E$ (7%), no change in $\dot{V}O_2$
yes	no	— yes	no	—	—	decreases in $\dot{V}_{EQ}O_2$ (14%) and La (1 mEq/L)
no	no	outpatient yes	no	yes	yes	no decrease in La
yes	yes	outpatient yes	no	yes	yes	no change in $\dot{V}O_2$ or La
no	no	outpatient no	no	yes	—	decreases in $\dot{V}O_2$ (22%) and $\dot{V}_{E2}$ (17%)
no	yes	outpatient no	no	yes	no	no change in $\dot{V}_E$ or $\dot{V}O_2$
no	yes	inpatient yes	no	yes	—	lower $\dot{V}O_2$ and $\dot{V}_E$ on treadmill but not on cycle
no	no	outpatient no	no	yes	—	no decrease in $\dot{V}O_2$ or $\dot{V}_E$
no	yes	outpatient no	no	yes	—	—
no	no	inpatient and outpatient, yes and no	—	yes	—	decreases in $\dot{V}O_2$ (13%) and $\dot{V}_E$ (18%)

Table continued on following page

TABLE 16–1. SUMMARY OF STUDIES INVESTIGATING RESPONSES

Reference	Total No. of Subjects Males (%) Average Age	Average FEV_1 Pao_2 (or Sao_2) and $Paco_2$	Program Duration Session Frequency Daily Duration	Exercise Intensity	Mode of Exercise During Program/During Testing
Mungall and Hainsworth[84] (1980)	10 100 57 yr	1.5 L Pao_2 = 67 mm Hg $Paco_2$ = 39 mm Hg	12 wk 1 per day 12 min/day	"as tolerated"	calisthenics/treadmill
Unger et al.[85] (1980)	30 — 60 yr	0.9 L Pao_2 = 72 mm Hg $Paco_2$ = 38 mm Hg	5 wk 3 per day 30 min/day	"highest level tolerated"	walking/treadmill
Cockcroft et al.[86] (1981)	18 100 61 yr	1.5 L — —	16 wk daily —	"graduated"	cycle, walking, etc./walking and treadmill
Alison et al.[87] (1981)	10 60 60 yr	1.5 L — —	12 wk 3 per wk 5–30 min/day	increasing per cent of highest work rate tolerated	cycle/walking and cycle
Belman and Kendregan[88] (1981)	7 71 60 yr	1.2 L — —	6 wk 4 per wk 40 min/day	maximum work rate sustained for 20 min	cycle/cycle
Mohsenifar et al.[89] (1983)	15 67 55 yr	42% pred Pao_2 = 70 mm Hg $Paco_2$ = 43 mm Hg	6 wk 3 per wk 20 min/day	75% pred maximum HR	treadmill or cycle/cycle
Tydeman et al.[90] (1984)	16 100 64 yr	0.7 L — —	36 wk 1 per day 30 min/day	"as tolerated"	stepping and walking/walking
Zack and Palange[91] (1985)	63 65 64 yr	1.3 L — —	12 wk 3 per week 25 min/day	"advanced as tolerated"	treadmill and walking/cycle
Jones et al.[92] (1985)	8 75 64 yr	0.8 L — —	10 wk 1 per day 20 min/day	"advanced as tolerated"	walking and calesthenics/cycle
Madsen et al.[93] (1985)	10 20 62 yr	0.8 L — —	6 wk 3 per day 15 min/day	"as tolerated"	stairs/treadmill
Ries and Moser[94] (1986)	7 29 67 yr	1.0 L — —	6 wk 3 per day 5–20 min/day	"pace increased as tolerated"	walking/cycle and treadmill
Ries and Archibald[95] (1987)	50 54 66 yr	1.1 L Pao_2 = 68 mm Hg $Paco_2$ = 41 mm Hg	6 wk 3 per day duration increased as tolerated	"approaching maximal exercise tolerance"	walking/cycle and treadmill
Corriveau et al.[96] (1988)	49 90 —	1.7 L Pao_2 = 71 mm Hg $Paco_2$ = 40 mm Hg	6 wk 2 per day 40 min/day	HR at anaerobic threshold	cycle/treadmill
Carter et al.[97] (1988)	59 68 62 yr	1.3 L — —	12 days 2 per day 30–40 min/day	"near the ventilatory limits"	treadmill and cycle/cycle
Busch and McClements[98] (1988)	7 71 65 yr	0.8 L — —	18 wk 5 days/wk 5 min/day	"symptom limited"	walking or stair stepping/cycle and stair stepping
Mall and Medeiros[99] (1988)	134 — —	— — —	6 wk 3 per wk 20 min/day	80% pred maximum HR	treadmill/treadmill
Holle et al.[100] (1988)	44 68 58 yr	33% pred — —	6 wk 3 per wk 20 min/day	80% of peak exercise level	treadmill/treadmill
Casaburi et al[101] (1991)	19 100 51 yr	1.8 L Pao_2 = 83 mm Hg $Paco_2$ = 40 mm Hg	8 wk 5 per wk 45–120 min/day	60% of difference between AT and $\dot{V}o_2$ max or 90% of AT	cycle/cycle

Key: HR: heart rate; $\dot{V}_E$: minute ventilation; pred: predicted; So_2: oxygen saturation of blood; La: blood lactate level; MVV: maximum voluntary ventilation; V_{EQO_2}: ventilatory equivalent for oxygen.

OF PATIENTS WITH COPD TO EXERCISE PROGRAMS Continued

Routine O_2 Supplementation	Control Group	Inpatient or Outpatient Program Supervised Exercise	Improved Spirometry	Increased Exercise Endurance	Increased $\dot{V}O_2$max	Change in Response to Identical Work Rate
no	no	outpatient no	FEV_1 increased 3.9%	yes	—	no change in HR or $\dot{V}_E$ at a given $\dot{V}O_2$
no	no	outpatient no	no	—	—	decreases in $\dot{V}O_2$ (13%) and $\dot{V}_E$ (12%)
no	yes	6 wk inpatient, yes; 10 wk outpatient, no	no	yes	no	no decrease in $\dot{V}O_2$ and $\dot{V}_E$
no	no	outpatient yes	no	yes	no	decrease in $\dot{V}_E$ (11%)
no	no	outpatient yes	no	yes	—	no change in $\dot{V}_E$ at a given $\dot{V}O_2$
no	no	outpatient yes	no	yes	no	decrease in La (12%), no change in $\dot{V}_E$ or HR
no	no	outpatient no	—	yes	—	—
yes	no	outpatient yes	—	yes	no	—
no	yes	outpatient no	no	yes, but no greater than that for control group	no	no change in $\dot{V}_E$, $\dot{V}O_2$, or HR
no	no	outpatient no	no	yes	yes	no change in $\dot{V}O_2$
no	no	outpatient no	no	yes	no	—
no	no	outpatient no	—	—	—	—
no	no	inpatient yes	—	—	yes	—
no	no	inpatient yes	no	yes	yes	—
no	yes	outpatient no	—	no	—	—
no	no	outpatient yes	—	yes	no	—
no	no	outpatient yes	no	yes	yes	—
no	no	inpatient yes	no	only for high-intensity training group	—	in high-intensity group decreases in La (31%), $\dot{V}_E$ (15%), and $\dot{V}O_2$ (6%)

TABLE 16–2. DISTRIBUTION OF EXERCISE PROGRAM DURATIONS IN 37 STUDIES OF PULMONARY REHABILITATION

Program Duration (wk)	No. of Programs
1–3	2
3–5	3
5–7	12
7–9	3
9–12	7
>12	10

oxygen therapy tends to allow even nonhypoxemic obstructed patients to exercise at higher work rates.[73, 91, 109–114] This effect might be mediated by the beneficial effects of pulmonary vasodilation or by the reduction of dyspnea through carotid chemoreceptor inhibition. However, it could be argued that if the training stimulus is linked to tissue hypoxia, then supplemental oxygen might reduce the probability that a training effect will be achieved. A well-controlled study is needed to determine whether supplemental oxygen therapy is an important element of rehabilitative exercise.

Control Groups. It is almost tautologic to assert that a well-controlled experiment is a necessary component of any scientific investigation. Since pulmonary rehabilitation programs offer multimodal therapy, it may be hazardous to ascribe any benefit specifically to the exercise component. A control group exposed to all elements of the program other than the exercise component obviates this problem.

However, a control group cannot be considered an absolute requirement unless we believe that all but 7 of the 37 studies were a waste of time. It can be strongly asserted that since the rehabilitative process seeks to increase the motivation of patients, any exercise test that is markedly dependent on motivation tends to show patient improvement even if the rehabilitation program does not have an exercise component. This is well demonstrated in the study of Jones and colleagues,[92] in which an increase in exercise endurance was observed in patients who participated in an exercise program; however, this improvement was matched by a control group that did not participate in an exercise program. In studies using exercise tests in which patient response does not depend on motivation, the need for a control group is less clear. Muscle ultrastructure or physiologic responses to a given exercise task are not dependent on motivational factors, and changes in these variables may be interpretable without a control group.

Setting and Supervision of the Exercise Program. Of the exercise programs for COPD patients represented in Table 16–1, 10 were inpatient programs and 22 were outpatient programs. At present, most inpatient programs in the United States cater to the patient requiring more intensive care (i.e., to the sicker patient). Despite this fact, the average FEV_1 of patients in the inpatient and outpatient studies listed in Table 16–1 (roughly 1 L/min in each group of studies) did not differ. This is likely because a number of the inpatient studies were performed at a time when inpatient programs were more readily funded. At least one recent study performed on the European continent[101] reflects the prevailing philosophy there that patients should be rehabilitated early, that is, when their rehabilitation will enable them to return to work rather than merely to get out of bed.

Among the outpatient programs, 13 of 22 featured exercise sessions that were largely or completely unsupervised and in which exercise was primarily performed in the home. Compliance with exercise prescription is probably lower in unsupervised programs than in supervised ones. Furthermore, the unsupervised patient is deprived of interaction with other patients and with staff, a factor that has been shown to contribute to dyspnea desensitization (see Chapter 18).

Results of the Exercise Programs

In many of these 37 studies, the authors stated that the patients derived subjective benefits from their exercise programs. Patients often stated that they felt better and that they believed they could tolerate more exercise. However, these subjective benefits may be the result of other components of the rehabilitation program, and it is better to rely on the objective benefits that are derived to demonstrate the value of exercise.

Improved Spirometry. It is probably unreasonable to expect that exercise would be able to reverse the structural deterioration in the lung that accompanies COPD. Indeed, FEV_1 improved significantly in patients of only 2 of the 29 studies presented in Table 16–1 in which resting spirometric data were recorded before and after the exercise program.[65, 84] These two studies included relatively few patients, and the absolute increases in FEV_1 observed in them were small. Besides, it is quite predictable that a few of these studies reject the null hypothesis (that is, exercise does not improve FEV_1) with 95% confidence, even if the null hypothesis is in fact true. Thus, any benefit attained in an exercise program cannot be ascribed to improvements in lung mechanics.

A related issue is whether a program of whole-body exercise is capable of strengthening the respiratory muscles to the extent that an improvement in the ability to ventilate the lungs is produced. This issue was specifically addressed by Belman and Kendregan,[115] who found that a program of exercise was not successful in improving measures of respiratory muscle strength.

TABLE 16–3. DISTRIBUTION OF EXERCISE SESSION DURATIONS IN 37 STUDIES OF PULMONARY REHABILITATION

Session Duration (min)	No. of Studies
10–20	11
20–30	7
30–40	5
40–60	2
>60	5
unclear or not stated	7

Improved Exercise Endurance. In the studies listed in Table 16–1, improved endurance was judged either by an ability to tolerate a higher level of exercise or by an ability to exercise at a given level for a longer period of time. In 31 of the 32 studies in which exercise tolerance was determined, tolerance was found to increase after a program of exercise. The only study that did not find such an increase was relatively small[98]; in another study, exercise tolerance increased but only by as much as was observed in the control group.[92]

There are several ways of evaluating the finding that exercise tolerance is increased after an exercise program. The overwhelming prevalence of improved exercise tolerance is evidence to support that exercise programs are effective therapy for lung disease patients. On the other hand, there is no question that exercise endurance is subject to motivational factors. Furthermore, performance of some tasks improves with practice[80, 103] (see Chapter 24); it seems unlikely that improvement that results from practice translates into improvement in the tolerance of everyday tasks.

Improved $\dot{V}O_2$max. The change in peak $\dot{V}O_2$ was measured in only about one half of the studies listed in Table 16–1. Of the 18 studies in which it was measured, $\dot{V}O_2$max improved in 10 studies but not in 8 others. It seems reasonable to look for differences among studies that might explain this disparity; unfortunately, no such differences emerge. It was observed that studies that utilized treadmill or walking tests demonstrated an improvement in $\dot{V}O_2$max more often (5 of 7 studies) than studies that employed bicycle ergometer tests (4 of 10 studies). It is interesting to note that all 6 of the studies that measured $\dot{V}O_2$max performed before 1977 found increases in $\dot{V}O_2$max, whereas only 4 of 12 studies performed since 1977 showed an increase in this value. The importance of this observation is unclear.

Although it is tempting to interpret an increase in $\dot{V}O_2$max as an indication of improved physiologic ability to perform exercise, such a conclusion would be inappropriate. Only in patients in whom $\dot{V}O_2$ fails to increase with increasing work rate does $\dot{V}O_2$max indicate that the peak rate of oxygen transport has been reached. However, a plateau in $\dot{V}O_2$ is seen regularly only in athletes and in some patients with cardiovascular disease. In all other patients, measured $\dot{V}O_2$max must be considered to be influenced by motivation and effort.

Reduced Responses to Identical Exercise Tasks. Twenty-five of the 37 studies compared patients' physiologic responses to identical exercise tests before and after exercise programs. Measured physiologic variables included heart rate, $\dot{V}O_2$, minute ventilation ($\dot{V}E$), and blood lactate level. It should not be implied that changes in these responses can be unequivocally interpreted as representing an increased physiologic ability to perform work (i.e., a training effect).

In this respect, three considerations deserve mention. First, decreases in heart rate are not necessarily a sign that the exercising muscles have been trained. Heart rates respond to decreases in the levels of circulating catecholamines. Levels of these "fight or flight" hormones can be reduced by a subject's perception of the difficulty of an exercise test, which may decrease with time.

Second, exercise tests that are subject to "learning effects" may yield a reduced metabolic requirement for a given task that a subject has practiced; this result may not be a sign of a physiologic training effect. This has especially been shown to be the case for treadmill exercise and may explain why decreased responses to a given rate of treadmill work were seen in 7 of 10 studies. In contrast, decreased responses to bicycle ergometer exercise were seen in only 4 of 10 studies.

Third, a large reduction in $\dot{V}O_2$ in response to a given exercise task is unlikely to be the result of a physiologic training effect. Rather, it may be the result of a better performance strategy. Four studies in which $\dot{V}O_2$ fell by 15%, 22%, 23%, and 24%[69, 78, 64, 65] probably fall into this category (all but one were treadmill studies). In fact, Belman has posited that any decrease in $\dot{V}O_2$ must mean that less work is performed.[103] This is likely to be true for moderate work rates for which the $\dot{V}O_2$ response to exercise is directly proportional to the adenosine triphosphate requirement for the exercise.[104] However, at work rates above the anaerobic threshold, training is associated with reduced lactate production; this apparently results in a slightly lower $\dot{V}O_2$ requirement[25, 29] (up to approximately 10%) (see Fig. 16–4). Thus, a mildly reduced $\dot{V}O_2$ at heavy work rates is one sign of a physiologic training effect.

The four studies discussed earlier in which a reduced physiologic response to bicycle ergometer exercise was observed deserve special attention. Do these studies present clear evidence of physiologic training effects? Holten[74] found a reduction in the ventilatory equivalent for $\dot{V}O_2$ ($\dot{V}E/\dot{V}O_2$) coupled with an average reduction of 1 mEq/L in blood lactate level. It is surprising that this response was obtained in patients exercising only 12 minutes per day for 4 weeks. Similarly, Alison and colleagues[87] found that $\dot{V}E$ decreased by 11% in response to identical exercise tasks performed before and after a program consisting of 5- to 30-minute sessions three times per week. On the other hand, the small group studied by Alpert and coworkers[78] exercised 60 minutes per day for 18 weeks. The 22% reduction in $\dot{V}O_2$ observed by these investigators is difficult to interpret as a training response. Finally, Casaburi and associates[101] found substantial reductions in ventilation and blood lactate levels and small reductions in $\dot{V}O_2$ in response to work rates engendering lactic acidosis. These changes were elicited by an exercise regimen designed to mimic exercise programs shown to be effective in young, healthy subjects; a low-intensity training regimen was found to be much less effective. The results of this study are discussed more fully later in this chapter.

The study of Belman and Kendregan[88] examining the ability of COPD patients to achieve a physiologic training effect deserves special mention. These investigators collected biopsies of muscle from patients before and after the patients participated in an exercise program. It is arguable that muscle biopsy is the gold standard for determining whether a training effect has been achieved. The study of Belman and Kendregan did not find changes in the muscle biopsy material that were consistent with a training response. However, this study has been criticized as possibly utilizing an inadequate training stimulus.[116] Further research in this area seems warranted.

RESPONSES TO EXERCISE TRAINING IN CHRONIC OBSTRUCTIVE PULMONARY DISEASE

Patients with COPD would indeed benefit if they could reduce their ventilatory requirement for exercise through a program of exercise training as healthy subjects do (see Fig. 16–5). Although healthy subjects are not limited in their exercise tolerance by the level of ventilation they can sustain, patients with COPD often are.[117] However, exercise programs for COPD patients have seldom focused on this physiologic rationale. There are two related but distinct reasons why this is so.

First, it has been posited that most patients with COPD are unable to stress the exercising muscles sufficiently to obtain a physiologic training effect.[88, 102, 103] This proposition has intuitive appeal because the symptom that usually results in the discontinuation of exercise is not muscle discomfort but dyspnea. It would not be unreasonable to suppose that many patients with COPD would be unable to exceed the critical training intensity and thus would be unable to train their muscles no matter what duration and frequency of exercise sessions were used. However, the logic of this supposition may be flawed. As discussed earlier, the determinants and even the existence of a critical training intensity are uncertain. Furthermore, it is quite possible that COPD patients train their muscles at lower intensities than do healthy subjects. Many patients accommodate to their disease by becoming extremely sedentary. Even low exercise intensities might serve as a conditioning stimulus. Also, the pulmonary vascular disease that often accompanies COPD may reduce oxygen delivery to the exercising muscles; this reduction might yield a greater than expected training stimulus at low work rates.

The second reason why it was supposed that patients with COPD might be unable to reduce their ventilatory requirement by training is that they are often unable to sustain work rates associated with lactic acidosis. As can be seen in Figure 16–5, work rates that are not associated with lactic acidosis (i.e., those below the anaerobic threshold) do not have a reduced ventilatory requirement after training. Thus, even if a physiologic training effect could be achieved, the ventilatory requirement for exercise might not be reduced.

Review of the literature, however, gives reason to believe that many (if not most) patients with COPD are able to exceed their anaerobic thresholds. Table 16–4 is a list of selected studies in which exercise-induced increases in blood lactate level (or, equivalently, decreases in standard bicarbonate level) were observed in COPD patients. It can be noted that the patients studied were able on average to raise their blood lactate levels appreciably; it is also notable that these lactate levels were observed at work rates that would not engender lactic acidosis in healthy subjects.

Predicting which patients will have increased blood lactate levels during exercise seems to be impossible if the patients do not actually perform exercise. Lung function at rest does not appear to be a strong determinant of blood lactate level, probably because the disease process produces a parallel decline in exercise tolerance and a tendency for the early onset of lactic acidosis. Spiro and coworkers[119] found that average peak lactate levels differed only modestly (3.6 mEq/L versus 2.6 mEq/L) in two groups of 20 COPD patients whose FEV_1 averaged 1.45 L and 0.62 L, respectively. Sue and associates[122] found no significant correlations between either resting FEV_1 or carbon monoxide diffusing capacity and the amount that standard bicarbonate falls with exercise. Casaburi and associates[101] found no significant correlations between FEV_1 and either the lactate threshold (the $\dot{V}O_2$ at which the lactate level begins to rise) or peak lactate levels.

Based on the foregoing considerations, it seems reasonable to contend that at least some COPD patients are able to achieve a physiologic training effect from a well-designed training program. Furthermore, these physiologic changes should have salutary effects on exercise tolerance.

We recently published a study designed to validate these concepts.[101] Nineteen male patients with COPD of mostly moderate severity who were found to have increased blood lactate levels during exercise underwent a program of stationary bicycle training. We took into consideration the design parameters of training programs for healthy subjects, and thus our patients trained 45 minutes per day and 5 days per week for 8 weeks. The exercise intensity was selected so as to increase blood lactate level substantially at the training work rate. To determine whether exercise intensity was a crucial variable, one half of the patient group trained at a lower work rate (below anaerobic threshold) than the other but exercised for a proportionately longer time each day. Before and after the training program, the participants underwent exercise testing that featured measurement of ventilation and gas exchange as well as sampling of arterial blood. Each subject performed incremental exercise tests as well as constant work rate tests at high (above anaerobic threshold) and low (below anaerobic threshold) work rates.

Figure 16–6 compares the physiologic responses to identical exercise stimuli in one of the patients in our study. It can be seen that the increase in blood lactate level is both delayed and attenuated after exercise training. Presumably as a consequence of this, ventilation, carbon dioxide output, and oxygen uptake were modestly but distinctly reduced. In association with this, greater exercise tolerance was observed during the incremental and heavy exercise tests. A reasonably good correlation was seen between the decrease in ventilation produced by training and the decrease in blood lactate level (Fig. 16–7); this correlation suggests a cause-and-effect relationship. We searched for predictors of which patients would be able to obtain the greatest physiologic

TABLE 16-4. SELECTED STUDIES IN WHICH LACTIC ACIDOSIS WAS OBSERVED IN COPD PATIENTS DURING EXERCISE

Reference	Total No. of Subjects / Males (%) / Average Age	Average FEV$_1$ / Pao$_2$ and Paco$_2$	Mode of Exercise	Exercise Intensity	Peak Lactate Level or Bicarbonate Level Change
Shuey et al.[118] (1969)	4 / — / 53 yr	1.2 L / — / —	treadmill, zero grade, and constant speed	maximum sustained	7.2 mEq/L
Vyas et al.[73] (1971)	11 / — / 61 yr	0.9 L / Pao$_2$ = 72 mm Hg / Paco$_2$ = 39 mm Hg	incremental bicycle ergometer	maximum (average = 100 watts)	4.2 mEq/L
Holten[74] (1972)	15 / 80 / 56 yr	MVV = 39 L/min / Pao$_2$ = 67 mm Hg / Paco$_2$ = 45 mm Hg	constant work rate bicycle ergometer	one half pred exercise tolerance	3.9 mEq/L
Brundin[76] (1974)	24 / 100 / 61 yr	0.8 L / Pao$_2$ = 60 mm Hg / Paco$_2$ = 48 mm Hg	constant work rate bicycle ergometer (supine)	greatest load tolerated (average = 22 watts)	4.8 mEq/L
Degre et al.[77] (1974)	11 / 100 / 50 yr	42% pred / Pao$_2$ = 76 mm Hg / Paco$_2$ = 38 mm Hg	constant work rate bicycle ergometer	submaximum work rate for 6 min (75 watts)	3.6 mEq/L
Spiro et al.[119] (1975)	40 / 100 / 61 yr	1.0 L / Pao$_2$ = 73 mm Hg / Paco$_2$ = 40 mm Hg	incremental bicycle ergometer	85% of maximum pred HR (average = 85 watts)	3.1 mEq/L
Kanarek et al.[120] (1979)	12 / — / 59 yr	1.0 L / Pao$_2$ = 80 mm Hg / Paco$_2$ = 34 mm Hg	incremental bicycle ergometer	maximum (average = 85 watts)	decrease in bicarbonate level of 1.7 mEq/L
Raffestin et al.[121] (1982)	20 / — / 67 yr	1.0 L / Pao$_2$ = 60 mm Hg / Paco$_2$ = 44 mm Hg	incremental bicycle ergometer	maximum (average = 70 watts)	5 mEq/L
Mohsenifar et al.[89] (1983)	8 / 67 / 55 yr	42% pred / Pao$_2$ = 70 mm Hg / Paco$_2$ = 43 mm Hg	incremental bicycle ergometer	30 watts (submaximum in most patients)	3.4 mEq/L
Sue et al.[122] (1988)	22 / — / 62 yr	45% pred / Pao$_2$ = 71 mm Hg / Paco$_2$ = 43 mm Hg	incremental bicycle ergometer	maximum (average $\dot{V}O_2$max = 1.2 L/min)	decrease in standard bicarbonate level = 3.0 mEq/L
Holle et al.[100] (1988)	44 / 68 / 58 yr	33% pred / — / —	incremental treadmill	maximum (average = 4 METS)	decrease in bicarbonate level >5 mEq/L in 41% of subjects
Casaburi et al.[101] (1991)	19 / 100 / 51 yr	1.8 L / Pao$_2$ = 83 mm Hg / Paco$_2$ = 40 mm Hg	incremental bicycle ergometer	maximum (average $\dot{V}O_2$max = 1.5 L/min)	6.5 mEq/L

Key: METS: multiple of resting metabolic rate; pred: predicted.

effect from training (indicated by decreases in blood lactate level and in ventilation in response to a heavy exercise task). Spirometric measurements made at rest were not good predictors; of the patients studied, those with a high or low FEV$_1$ were equally likely to have a training effect. However, those with high pretraining peak lactate levels had significantly greater decreases in ventilation and lactate levels as a result of training, suggesting that a prerequisite for triaging patients to this mode of therapy would include a test of maximum exercise and measurement of blood lactate level.

Other findings of this study require further investigation. The group that trained at a lower exercise intensity manifested a smaller training effect, even though the total work performed per session was the same as that performed by those who trained at the higher exercise intensity. This observation has implications for exercise prescription for COPD patients (see Chapter 24). Another interesting issue relates to the magnitude of the ventilatory decrease that accompanies the training-induced decrease in blood lactate level. On average, ventilation decreased 2.5 L/min for each 1 mEq/L decrease in blood lactate level in these 19 COPD subjects as opposed to an average reduction of 7.2 L/min per 1 mEq/L seen in training studies of healthy subjects.[29] Apparently, some COPD patients (those with very low breathing reserves) use the "benefit" of decreased metabolic acidosis to decrease ventilation, whereas others use this benefit to decrease carbon dioxide retention and systemic acidosis[123] (see Chapter 5).

Before this "physiologic strategy" can be incorporated routinely into programs of pulmonary rehabilitation, several questions need to be answered. Are most patients willing to undergo the rigorous exercise program required? Can "maintenance programs" be designed to ensure lasting benefits? Can practical selection criteria

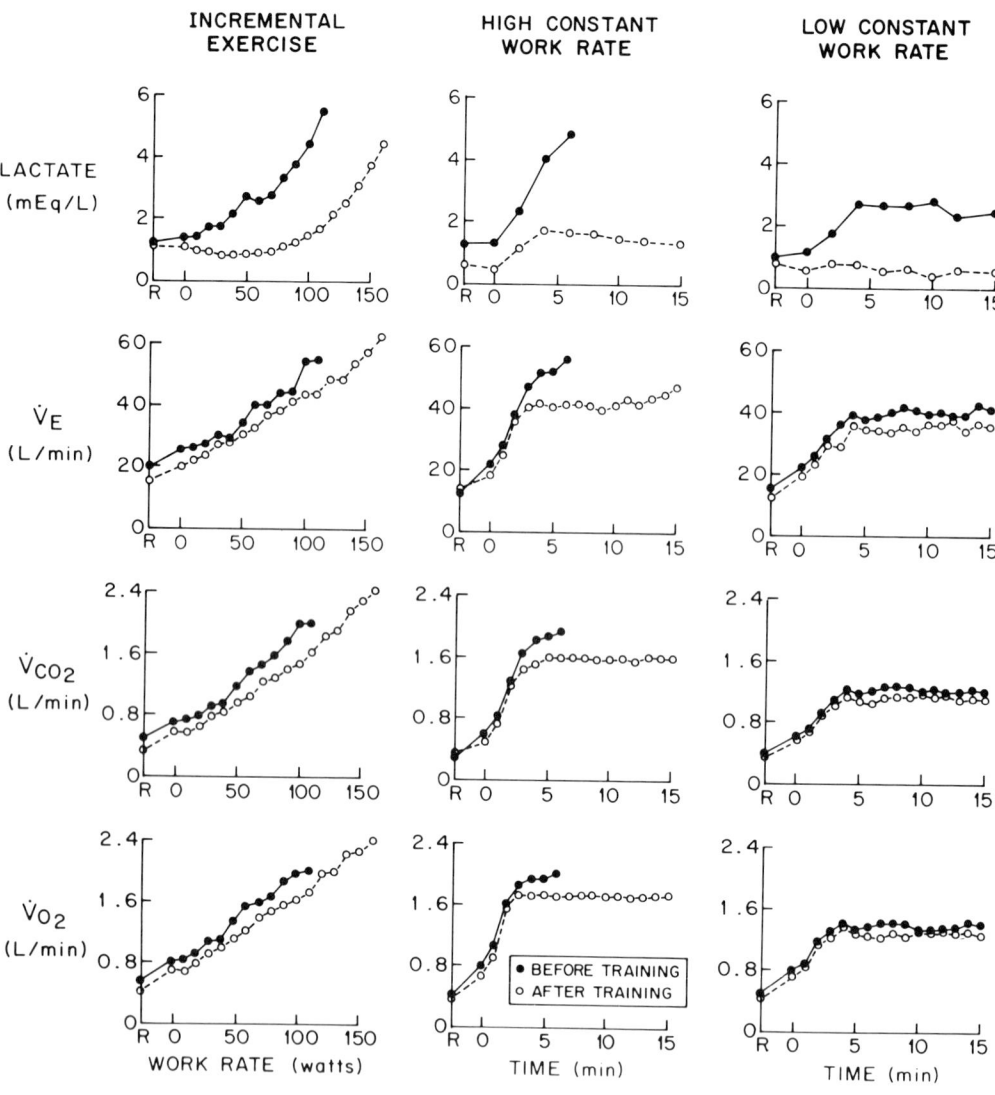

FIGURE 16-6. The time course of arterial lactate concentration, $\dot{V}_E$, $\dot{V}_{CO_2}$, and $\dot{V}_{O_2}$ before (*closed circles*) and after (*open circles*) a program of exercise training in a patient with chronic obstructive pulmonary disease (COPD). (Forced expiratory volume in 1 second [FEV_1] is 54% of predicted.) (*Left panels:* responses to incremental exercise [10 watts per minute]; *middle panels:* responses to high constant work rate [90 watts]; *right panels:* responses to low constant work rate test [50 watts].) A physiologic training effect is evidenced by a reduction in both blood lactate and in ventilation after the training program. Exercise duration is also improved. (From Casaburi R, Patessio A, Ioli F, et al. Reductions in exercise lactic acidosis and ventilation as a result of exercise training in patients with obstructive lung disease. Am Rev Respir Dis 1991; 143:9–18.)

be developed, and will the presence of frailty or of very severe lung disease be an exclusion criterion? We will probably not have to wait long before these questions can be answered.

EXERCISE TRAINING FOR THE UPPER EXTREMITIES

The upper extremities are quite often involved in activities of daily living. Patients with obstructive lung disease tolerate upper extremity exercise quite poorly because some of the muscles utilized are also accessory muscles of respiration. Activities involving the arms tend to produce dyspnea and discoordination of the respiratory muscles. Thus, strengthening of the upper extremities may be especially advantageous for pulmonary patients.

In humans, the histologic characteristics of the arm muscles are not much different from those of the leg muscles.[124] Yet, the muscle mass of the arms is smaller and, in almost all subjects, the arms are relatively untrained because they do not bear weight during ambulation. This fact has important metabolic implications. Healthy subjects can perform only low-level exercise without resorting to anaerobic energy sources. Furthermore, exercise tolerance is distinctly lower when the arms are unsupported during exercise, especially when they are elevated above the head.[125]

The consequences of the early onset of lactic acidosis are appreciable. $\dot{V}_{O_2}$, carbon dioxide output, and, in particular, ventilatory requirements are higher than if the exercise were to be performed totally aerobically. The concept that exercise with the arms is inherently "inefficient" (i.e., it requires more than the expected oxygen uptake to produce a given power output) is probably wrong; most investigators have simply studied exercise levels that are associated with lactic acidosis. This is not particularly surprising; the anaerobic threshold of sedentary healthy subjects for arm cranking exercise is typically around 20 watts.[126] In contrast, elite athletes who have trained for arm cranking tasks can manifest an anaerobic threshold of about 150 watts.[127]

The response of the upper body musculature to training regimens has been less well studied than that of the

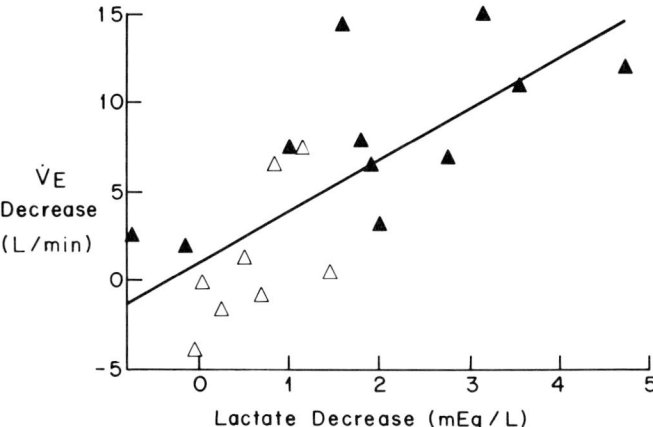

FIGURE 16-7. Relationship between the decrease in $\dot{V}_E$ and the decrease in arterial lactate levels in response to identical exercise tasks (high constant work rate tests) as a result of exercise training in 19 patients with COPD. (*Closed triangles:* high work rate training group; *open triangles:* low work rate training group.) The decrease in ventilation is highly correlated with the decrease in lactate ($r = .73$). The *solid line* is obtained by linear regression: $\Delta\dot{V}_E = 2.84 \Delta\text{lactate} + 1.19$. (From Casaburi R, Patessio A, Ioli F, et al. Reductions in exercise lactic acidosis and ventilation as a result of exercise training in patients with obstructive lung disease. Am Rev Respir Dis 1991; 143:9–18.)

lower body musculature, but the same principles seem to hold true in both areas. The principle of training specificity applies, that is, only upper body exercise trains the upper body muscles. Session duration, the number of sessions per week, and the length of an upper-body training program need to be approximately the same as those for a lower-body training program.[128, 129] Training intensity is necessarily lower but should be scaled to reflect the lower exercise tolerance of the arms.[128–130] The mode of exercise in an upper-body training program is usually arm cranking, but dynamic arm exercise designed to simulate the activities of daily living is also useful.

Training of the arms in healthy subjects increases $\dot{V}_{O_2}$max.[128] Furthermore, at identical work rates, lower levels of both blood lactate and ventilation are observed.[131] Although studies in COPD patients that attempt to confirm that arm exercise can produce lower blood lactate levels and can reduce ventilation have yet to be performed, it seems intuitively probable that these changes would be of benefit to such patients.

In fact, only a few studies have examined the responses of COPD patients to upper body exercise. Celli and coworkers[132] found that patients with severe COPD had very limited endurance for arm exercise. Exercise was limited by dyspnea, and in several patients dyssynchronous thoracoabdominal breathing was observed. It was postulated that the increased burden on the accessory muscles of respiration leads to dyssynchrony, early fatigue, and dyspnea. In another study, Criner and Celli[133] found that unsupported arm exercise leads COPD patients to depend on the diaphragm for breathing rather than on the inspiratory muscles of the rib cage, which are needed to support the arms.

Ries and associates[134] recently reported provocative results from a comparison of patients who participated in a multidisciplinary pulmonary rehabilitation program. Compared with a group that performed no upper extremity exercise, a group that did undergo such exercise exhibited increases in the endurance of arm cranking exercise but not in that for simulated activities of daily living.

The physiologic rationale for utilizing exercise training to enable COPD patients to reduce their ventilatory requirement for exercise is compelling. This form of therapy aims to relieve the stress on a sick organ system and may improve patient functional capacity. Since exercise programs are already an integral part of pulmonary rehabilitation, it is tempting to conjecture that fine-tuning these exercise regimens in order to improve their physiologic basis will yield a more effective program of pulmonary rehabilitation.

ACKNOWLEDGMENT

The author thanks Mrs. Maclovia Wallace for her excellent secretarial support in the preparation of this manuscript.

REFERENCES

1. Stark RD. Dyspnoea: Assessment and pharmacological manipulation. Eur Respir J 1988; 1:280–287.
2. Woodcock AA, Gross ER, Gellert A, et al. Effects of dihydrocodeine, alcohol, and caffeine on breathlessness and exercise tolerance in patients with chronic obstructive lung disease and normal blood gases. N Engl J Med 1981; 305:1611–1616.
3. Woodcock AA, Gross ER, Geddes DM. Drug treatment of breathlessness: Contrasting effects of diazepam and promethazine in pink puffers. BMJ 1981; 283:343–346.
4. Sue DY, Chung MM, Grosvenor M, Wasserman K. Effect of altering the proportion of dietary fat and carbohydrate on exercise gas exchange in normal subjects. Am Rev Respir Dis 1989; 139:1430–1434.
5. Theodore J, Robin ED, Morris AJR, et al. Augmented ventilatory response to exercise in pulmonary hypertension. Chest 1986; 89:39–44.
6. McArdle WD, Katch FI, Katch VL. Exercise physiology: Energy, nutrition and human performance. Philadelphia: Lea & Febiger, 1986.
7. Lamb DR. Physiology of exercise: Responses and adaptations. 2nd ed. New York: MacMillan Publishing Company, 1984.
8. Saltin B, Gollnick PD. Skeletal muscle adaptability: Significance for metabolism and performance. In: Peachey LD (ed). Handbook of Physiology: Skeletal muscle. Washington, DC: American Physiological Society, 1986, pp 555–631.
9. Komi PV, Viitasalo JHT, Havu M, et al. Skeletal muscle fibers and muscle enzyme activities in monozygous and dizygous twins of both sexes. Acta Physiol Scand 1977; 100:385–392.
10. Gollnick PD, Armstrong RB, Saltin B, et al. Effect of training on enzyme activity and fiber composition of human skeletal muscle. J Appl Physiol 1973; 34:107–111.
11. Anderson P, Henriksson J. Training induced changes in the subgroups of human type II skeletal muscle fibers. Acta Physiol Scand 1977; 99:123–125.
12. Holloszy JO. Adaptation of skeletal muscle to endurance exercise. Med Sci Sports 1975; 7:155–164.
13. Pattengale PK, Holloszy JO. Augmentation of skeletal muscle myoglobin by a program of treadmill running. Am J Physiol 1967; 213:783–785.
14. Saltin B, Henriksson J, Nygaard E, Andersen P. Fiber types

and metabolic potentials of skeletal muscles in sedentary man and endurance runners. Ann N Y Acad Sci 1977; 301:3–29.
15. Henriksson J. Training induced adaptation of skeletal muscle and metabolism during submaximal exercise. J Physiol 1977; 270:661–675.
16. Saltin B. Cardiovascular and pulmonary adaptation to physical activity. In: Bouchard C, Shephard RJ, Stephens T, et al. (eds). Exercise, Fitness and Health. Champaign, IL: Human Kinetic Books, 1990, pp 187–203.
17. Clausen JP, Klausen K, Rasmussen B, Trap-Jensen J. Central and peripheral circulatory changes after training of the arms or legs. Am J Physiol 1973; 225:675–682.
18. Pollock ML, Wilmore JH. Exercise in health and disease. 2nd ed. Philadelphia: W.B. Saunders Co., 1990.
19. Pollock ML, Miller HS, Janeway R, et al. Effects of walking on body composition and cardiovascular function of middle-aged men. J Appl Physiol 1971; 30:126–130.
20. Gaesser GA, Wilson LA. Effects of continuous and interval training on the parameters of the power-endurance time relationship for high-intensity exercise. Int J Sports Med 1988; 9:417–421.
21. Yoshida T, Suda Y, Takeuchi N. Endurance training regimen based upon arterial blood lactate: Effects on anaerobic threshold. Eur J Appl Physiol 1982; 49:223–230.
22. Henritze J, Weltman A, Schurrer RL, Barlow K. Effects of training at and above the lactate threshold on the lactate threshold and maximal oxygen uptake. Eur J Appl Physiol 1985; 54:84–88.
23. Gaesser GA, Poole DC. Lactate and ventilatory thresholds: Disparity in time course of adaptations to training. J Appl Physiol 1986; 61:999–1004.
24. Davis JA, Frank MH, Whipp BJ, Wasserman K. Anaerobic threshold alterations caused by endurance training in middle-aged men. J Appl Physiol 1979; 46:1039–1046.
25. Casaburi R, Storer TW, Ben-Dov I, Wasserman K. Effect of endurance training on possible determinants of $\dot{V}O_2$ during heavy exercise. J Appl Physiol 1987; 62:199–207.
26. Wasserman K, Hansen JE, Sue DY, Whipp BJ. Principles of exercise testing and interpretation. Philadelphia: Lea & Febiger, 1987.
27. Hansen JE, Casaburi R, Cooper DM, Wasserman K. Oxygen uptake as related to work rate increment during cycle ergometer exercise. Eur J Appl Physiol 1988; 57:140–145.
28. Wasserman K, Whipp BJ, Koyal SN, Cleary MG. Effect of carotid body resection on ventilatory and acid-base control during exercise. J Appl Physiol 1975; 39:354–358.
29. Casaburi R, Storer TW, Wasserman K. Mediation of reduced ventilatory response to exercise after endurance training. J Appl Physiol 1987; 63:1533–1538.
30. Fox EL, Bartels RL, Klinzing J, Ragg K. Metabolic responses to interval training programs of high and low power output. Med Sci Sports 1977; 9:191–196.
31. Taylor R, Jones NL. The reduction by training of CO_2 output during exercise. Eur J Cardiol 1979; 9:53–62.
32. Winder WW, Hickson RC, Hagberg JM, et al. Training-induced changes in hormonal and metabolic responses to submaximal exercise. J Appl Physiol 1979; 46:766–771.
33. Sutton JR, Farrell PA, Harber VJ. Hormonal adaptation to physical activity. In: Bouchard C, Shephard RJ, Stephens T, et al. (eds). Exercise, Fitness, and Health. Champaign, IL: Human Kinetics Books, 1990.
34. Gisolfi C, Robinson S. Relations between physical training, acclimatization and heat tolerance. J Appl Physiol 1969; 26:530–534.
35. Hill DW, Cureton KJ, Grisham SC, Collins MA. Effect of training on the rating of perceived exertion at the ventilatory threshold. Eur J Appl Physiol 1987; 56:206–211.
36. American College of Sports Medicine Position Stand. The recommended quantity and quality of exercise for developing and maintaining cardiorespiratory and muscular fitness in healthy adults. Med Sci Sports Exerc 1990; 22:265–274.
37. Wenger HA, Bell GJ. The interactions of intensity, frequency and duration of exercise training in altering cardiorespiratory fitness. Sports Med 1986; 3:346–356.
38. Dwyer J, Bybee R. Heart rate indices of the anaerobic threshold. Med Sci Sports Exerc 1983; 15:72–76.
39. Casaburi R, Storer T, Sullivan C, et al. Influence of training intensity on the physiologic responses to heavy exercise (abstract). FASEB J 1990; 4:A1073.
40. Sharkey BJ. Intensity and duration of training and the development of cardiorespiratory endurance. Med Sci Sports Exerc 1970; 2:197–202.
41. Shephard RJ. Intensity, duration and frequency of exercise as determinants of the response to a training regime. Int Z Angew Physiol 1968; 26:272–278.
42. Gaesser GA, Rich RG. Effects of high- and low-intensity exercise training on aerobic capacity and blood lipids. Med Sci Sports Exerc 1984; 16:269–274.
43. Katch V, Weltman A, Sady S, Freedson P. Validity of the relative percent concept for equating training intensity. Eur J Appl Physiol 1978; 39:219–227.
44. Kindermann W, Simon G, Keul J. The significance of the aerobic-anaerobic transition for the determination of work load intensities during endurance training. Eur J Appl Physiol 1979; 42:25–34.
45. Casaburi R, Wasserman K. Exercise training in pulmonary rehabilitation. N Engl J Med 1986; 314:1509–1511.
46. Hansen JE, Sue DY, Wasserman K. Predicted values for clinical exercise testing. Am Rev Respir Dis 1984; 129(Suppl):S49–S55.
47. Sady S, Katch V, Freedson P, Weltman A. Changes in metabolic acidosis: Evidence for an intensity threshold. J Sports Med 1980; 20:41–46.
48. Poole DC, Gaesser GA. Response of ventilatory and lactate thresholds to continuous and interval training. J Appl Physiol 1985; 58:1115–1121.
49. Davies CTM, Knibbs AV. The training stimulus. Int Z Angew Physiol 1971; 29:299–305.
50. Gaesser GA, Poole DC. Blood lactate during exercise: Time course of training adaptation in humans. Int J Sports Med 1988; 9:284–288.
51. Hickson RC, Hagberg JM, Ehsani AA, Holloszy JO. Time course of the adaptive responses of aerobic power and heart rate to training. Med Sci Sports Exerc 1981; 13:17–20.
52. Pollock ML, Dimmick J, Miller HS, et al. Effects of mode of training on cardiovascular function and body composition of middle-aged men. Med Sci Sports Exerc 1975; 7:139–145.
53. Pollock ML. The quantification of endurance training programs. Exerc Sports Sci Rev 1973; 1:155–188.
54. Hagberg JM, Graves JE, Limacher M, et al. Cardiovascular responses of 70- to 79-yr-old men and women to exercise training. J Appl Physiol 1989; 66:2589–2594.
55. Seals DR, Hurley BF, Schultz J, Hagberg JM. Endurance training in older men and women: II. Blood lactate response to submaximal exercise. J Appl Physiol 1984; 57:1030–1033.
56. Tzankoff SP, Robinson S, Pyke FS, Brawn CA. Physiological adjustments to work in older men as affected by physical training. J Appl Physiol 1972; 33:346–350.
57. Coyle EF, Martin WH, Sinacore DR, et al. Time course of loss of adaptations after stopping prolonged intense endurance training. J Appl Physiol 1984; 57:1857–1864.
58. Coyle EF, Martin WH, Bloomfield SA, et al. Effects of detraining on responses to submaximal exercise. J Appl Physiol 1985; 59:853–859.
59. Hickson RC, Rosenkoetter MA. Reduced training frequencies and maintenance of increased aerobic power. Med Sci Sports Exerc 1981; 13:13–16.
60. Hickson RC, Kanakis C, Davis JR, et al. Reduced training duration effects on aerobic power, endurance and cardiac growth. J Appl Physiol 1982; 53:225–229.
61. Hickson RC, Foster CC, Pollock ML, et al. Reduced training intensities and loss of aerobic power, endurance and cardiac growth. J Appl Physiol 1985; 58:492–499.
62. Barach AL, Bickerman HA, Beck G. Advances in the treatment of non-tuberculous pulmonary disease. Bull N Y Acad Med 1952; 28:353–384.
63. Miller WF, Taylor HF. Exercise training in the rehabilitation of patients with severe respiratory insufficiency due to pulmonary emphysema. South Med J 1962; 55:1216–1221.
64. Pierce AK, Taylor HF, Archer RK, Miller WF. Responses to

exercise training in patients with emphysema. Arch Intern Med 1964; 113:28–36.
65. Pierce AK, Paez PN, Miller WF. Exercise training with the aid of a portable oxygen supply in patients with emphysema. Am Rev Respir Dis 1965; 91:653–659.
66. Paez PN, Phillipson EA, Masangkay M, Sproule BJ. The physiologic basis of training patients with emphysema. Am Rev Respir Dis 1967; 95:944–953.
67. Christie D. Physical training in chronic obstructive lung disease. BMJ 1968; 2:150–151.
68. Woolf CR, Suero JT. Alterations in lung mechanics and gas exchange following training in chronic obstructive lung disease. Dis Chest 1969; 55:37–44.
69. Petty TL, Nett, LM, Finigan MM, et al. A comprehensive care program for chronic airway obstruction. Ann Intern Med 1969; 70:1109–1119.
70. Nicholas JJ, Gilbert R, Gabe R, Auchincloss JH. Evaluation of an exercise therapy program for patients with chronic obstructive pulmonary disease. Am Rev Respir Dis 1970; 102:1–8.
71. Bass H, Whitcomb JF, Forman R. Exercise training: Therapy for patients with chronic obstructive pulmonary disease. Chest 1970; 57:116–121.
72. Vyas MN, Banister EW, Morton JW, Grzybowski S. Response to exercise in patients with chronic airway obstruction: I. Effects of exercise training. Am Rev Respir Dis 1971; 103:390–400.
73. Vyas MN, Banister EW, Morton JW, Grzybowski S. Response to exercise in patients with chronic airway obstruction: II. Effects of breathing 40 per cent oxygen. Am Rev Respir Dis 1971; 103:401–412.
74. Holten K. Training effect in patients with severe ventilatory failure. Scand J Respir Dis 1972; 53:65–76.
75. Brundin A. Physical training in severe chronic obstructive lung disease: I. Clinical course, physical working capacity and ventilation. Scand J Respir Dis 1974; 55:25–36.
76. Brundin A. Physical training in severe chronic obstructive lung disease. II. Observations on gas exchange. Scand J Respir Dis 1974; 55:37–46.
77. Degre S, Sergysels R, Messin R, et al. Hemodynamic responses to physical training in patients with chronic lung disease. Am Rev Respir Dis 1974; 110:395–402.
78. Alpert JS, Bass H, Szucs MM, et al. Effects of physical training on hemodynamics and pulmonary function at rest and during exercise in patients with chronic obstructive pulmonary disease. Chest 1974; 66:647–651.
79. McGavin CR, Gupta SP, Lloyd EL, McHardy GJR. Physical rehabilitation for the chronic bronchitic: Results of a controlled trial of exercises in the home. Thorax 1977; 32:307–311.
80. Chester EH, Belman MJ, Bahler RC, et al. Multidisciplinary treatment of chronic pulmonary insufficiency: 3. Effect of physical training on cardiopulmonary performance in patients with chronic obstructive pulmonary disease. Chest 1977; 72:695–701.
81. Mertens DJ, Shephard RJ, Kavanagh T. Long-term exercise therapy for chronic obstructive lung disease. Respiration 1978; 35:96–107.
82. Sinclair DJM, Ingram CG. Controlled trial of supervised exercise training in chronic bronchitis. BMJ 1980; 1:519–521.
83. Moser KM, Bokinsky GE, Savage RT, et al. Results of a comprehensive rehabilitation program. Arch Intern Med 1980; 140:1596–1600.
84. Mungall IPF, Hainsworth R. A objective assessment of the value of exercise training to patients with chronic obstructive airways disease. Q J Med 1980; 193:77–85.
85. Unger KM, Moser KM, Hansen P. Selection of an exercise program for patients with chronic obstructive pulmonary disease. Heart Lung 1980; 9:68–76.
86. Cockcroft AE, Saunders MJ, Berry G. Randomised controlled trial of rehabilitation in chronic respiratory disability. Thorax 1981; 36:200–203.
87. Alison JA, Samios R, Anderson SD. Evaluation of exercise training in patients with chronic airway obstruction. Phys Ther 1981; 61:1273–1277.
88. Belman MJ, Kendregan BA. Exercise training fails to increase skeletal muscle enzymes in patients with chronic obstructive pulmonary disease. Am Rev Respir Dis 1981; 123:256–261.
89. Mohsenifar Z, Horak D, Brown HV, Koerner SK. Sensitive indices of improvement in a pulmonary rehabilitation program. Chest 1983; 83:189–192.
90. Tydeman DE, Chandler AR, Graveling BM, et al. An investigation into the effects of exercise tolerance training on patients with chronic airways obstruction. Physiotherapy 1984; 70:261–264.
91. Zack MB, Palange AV. Oxygen supplemented exercise of ventilatory and nonventilatory muscles in pulmonary rehabilitation. Chest 1985; 88:669–674.
92. Jones DT, Thomson RJ, Sears MR. Physical exercise and resistive breathing training in severe chronic airways obstruction: Are they effective? Eur J Respir Dis 1985; 67:159–165.
93. Madsen F, Secher NH, Kay L, et al. Inspiratory resistance versus general physical training in patients with chronic obstructive pulmonary disease. Eur J Respir Dis 1985; 67:167–176.
94. Ries AL, Moser KM. Comparison of isocapnic hyperventilation and walking exercise training at home in pulmonary rehabilitation. Chest 1986; 90:285–289.
95. Ries AL, Archibald CJ. Endurance exercise training at maximal targets in patients with chronic obstructive pulmonary disease. J Cardiopulmon Rehabil 1987; 7:594–601.
96. Corriveau ML, Harris CM, Chun DS, et al. Relationship between multiple physiologic variables and change in exercise capacity after a pulmonary rehabilitation program. J Cardiopulmon Rehabil 1988; 8:303–308.
97. Carter R, Nicotra B, Clark L, et al. Exercise conditioning in the rehabilitation of patients with chronic obstructive pulmonary disease. Arch Phys Med Rehabil 1988; 69:118–122.
98. Busch AJ, McClements JD. Effects of a supervised home exercise program on patients with severe chronic obstructive pulmonary disease. Phys Ther 1988; 68:469–474.
99. Mall RW, Medeiros M. Objective evaluation of results of a pulmonary rehabilitation program in a community hospital. Chest 1988; 94:1156–1160.
100. Holle RHO, Williams DV, Vandree JC, et al. Increased muscle efficiency and sustained benefits in an outpatient community hospital-based pulmonary rehabilitation program. Chest 1988; 94:1161–1168.
101. Casaburi R, Patessio A, Ioli F, et al. Reductions in exercise lactic acidosis and ventilation as a result of exercise training in patients with obstructive lung disease. Am Rev Respir Dis 1991; 143:9–18.
102. Weg JG. Therepeutic exercise in patients with chronic obstructive pulmonary disease. In: Wenger NK (ed). Cardiovascular Clinics: Exercise and the Heart. 2nd ed. Philadelphia: F.A. Davis Co., 1985, pp 261–275.
103. Belman MJ. Exercise in chronic obstructive pulmonary disease. Clin Chest Med 1986; 7:585–597.
104. Whipp BJ, Wasserman K. Efficiency of muscular work. J Appl Physiol 1969; 26:644–648.
105. Noctural Oxygen Therapy Trial Group. Continuous or nocturnal oxygen therapy in hypoxemic chronic obstructive lung disease. Ann Intern Med 1980; 93:391–398.
106. Medical Research Council Working Party. Long term domiciliary oxygen therapy in chronic hypoxic cor pulmonale complicating chronic bronchitis and emphysema. Lancet 1981; i:681–685.
107. Sue DY, Oren A, Hansen JE, Wasserman K. Diffusing capacity for carbon monoxide as a predictor of gas exchange during exercise. N Engl J Med 1987; 316:1301–1306.
108. Ries AL, Farrow JT, Clausen JL. Pulmonary function tests cannot predict exercise-induced hypoxemia in chronic obstructive pulmonary disease. Chest 1988; 93:454–459.
109. Cotes JE, Gilson JC. Effect of oxygen on exercise ability in chronic respiratory insufficiency: Use of portable apparatus. Lancet 1956; i:872–876.
110. Barach AL, Petty TL. Is chronic obstructive lung disease improved by physical exercise? JAMA 1975; 234:854–855.
111. Woodcock AA, Gross ER, Geddes DM. Oxygen relieves breathlessness in "pink puffers". Lancet 1981; i:907–909.
112. Stein DA, Bradley BL, Miller WC. Mechanisms of oxygen effects on exercise in patients with chronic obstructive pulmonary disease. Chest 1982; 81:6–10.
113. Raimondi AC, Edwards RHT, Denison RM, et al. Exercise tolerance breathing a low density gas mixture, 35% oxygen and

113. air in patients with chronic obstructive bronchitis. Clin Sci 1970; 39:675–685.
114. Barach AL. Oxygen supported exercise and rehabilitation of patients with chronic obstructive lung disease. Ann Allergy 1966; 24:51–57.
115. Belman MJ, Kendregan BA. Physical training fails to improve ventilatory muscle endurance in patients with chronic obstructive pulmonary disease. Chest 1982; 81:440–443.
116. Haber P. Exercise training fails to increase skeletal muscle enzymes in patients with chronic obstructive pulmonary disease (letter to the editor). Am Rev Respir Dis 1981; 124:347.
117. Pardy RL, Hussain SNA, Maclem PT. The ventilatory pump in exercise. Clin Chest Med 1984; 5:35–49.
118. Shuey CB, Pierce AK, Johnson RL. An evaluation of exercise tests in chronic obstructive lung disease. J Appl Physiol 1969; 27:256–261.
119. Spiro SG, Hahn HL, Edwards RHT, Pride NB. An analysis of the physiological strain of submaximal exercise in patients with chronic obstructive bronchitis. Thorax 1975; 30:415–425.
120. Kanarek D, Kaplan D, Kazemi H. The anaerobic threshold in severe chronic obstructive lung disease. Bull Eur Physiopathol Respir 1979; 15:163–169.
121. Raffestin B, Escourrou P, Legrand A, et al. Circulatory transport of oxygen in patients with chronic airflow obstruction exercising maximally. Am Rev Respir Dis 1982; 125:426–431.
122. Sue DY, Wasserman K, Moricca RB, Casaburi R. Metabolic acidosis during exercise in patients with chronic obstructive pulmonary disease. Chest 1988; 94:931–938.
123. Casaburi R, Patessio A, Ioli F, et al. Physiologic adaptations to reduced blood lactate levels after exercise training in patients with COPD. Am Rev Respir Dis 1991; 143:A168.
124. Johnson MA, Polgar J, Weightman D, Appleton D. Data on the distribution of fibers in thirty-six human muscles: An autopsy study. J Neurol Sci 1973; 18:111–129.
125. Astrand I, Guharay A, Wahren J. Circulatory responses to arm exercise with different arm positions. J Appl Physiol 1968; 25:528–532.
126. Casaburi R, Barstow TJ, Robinson T, Wasserman K. Dynamic and steady-state ventilatory and gas exchange responses to arm exercise. Med Sci Sports Exerc (in press).
127. Casaburi R, Soll B. Dynamics of ventilation and gas exchange in athletes trained for upper body exercise. Sports Training Exerc Rehabil (in press).
128. Franklin BA. Exercise testing, training and arm ergometry. Sports Med 1985; 2:100–119.
129. Franklin BA. Aerobic exercise training programs for the upper body. Med Sci Sports Exerc 1989; 21:S141–S148.
130. Sawka MN. Physiology of upper body exercise. Exerc Sports Sci Rev 1986; 14:175–211.
131. Rasmussen B, Klausen K, Clausen JP, Trap-Jensen J. Pulmonary ventilation, blood gases, and blood pH after training of the arms or the legs. J Appl Physiol 1975; 38:250–256.
132. Celli BR, Rassulo J, Make BJ. Dyssynchronous breathing during arm but not leg exercise in patients with chronic airflow obstruction. N Engl J Med 1986; 314:1485–1490.
133. Criner GJ, Celli BR. Effect of unsupported arm exercise on ventilatory muscle recruitment in patients with severe chronic airflow obstruction. Am Rev Respir Dis 1988; 138:856–861.
134. Ries AL, Ellis B, Hawkins RW. Upper extremity exercise training in chronic obstructive pulmonary disease. Chest 1988; 93:688–692.

Chapter 17

Ventilatory Muscle Training and Unloading

MICHAEL J. BELMAN, M.D.

At the conclusion of their paper in 1976, Leith and Bradley stated "that ventilatory muscle training (VMT) might improve performance, and that this VMT may have an application in human disease in which ventilatory loads are increased, or the capacity for sustaining them is decreased."[1] An increase in ventilatory load with a decrease in the capacity for sustaining that load is clearly the major pathophysiologic abnormality in patients with chronic obstructive pulmonary disease (COPD). During the 16 years since the publication of this paper, which was the first to address the question of specific VMT, a large number of studies of VMT have been performed in patients with chronic airflow limitation.[2] In the first part of this chapter, these studies are addressed, and an attempt to critically evaluate the validity of the benefits attributed to VMT is made. Several questions have been answered with regard to acceptable methods of VMT, but even after one and a half decades of relatively intense investigation, we are not yet at a stage where we can unequivocally recommend VMT for all patients with COPD. The issues that are yet unresolved are also highlighted in this chapter, and it is hoped that within the next few years further research will clarify these issues and that the appropriate indications for VMT will be defined. This chapter concerns the use of VMT in patients with obstructive airway disease, although this technique has also been used in patients with primary neuromuscular disorders in whom muscle weakness is the main abnormality.[2] Although muscle weakness may be a component of impaired muscle function in patients with COPD, it is generally a secondary result of altered ventilatory mechanics, malnutrition, or both.[2] The primary pathophysiologic defect is the expiratory airway obstruction.

RESPIRATORY MUSCLES IN CHRONIC OBSTRUCTIVE PULMONARY DISEASE

COPD has a major impact on the respiratory muscles with respect to (1) functional residual capacity (FRC) and (2) ventilatory and energy demands. This impact has been summarized.[3]

Functional Residual Capacity

A characteristic feature of COPD is hyperinflation, which is present chronically in patients with this disease, even at rest. Hyperinflation is aggravated by either voluntary hyperpnea or exercise. During exercise, dynamic hyperinflation occurs; this further increases end-expiratory lung volume (Fig. 17–1). Hyperinflation acts to reduce diaphragm strength. The effect is secondary to the shortening of diaphragm fibers, which places the diaphragm muscle at a suboptimal point on its length-tension curve. In addition, because of the increased radius of the diaphragm's curvature, there is a reduction in force that this muscle can produce (Laplace's law). Furthermore, hyperinflation results in a marked decrease in the size of the zone of apposition between the costal fibers of the diaphragm and the rib cage; this zone is important in the elevation of the lower ribs during inspiration. In extreme cases of COPD, the

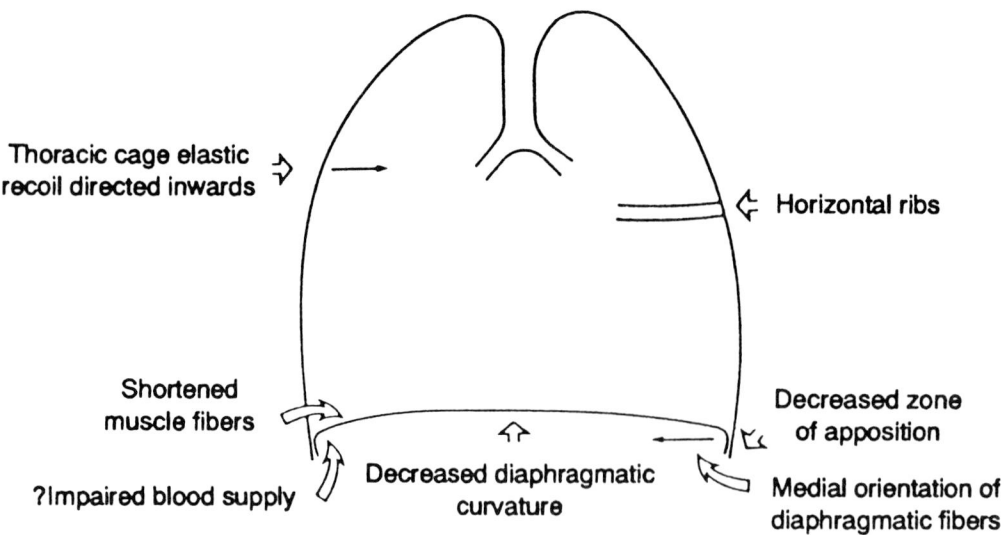

FIGURE 17-1. The detrimental effects of hyperinflation on respiratory muscle function. See text for discussion. (From Tobin MJ. Respiratory muscles in disease. Clin Chest Med 1988; 9:263-286.)

diaphragm may be so shortened that the orientation of the muscle fibers is almost horizontal, and thus inspiratory contraction results merely in an indrawing of the lower ribs (Hoover's sign).[3]

Ventilatory and Energy Demands

Several studies have clearly established that a rapid increase in energy consumption occurs during hyperpnea in patients with COPD compared with normal individuals.[4] This is consistent with the fact that the work of breathing is greatly increased in COPD patients not only at rest but also during exercise.[2] The increased energy consumption may also be relevant with respect to the weight loss frequently observed in COPD patients. Weight loss has even been documented in patients whose caloric intake is adequate. This weight loss may be secondary to the increased energy demands of breathing, that is, energy consumption is in excess of the energy supplied by the diet. Weight loss may further aggravate diaphragmatic function because it can lead to atrophy of muscle fibers and reduce the substrate for energy supply.[5]

Because of the impaired ventilatory muscle function that occurs in COPD, several investigators have proposed that specific training directed at improving the strength and endurance of the ventilatory muscles can be of benefit to COPD patients. It should be emphasized at the outset that this type of training is directed at improving intrinsic muscle function either through the hypertrophy of muscle fibers (i.e., increasing their strength) or through an increase in the oxidative enzyme profile (i.e., an improvement in endurance). This is distinct from the techniques designed to improve breathing strategies (such as pursed-lip breathing or diaphragmatic breathing), which are discussed elsewhere in this book. An additional point that should be emphasized is that expiratory airway obstruction has been recognized as the primary pathophysiologic defect in COPD. Dynamic hyperinflation occurs as a result of the limitation of expiratory time[6]; it results in an increased inspiratory load because (1) tidal breathing now occurs in a less compliant range of the pressure-volume curve and because (2) inspiration begins before the respiratory system has had time to return to passive FRC. This inspiratory load acts as a threshold load at the onset of inspiration. Thus, although the primary defect in COPD is increased expiratory resistance, its primary consequence is encountered during inspiration and is restrictive in nature.[6]

SKELETAL MUSCLES AND THEIR RESPONSE TO TRAINING

Skeletal muscles consist of several types of muscle fibers. Based on the results various histochemical staining tests, these fibers are most frequently divided into types I, IIa, and IIb.[7-9] In general, type I fibers have a high oxidative capacity and a relatively low concentration of glycolytic enzymes. Physiologically, they are activated by slow-twitch motor units. These units are the first to be recruited during muscle activation, they produce relatively low levels of force, and they are fatigue-resistant. Type IIb fibers are low in oxidative capacity, have high concentrations of glycolytic enzymes, produce the greatest level of force when activated, are the last to be recruited in motor efforts, and fatigue rapidly when activated repeatedly. Type IIa fibers are intermediate in oxidative capacity and glycolytic enzyme concentrations; they are also intermediate with respect to fatigability. Respiratory muscles are mixed skeletal muscles and contain mixtures of the fiber types discussed. The human diaphragm, for example, comprises approximately 50% type I fibers and 50% type II fibers.[10]

Adaptation of Skeletal Muscle Types to Training

The previously described properties of skeletal muscle are highly relevant to the study of training.[11] As ventilatory efforts increase, more motor units are recruited. As the firing rates of motor neurons increase, type I, IIa, and IIb fibers are recruited in a sequential fashion.[12] In order to obtain a training response in skeletal muscle, an appropriate stimulus must be applied. Faulkner has defined three basic principles of skeletal muscle training: overload, specificity, and reversibility.[10] The overload principle states that for skeletal muscle fibers to change their structure, improve their function, or both, they must be taxed beyond some critical level. This, in essence, is the concept of *intensity of exercise training*. It is clear that the stimulus for adaptation determines the nature of the changes in skeletal muscles in that it acts on specific elements of that muscle. The practical implication of this is that optimal results are achieved when subjects train using a specific modality of exercise to enhance a specific performance component (hence, the "principle of specificity"). This implies that strength training improves strength, and endurance training improves endurance. The reversibility principle states that the effects of conditioning decline after training ceases. Thus, based on these principles, VMT should include a load of appropriate intensity and should be conducted at least until true conditioning of the skeletal muscle occurs. The manner in which the ventilatory muscles are loaded is probably important in determining the specificity of the response. In endurance training, the classic training effect comprises an increase in myoglobin content, an increase in capillary density, an increase in mitochondrial density, and an increase in oxidative enzyme capacity. In strength training, the major development is increased fiber size (i.e., muscle hypertrophy); but unlike endurance training, there is little effect on enzyme concentrations.[11]

Ventilatory muscle biopsy specimens are obviously difficult to obtain in living humans, and, thus, there is no evidence to prove that the classic training effects develop after VMT in normal subjects and in patients with obstructive airway disease. However, extensive evidence from animal studies suggests that overloading of the ventilatory muscles does produce the expected training effects in the diaphragm and other inspiratory muscles.[13, 14]

METHODS OF VENTILATORY MUSCLE TRAINING

In general, specific ventilatory muscle training has been used to improve ventilatory muscle endurance. However, it has been noted in normal subjects and in patients with cystic fibrosis[15, 16] (but not in patients with COPD[17]) that whole-body exercise also improves ventilatory muscle endurance. Specifically, in the study of patients with cystic fibrosis, arm exercise (such as canoeing) was sufficient to improve ventilatory muscle endurance.[16] This effect was not seen in a study of patients with COPD.[17] In this study, two groups of patients exercised—one group performed arm exercise, and the other performed leg exercise. Neither group showed an increase in sustained ventilatory capacity. A possible explanation for this is the fact that whole-body exercise in COPD is usually carried out at levels of ventilation that are lower than those observed when specific endurance exercise of the ventilatory muscles is performed (50% maximum voluntary ventilation [MVV] versus 90% MVV). The intensity of whole-body exercise is inadequate to generate the appropriate increase in ventilatory endurance.

The three major methods that have been used for VMT in both normal subjects and lung disease patients are (1) voluntary isocapneic hyperpnea, (2) inspiratory resistive loading, and (3) inspiratory threshold loading.

Voluntary Isocapneic Hyperpnea

In this form of VMT, the patient maintains as high a level of minute ventilation as possible for periods of 10 to 15 minutes usually twice daily.[1, 16, 17] These prolonged periods of hyperpnea provide low tension and a high level of repetitive activity for the diaphragm and other inspiratory muscles. This particular pattern is the same as that used for promoting improved endurance in whole-body exercise (i.e., in running or swimming). The key index used to measure the level of hyperpnea is the maximum sustained ventilatory capacity (MSVC), which is defined as the maximum level of ventilation that can be sustained under isocapneic conditions for 15 minutes.[1, 16, 17] Because of the complexity of the rebreathing circuit required for this form of exercise, relatively few studies of this technique have been performed. One study has been done in normal subjects,[1] one in patients with cystic fibrosis,[16] and three in adults with obstructive airway disease.[18–20] The results of these studies are summarized in Table 17–1. Without exception, ventilatory muscle endurance determined by the MSVC improved from 20 to 55%. Belman and Mittman[20] were the first to examine the effect of this form of training on exercise endurance in patients with COPD. Their study showed an improved ability to perform both arm and leg exercise. However, this study had no control group, and in a subsequent study, Levine and coworkers[18] showed that although the MSVC improved in the group that underwent training, a second group that underwent a sham treatment (intermittent positive-pressure breathing) did not show improvement during treadmill or bicycle exercise. In addition, there was no difference in the second group's ability to perform activities of daily living.

Thus, although ventilatory muscle endurance can most certainly be improved by isocapneic hyperpnea, the use of this technique does not result in improvements in functional capacity. However, this form of training may provide benefits in other areas. For example, it may lead to increased resistance to respiratory failure or contribute to the weaning of patients from ventilatory support. In one study in which this technique was used during such weaning,[21] improvement in ventilatory function occurred. However, this study included few patients and did not have control subjects; thus, further verification is required.

TABLE 17-1. EFFECT OF HYPERPNEIC TRAINING ON VENTILATORY MUSCLES

Reference	No. of Subjects	Endurance Duration	Endurance Frequency	Course	Response*	Better than Control Subjects? (Yes or No)
Leith and Bradley[1] (1976)	4 normal	20–30 min	5 wk	5 wk	19%	yes
Keens et al.[16] (1977)	4 normal	25 min	5 wk	4 wk	22%	—
	4 with cystic fibrosis	25 min	5 wk	4 wk	55%	yes
Belman and Mittman[20] (1980)	10 with COPD	30 min	5 wk	6 wk	33%	—
Levine et al.[18] (1986)	15 with COPD	15 min	5 wk	6 wk	41%	yes
Reis and Moser[19] (1986)	5 with COPD	30 min	5 wk	6 wk	16%	no

*Increase in maximum sustained ventilatory capacity.

Inspiratory Resistive Loading

The complexity of the isocapneic hyperpneic technique led to the development of simple resistive devices for the loading of the respiratory muscles. Patients are required to breathe through inspiratory orifices of progressively decreasing diameter with the goal of increasing the load on the respiratory muscles. Breathing frequency during this type of training is generally kept within the range of 10 to 20 breaths per minute; this is in contrast to isocapneic hyperpnea, in which breathing frequencies are between 30 and 60 breaths per minute. A large number of studies incorporating this technique have been performed, but as will be described later, many of the early studies failed to account for changes in breathing strategy, and their results are therefore in question.[22]

The response to resistive training is generally evaluated by the measurement of maximum inspiratory pressure (PImax) and by the endurance time for loaded breathing. A common technique is to establish the pressure target as 60% of the baseline PImax and to record the time during which the patient can maintain this target. Failure is defined as the inability to achieve the pressure target for three successive breaths. An alternative method is to set the endurance time (e.g., 10 min) and then to record the mean maximum mouth pressure that can be developed with each breath. With the exception of a study by Clanton and associates,[23] most of the early studies failed to control the breathing strategy during training.[17] The ability of the patients to breathe through a smaller orifice was equated with improved inspiratory muscle endurance. Without information on the breathing strategy, it is difficult to know whether the ability to breathe through a smaller orifice represents a true training response or just a more favorable breathing strategy. In this regard, it is important to remember that a breathing pattern characterized by slow, deep inspirations is tolerated more easily (Fig. 17-2). This is because the inspiratory mouth pressure—the primary determinant of the effort sensation—is reduced.[24] In fact, in one study,[17] a change from the regular breathing pattern used by inexperienced patients to a pattern of long, slow breaths resulted in immediate improvement in endurance despite the use of a smaller orifice. This latter breathing pattern is also self-defeating because it reduces the inspiratory load on the respiratory muscles, probably to below the threshold required to induce a training response in some patients. It has become apparent, therefore, that control of the breathing strategy during training and testing is essential to ensure that improvements in endurance are not ascribed to changes in breathing strategy and that training stimuli of adequate intensity can be achieved.

More recent studies have taken these factors into account (Table 17-2). Belman and Shadmehr[25] showed that resistive devices could be used under controlled conditions. In their study, a target feedback device was connected to a resistor. This device provided feedback on both breathing frequency and inspiratory pressure. The target pressure was increased by having the patient aim for progressively higher peak pressures; however, the inspiratory orifice and breathing frequency were not changed. This required that the tidal volume and minute ventilation increase so that the new pressure target could be met. Patients in this study were randomized into a high-intensity training group or a low-intensity training group. After 6 weeks of training, the high-intensity group showed improvements in respiratory muscle strength and demonstrated increased endurance for

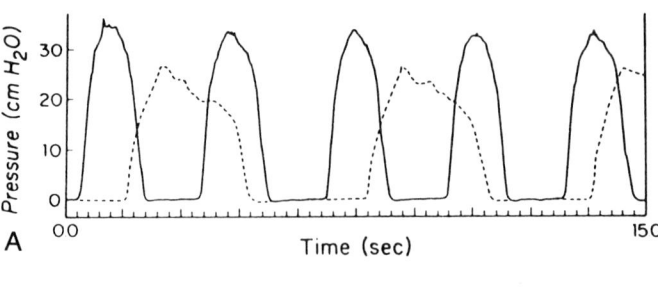
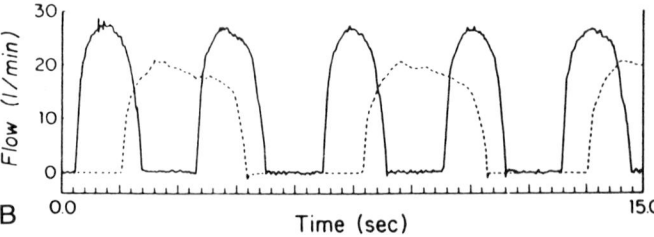

FIGURE 17-2. Fifteen-second records of pressure (A) and flow (B) patterns, respectively, in one patient breathing in the presence of inspiratory resistance. Uncoached and coached tracings are superimposed (*dotted line:* coached; *solid line:* uncoached). With coaching, reduced mouth pressure, peak inspiratory flow rate, and breathing frequency occur. (From Belman MJ, Thomas SG, Lewis MI. Resistive breathing training in patients with COPD. Chest 1986; 90:662–669.)

TABLE 17-2. RESISTIVE VENTILATORY MUSCLE TRAINING IN COPD*

Reference	Training	Strength	Endurance	Exercise Capacity	Better than Control Group? (Yes or No)
Belman and Shadmehr[25] (1988)	HI versus LI	Increased in HI group	Increased in HI group	Not studied	yes (HI group showed greater improvement than LI group)
Harver et al.[26] (1989)	30 min/day for 8 wk	Increased 32%	—	Reduction in dyspnea on exercise	yes
Dekhuizen et al.[28] (1991)	Rehabilitation versus rehabilitation with VMT	Increased in rehabilitation with VMT group only	Increased in rehabilitation with VMT group only	12-min walking distance, bicycle ergometer	yes

*Resistive training with target feedback.
Key: HI: high-intensity; LI: low-intensity.

loaded breathing as measured by the ability to reach higher peak mouth pressures with each breath over a period of 10 minutes. The low-intensity group, which essentially trained at very low target pressures, served as a control group and did not show significant improvement. Also observed in this study was a small increase (10%) in the MSVC in the high intensity group. As noted above, the MSVC is a measure of low-tension, high-repetition endurance activity, whereas the training in this study consisted of high-tension, low-repetition activity. Thus, the degree of improvement with loaded breathing was considerably better than that with hyperpnea. This fact underscores the importance of the specificity of training with respect to the respiratory muscles (Fig. 17-3).

Two more studies have also supported the use of resistive inspiratory loading. The study by Harver and colleagues[26] employed a control group and a treatment group. The treatment group aimed to reach progressively higher target pressures, whereas the control group breathed using an unloaded system. In this study, the patients received feedback on the inspiratory pressure they achieved, although there was no direct control of breathing frequency. In comparison to the control group, the treated patients showed improvements in respiratory muscle strength and endurance. It is also interesting to note that in this study a detailed evaluation of dyspnea was performed by means of a patient questionnaire.[27] The investigators found a significant reduction in dyspnea in the treated group only (Fig. 17-4). In a study from the Netherlands, Dekhuizen and coworkers[28] also showed improved ventilatory muscle strength, endurance, and exercise capacity in patients who underwent ventilatory muscle training. This study compared patients who underwent rehabilitation only with patients who performed ventilatory muscle training in addition to their participating in the rehabilitation program. Patients in the training group showed improvement in symptoms, a reduction in dyspnea, and an improvement in their ability to perform activities of

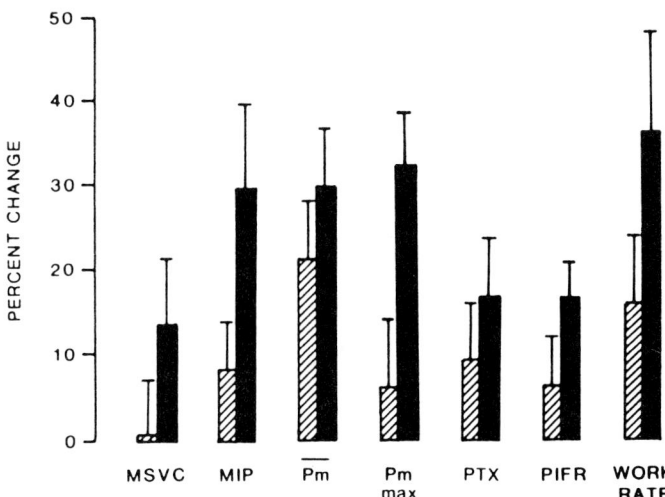

FIGURE 17-3. Per cent change (mean ± SE) in tests of ventilatory muscle function and indices of breathing strategy in high-intensity and low-intensity groups before and after ventilatory muscle training. (MSVC: maximum sustained ventilatory capacity; MIP: maximum inspiratory pressure; Pm: mean mouth pressure; Pmmax: peak mouth pressure; PTX: pressure time index; PIFR: peak inspiratory flow rate; *shaded bar*: low-intensity group; *solid bar*: high-intensity group.) (From Belman MJ, Shadmehr R. Targeted resistive ventilatory muscle training in chronic obstructive pulmonary disease. J Appl Physiol 1988; 65:2726–2735.)

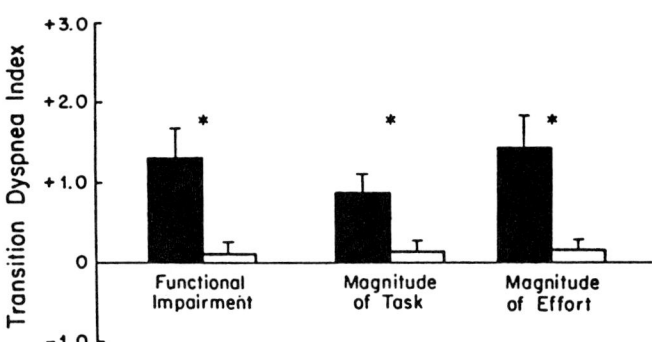

FIGURE 17-4. Mean scores for each category of the transition dyspnea index for both experimental (*closed bars*) and control (*open bars*) subjects (*bar*: one standard error;*: significant difference between experimental and control conditions). (From Harver A, Mahler DA, Daubenspeck JA. Targeted inspiratory muscle training improves respiratory muscle function and reduces dyspnea in patients with chronic obstructive disease. Ann Intern Med 1989; 111:117–124.)

daily living. Thus, in contrast to the earlier studies, which were largely inconclusive, the studies of Harver and colleagues and of Dekhuizen and coworkers have shown more impressive benefits for inspiratory resistive loading. The key to success may be the close monitoring of breathing strategy to ensure that the ventilatory muscles are appropriately and progressively loaded.

Inspiratory Resistive Training and Weaning

The technique of resistive VMT has also been used in patients with respiratory failure who are difficult to wean.[29] Of the 30 patients who were studied, 20 suffered from chronic respiratory disease. The results of VMT showed that 12 patients were ultimately weaned from ventilation completely, 5 were weaned to nocturnal ventilation, and 13 either failed to be weaned or died. Unfortunately, no randomized study comparing VMT with other weaning practices is available. These preliminary data indicate that VMT may be able to play a role in patients who are difficult to wean.

Inspiratory Threshold Loading

In 1982, Nickerson and Keens[30] developed a threshold loading device that permitted inspiration to commence only after a threshold mouth pressure was reached. The threshold pressure could be set by means of a weighted plunger. The potential advantage of the resistance produced by this device over alinear resistances is that inspiratory pressure is independent of the inspiratory flow rate. It was hoped that the dependence of inspiratory load on inspiratory flow rate could be avoided. Several investigators have now completed studies using this inspiratory threshold loading device. Larson and colleagues[31] are responsible for devising a simplified version of the original loading device. In their study, they utilized a simple spring-loaded valve. By adjusting the tension of the spring, threshold pressure could be varied. In their study, they incorporated high-intensity and low-intensity training at 30% and 15% of the PImax, respectively. In the high-intensity training group, improvements in respiratory muscle strength and endurance were observed, as was improved exercise ability (measured as an increase in the 12-minute walking distance). Changes in the low-intensity training group were not significant. In contrast, studies of Goldstein and coworkers[32] and of Flynn and associates[33] failed to show an improvement in exercise capacity, although both research groups, like Larson and colleagues, did show improvement in ventilatory muscle function (Table 17–3). It is interesting to note that Flynn and associates[33] observed a change in inspiratory timing in patients at rest after VMT. They demonstrated a reduction in inspiratory time and, as a result, a decrease in the ratio of inspiratory time to total respiratory cycle time. This effect could theoretically be beneficial to patients with COPD in that it provides more time for expiration; it also may allow patients to reach a lower end-expiratory lung volume and to increase the power output of their ventilatory muscles during exercise.[34] Although a change in breathing pattern was observed during loaded breathing at rest, this change was not demonstrated to occur during exercise (Fig. 17–5).

In the studies of Larson and colleagues[31] and of Goldstein and coworkers,[32] it was well documented that varying inspiratory flow rates did not appreciably alter inspiratory pressures, and thus the threshold loading devices functioned effectively.

Conclusions

From the studies discussed, several conclusions appear justified. First, ventilatory muscle function can be improved, but the improvement appears to be mode-specific.[1, 2, 6] This means that endurance training improves the ability to increase sustained hyperpnea, whereas pure strength training improves inspiratory pressures. Furthermore, loads found to occur with the use of threshold devices and with the use of moderately small inspiratory orifices appear to have a combined effect.

Second, it has been demonstrated that the most impressive benefits with respect to symptoms and exercise capacity have been obtained with resistance training. In the study by Harver and colleagues,[26] the effect was measured by means of a questionnaire, but in the study of Dekhuizen and coworkers,[28] the effect was documented using exercise testing. On the basis of these two studies, it would seem appropriate to recommend VMT that includes the use of resistive devices to stable nonhypercapnic patients with COPD. Breathing pattern and target pressures must be monitored and regulated during such training. However, this type of training requires a great deal of motivation and effort on the part of patients; whether they are willing to participate in such training on a large scale is not certain. More impressive

TABLE 17–3. THRESHOLD VENTILATORY MUSCLE TRAINING IN COPD

Reference	Training	Strength	Endurance	Exercise Capacity
Larson et al.[31] (1988)	At 15% of PImax or at 30% of PImax	Increased 15% Increased 19%	Increased 4% Increased 12.2%	Increased 2% Increased 7.6%*
Goldstein et al.[32] (1989)	20 min/day, control group versus trained group	Not studied	Increased 51% in control group and 174% in trained group	No difference between two groups
Flynn et al.[33] (1989)	30 min/day for 3 wk	Increased	Increased	Unchanged

*12-minute walking distance.

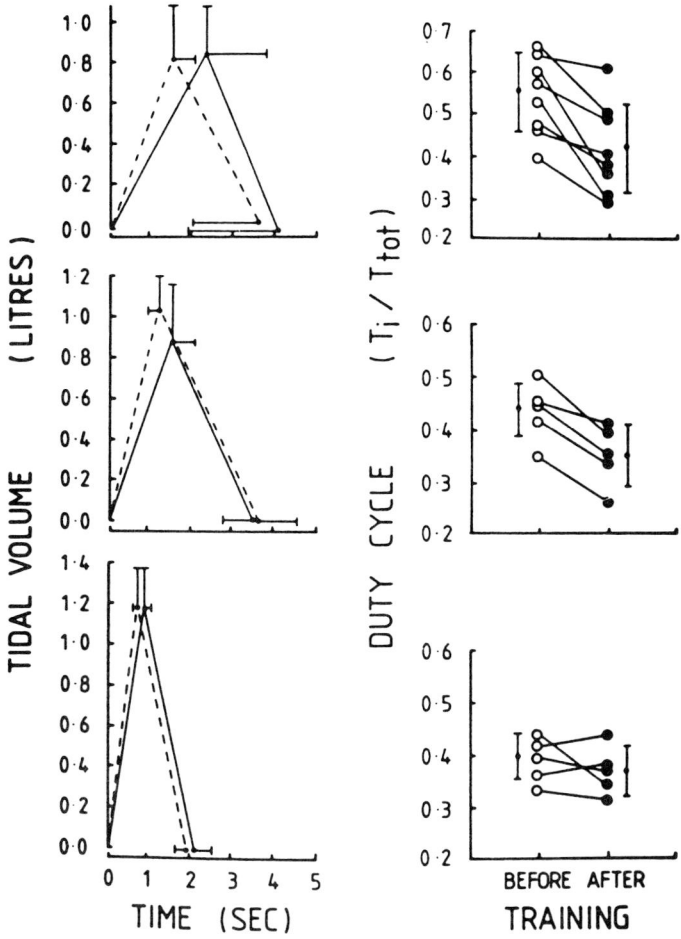

FIGURE 17-5. *Left column,* Average respiratory cycle with the ratio of tidal volume to inspiratory time (VT/Ti) represented by the slope of the ascending limb of the schematic spirogram, and end-expiratory lung volume understood to be zero. (*Continuous lines*: before training; *dashed lines*: after inspiratory muscle training [IMT]; *bars*: 1 SD from the mean.) *Right column,* duty cycle (Ti/Ttot) before (*open circles*) and after (*closed circles*) 6 weeks of IMT. (*Top row*: during threshold breathing; *middle row*: at rest; *bottom row*: during maximum cycle exercise. The *bars* indicate 1 SD either side of the mean.) (From Flynn MG, Barter CE, Nosworthy JC, et al. Threshold pressure training, breathing pattern, and exercise performance in chronic airflow obstruction. Chest 1989; 95:535–540.)

benefits would have to be demonstrated for this to occur. In view of the importance of the specificity of training and of the value of both improved strength and endurance, future studies evaluating combination forms of training (including both volume and pressure loading) are certainly indicated (see discussion later in this chapter).

RESPIRATORY MUSCLE REST

In a study published in 1977, Rochester and associates[35] concluded that "the demonstration that body respirators diminish inspiratory muscle electrical activity indicates that these respirators assume the work of breathing and provide rest for the overburdened inspiratory muscles. The immediate benefit is relief of dyspnea. It is also possible that the reduction of inspiratory muscle energy expenditure, which results from body respirator therapy, improves the function of these muscles and thus contributes to clinical improvement in patients with chronic progressive respiratory failure." Shortly after publication of this paper, several reports appeared that indicated that respiratory muscle fatigue could occur. A hypothesis was put forward that chronic fatigue might develop in the ventilatory muscles of patients with COPD. This was considered to be an inevitable consequence of the chronic increase in airway resistance.[36, 37]

In 1984, a report appeared that demonstrated that a period of several months of intermittent noninvasive ventilatory support provided to a group of mostly COPD patients resulted in improvement in these patients' arterial blood gas parameters and pulmonary function as well as in an increase in their respiratory muscle strength.[38] In addition, a reduction in dyspnea and in both the number of hospitalizations and of hospital days per year was observed. These preliminary results were enthusiastically embraced, and the notion that ventilatory muscle rest therapy (provided using intermittent ventilatory support) was effective in reversing chronic respiratory muscle fatigue quickly became widespread.[35] This section reviews the studies performed to date that have attempted to show improvement of ventilatory muscle function and pulmonary function in patients with severe chronic airways obstruction.

RATIONALE FOR REST THERAPY

Fatigue has been defined as the inability to sustain muscle tension with repeated activity. The failure to maintain force might result from a lack of effort on the part of the patient or from a defect in the train of events that occur from the central nervous system to the muscle contractile apparatus. The source of the fatigue may be central or peripheral.[39, 40]

Central Fatigue

The presence of central fatigue can be demonstrated by the technique of twitch interpolation.[41] In the presence of progressively greater voluntary activation of a muscle, superimposed electrical stimulation of the nerve produces a progressively smaller muscle twitch. At maximum voluntary activation, the electrical stimulus now no longer produces an added twitch because all muscle fibers are maximally activated. Thus, in the presence of central fatigue, an added stimulus produces a twitch. However, when central fatigue is absent, twitch occlusion occurs; that is, the twitch is not visible. Although this central fatigue has been documented in normal subjects after inspiratory muscle loading, there is still no documentation that it occurs in patients in chronic or acute respiratory failure.[39, 40] Furthermore, previous studies did not show this phenomenon in limb muscles, and therefore the importance of central fatigue in respiratory failure still remains somewhat speculative.

Peripheral Fatigue

Peripheral fatigue can be divided into two types: high-frequency fatigue and low-frequency fatigue.[42] It has been documented that the rapid loss of force that occurs with high-frequency stimulation is the result of transmission failure at the neuromuscular junction and muscle cell membrane. Paradoxically, although high-frequency stimulation produces forces that are initially large, muscle force rapidly decreases and is soon exceeded by the muscle force that can be produced with low-frequency stimulation. In fact, the nature of the decrease in muscle force during sustained voluntary maximum contractions indicates that there is probably a progressive decrease in neuronal firing rate from high to low frequencies as the muscle contraction is maintained. It has been suggested that this is an example of central wisdom "where the central nervous system avoids the adverse effect of high-frequency stimulation by gradually reducing the frequency of stimulation as to optimize the force generation."[39] It is conceivable that the pattern of rapid, shallow breathing seen in hypercapnic respiratory failure may in fact be the result of this reduced frequency of stimulation. By favoring rapid, shallow breathing, the "central wisdom" may avoid damage to the respiratory muscles as a result of excessive drive, even though this breathing pattern causes hypercapnia.[40,41]

Low-Frequency Fatigue

After prolonged muscular effort against high loads, the frequency force curve shifts to the right, so that a low-frequency stimulus to the muscle results in a reduction in force (Fig. 17–6A). This phenomenon has been termed *low-frequency fatigue* and may persist for several hours after the work episode (see Fig. 17–6B). It has been suggested that this low-frequency fatigue is in fact an important component of the chronic fatigue seen in hypercapnic respiratory failure.[37] After prolonged periods of working to overcome the high ventilatory loads of chronic airflow limitation, the muscles ultimately develop low-frequency fatigue and are no longer able to generate adequate forces. This type of fatigue requires several hours of rest to be resolved. The concept of low-frequency fatigue formed the basis of the idea that rest therapy might be efficacious.

Further clarification of the interaction between central fatigue and peripheral fatigue is important in determining optimal therapy. Both types of fatigue may coexist, and it has been observed that central motor output may be reduced in response to feedback from fatiguing peripheral muscle.[43] In this case, rest therapy might be efficacious in reversing the fatigue of the peripheral muscles and thus reflexly permit recovery from central fatigue. Conversely, if central neural drive is reduced and unrelated to peripheral fatigue, then rest treatment would not be expected to improve muscle function. However, it should be emphasized that it has been extremely difficult (if not impossible) to actually document the presence of low-frequency fatigue in the setting of acute or chronic respiratory failure, and therefore this supposition remains conjectural.

Simple and accurate diagnostic tests of central and peripheral fatigue are needed before it will be possible to determine if the failure of rest therapy in COPD is due to the inadequate application of muscle rest treatment or to the possibility that the underlying assumptions of chronic fatigue are false.[40,41,43]

Chronic Fatigue or Weakness: Which Is More Important?

In a recent editorial, Rochester[44] concluded that weakness, not fatigue, was the principal cause of hypercapnia in COPD patients with respiratory failure. Several lines of evidence formed the basis of this conclusion. First, the pressure-time integral of the diaphragm does not lie within the "fatigue zone" in COPD patients.[45] Second, few COPD patients with exacerbations of their disease demonstrate fatigue of the respiratory muscles as measured by the force frequency curve of the sternomastoid muscle.[46] Finally, the best predictor of hypercapnia in moderate to severe COPD was found to be R_L/P_{Imax} (where $r = 0.57$ and R_L is the load).[47] This last finding indicates that hypercapnia may represent an imbalance between load and capacity (P_{Imax}), a possibility that emphasizes weakness rather than fatigue as the main problem in respiratory muscle failure. The current hypothesis states that a breathing pattern characterized by rapid, shallow breathing minimizes the inspiratory load and reduces dyspnea, a key determinant of which is the ratio of breath pressure to P_{Imax}. In the presence of an abnormally high ratio of dead space to tidal volume, as occurs in COPD, small decreases in tidal volume result in the elevation of $Paco_2$. Treatment that reduces load or increases P_{Imax} is thus likely to be of benefit. This hypothesis has important implications for future therapy as it implies that training to improve the strength of the ventilatory muscles may be of value even in the hypercapnic patient. This approach is in direct contradiction to the previously held belief that chronic fatigue is the culprit and that muscle rest is crucial to the recovery of fatigued respiratory muscles.[36] This approach also has an impact on the type of ventilatory muscle training that should be performed and suggests that the emphasis should be on techniques that primarily improve strength rather than endurance (see discussion earlier in this chapter). This is clearly an area for future investigation.

The description of intermittent ventilatory support as "rest" therapy may be incorrect.[39,40] This terminology resulted from the the concept of chronic respiratory muscle fatigue. Now that this concept is being questioned and evidence has been established (certainly in other diseases, such as kyphoscoliosis) that improvement in respiratory function is not necessarily related to

FIGURE 17–6. *A,* Time-course of changes in pressure frequency curves of the diaphragms of four subjects at intervals of 2 to 4, 8 to 10, 14 to 17, and 25 to 30 minutes after fatigue. The *solid curves* represent the average of three curves before fatigue (control). The *dotted curves* represent the average of three curves at different times during the recovery period. Diaphragmatic pressure (Pdi) is expressed as a percentage of the Pdi generated for a stimulation frequency of 100 Hz (Pdimax). The *bars* indicate 1 SE. (From Aubier M, Farkas G, De Troyer A, et al. Detection of diaphragmatic fatigue in man by phrenic stimulation. J Appl Physiol 1981; 50:538–544.) *B,* Time-course of recovery of the sternomastoid from low-frequency fatigue in subject No. 1, a 34-year-old male. (*Open circles*: control; *closed circles*: after inspiratory loading.) (From Moxham J, Wiles CM, Newham D, et al. Sternomastoid muscle function and fatigue in man. Clin Sci 1980; 59:463–468.)

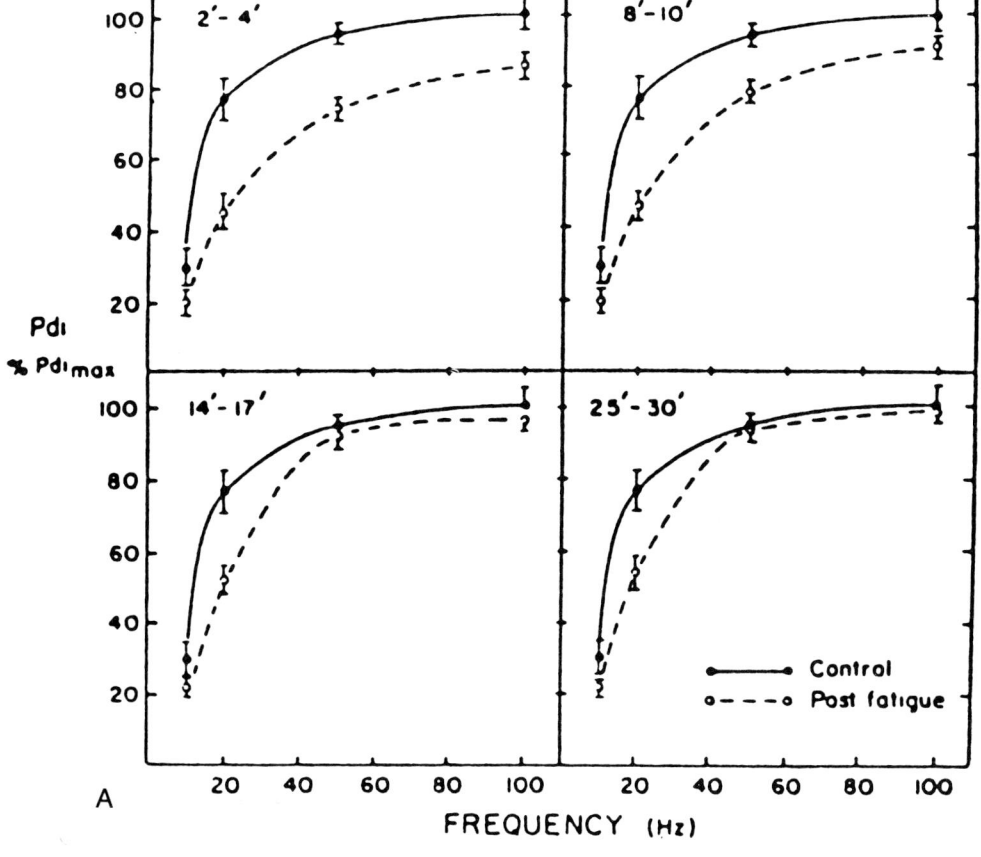

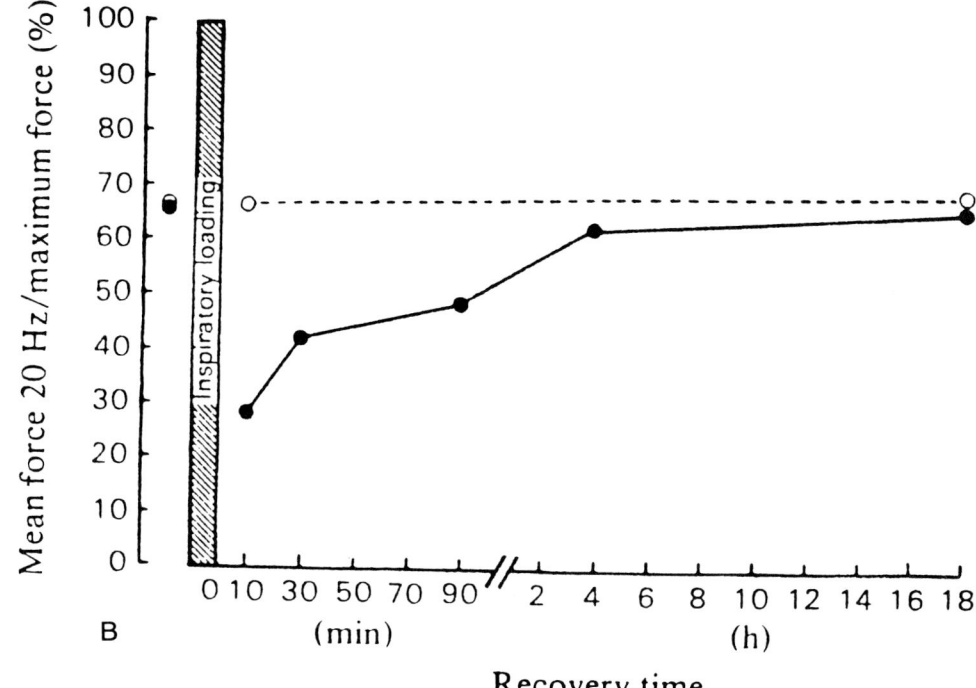

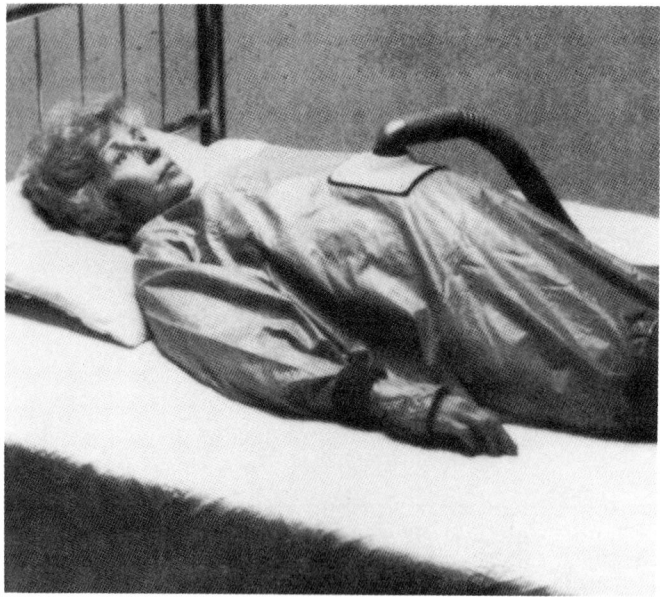

FIGURE 17–7. A patient wearing an airtight suit that is connected to a negative pressure ventilator. A rigid cage attached to a board surrounds the chest to provide support. Within the cage the pump creates the negative pressure. This negative pressure results in chest expansion.

several other studies (Table 17–4). Cropp and DiMarco[53] examined the effect of short-term ventilatory support (3–6 hr/day) using a negative-pressure ventilator on ventilatory muscle function measured specifically as MSVC. The eight patients in the study group showed significant increases in PImax and MSVC, and five of the eight who had arterial PCO_2 values greater than 43 mm Hg showed significant decreases in these values after treatment. The control group did not demonstrate any of these changes. This work was followed in 1988 by the intriguing demonstration of Gutierrez and colleagues[54] that an 8-hour regimen of cuirass ventilation once per week in five patients with advanced COPD and hypercapnia resulted in an improvement in blood gas parameters and exercise capacity as well as in the improvement of quality of life as measured by a questionnaire (Table 17–5). A reduction in the chronic hypercapnia in these patients also occurred. It should be emphasized that this study included a very small number of patients and no control group. More recent work from the United Kingdom has failed to show the same results using the same therapeutic regimen.[55]

Two subsequent controlled studies provided valuable information. In the first study, 20 stable patients with severe COPD were randomized to receive standard care

ventilatory muscle rest, it is probably more appropriate to describe this form of therapy generically as *noninvasive intermittent ventilatory support*. In this way, we avoid emphasizing that the ventilatory muscles are in fact being rested or that ventilatory muscle fatigue is the cause of the respiratory failure.

METHODS OF PROVIDING NONINVASIVE VENTILATORY MUSCLE SUPPORT

Ventilatory Muscle Rest Therapy

Extensive reviews of the equipment and techniques used in ventilatory muscle rest therapy have recently been published.[48, 49] In general, both negative-pressure and positive-pressure methods have been employed (Figs. 17–7 and 17–8). Early studies were performed using the tank respirator (or "iron lung"), but recent developments have simplified the application of negative-pressure therapy. These developments include the cuirass shell and various types of airtight body suits that, together with negative-pressure generators, provide effective methods of mechanical ventilation. Intense interest has developed recently in the application of positive-pressure ventilation in a noninvasive fashion. This can be done by using nasal masks with either volume-cycled or pressure-cycled ventilators.[50–52]

Noninvasive Ventilatory Support in Chronic Obstructive Pulmonary Disease

The 1984 publication of the work of Braun and Marino[38] on respiratory muscle fatigue was followed by

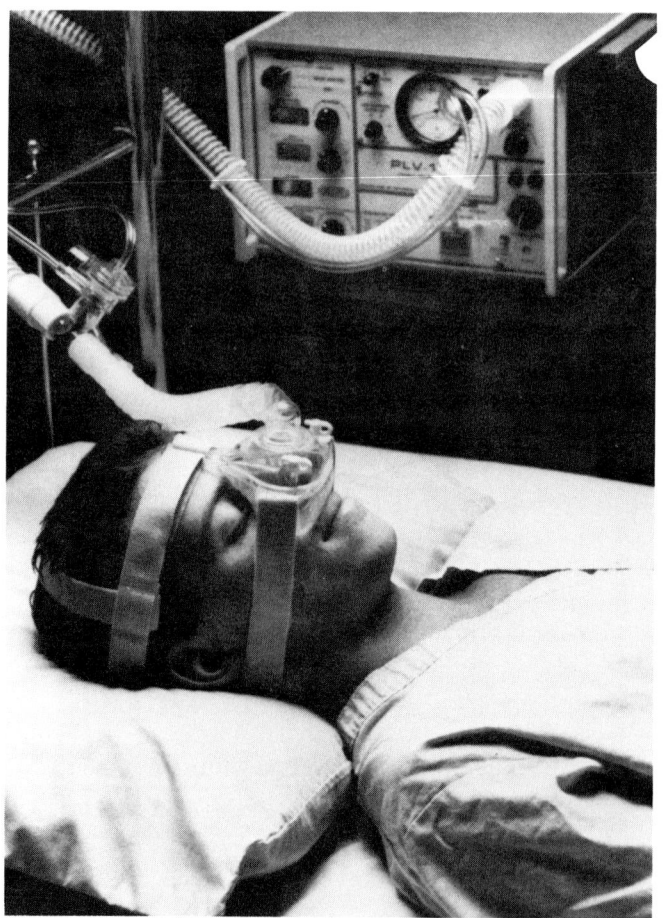

FIGURE 17–8. Positive-pressure ventilation can be applied noninvasively using a nasal mask secured firmly over the nose. The positive pressure can be delivered by employing various types of pressure or volume ventilators.

TABLE 17-4. CHARACTERISTICS OF COPD IN PATIENTS WHO RECEIVED INTERMITTENT NEGATIVE-PRESSURE VENTILATION THERAPY

Reference	No. of Patients	Age (yr)	FEV_1 (L)	P_{Imax} (cm H_2O)	$PaCO_2$ (mm Hg)
Braun and Marino[38] (1984)	14	—	—	36 ± 4	54 ± 1
Gutierrez et al.[54] (1988)	5	57 ± 8	—	47 ± 3	59 ± 5
Cropp and DiMarco[53] (1987)	8	58 ± 3	0.8 ± 0.1	67 ± 9	60 ± 7
Zibrack et al[56] (1988)	20	64 ± 2	0.6 ± 0.0	35 ± 3	48 ± 2
Celli et al.[57] (1989)	9	61 ± 4	0.6 ± 0.1	—	45 ± 2

or negative-pressure ventilation.[56] After 6 months, the treatment regimens were switched. At 6 months, no clinical differences between the treatments were found for flow rates, blood gas parameters, or maximum inspiratory and expiratory pressures. In addition, no improvement in exercise capacity was found. It is interesting to note, however, that 11 of the patients dropped out of the study because they were unable to tolerate ventilator use. Furthermore, even those patients who finished the study expressed dissatisfaction with the ventilator and complained of frequent musculoskeletal pain as well as of the inconvenience associated with the use of the device. The investigators concluded that negative-pressure ventilation via the ponchowrap body suit was poorly tolerated and that if this therapy was to be further investigated, more effective means would be needed for its provision. They also emphasized the fact that they did not document "rest" of the ventilatory muscles, and it should be noted that neither did previous investigators. In the study of Celli and coworkers published in 1989,[57] the additive effect of intermittent negative-pressure ventilation to a program of pulmonary rehabilitation was compared with the results of rehabilitation alone. Those patients who underwent electromyographic measurement of the diaphragm showed a significant reduction in the electromyographic signal that was consistent with rest or with capture of the respiratory muscles. However, this study failed to show that negative-pressure ventilation provided an additional benefit to the standard rehabilitation program. The authors emphasized that one patient who had an extremely high PCO_2 benefitted the most, suggesting that negative-pressure therapy might be efficacious if directed at patients with severe hypercapnia.

The most comprehensive study to date was a large randomized trial performed in Montreal, Canada, in 1989.[58] Preliminary data have been presented at several meetings.[43] The study was designed to test the efficacy of "rest" therapy in stable patients with advanced COPD. In general, patients with severe obstruction (FEV_1 < 50% of that predicted) and severe dyspnea (grade 4 or 5) based on an American Thoracic Society questionnaire were eligible for the study. One hundred eighty-four patients were randomized to receive either active or sham negative-pressure ventilation. It is very important to note that diaphragmatic electromyographic data were recorded in all patients in order to document the suppression of muscle activity during the ventilator therapy. The goal of the project was to ventilate the patients for 8 hours per day. The effects of the treatment on dyspnea, blood gas parameters, inspiratory and expiratory pressures, 6-minute walking distance, bicycle ergometer endurance, and quality of life were all recorded. As a result of the study, it appeared that therapy was not effective in regard to any of these measures. Furthermore, when subanalyses were performed with emphasis on the more severely hypercapnic patients, again no differences were found. In addition, no dose response effect was found in that those patients who used the ventilator for more than 28 hours per week also showed no benefit in comparison with those who used it minimally.

It was observed in this study that it was difficult for patients to acclimate to this form of therapy. Although nocturnal ventilatory support was intended, a major problem that plagued this study as well as many previous studies was the occurrence of nocturnal desaturation as a result of upper airway obstruction. During sleep, there is loss of activation of the upper airway (including that of the laryngeal muscles); as a result, the negative pressure that develops in the chest causes or aggravates upper airway collapse. This is obviously a serious problem that limits the use of negative-pressure ventilation in advanced COPD patients. Treatment of this problem

TABLE 17-5. RESULTS OF INTERMITTENT NEGATIVE-PRESSURE VENTILATION THERAPY IN COPD

Reference	Frequency	Diaphragm Capture	Blood Gas Parameters
Gutierrez et al.[54] (1988)	8 hr/wk	2/5 Pdi* measured	PCO_2 decreased, PO_2 increased
Zibrak et al.[56] (1988)	6–8 hr/day for 6 mo	Not measured	No improvement
Celli et al.[57] (1989)	3–11 hr/day for 3 wk	50% reduction in EMG† of the diaphragm	No improvement in Pdimax in treated group
Martin and Levy[43] (1989)	8 hr/day for 3 mo	Documented by EMG of the diaphragm	No benefit to treated group with respect to dyspnea, P_{Imax}, and exercise capacity

*Transdiaphragmatic pressure.
†Electromyogram.

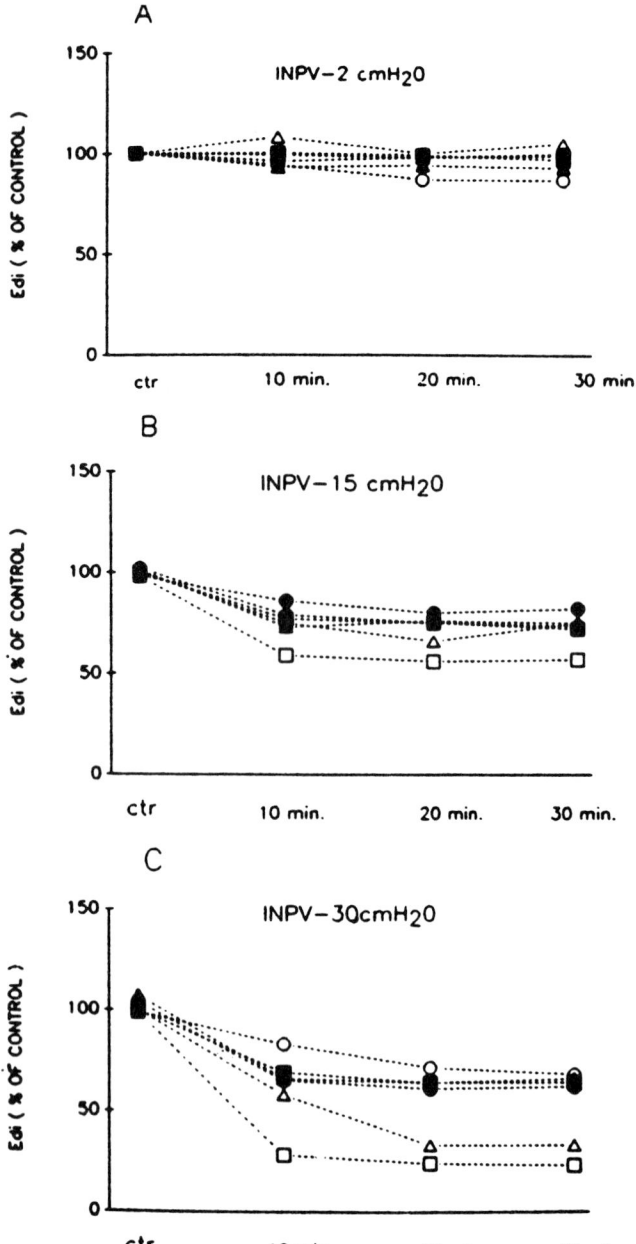

FIGURE 17-9. Time-course of diaphragmatic elastance (Edi), expressed as individual values, during intermittent negative pressure ventilation (INPV) trials at −2 cm H₂O (upper graph), −15 cm H₂O (center graph), and −30 cm H₂O (lower graph) in patients with COPD. (From Nava S, Ambrosino N, Zocchi L, et al. Diaphragmatic rest during negative pressure ventilation by Pneumowrap. Chest 1990; 98:857–865.)

investigators have successfully ventilated COPD patients (Fig. 17-9). This was demonstrated in an Italian study[61] in which negative-pressure ventilation using both 15 and 30 cm H_2O of pressure was effective in significantly reducing diaphragm electromyographic activity. With sufficient instruction and a great deal of practice, it appears that some patients can be ventilated using negative-pressure devices. This study also emphasized the need for relaxation on the part of the subject as well as for long periods of acclimatization to the ventilator. As noted earlier, however, many patients are not able to adapt to the ventilator.

Noninvasive Positive-Pressure Ventilation

The difficulties with negative-pressure ventilation have paved the way for the application of noninvasive nasal positive-pressure ventilation via continuous positive airway pressure masks.[51,52] Preliminary studies that have explored the utility of positive-pressure ventilation in COPD have shown great promise for this modality. These studies have shown impressive reductions in diaphragm electromyographic activity when positive-pressure ventilation is applied (Fig. 17-10). In the study by Belman and coworkers,[51] integrated electromyographic activity of the diaphragm was reduced by approximately 25% compared with pretherapy values. The reduction was considerably greater than that achieved with negative-pressure ventilation. Furthermore, the transdiaphragmatic pressure was reduced almost to zero during positive-pressure ventilation. This form of ventilation has also been successfully used in the treatment of several neuromuscular disorders, indicating that patients

in the past has been accomplished by the use of drugs, such as protriptyline, or by the administration of continuous positive airway pressure via nasal mask.[59] The problems of negative-pressure ventilation and of its effect on sleep were studied in normal subjects by Levy and associates.[60] They showed that normal subjects developed an increased number of apneas and hypopneas and experienced decreased sleep efficiency, sleep fragmentation, and altered sleep architecture. Despite the difficulties of negative-pressure ventilation, some

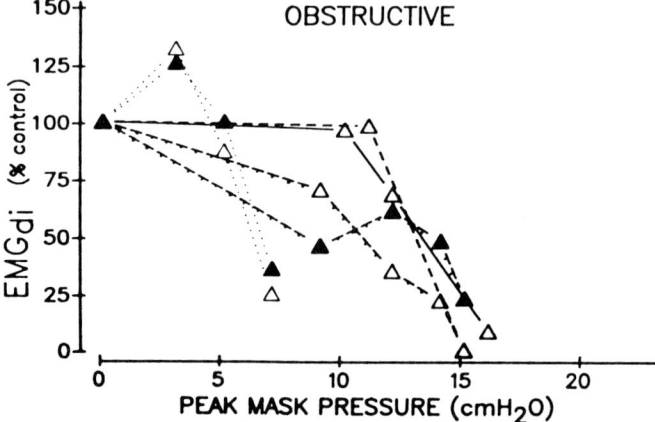

FIGURE 17-10. The relationship between the mean amplitude of the diaphragm electromyelogram (EMGdi) and the level of mask pressure (Pmask) during nasal ventilation. Results for individual subjects are expressed as a percentage of control values obtained for each subject during spontaneous breathing. The open and closed triangles represent diaphragm activity recorded from surface and esophageal electrodes, respectively. In all subjects, nasal ventilation resulted in substantial reductions of EMGdi amplitude. Surface and esophageal EMGdi amplitudes decreased in a similar fashion in those subjects in whom both signals were recorded. (From Carrey Z, Gottfried SB, Levy RD. Ventilatory muscle support in respiratory failure with nasal positive pressure ventilation. Chest 1990; 97:150–158.)

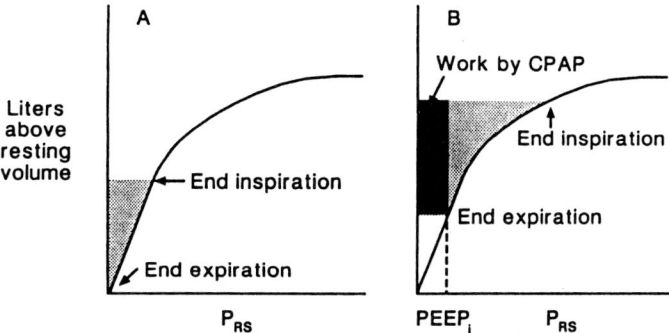

FIGURE 17-11. The relationship between the elastic recoil of the respiratory system (PRS) and the volume in liters above resting volume is illustrated in the absence (A) and in the presence (B) of intrinsic positive end-expiratory pressure (PEEPi). The *total shaded area* in both panels depicts the elastic work required to inflate the respiratory system with the same tidal volume. The *darkly shaded area* represents the theoretic reduction of elastic work that could be supplied by continuous positive airway pressure (CPAP), which would in turn reduce the burden imposed by the presence of PEEPi. (From Gay PC, Rodarte JR, Hubmayr RD. The effects of positive expiratory pressure on isovolume flow and dynamic hyperinflation in patients receiving mechanical ventilation. Am Rev Respir Dis 1989; 139:621–626.)

can adapt to long-term use.[50] Extensive experience with positive-pressure ventilation has been gained in France, where over 100 patients have received this form of treatment in the long term.[62] Although the French study very effectively documented that such ventilation can be delivered on a large scale on an outpatient basis, the patients were not randomized to treatment and to control groups; therefore, at this stage, it is difficult to critically assess this study's results.[62] Reports of controlled randomized studies of noninvasive positive-pressure ventilation in patients with COPD have yet to be published.

Conclusion

Although doubt has been expressed as to the existence of chronic fatigue of the respiratory muscles,[39, 40, 43] there is still great interest in the potential benefits of intermittent noninvasive ventilatory support. Experience in the treatment of neuromuscular disorders, particularly of kyphoscoliosis, is an incentive to more effectively evaluate the effects of this form of therapy in COPD. In kyphoscoliosis, significant benefits with respect to both lung function and quality of life have been achieved.[50] According to the work of Ellis and colleagues, a major mechanism of the decrease in hypercapnia may be the restoration of central drive together with an increase in carbon dioxide chemoresponsiveness. Whether this mechanism is important in COPD or other potential mechanisms such as rest of the muscles or improved sleep structure is not certain. Nevertheless, the relative ease with which ventilatory support can now be achieved by means of positive-pressure ventilation has spawned several new studies, the results of which should answer these questions in the near future.

UNLOADING OF THE RESPIRATORY MUSCLES

Expiratory flow rates during tidal breathing in patients with severe COPD are close to or equal to the maximum expiratory flow-volume relationship.[63, 64] COPD patients can increase their expiratory flow rates during hyperpnea and exercise through dynamic hyperinflation and an increase in end-expiratory lung volume.[64] The improvement in expiratory flow rates is offset by the increase in inspiratory work caused by the dynamic hyperinflation. This is the result of several factors that come into play during dynamic hyperinflation. First, during dynamic hyperinflation, tidal volume oscillates in a less compliant range of the pressure-volume relationship, whereas the tachypnea that results from exercise causes a decrease in dynamic compliance.[6] Second, the patient is required to generate additional inspiratory pressure at the initiation of inspiration in order to overcome the increased elastic recoil of the respiratory system. This increased threshold load at the start of inspiration has been referred to as *intrinsic positive end-expiratory pressure*, and although it was originally described in patients receiving mechanical ventilation, it has now been well documented in COPD patients breathing spontaneously during exercise and at rest.[65, 66] Thus, dynamic hyperinflation results in an increased inspiratory load that

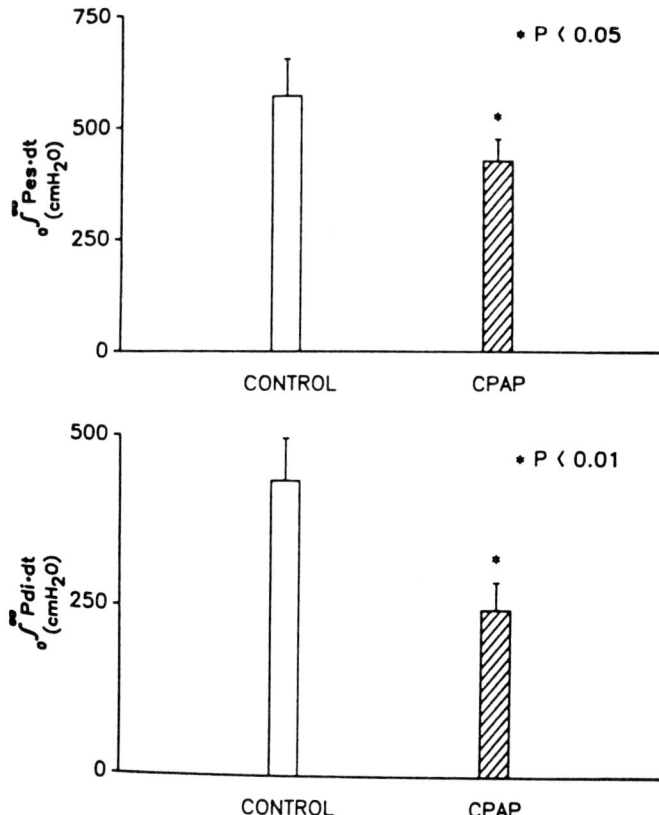

FIGURE 17-12. Time integral of pressure for the respiratory muscles ($\int Pes \cdot dt$) and for the diaphragm ($\int Pdi \cdot dt$) before and during the application of CPAP. Values are expressed as mean ± SE. (From Petrof BJ, Calderini ED, Gottfried SB. Effect of CPAP on respiratory effort and dyspnea during exercise in severe COPD. J Appl Physiol 1990; 69:179–188.)

comprises both elastic and threshold components. As has been pointed out earlier,[6] in COPD "the mechanical defect is primarily resistive in expiration, the mechanical consequences are encountered in inspiration and are primarily restrictive in nature."

EFFECT OF CONTINUOUS POSITIVE AIRWAY PRESSURE

After it was demonstrated in one study that low levels of positive end-expiratory pressure improved lung mechanics in ventilated patients with COPD,[67] a subsequent study showed that continuous positive airway pressure (CPAP) reduced work of breathing and dyspnea in COPD patients with respiratory failure during weaning from mechanical ventilation.[68] It is believed that CPAP counterbalances the increased recoil pressure of the respiratory system at end-expiration (Fig. 17–11). In a more recent study, Petrof and colleagues[69] examined respiratory effort and dyspnea during exercise in patients with obstructive airway disease. Approximately 7.5 to 10.0 cm H_2O of CPAP was applied during single-stage exercise in these patients. The level of dyspnea and respiratory mechanics were measured during the application of CPAP as well as during a control period. Although the application of CPAP produced more positive values of the maximum expiratory and minimum expiratory levels of esophageal pressure, total tidal excursion of esophageal pressure was significantly reduced, whereas tidal volume remained unchanged. Similar effects were noted for transdiaphragmatic pressure (Fig. 17–12). Associated with these changes was a more positive value of maximum expiratory gastric pressure. All of the pressure changes resulted in significant reductions of the pressure-time integrals of both esophageal and diaphragmatic pressures but in an increase of the pressure-time integral of gastric pressure. Of the eight patients studied, five indicated a subjective improvement in dyspnea, whereas three experienced a worsening of this sensation. It is interesting to note that the improvement in dyspnea was directly related to the reduction in the time integrals of the esophageal and diaphragmatic pressures but inversely related to the increase in the gastric pressure-time integral.

This study clearly showed that reduction in dyspnea is possible with the use of CPAP, although the effects of CPAP in different patients were not consistent. In some patients, worsening of dyspnea and significant increases in gastric pressure occurred, suggesting that excessive abdominal muscle recruitment during expiration took place and nullified the benefit of the reduction in inspiratory pressure. Further work in this area is required to estimate correctly and supply the appropriate level of CPAP to consistently provide benefit to these patients.

Two subsequent studies have provided further support for the use of CPAP. O'Donnell and associates found that the application of CPAP resulted in a reduction in dyspnea during exercise in eight patients (Fig. 17–13).[70] In addition to CPAP, they studied the separate effects of continuous positive inspiratory pressure and continuous positive expiratory pressure. Only the former was effective in reducing symptoms of dyspnea; this emphasizes the importance of inspiratory unloading and suggests that the effect of the latter on dynamic compression is not helpful. In a follow-up study by the same group of investigators,[71] the administration of CPAP to exercising patients with COPD resulted in significant improvement in exercise endurance. The mean increase in endurance during a single-stage test was from 5.98 minutes to 8.82 minutes. The application of positive airway pressure during exercise offers a novel means of reducing symptoms and increasing exercise endurance.

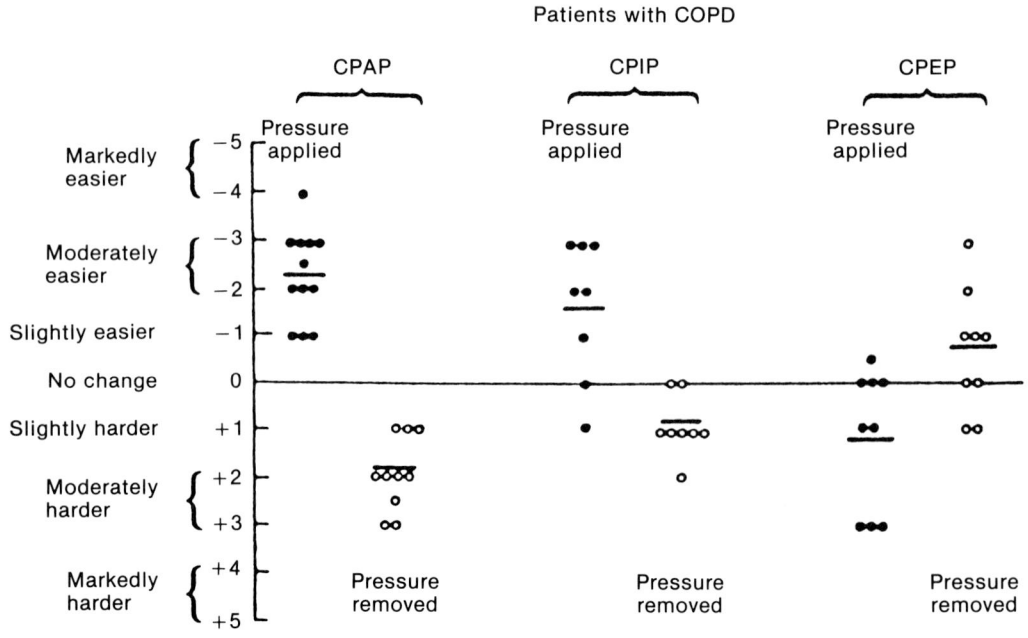

FIGURE 17–13. Category scale and ratings selected by the COPD group. Each *closed circle* represents the subject's perception of change in breathing effort during a given pressure application compared with his or her perceptions immediately preceding the unloaded time period. The *open circles* represent perceived change in breathing effort after removal of the various pressures as compared with patient perceptions when they were applied. (CPAP: continuous positive airway pressure; CPIP: continuous positive inspiratory pressure; CPEP: continuous positive expiratory pressure.) (From O'Donnell DE, Sanii R, Giesbrecht G, Younes M. Effect of continuous positive airway pressure on respiratory sensation in patients with chronic obstructive pulmonary disease during submaximal exercise. Am Rev Respir Dis 1988; 138:1185–1191.)

The wider application of CPAP can be facilitated by the use of battery-powered units to generate positive pressure. If successful, the benefits of CPAP will be able to be attained without the need for prolonged therapy or exercise training.

REFERENCES

1. Leith DE, Bradley M. Ventilatory muscle strength and endurance training. J Appl Physiol 1976; 41:508–516.
2. Pardy RL, Reid WD, Belman MJ. Respiratory muscle training. Clin Chest Med 1988; 9:287–297.
3. Tobin MJ. Respiratory muscles in disease. Clin Chest Med 1988; 9:263–286.
4. Cherniack RM. The oxygen consumption and efficiency of the respiratory muscles in health and emphysema. J Clin Invest 1959; 38:494–499.
5. Lewis MI, Belman MJ. Nutrition and the respiratory muscles. In: Tobin MJ (ed). Respiratory Muscles: Function in Health and Disease. Philadelphia: J. B. Lippincott Co., 1990, pp 343–359.
6. Younes M. Load responses, dyspnea and respiratory failure. Chest 1989; 3:595–685.
7. Dubowitz V, Brooke MH. Muscle biopsy: A modern approach. Philadelphia: W. B. Saunders Co., 1973.
8. Green HJ, Reichmann H, Pette D. Inter- and intraspecies comparisons of fiber type distribution and succinate dehydrogenase activity of type I, IIA, and IIB fibers of mammalian diaphragms. Histochem J 1984; 81:67–73.
9. Burke RE, Levine DN, Azjac FE, et al. Mammalian motor units: Physiological-histochemical correlation in three types in cat gastrocnemius. Science 1971; 174:709–712.
10. Faulkner JA. Structural and functional adaptations of skeletal muscle. In: Roussos C, Macklem PT (eds). The Thorax. New York: Marcel Dekker, Inc., 1985, pp 1324–1352.
11. Holloszy JO, Coyle EF. Adaptations of skeletal muscle to endurance exercise and their metabolic consequences. J Appl Physiol 1984; 56:831–838.
12. Sieck GC. Diaphragm muscle: Structural and functional organization. Clin Chest Med 1988; 9:195–209.
13. Keens TG, Chen V, Patel P, et al. Cellular adaptations of the ventilatory muscles to a chronic increased respiratory load. J Appl Physiol 1978; 44:905–908.
14. Akabas SR, Bazzy AR, Di Marco S, et al. Metabolic and functional adaptations of the diaphragm to training with resistive loads. J Appl Physiol 1989; 66:529–535.
15. Robinson EP, Kjeldgaard JM. Improvement in ventilatory muscle function running. J Appl Physiol 1982; 52:1400–1406.
16. Keens TG, Krastins IRB, Wanamaker EM, et al. Ventilatory muscle endurance training in normal subjects and patients with cystic fibrosis. Am Rev Respir Dis 1977; 116:853–860.
17. Belman MJ, Kendregan BA. Exercise training fails to increase skeletal muscle enzymes in patients with chronic obstructive pulmonary disease. Am Rev Respir Dis 1981; 123:256–261.
18. Levine S, Weiser P, Gillen J. Evaluation of a ventilatory muscle endurance training program in the rehabilitation of patients with COPD. Am Rev Respir Dis 1986; 133:400–406.
19. Reis AL, Moser KM. Comparison of isocapnic hyperventilation and walking exercise training in pulmonary rehabilitation. Chest 1986; 90:285–289.
20. Belman MJ, Mittman C. Ventilatory muscle training improves exercise capacity in chronic obstructive pulmonary disease patients. Am Rev Respir Dis 1980; 121:273–280.
21. Belman MJ. Respiratory failure treated by ventilatory muscle training. Eur J Respir Dis 1981; 62:391–395.
22. Belman MJ, Gaesser GA. Ventilatory muscle training in the elderly. J Appl Physiol 1988; 64:899–905.
23. Clanton TL, Dixon G, Drake J, et al. Inspiratory muscle conditioning using a threshold loading device. Chest 1985; 87:62–66.
24. Killian KJ, Jones NL. Respiratory muscles and dyspnea. Clin Chest Med 1988; 9:237.
25. Belman MJ, Shadmehr R. Targeted resistive muscle training in chronic obstructive pulmonary disease. J Appl Physiol 1988; 65:2726–2735.
26. Harver A, Mahler DA, Daubenspeck JA. Targeted inspiratory muscle training improves respiratory muscle function and reduces dyspnea in patients with chronic obstructive disease. Ann Intern Med 1989; 111:117–124.
27. Mahler DA, Weinberg DH, Wells CK, et al. The measurement of dyspnea. Chest 1984; 85:751–758.
28. Dekhuizen PNR, Folgering HTM, van Herwaarden CLA. Target flow inspiratory muscle training during pulmonary rehabilitation in patients with COPD. Chest 1991; 99:128–133.
29. Aldrich TK, Karpel JP, Uhrlass RM, et al. Weaning from mechanical ventilation. Crit Care Med 1989; 17:143–147.
30. Nickerson BG, Keens TG. Measuring ventilatory muscle endurance as sustainable inspiratory pressure. J Appl Physiol 1982; 52:768–772.
31. Larson JL, Kim MJ, Sharp JT, et al. Inspiratory muscle training with a pressure threshold breathing device in patients with chronic obstructive pulmonary disease. Am Rev Respir Dis 1988; 138:689–696.
32. Goldstein R, De Rosie J, Long S, et al. Applicability of a threshold loading device for inspiratory muscle training in patients with COPD. Chest 1989; 96:564–571.
33. Flynn MG, Barter CE, Nosworthy JC, et al. Threshold pressure training, breathing pattern and exercise performance in chronic airflow obstruction. Chest 1989; 95:535–540.
34. Flenley DC. Short Review: Inspiratory muscle training. Eur J Respir Dis 1985; 67:153–158.
35. Rochester DF, Braun NMT, Lane S. Diaphragmatic energy expenditure in chronic respiratory failure: The effect of assisted ventilation with body respirators. Am J Med 1977; 63:223–232.
36. Macklem PT. The clinical relevance of respiratory muscle research. J. Burns Amberson lecture. Am Rev Respir Dis 1986; 134:812–815.
37. Macklem PT. Respiratory muscles: The vital pump. Chest 1980; 78:753–758.
38. Braun NMT, Marino WD. Effect of daily intermittent rest of respiratory muscles in patients with severe chronic airflow limitation. Chest 1984; 85:59S.
39. Moxham J. Respiratory muscle fatigue, mechanisms, evaluation and therapy. Br J Anesth 1990; 65:43–53.
40. La Rouche CM, Moxham J, Green M. Respiratory muscle weakness and fatigue. Q J Med 1989; 71:373–397.
41. Bellemare F, Bigland-Ritchie B. Assessment of human diaphragm strength and activation using phrenic nerve stimulation. Respir Physiol 1984; 58:263–277.
42. Edwards RHT, Hill DK, Jones DA, et al. Fatigue of long duration in human skeletal muscle after exercise. J Physiol (Lond) 1977; 272:769–778.
43. Martin JG, Levy RD. Ventilatory muscle rest and problems in respiratory care. In: Tobin MJ (ed). The Respiratory Muscles. Philadelphia: J. B. Lippincott Co., 1989, pp 535–541.
44. Rochester DF. Respiratory muscle weakness, pattern of breathing, and CO_2 retention in chronic obstructive pulmonary disease. Am Rev Respir Dis 1991; 143:901–903.
45. Bellemare F, Grassino A. Force reserve of the diaphragm in patients with chronic obstructive pulmonary disease. J Appl Physiol 1983; 55:8–15.
46. Efthimiou J, Fleming J, Spiro SG. Sternomastoid muscle function and fatigue in breathless patients with severe respiratory disease. Am Rev Respir Dis 1987; 136:1099–1105.
47. Begin P, Grassino A. Inspiratory muscle dysfunction and chronic hypercapnia in chronic obstructive pulmonary disease. Am Rev Respir Dis 1991; 143:905–912.
48. Levine S, Henson D, Levy S. Respiratory muscle rest therapy. Clin Chest Med 1988; 9:297–309.
49. Hill NS. Clinical applications of body ventilators. Chest 1986; 90:897–905.
50. Ellis ER, Grunstein RR, Chan S, et al. Noninvasive ventilatory support during sleep improves respiratory failure in kyphoscoliosis. Chest 1988; 94:811–815.
51. Belman MJ, SooHoo G, Kuei J, et al. Efficacy of positive vs. negative pressure ventilation in unloading the respiratory muscles. Chest 1990; 98:850–856.
52. Carrey Z, Gottfried SB, Levy RD. Ventilatory muscle support in

respiratory failure with nasal positive pressure ventilation. Chest 1990; 97:150–158.
53. Cropp A, DiMarco AF. Effects of intermittent negative pressure ventilation on respiratory muscle function in patients with severe chronic obstructive pulmonary disease. Am Rev Respir Dis 1987; 135:1056–1061.
54. Gutierrez M, Beroiza T, Contreras G, et al. Weekly cuirass ventilation improves blood gases and inspiratory muscle strength in patients with chronic air-flow limitation and hypercarbia. Am Rev Respir Dis 1988; 138:617–623.
55. Bott J, Keildy SEJ, Jenkins SC, et al. Weekly nasal positive pressure ventilation does not improve function in patients with stable severe COPD. Am Rev Respir Dis 1991; 143:A74.
56. Zibrak JD, Hill NS, Federman EC, et al. Evaluation of intermittent long-term negative pressure ventilation in patients with severe chronic obstructive pulmonary disease. Am Rev Respir Dis 1988; 138:1515–1518.
57. Celli B, Lee H, Criner G, et al. Controlled trial of external negative pressure ventilation in patients with severe chronic airflow limitation. Am Rev Respir Dis 1989; 140:1251–1256.
58. Shapiro SH, Macklem PT, Gray DK, et al. A randomized controlled clinical trail of intermittent negative pressure in severe COPD. J Clin Epidemiol 1991: 44:483–496.
59. Goldstein RS, Molotiu H, Skrastins R, et al. Reversal of sleep induced hypoventilation and chronic respiratory failure by nocturnal negative pressure ventilation in patients with restrictive ventilatory impairment. Am Rev Respir Dis 1987; 135:1049–1055.
60. Levy RD, Bradley TD, Newman SL, et al. Negative pressure ventilation: Effects on ventilation during sleep in normal subjects. Chest 1989; 95:95–99.
61. Nava S, Ambrosino N, Zocchi L, et al. Diaphragmatic rest during negative pressure ventilation by pneumowrap. Chest 1990; 98:857–865.
62. Leger P, Bedicam JM, Cornette A, et al. Long term follow up of severe chronic respiratory insufficiency patients (n=373) treated by home nocturnal noninvasive nasal IPPV. Am Rev Respir Dis 1991; 143:A73.
63. Potter WA, Olafsson S, Hyatt RE. Ventilatory mechanics and expiratory flow limitation during exercise in patients with obstructive lung disease. J Clin Invest 1971; 50:910–919.
64. Stubbing DG, Pengelly LD, Morse JLC, Jones N. Pulmonary mechanics during exercise in subjects with chronic airflow obstruction. J Appl Physiol 1980; 49:511–515.
65. Fleury B, Murciano C, Talamo C, et al. Work of breathing in patients with chronic obstructive pulmonary disease in acute respiratory failure. Am Rev Respir Dis 1985; 131:822–827.
66. Haluszka J, Chartrand DA, Grassino AE, Milic-Emili J. Intrinsic PEEP and arterial PCO_2 in stable patients with chronic obstructive pulmonary disease. Am Rev Respir Dis 1990; 141:1194–1197.
67. Smith TC, Marini JJ. Impact of PEEP on lung mechanics and work of breathing in severe airflow obstruction. J Appl Physiol 1988; 65:1488–1499.
68. Petrof B, Legaré M, Goldberg P. Continuous positive airway pressure and dyspnea during weaning from mechanical ventilation in severe chronic obstructive pulmonary disease. Am Rev Respir Dis 1990; 141:281–289.
69. Petrof BJ, Calderini E, Gottfried SB. Effect of CPAP on respiratory effort and dyspnea during exercise in COPD. J Appl Physiol 1990; 69:179–188.
70. O'Donnell DE, Sanii R, Greslnecht G, et al. Effect of continuous positive airway pressure on respiratory sensation in patients with chronic obstructive pulmonary disease during submaximal exercise. Am Rev Respir Dis 1988; 138:1185–1191.
71. O'Donnell DE, Sanii R, Younes M. Improvement in exercise endurance in patients with chronic airflow limitation using continuous positive airway pressure. Am Rev Respir Dis 1988; 138:1510–1514.

Chapter 18

Desensitization to Dyspnea in Chronic Obstructive Pulmonary Disease

FRANCOIS HAAS, Ph.D
JOHN SALAZAR-SCHICCHI, M.D.
KENNETH AXEN, Ph.D.

Dyspnea is the unpleasant awareness of labored breathing. In chronic pulmonary disease, dyspnea can eventually result in severe physical deconditioning to the extent that activities of daily living are compromised out of proportion to the patient's actual cardiorespiratory deficit (Fig. 18–1).

Dyspnea arises from the various sensory systems associated with the act of breathing. Chapter 9 details the generation of respiratory sensation and the pathophysiologic factors that contribute to dyspnea. Figure 18–2A is a schematic representation of the various components purported to be associated with the genesis of dyspnea.

The large body of research addressing the effect of physiologic cues on dyspnea, however, reveals that only 10% of the variance in chronic dyspnea can be accounted for by reduction in pulmonary function.[1] Such psychologic factors as anxiety and depression have been shown to modulate the perception of dyspnea.[2] In accordance with this, chronic obstructive pulmonary disease (COPD) patients have been in part characterized as depressed, anxious, excessively preoccupied with their bodies,[3] and predisposed to somatization.[4]

Because dyspnea is usually triggered by a ventilation increase in response to increased energy demands, traditional dyspnea management focuses on reducing the stimulus that leads to this increase. The wide variety of methods for accomplishing this (e.g., energy-conservation techniques, supplemental oxygen therapy, and relaxation techniques) are discussed elsewhere in this book. In contrast, desensitization to dyspnea (defined here as the reduction or abolition of the sensation to a given dyspneic stimulus*) suggests the application of management techniques designed to attenuate the sensation without altering the external stimulus. Because dyspnea is a psychophysiologic phenomenon involving perceptual modalities and their integration, desensitization could, in theory, be accomplished either (1) by manipulating psychologic or physiologic factors (see Fig. 18–2A) so as to alter the perception of a dyspneic stimulus or (2) by reducing peripheral receptor sensitivity, central receptor sensitivity, or both (see Fig. 18–2B to F). This chapter considers theoretical aspects of alternatives for achieving these ends. These alternatives include exercise, hypnosis, the use of neurochemicals, and peripheral receptor intervention.

---

*Because of the complexity of stimuli involved in the genesis of dyspnea, and for the purpose of simplicity, we have consolidated all such stimuli under the term *dyspneic stimulus*.

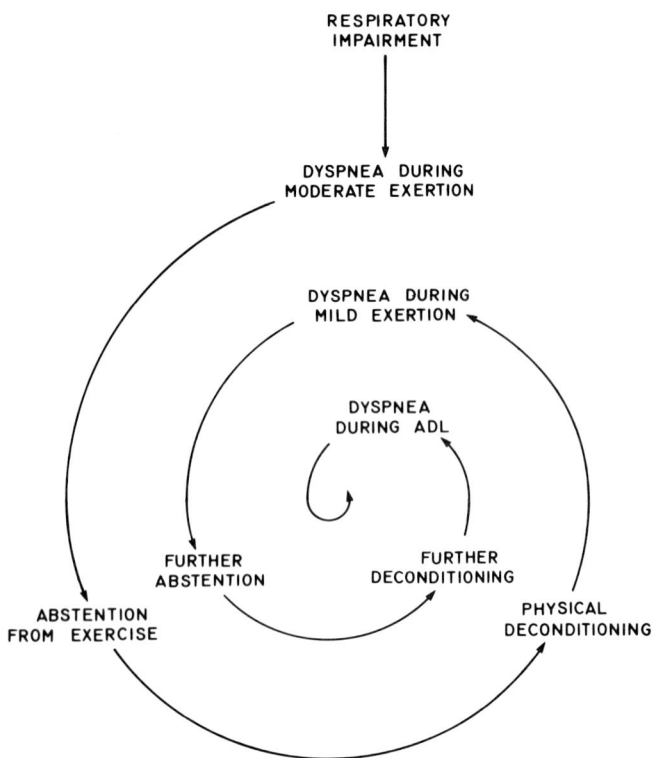

FIGURE 18–1. The dyspnea spiral. (ADL: activities of daily living.) (From Haas F, Axen K. Pulmonary Therapy and Rehabilitation: Principles and Practice. 2nd ed. Baltimore: Williams & Wilkins, 1991.)

EXERCISE

Several studies of patients with severe COPD have shown an improved sense of well-being and reduced breathlessness after exercise training[5, 6] despite little or no improvement in cardiopulmonary function. A report by Sinclair and Ingram[6] is typical. Exercise training that involved daily 12-minute walks and simple stair climbing exercises conducted under close medical supervision increased 12-minute walking distance time by 24% in 15 patients with severe chronic bronchitis after 8 to 12 months. In addition, all 15 patients indicated diminished dyspnea, 12 reported an improved sense of well-being, and 10 reported an increase in daily activity. The exercising patients showed significantly greater improvement than patients in a nonexercising control group, even though they did not have measurable cardiopulmonary changes that are normally associated with training.

The lack of cardiopulmonary response to training among severe COPD patients supports the view that they experience significant benefit from exercise even though they are unable to exercise with sufficient intensity to achieve appreciable cardiopulmonary training effects. Patients with severe COPD who exercise regularly can increase their exercise capacity.[7] However, the lack of a typical cardiopulmonary response to training suggests that these observed improvements in endurance and dyspnea are primarily a function of psychologic factors rather than of physiologic factors.[8] Several hypotheses (most with supportive data) have been proposed to explain these effects (see Fig. 18–2B).

Antidepressant Hypothesis

North and coworkers[9] recently reviewed the literature on the effect of regular exercise on depression. Their overall conclusion indicates that exercise significantly decreases depression, and that this antidepressant effect continues for some time after exercise stops. Aerobic exercise and anaerobic exercise are equally effective as antidepressants. The important variables are duration and frequency. Longer higher-frequency exercise programs are more effective than shorter, low-frequency programs. Therefore, to the extent that depression is one of the modulators of dyspnea, decreased depression stemming from the exercise schedule of a pulmonary rehabilitation program could in part account for the characteristically diminished dyspnea.

One of the proposed mechanisms for the antidepressant effect of exercise has been put forth by Bandura,[10] who suggested that people who master something that they perceive as difficult experience positive psychologic feedback that significantly improves their self-confidence and their ability to cope with personal problems. Because COPD patients see exercise as a difficult task, becoming a regular exerciser can initiate this psychologic chain of events (Fig. 18–3). This in turn can break the negative cognitive mindset of depression, that is, it can ameliorate the automatic cycle of negative thoughts that produces the systematic errors in logical thought that in turn perpetuate the depression.[11]

Social Interaction Hypothesis

Agle and associates[12] suggested that the process of graduated exercise training in a safe environment and in the presence of trained medical personnel "inadvertently functions as a desensitizing form of behavior therapy." That is, patients with severe COPD who performed progressive exercise in a well-supervised environment reduced their unrealistic fear of activity and dyspnea. Therefore, this means of the desensitization to dyspnea may be a key component of improved endurance after exercise. Although this view has not yet been documented with objective measures of exercise endurance, it is consistent with anecdotal reports. The following comments of a COPD patient in an exercise program are typical:

"I was always afraid of pushing myself with physical exercise. I would never take a challenge because, when the going literally got rough (i.e., when dyspnea occurred)* the tape would go off in my head and I

---
*Author's note.

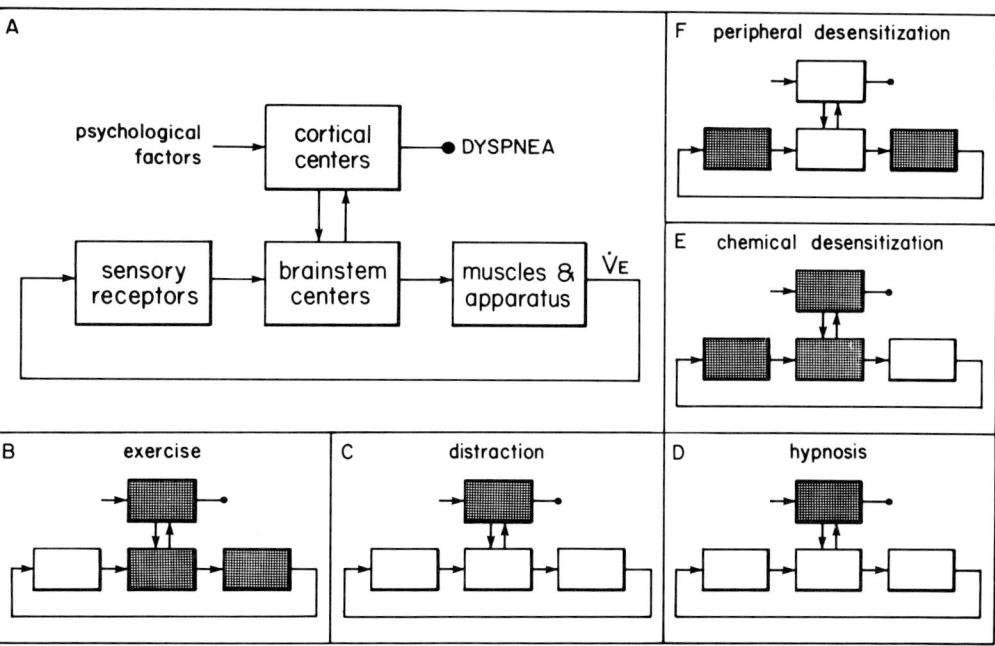

FIGURE 18–2. A, Schema of components associated with dyspneagenesis, and points where appropriate intervention might result in desensitization. B–F, The shaded area indicates the component affected by the intervention indicated. Hypnosis (D), for example, affects the cortical centers, whereas chemical desensitization (E) effects sensory, cortical, or brain stem centers, or any combination of these centers. ($\dot{V}E$: expired minute ventilation).

would quit rather than pushing through. Through this exercise program and the progress I see myself making, I now have the confidence to push through difficulties."

One possible explanation for the fourfold improvement in COPD patients who perform supervised exercise[6] compared with those who exercise unsupervised at home[13] is that patients are far more confident to push themselves in the safety of a supervised setting than in an unsupervised environment at home. The supervised rehabilitation environment may actually be desensitizing these patients to the dyspnea they experi-

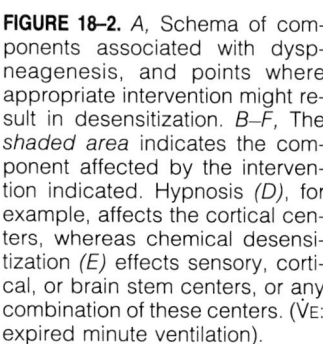

FIGURE 18–3. The depression cycle proposed by Bandura can be interrupted by exercise. (From Bandura A. Self-efficacy: Towards a unifying theory of behavioral change. Psychol Rev 1977; 2:191–215.)

ence at the higher workloads demanded by a reconditioning program.

Distraction Hypothesis

Desensitization implies a change in baseline stimulus threshold. One way to accomplish this is by decreasing the ratio of signal (dyspneic stimulus) to noise (nondyspneic stimulus) that reaches the higher centers of the central nervous system. Traditional therapies attempt this by decreasing the dyspnea signal, whereas distraction strategies increase the noise component.

Rejeski's[14] adaptation of the parallel information processing model developed in pain research by Levanthal and Everhart[15] can be used to explain how distraction may attenuate dyspnea. Since dyspnea, like pain, has an important affective dimension of unpleasantness or distress that is shaped by cognitive and contextual factors, adoption of this model is justified. The model suggests that a range of sensory and emotional information is preconsciously processed in parallel (Fig. 18–4). This preconscious processing selectively filters information to conscious awareness. Thus, sensory information (e.g., the sensing of length-tension appropriateness), affective information (e.g., apprehension as a result of increased ventilatory demand), or both, can become the focus of attention and intensify dyspnea perception.

As it is difficult to focus attention on multiple sources simultaneously, only a limited amount of information is processed at one time. This information processing model suggests that the presentation of an unrelated second stimulus can influence both perceived effort and affect by occupying attention channels that normally carry dyspneagenic information. Thus, factors that direct

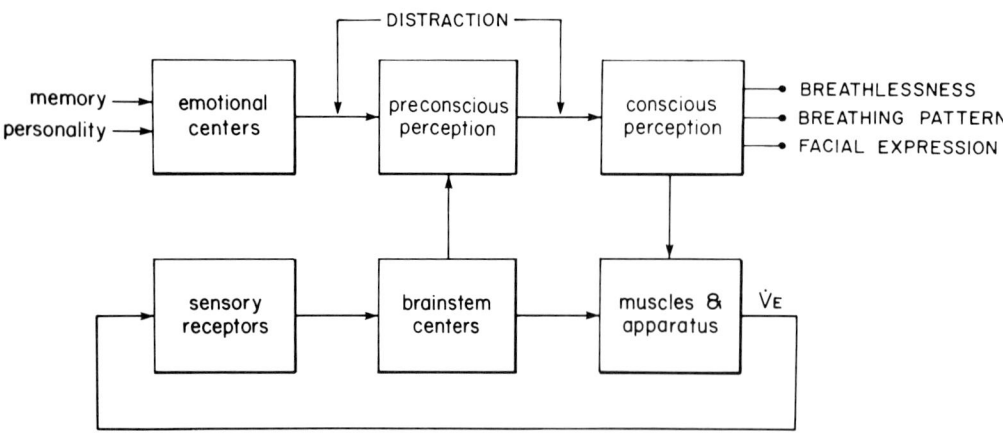

FIGURE 18–4. Dyspneic stimuli information passing through sensory and emotional channels are processed preconsciously. The presence of limited channels results in only some of this information reaching conscious perception. If sufficient dyspneagenic information reaches consciousness, it is interpreted as dyspnea and distress. This is manifested in breathlessness (as indicated by high Borg scale scores), a labored breathing pattern, and facial expressions that indicate distress. Flooding the preconscious and attentional channels with distractive stimuli (e.g., noise) reduces the amount of dyspneagenic information reaching consciousness and thus reduces dyspnea. (Based in part on Levanthal H, Everhart D. Emotion, pain, and physical illness. In: Izard CE (ed). Emotions in Personality and Psychopathology. New York: Plenum Publishing Corp., 1979, pp 263–298.)

attention externally lessen dyspnea by reducing the awareness of relevant internal sensations and by minimizing the negative affect accompanying them.

This explains why many exercisers listen to music. This self-distracting strategy allows the exerciser to avoid attending to internal feelings associated with discomfort. In fact, distraction in the form of music has been used to decrease pain perception during dental procedures[16] and during administration of electric shocks.[17] Support for the benefits of attentional distraction during exercise has been demonstrated by Pennebaker and Lightner.[18]

The distraction model is also consistent with anecdotal reports from COPD patients who claim to be less dyspneic when they walk with others than when they walk unaccompanied.* It may also explain why supervised exercise appears to be more effective than unsupervised home exercise. Perhaps the supervised rehabilitation environment provides more distraction than the home setting.

Although there has been no formal study of the factors that influence the perception of dyspnea, studies of the effect of distraction strategies on perceived effort in healthy people support the distraction hypothesis. Boutcher and Trenske[19] recently demonstrated that perceived exertion decreased when patients listened to music and that it increased during periods of sensory deprivation.

Summary

These findings and observations regarding the antidepressant effect, the feedback from social interaction, and the distractive influence that regular supervised exercise can provide (none of which are dependent on cardiopulmonary training effects) strongly support its ability to tap psychologic factors to improve endurance and decrease dyspnea in patients with severe COPD.

---
*Unpublished observation.

HYPNOSIS

The hypothesis that desensitization may be brought about by cortical modification of central chemoreceptor sensitivity has also been advanced and supported (see Fig. 18–2D). Hypnosis is a trance state that combines a heightened inner awareness with a diminished awareness of one's surroundings. It can be induced artificially (e.g., by hypnotism), but it also occurs naturally in the appropriate circumstances. For example, a hypnotic state is reached during daydreaming. It also describes the experience of being so completely engrossed (such as by music or a theatrical performance) that awareness of one's surroundings temporarily disappears.

Hypnosis has become a therapeutic tool because a person in this state is highly susceptible to positive, reasonable suggestions. For example, it has been successfully applied in the clinical treatment of asthma.[20–22] In general, relevant studies have demonstrated improved resting[20, 21] and postexercise[22] pulmonary function as well as an improved subjective rating of dyspnea (Table 18–1) following hypnotic induction or posthypnotic suggestion.

More recently, hypnosis was shown to diminish carbon dioxide sensitivity in healthy people.[23] Hypercapnic ventilatory response, oxygen consumption, breathing pattern (i.e., tidal volume and frequency), inspiratory flow rate, inspiratory timing, and mouth occlusion pressure were measured in 20 COPD patients both before and during the hypnotic state and both with and without suggestion to maintain normal ventilation (Fig. 18–5). Although there was no apparent metabolic change with hypnosis, the shift to the right of the hypercapnic ventilatory response curve during hypnosis suggests that the central chemoreceptor sensitivity threshold was raised. Suggestion to maintain normal ventilation significantly reduced the slope of the hypercapnic ventilatory response curve both during wakefulness and during hypnosis, but the response was attenuated to a significantly greater extent during hypnosis. The authors suggested that patients can voluntarily modulate cortical

TABLE 18–1. EFFECT OF HYPNOSIS ON PATIENT RATING OF DYSPNEA*

Patient	Patient Sensation of Dyspnea			
	Prehypnosis	Immediately After Hypnosis	15 min After Hypnosis	30 min After Hypnosis
1	severe	slight	slight	slight
2	slight	slight	slight	none
3	severe	none	none	none
4	moderate	none	none	none
5	moderate	none	none	none
6	slight	slight	none	none
7	moderate	slight	none	none
8	moderate	slight	none	none
9	slight	slight	slight	slight
10	moderate	slight	none	none
11	moderate	slight	none	none
12	severe	slight	none	none
13	moderate	slight	slight	slight
14	moderate	slight	none	none
15	moderate	none	none	none
16	moderate	slight	slight	slight

*Data from Aronoff GM, Aronoff S, Peck LW. Hypnotherapy in the treatment of bronchial asthma. Ann Allergy 1975; 34:356–361.

input to decrease central chemoreceptor threshold and sensitivity. Although this study did not evaluate the effects of posthypnotic suggestion or the use of self-hypnosis, results suggest that hypnosis may be clinically relevant in dyspnea desensitization for COPD patients with dyspnea-based exercise intolerance.

PHARMACOLOGIC AND NEUROCHEMICAL DESENSITIZATION

With the understanding that psychologic and physiologic effects are not as easily separated as might appear to be the case based on the literature, this section discusses the desensitization to dyspnea through the use of exogenous or endogenous chemical means (see Fig. 18–2C).

Because anxiety and panic are common psychologic characteristics of dyspneic COPD patients, it has been suggested that tranquilizers (to the extent that they can modify these reactions) might be capable of reducing dyspnea in these patients. Despite the scarcity of data in this area, some relevant information does exist on a variety of tranquilizing drugs.

In 1980, Mitchel-Heggs and colleagues[24] reported the use of diazepam for this purpose in a single-blind, placebo-controlled trial that included four patients incapacitated by dyspnea. The authors described dramatic improvement in the functional capacity of all of these patients; they associated this improvement with an attenuation of carbon dioxide sensitivity as assessed by the carbon dioxide rebreathing response. However, subsequent observations made during the use of benzodiazepines, diazepam, alprazolam, or promethazine have not corroborated this earlier report. Although these later studies did not demonstrate appreciable improvement in dyspnea level in patients as a group, some individuals did appear to gain significant relief.

In contrast, opioid drugs have generally shown more consistent benefits. For example, Woodcock and coworkers[25] observed a 20% decrease in subjective breathlessness along with an 18% increase in exercise tolerance in 12 COPD patients after ingestion of a single dose of dihydrocodeine. A follow-up study was performed in 16 COPD patients with normal blood gas parameters who were given 30 to 60 mg dihydrocodeine three times daily. Although results similar to those of the original study were observed, five patients could not complete the protocol because of nausea, constipation, or drowsiness.[26]

A recent report[27] of the effects of a single dose of morphine in 13 COPD patients with normal arterial blood gas parameters and a mean forced expiratory volume in 1 second (FEV_1) of 1 L described a 19% increase in maximum workload and peak oxygen consumption compared with the results from a placebo-treated group. At the maximum workload obtained with the placebo, the morphine-treated patients had significantly lower subjective dyspnea scores (8.6 versus 7.1 on the Borg scale) despite a 10% increase in ventilation (Fig. 18–6). At the maximum work rate, the morphine-treated group also had significantly lower levels of PaO_2 (65.8 ± 11.6, mean ± SD) and higher levels of $PaCO_2$ (43.5 ± 8.34) compared with the levels in the placebo-treated group (71.9 ± 15.5 and 38.3 ± 8.51, PaO_2 and $PaCO_2$, respectively). The only problem encountered was that some of the morphine-treated patients became drowsy and two became hypotensive after the exercise test. In another study,[28] low-dose nebulized morphine increased endurance by an average of 65 seconds as opposed to 9 seconds with placebo use. This increase was attributed to a decrease in dyspnea that resulted from morphine's attenuation of peripheral neural activity in the lung.

Thus, although opioids are effective in desensitizing the COPD patient to dyspnea, their reported side effects as well as their tendency to lead to tolerance and addiction limit their use in the treatment of highly specific cases of severe dyspnea.

Endogenous opioids (e.g., beta-endorphin) and their

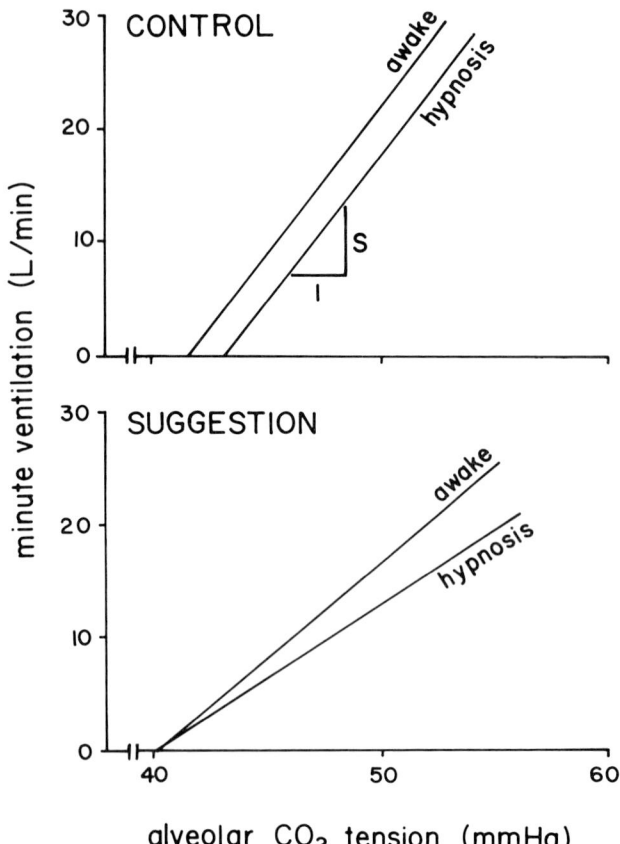

FIGURE 18–5. Hypercapnic ventilatory response plotted as minute ventilation versus alveolar $P{CO_2}$. Hypnosis with suggestion demonstrates a CO_2 sensitivity (S) that is significantly less than the other three conditions ($P<.001$ for the two control states, and $P<.01$ for the awake suggestive state). (From Sato P, Sargur M, Schoene RB. Hypnosis effect on carbon dioxide chemosensitivity. Chest 1988, 89:828–831.)

by the innate ability of humans to activate endogenous opioid mechanisms.[30]

Although the effects of both external and endogenous opioids on respiration are well established, attempts to define when and why endogenous opioids participate in the normal control of ventilation have produced conflicting hypotheses.[28] However, much of the existing evidence indicates that beta-endorphins do not modulate breathing at rest in healthy subjects.[28] Their suggested role is as an inhibitory influence on ventilation in patients with chronic airflow limitation. In the clinical setting, beta-endorphin production represents one aspect of a compensatory response to the persistent increase in the work of breathing characteristic of COPD.[31]

This hypothesis assumes a parallel between the effect of endogenous opioids on breathing and their effect on the psychophysiologic response to pain. Endogenous opioids contribute to the mediation of the pain perception system.[32-34] Their influence on pain receptors is activated by prolonged noxious stimuli above a specific threshold. Similarly, beta-endorphins do not tonically mediate breathing, but they participate upon their acti-

receptors have been histochemically demonstrated in the carotid bodies, medulla, and vagi—structures that are intimately linked with the control of breathing. The effects of endogenous opioids on respiration are similar to the well-known effects of exogenously administered drugs. In general, endogenous opioids diminish both ventilation and the ventilatory response to hypoxia and hypercapnia. This depressant effect appears to be moderated by their action on the chemosensitive structures in the brain stem and carotid bodies. In addition, an action on the neuronal pools that are rostral to the medulla, which are involved in respiratory timing, has been postulated.[29]

Many of the experiments on endogenous opioids involve the use of placebo controls. However, the use of placebos in situations where the existence of endogenous opioids is postulated lacks its usual clarifying power. Stress—a potential agent of the testing experience for all patients—can generate the release of endorphins creating difficulty in interpreting the data. Although placebo controls are very useful in avoiding the misinterpretation of possible nonspecific postdrug responses, their use in conscious subjects is complicated

BORG SCALE AT HEWL FOLLOWING PLACEBO AND MORPHINE

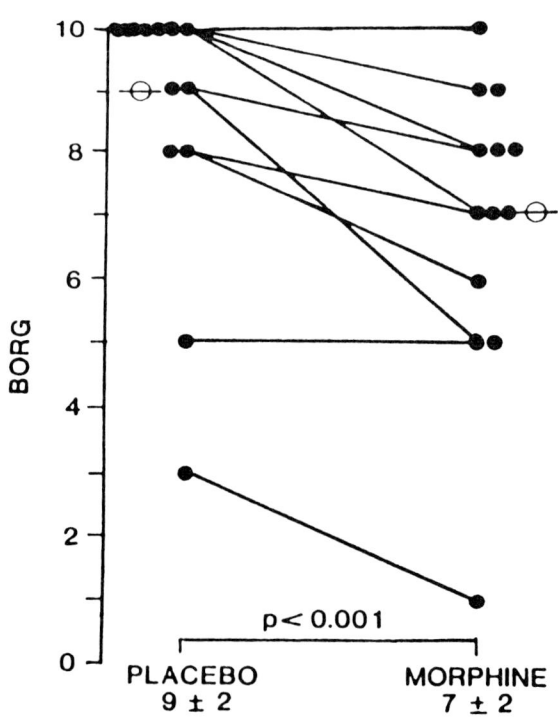

FIGURE 18–6. Borg scale scores recorded at the highest equivalent workload (HEWL) after placebo administration were significantly higher than those recorded after morphine administration. (From Light RW, Muro JR, Sato RI, et al. Effects of oral morphine on breathlessness and exercise tolerance in patients with chronic obstructive pulmonary disease. Am Rev Respir Dis 1989, 139:126–133.)

TABLE 18-2. MEAN BETA-ENDORPHIN LEVELS AT REST AND DURING EXERCISE IN COPD PATIENTS*

Patients	No. of Patients	Beta-Endorphin Levels (ng/L)	
		At Rest†	During Exercise
Pink puffers	6	877	775
Blue bloaters	6	437	607
Explosive athletes	6	254	459
Endurance athletes	6	299	1693

*Data from Woodcock AA, Johnson MA, Geddes DM. Catecholamines and endogenous opiates at rest and exercise in athletes and patients with chronic airflow obstruction (abstract). Am Rev Respir Dis 1983; 127:249.
†Normal values at rest < 200 ng/L.

vation by prolonged or intense noxious stimuli (e.g., increased airway resistance or dyspnea).

Use of naloxone, for example, increases the compensatory response to added inspiratory resistance in COPD patients,[35] suggesting that load compensation is inhibited by opioids. After Bellofiore and associates[36] demonstrated that pretreatment with naloxone increased the sensation of dyspnea during severe methylcholine-induced bronchoconstriction, they concluded that the level of endogenous opioids increases during severe bronchoconstriction to mitigate the stress of impaired ventilation. The stress from chronic dyspnea has also been postulated as a stimulus for endogenous opioid elaboration in COPD. This contention is based on the finding that the depressed ventilatory response to chemical (e.g., carbon dioxide sensitivity) and mechanical (e.g., added inspiratory resistance) loads that has been observed in some COPD patients could be restored by naloxone administration.[35]

In sum, these findings strongly suggest that COPD patients elaborate endogenous opioids, most likely in response to the stress that is caused by increasing constraints from the variety of mechanical, chemical, and neural consequences of the pathologic changes in COPD.

Opioid elaboration in patients with COPD may serve a doubly protective function. First, it reduces the stress of prolonged dyspnea. Second, by inhibiting ventilation it minimizes peripheral muscle fatigue (which is consistent with the observed attenuation of resistive load compensation in some COPD patients.[35] Therefore, endogenous opioid elaboration could be of symptomatic benefit to patients manifesting this adaptive response, especially in advanced COPD in which gas exchange is not expected to improve significantly during hyperventilation.

Although endogenous opioids are not typically measured in COPD patients, a preliminary study found elevated beta-endorphin levels in both pink puffers and blue bloaters (Table 18-2). Although no statistics of relationships between these two groups were published, the highest beta-endorphin levels were manifested by the pink puffers, that is, by those patients expected to be the most dyspneic. With exercise,[37] the blue bloaters' beta-endorphin levels increased further; no such change was observed in the pink puffers.

To the extent that blue bloaters resemble the postmorphine COPD patients described previously (i.e., they are hypoxemic, hypercapnic, and comparatively less dyspneic), they would be expected to have shown the highest beta-endorphin levels. The observation of higher levels in pink puffers (who were characterized by the maintenance of normal arterial blood gas parameters and by relatively more severe dyspnea than the blue bloaters) suggests that dyspnea is the direct stimulus for endorphin release, that these patients have an abnormal endorphin response, or both. The fact that beta-endorphin levels did not increase with exercise in pink puffers is consistent with impaired release.

Another possibility is that some patients are susceptible to a paradoxical response to beta-endorphins similar to that seen in pain adaptation.[38] Applying signal detection theory to integrate sensory-discriminatory factors and response factors, naloxone was used to assess change in sensitivity to radiant heat. Two response groups were identified: one pain-sensitive and the other pain-insensitive. Pain-insensitive individuals reacted to naloxone with an expected increase in pain sensitivity. Paradoxically, pain-sensitive individuals reacted with a decrease in pain sensitivity (Fig. 18-7). Naloxone's effect on the evoked potential response pattern also differed between the two groups. Naloxone markedly changed the evoked potential response pattern of the pain-insensitive group in the direction of sensitization. The trend in the pain-sensitive group was opposite, that is, toward desensitization. Bidirectionality effects may reflect individual differences in the functional activity of the pain modulating system.

To the extent that dyspnea and pain reflect similar psychophysiologic processes, the difference in endorphin levels may, by analogy, reflect differences in the functional dyspnea modulation systems of *dyspnea-sensitive* patients (pink puffers) and *dyspnea-insensitive* patients (blue bloaters). If this model is accurate, naloxone

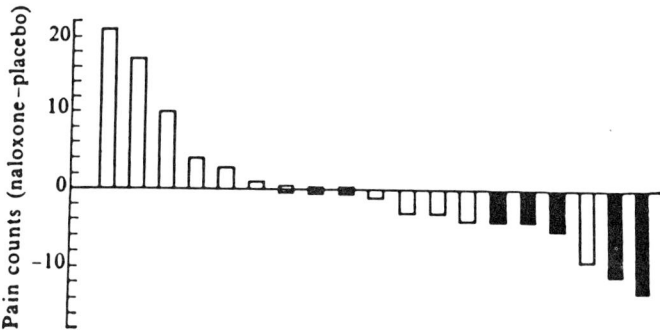

FIGURE 18-7. Pain counts (unpleasant plus very unpleasant subjective ratings) illustrated as the difference between naloxone days and placebo days for each individual studied. Positive differences indicate that more stimuli were rated as unpleasant or worse during naloxone administration. Subjects were categorized as pain-insensitive (open bars) or pain-sensitive (solid bars) on the basis of a sensitivity measure derived from signal detection analysis during a predrug trial session. Note that no pain-sensitive subjects became more sensitive during naloxone administration, whereas most pain-insensitive individuals did ($P<.05$). (From Buchsbaum MS, Davis GC, Bunney WE Jr. Naloxone alters pain perception and somatosensory evoked potentials in normal subjects. Nature 1977, 270:620–623.)

would be predicted to decrease dyspnea in the sensitive (pink puffer) group, whereas it would be expected to increase dyspnea in the insensitive (blue bloater) group. This hypothesis remains to be experimentally evaluated.

Altose and colleagues[39] demonstrated that hypercapnic patients were less chemosensitive than eucapnic patients. Mountain and coworkers[40] showed that this variation in ventilatory response to carbon dioxide may be in part genetically determined. Genetics may also determine whether a patient becomes hypercapnic. Similarly, studies of the parents of children who died of sudden infant death syndrome show that these parents appear to have a genetically transmitted variation in flow-resistive load compensation.[41] Thus, the difference between patients with and without dyspnea may reflect the existence of a genetically determined mechanism that controls beta-endorphin release.

In addition to directly attenuating dyspnea, increased levels of endogenous opioids may serve to indirectly reduce dyspnea by reducing contributing factors such as anxiety.[42] As we noted previously, increased levels of endogenous opioids could provide symptomatic benefit to those patients for whom hyperventilation is not expected to improve gas exchange.

Although it is unclear how endogenous opioids are modulated, regular exercise training has been shown to increase endorphin levels in healthy subjects. Moderately high-intensity exercise (>75% of maximum oxygen consumption) has been shown to stimulate the release of beta-endorphins.[43] The postulated mechanism is that physical training promotes adaptations within the opioid system, such as an altered peptide response to exercise or an increase in the number of receptors.[43] In support of the first possibility, training has been shown to facilitate the exercise-induced secretion of both beta-endorphins and beta-lipotropin.[44,45] More recent evidence[46] indicates that this facilitation is related to the degree of anaerobic rather than of aerobic training.[47]

Although it is clear that most asthmatic patients can exercise at a sufficiently high intensity to elicit a marked training effect[48,49] (Table 18–3) and thus presumably affect endogenous opioid function, most patients with severe COPD cannot achieve this intensity. This raises the question as to whether the maximum exercise level of these COPD patients is sufficient to stimulate modification in their endogenous opioid system. There are at least two reasons to expect that the level is sufficiently high.

First, since preliminary data on blue bloaters (see Table 18–2) suggest that COPD patients can perform a level of exercise sufficiently intense to stimulate beta-endorphin release,[37] this level of exercise presumably would perform the same function in a training context. Second, it has not been established that opioid modification requires the same training intensity as cardiovascular adaptation. To the extent that the opioid response is stress-related, we would expect blue bloaters to reach the necessary threshold at relatively low levels of exercise. Furthermore, Ekdahl and associates[50] have demonstrated modification of the opioid system in rheumatoid arthritis patients after 1 year of low-intensity exercise training.

PERIPHERAL DESENSITIZATION

Much experimental evidence exists to indicate that afferent input from peripheral mechanical and chemical receptors is important in the genesis of dyspnea (see Chapter 10). Thus, in theory, dyspnea desensitization could occur through a reduction in the amount of peripheral information reaching higher centers of the central nervous system (see Fig. 18–2B). Interestingly, many of the effects of endogenous opioids discussed earlier may be modulated at the level of peripheral receptors (e.g., in the carotid bodies).[29]

One possible peripheral source of information is inspiratory muscle function, which has been postulated to be intimately associated with dyspnea.[51] In addition, weak or fatigued inspiratory muscles (which decrease the force associated with a given neural drive) have been shown to increase dyspnea sensations.[52] Therefore, one way to achieve dyspnea desensitization may be by strengthening or relieving fatigue in these muscles prior to an increase in ventilatory demand. Theophylline not only has a bronchodilator effect but also increases muscle strength and decreases the potential for fatigue. Experimental results vary, however, with no consensus that these effects are of any clinical consequence.[53]

In contrast, data from studies of resistive inspiratory muscle training suggest that dyspnea ratings decrease after training.[54,55] For example, Harver and coworkers[55] quantified the effects of targeted inspiratory muscle training in 19 COPD patients using a commercially available resistive device twice daily for 15-minute sessions. After 8 weeks significant increases in muscle strength were observed. Although pulmonary function (including maximum voluntary ventilation) did not change, dyspnea scores were significantly reduced (Table 18–4). In contrast, Braun and Marino[56] described

TABLE 18–3. EFFECT OF TRAINING ON HEART RATE RESPONSE AND EXTERNAL WORK PERFORMANCE IN ASTHMATIC PATIENTS*

	Heart Rate (beats/min)	Peak Minute Ventilation (L/min)	Work (kcal)	Maximum O$_2$ Consumption (ml/kg/min)
Before training	165.0 ± 2.8	70.7 ± 6.6	4.85 ± 0.33	33.8 ± 2.25
After training	169.8 ± 2.7	73.3 ± 5.4	6.44 ± 0.39†	38.8 ± 3.02†

*From Haas F, Pasierski S, Axen K, et al. Effect of aerobic training on forced expiratory airflow in exercising people with asthma. J Appl Physiol 1987; 63:1230–1235.
†$P < .001$

TABLE 18-4. MEAN CLINICAL DYSPNEA RATINGS AND MAGNITUDE SCALING EXPONENTS FOR EXPERIMENTAL AND CONTROL GROUPS*

Variables	Experimental Group		Control Group	
	Baseline	At 8 Wk	Baseline	At 8 Wk
Baseline dyspnea index				
Functional impairment	1.8 + 1.0		1.8 ± 1.2	
Magnitude of task	1.9 ± 0.9		1.6 ± 0.5	
Magnitude of effort	1.7 ± 0.8		1.6 ± 0.5	
Focal score	5.4 ± 2.5		4.9 ± 2.1	
Transition dyspnea index				
Functional impairment		+1.3 ± 0.9†		+0.1 ± 0.3†
Magnitude of task		+0.8 ± 0.8†		+0.1 ± 0.3†
Magnitude of effort		+1.4 ± 1.1†		+0.1 ± 0.3†
Focal score		+3.5 ± 2.5†		+0.3 ± 1.0†
Magnitude scaling exponents				
Resistive loads	0.3 ± 0.2	0.4 ± 0.3	0.5 ± 0.4	0.6 ± 0.2
Line length	0.8 ± 0.1	0.8 ± 0.2	0.8 ± 0.2	0.8 ± 0.1

*From Harver A, Mahler DA, Daubenspeck JA: Targeted inspiratory muscle training improves respiratory muscle function and reduces dyspnea in patients with chronic obstructive pulmonary disease. Ann Intern Med 1989; 111:117–124. Values are mean ±SD.
†Subjects showed significantly greater improvement in each category of the Transition Dyspnea Index at week 8 ($P = .003$).

the benefits of daily intermittent respiratory muscle rest in severe COPD patients. Although these authors reported improved lung function and functional status, further study is needed to evaluate the effect of intermittent respiratory muscle rest on dyspnea before it can be used as a treatment modality.

Bilateral Carotid Body Resection

Bilateral carotid body resection, the most radical approach to modifying peripheral receptor information, has been recommended for the treatment of dyspnea by Winter.[57] The unilateral procedure was initially enthusiastically reported in the literature,[58] but controlled studies later showed it to be no more effective than sham surgery.[59]

Although bilateral carotid body resection has been reported to be effective, the deterioration in blood gas values that often follows this procedure leads one to question the safety of this operation. A study of three patients who underwent bilateral carotid body resection demonstrated a marked postsurgical decrease in PaO_2 from 57 to 45 mm Hg and a significant increase in $PaCO_2$ from 45 to 57 mm Hg.[58] All three patients died within three years of the procedure, but it is unclear to what extent it shortened their life span. A more positive report on 27 COPD patients who had undergone bilateral carotid body resection showed their 5-year mortality rate of 44% to be no different than that predicted for the entire COPD population.[60] Only a slight decrease in resting PaO_2 was observed in these patients; furthermore, no unacceptable side effects or signs of right-sided heart failure were seen. The incidence of nocturnal desaturation was the same in both treated and control COPD patients. All surviving patients continued to claim an improvement in dyspnea.

Despite the risk of significantly exacerbated pulmonary insufficiency, this procedure should not be abandoned entirely. Wasserman[61] has suggested that in certain individuals a tradeoff between relief from suffering and increased pulmonary insufficiency may be warranted. Because of the potential benefit of this tradeoff, a National Institutes of Health task force has recommended that a controlled study be done to assess both the efficacy and dangers of this operation.[62] However, no such study has yet been undertaken, and Medicare reimbursement for bilateral carotid body resection has been withdrawn.[63]

The three possible mechanisms that would explain why bilateral carotid body resection relieves dyspnea include (1) a reduction in ventilation caused by the removal of peripheral stimulation that would increase ventilatory drive, (2) a reduction in ventilation caused by the direct removal of sensory impulses to the brain, and (3) the psychologic effects of surgical placebo. In support of the first possibility, the procedure has repeatedly been shown to cause a decrease in ventilation.[64-67] A consequent reduction in reported dyspnea is consistent with the theory of Campbell and colleagues[51] and of Killian and coworkers,[68] which states that a reduction in total ventilation for a given workload results in less dyspnea. Vermeire and associates[64] have suggested that bilateral carotid body resection might reduce dyspnea directly by removing hypoxic sensory impulses to the brain. This would also explain the prolongation of breathholding that occurs after this procedure as well as that which can be temporarily produced in patients with intact carotid bodies who breathe 100% oxygen.[69] Finally, a psychologic effect cannot be ruled out. For example, one patient was able to lie flat without experiencing dyspnea for the first time in years following a sham carotid body resection procedure.[70]

CONCLUSION

Dyspnea is a complex psychophysiologic phenomenon. The quality of the sensation of breathlessness differs from person to person and from circumstance to circumstance. The expression of dyspnea is shaped not only by afferent receptor feedback (primarily in the respiratory muscles) but also by individual behavior, personality, and emotional state.

Although we have attempted to categorize potential approaches to dyspnea desensitization, it is important to realize that all these approaches are interrelated. Modification in one area of treatment eventually creates perturbation in others. Of the potential approaches discussed, physical exercise appears to be the most profitable intervention (see Fig. 18–2), in part because it affects both the psychologic and the physiologic aspects of dyspnea. It can be an antidote to depression, provide a sense of mastery, involve social interaction and distraction, and achieve an improvement in aerobic conditioning. This may lead to a reduction in ventilation at a given workload, an alteration in endogenous opioid production, and, as dyspnea diminishes, a reduction in anxiety. To the extent that each of these factors contributes to the sensation of dyspnea, their amelioration through exercise can reverse the dyspnea spiral (see Fig. 18–1).

REFERENCES

1. Fuhs MF. Correlates of dyspnea in individuals with chronic obstructive pulmonary disorders. Washington, D.C.: The Catholic University of America; 1980. Doctoral dissertation.
2. Suess WH, Alexander AB, Smith DD, et al. The effects of psychological stress on respiration: A preliminary study of anxiety and hyperventilation. Psychophysiology 1980; 17:535.
3. Agle DP, Baum GL. Psychological aspects of chronic obstructive pulmonary diseases. Med Clin North Am 1977; 61:749–758.
4. Gift AG, Plaut M, Jacox A. Psychologic and physiologic factors related to dyspnea in subjects with chronic obstructive pulmonary disease. Heart Lung 1986; 15:595–601.
5. Cockroft AE, Saunders MJ, Berry G. Randomized controlled trial of rehabilitation in chronic respiratory disability. Thorax 1981; 36:200–203.
6. Sinclair DJM, Ingram CG. Controlled trial of supervised exercise training in chronic bronchitis. BMJ 1980; 1:519–521.
7. Pineda H, Haas F, Axen K, Haas A. Ability of standard pulmonary function tests to predict exercise capability. Chest 1984; 86:564–567.
8. Rosser R, Guz A. Psychological approaches to breathlessness and its treatment. J Psychosom Res 1981; 25:439–447.
9. North TC, McCullagh P, Tran ZV. Effect of exercise on depression. Exerc Sport Sci Rev 1990; 18:379–415.
10. Bandura A. Self-efficacy: Towards a unifying theory of behavioral change. Psychol Rev 1977; 2:191–215.
11. Beck AT. The Diagnosis and Management of Depression. Philadelphia: University of Pennsylvania Press, 1973.
12. Agle DP, Baum GL, Chester EH, et al. Multidisciplinary treatment of chronic pulmonary insufficiency: Functional status at one year follow-up. In: Johnston RF (ed). Pulmonary Medicine: A Hahnemann Symposium. New York: Grune & Stratton, Inc., 1973, p 355.
13. McGavin CR, Gupta SP, Lloyd EL, McHardy GJR. Physical rehabilitation for the chronic bronchitic: Results of a controlled trial of exercises in the home. Thorax 1977; 32:307–311.
14. Rejeski WJ. Perceived exertion: An active or passive process? J Sport Psychol 1985; 1:371–378.
15. Levanthal H, Everhart D. Emotion, pain, and physical illness. In: Izard CE (ed). Emotions in Personality and Psychopathology. New York: Plenum Publishing Corp. 1979, pp 263–298.
16. Corah NL, Gale EN, Pacc LF, Seyrek SK. Relaxation and musical programming as means of reducing psychological stress during dental procedures. J Am Dent Assoc 1981; 103:232–234.
17. Lavine R, Buchsbaum MS, Poncy M. Auditory analgesia: Somatosensory evoked response and subjective pain. Psychophysiology 1976; 13:140–148.
18. Pennebaker JW, Lightner JM. Competition of internal and external information in an exercise setting. J Pers Soc Psychol 1980; 39:165–174.
19. Boutcher SH, Trenske M. The effect of sensory deprivation and music on perceived exertion and affect during exercise. J Sport Exerc Psychol 1990; 12:167–176.
20. A Report to the Research Committee of the British Tuberculosis Association: Hypnosis for asthma: A controlled trial. BMJ 1968; 4:71–76.
21. Aronoff GM, Aronoff S, Peck LW. Hypnotherapy in the treatment of bronchial asthma. Ann Allergy 1975; 34:356–361.
22. Ben-Zvi Z, Spohn WA, Young SH, Kattan M. Hypnosis for exercise-induced asthma. Am Rev Respir Dis 1982; 125:392–395.
23. Sato P, Sargur M, Schoene RB. Hypnosis effect on carbon dioxide chemosensitivity. Chest 1988; 89:828–831.
24. Mitchel-Heggs P, Murphy K, Minty K, et al. Diazepam in the treatment of dyspnoea in the "pink puffer" syndrome. Q J Med 1980; 49:9–20.
25. Woodcock AA, Gross ER, Gellert A, et al. Effects of dihydrocodeine, alcohol, and caffeine on breathlessness and exercise tolerance in patients wtih chronic obstructive lung disease and normal blood gases. N Engl J Med 1981; 305:1611–1616.
26. Woodcock AA, Gross ER, Gellert A, et al. Breathlessness, alcohol and opiates. N Engl J Med 1982; 306:1363–1364.
27. Light RW, Muro JR, Sato RI, et al. Effects of oral morphine on breathlessness and exercise tolerance in patients with chronic obstructive pulmonary disease. Am Rev Respir Dis 1989; 139:126–133.
28. Young IH, Daviskas E, Kenna VA. Effect of low dose nebulized morphine on exercise endurance in patients with chronic lung disease. Thorax 1989; 44:387–390.
29. Santiago TV, Edelman NH. Opioids and breathing. J Appl Physiol 1985; 59:1675–1685.
30. Clement-Jones V, Besser GM. Clinical perspectives in opioids and peptides. Br Med Bull 1983; 39:95–100.
31. Tabona MVZ, Ambrosino N, Barnes PJ. Endogenous opiates and the control of breathing in normal subjects and patients with chronic airflow obstruction. Thorax 1982; 38:834–839.
32. Fields HL. Neurophysiology of pain and pain modulation. Am J Med 1984; 77:2–8.
33. Lewis JW, Cannon JT, Liebeskind JC. Opioid and non-opioid mechanisms of stress analgesia. Science 1980; 208:623–625.
34. Watkins LR, Mayer DJ. Organization of endogenous opiate and non-opiate pain control systems. Science 1982; 216:1185–1192.
35. Santiago TV, Remolina C, Scoles V III, Edelman NH. β-endorphins and the control of breathing: Ability of naloxone to restore flow-resistive load compensation in chronic obstructive pulmonary disease. N Engl J Med 1981; 304:1190–1195.
36. Bellofiore S, DiMaria GU, Privitera S, et al. Endogenous opioids modulate the increase in ventilatory output and dyspnea during severe acute bronchoconstriction. Am Rev Respir Dis 1990; 142:812–816.
37. Woodcock AA, Johnson MA, Geddes DM. Catecholamines and endogenous opiates at rest and exercise in athletes and patients with chronic airflow obstruction (abstract). Am Rev Respir Dis 1983; 137: 249.
38. Buchsbaum MS, Davis GC, Bunney WE Jr. Naloxone alters pain perception and somatosensory evoked potentials in normal subjects. Nature 1977; 270:620–623.
39. Altose MD, McCauley WC, Kelsen SG, Cherniack NS. Effects of hypercapnia and inspiratory flow-resistive loading on respiratory activity in chronic airway obstruction. J Clin Invest 1977; 59:500–507.
40. Mountain R, Zwillich C, Weil J. Hypoventilation in obstructive lung disease: The role of familial factors. N Engl J Med 1978; 298:521–525.
41. Schiffman PL, Westlake RE, Santiago TV, Edelman NH. Ventilatory control in parents of victims of sudden-infant-death syndrome. N Engl J Med 1980; 302:486–491.
42. Ransford CP. A role for amines in antidepressant effect of exercise: A review. Med Sci Sports Exerc 1982; 14:1–10.

43. Sforzo GA. Opioids and exercise: An update. Sports Med 1989; 7:109–124.
44. Carr DB, Bullen BA, Skrinar GS, et al. Physical conditioning facilitates the exercise-induced secretion of beta-endorphin and beta-lipotropin in women. N Eng J Med 1981; 305:560–563.
45. Howlett TA, Tomlin S, Hgahfoong, et al. Release of β-endorphins and met-enkephalin during exercise in normal women: Response to training. BMJ 1984; 288:1950–1952.
46. Kraemer WJ, Fleck SJ, Callister R, et al. Training responses of plasma beta-endorphin, adrenocorticotropin, and cortisol. Med Sci Sports Exerc 1989; 21:146–153.
47. Farrell PA, Garthwaite TL, Gustafson AB. Plasma adrenocorticotropin and cortisol responses to submaximal and exhaustive exercise. J Appl Physiol 1983; 55:1441–1444.
48. Haas F, Pasierski S, Axen K, et al. Effect of aerobic training on forced expiratory airflow in exercising people with asthma. J Appl Physiol 1987; 63:1230–1235.
49. Haas F, Pineda H, Axen K, et al. Effects of physical fitness on expiratory airflow in exercising asthmatic people. Med Sci Sports Exerc 1985; 17:585–592.
50. Ekdahl C, Ekman R, Andersson SI, et al. Dynamic training and circulating levels of corticotropin-releasing factor, beta-lipotropin and beta-endorphin in rheumatoid arthritis. Pain 1990; 40:35–42.
51. Killian KJ, Gandevia SC, Summers E, Campbell EJM. Effect of increased lung volume on perception of breathlessness, effort and tension. J Appl Physiol 1984; 57:686–691.
52. Mahler DA. Dyspnea: Diagnosis and management. Clin Chest Med 1987; 8:215–230.
53. Sweer L, Zwillich CW. Dyspnea in the patient with chronic obstructive pulmonary disease: Etiology and management. Clin Chest Med 1990; 11:417–443.
54. Falk P, Eriksen A-M, Kolliker K, Andersen JB. Relieving dyspnea with an inexpensive and simple method in patients with chronic airflow limitations. Eur J Respir Dis 1985; 66:181–186.
55. Harver A, Mahler DA, Daubenspeck JA. Targeted inspiratory muscle training improves respiratory muscle function and reduces dyspnea in patients with chronic obstructive pulmonary disease. Ann Intern Med 1989; 111:117–124.
56. Braun NMT, Marino WD. Effect of daily intermittent rest of respiratory muscles in patients with severe chronic airflow limitation. Chest 1984; 85:59S–60S.
57. Winter B. Bilateral carotid body resection for asthma and emphysema: A new surgical approach without hypoventilation or baroreceptor dysfunction. Int Surg 1972; 57:458–466.
58. Stulbarg MS, Winn WR. Bilateral carotid body resection for the relief of dyspnea in severe chronic obstructive pulmonary disease. Chest 1989; 95:1123–1128.
59. Curran WS, Graham WGB. Long term effects of glomectomy: Follow-up of a double blind study. Am Rev Respir Dis 1971; 103:566–568.
60. Vermeire P, de Backer W, van Maele R, et al. Bilateral carotid body resection for severe chronic airway obstruction: A 6 year follow-up (abstract). Am Rev Respir Dis 1988; 137:443.
61. Wasserman K. The carotid bodies: Pathologic or physiologic? Chest 1978; 73:564–566.
62. Report of Task Force on Bilateral Carotid Body Resection. Federal Register 1980; 45:71427–71431.
63. Health Care Financing Administration. Exclusion from Medicare coverage of bilateral carotid body resection to relieve pulmonary distress. Federal Register 1980; 210:71426–71432.
64. Vermeire P, de Backer W, van Maele R, et al. Carotid body resection in patients with severe chronic airflow limitation. Clin Respir Physiol 1987; 23:165S–166S.
65. Whipp BJ. Physiological consequences of bilateral carotid body resection in man: A frame of reference. Respir Ther 1975; 5:29–31.
66. Whipp BJ, Wasserman K. Carotid bodies and ventilatory control dynamics in man. Fed Proc 1980; 39:2663–2673.
67. Honda Y, Myojo S, Hasegawa T, Severinghaus JW. Decreased exercise hypercapnia in patients with bilateral carotid chemoreceptor resection. J Appl Physiol 1979; 46:908–912.
68. Killian KJ, Campbell EJM. Dyspnea and exercise. Ann Rev Physiol 1983; 45:465–479.
69. Davidson JT, Whipp BJ, Wasserman K, et al. Role of the carotid bodies in breath holding. N Engl J Med 1974; 290:819–822.
70. Marschke G, Bealle GN, Stern WE, Murray JF. Carotid-body removal in asthma. JAMA 1965; 191:125.

Chapter 19

Psychobiologic Evaluation and Rehabilitation in Pulmonary Disease*

DONALD L. DUDLEY, M.D.
JUDITH SITZMAN, Ph.D.

The treatment of psychobiologic aspects of chronic obstructive pulmonary disease (COPD) is best considered in the light of factors that influence the development of disease and the continuation of disability and insufficiency. Disability is the decrease in the patient's productivity and comfort, and insufficiency is the loss of organ function. We find it instructive to differentiate acute and chronic disease in discussions of COPD and its treatment.

ACUTE TREATMENT MODEL

The acute treatment model takes into consideration the self-limiting aspects of many disease processes. The patient is ill for a period of days, weeks, or, at the most, months, and then returns to an acceptable level of physiologic and psychologic functioning. The physician is congratulated on the "cure," and the patient has an increasing respect for the physician.

Acute treatment is best accomplished in an efficient, competent manner that is reassuring and supportive and that decreases the dramatic, excited nature of an emergency. A relaxed, unhurried approach to the patient conveys a sense of concern and facilitates interaction. The importance of the patient should be emphasized, and the importance of medical equipment should be deemphasized. Highly verbal patients can tolerate longer interviews, whereas very anxious or physically weak, debilitated patients require brief interactions.

Reassurance and support in the form of information regarding the condition should be given to the patient early in the course of treatment and should be shared with important family members. If the patient has a stable pulmonary embolus, a statement such as "You have a blockage of a small vessel in your lung that is clearing and will now heal like a broken arm or leg" is important. It is helpful to provide the patient with an easily understood reference from everyday life. Patients hospitalized for diagnostic tests should be informed by the physician of the purpose and nature of each test, when it will be scheduled, where it will take place, and generally what he or she may experience during and after the procedure. For example, patients who are to undergo routine pulmonary function testing often feel more comfortable knowing they will not experience pain and will simply be breathing in and out through a mouthpiece. It may be important to have a close family member with the patient during the acute phases of treatment.

---

*Adapted from Dudley, DL, Sitzman, J. Psychobiological Evaluation and Treatment of COPD. In: McSweeny, AJ, Grant, I (eds.). Pulmonary Disease: A Behavioral Perspective. New York: Marcel Dekker, Inc., pp 183–236, by courtesy of Marcel Dekker, Inc.

The patient, family, and staff should be assured that the patient will receive all the help that can be provided. However, it is important to decrease dependency early in treatment. What is desirable during an emergency (passive cooperation) becomes undesirable during the rehabilitation phase. The patient and family should have the feeling that they need to help the staff. This will help the patient to avoid passivity, depression, and fright when faced with the need for emotional and physical activity as he or she returns to productive life.

In selected patients, once the emergency is over, angina pectoris, hypertension, dyspnea, or congestive heart failure may respond only to treatment of psychiatric problems using appropriate psychoactive medications. Above all, it is important to treat in a setting that is nonaversive to the patient. Treatment instructions should not be coupled with threats of the dire consequences of noncompliance. They should be coupled with an explanation of the positive consequences. This avoids making treatment directly related to negative feelings or fright and thus increases the probability of compliance.

CHRONIC TREATMENT MODEL

The chronic treatment model takes into consideration the long-term effects of continued organ insufficiency and bodily disability. The patient is continuously ill and may never return to an acceptable level of physiologic and psychiatric functioning. The physician is confronted with a patient and family members who have learned that modern medicine will not cure the patient's condition. They may be disillusioned, angry, depressed, or frightened. They need to be congratulated on their ability to deal with the problem and assured that professional help will be available to them regardless of how bad things get. The physician often finds that the patient and family feel cheated by life and that they are not capable of expressing appreciation, regardless of the physician's interest and dedication. This is obviously a difficult social situation in which to practice medicine.

It is useful to arrange the treatment plan around positive attainable rewards and goals. The reward may be added attention by the physician, increased attention by the family, material objects, and so on. The goal may be, for example, increased independence or increased exercise tolerance. With this approach, the emphasis is not on eliminating the disease but on gradually increasing understanding and the ability to deal with the disease and the surrounding environment. To accomplish this task, it may be necessary to use the usual clinical treatment method in combination with education, group psychotherapy, psychoactive medications, or any other useful method of increasing the patient's and his or her significant others' ability to cope with life.

DISCUSSION

In the acute disease situation, the patient and physician are seen as rewarding each other. In the chronic disease situation, both physician and patient are faced with their own relative impotence. The patient is often seen as weak or as lacking drive and spirit, or both; the physician may be seen as lacking clinical competence. Since the patient never gets well, there is often little reason for the patient and family to reward the physician with the positive feedback needed for him or her to be able to deal with chronic disease. For many physicians, this is sufficient reason not to deal with such patients. In addition, friends may encourage the patient to "See my doctor—his patients get well," and thereby actually undermine treatment. Patients with chronic respiratory disease often try a number of physicians before realizing that no one is going to cure them and that they must learn to live with the disorder and with the doctors.

PSYCHOSOCIAL AND PSYCHOPHYSIOLOGIC ISSUES IN CHRONIC OBSTRUCTIVE PULMONARY DISEASE: ENVIRONMENT AND THE PATIENT[1]

The interaction between environment and disease can be illustrated in a number of ways:[2, 3]

1. The lag between reactions of different organ systems[4-6]
2. The overload on an impaired organ system[4, 7, 8]
3. The accumulation of disruptive life changes[9, 10]
4. The use of psychosocial assets[11, 12]
5. The social indicators of disease[3]

Lag Between Organ Systems

The lag between the responses of the skeletal muscle system and those of the pulmonary system is responsible for both the hyperventilation and hypoventilation syndromes. The central nervous system, when activated or inactivated from a steady state, increases and decreases alveolar ventilation or the activity of the skeletal muscles in preparation for action or for inaction, respectively. Normally, the pulmonary system, when activated or inactivated from a steady state, increases or decreases the supply of air faster than the skeletal muscles increase or reduce oxygen consumption and carbon dioxide output, respectively. When the lag is abnormally long and severe, acute hyperventilation and hypoventilation syndromes occur. These syndromes occur when the lag between the response of the skeletal muscle system and that of the respiratory system is more severe than usual; as a result, patients experience symptoms. It is important to recognize that both hyperventilation and hypoventilation syndromes are commonly seen in emergency rooms. The symptoms of these two syndromes can be very similar in some patients, and, unfortunately, acute hypoventilation is rarely recognized.

Overload of an Impaired Organ System

With this problem, the importance of psychosocial factors is not in the triggering of the disease but in increasing or producing disability and insufficiency once the disease has developed. The normal lag between the reactions of the skeletal muscle and pulmonary systems is gone. A patient with emphysema and a maximum alveolar ventilation of 10 L/min cannot afford to participate in overly active situations, whether they be exercise, anger, anxiety, euphoria, or general excitement. The muscular system is not impaired in such a patient. It can consume normal amounts of oxygen and produce normal amounts of carbon dioxide. The more active the patient becomes and the greater the work of breathing, the more tense the skeletal muscles become. The more oxygen is used and the more carbon dioxide is produced, the less effective the pulmonary system is at coping. The 10-L maximum alveolar ventilation is soon reached, and the patient becomes increasingly hypoxic and dyspneic, or hypoxic, hypercarbic, and dyspneic, depending on the amount of pulmonary insufficiency present. If the dyspnea frightens the patient, a vicious circle may be produced that is characterized by dyspnea, which leads to fright, which in turn leads to increasing activation and physiologic insufficiency. This further leads to increasing dyspnea that may be very difficult to stop. By the same process, a patient with a maximum cardiac output of 7 L/min can be disabled. Depression can lead to similar problems, since it is often associated with a drop in ventilation below the level that is necessary to supply oxygen and remove carbon dioxide.

Patients usually learn by trial and error to avoid experiencing emotions, to isolate themselves from psychosocial stimuli, and to deny and suppress emotions to reduce their physiologic impact. The physician must be careful to avoid inducing sudden emotional changes, since they can lead to increasing disability and insufficiency in the patient with pulmonary disease.

Accumulation of Life Change

It is generally agreed that causative factors in the development of a given disease are multifactorial and involve a complex interplay between humans as psychobiologic units and the environment. There is little controversy regarding the importance of physical factors in the development of disease. The importance of the concept that psychosocial variables play a similar role has generally not been well accepted despite emphasis on multiple causative factors.

Part of the problem in dealing with psychosocial variables has been related to the inability to quantify them in a way that would allow different investigators to directly compare results, much as they do for white blood cell count, measurement of blood urea nitrogen, serum iron determination, and so on. The meaning and impact of psychosocial factors were thought to be too variable among individuals to be quantified. Recent studies have indicated that although the reactions to psychosocial stimuli may differ from person to person, the perceptions of the amount of impact that the stimulus carries are remarkably similar. This has allowed the development of techniques for quantifying psychosocial phenomena.

The Schedule of Recent Experience was developed to provide a "yardstick" for quantifying life change. It uses *life change units* as the basic measurement of life change. The 42 life changes contained in the Schedule include those judged to be socially acceptable or good, such as job promotion, marriage, and outstanding personal achievement. These items were included because they generally occur before disease onset in the same context as do socially undesirable items, such as divorce, the death of a close friend, and being fired from work. Change, rather than desirability or undesirability, was the characteristic of life events that contributed to their association with psychologic adjustment and, hence, disease. Using the same techniques that allowed the quantification of psychosocial events in life change units, disease has been measured in *seriousness of illness units*.[13, 14] In all, 126 diseases were quantified. These ranged from dandruff (number 1) with a value of 21 to leukemia (number 126) with a value of 1080. Using this system, the diseases commonly encountered by the clinical pulmonary specialist spanned the entire spectrum of possible diseases.

The quantification of disease in this manner can be used by the clinician in two ways. First, it provides some appreciation of people's perception of the seriousness of a given disease and thus of the amount of time, effort, and dedication the patient expects to be given. An asthmatic patient, for example, may give asthma a value of 1000, whereas his or her family may give it a value of 413. It may be difficult to treat such a patient until there is agreement among family members regarding the seriousness of the disease and the amount of their lives it should justifiably control. Second, there is a relationship between life change (as measured in life change units) and the seriousness of the disease. Specifically, there is a positive relationship between life change units and seriousness of illness units. Thus, people who have 1000 life change units are more likely to develop a disease such as heart failure or a blood clot in the lung, and those with 100 life change units are more likely to develop the common cold or hay fever. Not only is the probability of getting sick increased with life change, but the probability of getting a serious disease or of dying is also increased.

Use of Psychosocial Assets

With the advent of the Schedule of Recent Experience for the quantification of psychosocial input, measurements of the ability to deal with this input became essential. In this regard, a person's overall ability to deal with the environment can be called his or her "psychosocial assets." There are three categories of psychosocial assets:

I. Social Support
   1. Being in a setting in which the patient receives love.

2. Being in a setting in which the patient is esteemed.
   3. Being in a mutually defensive system (e.g., if the patient is attacked, those around him or her will come to his or her aid).
II. Coping Ability
   1. The patient's ability to change environments to meet needs.
III. Adaptive Ability
   1. The patient's ability to adapt to existing environments.

A patient who rates strongly in all of the categories is considered to have good psychosocial assets. Currently, the only test that takes all of the above factors into consideration is the Berle Index. In general, patients who score above the 80th percentile on this test get well, control their disease without a great deal of difficulty, and seldom get sick. Patients who score below the 60th percentile tend to do poorly. It is usually not possible to predict health status if the score is between the 61st and 79th percentiles.

The essential explanation for why life change induces illness is that life change requires one to adapt to or cope with a stressful life event. The adaptation requires use of the body and its organ systems. A few individuals display a nearly fathomless ability to muster coping behaviors and coping mechanisms to deal with life changes. These people probably never get sick. A few people rely only on one or two coping behaviors and are sick all the time. Most of us fall somewhere in between these two extremes in the number of coping behaviors we utilize.

Coping behaviors include emotional responses (e.g., anger, sorrow, and elation), personal habits (e.g., eating, smoking, physical activity, and sex), and unconscious habits (e.g., nail biting, sighing, and finger drumming). Devoting attention to one's job and hobbies is a coping behavior, as is spending time with one's family.

Initial interviews with patients should involve a comprehensive psychologic screening. Quantitative measurements may include the Schedule of Recent Experience, the Berle Index, and a self-rating scale for depression. Interviews should cover the patient's perception of his or her illness and how it has affected relationships with significant others and occupational and recreational activities. How a patient adjusts to an illness depends on his or her inner resources and outside support systems, as well as on the existence of adequate finances and housing. Since significant relationships may be affected by the patient's illness, it is important to interview spouses or people that the patient identifies as close to him or her. Understanding the nature of these relationships and the perceptions and reactions of significant others to the patient's illness guides staff in defining problem areas and in setting realistic treatment goals.

Social Indicators of Disease

Laymen and physicians alike tend to confuse the symptoms of disease with the disease itself. However, symptoms and disease are not the same. A patient can be terribly sick and have no outward manifestations of disease. The explanation for this paradox is that culturally we interpret being sick or ill as experiencing a loss of comfort, productivity, or both. A patient may have hypertension, a disease that is not characterized by loss of comfort or productivity. During a smog alert, another person may wheeze, feel miserably ill, uncomfortable, and unproductive while having no disease. The schizophrenic patient may be very comfortable but is wholly unproductive. In order to live with disease and sickness, it is essential to understand that the disease and being sick are not the same thing. On the other hand, this complicates the interaction of the disease with our culture, since people with recognizable disease entities who do not fit the cultural definition of illness may be seen as malingerers and be treated with hostility. This is true for many chronic diseases.

Another cultural problem is related to the laboratory diagnosis of diseases. It is easy for a patient to understand that he or she is ill if there is severe leg pain and if the leg is bent at an unusual angle; it is obviously broken. However, this may be difficult for a patient to understand if he or she feels well, comfortable, and productive but has an electrocardiogram that indicates heart disease, has a chest x-ray that indicates pulmonary carcinoma, or undergoes pulmonary function testing that indicates COPD. Subsequently, the patient is told that he or she has a devastating disease. The patient must take the physician's word for this and submit to treatment that may be well beyond his or her understanding. In these circumstances, patients who feel "well" are subjected to medical and surgical procedures that may radically change their lives. Few patients adjust easily to this. They need to "feel sick" if something is physically wrong, and in this kind of setting, many people begin to act sick simply to communicate the severity of their disease. The development of a carcinoma is a frightening and life-threatening event, but others will not understand this unless the patient acts sick. Without this cultural expression of illness, the carcinoma patient must face a potentially devastating situation alone. Few of us in such situations choose to do this.

Another clinical situation can be equally distressing. The patient may find himself or herself with a symptom but no sign of disease; for example, he or she may have early COPD with dyspnea but no "significant" reduction in pulmonary function variables. Examination after examination is performed without positive findings. There is simply "no reason" for the dyspnea. What can the patient do? Should he or she endure the dyspnea while awaiting the occurrence of some sign that will make the symptoms socially significant? Should such a sign occur, the patient can be considered "appropriately ill." If it does not, the patient may find that people do not believe that he or she experiences dyspnea; alternatively, people might suggest that the dyspnea is "all in the head." In this situation, it is helpful to remember that all symptoms are "in the head."

Unfortunately, dyspnea without an appropriate sign may lead the patient to alienate himself or herself from the physician or to increasingly rely on less traditional or even phony treatment. When this occurs, it is essential that the physician be understanding and tolerant. The patient may need to try different and even unorthodox treatments and needs a physician who will stand by him or her and provide care for any serious trouble that results from the dyspnea or the treatments. Situations in which incurable symptoms are encountered should be met maturely, and the limitations of treatment of these symptoms should be spelled out. The physician and patient can then relate comfortably to each other and arrange the best possible clinical management.

Pain and Dyspnea Compared

Pain is a symptom that all agree is closely associated with the need for medical attention. Pain is always analyzed as uncomfortable and dangerous. Still, no matter how articulate the patient or sophisticated the diagnostician, the only test of pain's severity is the patient's report. Avoidance of pain has played a profound role in our evolution. Since prehistoric times, we have searched for ways to deal with pain and pain-producing situations. The belief that pain is a danger signal is so instilled in us that its presence in even small and innocent amounts triggers massive physiologic reactions throughout our nervous system. Despite the massive problem of chronic pain, physicians and patients feel comfortable dealing with pain. Pain is a traditional symptom; its pathways are known and treatment modalities for it have been described.

Dyspnea, like pain, is a common symptom. Unlike pain, it is not a generalized danger signal. It specifically alerts the physician to the cardiopulmonary system, and as a symptom it is localized to that system. Like pain, its identification is based on the subjective judgment of the patient and is generally not definable in terms of blood gas or ventilatory abnormalities.

Patients vary in their descriptions of dyspnea, but the general complaint is of uncomfortable sensations arising in the chest or airways that are interpreted as interfering with normal breathing. The patient feels smothered and breathless and as if not enough air is available. Some patients experience severe dyspnea with little or no structural change in the cardiopulmonary system, whereas others experience mild or no dyspnea with severe structural change. Dyspnea is sometimes experienced by normal, healthy people during strenuous exercise and periods of emotion.

When people prone to dyspnea attacks are studied in detail, dyspnea is found to be associated with both activating and nonactivating emotions. With nonactivating emotions, such as depression, dyspnea is associated with decreased ventilation or hypoventilation. With action-oriented emotions, such as anger or anxiety, dyspnea occurs in association with hyperpnea or hyperventilation. Thus, emotionally triggered dyspnea is associated with both increased and decreased ventilation.

Since healthy people and cardiopulmonary patients both experience dyspnea and since either a relative increase or decrease in ventilation may act as a trigger of dyspnea, it can be a confusing symptom. The best explanation for this is that dyspnea can be learned. It can depend on past conditioning experiences. Events such as breathholding or excessive crying during childhood, congestive heart failure, allergic reactions, and bronchial infections apparently lead to physiologic reactions that are associated with emotion and in which dyspnea occurs. In other words, people who suffer dyspnea attacks may be sensitized or conditioned to respond with dyspnea to emotionally induced changes in their cardiopulmonary system. They experience a kind of psychobiologic drowning or respiratory short circuit. Other people are unaware of these changes and do not suffer the dyspnea symptoms. Also, as with so many other illness symptoms, emotional reactions to dyspnea attacks often trigger more and worse dyspnea attacks because of the same conditioning.

Since dyspnea is associated with danger in only two organ systems, unlike pain, it is not recognized as a general danger signal. Hence, a patient with dyspnea is more likely to be called a malingerer. People tend not to understand the reason for the patient's inability to work or play; this produces difficult social relations unless the patient's dyspnea becomes severe enough to be interpreted by others as being painful.

In summary, there are three important differences between dyspnea and pain: (1) dyspnea is not a generalized danger signal; (2) there are no specific nerve pathways that have been reliably demonstrated to produce dyspnea (i.e., dyspnea must be learned, or there must be cardiac or pulmonary disease present to initiate it); and (3) dyspnea is closely associated with physical and emotional activity.

The patient with dyspnea should remain physically active unless there is a medical problem that prohibits activity. As patients with dyspnea exercise to tolerance, they learn that the dyspnea is not life-threatening. The more they exercise, the more control is learned, and the less threatening the symptom becomes. Thus, the patient is "deconditioned" or "desensitized."

There are many other symptoms that patients with pulmonary disease may exhibit, such as fatigue, anxiety, and depression. It is important that each symptom be understood by the patient in terms of its effect on emotion and behavior and that the patient learn to quantify the symptoms and the degree of "cultural impairment." For any given symptom, 100 can stand for the most the patient has ever experienced and 0 for the absence of the symptom. The patient can then report a definite number as representing the current symptom level. In addition, the patient can specify the amount of the symptom that is tolerable; making such a judgment can be one of the goals of treatment. Such psychophysical judgments regarding subjective phenomena are clinically accurate.

Psychophysical Assessment

Psychophysical assessments provide an indication of how sick the patient thinks he or she is. They are important in quantifying this for the physician. Most patients who use this method find that they are not as sick as they thought they were and are reassured. In addition, this method gives the physician an indication of what the patient's treatment goals are. If goals have been reached, there may be no reason to pursue aggressive treatment, since the physician may be met with passive resistance. On the other hand, a patient may insist on a 100% return of normal function, although the physician knows that only a 50% return is possible, even with very aggressive treatment. Such a patient may need assistance in readjusting his or her goals downward, whereas another patient whose goals are too unambitious may need to adjust his or her goals upward.

Nonverbal Communication.[3] It is always constructive to understand what a situation means to the patient. Understanding can lessen tension for both the patient and the physician. The physician can ease potentially stressful circumstances by understanding what is being communicated by the patient. Since as much as 50% of what is communicated in any person-to-person transaction is nonverbal, some knowledge of this nonverbal behavior is essential if the physician is to deal with patients in a systematic and reasonable manner.

All of us recognize certain nonverbal cues. When meeting people, we automatically notice their facial expressions, their body posture, and whether their speech is rapid or slow. We notice if they are tense or relaxed. Few of us, however, do this in a systematic manner or use the information to benefit the interpersonal transaction.

The Telltale Handshake. When first meeting a patient, the physician should notice how far away the patient stands and the temperature of the patient's hand when he or she shakes it. Hand temperature and body distance are important indicators of emotional depression in our culture.

Hand temperature tends to be cool or cold during three emotional states: anger, anxiety, and depression. Hand temperature increases to warm or hot during periods of resentment and during periods of comfort and contentment. By shaking the patient's hand, the clinician can obtain a general idea of the patient's emotional state.

In some situations, it is appropriate to have cold hands (e.g., before a traumatic procedure). If the patient's hands are warm and his or her face is flushed, the physician might consider the presence of resentment and the possibility of legal and interpersonal difficulties with the patient should anything go wrong. On the other hand, cold hands could mean that the patient is angry rather than anxious about the procedure; this could also lead to problems.

Facial Expression and Physical Appearance.[15] Nonverbal communication is an inseparable part of the communication process. Under some circumstances, it may contradict, modify, or elaborate verbal messages. Frequently, it regulates the flow of communication between people. For example, a head nod, eye movement, or shift in position may signal someone to speak or to stop speaking.

Since we are concerned about how people react to their illness, it is important to understand the patient's emotional state. Facial expressions often reflect one or several emotions. Rapidly changing facial expressions may reflect repressed affective states. These states may be fleeting and go unnoticed during an interview. Facial expressions may also conflict with verbal messages. A typical example is that of a patient who smiles when telling someone that he or she is upset. His or her words say, "I'm angry." However, his or her smile says, "Not really," or "I'm not serious." The smile may serve to reduce the tension or anxiety experienced when anger is expressed. When nonverbal and verbal messages are incongruent, therapeutic communication between staff and patient is disrupted. Whenever possible, it is important during interviews to acknowledge and clarify incongruent messages.

What we think of ourselves—that is, our self-image—may also be communicated through our physical appearance. Clothes may convey such personal attributes as sex, age, nationality, socioeconomic status, identification with a specific group, occupation, mood, interests, and values. For example, depressed people often perceive themselves as unattractive, and thus their dress may reflect this attitude.

Body Space.[3] The distance at which someone stands while talking with others is another index of emotional condition. In American society, we normally hold people at a "handshake's" distance away, that is, at the distance needed to reach out and shake someone's hand. Most people feel uncomfortable when anyone either gets closer than handshake distance or farther away than it during normal conversation. Thus, the handshake distance (about 3 ft) is the optimal distance for good communication. If the physician knows a patient is feeling depressed or dependent, however, moving in (while standing or sitting) and touching the patient at a distance of 1 or 2 ft is best, because a depressed or dependent person is acutely aware of a space immediately around his or her body but does not pay much attention to things that occur beyond that distance (i.e., he or she has reduced body space). However, if the practitioner notices that someone is shy, uncomfortable, hostile, or suspicious, it will be easier to communicate while standing or sitting 4 to 6 ft away (i.e., the patient has expanded body space). Suspicious people have a body space that exceeds 4 ft. When someone approaches closer than 4 to 5 ft, the suspicious person feels the way one normally does when someone comes closer than 3 ft and literally talks into one's face. To maintain good communication, it may sometimes be necessary to establish a distance that is not comfortable for the physician but that is for the other person.

Being an Aversive Stimulus. Observations of the kinds previously discussed are helpful in dealing with patients, but they only scratch the surface of nonverbal clues. A primary issue with which the physician must learn to deal is that of becoming an aversive stimulus. For example, a patient may get dyspneic each time he or she is anxious. If the physician's manner makes the patient feel uncomfortable and anxious, the patient may become dyspneic. This may be of serious concern if dyspnea occurs, for example, during weekly or monthly visits to the physician over a period of 1 year. The physician becomes an aversive stimulus. Simply looking at or thinking about the physician may produce dyspnea in such a patient. This patient can then easily become a problem in terms of medical management. The physician must learn to be a positive element in the patient's life, one whose presence is associated with comfort and help. Otherwise, the patient's well-being and compliance with treatment are sacrificed.

The physician should avoid only seeing the patient in crisis situations or during exacerbations of the illness. He or she should schedule the patient for occasional meetings at which progress is reviewed and additional information that adds to the understanding of the disease is transmitted to the patient. It is often appropriate for the physician to write the patient a letter that explains the latest laboratory findings and expresses continued interest in the patient's safety and well-being. In all events, the physician should avoid becoming an aversive stimulus.

Loss and Depression

Losses may be sudden or gradual. Some are predictable; others are unpredictable. Chronically ill respiratory patients experience varied losses. Their positive feelings associated with health are often replaced by fatigue, dyspnea, and reduced exercise tolerance. Knowing that their illness is irreversible may create feelings of hopelessness and fear of losing control in these patients. When their illnesses progress, positive self-attitudes often diminish. Independence and pride are lost as patients are forced to retire, change their recreational activities, and rely on others for assistance in performing household tasks or in meeting personal needs such as dressing or bathing. Feelings of inadequacy may result when social roles change.

A major part of our self-image is our body image—that is, the perceptions, attitudes, and feelings we have toward our body. Alterations in our body image may be a major source of frustration and stress. Body image changes occur in respiratory patients when they begin to notice and feel uncomfortable about the barrel chest that results from hyperinflation or about the ankle swelling that is caused by congestive failure. People who value trimness react unfavorably to the weight gain and facial changes that accompany long-term steroid therapy. Continuous use of oxygen at home not only affects one's social situation but can create feelings of unattractiveness.

People react to the same stressor in various ways. Minor emergency responses include fantasy, swearing, weeping, laughing, talking it out, and walking it off. In the presence of major stress, the ego is more taxed, and people may resort to the extended use of repression, depression, excessive fantasy, somatic reactions, and detachment from reality.

Reactions to loss are called *bereavement states*—they are the thoughts, feelings, and actions that are consequences of the loss. Generally, such states are limited in intensity and duration. However, some are maladaptive and last for years. The most adaptive response to loss is the grief and mourning process. Families of dying patients may be deprived of their relationship unless medical personnel intervene to prevent their withdrawal. Less adaptive responses to loss include delayed or absent grief, depression, hypochondriasis, acting-out behavior, or neurotic and psychotic states.

Depression appears to be a common problem in chronically ill respiratory patients. This may be caused by the accumulation of losses they experience as a result of their illness. Health personnel need to recognize signs of depression so that appropriate treatment can be instituted early. When uncertainty exists about the presence of depression, its severity, or its management, psychiatric consultation is necessary.

The behavior of depressed people has been described as falling into four categories: physical, emotional, cognitive, and motivational. Physical symptoms often experienced by depressed people are decreased appetite, difficulty in sleeping, and increased fatigue. Since respiratory patients usually experience fatigue as a result of the increased work of breathing and sometimes experience difficulty in falling asleep because they are taking bronchodilators, physical symptoms of depression may be masked.

Feelings of hopelessness and helplessness characterize the emotional state of depressed people. Some patients experience fluctuating mood, whereas the severely depressed express more persistent feelings of hopelessness. Crying spells may be frequent or absent. The sense of humor is usually decreased. Relationships suffer as patients experience less concern and affection from those close to them. Diminished interaction occurs as they focus more on themselves than on others. Sexual activity may be limited. Therefore, it is imperative for the physician to understand the reactions of spouses or significant others, to discuss the patient's depression with them, and to suggest how they may be of support to the patient.

The cognitive state is marked by indecisiveness and low self esteem. Because they have perfectionist standards, many depressed people engage in self-criticism and overreact to errors. These patients are drawn to activities that are less demanding and involve less responsibility. They prefer passivity to activity, dependence to independence. Suicidal ideation may take various forms, such as obsessive thoughts, daydreams, and passive or active wishes.

Several brief screening measures may be used to evaluate patients for depression. The Beck Depression Inventory,[16] the Zung Self-Rating Scale,[17] and scales derived from the *Diagnostic and Statistical Manual of Mental Disorders* (DSM-III-R) are particularly recommended. Management of the depressed patient involves alleviation of guilt and suffering, stimulation of hope, and protection from self-injury. This is accomplished through psychotherapy and, in some cases, the use of antidepressant medication. Some patients who refuse referrals to mental health facilities may be willing to meet with social workers or nurses prepared to do supportive counseling. Office visits can also have a counseling value.

Patient interviews that show serious concern on the part of the physician should be considered. Since spontaneity of speech is decreased, the professional must be more active in the interview. Humor should be avoided. Commenting on the patient's mood may elicit various emotional reactions that can be acknowledged and discussed. For example, some patients may deny that they are depressed but acknowledge that they are discouraged. In this instance, discussion of their discouragement is more helpful than telling them they are depressed. Daily routines should be investigated, since structure is often absent in these patients' lives and may need to be part of the treatment plan. Inquiring about any suicidal wishes or thoughts shows concern and conveys the message that suicide is not a taboo topic.

Muddling Through

In our culture, muddling through is expected. Those among us who are terrified of flying in airplanes, frightened of swimming, or intimidated by crowds are expected from early childhood to "grow up," "bite the bullet," or "get a grip" on themselves. Since our society admires feats of overcoming anxiety and fear, most of us do "tough it out" and endure the subsequent jolts to organ systems we recognize as discomfort or sometimes severe discomfort. We try, and we somehow "hang on."

Despite popular opinion, why should anyone who reacts with severe stress to public speaking force himself or herself to accept public speaking invitations? To be sure, in a job in which public speaking is expected, one might seek professional counseling to help overcome the problem. But "toughing out" such events on a regular basis, whether part of the job or not, is nothing more than a sure way to get sick. It is one thing if a person can learn to stop reacting with stress to public speaking. It is certainly worth some effort to do so. However, if one cannot overcome the phobia, one should avoid public speaking. Continuing to engage in an activity that is overtly and continuously distressing makes as much sense as forsaking sleep or giving up food.

This does not mean one should avoid everything that might lead to uneasiness. Often the anticipation of an event will cause some discomfort or even considerable discomfort. Inevitably, a sprinter feels ill at ease before the gun goes off for an important track race. Likewise, it is natural for actors to have opening-night "butterflies" before the curtain rises. But when the curtain rises, they can go on like the professionals they are. When the gun fires, the sprinter takes off with practiced fluid strides. There is, however, a considerable difference between some nervousness preceding a great performance and the clutching of one's seat for the duration of a 2-hour airplane flight, feeling panic in crowded rooms, or experiencing terror upon entering an elevator. In essence, these kinds of stress reactions represent your effort to communicate nonverbally with yourself. You are saying to yourself, "I shouldn't be here because this is not good for me." For a number of patients, avoiding life events that trigger discomfort is good business. There is no reason for everyone to "muddle through," particularly if their heart and lungs are failing them.

PSYCHOSOCIAL AND PSYCHOPHYSIOLOGIC TREATMENT

Intensive Care Unit

The management of patients with severe COPD who require treatment in the intensive care unit is difficult at best. There is recognition by the patient and staff that the unit is bringing only temporary relief. Patients' lives may or may not be extended, but they will not become more functional even if treatment is "successful." In this setting, it is difficult for either the patient or the medical team to maintain an optimistic, hopeful outlook. The grim reality of the situation makes it difficult to maintain staff morale and can lead to perfunctory and dehumanized treatment of the patient. The treatment of these patients during their intensive care unit stay can be greatly facilitated by understanding their psychosocial and psychophysiologic situations as outlined in this chapter.

The path that leads the patient to the intensive care unit may be a long one of gradually increasing disability, and the patient may arrive with an acutely failing pulmonary system superimposed on his or her chronically disabled state. The patient's level of pulmonary function is usually such that it marginally sustains him or her during quiet rest. Any change in metabolic demand leads to the rapid onset of symptoms. One way that metabolic demand, and thus symptoms, are increased is by placing the patient in a situation in which he or she is unable to avoid emotional stress. Patients who are severely ill with a pulmonary crisis are rarely able to tolerate emotional stresses of even a routine nature.

Most of these problems with emotional stress may change when assisted breathing therapy is prescribed for the patient. If completely successful, for the first time in years the patient is receiving a sufficient amount of oxygen to supply his or her metabolic needs totally. The patient is then able to allow himself or herself to participate in emotional expression, which was denied previously because of potential respiratory embarrassment secondary to the physiologic results of emotional change. There is little doubt that this type of experience leads to dependence on the machinery that is required to assist breathing. The dependence often is not related to the patient's lack of drive or determination to breathe on his or her own but rather to the reluctance to give up feeling emotionally normal or near normal.

The intensive care unit staff is presented with a person who will in all probability not reward it by becoming symptom-free and who will continue to complain of discomfort after the staff has done its best. For reasons noted above, these patients often lack warmth and the capacity to relate; thus, they will frequently seem to lack emotional involvement with the staff no matter how hard the staff works. It takes a highly motivated staff to absorb the emotional punishment of caring for these patients when the rewarding admiration of a grateful patient is absent. The staff seldom feels adequately rewarded for its hard work and dedication to patient care. Staff members are often left with only the satisfaction that their clinical expertise has given the patient additional time to live.

Acutely ill patients suffer from some sleep deprivation, sensory overstimulation, and isolation. Death may be an imminent concern. Besides investigating the patient's immediate concerns, the staff can reduce stress by:

1. Orienting patients to their environment and daily activities.
2. Planning activities to minimize fatigue and the work of breathing.
3. Maintaining an attitude of competence in the patient's presence.
4. Controlling the environment for traffic and noise.
5. Utilizing resources for patient and staff support.

Too frequently, families are neglected in the acute care setting. Families should be familiarized with the physical surroundings and visiting hours and should be informed as to when they can receive progress reports. For example, spouses may be told that flexible visiting hours are allowed while the patient is in critical condition but that the usual schedule for visiting will be reinforced once his or her condition stabilizes. Guidelines for family involvement in patient care should be clarified by the nursing staff.

Patients often become increasingly independent as the crisis begins to resolve. However, some patients show increased dependence in the recovery phase or in the ambulatory care setting when it is time for them to begin doing more for themselves. This helpless-dependent position may be reflected in a patient's unwillingness to cooperate with a treatment program. He or she may express feelings of helplessness and resentment. Staff may also be pitted against each other by such a patient. A patient's dependent attitude may also be manifested in the clinging nature of his or her relationships and in his or her lack of initiative in seeking instructions.

Too often, patients alienate others by their self-preoccupation. Staff members become irritated and may unintentionally ignore patients or express frustration and resentment. Rather than avoid a patient, staff members should agree upon a consistent treatment approach. Reflecting on the patient's behavior during an interview may reveal particular fears and anxieties related to his or her illness, treatment program, or hospital discharge that can be discussed and sometimes alleviated. When a patient's anxiety is decreased, his or her dependent behavior may decrease. Management also includes clarifying the amount of time spent in interviews, introducing patients to other resource staff in a given setting, and reinforcing independent behavior. Maintaining a nonjudgmental attitude is essential, since some patients are highly sensitive to criticism and unable to express anger because they fear rejection by others.

Group Psychotherapy

Reports in the literature have indicated the salutary effects of group treatment on both patient status and staff-patient relations. However, patients with COPD present a complex therapeutic problem. The patients most likely to need this type of therapy are the same ones who would need it if they did not have COPD. The intimate interdependence between the emotional state of the patient and pulmonary function creates special problems. Emotional states of action-orientation, such as anger and anxiety, increase respiratory and metabolic activity. Conversely, emotional states of action-inhibition, such as depression or apathy, decrease respiratory and metabolic activity. In normal subjects or minimally diseased persons, such shifts in affect and behavior and the concomitant shifts in pulmonary function may be uncomfortable and result in dyspnea, but there is adequate physiologic reserve for the maintenance of pulmonary compensation. However, the patient with severe COPD has a very narrow range within which he or she can maintain pulmonary balance. A rapid shift to either action-activation or action-inhibition may set the stage for the production of pulmonary embarrassment.[8, 18]

Patients who need group psychotherapy have a history of precarious psychosocial balance that has left them ill-prepared for the stress of severe debilitating disease and its concomitant need for continuous medical care and intermittent hospitalization. Their inability to deal with emotions is further compromised by the precarious pulmonary balance. When faced with emotional conflicts, they may be unable to deal with the affect involved without precipitating pulmonary decompensation and disabling symptoms.

Patients who have reasonable interpersonal and social resources and some physiologic reserve have the capacity to respond to the frustrations of their illness without upsetting their pulmonary balance. These types of patients are able to participate in group discussions involving insight-oriented therapy and to profit from them.

Observations of the relationship between physiologic and psychologic factors highlight the importance of structuring group methods to the needs of the patient population. Physiologic limitations and particular psychologic defense mechanisms make it impossible for some patients to participate in group treatment that focuses on the exploration of affect and conflict.

In general, patients with higher psychosocial assets and good pulmonary function demonstrate successful participation in group treatment. Unsuccessful patients have low psychosocial assets and severe physiologic limitations. These patients' reactions to group treatment are characterized by a guarded pose and the avoidance of emotionally charged or personally related topics. It is not uncommon to observe them react to emotionally charged topics with anxiety, anger, depression, dyspnea, and physiologic insufficiency. Supportive didactic discussions or activity and social groups that are task-oriented are usually positive experiences, regardless of the degree of physiologic insufficiency.

Relation of Variables Affecting Group Participation

Two hypotheses can be advanced concerning the severe repression, denial, and isolation that characterize severely incapacitated COPD patients. The first suggests that these patients had reasonably adequate coping mechanisms prior to their disease and that the emotional crippling is an adaptive response to the severe physiologic limitation. In support of this is the fact that most patients had been self-sufficient throughout their lives and did not experience prior known psychiatric symptoms or complaints. However, many also had a history of unsuccessful marital relations, suggesting difficulties in interpersonal relations.

The second hypothesis suggests that these patients had always overutilized the psychologic defenses of denial, suppression, repression, and isolation and that the disease process was superimposed on this pattern of defense. Observations by other workers on the premorbid personality of the tuberculosis patient lend support to this hypothesis.

In either case, the end result is that the only psychologic mechanisms available to these patients for handling affect and interpersonal conflict are gross denial, suppression, repression, and isolation. This, of course, becomes a vicious circle, for as patients face the realistically severe problems associated with an incapacitating disease and chronic treatment, they cannot face their feelings or deal with interpersonal conflicts without literally endangering their lives. The rigid avoidance of affect and conflicts only perpetuates the problems and increases frustration, anger, and despair, which cannot be dealt with by the patient.

These observations are pertinent to the development and prescription of group methods for the treatment of patients with chronic lung disease as well as other medically disabling diseases. Based on these observations, significant questions should be raised by therapists regarding selection and outcome criteria for group treatment.

Selection criteria for group treatment usually depend on the structure, procedures, and goals of the therapy group. Admission of a patient to a group is also influenced by the theoretical orientation, experience, and professional background of the therapist. Standard psychologic diagnostic tests have failed to yield valid predictions as to how patients may behave in group treatment. The relationship among interpersonal behavior, expression of affect, and pathophysiology may prove an effective predictor when selecting medical patients for group treatment. It has been questioned whether group treatment should be undertaken with any severely disabled medical patient who may compromise a physiologic system temporarily when confronted with the exploration of affect and interpersonal conflict. Usual group methods may not be applicable to such a patient, and new group approaches may need to be developed and tested. Further clinical and research evidence is also needed that will support the indications and contraindications for varied group treatment approaches with varying medical populations experiencing varying degrees of disability. Since families are often affected by patients' illnesses, under what circumstance should they be included in group treatment? It is often assumed by therapists that families or spouses should be directly involved. Yet, it is important to consider what characteristics may contraindicate their inclusion.

There is also a need to establish successful outcome criteria. Patients may perceive improvement in different ways. For example, respiratory patients who associate expression of affect with dyspnea may learn that expressing emotions does not consistently produce dyspnea. Socially isolated patients may learn what they fear about intimacy, and the group may further the socialization process for them.

Insight gained in group treatment may occur on at least four levels: (1) patients learn how they are seen by others, (2) some patients learn what they are doing to and with other people, (3) others learn why they behave in certain ways and why they have not been able to behave differently, and, last, (4) some gain an understanding of the cause of their present interpersonal behavior.

Discussion

The use of educational, psychotherapeutic, and medical principles in a unified approach to the treatment of patients with chronic pulmonary disease has a long history in the United States. Joseph Hersey Pratt, a Boston internist, developed the first such treatment method in 1905 for tuberculosis patients. This early program consisted of a combination of group psychotherapy, didactic teaching, and medical treatment. It was referred to as the Thought Control Clinic, and a derivation of it was called the Class Method of Treatment. The results of this early work were impressive, and Pratt and his colleagues extended use of the method to patients with diabetes and cardiac disease. Other groups of researchers extended his work to patients with hypertension and peptic ulcers. Around 1921, as a direct result of Pratt's work, St. Elizabeth's Hospital in Washington, D.C., instituted group therapy for the treatment of chronic schizophrenia patients. Despite the intent of Dr. Pratt and his colleagues and the treatment's demonstrated effectiveness, the integrated use of group therapy and teaching in the treatment of chronic diseases had almost disappeared from the field of internal medicine by the 1940s, except in tuberculosis sanatoriums. With the closing of these institutions in the 1960s and 1970s, the technique disappeared as an organized treatment method in internal medicine.

In the past decade, the increasing emphasis on the treatment of chronic disease and the acceptance of a chronic disease model have resulted in increased interest in such an integrated approach to patient care. In addition, in many instances treatment techniques have become too much for the patient to handle without special instruction and support. Some hemodialysis programs utilize a programmed text in self-care for patients to overcome some of these difficulties. In other programs, manuals or textbooks have been developed for use by diabetics and patients with chronic airway disease and arthritis. These techniques all appear to be effective in aiding the patient to adapt better to disease. Work in the Netherlands on the use of group education and group therapy for the treatment of asthma and diabetes is of particular importance because it has demonstrated a significant reduction in morbidity. Dutch studies recommend a treatment program model unlike that followed by most American programs in that the integrative process is directed by a skilled internist and the emphasis is not limited to the giving of information. Emphasis is placed on the integration of the patient's degree of incapacity with the pattern of life.

These observations are pertinent for the development and prescription of group methods for the treatment of patients with severe chronic lung disease. Programs conducted on the wards, which include various group treatments, have been developed in many hospital tuberculosis wards. Group treatment has been used successfully to manage outpatients with tuberculosis, bronchial asthma, and emphysema.

However, some authors report that they avoid involving patients in group programs who are severely debilitated, are so seriously ill that death is an imminent possibility, or are severely immobilized by physical illness. Thus, the usual group methods described do not seem directly applicable to the most severely ill patient population. The few exceptions include group work with patients such as those in poliomyelitis respiratory wards.

Yet, even in less physically handicapped patients, group leaders report that they have found it necessary to modify discussion groups and joint group social and vocational activities. Furthermore, they report that group techniques that focus on immediate exploration of affect and interpersonal conflict have not been successful with patients with moderate to severe lung disease or with debilitated, aged patients.

In this light, it is pertinent to report two group methods that seem to have been uniformly successful. Most patients and staff who participated concluded that these two group activities did have a salutary effect.

The first is a discussion group conducted by a physician and a well-trained paramedical professional. It is important that the physician and the family be directly involved. Pertinent aspects of pulmonary and cardiac physiology and pathology are reviewed, and effects of chronic lung disease on patterns of life activity are described. All information is provided to the group in a neutral manner. The talks are didactic, and time is provided for questions and discussion. There is no forced emotional intervention. The second is a physical therapy or rehabilitation group. This should be prescribed treatment in which six to eight patients (and families, if appropriate) assemble to exercise, practice breathing, or share experiences they have had with their disease. It is useful to have the sessions conducted by outgoing, energetic people with whom the patients can identify. There is generally joking, exchange of experiences, and friendly competition over the adequacy of their performance. The patients perceive these group experiences as positive because their disease, and not themselves, is in question. These groups play in part into patients' denial mechanisms, but they also afford some measure of secondhand intervention in patterns of interpersonal relations.

Ambulatory Care

Patient and Family Education

The goals of patient and family education are to maintain health, prevent complications, and maximize individual growth. Success or failure of educational programs depends on many interrelated factors, such as:

1. The teaching skills of the educator
2. The patient's or family's involvement in planning the program
3. The adequacy of program objectives
4. The identification of resources and barriers
5. The effectiveness of the evaluation process

Teaching Skills. Professionals who are successful at teaching use teaching and learning principles and strategies that optimize the learning situation. Since the physical environment influences learning, teachers can achieve a suitable atmosphere by regulating room size, ventilation, heat, and light. Respiratory patients in particular are sensitive to crowded rooms and ventilation changes. Learning is also enhanced through the clarification of guidelines on attendance and participation and the selection of material best suited for the learner. If information is presented at too high a level of comprehension, patients become frustrated, whereas if the material presented is too simplified, they lose interest and become annoyed. Increased anxiety can also result when patients' questions are ignored or when too much information is given to a patient too rapidly.

If you wish to create an atmosphere of self-expression and shared problem-solving, small groups of patients who are arranged in circular fashion without a table are more effective than are large groups of patients who are seated in rows of chairs facing the educator. Guided discussion in small groups places increased responsibility on the learners. They become active participants and more aware of their communication styles and problem-solving skills; as a result, they may eventually increase interpersonal skills.

When the paramedical professional functions as a leader of a discussion group, the learning objectives may be facilitated through various techniques. For example, he or she may use inductive learning to help patients and families understand the principles related to anxiety by asking them to describe anxiety-provoking situations and how they have coped with them. Principles and generalizations may then be drawn from their observations and experiences. Questions may also be used to seek more information, clarify behavior, and compare and contrast different patient situations.

Positive reinforcement strengthens behavior and can be achieved by giving patients feedback about the nature of their performance. When patients present incorrect information, they can be rewarded for their effort while they are informed of correct information. In any learning situation, the educator must decide what behavior to reinforce. He or she may wish to reinforce the participation of a withdrawn patient in a discussion group or to emphasize one patient's willingness to tackle a problem or another's performance of a task. In group situations, it is important for each patient to recognize the achievements of the others.

Patient and Family Participation. Active participation in the learning process enhances learning and increases autonomy. Patients and families should have some control over the information they receive and when it is presented. Too frequently, educational programs are planned for them without assessing their learning needs, their readiness to learn, and how their cultural backgrounds may affect the learning process. Educators must also set realistic expectations. For example, anxious, depressed, or dependent patients may not be able to participate fully in initial planning sessions.

Adequacy of Program Objectives. Perhaps one of the most difficult tasks is the clear definition of learning objectives. When goals are hazy, it is impossible to select appropriate content and evaluate a program efficiently. Useful objectives are statements that identify the kind of performance desired and that demonstrate what someone must do to achieve that performance level. They establish conditions under which certain behavior is expected to occur, and they specify how well the educator wants the learner to perform the behavior (i.e., the minimal level of acceptable performance).

Identification of Resources and Barriers. Educators need to evaluate the following resources prior to planning any educational program: the support within the organization, financial support, time, space, and the personnel affected by the program. Such assessments prevent unnecessary conflicts that may occur at a later date; they help the educator analyze the factors that may oppose or strengthen an educational program. Awareness of the constraints and strengths of a program helps educators plan strategies to weaken the opposing forces.

Effectiveness of the Evaluation Process. Evaluation is a continuous process in any educational program. Educators evaluate program objectives, instructional materials, and patients' progress in achieving objectives. Generally, evaluation measurements are used to determine the effectiveness in attaining program goals and objectives. Educators need to decide whether clinical observations should be used alone or in conjunction with evaluation measurements that are valid and reliable. Evaluation resources may also be limited to clinical settings because of inadequate funds, staff, or time.

In summary, patient education is often considered to be a viable part of any pulmonary rehabilitation program. Clinicians planning these programs may want to consider the following factors that contribute to an improved psychologic state and to improved performance in a rehabilitation program:

1. Progressive exercise that leads to decreased fear of activity
2. Education in self-care that leads to increased autonomy in the control of symptoms
3. Staff attitudes that stress that the patient is worth the effort
4. Setting of realistic goals that lead to improvement in self-esteem
5. Monthly follow-up to consolidate gains
6. Mutual support from group interaction
7. Factors within patients that lead to strong motivation

DEALING WITH PSYCHIATRIC DISEASE

In contrast to the previously discussed psychosocial and psychophysiologic problems and the accompanying emotions that afflict many or most patients with severe pulmonary disease, psychiatric disease is probably no more frequent in these patients than in patients without pulmonary disease. The distinction between psychophysiologic and psychosocial problems and significant psychiatric disease is a critical issue. The treatment of the former can often be with various psychotherapies, behavioral therapies, and social support systems, and, *when necessary*, with medication as an adjunct therapy; however, treatment of the latter should initially be primarily with medications. Other types of therapy may be needed in the recovery period, but there likely will be no recovery period without the use of medications.

In general, the psychiatric diseases to be concerned about are the schizophrenias, manic-depressive illness (unipolar and bipolar types), major depression, and delirium (acute brain syndromes). Specific pharmacologic treatments are also available for anxiety and depression not classified in the above categories. A review of psychiatric diseases can be obtained from any of the current textbooks of psychiatry.

Patients with combined psychiatric and pulmonary disease are more likely to have serious problems than patients without such a combination. A good way to screen for possible psychiatric disease can be to identify (1) patients with marked pulmonary disease but with no complaints or no response to the reality of the disease, (2) those with limited pulmonary disease who are incapacitated, and (3) patients who overreact and feel little hope for coping with the concomitant problems. This clinical information suggests an increased probability that a given patient has a psychiatric problem but does not necessarily confirm the diagnosis.

In early stages of pulmonary disease, changes in psychologic activation are often associated with dyspnea only. As the disease progresses in severity, a point may be reached at which increases in emotional activation of any type produce elevations in oxygen consumption and carbon dioxide production that cannot readily be compensated for physiologically because of the patient's impaired ventilation. Thus, even minimal changes in alveolar ventilation become difficult to accommodate. With psychologic activation, the patient with an unimpaired muscular system (that is, one who is not paralyzed and who thus can contract muscles) is likely to then develop hypoxia and possible hypercarbia. When psychologic activation decreases, there is a drop in the amount of air the patient breathes but no equivalent drop in the oxygen needs and nutritional requirements of the skeletal muscles. Thus, any and all emotional change may be associated with uncomfortable symptoms because during such change the pulmonary system tends to deliver less oxygen than is required to meet metabolic demand.

The secondary reaction to the dyspnea, wheezing, cough, sputum production, and pain that occur can be anxiety, fear, or depression, or any combination of these. These emotional responses in turn serve as another emotional stimulus to further compromise the patient's physiologic and emotional states.

It is understandable that such a patient tends to avoid interpersonal contact because of the psychologic stress involved. He or she thereby decreases the number of psychologic stressors. By using denial and repression, the patient lessens the impact of emotionally loaded events. The psychologic defenses used to protect a failing organ system, however, are often regarded by others as socially inappropriate, that is, the patient may be perceived as rejecting, bland, and unresponsive. The previously noted problems can be magnified many times by patients with coexisting psychiatric disorders.[19-23]

Psychoactive Medications

In contrast to psychosocial and psychophysiologic problems and the accompanying emotions that affect many or most patients with severe COPD, psychiatric disease is probably no more frequent in these patients than in patients without COPD.[24] It is necessary to be positive about the diagnosis. The medications to be reviewed are not substitutes for counseling and psychotherapy. On the other hand, counseling and psychotherapy are not substitutes for psychotropic medications. A strong effort should be made to establish a positive diagnosis and to tailor the treatment to the diagnosis and the patient. It is necessary to know what is being treated and, therefore, the reason for the use of psychoactive agents.

The distinction between psychophysiologic and psychosocial problems and psychiatric disease is critical. The treatment of the former can often be done with various psychotherapies, behavioral therapies, and social support systems, with medication as an adjunct when necessary, whereas treatment of the latter should be initiated with medications along with psychotherapy.

It should be remembered that the role of psychoactive medications in the treatment of COPD patients is of considerable importance, since many patients lack the ability to utilize other treatment techniques. In other words, some patients reject or cannot respond to any treatment of a "psychologic" nature, and thus the clinician is left with the use of either medications or nothing. Also, in a number of these patients, counseling and psychotherapy may not be possible because of time limitations, finances, or the physiologic and psychologic states of the disease.

If a patient fulfills the major and minor criteria for depression as indicated in the *DSM III–R*,[25] administration of an antidepressant is indicated. If counseling or psychotherapy is to be utilized, it is as an adjunct to the antidepressant medication. However, if a patient fulfills the *DSM III–R*'s criteria for a traumatic stress reaction, narcotherapy is indicated, and both medications and counseling or psychotherapy are seen as adjuncts. Treatment should be tailored to the patient and the diagnosis.

Some General Guidelines

The age of the patient, the chronicity of the disease, and individual variations in metabolism determine the dosage of the psychoactive medication utilized. It should be remembered that the rate of metabolism of psychoactive medications by different people can vary by as much as 30 times. In other words, one patient may need a dose of 30 mg and another a dose of 900 mg. However, a good general rule is that the dose of psychoactive medication is inversely related to the age of the patient and the chronicity of disease. It is important to select medications that do not depress, overly stimulate, or interfere with the respiratory center or with respiratory movement. The psychoactive medication should also minimally interfere with existing pulmonary medications. Knowledge of the blood levels of psychoactive agents is essential for adequate treatment of the COPD patient. As a general rule, psychoactive agents are greatly beneficial when used discriminately and with awareness of their indications, contraindications, and side effects in a given patient.

Neuroleptics

The neuroleptics (also called *major tranquilizers* or *antipsychotics*) are used in the treatment of psychiatric diseases such as schizophrenia, mania, acute psychotic reactions, and delirium (Table 19–1). In common with the antidepressants, they tend not be habit-forming or addictive and are generally well tolerated if their side effects are understood. Neuroleptics and antidepressants are generally seen as powerful and dangerous, whereas the anxiolytic agents are considered innocuous. However, all three types of medications can have side effects in some patients, and they should be seen as equally powerful. The adverse consequences to the patient may be equally severe if breathing is compromised because he or she has been too stimulated by protriptyline, has had the respiratory center drive reduced by chlordiazepoxide, or cannot move the chest muscles as a result

TABLE 19–1. PROPERTIES AND DOSAGE OF NEUROLEPTIC DRUGS

Specific Medication	Special Properties	Usual Daily Dosage	Daily Dosage in Moderate to Severe COPD
Phenothiazines Thioridazine HCl (Mellaril)	Similar to chlorpromazine, but it has been reported to produce pigmented retinitis in doses over 800 mg. Mild D-2, highest alpha$_1$, moderate alpha$_2$ and high cholinergic receptor blocking.	Oral: 50–800 mg	Oral: 5–200 mg
Chlorpromazine (Thorazine)	Older dose forms may contain tartrazine and should be avoided if this medication is used in asthmatics. Current dose forms should be free of tartrazine. Can be very sedating. Associated with the production of antinuclear antibodies. Mild to moderate D-2, high alpha$_1$, moderate alpha$_2$, high H-1, and high cholinergic receptor blocking effect.	Oral: 500–2000 mg IM: 50–100 mg every 30–60 min until symptoms are under control to a total dose of 200 mg	Oral: 5–200 mg IM: 25 mg every 30–60 min until symptoms are under control to a total dose of 100 mg
Trifluoperazine HCl (Stelazine)	Can be activating. Moderate D-2, low alpha$_1$, low alpha$_2$, moderate H-1, and moderate cholinergic receptor blocking effect.	Oral: 10–40 mg	Oral: 2–5 mg
Dihydroindolones Molindone HCl (Moban)	Apparent low cardiovascular toxicity. Does not block guanethidine. Mild D-2, low alpha$_1$, moderate alpha$_2$, low H-1, and low cholinergic receptor blocking effect. There is little experience with this medication in COPD.	Oral: 30–100 mg	Oral: 10–30 mg
Thiothanxenes Thiothixene (Navane)	No tartrazine. Low anticholinergic effect. May have significant antidepressant effect. Decreases sensory input. Can be nonsedating or sedating. Strong D-2, moderate to low alpha$_1$, moderate alpha$_2$, high H-1, and low cholinergic receptor blocking effect. (D-2 receptor blocking refers to antipsychotic effect. Higher D-2 blockade is thought to be synonymous with greater antipsychotic effect.)	Oral: 5–80 mg IM: 5–20 mg every 30–60 min to a total dose of 80 mg	Oral: 2–20 mg IM: 5 mg every 30–60 min to a total dose of 40 mg
Butyrophenones Haloperidol (Haldol)	1-, 5-, and 10-mg tablets of haloperidol contain tartrazine. These dose forms should be avoided if this medication is used in patients with asthma. Can be nonsedating. Decreases sensory input. Likely to produce movement disorders that can interfere with chest movement. Moderate D-2, moderate alpha$_1$, low alpha$_2$, low H-1, and low cholinergic receptor blocking effect.	Oral: 2–40 mg IM: 5–10 mg every 30–60 min to a total dose of 40 mg IV: 2 mg every 6–8 hr	Oral: 1–10 mg IM: 2–5 mg every 30–60 min to a total dose of 20 mg IV: 2 mg every 6–8 hr

From thioridazine to haloperidol, extrapyramidal symptoms increase, and, moving backward, alpha-adrenergic blocking, allergic responses, sedation, atropine-like effects, seizures, and orthostatic hypotension generally increase. For all neuroleptics listed, drowsiness or lack of attention may make operation of machinery dangerous, particularly during initial treatment. Selected patients may need the usual daily dose. Respiratory depression with aggravation or onset of hypoxia and hypercarbia is always a possible complication when the neuroleptics are used in the COPD population.

Neuroleptics in general can alter sexual function and drive. Each medication in this class can produce specific types of problems. For example, thioridazine may contribute to delayed or inhibited ejaculation, and chlorpromazine may contribute to a simple reduction in sexual drive. On the other hand, both may increase sexual drive and performance in specific patients. In addition, sexual dysfunction is so common in patients who need to be treated with neuroleptics that it is often difficult to know what the cause of the change in sexual function is secondary to.

Common side effects	Precautions with	Contraindications
Blurred vision Dysuria Constipation Nasal congestion Postural hypotension Photosensitivity Drowsiness Fatigue Weight gain Extrapyramidal side effects Respiratory depression Potential difficulty handling secretions Changes in temperature control	Seizures Depression Pregnancy Respiratory disease Cardiac disease Respiratory depression May reverse the hypertensive action of medications such as epinephrine and block the antihypertensive effect of guanethidine	Comatose states Central nervous system depression Bone marrow depression Subcortical brain depression Seriously impaired liver function Hypersensitivity Uncontrolled epilepsy Severe retarded depression

Key: IM: intramuscularly; IV: intravenously.

TABLE 19–2. RECEPTOR-BLOCKING PROPERTIES OF SELECTED NEUROLEPTICS*†

	D-2 (Haloperidol)	Cholinergic (Atropine)	H-1 (Diphenhydramine)	Alpha$_1$ (Prazosin)	Alpha$_2$ (Yohimbine)
Thiothixene	8.88	0.00081	2.5373	0.00827	0.0081
Haloperidol	1.00	0.00010	0.0079	0.01455	0.0004
Chlorpromazine	0.21	0.03333	1.6418	0.03455	0.0021
Thioridazine	0.14	0.1333	0.9254	0.18182	0.0019
Molindone	0.03	0.00001	0.0001	0.00004	0.0026
Haloperidol	1				
Atropine		1			
D-Chlorpheniramine			1		
Prazosin		0.1		1	
Yohimbine		8.0			1

*From Richelson E. Pharmacology of neuroleptics in use in the United States. J Clin Psychiatry 1985; 46:8–14 and personal communication, 1986.
†Figures represent the number of milligrams of the reference blocking agent effect represented by 1 mg of the psychotropic agent. For example: 1 mg of thiothixene = 8.88 mg of haloperidol in terms of D-2 blocking effect, 0.00081 mg of atropine in terms of anticholinergic effect, 2.54 mg of diphenhydramine in terms of H-1 blocking effect, 0.008 mg of prazosin in terms of alpha$_1$-blocking effect, and 0.008 mg of yohimbine in terms of alpha$_2$-blocking effect. Receptors are cellular recognition sites for neurotransmitters and neurotransmitter blockers. They are generally membrane-bound proteins on the outside of the cell and have the ability to recognize specific molecular structures. The names of the receptor recognition sites are usually related to the function of the site. For example, D-1 and D-2 are recognition sites for dopamine. The D-2 site seems to be the one that decreases psychotic activity when blocked. Histamine recognition sites are called H-1 and H-2 sites. The antihistamine action of diphenhydramine and D-chlorpheniramine is secondary to their ability to block H-1 cellular recognition sites. Similarly, there are two subclassifications of alpha-adrenergic receptors called alpha$_1$ and alpha$_2$ sites, found in both the central and peripheral nervous systems. These play important roles in the regulation of blood pressure. Blocking alpha$_1$ recognition sites lowers blood pressure, while blocking alpha$_2$ recognition sites increases blood pressure.

of a respiratory extrapyramidal reaction secondary to haloperidol.

Two drugs that provide reasonable examples of the benefits and problems of this class of medications are thiothixene and thioridazine. They are considered to be good neuroleptics, that is, they do the job the psychiatrist needs to have done. Both have side effects that lessen their usefulness in COPD. The major side effects are extrapyramidal symptoms (drug-induced parkinsonism), acute dyskinesias (acute dystonic reactions), akathisias, tardive dyskinesias, and the neuroleptic malignant syndrome.

Regardless of the neuroleptic compound used, side effects interfere with functioning in about 50% of patients. It is important to know the possible side effects when the kind and dose of an agent are selected. In general, thiothixene has been utilized in COPD and seems well tolerated. As with other neuroleptics, it can be administered orally, intramuscularly, or intravenously. Although the intravenous route is not recommended and has not been approved by the Food and Drug Administration, it may prove to be the route of choice in certain patients in the future. To judge the relative usefulness of neuroleptics to achieve a clinical effect, the reader is referred to Table 19–2 and Table 19–3. When these tables are used as a guide, thiothixene is found to be the best D-2 blocker as it is almost nine times more effective than haloperidol. Since D-2 receptor blocking is an indication of antipsychotic activity, this agent may be the best antipsychotic on the market. One hundred milligrams of thiothixene is the equivalent of 888 mg haloperidol in D-2 receptor blocking effect, 0.08 mg atropine in anticholinergic activity, 254 mg diphenhydramine in H-1 blocking effect, and 0.8 mg prazosin in alpha$_1$-blocking effect.

Similar values for thioridazine are 14.0 mg, 93 mg, 13.3 mg, and 18.2 mg, respectively. In other words, by using Tables 19–2 and 19–3, one can choose a neuroleptic (such as thioridazine) that provides a high-dose (low D-2) effect and that has high anticholinergic and high alpha$_1$-blocking action. If low-dose (high D-2) effect, low anticholinergic activity, and relatively low alpha$_1$-blocking action are desired, thiothixene might be chosen. These data have been provided by Richelson[26, 27] and are based on receptor studies performed on the human brain. The relationships listed serve as rough guides. Much information of this nature is based on data from studies of rat or other nonhuman brains, and the technology used in such studies varies. Richelson's data were used for Tables 19–2 and 19–3 because they seemed to parallel clinical experience and because they were translatable in terms of milligrams of standard blocking agents.

Rapid treatment of extrapyramidal reactions is important in maintaining unimpaired respiratory movements. These reactions to neuroleptics can be treated with benztropine mesylate, 1 to 2 mg, or with 50 to 100 mg intravenous diphenhydramine hydrochloride in most cases of respiratory impairment. Oral maintenance therapy can be accomplished with any of the antiparkinson-

TABLE 19–3. RECEPTOR-BLOCKING CHARACTERISTICS OF FOUR PSYCHOTROPIC MEDICATIONS*†

	D-2 (Haloperidol)	Cholinergic (Atropine)	H-1 (Diphenhydramine)	Alpha$_1$ (Prazosin)
Thiothixene	888.0	0.08	254	0.8
Haloperidol	100.0	0.01	1	1.5
Doxepin	0.2	2.30	77,500	0.3
Amitriptyline	0.4	10.00	19,250	0.2

*From Richelson E. Pharmacology of neuroleptics in use in the United States. J Clin Psychiatry 1985; 46:8–14, Richelson E. Pharmacology of antidepressants in use in the United States. J Clin Psychiatry 1982; 43:4–11 and 1983; 44:4–9, and personal communication, 1988.
†Figures represent the approximate number of milligrams of the reference blocking agent effect represented by 100 mg of psychotropic agent. For example: 100 mg of thiothixene = 888 mg of haloperidol in terms of D-2 blocking, 0.08 mg of atropine in terms of anticholinergic effect, 254 mg of diphenhydramine in terms of H-1 blocking effect, and 0.8 mg of prazosin in terms of alpha$_1$-blocking effect.

TABLE 19–4. RECEPTOR-BLOCKING PROPERTIES OF SELECTED ANTIDEPRESSANTS*†

	H-1	Cholinergic	Alpha$_1$	Alpha$_2$	S-1	S-2	D-2
Doxepin	775.0	0.02708	0.00257	0.040	0.200	0.267	0.002
Triimipramine	250.0	0.03542	0.00256	0.065	0.007	0.207	0.022
Amitriptyline	192.5	0.11458	0.00236	0.050	0.312	0.227	0.004
Maprotiline	25.0	0.00416	0.00067	0.005	0.005	0.055	0.012
Amoxapine	3.8	0.00208	0.00122	0.017	0.271	11.333	0.025
Nortriptyline	3.5	0.01458	0.00098	0.017	0.189	0.153	0.003
Imipramine	2.5	0.02292	0.00067	0.014	0.006	0.080	0.002
Protriptyline	0.7	0.08333	0.00050	0.007	0.007	0.100	0.002
Trazodone	0.4	0.00001	0.00171	0.087	1.000	0.867	0.001
Desipramine	0.1	0.01042	0.00045	0.006	0.006	0.240	0.001
Fluoxetine	0.0	0.00120	0.00250	0.000	0.003	0.032	0.000
Bupropion	0.0	0.00010	0.00330	0.000	0.004	0.000	0.000
Diphenhydramine	1						
Atropine		1					
Prazosin			1				
Phentolamine				1			
Trazodone					1		
Methysergide						1	
Haloperidol							1

*From Richelson E. Pharmacology of neuroleptics in use in the United States. J Clin Psychiatry 1985; 46:8–14, Richelson E. Pharmacology of antidepressants in use in the United States. J Clin Psychiatry 1982; 43:4–11 and 1983; 44:4–9, Dudley DL, Schacher S. Depression in patients with respiratory disease. Chest Clin North Am 1989; 319–324.

†Figures represent the approximate number of milligrams of the reference blocking agent effect represented by 1 mg of the psychotropic agent. These data may vary with differing studies.

ian medications, such as benztropine mesylate or procyclidine hydrochloride.

Antidepressants

In the treatment of depression, it is helpful to have information on the clinical application of antidepressants that can be used to produce sedation and activation. Since nomifensine has been removed from the market, it is hoped that an activating compound such as fluoxetine or bupropion will be made available and that such compounds will be compatible with COPD treatment.

Doxepin is the antidepressant of choice in agitated, depressed patients with COPD. In addition to its antidepressant characteristics, it is sufficiently sedating to reduce or eliminate agitation. The sedative effect is apparent in minutes or hours, whereas the antidepressant effect may take days or weeks to be apparent. Like other antidepressants, doxepin appears to have little or no effect on the respiratory center and seems to act as a bronchodilator.[28,29] It should be noted that doxepin and other psychotropic agents have been found to decrease the number of seizures in patients with seizure disorders. One hundred milligrams of doxepin contains the equivalent of 0.2 mg haloperidol in D-2 blocking action, 2.3 mg atropine in anticholinergic effect, 77,500 mg diphenhydramine in H-1 blocking action, 0.3 mg prazosin in alpha$_1$-blocking action, and 4.0 mg yohimbine in alpha$_2$-blocking activity (Table 19–4; see also Table 19–3).

Fluoxetine or bupropion is probably the antidepressant of choice in retarded, depressed patients with low drive and motivation. An activating effect can appear within hours of administration, and an antidepressant effect can occur within days or weeks. The most common side effects are sleep disturbance, restlessness, and diaphoresis. These medications are under consideration for commercial use, but information obtained from clinical trials is needed before they can be released. They reportedly have little or no anticholinergic effect and are not cardiotoxic. A reliable receptor blocking profile for fluoxetine and bupropion should be available soon.

Doxepin has a relatively low incidence of side effects if it is used in patients with the appropriate indications. It is generally not advisable to utilize doxepin in the morning or use fluoxetine or bupropion at night because patients do not adapt well to such regimens. To obtain optimal therapeutic effect, advantage should be taken of these agents' initial sedating or activating characteristics by prescribing them when sedation or activation does not interfere with the patient's life.

In utilizing antidepressants and neuroleptics, it is important to remember that blood levels of these drugs may have little relationship to oral dose, and cellular levels may be poorly related to either of these values. Since these compounds may have therapeutic windows above or below which no positive clinical effects are observed, it is essential to maintain optimal blood levels of the medications. This is particularly true for the antidepressants. The desired clinical response can be associated with a specific blood level of an antidepressant, and this level should be maintained. This is the preferred method of dosage in patients with combined psychiatric and pulmonary disease. Since metabolism varies greatly among individuals, major side effects, such as cardiotoxicity, can be avoided by the measurement of drug blood levels and by appropriate adjustment in dosage.

Although it is important for the clinician to deal with the side effects of individual psychoactive agents, it is also important to understand that certain medications are converted to known psychoactive agents in the course of their metabolism in the human body. For example, imipramine is broken down to desipramine, and amitriptyline is broken down to nortriptyline. The metabolites differ from the parent compounds in that they have different receptor-blocking characteristics and different side effects (Table 19–5; see also Table 19–4). The issue is complicated by the fact that once a steady state is reached (7–10 days), the ratio of desipramine to imipramine is about 2:1, and the ratio of nortriptyline to amitriptyline is about 1.2:1.

Lithium

Understanding lithium therapy has been increasingly important as clinical studies continue to demonstrate its effectiveness in controlling mania, depression, or cyclic swings from mania to depression. Mania may be treated initially with a neuroleptic, and depression can be treated with an antidepressant. However, lithium therapy should be started concomitantly if mood swings are a serious problem. The starting dosage of lithium is generally 150 to 450 mg/day. The dosage may require modification if the patient is taking theophylline or a diuretic because theophylline tends to cause an increase in the excretion of lithium and because most diuretics decrease the excretion of lithium. In addition, lithium excretion may vary with salt intake, which should be kept stable during lithium administration. A fasting, morning level of lithium (9–10 hr after the evening dose) of 0.5 to 1.0 mEq/L (or lower) is usually therapeutic in patients with moderate to severe lung disease. It may take 3 to 10 days to equilibrate the therapeutic blood level of lithium. Lithium usually has a 7- to 10-day lag between the onset of therapy and the therapeutic response. When the maintenance dose is reached, the neuroleptic or antidepressant can often be withdrawn. Note that some COPD patients obtain good therapeutic effects with lithium blood levels of less than 0.5 mEq/L.

Patients should be monitored carefully for signs of toxicity (particularly hyperthermia), and alternative treatment should be planned in advance. Lithium carbonate occasionally produces severe depression. If this occurs, it is necessary to treat the patient using an antidepressant with or without lithium carbonate.

It should be noted that increasing experience is being gained with the use of carbamazapine, valproic acid, lecithin, and other agents in the treatment of the approximately 25% of patients who cannot tolerate or do not respond to lithium (Table 19–6).

Anxiolytic Agents

These psychopharmacologic agents are often overused. They tend to be given in sympathy for a patient's condition and as a result of our inability to cure him or her rather than for specific indications. As with any medication, it is better not to prescribe anxiolytic agents if clinical indications for their administration are unclear. They are potent compounds, and prescribing them indiscriminately (i.e., to a patient who may not need them or who needs some other type of medication, such as an antidepressant or neuroleptic) can be antitherapeutic and even dangerous in the COPD patient. Without a positive diagnosis, it is likely that their only effect will be sedation, the potentiation of depression, or behavioral disorganization (or any combination of these factors), which can further aggravate problems with COPD. Generally, these agents should be used to attain short-term goals, such as overcoming an acute stress reaction. The statement that taking them over long periods of time leads to significant problems with habituation and addiction needs to be studied. In particular, some newly released, some not yet released, and probably some older compounds in this category may carry roughly the same probability of causing habituation and addiction as do digitalis or hydrochlorothiazide. If an anxiolytic agent has been administered in high doses over a period of months, withdrawal should be carried out by gradual reduction of the dose rather than by abrupt withdrawal. A reasonable schedule includes the gradual reduction of the current dosage by 10% each week. In some cases, it may be desirable to replace one type of anxiolytic with another rather than to withdraw the medication and have the patient experience recurrence of the symptoms for which it was originally prescribed. Abrupt withdrawal is not desirable for any medication, and anxiolytic agents are no exception. Sudden withdrawal often results in such symptoms as nervousness, anxiety, tremor, and insomnia.

Commonly used anxiolytic agents include diazepam, chlordiazepoxide, chlorazepam, alprazolam, triazolam, and hydroxyzine (Table 19–7).

Anticholinergic Problems

Medications with high anticholinergic properties, such as antiparkinsonian agents, thioridazine, and amitriptyline, occasionally produce an anticholinergic psychosis (delirium). The use of multiple medications increases the probability of this reaction. The reaction is characterized by the signs and symptoms of atropine ingestion, including mild temperature elevation, flushed, warm skin, an increased heart rate, decreased sweating, mydriasis, and an acute brain syndrome. It is important that the reaction be recognized early, since increasing the dosage of the offending agents increases the severity of the psychosis. Treatment with intramuscular or intravenous physostigmine (1 mg) is recommended, if necessary, for the patient's well-being and survival.[30, 31] Reversal of the reaction is rapid (i.e., it occurs within minutes). Only physostigmine crosses the blood-brain barrier; neostigmine simply produces symptoms of peripheral cholinergic action. Methscopolamine (0.5–1.0 mg intramuscularly) can be used to block the peripheral effects of physostigmine and to help avoid respiratory problems, if necessary.

Summary

Four primary types of medications are useful in the treatment of psychiatric disease or sustained emotional upsets in patients with COPD:

TABLE 19–5. HETEROCYCLIC ANTIDEPRESSANTS

Specific Medication	Special Properties	Usual Daily Dosage	Daily Dosage in Moderate to Severe COPD
Tricyclic Agents			
Amitriptyline HCl (Elavil)	Information uncertain. May act as a mild bronchodilator and may depress ventilation. Generally not recommended in COPD patients with arrhythmias. Metabolically converted to nortriptyline (Aventyl or Pamelor); thus may begin as sedating and end up in 7–14 days as nonsedating or activating. Low D-2, moderate H-1, high cholinergic, low alpha$_1$, and moderate serotonin receptor blocking effect.	Oral: 50–300 mg	Oral: 10–100 mg
Doxepin HCl (Adapin, Sinequan)	Low cardiac toxicity; little or no effect on respiratory center; may act as a mild bronchodilator. Particularly effective in treatment of panic attacks associated with depression. Antidepressant of choice for agitated/depressed patients. Major side effects may be sedation and weight gain. Acts as an antiseizure agent in patients with a seizure disorder. Unlikely to inhibit guanethidine in doses under 150 mg. Initially may be sedating. May produce rapid remission in steroid-dependent intractable asthma. Low D-2, high H-1, low to moderate cholinergic, low alpha$_1$, and moderate serotonin receptor–blocking effect.	Oral: 50–300 mg	Oral: 10–100 mg
Imipramine HCl (Janimine, SK-Pramine, Tofranil)	Similar to amitriptyline HCl, but more activating. Metabolically converted to desipramine (Pertofrane or Norpramine), thus may begin as sedating or activating and end up in 7–14 days as more activating. Low D-1, low H-1, moderate cholinergic, low alpha$_1$, and low serotonin receptor blocking.	Oral: 50–300 mg	Oral: 10–100 mg
Desipramine (Pertofrane, Norpramin)	Metabolic product of imipramine. Clinically less cardiotoxic than protriptyline, but probably not as activating. Low D-1, low H-1, low to moderate cholinergic, low alpha$_1$, and low serotonin receptor blocking.	Oral: 50–200 mg	Oral: 10–100 mg
Nortriptyline (Aventyl, Pamelor)	Clinically similar to desipramine. Unknown D-2, low H-1, low to moderate cholinergic, low alpha$_1$, and low serotonin receptor blocking.	Oral: 50–100 mg	Oral: 10–50 mg
Protriptyline (Vivactil)	May stimulate ventilation. Generally antidepressant of choice for retarded depressed patients with low motivation. Similar cardiotoxicity to amitriptyline. New generation antidepressants may substitute for this medication. Low D-2, low H-1, moderate cholinergic, low alpha$_1$, and low serotonin receptor blocking.	Oral: 5–60 mg	Oral: 2.5–20 mg
Tetracyclic Amines			
Maprotiline (Ludiomil)	Generally similar to protriptyline and desipramine with the exception that it appears to have the highest incidence of seizures of any antidepressant on the United States market. D-2 blocking unknown, H-1 blocking low to moderate, cholinergic blocking low, alpha$_1$ blocking low, and unknown serotonin receptor blocking.	Oral: 75–225 mg	Oral: 10–100 mg
Triazolopyridines			
Trazodone (Desyrel)	Associated with priapism and impotence subsequent to treatment of the priapism. Generally sedating. Low D-2, low H-1, low cholinergic, low alpha$_1$, and unknown serotonin receptor blocking.	Oral: 150–400 mg	Oral: 50–150 mg
Dibenzoxazepines			
Amoxapine (Asendin)	Useful in psychotic, depressed patients (in roughly the group of patients treated with combinations of antidepressants and neuroleptics). Has some of the side effects of neuroleptics, including extrapyramidal symptoms. Generally sedating. High D-2 (for an antidepressant), low H-1, low cholinergic, low alpha$_1$, and unknown serotonin receptor blocking.	Oral: 75–400 mg	Oral: 25–100 mg

TABLE 19–5. HETEROCYCLIC ANTIDEPRESSANTS *Continued*

Specific Medication	Special Properties	Usual Daily Dosage	Daily Dosage in Moderate to Severe COPD
Benzodiazepines (Triazolobenzodiazepine) Alprazolam (Xanax)	An anxiolytic with what may prove to be reasonable antidepressant characteristics.	Oral: 0.25–1 mg	Oral: 0.125–2 mg
Phenylpropylamines (Bicyclic) Fluoxetine (Prozac)	A bicyclic unrelated to the tricyclic antidepressants. A relatively specific serotonin reuptake blocker with little effect on other receptors. It is not a serotonin agonist. It is usually superior to protriptyline in retarded, depressed patients with low drive and motivation. Initial experience indicates that it is well tolerated and has few side effects in patients with pulmonary disease. The most frequent problems are nervousness, headache, insomnia, dry mouth, and diarrhea. The dose varies from 20–80 mg, with the average being 20–40 mg. It is important to note that many pulmonary disease patients do well with 20 mg every other or every third day. Occasionally, patients do well on 20 mg/wk. The intermittent dosing is possible because of the half-life of norfluoxetine (the major metabolite), which ranges from approximately 7 to 15 days. It has no D-2, no H-1, almost no cholinergic, low to no alpha, and low serotonergic receptor blocking.	Oral: 20–80 mg	Oral: From 20 mg every 7 days to 40 mg each day
Chloropropiophenones (Monocyclic) Bupropion (Wellbutrin)	A monocyclic that is structurally related to the amphetamines. The author is not aware of any publications on bupropion and chronic lung disease. It has no significant cardiac and (presumably) pulmonary effects. From basic and clinical literature on the medication, it should be superior to both protriptyline and fluoxetine in treatment of depressed, retarded pulmonary patients with low drive and motivation. The compound may cause weight loss and increased sexuality in pulmonary patients. The most frequent side effects are excitement and insomnia. It has no D-2, no H-1, no cholinergic, low to no alpha, and low to no serotonergic blocking. The half-life is approximately 14 hr, and it can usually be given in single or divided doses. Single doses of over 150 mg are not recommended.	Oral: 300 mg/day	Experience with patients who have chronic disease supports the use of from 75 mg/day to the rare use of 300 mg/day.

For all antidepressants listed, drowsiness or lack of attention may make operation of machinery dangerous, particularly during initial treatment.

A beneficial side effect of these medications in COPD patients may be mild bronchodilation. Selected patients may need the usual daily dose.

Common Side Effects	Precautions with	Contraindications
Dry mouth	Urinary retention	Acute myocardial infarction
Potential difficulty handling secretions	Cardiovascular disorders	Hypersensitivity
Blurred vision	Narrow angle glaucoma	Acute schizophrenia
Constipation	Organic brain syndrome	Mania
Nausea	Schizophrenia	Monoamine oxidase inhibitors
Heartburn	Mania	
Hypotension	Convulsive disorders	
Weight gain	Thyroid disease	
	Pregnancy	
	Potentiation of sympathomimetic amines	
	Blocking guanethidine	

TABLE 19-6. MANIC-DEPRESSIVE AGENTS

Specific Medication	Special Properties	Usual Daily Dosage	Daily Dosage in Moderate to Severe COPD
Lithium carbonate* (Eskalith, Lithane)	Reduces or stops cyclic mood swings. Prophylactic against recurrent mania or depression. Often takes 7–14 days for therapeutic effect to be seen. Give with psychiatric supervision. 20% or more of the population with manic-depressive disease do not respond or have unacceptable side effects, and other agents need to be utilized. Can produce diabetes insipidus.	Oral: 900–1800 mg/day until blood level of 0.8–1.2 mEq/L is attained; may have to be reduced to ½ to ⅔ of starting dosage for maintenance	Oral: Same dosage; aim for serum level of 0.6–1.0 mEq/L (stay on low side)
Carbamazapine (Tegretal)	An iminodibenzyl derivative with a tricyclic structure similar to that of the tricyclic antidepressants. For treatment of acute episodes, it is particularly efficacious in mania. It has a growing use in bipolar or schizoaffective patients who do not respond to or tolerate lithium. It has also been used in treatment of lithium-induced diabetes insipidus. Usually used as an antiseizure agent, but has growing applications as a psychotropic medication. The feared adverse effect of aplastic anemia is rare, but white blood cell count suppression early in treatment is common. Regular hematologic monitoring is recommended. Common side effects are dizziness, ataxia, and clumsiness. Use only under the supervision of those familiar with the medication.	Oral: 400–1400 mg/day until blood level of 4–12 mg/L is attained	Oral: Same dosage; aim for serum level of 2–10 mg/L (preferable to maintain lower levels)
Valproic acid (Depakote)	A GABA-ergic drug, strong antiseizure agent. Preliminary studies indicate that this medication may have antimanic characteristics. It should be used only by those familiar with its action and with the failure of other methods of controlling manic depressive disease.	Oral: 20–50 mg/kg/day until blood level of 20–100 mg/L is attained	Oral: Same dosage (check for carnitine deficiency)
Lecithin and Choline	Lecithin in doses between approximately 20 and 40 g has been shown to exert some antimanic activity. Adverse side effects seem to be onset of depression and diarrhea. Choline can produce an unpleasant body smell in about 20% of those who take it and is not recommended for those individuals.	Oral: 20–40 g	Oral: 20–40 g

*Blocks release of T-4; likely to precipitate depression; contraindicated with brain damage or significant cardiovascular or renal disease.
Considerable caution should be used with diuretics since lithium carbonate may be substituted for sodium and toxic levels of lithium rapidly produced, leading to potentially fatal cardiac arrhythmias. Caution should also be used when it is utilized in hot weather and the patient is losing salt.
Contraindicated in comatose states, presence of a large amount of CNS depressants, hypersensitivity, and history of addiction or habituation.

1. Neuroleptics, previously called major tranquilizers or antipsychotic agents. They are used in the treatment of diseases such as schizophrenia, mania, acute psychotic reactions, and, in some cases, delirium and dementia.
2. The heterocyclic antidepressants, called tricyclic antidepressants before the introduction of molecular structures that were not tricyclic in origin. They are used in the treatment of recurring or single episodes of depressive disease (bipolar or unipolar).
3. Medications for the control of swings in mood from depression to mania, from depression to a normal mood, or from mania to a normal mood. The only medication in this group recognized in the past was lithium carbonate. Increasing evidence indicates that there is a role for carbamazepine, lecithin, valproic acid, and other compounds.
4. Anxiolytic agents. These medications can be used for the control of anxiety in conjunction with any of the above compounds. They vary and include medications used to treat panic, seizures, and anxiety, or to induce sleep. They are safe if they are not abused. In general, when used alone, they have little effect on major psychiatric problems, and, in patients with

TABLE 19-7. ANXIOLYTIC AGENTS (MINOR TRANQUILIZERS OR SEDATIVE HYPNOTICS)

Specific Medication	Special Properties	Usual Daily Dosage	Daily Dosage in Moderate to Severe COPD
Benzodiazepines			
Chlordiazepoxide HCl (Librium)	May be drug of choice in alcohol withdrawal. Poor absorption by intramuscular route.	Oral: 10–20 mg IV: for treatment of acute reactions, including seizures and delirium tremens; 0.5 mg/kg at rate of 5 mg/min to total dose of 50 mg every 4–6 h	Oral: 10–50 mg IV: one-half the usual dose
Diazepam (Valium)	Good muscle relaxant. Poor absorption by intramuscular route.	Oral: 5–50 mg IV: For treatment of acute reactions, including seizures and delirium tremens: 0.1 mg/kg at a rate of 1 mg/min to a total dose of 5–10 mg every 4–6 h	Oral: 5–10 mg IV: one-half the usual dose
Chlorazepate dipotassium (Tranxene)	Antiseizure agent.	Oral: 3.75–45 mg	Oral: 3.75–15 mg
Alprazolam (Xanax)	Often recognized as the medication of choice in panic attacks and similar conditions. Also noted by some to have antidepressant properties (see Table 19–5).	Oral: 0.25–4.0 mg	Oral: 0.125–2.0 mg
Triazolam (Halcion)	Short half-life: approximately 2.5 h. Usually well-tolerated sleep medication. Can be utilized in low doses as a temporary treatment for anxiety (0.0625–0.125 mg) with low risk of sedation. Has reportedly been given in a dose of 0.125 mg daily for up to a year without producing habituation.	Oral: 0.125–0.5 mg	Oral: 0.0625–0.25 mg

Barbiturates produce unacceptable central nervous system depression, sedation, dependency, and addiction risk and have a low safety margin compared to the medications listed above, with the exception of meprobamate. For all anxiolytics listed, drowsiness or lack of attention may make operation of machinery dangerous, particularly during initial treatment. Selected patients may need the usual daily dose. Respiratory depression with aggravation or onset of hypoxia and hypercarbia is always a possible complication when the anxiolytic agents are used in the COPD population.

In selected patients with high anxiety levels, there may be no effect on respiratory drive, sedation, or habituation, and the primary effects may be symptom-reducing and lifesaving.

Common Side Effects	Precautions with	Contraindications
Drowsiness Ataxia Confusion Slurred speech Headache Dizziness Impaired visual accommodation Dependency Dry mouth Potential difficulty handling secretions	Glaucoma Anticoagulants Renal impairment Respiratory depression Hepatic impairment Pregnancy Withdraw slowly when used long-term to avoid problems such as convulsions Breast-feeding mothers: medication may be transferred via milk May occasionally produce paradoxical rage, anxiety, or depression	Hypersensitivity Porphyria (do not use meprobamate) Comatose states Severe dependency or addiction

psychiatric disorders, they should be used as an adjunct to the primary neuroleptic, antidepressant, or mood-controlling medication. They are most useful in the patient who is acutely or chronically emotionally upset.

With the availability of receptor-blocking profiles (see Tables 19–2 to 19–4) for many of these agents, the clinician can look up a particular medication and estimate the extent of its specific receptor-blocking characteristics. For example, if there is concern about anticholinergic effect, it is possible to find out how much of this characteristic the medication has in comparison with atropine, a familiar blocking agent. This is an area of medicine with a number of unanswerable questions, but the information is of undoubted use to the clinician.

REFERENCES

1. Dudley DL, Sitzman J. Psychobiologic evaluation and treatment of chronic obstructive pulmonary disease. In: McSweeny RJ, Grant I (eds). COPD: A Behavioral Perspective. Philadelphia: W. B. Saunders Co., 1988.
2. Dudley DL, Martin CJ, Masuda M, et al. The Psychophysiology of Respiration in Health and Disease. New York: Appleton-Century-Crofts, 1969.
3. Dudley DL, Welke E. How to Survive Being Alive. New York: Doubleday & Co., 1977.
4. Dudley DL, Holmes TH, Martin CJ, Ripley HA. Changes in respiration associated with hypnotically induced emotion, pain and exercise. Psychosom Med 1964; 26:46–57.
5. Dudley DL, Martin CJ, Holmes TH. Psychophysiologic studies of pulmonary ventilation. Psychosom Med 1964; 26:645–660.
6. Dudley DL, Martin CJ, Holmes TH. Dyspnea: Psychologic and physiologic observations. J Psychosom Res 1968; 11:325–339.
7. Dudley DL, Verhey JW, Masuda M, et al. Long term adjustment, prognosis and death in irreversible diffuse obstructive pulmonary syndromes. Psychosom Med 1969; 91:310–325.
8. Dudley DL, Pattison EM. Group psychotherapy in patients with severe diffuse obstructive pulmonary syndrome. Am Rev Respir Dis 1969; 100:575–576.
9. de Araujo G, Van Arsdel PP Jr, Holmes TH, Dudley DL. Life changes, coping ability and chronic intrinsic asthma. J Psychosom Res 1973; 17:359–363.
10. Petrich J, Holmes TH. Life change and illness onset. Med Clin North Am 1977; 61:825–838.
11. de Araujo G, Dudley DL, Van Arsdel PP Jr. Psychosocial assets and severity of chronic asthma. J Allergy Clin Immunol 1972; 50:257–263.
12. Dudley DL, Aickin M, Martin CJ. Cigarette smoking in a chest clinic population: Psychophysiologic variables. J Psychosom Res 1977; 21:367–375.
13. Wyler AR, Masuda M, Holmes TH. The seriousness of illness rating scale reproducibility. J Psychosom Res 1970; 14:59–64.
14. Wyler AR, Masuda M, Holmes TH. Magnitude of life events and seriousness of illness. Psychosom Med 1971; 33:115–122.
15. Knapp ML. Nonverbal Communication in Human Interaction. New York: Holt, Rinehart & Winston, Inc., 1972.
16. Beck AT, Ward CH, Mendelson M, et al. An inventory for measuring depression. Arch Gen Psychiatry 1961; 4:561–571.
17. Zung WW. A self-rating depression scale. Arch Gen Psychiatry 1965; 12:63–70.
18. Pattison EM, Rhodes RJ, Dudley DL. Response to group treatment in patients with severe chronic lung disease. Int J Group Psychother 1971; 21:214–225.
19. Dudley DL, Glaser EM, Jorgenson B, Logan DL. Psychosocial concomitants to rehabilitation in chronic obstructive pulmonary disease. Part I: The psychosocial and psychophysiologic format. Chest 1980; 77:413–420.
20. Dudley DL, Glaser EM, Jorgenson B, Logan DL. Psychosocial concomitants to rehabilitation in chronic obstructive pulmonary disease. Part II: The psychosocial and psychophysiologic treatment. Chest 1980; 77:544–551.
21. Dudley DL, Glaser EM, Jorgenson B, Logan DL. Psychosocial concomitants to rehabilitation in chronic obstructive pulmonary disease. Part III: Dealing with psychiatric disease. Chest 1980; 77:677–684.
22. Dudley DL, Pitts-Poarch AR. Psychophysiologic concepts of respiratory control. Clin Chest Med 1980; 1:131–143.
23. Dudley DL, Sitzman J. Psychosocial and psychophysiologic approach to the patient. Semin Respir Med 1979; 1:59–83.
24. Dudley DL, Sitzman J, Rugg M. Psychiatric aspects of patients with chronic obstructive pulmonary disease. Adv Psychosom Med 1985; 14:64–77.
25. American Psychiatric Association. Diagnostic and Statistical Manual of Mental Disorders. 3rd ed (revised). Washington, D.C.: The American Psychiatric Association, 1987.
26. Richelson E. Pharmacology of neuroleptics in use in the United States. J Clin Psychiatry 1985; 46:8–14.
27. Richelson E. Pharmacology of antidepressants in use in the United States. J Clin Psychiatry 1982; 43:4–11 and 1983; 44:4–9.
28. Knapp PH, Mathe AA, Vachon L. Psychosomatic aspects of bronchial asthma. In: Reiss EB, Segal M (eds). Bronchial Asthma: Mechanisms and Therapeutics. Boston: Little, Brown & Co., Inc., 1976.
29. Steen SN. The effects of psychotropic drugs on respiration. Pharmacol Ther 1976; 2:717–741.
30. Burks JS, Walter JE, Rumach BH. Tricyclic antidepressant poisoning. JAMA 1974; 230:1405–1407.
31. El-Yousef KM, Janowsky DS, Davis HM. Reversal of anti-parkinsonian drug toxicity by physostigmine: A controlled study. Am J Psychiatry 1973; 130:141–145.
32. Dudley DL, Schacher S. Depression in patients with respiratory disease. Chest Clin North Am 1989; 319–324.

Chapter 20

Home Ventilator Care

DAVID J. PIERSON, M.D.
ROBERT M. KACMAREK, Ph.D., R.R.T.

Long-term mechanical ventilation (LTMV) is the application of chronic ventilatory support to patients who are not in acute respiratory failure and who do not need the diagnostic, therapeutic, and monitoring capabilities of the intensive care unit (ICU). The first application of LTMV was during the polio epidemics of a half-century ago.[1, 2] Negative-pressure ventilation (NPV) via the "iron lung"[3-5] was successful in maintaining normal alveolar ventilation in persons with ventilatory muscle paralysis who otherwise would have died; some of these same individuals survive today. Intermittent positive-pressure ventilation (IPPV) via tracheostomy was introduced in France[6] and elsewhere[2, 7, 8] in the 1960s[2] and achieved success in managing not only paralyzed patients but also those with muscular dystrophy, kyphoscoliosis, and, in some cases, chronic obstructive pulmonary disease (COPD).[6] Variations for administering these therapies were introduced, such as the chest cuirass[5, 9] and other partial body enclosures[11-14] for NPV, the pneumobelt,[15, 16] the rocking bed,[11, 17] and the mouthpiece[18] and, more recently, the nasal mask[19-24] for IPPV.

Developments during the last decade have led to the emergence of two distinct concepts, or clinical settings, for LTMV: life support and elective therapy.[25-27] For patients with ventilatory muscle paralysis and other conditions that render their lungs incapable of sustaining normal gas exchange, LTMV constitutes a life support system; that is, such patients would die within minutes or hours without it. In a newer, more controversial application, LTMV is used electively in patients with progressive chronic respiratory insufficiency in an attempt to forestall the development of acute respiratory failure, to preserve function, and possibly to increase survival.

This chapter reviews the published experience with LTMV in these two clinical settings. It offers guidelines for the selection and discharge preparation of hospitalized ventilator-dependent patients, describes the skills and facilities necessary for carrying out LTMV in the home, and reviews the ventilators and other equipment currently available for this specialized form of therapy.

LONG-TERM MECHANICAL VENTILATION AS LIFE SUPPORT

As described above, this was the original setting for prolonged ventilatory support in persons who had recovered from acute respiratory failure but who could not breathe on their own. Life support remains the most common clinical purpose for LTMV. Figure 20–1 depicts the clinical sequence that typically leads to initiation of LTMV. A traumatic injury, acute illness, or progressive chronic condition causes the patient to be admitted to the ICU, intubated, and ventilated for acute respiratory failure. The patient survives this acute episode, but multiple attempts at ventilator weaning are unsuccessful.[28, 29] In this setting, usually after a prolonged ICU stay, the patient is considered for LTMV as a result of increasing pressure to move him or her out of the ICU.

Incentives for Moving the Patient Out of the Intensive Care Unit

Inpatient care has changed drastically in the United States during the 1980s with the advent of prospective

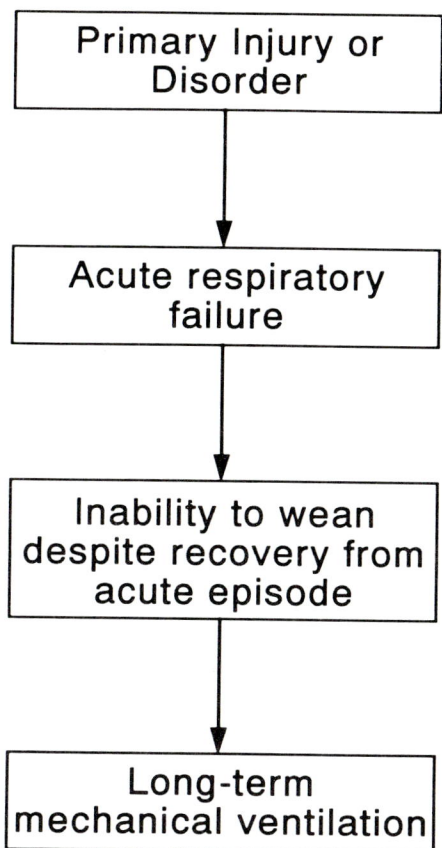

FIGURE 20-1. Usual clinical scenario for initiation of long-term mechanical ventilation (LTMV) as life support. See text for details.

payment and of other changes in the financing of hospital stays. These changes favor short-term stays and penalize hospitals for prolonged inpatient care, especially when this care is very expensive, as it is in the ICU. There is thus powerful economic motivation to discharge long-term, high-cost patients, the most glaring example of whom are perhaps those requiring mechanical ventilation.[30-32]

A stay in an ICU, especially when this includes mechanical ventilation through an artificial airway, predisposes patients to nosocomial infections and a host of other potentially life-threatening complications. The ICU environment also poses serious psychosocial threats to both patients and families.[33-36]

More compelling from the humanitarian point of view is the possibility of improving the lives of such patients. Once acute respiratory failure and other medical conditions have been reversed or controlled, movement out of the acute hospital setting to home or other stable environment offers the patient an opportunity to achieve at least some aspects of normal life.[30, 34]

Balanced against these motivations to discharge the patient from the hospital are several potential disadvantages that must be considered. They include adverse effects on family relationships,[34] less intense observation in the case of medical or mechanical problems, physical distance from the hospital or other medical care, and crushing financial costs if adequate insurance coverage cannot be obtained.[30]

Appropriate Diagnoses and Other Medical Considerations

Not all patients who stabilize but remain unweanable from the ventilator should be considered for LTMV, either in the home or elsewhere.[1] Clinical experience with thousands of patients over the last quarter century has demonstrated that certain diagnostic categories are more suitable to successful LTMV (i.e., survival, medical stability, manageable logistics, and acceptable quality of life) than are others. Table 20-1 lists the conditions that have been associated with favorable results along with those in which LTMV has tended to be much less successful.

In general, appropriate diagnoses are those that affect only the respiratory systems of individuals who are otherwise healthy, those that occur either in young people or in patients who have had years to prepare for possible LTMV while coping with a slowly and progressively deteriorating condition, and those whose effects on the respiratory system are static or only slowly progressive. The classic examples of such diagnoses are poliomyelitis and traumatic high cervical spinal cord injury. On the other hand, ventilatory insufficiency that occurs in the setting of progressive or multisystem disease (particularly in older individuals) or in primary lung disease that remains active and requires ongoing management (e.g., COPD) is not well suited to this form of therapy, and published results of the management of such conditions with LTMV have been disappointing.[7, 37-41]

Coexisting medical conditions can make LTMV less feasible if these conditions are debilitating or necessitate ongoing management. Examples are severe cardiac disease, psychiatric disorders, and cancer. As discussed later, discharge to the home setting can only be accomplished when the patient is emotionally prepared for this event; the same is true for medical stability and preparation. The following conditions should be met by the patient:[1]

- The absence or control of sustained dyspnea
- An oxygen requirement of less than 40%
- Stable ventilatory needs (e.g., ventilatory mode, tidal volume, ventilatory rate, and inspired oxygen fraction)
- Absence of acute infection
- Stability in other organ systems
- Stable metabolic, acid-base, and electrolyte status
- Adequate nutrition
- Ability to clear secretions and protect the airways

In addition, the patient's overall medical condition should be such that the need for readmission to the hospital is not foreseen for at least 1 month.[1]

Clinical Experience with Long-term Mechanical Ventilation as Life Support

Reported experience from several medical centers[37, 41-43] bears out the observation that LTMV is more

TABLE 20-1. LONG-TERM MECHANICAL VENTILATION AS LIFE SUPPORT: DIAGNOSES

Site or Type of Defect	Favorable Diagnoses	Unfavorable Diagnoses
Ventilatory drive	Central hypoventilation syndromes Ondine's curse Arnold-Chiari malformation	Cerebrovascular accident (stroke) Malignancy
Neural transmission to the ventilatory muscles	High cervical spinal cord injury Poliomyelitis Guillain-Barré syndrome Bilateral phrenic nerve paralysis	Amyotrophic lateral sclerosis Multiple sclerosis
Ventilatory muscles	Muscular dystrophy Congenital myopathies	
Bony thorax	Kyphoscoliosis Post-thoracoplasty	
Lungs and airways	Bronchopulmonary dysplasia	Chronic obstructive pulmonary disease Bronchiectasis Cystic fibrosis Interstitial lung disease Adult respiratory distress syndrome

successful in some patient populations than in others. Patients with neuromuscular and skeletal disorders generally do well, whereas those with primary pulmonary disease do not. In the largest series reported to date,[37] Robert and colleagues followed 222 patients for up to 20 years in Lyon, France. In this series, 41 patients with sequelae of poliomyelitis had a 5-year survival rate of 95%, and 87% of the patients were alive at 10 years; 73% and 61% of a smaller number of individuals were alive at 20 and 25 years, respectively.[37] At the other extreme, of 50 patients with COPD, 28% died during the first 2 years of LTMV, and only 18% survived for 5 years; experience was similar with 10 patients with bronchiectasis, none of whom survived for 5 years. Survival rates for the different diagnostic groups in the Lyon series are shown in Figure 20–2.[37] The experience at other centers has been similar.[39,41]

The differences among diagnoses extend beyond survival and include day-to-day morbidity, the need for recurrent acute hospitalization, the ability to leave the home on a regular basis, and other aspects related to quality of life. Table 20–2 summarizes these and other aspects of the experience from Lyon.[37]

LONG-TERM MECHANICAL VENTILATION AS ELECTIVE THERAPY TO REST THE VENTILATORY MUSCLES

History and Rationale

Muscle fatigue may be defined as a condition in which there is a loss in the capacity for developing force, the velocity of muscle contraction, or both, resulting from muscle activity under load, which is reversible by rest.[44] Since the early 1980s, much attention has been focused on the ventilatory muscles, and it is currently believed by many investigators that progressive muscle fatigue is an important contributor to the development of acute ventilatory failure in patients with chronic respiratory insufficiency. It is further believed, although it has not been proved, that resting the ventilatory muscles enables them to recover from the fatigued state, thus improving their contractility and endurance.

Studies have shown that signs of ventilatory muscle fatigue can be reduced or eliminated following a period of controlled ventilation.[45] In view of this, there is considerable current interest in the use of elective resting of the ventilatory muscles for several hours on a daily basis in an effort to improve ventilatory function between periods of rest.[25] If such were the case and if ventilatory muscle fatigue were important in the genesis of progressive deterioration in patients with chronic ventilatory insufficiency, then LTMV might improve function, reduce the need for hospitalization, forestall the development of acute ventilatory failure, and even increase survival (Fig. 20–3). Although convincing proof of these beneficial effects is not yet available, a number of investigators have obtained encouraging results in certain patient groups,[14, 22-24, 26, 46-48] and recommendations can be made as to which patients would be expected to benefit most from this therapy.

Appropriate Diagnoses and Other Medical Considerations

With the exception of acute cervical spinal cord transection and other paralytic states, the patient groups best suited to LTMV as elective therapy are the same ones who were discussed previously as best suited for LTMV for life support (e.g., patients with muscular dystrophy, postpolio chronic respiratory insufficiency, kyphoscoliosis, and the late sequelae of thoracoplasty). Such patients have respiratory insufficiency in the setting of restrictive disease, which does not primarily affect the lung parenchyma. Individuals with obstructive lung disease (e.g., COPD and cystic fibrosis) or with primary restrictive pulmonary disease (e.g., interstitial pulmonary fibrosis) are not good candidates, and clinical

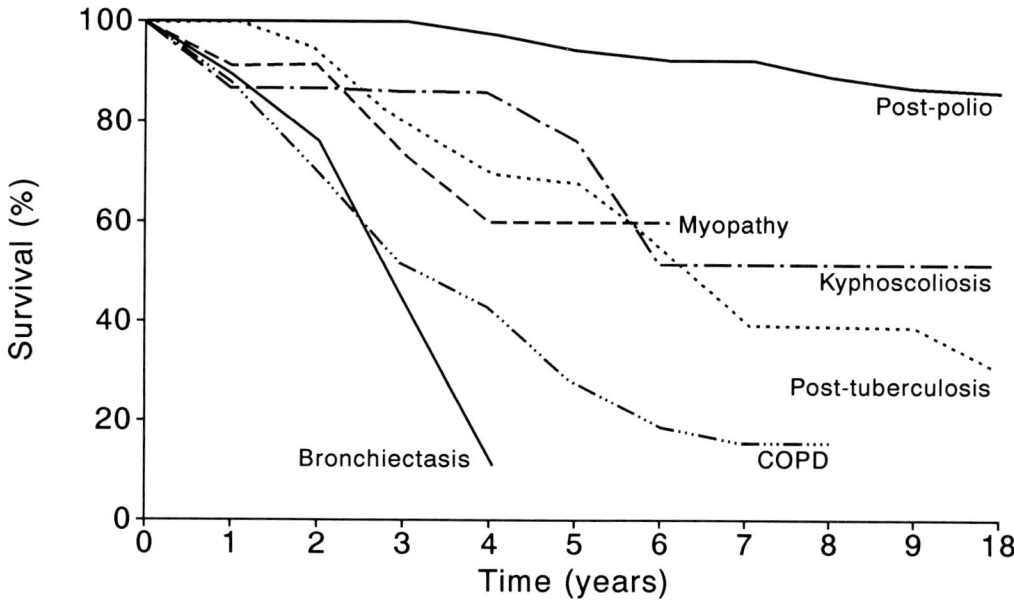

FIGURE 20–2. Actuarialized survival among 222 patients with various respiratory diseases ventilated at home via tracheostomy and positive-pressure ventilation from 1960 to 1982. (From Robert D, Gerard M, Leger P, et al. Domiciliary mechanical ventilation by tracheostomy for chronic respiratory failure. Rev Fr Mal Respir 1983; 11:923–936.)

experience with this therapy in such settings has been disappointing.

Because part-time ventilatory assistance is an elective treatment applied to patients who are less seriously ill than those discussed in the preceeding section, it does not require such extensive resources and training as LTMV for life support. Since patients can usually initiate and terminate the session of mechanically-assisted breathing by themselves, it is unnecessary to have a caregiver in attendance, and no back-up ventilator is required. In most instances, the period of ventilatory assistance is timed to coincide with or include the patient's hours of sleep.

Clinical Experience with LTMV as Elective Therapy

Clinical experience with LTMV as elective therapy to rest the ventilatory muscles is rapidly accumulating.* More than 15 years ago, Rochester and associates[51] demonstrated that the ventilatory muscles of hypercapnic COPD patients could in fact be rested using NPV, and other investigators have subsequently confirmed these observations.[13] Different techniques of ventilatory assistance and different types of apparatus vary in the degree to which they can achieve true muscle rest,[44] and a recent study found that IPPV via nasal mask was more effective in this respect than NPV via Pneumowrap.[52]

Whether elective LTMV can actually produce the results implied in Figure 20–3 (i.e., the preservation of physiologic and clinical function and the avoidance of

---
*See references 12, 14, 18–20, 22–24, 26, and 47–50.

acute respiratory failure) is less certain, particularly in COPD. However, encouraging results have been reported in patients with neuromuscular and restrictive disorders. The Lyon group[23] recently reported on 29 such patients (5 with neuromuscular disease, 15 with kyphoscoliosis, and 9 who had had tuberculosis) on whom clinical and physiologic data were available prior to and after 1 year of elective LTMV using IPPV via nasal mask. All patients had been followed by the investigators for more than 1 year prior to the institution of nocturnal ventilation and had progressive chronic respiratory insufficiency. Total lung capacity in these patients averaged 45% of predicted values; they also had progressive hypoxemia and hypercapnia. Figure 20–4 shows their Pa_{O_2} and Pa_{CO_2} values 1 year before LTMV was begun, at the time it was started, and while they breathed spontaneously for several hours after 1 year of nocturnal ventilatory assistance.[23]

The patients in this study tolerated the nasal mask ventilation well and experienced no serious adverse effects. Subjectively, they noted the disappearance of morning headaches, improved quality of sleep, and increased social activity (i.e., 17 of the 29 were able to leave the house more than three times per week, 8 resumed driving, and 6 returned to work[23]). The results of this study need to be confirmed and extended by other groups and in other patient populations, but it would appear that elective LTMV can produce both physiologic and symptomatic benefits in at least some patient populations.

PLACEMENT ALTERNATIVES OUTSIDE THE HOSPITAL

Home is the preferred discharge destination for the majority of patients, and in many communities it is the

TABLE 20–2. CLINICAL STATUS OF 222 PATIENTS RECEIVING HOME POSITIVE-PRESSURE VENTILATION VIA TRACHEOSTOMY*

Diagnosis	Polio	Myopathy	Kyphoscoliosis	Sequelae of Tuberculosis	COPD	Bronchiectasis
Number of patients	41	13	53	55	50	10
H/day on ventilator (mean)	15	17	11	12	12	20
Frequency of suctioning (times/day)	<1	<1	4	10	15	50
Days of acute illness at home per year	7	7	13	18	23	66
Days of hospitalization per year	3	7	6	8	12	22
Per cent of patients able to leave home more than 3 times/wk	38	—	33	24	25	0
Five-year survival rate (%)	95	62	77	70	18	0

*Adapted from Robert D, Gerard M, Leger P, et al. Domiciliary mechanical ventilation by tracheostomy for chronic respiratory failure. Rev Fr Mal Respir 1983; 11:923–936.

only available alternative to an acute care hospital.[53, 54] However, depending on local resources and funding, there are several other potential sites for long-term ventilator care. Skilled nursing facilities may include extended care facilities, chronic care hospitals, convalescent centers, or nursing homes.[1, 53, 54] Care in such facilities is still impossible for many patients in the United States because of inadequate financial reimbursement; however, it is being made available to an increasing number of individuals in some areas. Some hospitals own or contract with a nursing home and can utilize part of the nursing home for ventilator patients, thus realizing large financial savings in comparison with care in an ICU, a step-down unit, or an acute medical-surgical ward.

Specialized respiratory care centers exist in some areas.[1, 53, 54] Some of these are facilities that formerly managed polio survivors and have recently expanded their patient populations to include other disorders requiring LTMV. More recently, the United States Health Care Financing Administration has established demonstration units for ventilator-assisted patients in hospitals.[55–57] These units are not primarily for long-term ventilator patients, but they may yield important cost-effectiveness data to facilitate the federal funding of other types of units for LTMV in the future.

In some areas, congregate living centers have been established. These centers are adaptations of private homes for the care of several ventilator-dependent individuals.[53, 54] In several such facilities, patients have

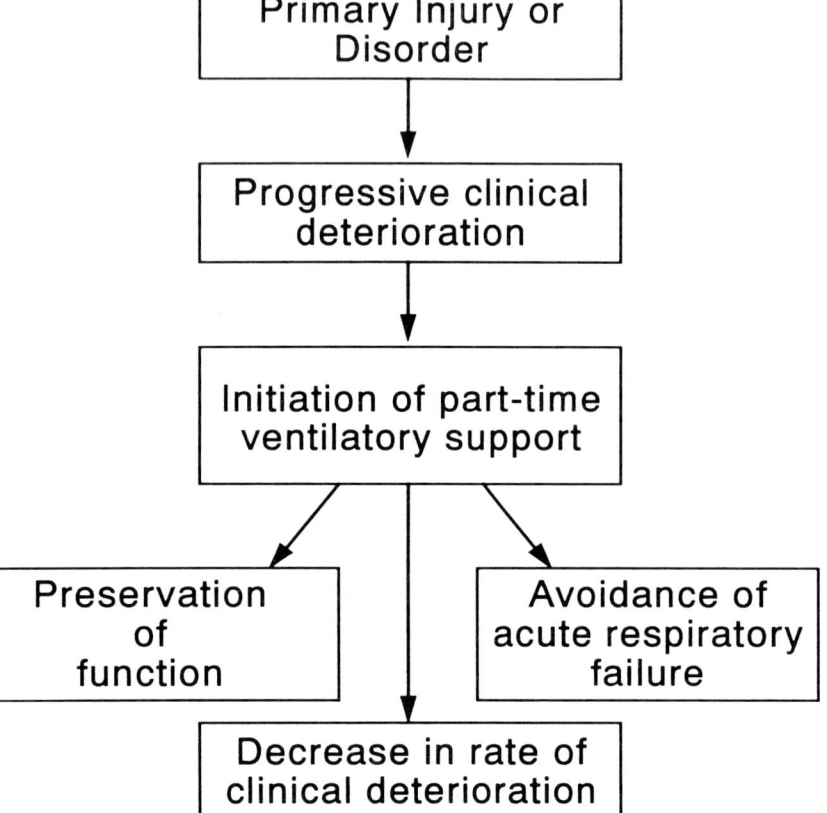

FIGURE 20–3. Clinical setting and rationale for initiation of LTMV as an elective therapy rather than as a life-support system. See text for details.

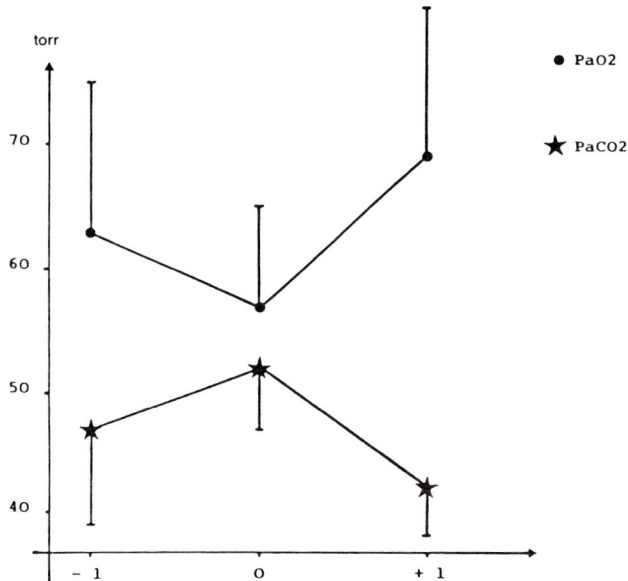

FIGURE 20–4. Changes in PaO_2 and PaCO_2 with elective nocturnal intermittent positive-pressure ventilation (NIPPV) via nasal mask in 29 patients with neuromuscular or restrictive disease. Data are compared from 1 year prior to initiation of LTMV (−1), from the onset of LTMV (0), and after 1 year of LTMV (+1). Arterial blood gases were drawn while the patients were spontaneously breathing air, and in the last two data sets, after they were off the ventilator for at least 4 hours. (From Leger P, Jennequin J, Gerard M, et al. Home positive-pressure ventilation via nasal mask for patients with neuromuscular weakness or restrictive lung or chest wall disease. Respir Care 1989; 34:73–77.)

more autonomy (e.g., single rooms, a greater degree of decision-making, and regular chores and responsibilities) than in other long-term care centers. However, substantial changes in funding regulations would be required before this type of facility could be made more widely available to ventilator-dependent patients.

PATIENT SELECTION FOR HOME VENTILATOR CARE

Ventilator care in the home is a complicated, multidisciplinary activity requiring that each of numerous individual aspects be considered and satisfactorily carried out.[1, 30, 41, 58, 59] These aspects can be summarized in the eight categories listed in Table 20–3.[30] The nonmedical aspects of patient selection for LTMV have been reviewed by Gilmartin.[1] It is important to remember that much more than biomedical data is required for successful selection. Table 20–4[1] summarizes the personality traits and other personal factors that determine whether a given individual is a good candidate for LTMV.

Many of the characteristics listed in Table 20–4 can be assessed through psychologic testing and the taking of a thorough history.[1, 60] A person's ability to cope with stressors in the past is a good indicator of how he or she will likely cope with the stress of LTMV. Optimism is a crucial factor; the patient who is well suited for LTMV looks forward to leaving the hospital and has plans for the future. The patient must be motivated and an active participant in the process of discharge planning; those who passively accept the direction of others and take no active part in directing their care are less likely to do well in the home setting. A sense of humor in such a patient is extremely helpful.

As shown in Table 20–4, the ideal patient has a close, supportive family, a college education, and a certain degree of financial security in addition to the personality characteristics just mentioned. Unfortunately, many candidates for LTMV do not meet these requirements. However, the characteristics listed in the middle column in Table 20–4 can be considered minimum qualifications for LTMV. Too often, patients lacking these characteristics are referred for discharge to the home; in the presence of those aspects shown in the right-hand column, it is most unlikely that home ventilator care will succeed.

DISCHARGE PLANNING

The key to successful placement of a ventilator-dependent patient in the home is a well-coordinated discharge process.[1] Generally, involvement in this process is required by the discharging physician, the primary nurse, the respiratory therapist caring for the patient, and the agencies providing care in the home. However, numerous other individuals (Table 20–5) may also be necessary, depending on the particular needs of the patient and the professional role delineations within an institution. The most effective discharges are those coordinated by an assigned case manager who may be the primary nurse, a respiratory therapist, the continuing care nurse, or a social worker. Generally, it is the case manager's responsibility to see that all aspects of care are appropriately coordinated and that individual aspects of the discharge are followed to completion.[1] It is critically important that all discharge planning meetings be attended by all involved in the process, including the patient (if he or she is capable of managing his or her own care) or the family member who functions as the primary caregiver in the home. At these meetings, a thorough assessment of all potential needs of the patient is performed. This assessment should address home care equipment, the need for continuing nursing care, rehabilitation services, and reimbursement.[58]

The insurance coverage and financial capability of the family need to be carefully assessed early in the discharge process. Many families are unaware of the costs associated with LTMV, nor are they aware of the coverage that is provided by their insurer. Normally, the social worker or continuing care nurse reviews this aspect of care and establishes guidelines before the discharge process has progressed significantly.

Assessment and input by rehabilitative services personnel (e.g., physical and occupational therapists) are essential in determining the types of nonventilatory assistive devices required (e.g., wheelchairs and bathing aids) as well as the rehabilitative potential of the patient.

TABLE 20–3. FACTORS DETERMINING WHETHER A VENTILATOR-DEPENDENT PATIENT CAN LEAVE THE HOSPITAL

Aspect	Factors
Illness	Primary diagnosis; coexisting disease; medical stability
Patient	Mental status; psychologic profile; motivation (see Table 20–4)
Family	Relationship to patient; strengths/weaknesses; motivation
Home	Physical and psychologic environment; alternative care sites
Ventilator	Capabilities in relation to patient's needs; simplicity; reliability
Funding	Reimbursement for professional services and equipment
Team	Physicians; primary caregivers; home care providers; equipment maintenance and supply
Plan	Specific goals; stepwise approach; continuity

Strength- and endurance-building programs are normally developed to enhance activities of daily living. In patients requiring tracheostomy tubes, a skilled speech therapist is invaluable in establishing communication systems.[61]

The respiratory therapist and the provider of durable medical equipment are primarily involved in the selection, set-up, and instruction in the use of the respiratory care equipment that is to be employed in the home. It is essential that the specific equipment to be taken home be used in the hospital for a period of days to weeks to ensure appropriate operation, suitable adjustment, and complete operational understanding by the patient and primary caregivers in the home.

The primary nurse plays a central role in the discharge process by coordinating the daily activities of the patient, by assisting in the teaching of self-care and respiratory care techniques, and by ensuring that the stresses of the discharge process do not overwhelm the patient and family. The discharging physician has a key role in ensuring that the patient and family understand the limitations of LTMV and have realistic expectations of the outcome of the process. He or she must advise team members of the patient's overall medical status and provide leadership and guidance.

The Home Care Team

Key in the overall discharge process is the realization by all hospital-based personnel that they are preparing the patient to be managed by a *home care team,* which normally consists of the patient, the family, the supplier of the durable medical equipment, and, potentially, home nursing agencies, community service groups, and privately funded caregivers. Generally, the supplier of the durable medical equipment is responsible for the operation and care of all equipment used in the home. In the case of the LTMV patient, home respiratory therapy personnel are included in the service and provide home visits on a routine basis to evaluate both equipment function and patient status. Depending on the patient's overall medical status, the capabilities of the family, and the age of the patient, nursing personnel

TABLE 20–4. PATIENT CHARACTERISTICS THAT MAY DETERMINE SUCCESS IN HOME VENTILATOR CARE*

	Ideal	Acceptable	Unacceptable
Individual coping styles	Optimistic Motivated Resourceful Flexible Adaptable Sense of humor Directive	Optimistic Motivated Sense of humor	None
Support systems	Close family and social supports	Social supports	Lack of family and social supports
Education	College degree Ability to learn	Able to learn Mechanically astute	Altered mental status Unable to learn
Financial resources	Adequate personal assets Optimal health insurance coverage	Adequate health insurance coverage	Lack of personal assets Lack of health insurance
Medical condition	Stable neuromuscular disease Significant "free time" off the ventilator No other medical illnesses	Stable neuromuscular or obstructive airway disease Limited or no "free time" off the ventilator	Medically unstable
Self-care ability	Ability to provide self-care, to direct others, or both	Able to provide self-care	Unable to care for self or to direct others

*From Gilmartin, ME. Long-term mechanical ventilation outside the hospital. In: Pierson DJ, Kacmarek RM (eds). Foundations of Respiratory Care. New York: Churchill Livingstone, Inc., 1992, p 1189.

TABLE 20-5. DISCHARGE TEAM MEMBERS AND ROLES FOR HOME CARE OF THE VENTILATOR-DEPENDENT INDIVIDUAL

Primary Team Members	
Member	**Role**
Physician	Team leader; establishes medical stability
	Informs family and patient of limitations of LTMV
	Sets realistic expectations
Nurse	Coordinates bedside activities
	Teaches self-care
	Teaches respiratory care
	Prepares family for independence
Respiratory therapist	Selects respiratory care equipment
	Ensures that equipment functions properly
	Teaches operation
	Ensures that patient and family understand equipment's operation
Durable medical equipment supplier	Supplies all home care equipment
	Maintains and teaches operation
	Provides routine in-home evaluation
	Assesses home environment

Secondary Team Members	
Member	**Role**
Social worker/continuing care nurse	Coordinates overall discharge
	Ensures insurance coverage
	Assesses family financial capability
	Assists family in interactions with outside agencies
Physical therapist	Establishes rehabilitation program
	Enhances mobility
Occupational therapist	Determines need for nonventilatory assistance devices
	Assists in identification and correction of barriers to mobility in the home
Speech therapist	Develops communication systems
Nutritionist	Outlines dietary needs
	Establishes recommended diet
Psychiatric services	Assist with transitional adjustments
	Assess need for psychotropic medication
	Assess cognitive capability of patient

may be required as infrequently as once per month or continuously for 24 hours per day. The more limited the patient's ability to ventilate independently of the ventilator, the younger his or her age, and the more compromised the ability of the family to provide care, the greater the need for regular home nursing assistance. Of all the costs associated with home care, those for nursing assistance contribute most to monthly expenses.

The patient and family members are essential components of the home care team. Their desire to ensure that the home care experience is rewarding is the primary factor in its success. Ideally, patients should direct their own home care.

Assessment of the Home

Prior to discharge, a careful assessment of the home environment is performed, frequently by both the supplier of the durable medical equipment and by the hospital team. Of primary concern is the capability of the electrical system. Ideally, the ventilator should be operated from its own circuit.[62] Systems to provide backup electrical power in the event of a power failure must be developed. Barriers to access to the home must be modified. Ramps may need to be built for the wheelchair-dependent patient.

One of the primary barriers to successful discharge is fear and ambivalence on part of the patient about leaving the hospital. This is best averted by a well-coordinated discharge process in which communication is appropriate at all levels. Frequently, the process must be instituted weeks to months before the anticipated discharge.[1] As soon as the likelihood of LTMV is anticipated, the process should begin. The discharge process normally doomed to failure is the one that is begun on a Monday and plans discharge on Friday of the same week.

EQUIPMENT USED FOR HOME VENTILATORY CARE

Numerous specific types of equipment are currently available for use in home ventilatory assistance programs.[63] Most health care professionals immediately think of positive-pressure devices for the provision of ventilatory assistance; however, numerous approaches to noninvasive, nonpositive-pressure ventilation are available. Even with positive-pressure ventilation, both invasive and noninvasive approaches are currently used.

Approaches Other Than Positive-Pressure Ventilation

In this category, three specific approaches are currently available: NPV, the use of Pneumobelts, and the utilization of rocking beds. Each is effective in assisting with gas movement in select patient groups, although none is as effective as IPPV. However, these approaches should always be considered when a home ventilatory assistance program is established, especially if the patient's ventilatory problem has arisen from neurologic or neuromuscular abnormalities.[9–11, 13]

Negative-Pressure Ventilation

Negative-pressure ventilatory assist devices represent the oldest group of commercially available mechanical ventilators still available in the United States. Iron lungs have been used since the late 1920s to provide ventilatory support to patients with neuromuscular and neurologic disorders.[3] More recently, some authors have demonstrated limited success using negative-pressure nocturnal ventilation in patients with COPD and ventilatory muscle dysfunction associated with chronic ventilatory failure.[13, 52] Of primary concern with the use of negative-pressure ventilation is the fact that all except one of the negative-pressure generators is a controller. As a result, it is difficult to coordinate these units with the patient's ventilatory drive on a continual basis. In addition, no mechanisms are included to abort the development of negative pressure once the unit activates the inspiratory phase, regardless of what the patient desires. Few patients—particularly those with COPD—adjust to this controlled, nonflexible approach to ventilator support.

Negative-pressure systems are cumbersome and difficult for patients to assemble independently. They make it problematic for the patient to get out of bed in the middle of the night or to sleep in anything but the supine position. Patients also frequently complain of being cold during therapy, since the negative pressure causes air to be drawn across the patient's chest during inspiration. The sensation of cold adversely affects compliance. Finally, NPV is contraindicated in patients with upper airway obstruction.[1, 5] The enhanced development of negative intrathoracic pressure increases the frequency and severity of upper airway obstruction.[5] The use of negative pressure has been most successful in the management of children and young adults with neuromuscular or neurologic disorders.

Numerous approaches to NPV (Table 20–6) are currently available, and each has its own unique problems. It is our opinion that the use of a customized chest cuirass (Fig. 20–5) is better tolerated than any of the other available approaches.

Pneumobelts

The Pneumobelt (Fig. 20–6) is designed to provide periodic ventilatory assistance to patients requiring negative-pressure or positive-pressure assistance on an almost continuous basis.[15, 16] It functions by exerting a positive pressure on the abdomen that forces the abdomen cephalad, thus assisting exhalation (Fig. 20–7). Inspiration must proceed by means of the patient's own efforts. With proper application, the patient's functional residual capacity is reduced during assisted exhalation, and its re-expansion assists in increasing tidal volume and in decreasing the work of breathing. Tidal volumes of 300 to 500 ml are attainable with this device.[15]

To ensure proper function, the appropriate size Pneumobelt should be selected and fitted snugly over the abdomen from the xiphoid process to just above the pelvic arch.[63] Fit is important to prevent paradoxical movement of the rib cage during exhalation. Depending on patient size, pressures between 30 and 50 cm H_2O must be applied through the Pneumobelt.[16] In doing so, a volume of 1000 to 2000 ml is normally needed to inflate the belt.[15] In addition, the patient should ideally be seated at a 75-degree angle from the supine position. As the angle decreases, the effectiveness of the belt decreases. Any positive-pressure generator capable of generating in excess of 50 cm H_2O and of delivering a 2.0-L volume may be used to power the Pneumobelt.

Rocking Bed

As with Pneumobelts, rocking beds (Fig. 20–8) are usually used in conjunction with other approaches to ventilatory support. In the neuromuscularly or neurologically diseased patient of relatively normal body weight and with some abdominal girth, the rocking motion of the bed assists spontaneous breathing and the establishment of tidal volumes of 250 to 400 ml.[17] This device is best for patients who have diaphragm paralysis

TABLE 20–6. NEGATIVE-PRESSURE VENTILATION

Enclosure*	Description	Comments
Iron lung	Full-body enclosure	Heavy, immobile; requires assistance to enter or exit; costly
Porta lung	Full-body enclosure	Lightweight (about 50 lb), portable; requires assistance to enter or exit
Chest cuirass	Chest covering; mass-produced or customized	Customized units fit better than those mass-produced; patient can enter and exit without assistance; large air leak can occur if unit is poorly fitted
Raincoat	Poncho covering chest, part of arms, and torso to midhip level with shell-like grid over chest	Difficult to enter and exit without assistance; large air leak common; generally poorly tolerated
Pneumosuit	Full-body suit covering arms and legs with shell-like grid over chest	Difficult to enter and exit without assistance; air leakage is minimized by full-body covering.

*All enclosures except the iron lung require a separate negative-pressure generator for normal operation.

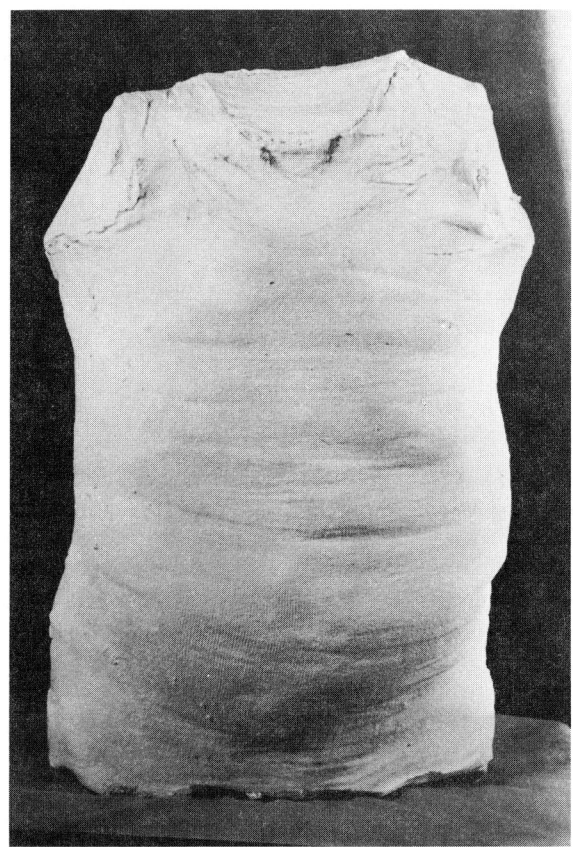

FIGURE 20–5. Cast of the thorax used to make a customized chest cuirass.

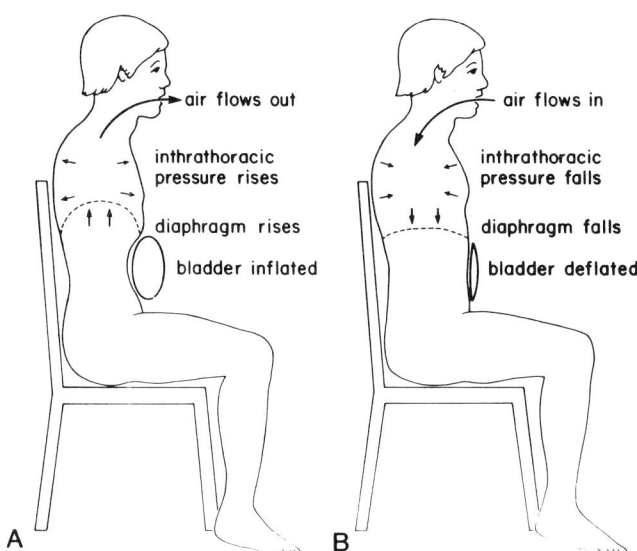

FIGURE 20–7. Illustration of the function of the Pneumobelt. The Pneumobelt functions by exerting pressure on the abdominal contents by means of the inflation of a rubber bladder, which forces the diaphragm upward and assists exhalation (*A*). When the bladder deflates, gravity pulls the diaphragm back down, thus assisting inhalation (*B*). (From Hill NS. Clinical application of body ventilators. Chest 1986; 90:897–905.)

but also some accessory muscle use and who do not have primary pulmonary disease.[1, 11] Its operation is based on the effect that gravity has on the abdominal contents; that is, as the bed rocks, the abdominal contents shift, which assists in the movement of the diaphragm. When the bed tilts head down, exhalation is assisted; when the head tilts up, inspiration is assisted.

The bed can move through a total arc of up to 60 degrees, a maximum of 30 degrees head down, and a maximum of 30 degrees head up. Generally, a 15-degree head-down tilt combined with a 30-degree head-up tilt is sufficient for most patients.[17, 63] The rate of tilt may be adjusted to between 8 per minute and 34 per minute, and a break at the knee can be established to prevent sliding. The rocking bed and the Pneumobelt function as controllers and may not be tolerated by anxious patients who frequently desire to change their ventila-

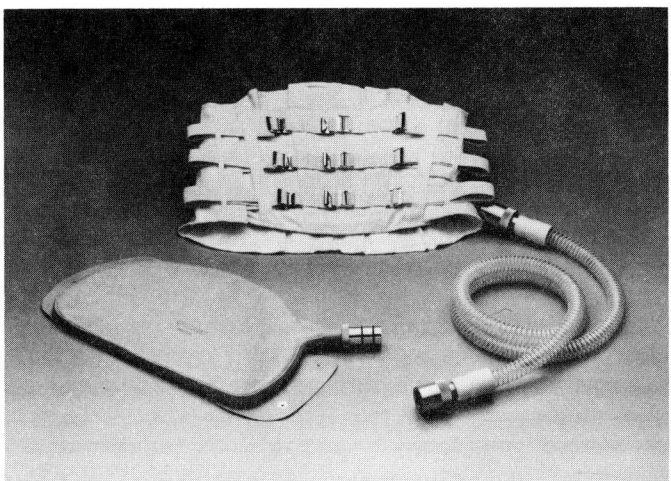

FIGURE 20–6. The Pneumobelt, a bladder, and an abdominal belt. (Provided by Lifecare, Boulder, CO.)

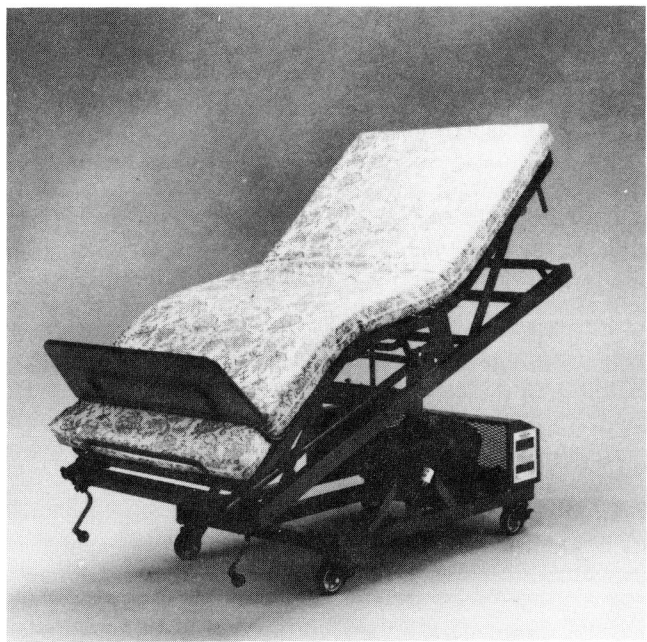

FIGURE 20–8. The Emerson rocking bed. (Provided by Lifecare, Boulder, CO.)

tory rate. In addition, motion sickness is common with the rocking bed.

Positive-Pressure Ventilation

Historically, positive-pressure ventilation (PPV) has been provided via a tracheostomy. However, recent data indicate successful administration of PPV via nasal mask, particularly in those circumstances where the institution of ventilatory assistance is elective.[19-26] All of the ventilators currently available for the application of positive pressure in the home care setting may be used to apply noninvasive nasal PPV. However, only the Respironics BiPAP unit has been designed especially for this purpose.[64]

Elective Nasal Positive-Pressure Ventilation

Successful use of nasal PPV requires a commitment from both the patient and the caregiver. Patients must be willing to tolerate a nasal mask strapped to the face for periods of 6 to 8 hours daily, whereas the caregivers must have the time and patience to sit with the patient for long periods to ensure the proper adjustment of the ventilator and to verify the achievement of the goals of elective nasal PPV. Most applications of nasal PPV are designed to allow ventilatory muscle rest and recovery to ensure maximum muscle capability when nasal PPV is not in use.[23, 25, 26] Proper setting of the ventilator ensures controlled ventilation during sleep. Assist/control back-up rates must be set high to eliminate the patient's need to trigger the ventilator, thus assuring complete rest of the ventilatory muscles. Optimal set-up results in mild hyperventilation and a decrease in ventilatory drive; this enhances the likelihood of patient/ventilator synchrony.[20, 22]

Invasive Positive-Pressure Ventilation

The provision of PPV via a tracheostomy normally implies the need for PPV to prevent acute ventilatory failure. As noted above, this is not the case with nasal PPV. Most patients receiving nasal PPV can function independently of ventilatory support for prolonged periods of time. The fact that the patient has a tracheotomy tube in place and requires mechanical ventilation also defines the need for additional equipment (e.g., airway care equipment, remote alarm systems, manual ventilators, and back-up mechanical ventilators) to be made available in the home (Table 20–7).

Positive-Pressure Ventilators

Numerous mechanical ventilators that are designed for home use are currently available. Each is capable of providing both invasive and noninvasive ventilatory support. The one exception is the Respironics BiPAP unit. It is not alarmed and does not provide any indication of patient respiratory rate, tidal volume, or pressure development during ventilation; as a result, it should only

TABLE 20–7. EQUIPMENT FREQUENTLY REQUIRED DURING INVASIVE POSITIVE-PRESSURE VENTILATION IN THE HOME

Primary ventilator
Back-up ventilator*
System humidifier
Ventilator circuits
Oxygen source
Suction apparatus
Suction equipment
Spare tracheostomy tube
Remote alarm
Battery
Battery charger
Manual ventilator
Compressor for aerosol medication
Small-volume nebulizer
Electrical generator*

*Only necessary if patient requires ventilatory support for longer than 16 h/day or is located more than a 4-h distance from a hospital.

be used for noninvasive nasal PPV. The ventilators most commonly used today for home mechanical ventilation are the Aequitron LP-6, Aequitron LP-10, Puritan Bennett 2800, Puritan Bennett 2801, Lifecare PLV-100, and Intermed Bear 33 (Table 20–8).

Modes of Ventilation. Figure 20–9 depicts the internal gas delivery system common to all of the above mentioned units except the Respironics BiPAP. As illustrated, all of the devices utilize a piston delivery system and do not have the capability of demand gas delivery.[65] It is important to appreciate the problems inherent in the intermittent mandatory ventilation/synchronized intermittent mandatory ventilation (IMV/SIMV) mode on all of these units. None of them functions as does an ICU ventilator because of the absence of demand or continuous flow.[65] As a result, during the spontaneous breathing phase of IMV/SIMV, the patient must draw gas (1) through the air intake valve of the piston chamber via the piston chamber itself (however, gas flow via this route is not available during the backstroke of the piston); (2) through an antisuffocation valve located within the machine between the piston and the exit port for gas flow from the ventilator; or (3) through the exhalation valve of the ventilator circuit. The workload experienced by the patient during the spontaneous breathing phase of IMV/SIMV is markedly elevated.[65] As a result, we only recommend the use of the assist/control mode during home mechanical ventilation. If IMV/SIMV is desired, we would recommend a modification of the inspiratory circuit (Fig. 20–10) that would allow spontaneous breathing via a one-way valve to atmosphere and the use of a passover humidifier.[65]

The Respironics BiPAP unit is unique in that it provides a continuous gas flow and allows for the setting of CPAP (continuous positive airway pressure, referred to as expiratory PAP) and an inspiratory pressure plateau (inspiratory positive airway pressure [IPAP], which is actually similar to pressure support or pressure control ventilation).[64] This unit's modes are labeled "spontaneous," "spontaneous/timed," and "timed" and are equivalent to the "assist," "assist/control," and "controlled" modes of other ventilators. The BiPAP also

TABLE 20-8. CAPABILITIES OF SELECTED HOME CARE POSITIVE-PRESSURE VENTILATORS

	Puritan Bennett 2800	Puritan Bennett 2801	Aequitron LP-6	Aequitron LP-10	Lifecare PLV-100	Intermed Bear 33	Respironics BiPAP
Modes	C, A/C, SIMV, press limited plateau	C, A/C, SIMV, press limited plateau	C, A/C, SIMV, press limited	C, A/C, SIMV, press cycled, press limited plateau	C, A/C, SIMV	C, A/C, SIMV	S, S/T, T, all press limited plateau
Tidal volume (ml)	50–2800	50–2800	100–2200	100–2200	50–3000	100–2200	Dependent on inspiratory pressure plateau
Breating rate/min	1–69	1–69	1–38	1–38	2–40	2–40	4–30
Sensitivity (cm H_2O)	−5–+10	−5–+10	−10–+10	−10–+10	−6–+3	−9–+19	Preset
Peak flow rate (L/min)	40–125	40–125	—	—	10–120	20–120	—
Inspiratory time (sec)	—	—	0.5–5.5	0.5–5.5	—	0.25–4.99	—
Per cent inspiratory time	—	—	—	—	—	—	10–90
Sigh volume (ml)	125–2800	125–2800	—	—	—	1.5 times set tidal volume	—
Sigh rate	3 per 10-min period	3 per 10-min period	—	—	—	6/hr	—
Peak inspire press alarm (cm H_2O)	20–60	20–60	25–100*	25–100*	5–95*	10–80*	—
Peak inspire press limit (cm H_2O)	20–70	20–70	25–100*	25–100*	5–95*	10–80*	2–20
Low inspire press limit (cm H_2O)	3–20	3–20	2–50	2–50	2–50	3–70	—
PEEP/CPAP (EPAP) level (cm H_2O)	—	—	—	—	—	—	2–20
Internal battery present (yes or no)	yes	yes	yes	yes	yes	yes	no

*One control simultaneously sets both the peak pressure alarm and peak pressure limit.
Key: C: controlled; A/C: assist/control; S: spontaneous; S/T: spontaneous/timed; T: timed.

permits the independent use of CPAP but always requires a minimum of about 2 cm H_2O CPAP when BiPAP is applied.

Fraction of Inspired Oxygen. None of these units is designed to provide precise fractions of inspired oxygen (FIO_2s).[63] Each establishes an elevated FIO_2 by mixing 100% oxygen via a flow meter with gas delivered to the patient. This is accomplished in some units by means of a mixing chamber and in others by the titration of oxygen into the respiratory limb of the ventilator circuit. Regardless of approach, FIO_2 variations on a breath-by-breath basis may be large (±5%).

Positive End-Expiratory Pressure/Continuous Positive Airway Pressure. The Respironics BiPAP is the only home care ventilator designed with positive end-expiratory pressure (PEEP)/CPAP as an integral part of the ventilator function.[64] None of the other units discussed earlier is designed for the application of PEEP/CPAP. A PEEP device can be easily affixed to any ventilator circuit, but unless true control ventilation is provided, the work of breathing is normally increased. With all of these units (except the Respironics BiPAP), during the assist/control ventilation mode, the sensitivity must be adjusted to decrease the pressure gradient necessary to trigger the unit. That is, if 5 cm H_2O PEEP is applied, the sensitivity must be set to about +4 cm H_2O (1 cm H_2O pressure gradient is required to trigger inspiration).

PEEP/CPAP should not be used in the IMV/SIMV mode.[65] Appropriate setting of the sensitivity may allow for triggering during positive-pressure breaths, but the work of breathing during spontaneous breaths is markedly increased. With these units, there is no reasonable method available to reduce the pressure gradient that is necessary for the patient to inspire spontaneously when PEEP/CPAP is applied. Fortunately, clinical indications for the use of PEEP in the population of patients sent home with mechanical ventilatory support are rare. However, if these indications do arise, the use of the assist/control mode (with the appropriate sensitivity setting) is recommended.

Humidification. Three basic humidification systems are available for use in the home: bubble-through systems, passover systems, and heat and moisture exchang-

286 THERAPEUTIC MODALITIES IN PULMONARY REHABILITATION

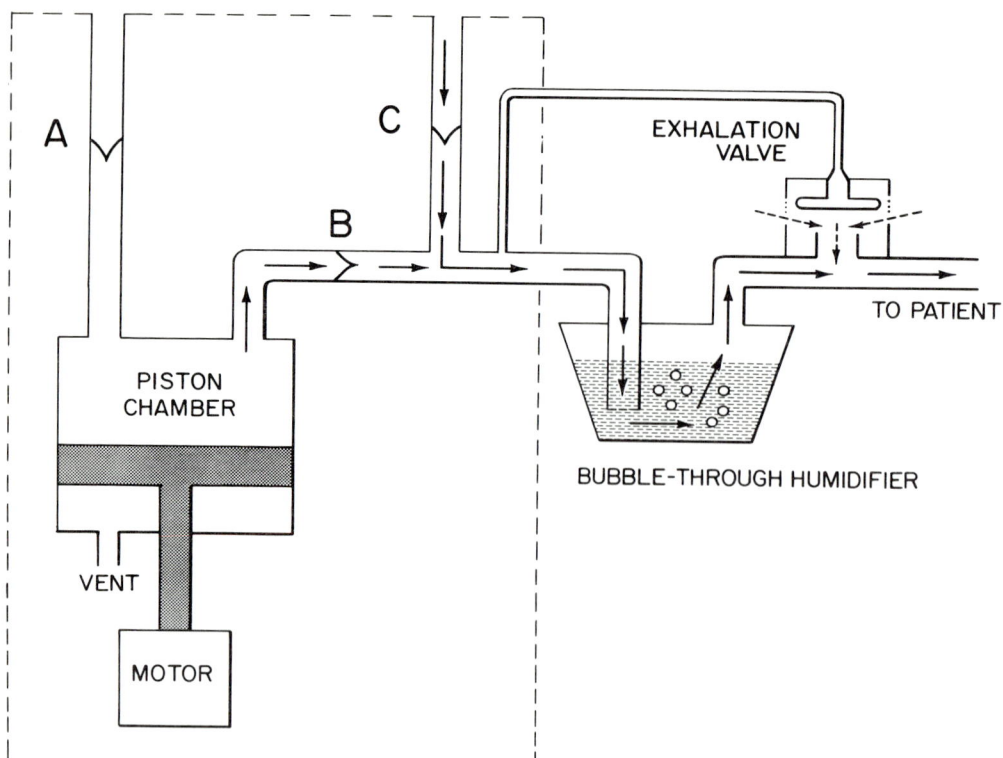

FIGURE 20-9. Diagram showing gas flow during spontaneous inspiration through a typical home care ventilator. *A*, A one-way check valve allows gas entry into the piston chamber during piston backstroke. *B*, A one-way check valve prevents subatmospheric pressure from developing in the ventilator circuit during piston backstroke. *C*, A one-way check valve allows the patient to inspire spontaneously during closure of the check valve at *B* when piston backstroke is in progress. Some gas may enter the system at the exhalation valve. The *arrows* depict gas flow during spontaneous inspiration. (From Kacmarek RM, Stanek KS, McMahon KM, Wilson RS. Imposed work of breathing during synchronized intermittent mandatory ventilation provided by five home care ventilators. Respir Care 1990; 35:405–414.)

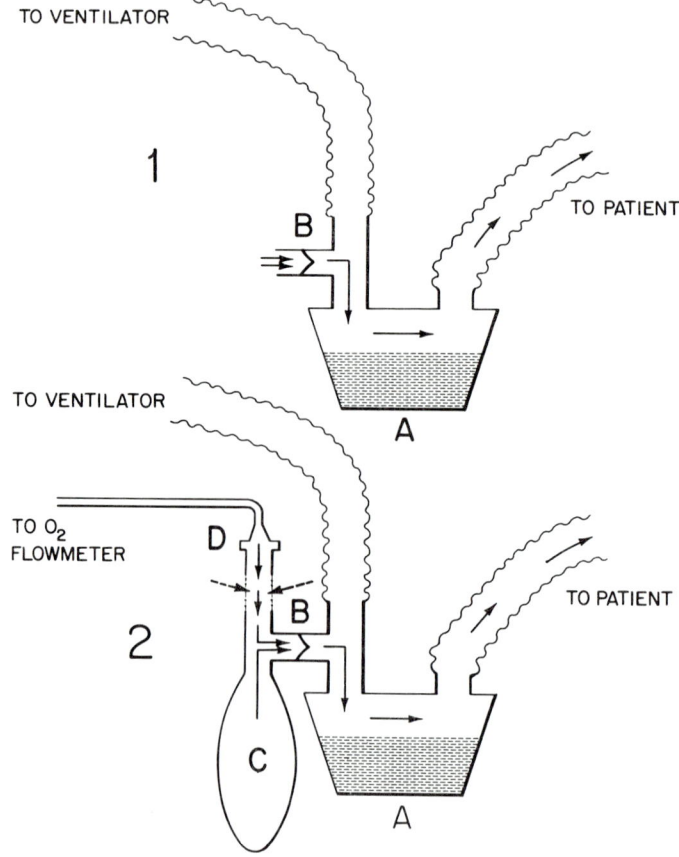

FIGURE 20-10. Diagram of one-way H-valve systems. *1,* Valve open to atmosphere. *2,* Valve with a 3-liter reservoir bag attached to a 28%-oxygen air entrainment device powered by 4 L/min of oxygen. (*A:* Passover humidifier; *B:* one-way valve; *C:* reservoir; *D:* 28% oxygen air entrainment valve.) The *arrows* depict gas flow during spontaneous inspiration. (From Kacmarek RM, Stanek KS, McMahon KM, Wilson RS. Imposed work of breathing during synchronized intermittent mandatory ventilation provided by five home care ventilators. Respir Care 1990; 35:405–414.)

ers. Since they further increase work of breathing, bubble-through humidifiers should never be used during SIMV. However, during control or assist/control modes, both bubble-through and passover units function quite well. Heat and moisture exchangers, although not recommended on a continuous basis, are very useful during patient transport and periods of time away from home. The use of heat and moisture exchangers greatly simplifies ventilator set-up on a wheelchair or in a car.

REFERENCES

1. Gilmartin ME. Long-term mechanical ventilation outside the hospital. In: Pierson DJ, Kacmarek RM (eds). Foundations of Respiratory Care. New York: Churchill Livingstone, Inc., 1992, pp 1185–1204.
2. Masferrer R, Dolan GK, Ward JJ. History of the respiratory care profession. In: Burton GG, Hodgkin JE, Ward JJ (eds). Respiratory Care: A Guide to Clinical Practice. 3rd ed. Philadelphia: J.B. Lippincott Co., 1991, pp 3–18.
3. Drinker P, Shaw LA. An apparatus for the prolonged administration of artificial ventilation. J Clin Invest 1929; 7:229–247.
4. Drinker PA, McKhann CF. The iron lung, first practical means of respiratory support. JAMA 1986; 255:1476–1480.
5. Hill NS. Clinical application of body ventilators. Chest 1986; 90:897–905.
6. Robert D, Fournier G, Thomas L, et al. Indications de la ventilation chronique a domicile par tracheotomie de l'insuffisance chronique non paralyttique. Rev Fr Mal Respir 1979; 7:353–355.
7. Gilmartin ME. Mechanical ventilation in the home: An overview. In: Gilmartin ME, Make BJ (eds). Problems in Respiratory Care. Philadelphia: J.B. Lippincott Co., 1988, pp 155–166.
8. Goldberg AI, Faure EAM. Home care for life supported persons in England: The responaut approach. Chest 1984; 86:910–914.
9. Collier CR, Affeldt JE. Ventilatory efficiency of the cuirass respirator in totally paralyzed chronic poliomyelitis patients. J Appl Physiol 1954; 6:531–538.
10. Holtackers TR, Loosbrock LM, Gracey DR. The use of the chest cuirass in respiratory failure of neurologic origin. Respir Care 1982; 27:271–275.
11. Goldstein RS, Molotiu N, Skrastins R, et al. Assisting ventilation in respiratory failure by negative pressure ventilation and by rocking bed. Chest 1987; 92:470–474.
12. Goldstein RS, Molotiu N, Skrastins R, et al. Reversal of sleep-induced hypoventilation in chronic respiratory failure by nocturnal negative pressure ventilation in patients with restrictive ventilatory impairment. Am Rev Respir Dis 1987; 135:1049–1055.
13. Nava S, Ambrosino N, Zocchi L, et al. Diaphragmatic rest during negative pressure ventilation by Pneumowrap: Assessment of normal and COPD patients. Chest 1990; 98:857–865.
14. Garay SM, Turino GM, Roldring RM. Sustained reversal of chronic hypercapnia in patients with alveolar hypoventilation syndromes: Long-term maintenance with non-invasive nocturnal mechanical ventilation. Am J Med 1981; 70:269–274.
15. Adamson JP, Stein JD. Application of abdominal pressure for artificial respiration. JAMA 1959; 169:1613–1617.
16. Miller JH, Thomas E, Wilmont CB. Pneumobelt use among high quadriplegic population. Arch Phys Med Rehabil 1988; 69:369–372.
17. Coville P, Shugg C, Ferris BG. Effects of body tilting on respiratory mechanics. J Appl Physiol 1956; 9:19–24.
18. Bach JR, Alba AS, Bohatuik G. Mouth intermittent positive pressure ventilation in the management of post polio respiratory insufficiency. Chest 1987; 91:859–864.
19. Bach JR, Alba A, Mosher R. Intermittent positive pressure ventilation via nasal access in the management of respiratory insufficiency. Chest 1987; 92:168–170.
20. Bach JR, Alba AS. Management of chronic alveolar hypoventilation by nasal ventilation. Chest 1990; 97:52–57.
21. Ellis ER, McCavley VB, Mellis C, et al. Treatment of alveolar hypoventilation in a six-year-old girl with intermittent positive pressure ventilation through a nose mask. Am Rev Respir Dis 1987; 136:188–191.
22. Kerby GR, Mayer LS, Pingleton SK. Nocturnal positive-pressure ventilation via nasal mask. Am Rev Respir Dis 1987; 135:738–740.
23. Leger P, Jennequin J, Gerard M, et al. Home positive pressure ventilation via nasal mask for patients with neuromuscular weakness or restrictive lung or chest wall disease. Respir Care 1989; 34:73–77.
24. Segall D. Noninvasive nasal mask-assisted ventilation in respiratory failure of Duchenne muscular dystrophy. Chest 1988; 93:1298–1300.
25. Goldstein RS, Pierson DJ. Long-term mechanical ventilation as elective therapy. Respir Care 1991; 36:288–289.
26. Goldstein RS, Avendano MA. Long-term mechanical ventilation as elective therapy: Clinical status and future prospects. Respir Care 1991; 36:297–304.
27. Luce JM, Tyler ML, Pierson DJ. Intensive Respiratory Care. 2nd ed. Philadelphia: W.B.Saunders Co. (In press.)
28. Marini JJ. The physiologic determinants of ventilator dependence. Respir Care 1986; 31:271–282.
29. Stoller JK. Establishing clinical unweanability. Respir Care 1991; 36:186–198.
30. Pierson DJ, George RB. Mechanical ventilation in the home: Possibilities and prerequisites. Respir Care 1986; 31:266–270.
31. Whitcomb ME. Care of the ventilator-dependent patient: Public policy considerations. Respir Care 1986; 31:283–287.
32. Plummer AL, O'Donohue WJ Jr, Petty TL, et al. Consensus conference on problems in home mechanical ventilation. Am Rev Respir Dis 1989; 140:555–560.
33. Clark K, Boltwood M. Psychosocial aspects of critical care. In: Zschoche DA (ed). Mosby's Comprehensive Review of Critical Care. St. Louis: C.V. Mosby Co., 1986, pp 93–121.
34. Clark KG. Psychosocial aspects of prolonged ventilator dependency. Respir Care 1986; 31:329–333.
35. McHugh LG, Clark KG, Pierson DJ. Psychosocial aspects of critical care. In: Pierson DJ, Kacmarek RM (eds). Foundations of Respiratory Care. New York: Churchill Livingstone, Inc., 1992, pp 1221–1236.
36. Cassem NH. Psychiatric problems of the critically ill patient. In: Shoemaker WC, Ayres S, Grenvik A, et al (eds). Textbook of Critical Care. 2nd ed. Philadelphia: W.B.Saunders Co., 1989, pp 1404–1414.
37. Robert D, Gerard M, Leger P, et al. Domiciliary mechanical ventilation by tracheostomy for chronic respiratory failure. Rev Fr Mal Respir 1983; 11:923–936.
38. Make B, Gilmartin M, Brody JS, et al. Rehabilitation of ventilator-dependent subjects with lung diseases: The concept and initial experience. Chest 1984; 86:358–365.
39. Make BJ, Gilmartin ME. Mechanical ventilation in the home. Crit Care Clin 1990; 6:785–796.
40. Make BJ, Gilmartin ME. Care of the ventilator-assisted individual in the home and alternate sites. In: Burton GG, Hodgkin JE, Ward JR (eds). Respiratory Care: A Guide to Clinical Practice. 3rd ed. Philadelphia: J.B. Lippincott Co., 1991, pp 669–690.
41. Make BJ, Gilmartin M. Rehabilitation of ventilator-assisted individuals. Clin Chest Med 1986; 7:679–691.
42. Sivak ED, Cordasco EM, Gipson WT, et al. Home care ventilation: The Cleveland Clinic experience from 1977 to 1985. Respir Care 1986; 31:294–302.
43. Peters SG, Viggiano RW. Home mechanical ventilation. Mayo Clin Proc 1988; 63:1208–1213.
44. Stoller JK. Physiologic rationale for resting the ventilatory muscles. Respir Care 1991; 36:290–296.
45. Goldstein RS, DeRosie JA, Avendano MA, et al. Influence of noninvasive positive pressure ventilation on inspiratory muscles. Chest 1991; 99:408–415.
46. Make BJ. Long-term management of ventilator-assisted individuals: The Boston University experience. Respir Care 1986; 31:303–310.
47. Curran FJ. Night ventilation by body respirators in chronic respiratory failure due to late stage Duchenne muscular dystrophy. Arch Phys Med Rehabil 1981; 62:270–274.
48. Delaubier A, Guillou C, Mordelet M, et al. Early respiratory

assistance by nasal route in Duchenne's muscular dystrophy. Agressologie 1987; 28, 7:737–738.
49. Ellis ER, Bye PTP, Bruderer JW, et al. Treatment of respiratory failure during sleep in patients with neuromuscular disease. Am Rev Respir Dis 1987; 135:148–152.
50. Hoeppner VH, Cockroft DW, Dosman JA, et al. Nighttime ventilation improves respiratory failure in secondary kyphoscoliosis. Am Rev Respir Dis 1984; 129:240–243.
51. Rochester DF, Braun NMT, Laine S. Diaphragmatic energy expenditure in chronic respiratory failure: The effect of assisted ventilation with body respirators. Am J Med 1977; 63:223–232.
52. Belman MJ, Soo Hoo GW, Kuei JH, et al. Efficacy of positive vs negative pressure ventilation in unloading the respiratory muscles. Chest 1990; 98:850–856.
53. Prentice WS. Placement alternatives for long-term ventilator care. Respir Care 1986; 31:288–293.
54. Prentice WS. Transition from hospital to home. Probl Respir Care 1988; 1:174–191.
55. O'Donohue WJ Jr. Patient selection and discharge criteria for home ventilator care. Probl Respir Care 1988; 1:167–174.
56. O'Donohue WJ Jr, Branson RD, Hoppough JM, et al. Criteria for establishing units for chronic ventilator-dependent patients in hospitals. Respir Care 1988; 33:1044–1046.
57. Nochomovitz ML, Montenegro HD, Parran S, et al. Placement alternatives for ventilator-dependent patients outside the intensive care unit. Respir Care 1991; 36:199–204.
58. Gilmartin ME. Long-term mechanical ventilation: Patient selection and discharge planning. Respir Care 1991; 36:205–216.
59. Kopacz MA, Moriarty-Wright R. Multidisciplinary approach for the patient on a home ventilator. Heart Lung 1984; 13:255–262.
60. LaFond L, Horner J. Psychological issues related to long-term ventilatory support. Probl Respir Care 1988; 1:241–256.
61. Weisinger W, Goldsmith T. Artificial ventilation: Its import on communication and swallowing problems. In: Gilmartin ME, Make BJ (eds). Problems in Respiratory Care. Philadelphia: J.B. Lippincott Co., 1988, pp 204–206.
62. Wilhelm L, Plummer A. Role of the home care practitioner. In: Gilmartin ME, Make BJ (eds). Problems in Respiratory Care. Philadelphia: J.B. Lippincott Co., 1988, pp 279–292.
63. Kacmarek RM, Spearman CB. Equipment used for ventilatory support in the home. Respir Care 1986; 31:311–328.
64. Strumpf DA, Carlisle CC, Millman RP, et al. An evaluation of the Respironics BiPAP Bi-Level CPAP device for delivery of assisted ventilation. Respir Care 1990; 35:415–422.
65. Kacmarek RM, Stanek KS, McMahon KM, Wilson RS. Imposed work of breathing during synchronized intermittent mandatory ventilation provided by five home care ventilators. Respir Care 1990; 35:405–414.

Chapter 21

Nicotine Addiction Treatment

LOUISE M. NETT, R.N., R.R.T.

PREPARING TO QUIT

Smokers with chronic obstructive pulmonary disease (COPD) who continue to smoke usually meet criteria for nicotine dependence. Nicotine-addicted persons use some form of tobacco (usually cigarettes) in a daily dosage schedule. Nicotine has powerful psychoactive effects. Some of the effects are pleasurable, even to the dependent smoker. The primary criteria for drug dependence are (1) highly controlled or compulsive drug use, (2) the presence of psychoactive effects, and (3) drug-reinforced behavior. Additionally, the use of drugs that lead to dependence is often continued by people even if these drugs have harmful effects. Cessation of smoking often causes severe withdrawal symptoms and is associated with recurrent and persistent nicotine craving, which often results in the resumption of smoking.[1]

Nicotine-dependent smokers who have made previous unsuccessful attempts to quit smoking need a systematic therapeutic program for their next effort. Most smokers with disease have made several attempts to quit. Every unsuccessful effort to quit is viewed by the smoker as an exercise in futility.

In preparing again to quit smoking, smokers should be informed of the specific benefits that may be realized after tobacco use cessation. The health professional should have a serious discussion with patients who smoke about the benefits of quitting. A good reference text on the positive aspects of cessation is the 1990 Surgeon General's Report, *The Health Benefits of Smoking Cessation*.[2] Health professionals should quote the benefits of quitting outlined in this report's major chapters. The major benefits of quitting to be gained by smokers with COPD are cited in Table 21–1.

It would be useful for the smoking intervention team to develop a list of publications that show the benefits of smoking cessation. For example, physicians might cite the health benefits of cessation described in the work of Calverly and colleagues.[3] These Scottish researchers discovered that smokers who quit smoking realized a decrease in red blood cell mass if they received continuous oxygen therapy. Patients who did not quit smoking had continued problems with polycythemia.

According to a British study,[4] patients who stop smoking may reduce their risk of respiratory morbidity. This 10-year study of 1445 male smokers aged 40 to 59 years found that those who quit had a reduction in nasal obstruction and showed improvement in bronchitis symptoms. Also noted was a slowing in the rate of loss of ventilatory function.

TABLE 21–1. BENEFITS OF QUITTING: SMOKING CESSATION AND NONMALIGNANT RESPIRATORY DISEASES*

1. Smoking cessation reduces rates of respiratory symptoms (such as cough, sputum production, and wheezing) and respiratory infections (such as bronchitis and pneumonia) compared with continued smoking.
2. For persons without overt COPD, smoking cessation improves pulmonary function about 5% within a few months after cessation.
3. Cigarette smoking accelerates the age-related decline in lung function that occurs among never-smokers. With sustained abstinence from smoking, the rate of decline in pulmonary function among former smokers returns to that of never-smokers.
4. With sustained abstinence, the COPD mortality rates among former smokers decline in comparison with those of continuing smokers.

*From Surgeon General's Report: The Health Benefits of Smoking Cessation. Rockville, MD: Centers for Disease Control, Office on Smoking and Health; 1990. U.S. Department of Health and Human Services publication (CDC) 90-8416.

Even a reduction in the number of cigarettes smoked per day may have beneficial effects. A reduction from 50 to 18 cigarettes per day resulted in improvement in bronchial inflammation in a pilot study of 15 heavy smokers by Rennard and associates.[5] This pilot study also measured a reduction in the number of inflammatory cells in the lungs as judged by bronchoalveolar lavage.[5] Thus, even a reduction in the number of cigarettes smoked may be of value to heavy smokers. After a smoker moves to a lower daily number of cigarettes, encouragement to quit smoking may be more successful. Complete cessation obviously results in the greatest health benefits.

Dudley and associates found that chest clinic patients quit smoking because of associated symptoms.[6] It is surprising that patients reported that the most important symptom that caused them to stop smoking was wheezing. Smokers with higher psychosocial assets and greater psychologic stability were more likely to be successful at quitting smoking.

USING BIOLOGIC TESTS TO MOTIVATE PATIENTS TO STOP SMOKING

Exhaled carbon monoxide and pulmonary function tests should be performed for all smokers. Carbon monoxide levels as high as 8 to 10 ppm are found in nonsmokers and are due to some endogenous production of this gas.[7] Higher levels are occasionally found in nonsmokers in heavily polluted cities.

Most smokers who smoke one pack of cigarettes per day have a level of exhaled carbon monoxide of 25 to 35 ppm.[8] This is equal to a carboxyhemoglobin level of 5 or 6%. This is an important consideration in the management of hypoxemic patients with COPD. In patients with a marginal oxygenation level, this amount of carbon monoxide can be a significant factor in oxygen uptake and delivery.

Exhaled carbon monoxide can be easily measured using an inexpensive hand-held instrument. There is a fairly good correlation between the level of exhaled carbon monoxide and the number of cigarettes smoked. The test should be performed in the late afternoon and one-half hour after a cigarette has been smoked if the most accurate results are to be obtained. For insurance reimbursement purposes, the fourth edition of *The Physicians' Current Procedure Terminology (CPT)* lists carbon monoxide testing under the chemistry and toxicology section and assigns it a code number of 82375.[9]

The exhaled carbon monoxide test can be used to verify whether a patient is a smoker or a nonsmoker. It may also be useful as a biofeedback tool to encourage cessation. The half-life of carbon monoxide in COPD patients is approximately 6.5 hours, compared with 2 to 5 hours in normal subjects.[10] The expected time for clearance from high levels to a normal level is 24 hours or less.

Carefully performed spirometric testing identifies smokers in the early stages of COPD. The measuring of pulmonary function may be a motivation for some smokers to quit. Petty and associates noted an 18% smoking cessation rate for smokers with abnormal pulmonary function compared with an 11% cessation rate for those with normal pulmonary function.[11] Hepper and colleagues found that 21% of participants with abnormal screening results stopped smoking within the following 2 to 3 years. Only 11.7% of smokers with normal pulmonary function test results quit.[12]

The concept of "lung age" may also be useful in motivating smoking cessation. Morris and Temple interpreted the pulmonary function test results of smokers according to the age at which the observed results would be normal.[13] For example, a 40-year-old male smoker who is 5 ft 11 in tall should have a forced expiratory volume (FEV_1) of approximately 4.29 L. If the observed value is 3.55 L, then the smoker has lungs that would normally be found in a 70-year-old body. Such an interpretation can be a real "attention grabber" for the smoker. Morris and Temple noted a 20% quit rate in smokers who were so informed.

Risser and Belcher immediately informed smokers of their carbon monoxide measurements and spirometric testing results as well as of their symptoms related to the use of cigarettes in a Veterans Administration Hospital screening clinic.[14] Those smokers who received immediate feedback (50% of smokers in the trial) had a 40% smoking cessation rate compared with those in a control group who had a 16% smoking cessation rate. After 12 months, 20% of those who received feedback had not resumed smoking, whereas only 7% of those in the control group did not continue to smoke. The authors found these smoking cessation rates especially encouraging because these smokers were not especially motivated for a smoking cessation trial. A substantial number of the smokers who eventually quit had no definite plans to stop and had not set a quit date immediately after they received initial intervention. Both groups were offered education and instruction in smoking cessation. This study supports the concept that sharing the results of carbon monoxide testing and spirometric testing can be motivations to quit smoking and to prevent relapse.

Other investigators have shown that there are improvements in pulmonary function following smoking cessation. Paxton and Scott noted that smokers who were successful at quitting had better pulmonary function at baseline than those who were not successful. Subjects who did not smoke cigarettes for 2 months showed greater improvement in lung function (in terms of FEV_1) measured during the subsequent 3 weeks than did subjects who had resumed smoking at 2 months.[15] McCarthy and coworkers noted that smokers with a long history of smoking had the worst pulmonary function compared with those who smoked less or who did not smoke.[16] Thirty per cent of the 131 persons who attended a stop smoking clinic had abnormal FEV_1 measurements. Repeat measurements taken at 25 and 48 weeks showed improvement in pulmonary function in smokers who quit and also in those who reduced their cigarette use but did not quit. These encouraging results should be used to motivate smokers at all stages of COPD to make an effort to quit smoking. It is never too late to stop smoking in COPD, but the greatest benefit occurs in patients who quit during the early or mild stages of disease and who are of a relatively young age.[17]

Buist and colleagues studied 75 cigarette smokers who attended a smoking cessation clinic.[18] Pulmonary function was assessed before cessation and four times thereafter. At follow-up, the participants were classified as smokers, intermittent smokers, or quitters. The smokers had the worst pulmonary function test results. At the end of the study, Buist and colleagues concluded that stopping smoking or reducing cigarette consumption by 25% results in improvement in pulmonary function and in symptoms. In the group of quitters, cough, expectoration, shortness of breath, and wheezing were the symptoms that were most improved. Patients who complain of these symptoms may find this a sufficient motivation to quit.

ENCOURAGING EFFORTS TO STOP SMOKING

Health care teams should develop a system to identify the smoker at each clinical encounter. Hospital, clinic, and office personnel should have a routine system to label the charts of all smokers. The entire health care team can then offer support and help to encourage smokers to quit.[19]

Documenting smoking status in a patient's record should be done for all smokers. The medical record should include information about specifics of the patient-physician discussion and whether a prescription for stopping smoking was given to the smoker. Such a record serves as medical and legal documentation in the event of morbidity or mortality from smoking-related diseases. The physician or designated physician extender should prescribe smoking cessation on a prescription form. This action signifies the importance of smoking cessation.

Smokers who have already experienced one or more unsuccessful attempts to quit smoking may have a fear of failure. Fear of failure can hold back an individual from taking the risk of attempting to stop smoking. Short-term quitters usually receive positive responses from friends and family. The inevitable "slip," which often leads to relapse, becomes a major source of embarrassment. The shame associated with relapse prevents the smoker from trying to quit again. An open, frank discussion about this vicious circle may pave the way for a new attempt at smoking cessation.

Smokers who have tried but have not succeeded at smoking cessation should be encouraged to view previous attempts as experience or practice sessions. It should be emphasized that repeated efforts may be required to attain any goal. Learning smoking cessation is no different than learning other new skills. "Practice makes perfect," a refrain from our childhood, applies to this situation.

The major factors that serve as a hindrance to the attempt to quit should be investigated. The smoker might be concerned about painful withdrawal symptoms. If so, it should be learned whether the patient was prepared for a previous cessation attempt and whether a pharmaceutical agent was used to reduce withdrawal symptoms. A surprising number of smokers have not made use of nicotine replacement in the form of nicotine-containing gum (nicotine polacrilex [Nicorette]). Others have used this gum inappropriately. Seriously addicted smokers should be encouraged to maximize their potential to quit successfully by using pharmaceutical aids.

It is possible that a smoker might hesitate to quit because his or her spouse also smokes. In this situation, the health professional should have a discussion with both parties. Success is increased when the spouse is supportive.[20] This support may necessitate that the spouse quit smoking with the patient.

A specific quit date is mandatory for success. Preparation is necessary, but it must culminate on a chosen or assigned date. The smoker should choose a date, not the health care professional. This leads the smoker to make a personal commitment and a personal contract.

Preparation for cessation includes making changes in the usual routine of smoking. Previously mentioned studies have shown the benefits of a reduction in smoking. A reduction in the number of cigarettes smoked may reduce the nicotine blood level. Nicotine replacement by gum or the recently available transdermal system (i.e., the nicotine patch) may be more easily achieved if smokers have already decreased their blood level of nicotine. Not all smokers are able to reduce their consumption of nicotine. Some smokers compensate by changing how they inhale the cigarette smoke. Deeper, longer inhalations can result in the increased extraction of nicotine from a cigarette. Smokers who change to cigarettes containing lower nicotine levels in preparation for quitting should be made aware that changes in the inhalation technique may negate the benefit of changing brands.[21]

Preparation for the smoking cessation effort can include self-imposed restrictions on when and where a cigarette is smoked. A useful exercise is to have the patient keep a daily diary of each cigarette consumed on a convenient pocket card. This simple tracking exercise alone usually causes a decrease in total consumption. Restricting smoking to only certain areas of the home or to in the car only when it is parked may encourage some smokers to decrease consumption. Holding the cigarette with the nondominant hand may reduce pleasure for some; this also results in a reduction in smoking. Substituting the cigarette with a lollipop or ordinary chewing gum works for some people.

PREPARING THE MIND FOR SMOKING CESSATION

Mental preparation is the most important factor in successful smoking cessation. The smoker should develop a list of reasons for smoking or quitting. Posting the list in a highly visible area makes it easy for the patient to add more reasons each day. Smokers who equivocate about stopping smoking find it difficult to add reasons to such a list. Smokers fighting a mental

TABLE 21-2. REASON FOR SMOKING DAILY DIARY

Cigarette No. / Time of day	1	2	3	4	5	6	7	8	9	10	11	12	13	14	15	16	17	18	19	20
Stimulation																				
Pleasure																				
Handling																				
Crutch or Tension Reduction																				
Craving, Psychologic Addiction																				
Habit																				

Stimulation

Stimulation smoking involves using smoking to give one a "lift," to become more awake, or to keep from slowing down.

Pleasure

Smoking is engaged in because it is a pleasurable and enjoyable activity. Smoking can be used to enhance an already pleasant mood, or it can be used to induce pleasure and enjoyment.

Sensorimotor Manipulation—Handling

Fiddling. The sensory and motor aspects of smoking motivate smoking. Examples include blowing smoke rings, flicking ashes, the steps in lighting up a cigarette, and fiddling with a lit cigarette.

Reduction of Negative Emotions—Crutch or Tension Reduction

Smoking is used to sedate or calm the smoker so as to reduce negative emotions such as anger, anxiety, shame, and embarrassment.

Psychologic Addiction—Craving

Psychologic addiction involves experiencing a craving (i.e., a gnawing hunger) for a cigarette that can only be reduced if a cigarette is smoked. Also, in this type of smoking, actually smoking a cigarette satisfies the craving.

Habit

Here, there is no true reason for smoking except that it has become automatic or habitual.

"civil war" find it difficult, if not impossible, to succeed at cessation. Smokers who decide to quit and want to quit are receptive to the learning of skills to prevent the resumption of smoking.

The "Why Do You Smoke Quiz" is a self-administered tool to quantify seven reasons for smoking.[22] This tool is intended to help the smoker understand possible future problem situations that might result from their smoking. The free government publication, *Why Do You Smoke?* includes an explanation for each reason and offers ideas for alternative behavior. The reasons for smoking are presented along with a daily diary form in Table 21-2.

Mind teasers may help the smoker develop a personal inventory of skills to quit and prevent relapse. In order to remain free of cigarette use, the smoker must depend on his or her personal resources. The health care professional could have the smoker perform the following "mind expanders" that demonstrate the need to prepare for cessation by learning relapse prevention skills. Under a time constraint of 1 or 2 minutes, the smoker lists on a blank sheet of paper all the things that he or she can do with a paper clip; alternatively, he or she might list all the things in the house that weigh less than 1 lb.[23] Usually, people get frustrated when they cannot think fast enough under pressure. When given adequate time, the smoker can list dozens of things that he or she can do with a paper clip or numerous items in the home that weigh less than 1 lb. It should be explained that in the presence of life's usual stresses, the smoker will have difficulty thinking up coping skills. Therefore, it is essential for the smoker to decide on coping techniques prior to the onset of a stressful event. It is necessary to develop a list of alternatives to smoking; these alternatives can be used automatically in the event of stress. A useful technique is to practice smoking alternatives before smoking cessation. The practicing of alternatives during the preparation time assures the smoker that he or she has developed natural techniques for coping with future urges to smoke.

The patient with chronic lung disease who has tried to quit smoking needs to understand that smoking cessation requires more than just will power. It requires "brain power" and strategies that work. Will power is usually referred to by smokers as "toughing it out." Reliance on will power suggests that the smoker does not use coping skills.[24] Smokers who are unable to list alternatives to smoking usually lapse and then relapse. Brain power suggests the selection of reasonable, usable, and natural coping techniques to deal with urges to smoke. Teaching smokers specific skills to prevent relapse can increase the success of efforts to cease smoking.[25]

Cigarette smoking has a powerful hold on smokers. It is both a physical and psychologic addiction. The psychologic addiction may be as hard to break as the physical addiction. For the lonely person, the cigarette becomes a best friend. It is always there to comfort in times of difficulty. Giving up cigarettes represents a significant loss to the smoker. The cigarette advertisements of the 1930s and 1940s suggested that the cigarette would be a "best friend" and it "would never let the smoker down"; in contrast, today all cigarette packs carry warning labels (Fig. 21–1). The smoker who has this personal relationship with the cigarette struggles to maintain cessation during personal crisis situations. In preparation for quitting, the smoker should be asked to describe his or her cigarette using every possible term. This exercise gives the interventionist clues to the psychologic significance of the cigarette to the smoker. Pharmaceutical support is unlikely to serve the same companionship function. Other coping strategies or replacement devices may be needed for these situations.

Not every smoker needs a lengthy preparation time. First-time quitters may be eager to quit without preparation. However, most pulmonary patients who continue to smoke have failed in such an attempt. COPD patients who still smoke need special help. They require a rehabilitation program as complex as the one used to improve muscle tone and general well-being. Continued smoking by a patient with COPD is a serious problem that requires a comprehensive therapeutic program. A rehabilitation program for smokers must have several components. Pulmonary rehabilitation patients learn new breathing techniques, how to use medication properly, the importance of an exercise program, and whom to call if they have trouble. In brief, they learn self-management techniques. These same principles apply to

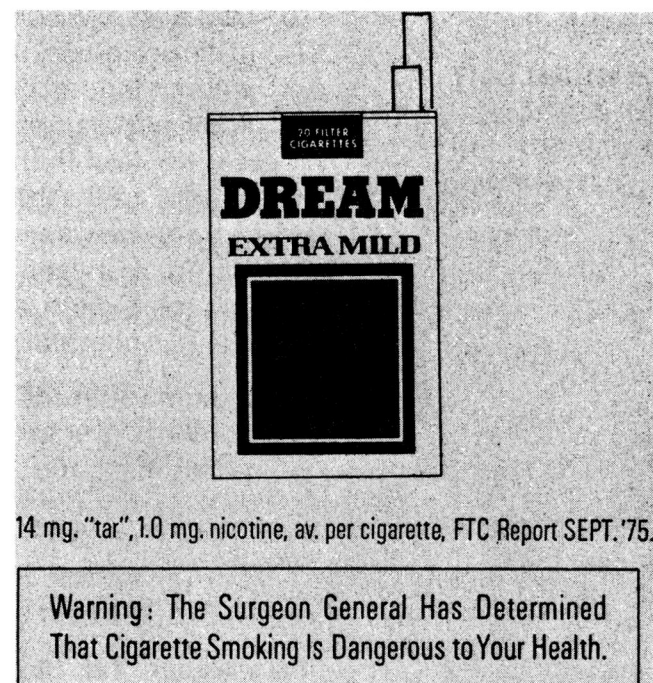

FIGURE 21–1. Cigarette advertising at one time promoted the benefits of smoking, but now all cigarette packs carry a warning label from the Surgeon General.

learning to live without tobacco. There is considerable need for the research of creative new ideas for smoking rehabilitation programs.

EVALUATING FOR NICOTINE DEPENDENCE

Nicotine dependence and nicotine withdrawal are medical diagnoses listed in the *International Classification of Diseases* and in the *Diagnostic and Statistical Manual of Mental Disorders, Third Edition–Revised (DSM III-R)*.[26] The health care team should view nicotine dependence as a medical problem. Medical problems require criteria for their definition and laboratory tests for confirmation of their diagnosis. Nicotine dependence criteria are listed in Table 21–3, and nicotine withdrawal symptoms are listed in Table 21–4.

Health professionals should use the *DSM III-R*'s criteria to define nicotine dependence disease. A simplified version of the criteria has been converted into a potential tool to evaluate for nicotine dependence (Tables 21–5 and 21–6). The medical record notations should follow the criteria for diagnosis. Most "sick smokers" meet the minimum criteria for the diagnosis of nicotine dependence. It may console the "sick smoker" to know that the reason for difficulty in quitting smoking and maintaining abstinence from cigarettes is related to a medical problem. An example of a proper notation that complies with the medical diagnosis is listed in Table 21–7.

The Fagerstrom Nicotine Tolerance Score is a frequently used test to evaluate a smoker's level of nicotine dependence.[27] There is some debate whether this tool measures physical or psychologic dependence.[28] Re-

TABLE 21–3. DIAGNOSTIC CRITERIA FOR PSYCHOACTIVE SUBSTANCE DEPENDENCE—NICOTINE DEPENDENCE 305.10*

A. At least three of the following:
   (1) substance often taken in larger amounts or over a longer period than the person intended
   (2) persistent desire or one or more unsuccessful efforts to cut down or control substance use
   (3) great deal of time spent in activities necessary to get the substance (e.g., theft), taking the substance (e.g., chain smoking), or recovering from its effects
   (4) frequent intoxication or withdrawal symptoms when expected to fulfill major role obligations at work, school or home (e.g., does not go to work because hung over, goes to school or work "high," intoxicated while taking care of his or her children), or when substance use is physically hazardous (e.g., drives when intoxicated)
   (5) important social, occupational, or recreational activities given up or reduced because of substance use
   (6) continued substance use despite knowledge of having a persistent or recurrent social, psychological, or physical problem that is caused or exacerbated by the use of substance (e.g., keeps using heroin despite family arguments about it, cocaine-induced depression, or having an ulcer made worse by drinking)
   (7) marked tolerance: need for markedly increased amounts of the substance (i.e., at least a 50% increase) in order to achieve intoxication or desired effect, or markedly diminished effect with continued use of the same amount

   Note: The following items may not apply to cannabis, hallucinogens, or phencyclidine (PCP):
   (8) characteristic withdrawal symptoms (see specific withdrawal syndromes under Psychoactive Substance–induced Organic Mental Disorders)
   (9) substance often taken to relieve or avoid withdrawal symptoms

B. Some symptoms of the disturbance have persisted for at least one month, or have occurred repeatedly over a longer period of time.

*From American Psychiatric Association: *Diagnostic and Statistical Manual of Mental Disorders. Third Edition, Revised.* Washington, DC, American Psychiatric Association, 1987.

cently, the tool has been revised to correspond to people's changing smoking patterns. Most experts agree that the most important question to ask a smoker is how soon after waking does he or she smoke. The smoker who has a cigarette immediately upon awakening usually gives a positive response to the other questions relating to dependence. The heavily dependent smoker needs to increase his or her blood level of nicotine immediately after several hours of sleep to avoid withdrawal symptoms. The smoker who delays the smoking of the first cigarette and who experiences no withdrawal with delay may be a so-called "habit smoker."

The physical signs of addiction to nicotine include a slight increase in heart rate after cigarette smoking and a decrease in body and skin temperature. Smokers who have a rapid heart rate after smoking a cigarette have not developed tolerance to the nicotine and are not considered physically dependent.[29]

PHARMACOLOGIC THERAPY

Nicotine-dependent smokers are the ones most likely to benefit from pharmacologic therapy. This is the conclusion of two recent studies reporting that addicted smokers were more successful at quitting when they used nicotine polacrilex than when they did not. The study of Tønnesen and associates separated 173 smokers into a high-dependence group and a low-dependence group.[30] These researchers used the less popular Horn-Russell dependence score instead of the Fagerstrom score. The highly dependent smokers received either 2- or 4-mg nicotine polacrilex. The smoking cessation rate among those receiving 4-mg nicotine polacrilex was 44.4% at 1 year and 33.3% at 2 years. The highly dependent smokers who received 2-mg nicotine polacrilex had abstinence rates of 12.1% at 1 year and 6.1% at 2 years. The lower cessation rate was likely a result of the inadequate relief of withdrawal symptoms owing to insufficient levels of nicotine replacement. The low-dependence group smokers who received 2-mg nicotine polacrilex had abstinence rates of 38.3% and 28.3% at 1 and 2 years, respectively. The low-dependence group smokers receiving placebo gum had abstinence rates of 22.6% and 9.4% at 1 year and 2 years of follow-up (Table 21–8).

The study program of Tønnesen and associates included six group support sessions in addition to the use of medication. This behavioral counseling probably accounted for the good smoking cessation rate in the nondependent smokers. The data showed a statistically significant positive result with the use of high-dose nicotine polacrilex in highly dependent smokers. These authors concluded that nicotine-containing gum should be used in appropriate doses to help smokers who want to quit. Fifteen per cent of abstainers continued to use the nicotine polacrilex at 2 years. A behavior counseling program should be used to wean these individuals from the nicotine replacement therapy.

Blöndal reported a study that included a 2-year follow-up program.[31] Participants in this study were all offered the same behavioral counseling therapy consisting of five 1-hour group sessions, although not all attended the sessions. In this double-blind, placebo-controlled study, participants were given either free nicotine polacrilex (4 mg) or placebo gum. Participants were instructed to use as much gum as they needed each day for 3 months. The smoking cessation rates were verified with exhaled carbon monoxide testing. The Fagerstrom nicotine tol-

TABLE 21–4. DIAGNOSTIC CRITERIA FOR 292.00 NICOTINE WITHDRAWAL*

A. Daily use of nicotine for at least several weeks.
B. Abrupt cessation of nicotine use, or reduction in the amount of nicotine used, followed within 24 hours by at least four of the following signs:
   (1) craving for nicotine
   (2) irritability, frustration, or anger
   (3) anxiety
   (4) difficulty concentrating
   (5) restlessness
   (6) decreased heart rate
   (7) increased appetite or weight gain

*From American Psychiatric Association: *Diagnostic and Statistical Manual of Mental Disorders. Third Edition, Revised.* Washington, DC, American Psychiatric Association, 1987.

TABLE 21–5. QUESTIONNAIRE BASED ON THE DSM III-R DIAGNOSTIC CRITERIA FOR NICOTINE DEPENDENCE (CODE NO. 305.10)*

Version I

Yes / No — At least three of the following:

(1) When you first began smoking, did you think you could quit smoking or reduce the amount you smoked whenever you wanted?
(2) Have you ever tried to quit smoking?
(3) Do you spend a great deal of time smoking each day? Number of hours: _____
(4) Have you ever experienced bothersome withdrawal symptoms when cigarette use was delayed for more than two hours?
(5) Do you ever avoid going places where smoking is not allowed, such as the homes of friends or relatives who do not allow smoking or public buildings where smoking is not allowed?
(6) If you have a health problem, has your doctor ever told you to quit smoking for your health, or do you think you should quit for your health?
(7) Do you sometimes need to smoke more cigarettes than you want to in order to feel the effect of the cigarettes?
(8) Have you ever experienced craving for a cigarette or felt nervous, irritable, or anxious when you couldn't have a cigarette for a while?
(9) Are these feelings relieved when you smoke a cigarette?

Total Score. A score of three or more "yes" answers indicates nicotine dependence.

Version II

Yes / No

(1) Teenage smokers think they can quit any time they want. Did you know that?
(2) Have you ever tried to quit?
(3) Do you spend more than a few minutes smoking each day?
(4) Do you feel uncomfortable when you go without a cigarette for 4 to 5 hours?
(5) Are you uncomfortable when you are not allowed to smoke?
(6) Do you have any medical condition made worse by smoking?
(7) Do you smoke more cigarettes now than when you were 18?
(8) If you feel awful or hungry, does smoking make you feel better?

*Adapted from American Psychiatric Association: *Diagnostic and Statistical Manual of Mental Disorders. Third Edition, Revised.* Washington, DC, American Psychiatric Association, 1987.

---

erance score was used to determine the dependence level. At 2 years, the 72 participants with high dependence scores were analyzed. The participants with high dependence scores who received the nicotine polacrilex 4 mg had a 45.5% cessation rate. The high dependence score participants who received the placebo had only a 3.6% cessation rate ($P<.001$). The smokers with low dependence scores (those having a Fagerstrom score of less than 7) were successful at cessation whether or not they received medication (Table 21–9). This indicates that behavioral counseling was helpful. The nicotine-treated subjects with low dependence scores had a 41.7% smoking cessation rate, and the placebo-administered subjects had a 37.1% success rate. There was no statistical difference in cessation rates among those in the low-dependence group.

There are many other reports in the literature that review the use of nicotine polacrilex and transdermal systems. Some have been performed using subjects in smoking cessation clinics or in the outpatient departments of hospitals, whereas others have recruited subjects from the community. The majority of studies

---

TABLE 21–6. QUESTIONNAIRE BASED ON THE DSM III-R DIAGNOSTIC CRITERIA FOR NICOTINE WITHDRAWAL (CODE NO. 292.00)*

Yes / No

A. Do you smoke cigarettes every day?
B. Have you ever had any of the feelings or symptoms addressed by the following questions when you stopped smoking (or have you had these symptoms when cigarette smoking has been delayed for several hours)?:
 (1) Did you have a craving for, need, or really want a cigarette?
 (2) Have you ever felt irritable, short tempered, or angry?
 (3) Have you ever felt anxious, nervous, or uncomfortable?
 (4) Have you had difficulty concentrating or been unable to stay focused on tasks?
 (5) Have you ever felt restless, edgy, or ill at ease?
 (6) Have you ever noticed a decreased heart rate?
 (7) Did you experience an increase in appetite, hunger, or food intake?
C. If you were off cigarettes for one month, did any of the symptoms last that long?

A score of four or more "yes" answers indicates nicotine withdrawal.

*Adapted from American Psychiatric Association: *Diagnostic and Statistical Manual of Mental Disorders. Third Edition, Revised.* Washington, DC, American Psychiatric Association, 1987.

TABLE 21–7. EXAMPLE OF PROPER DIAGNOSTIC NOTATION FOR NICOTINE DEPENDENCE

Mr. Jones, a 55-year-old male patient, was admitted to the hospital for chronic bronchitis. He began smoking at age 14 years and at age 18 years was smoking one pack of Camel cigarettes per day. He increased to two packs per day at approximately 30 years of age and had smoked this amount until this admission. He was advised to quit by his physician because of chronic bronchitis. He has attempted to quit on at least five occasions. His longest period of abstinence from cigarettes was 3 days in 1970, when his son was born. He resumed smoking because he "felt awful." Each attempt to quit was accompanied by irritability, difficulty concentrating, restlessness, and a craving for nicotine. His most recent attempt to quit was January 1st of this year.

Mr. Jones meets DSM III-R criteria for Nicotine Dependence—Code No. 305.10		Mr. Jones meets four DSM III-R criteria for nicotine withdrawal—Nicotine Withdrawal—Code No. 292.00	
DSM III-R No. 1	Substance taken in amount larger than that intended	DSM III-R No. 1	Craving for nicotine
No. 4	Withdrawal symptoms experienced on cessation	No. 2	Irritability
No. 6	Smoking continued in the presence of medical disease that is worsened by smoking	No. 4	Difficulty concentrating
		No. 5	Restlessness

indicate the effectiveness of nicotine replacement in smoking cessation. Unfortunately, not all studies validate the subjects' report of cessation. The use of the exhaled carbon monoxide testing should be standard in any treatment program. Most studies do not separate smokers by level of nicotine dependence. It is apparent from the reports of Tønnesen and associates and Blöndal that separating smokers by nicotine dependence level is important. The degree of nicotine dependence has significant implications for the treatment of "sick smokers."

Concerns relating to the cost of treating smokers have been reviewed. In a meta-analysis of data from published reports of the use of nicotine polacrilex, Oster and colleagues estimated the cost-effectiveness of nicotine gum as an adjunct to physician advice.[32] Their conclusion is that use of the gum in a medical care outpatient setting compares favorably with other health therapies. A follow-up study by Cummings and coworkers did not include the use of nicotine polacrilex in evaluating the cost effectiveness of counseling smokers to quit.[33] However, they concluded that advising smokers to quit should be a routine part of every health visit. Neither study addressed the special needs of nicotine-dependent smokers who have disease and may require more time and therapy but for whom intervention may be more cost-effective for the health care system in the long run.

Nicotine polacrilex has been used in many controlled trials in both the United States and Europe. Well over a dozen studies have reported on its clinical effectiveness since the early reports of its use in 1982. Nicotine replacement using this resin-based method (gum) can only be successful if the patient uses enough of the substance and uses it correctly. The nicotine is released from the resin base when it is chewed. The nicotine is absorbed in the buccal mucosa in a normal pH environment. An acidic environment in the mouth blocks absorption. Most drinks, such as coffee, teas, colas, and juices, as well as many foods, create an acidic oral environment. The pH of the mouth returns to normal within 10 to 15 minutes. This nicotine replacement therapy should be used either before or at least 15 minutes after the consumption of acidic food or drink.

The therapeutic value of any medication depends on the attainment of adequate blood levels. Therefore, it is important to use a sufficient quantity of the prescribed medication. Food and Drug Administration requires the package insert for nicotine polacrilex to state that the medication be used on an as-needed basis. Practitioners now realize that it is better to use the nicotine replacement gum on a scheduled dosing basis. It takes 20 to 30 minutes of correct chewing to achieve adequate blood nicotine levels. The ex-smoker should use the medication soon after awakening from sleep. Hourly dosing thereafter achieves the best maintenance blood levels of nicotine. If the ex-smoker is not relieved of withdrawal symptoms with hourly dosing, it is possible to use two pieces of 2-mg nicotine polacrilex or to use a fresh piece of the medication every 30 minutes. The dosage should be increased until it is adequate to relieve withdrawal symptoms. The lowest maintenance dose during the early stages of quitting is 10 pieces of gum per day.

TABLE 21–8. RESULTS OF THE STUDY BY TØNNESON AND ASSOCIATES*

	Smokers with a High Nicotine Dependence Level†		Smokers with a Low Nicotine Dependence Level†	
Nicotine polacrilex dose/placebo	4 mg	2 mg	2 mg	placebo
Smoking cessation rate at 1 yr (%)	44.4	12.1	38.3	22.6
Smoking cessation rate at 2 yr (%)	33.3	6.1	28.3	9.4

*From Tønneson P, Fryd V, Hansen M, et al. Effect of nicotine chewing gum in combination with group counseling on the cessation of smoking. N Engl J Med 1988; 318:15–18.
†N = 173

TABLE 21–9. RESULTS OF THE BLÖNDAL STUDY*

	Smokers with a High Nicotine Dependence Level†		Smokers with a Low Nicotine Dependence Level†	
Nicotine polacrilex dose/placebo	4 mg	placebo	4 mg	placebo
Smoking cessation rate at 2 yr (%)	45.5	3.6	41.7	37.1

*Data from Blöndal T. Controlled trial of nicotine polacrilex gum with supportive measures. Arch Intern Med 1989; 149:1818–1821.
†N = 72

Replacement therapy with the nicotine transdermal system is a simpler way to administer nicotine.[34] The dosage of nicotine via the transdermal system maintains a steady replacement amount. Experience in Europe and in the United States indicates that it is a safe and efficacious agent. Use of the nicotine transdermal system is particularly helpful for patients and individuals who have difficulty using a resin-based medication.

Daughton and colleagues reported on the use of the nicotine transdermal system (patch) in a 6-month study of 158 smokers. The study comprised three subject groups: one using a 24-hour nicotine patch, one using a nicotine patch during waking hours, and one using a placebo. At the end of 4 weeks of nicotine patch therapy, 39% of those receiving the 24-hour therapy had quit smoking, 35% of those using the patch only during working hours had quit, and 13.5% in the placebo group had quit. All had minimal intervention consisting of either guidance using a self-help book or two group lectures. All participants were seen weekly. At 6 months, the active nicotine patch users had a better smoking cessation rate than the placebo users.

Some smokers hesitate to use pharmaceutical aids and prefer to quit smoking on their own without medication. Since most of the addicted smokers have tried this "cold turkey" method (some repeatedly), it may not be a good idea for them to try to quit again without pharmacologic replacement therapy. Smokers cycle through stages of being ready to quit, of making the effort to quit, and, if they fail, of delaying for a period of time until they try again.[35] Another failure may reinforce the smoker's concept that he or she is unable to quit smoking. Health professionals should encourage addicted smokers to use every possible support to achieve success. For these smokers, it may be helpful to "wean into" nicotine replacement by using the nicotine polacrilex prior to quitting. By substituting a piece of nicotine polacrilex for a cigarette, they may learn the benefit of this therapy. It may convince the smoker to attempt another effort to cease smoking.

Since smoking is a complex behavior, it is no surprise that nicotine replacement as the sole intervention is usually not successful. This complex behavior requires a multicomponent approach to therapy. The more components used in the therapeutic program, the better the results.[36] For example, diabetes management and pulmonary rehabilitation programs incorporate many strategies for success, and thus so must the rehabilitation program for nicotine addiction.

BEHAVIORAL AND COGNITIVE TECHNIQUES TO PREVENT RELAPSE

Behavior modification techniques include substitution behaviors. They encourage the use of different behaviors as a substitute for cigarette smoking. The behavior changes include modifying the environment to avoid reminders of smoking. Seventy-five per cent of first-time quitters relapse into smoking.[37] Refraining from smoking requires practice and experience.

A "lapse" or "slip" in the abstinence from smoking usually precedes a complete relapse. How the smoker reacts to this mistake determines what happens next. The smoker who is self-forgiving can quickly correct the slip to prevent relapse. The smoker who regards having one cigarette as a serious fault usually resumes smoking.

Marlatt has presented the concept of the *abstinent violation effect*.[38] Some smokers believe that once they have stopped smoking, they must never again inhale a puff of smoke. To have even one puff "violates" his or her sacred personal truce. Once the smoker has a cigarette, he or she may view himself or herself as weak and incapable of abstinence and cessation. This perception often leads to the resumption of smoking.

The smoker who has been educated to be less severe with himself or herself during a lapse may be able to maintain abstinence. A slip should be viewed for what it is—an isolated smoking episode. It is not a return to smoking. The smoker can be educated to avert the resumption of smoking by positive self-talk.

Self-talk can be described as a personal, mental tape that is played in the mind. Self-talk can be positive or negative.[39] An example of positive self-talk to rationalize and correct a smoking lapse might be, "O.K., I knew there would be times like this, but I will not let it cause me to smoke again." In contrast, negative self-talk might be, "I know I'm weak; I'll never be able to stop smoking, so why should I try?"

Self-efficacy and smoking reduction were studied by Devins and Edwards in 45 COPD patients.[40] The greatest reduction in smoking was observed in smokers with the highest degree of self-efficacy. Individuals who believed they could avoid smoking by using self-selected coping strategies were able to reduce smoking. Smokers with low motivation to quit and weak self-efficacy expectancies continued to smoke. An example of a tool used to evaluate self-efficacy is shown in Table 21-10.

The self-efficacy tool is used by the smoker to rate the likelihood that he or she will not smoke in a given situation. Smokers who are insecure about abstinence from cigarettes need help. To prevent relapse, the smoker needs to identify practical and usable alternatives to smoking in high-risk situations. The health care professional can explore these areas with the smoker.

Other researchers have studied smokers' beliefs that they are able to avoid smoking in certain situations. Condiotte and Lichtenstein studied the relation between outcome and self-efficacy.[41] The authors observed that individuals with a higher initial level of perceived self-efficacy smoked fewer cigarettes than those with a lower level of self-efficacy. Smokers were asked to rate their confidence in their ability to use coping techniques when faced with a temptation to smoke. Techniques such as using a reward, meditation, or an alternative activity were rated on a nine-point scale whose descriptors varied from "not at all confident" to "very confident." The participants were aware of the health hazards of continued smoking, and most knew several behavioral techniques for stopping smoking. Future work should look at methods to enhance self-efficacy for improved compliance.

TABLE 21-10. SELF-EFFICACY RATING FOR SMOKERS*

If you were to try to stop smoking, how confident are you that you could use the following strategies?
Please circle the one number that best describes how you feel.
Please explain why you chose each rating.

Stop-Smoking Stategy	Confidence Level
a. Rewarding yourself or using incentives Why did you choose that rating? _____	1 2 3 4 5 6 7 8 9 not at all confident very confident
b. Imagining yourself smoking Why did you choose that rating? _____	1 2 3 4 5 6 7 8 9 not at all confident very confident
c. Meditation or muscle relaxation Why did you choose that rating? _____	1 2 3 4 5 6 7 8 9 not at all confident very confident
d. Engaging in alternate activity Why did you choose that rating? _____	1 2 3 4 5 6 7 8 9 not at all confident very confident
e. Having cigarettes handy Why did you choose that rating? _____	1 2 3 4 5 6 7 8 9 not at all confident very confident
f. Avoiding smokers and common smoking situations Why did you choose that rating? _____	1 2 3 4 5 6 7 8 9 not at all confident very confident
g. Thinking of the negative effects of smoking Why did you choose that rating? _____	1 2 3 4 5 6 7 8 9 not at all confident very confident
h. Associating with others to enjoy the smoke Why did you choose that rating? _____	1 2 3 4 5 6 7 8 9 not at all confident very confident

*Reproduced with permission of Gerald Devins, University of Calgary, Alberta, Canada.

Role playing with the smoker and his or her family and friends that involves self-efficacy situations may be a useful technique to teach relapse prevention. How to perform self-management at home for asthma, COPD, and cystic fibrosis is frequently incorporated in the teaching of pulmonary patients. The same educational principles can be used to teach smoking avoidance.

Maintaining a health program requires ongoing commitment and support. It is well known that pulmonary rehabilitation programs can help many patients improve their level of physical activity. The recovery of increased exercise function lasts as long as the patient actively participates. If the patient does not comply with the daily program, regression occurs. The same is true of the smoker's rehabilitation program. It is part of a lifelong process of participation in health maintenance.

Health professionals have successfully developed and implemented unique and sometimes personalized rehabilitation programs for pulmonary patients. The new frontier is the development of rehabilitation programs

TABLE 21-11. COMPONENTS OF A REHABILITATION PROGRAM FOR SMOKERS

Component	Explanation
1. Complete history and physical examination	A detailed fact-gathering history about health habits and unsafe health practices of the patient, including smoking. Smoking history should determine any symptoms related to tobacco use, age of onset, amount used, frequency of use, discomfort when discontinued, and number of attempts to quit. Use of DSM III-R criteria and Fagerstrom Nicotine Tolerance score to determine nicotine dependence.
2. Biologic tests	Exhaled carbon monoxide unit. Pulmonary function test. Urine or saliva cotinine test.
3. Pharmacologic therapy	Nicotine replacement for nicotine dependent smokers.
4. Behavioral counseling	Maximize amount of time spent educating smokers to quit and to remain free of smoking.
5. Home care and follow-up	See smoker at least monthly for the first year after quitting.

for smokers (Table 21-11). By incorporating the same basic components as pulmonary rehabilitation programs, including a complete history, a physical examination, biologic tests, pharmacologic therapy, behavioral counseling (education), home care, and long-term follow-up, smoking rehabilitation programs can help many smokers pursue a healthier lifestyle.

REFERENCES

1. Surgeon General's Report: The Health Consequences of Smoking: Nicotine Addiction. Rockville, MD: Centers for Disease Control, Office on Smoking and Health; 1988. U.S. Department of Health and Human Services, publication (CDC) 88-8406.
2. Surgeon General's Report: The Health Benefits of Smoking Cessation. Rockville, MD: Centers for Disease Control, Office on Smoking and Health; 1990. U.S. Department of Health and Human Services, publication (CDC) 90-8416.
3. Calverley PMA, Leggett RJ, McElderry L, Flenley DC. Cigarette smoking and secondary polycythemia. Am Rev Respir Dis 1982; 125:507-510.
4. Rose G, Hamilton PJ, Colwell L, Shipley MJ. A randomised controlled trial of anti-smoking advice: 10-year results. J Epidemiol Community Health 1982; 36:102-108.
5. Rennard SI, Daughton D, Fujita J, et al: Short-term smoking reduction is associated with reduction in measures of lower respiratory tract inflammation in heavy smokers. Eur Respir J 1990; 3:752-759.
6. Dudley DL, Aickin M, Martin CJ. Cigarette smoking in a chest clinic population: Psychophysiologic variables. J Psychosom Res 1977; 21:367-375.
7. Grabowski J, Bell CS (eds). Measurement in the Analysis and Treatment of Smoking Behavior. Washington, D.C.: National Institute of Drug Abuse; 1983. Research Monograph 48.
8. Henningfield JE. Nicotine: An old-fashioned addiction. (The Encyclopedia of Psychoactive Drugs). New York: Chelsea House Publishers, 1985.
9. American Medical Association. Physicians' Current Procedural Terminology 1991. Chicago: American Medical Association, 1990, pp 45, 47, 448, 454.
10. Crowley TJ, Andrews AE, Cheney J, et al: Carbon monoxide assessment of smoking in chronic obstructive pulmonary disease. Addict Behav 1989; 14:493-502.
11. Petty TL, Pierson DJ, Dick NP, et al: Follow-up evaluation of a prevalence study for chronic bronchitis and chronic airway obstruction. Am Rev Respir Dis 1976; 114:881-890.
12. Hepper NG, Drage CW, Davies SF, et al: Chronic obstructive pulmonary disease: A community-oriented program including professional education and screening by a voluntary health agency. Am Rev Respir Dis 1980; 121:97-104.
13. Morris JF, Temple W. Spirometric "lung age" estimation for motivating smoking cessation. Prev Med 1985; 14:655-662.
14. Risser NL, Belcher DW. Adding spirometry, carbon monoxide, and pulmonary symptom results to smoking cessation counseling: A randomized trial. J Gen Intern Med 1990; 5:16-22.
15. Paxton R, Scott S. Nonsmoking reinforced by improvements in lung function. Addict Behav 1981; 6:313-315.
16. McCarthy DS, Craig DB, Cherniack RM. Effect of modification of the smoking habit on lung function. Am Rev Respir Dis 1976; 114:103-113.
17. Peto R, Speizen FE, Cochrane AL, et al. The relevance in adults of airflow obstruction but not of mucus hypersecretion to mortality from chronic lung disease. Am Rev Respir Dis 1983; 128:491-500.
18. Buist AS, Sexton GJ, Nagy JM, Ross BB. The effect of smoking cessation and modification on lung function. Am Rev Respir Dis 1976; 114:115-122.
19. Kottke TE, Soldberg LI, Brekke ML, Maxwell P. Smoking cessation strategies and evaluation. J Am Coll Cardiol 1988; 12:1105-1110.
20. Hanson BS, Isacsson SO, Janzon L, Lindell SE. Social support and quitting smoking for good. Is there an association? Results from the population study, "Men Born in 1914," Malmö, Sweden. Addict Behav 1990; 15:221-233.
21. Benowitz NL, Hall SM, Herning RI, et al. Smokers of low yield cigarettes do not consume less nicotine. N Engl J Med 1983; 309:139-142.
22. Tate JC, Stanton AL. Assessment of the validity of the reasons for smoking scale. Addict Behav 1990; 15:129-135.
23. Oech R. A Whack on the Side of the Head: How You Can Be More Creative. New York: Warner Books, Inc., 1990.
24. Gritz ER, Carr CR, Marcus AC. Unaided smoking cessation: Great American Smokeout and New Year's Day Quitters. J Psychosoc Oncol 1988; 6:217-234.
25. Stevens VJ, Hollis JF. Preventing smoking relapse using an individually tailored skills-training technique. J Consult Clin Psychol 1989; 57:420-424.
26. American Psychiatric Association. Diagnostic and Statistical Manual of Mental Disorders. 3rd ed. Revised. Washington, D.C.: American Psychiatric Association, 1987.
27. Fagerstrom KO. Measuring the degree of physical dependence to tobacco smoking with reference to individualization of treatment. Addict Behav 1978; 3:235-241.
28. Lombardo TW, Hughes JR, Fross JD. Failure to support the validity of the Fagerstrom Tolerance Questionnaire as a measure of physiological tolerance to nicotine. Addict Behav 1988; 13:87-90.
29. Fagerstrom KO. Measuring the degree of physical dependence to tobacco smoking with reference to individualization of treatment. Addict Behav 1978; 3:235-241.
30. Tønnesen P, Fryd V, Hansen M, et al. Effect of nicotine chewing gum in combination with group counseling on the cessation of smoking. N Engl J Med 1988; 318:15-18.
31. Blöndal T. Controlled trial of nicotine polacrilex gum with supportive measures. Arch Intern Med 1989; 149:1818-1821.
32. Oster G, Huse DM, Delea TE, Colditz GA. Cost-effectiveness of nicotine gum as an adjunct to physician's advice against cigarette smoking. JAMA 1986; 256:1315-1318.
33. Cummings SR, Rubin SM, Oster G. The cost-effectiveness of counseling smokers to quit. JAMA 1989; 261:75-79.
34. Daughton DM, Heatley SA, Prendergast JJ, et al. Effect of transdermal nicotine delivery as an adjunct to low-intervention smoking cessation therapy: A randomized, placebo-controlled, double-blind study. Arch Intern Med 1991; 151:749-752.
35. DiClemente CC, Prochaska JO, Fairhurst SK, et al. The process of smoking cessation: An analysis of precontemplation, contemplation, and preparation stages of change. J Consult Clin Psychol 1991; 59:295-304.
36. Kottke TE, Battista RN, DeFriese GH, Brekke ML. Attributes of successful smoking interventions in medical practice: A meta-analysis of 39 controlled trials. JAMA 1988; 259:2883-2889.
37. Marlatt GA. Relapse prevention: A self-control program for the treatment of addictive behaviors. In: Stuart RB (ed). Adherence, Compliance and Generalization in Behavioral Medicine. New York: Brunner/Mazel, Inc., 1982, Chapters: 329-370.
38. Marlatt GA. Relapse prevention: Theoretical rationale and overview of the model. In: Marlatt GA, Gordon JR (eds). Relapse Prevention. New York: Guilford Press, 1985, Chapters 3-70.
39. Burns DD. Feeling Good: The New Mood Therapy. New York: William Morrow & Co., 1980.
40. Devins GM, Edwards PJ. Self-efficacy and smoking reduction in chronic obstructive pulmonary disease. Behav Res Ther 1988; 26:127-135.
41. Condiotte MM, Lichtenstein E. Self-efficacy and relapse in smoking cessation programs. J Consult Clin Psychol 1981; 49:648-658.

3

Components of the Pulmonary Rehabilitation Program

Chapter 22

Pulmonary Rehabilitation Program Organization

BRIAN L. TIEP, M.D.

Pulmonary rehabilitation applies art, skill, physiology, and multiple clinical disciplines to reverse the disability of patients with chronic lung disease. This disability stems from a combination of both reversible and irreversible pulmonary impairment, physical deconditioning, and a host of psychosocial factors.[1-3] Over the long process of physiologic deterioration, pulmonary patients learn to live lifestyles of progressive inactivity that is forged by dyspnea and anchored by the fear of dyspnea. In the latter stages of their disease—that is, by the time a referral for pulmonary rehabilitation is made—they have become dependent on others and have relinquished control of their lives. Reversing this process requires that patients accept their diagnosis and the fact that therapy necessitating serious personal involvement can help them to live more comfortable and enjoyable lives. Thus, pulmonary rehabilitation must optimally manage the reversible components of pulmonary impairment and improve patient strength, endurance, and stamina while at the same time attending to the myriad physiologic and psychologic factors that have woven the pattern of disability.[2]

The organization of pulmonary rehabilitation programs varies, depending on the personnel and logistics of the treatment facility.[4] Some programs are administered by a full team of medical and paramedical professionals and are performed in gyms and education centers dedicated to the programs; others are conducted by only one or two part-time therapists in a room within a hospital, in a physician's office, or at a community center. The success of a program is determined by the dedication and interactive clinical skills of the therapeutic team, since the overall goal of any program is to positively alter the patient's lifestyle or pattern of living. Life pattern changes are difficult and unnatural, especially for elderly patients who suffer from chronic lung disease. Thus, any program always has a strong psychologic orientation, regardless of whether or not a psychologist directly participates in it.

GOALS AND EXPECTATIONS OF PULMONARY REHABILITATION

For rehabilitation to be successful, the patient and the therapeutic team must have high but realistic goals and expectations. The work involved is difficult and arduous. The therapeutic team and the patient must believe that an excellent outcome for the patient is likely so that they can dedicate themselves to the task ahead. Patients should plan to feel better by the end of the program.[5] Typical goals and expectations of patients and team members are presented in Table 22-1.

Since most pulmonary patients enter rehabilitation programs because they are dyspneic, the reduction of dyspnea is a major goal of such programs.[6] Moreover, the programs attend to the patients' fear of dyspnea, which inhibits them from being active. Their exercise tolerance (particularly their endurance), strength, and stamina should be significantly improved as a result of rehabilitation. Patients should expect to become more active and independent in their self-care and in the care of their homes. When they are able to achieve this, they will be able to venture out of their homes and assume

TABLE 22-1. GOALS AND EXPECTATIONS OF PULMONARY REHABILITATION

Feeling Better
　Less reduced dyspnea
　Greater confidence
　Less depression, anxiety, and panic
　Less frequent insomnia

Greater Activity
　At home
　In the community
　During leisure time

Increased Endurance and Strength
　Muscles of ambulation
　Upper extremities
　Ventilatory muscles

Greater Range of Function
　Self-care
　Care of the home
　Shopping
　Sexual activity
　Leisure activity
　Work (if appropriate)

Self-Control and Self-Management
　Dyspnea
　Living situation
　Clearance of secretions
　Medications
　Oxygen
　Nutrition
　Family matters

Physician-Patient Communication
　More effective visits to the physician, with the understanding that the patient is an extension of the physician

---

a more active role in the community. They will be able to participate in their favorite leisure pursuits, such as bowling, golfing, traveling, visiting the theater, dining out, and performing volunteer work. Some patients will even be able to return to part-time or full-time work.

FACILITIES

Facilities for pulmonary rehabilitation should be friendly, comfortable, and accessible. Many pulmonary patients had been confined to their own homes because it was uncomfortable for them to venture out; thus, the accessibility of facilities is important. Parking should be near the facilities in order to provide easy access to the rehabilitation area. Space in the facilities should be planned so that it is able to accommodate patient therapy groups, which help patients to realize that they are not alone and that many of their concerns are shared by others. It is also helpful for the patients to be able to dine together.[2,4]

The rooms should be well ventilated and pleasant. Fans installed in the exercise areas often relieve patient claustrophobia. Respiratory patients require facilities that are free of dust and chemical odors such as those produced by cleaning agents or new paint. Consistently, the staff and patients should avoid perfumes. A large gym is unnecessary. However, an area for walking (i.e., a long hallway or an outdoor facility for use in good weather) should be provided. Areas in which to perform arm exercises (e.g., arm cranking and gravity-resistive exercises) as well as relaxation training mats should also be provided. A storage area for various respiratory equipment should be included as well.

Oxygen supply equipment must be available and include appropriate liquid systems for the refilling of portable units. Local oxygen suppliers can help in this regard. A nebulizer machine with an adequate supply of bronchodilators is needed in the event that a patient becomes dyspneic and requires respiratory assistance. Also, a crash cart and trained personnel must be available.

If available, activities of daily living (ADL) facilities are very useful for training patients to manage in the home by employing ADL and energy conservation techniques. Facilities might include an ADL kitchen and bedroom. If this type of facility is unavailable at a particular rehabilitation center, a field trip to one of the patients' homes or to a nearby facility may suffice. A summary of the equipment and facilities needed for an effective rehabilitation center is shown in Table 22-2.

MARKETING THE PROGRAM

Marketing is the means by which pulmonary rehabilitation programs make others aware of their presence and of the important function they perform.[4] The target audience includes referring physicians, nurses, discharge planners, other health care professionals (both inside and outside the hospital), and home respiratory equipment suppliers as well as patients with lung disease and their families. Methods of marketing must remain ethical and professional. Marketing can largely consist of providing educational services to patients and referring sources as well as speaking before community groups. Word-of-mouth and a good performance record contribute significantly to the solidification of a program's place in the community.

REIMBURSEMENT

Pulmonary rehabilitation programs are reimbursed differently depending on the reimbursement source, the part of the country in which they are conducted, and the type of center in which they take place. Many

TABLE 22-2. SUMMARY OF REHABILITATION FACILITIES

Classroom
Exercise areas and equipment (e.g., a hallway for walking and an arm cranking machine)
Exercise testing equipment
Relaxation areas with mats or comfortable recliners
ADL training facilities (e.g., kitchen)
Oxygen and respiratory therapy equipment
Crash cart and availability of trained personnel
Storage facilities for respiratory equipment and relaxation training mats
Easy access parking

pulmonary patients receive Medicare benefits, and reimbursement is determined by a *fiscal intermediary*. It is important for the rehabilitation team and the billing department of a facility to be familiar with the requirements of both Medicare and the fiscal intermediary. It is extremely unfortunate that most Medicaid systems (in contrast to Medicare) do not reimburse for pulmonary rehabilitation programs; this effectively denies many patients an important treatment.

Private insurance companies generally reimburse for pulmonary rehabilitation, although the amount and form of reimbursement vary greatly. Health maintenance organizations (HMOs) also vary widely with respect to their reimbursement for pulmonary rehabilitation. More and more frequently, HMOs are regarding pulmonary rehabilitation as a means of reducing the length of hospitalization and, therefore, specifically refer patients to rehabilitation programs.

Documentation is one of the most important factors in obtaining reimbursement. All members of the rehabilitation team are advised to document their services carefully as described in the next section.

DOCUMENTATION AND REPORTING

In accordance with the provision of quality care and with the necessity of patient chart review by reimbursement agencies, individual patient documentation should clearly express the specific goals of both the patient and the team and describe the progress made in pursuing those goals. Documentation begins with an initial assessment that describes the need for rehabilitation, the skill level of the therapists required, and the plan for attaining reasonable goals. Verification of the need for rehabilitation in terms of the patient's ability to function is made, and the patient's current limitations are compared with their previous level of functioning. The rehabilitation team must describe specific problems and consistently document in the progress notes how these problems are being managed. Descriptions should be specific and not include catchall phrases (e.g., ADL) that tend to suggest that the patient is receiving a program that is not individualized.

The documentation need not be voluminous. Rather, it should be clear as to the need for the high level of caregiver skill involved in rehabilitation and as to how the patient is progressing toward reasonable goals. Consistent documentation states goals, discusses problems, and describes the patient's progress toward the attainment of goals. A well-documented patient chart saves the time of the team and that of the reviewer. Also, the report to the referring physician should be included in any consideration of documentation because he or she is responsible for the patient's long-term management.

ORGANIZATION OF THE PROGRAM

Program organization includes not only the components of a successful pulmonary rehabilitation program but also the structure of the program. The structure of the rehabilitation program takes into account the patient population and the overall goal of rehabilitation (i.e., to change patients' lifestyles).

Most patients who enter pulmonary rehabilitation programs are in the geriatric age group, and many of these patients have decreased cognitive functioning. Thus, a program that requires patients to digest and distill a large amount of information may not bring forth a lasting lifestyle change. In such a program, the patients are left to interpret, modify, and adapt the information they receive to meet their own needs.

A preferable alternative is to introduce the patient to a living framework that includes a more active lifestyle and disease self-management. This living pattern is initiated on the very first day of rehabilitation and is practiced throughout the program under health care team supervision. It includes daily exercises, bronchial hygiene skills, and other disciplines of daily life. In the course of the program, the patients are helped to understand the logical basis for the pattern they are practicing. In this manner, the patients have the greatest possible opportunity to practice the program under professional observation and direction.

PRESENTATION

Presentation of information must be clear, concise, uncomplicated, and repetitive. Only a limited number of important "take-home messages" should be presented within a given time span. Disciplines and methods should be repeated and practiced throughout the program. As the program progresses, the patients learn the value of these practices through both training and positive experience. The patients' goal is to learn a more efficacious lifestyle and to manage their lung disease with a minimum of intrusion in their lives.

Inpatient Versus Outpatient Rehabilitation

The advantage of an inpatient program lies in its capacity to be intensive even for patients with severe impairment.[7, 8] However, outpatient programs afford patients the opportunity to practice their skills at home and to be more nearly independent earlier in the course of rehabilitation. The major factor that determines a patient's status (inpatient or outpatient) is whether he or she requires 24-hour nursing care. If the patient has just experienced an exacerbation of disease and is still too weak to return home from the hospital, an inpatient program may provide an excellent transition to a less expensive and more appropriate level of care. As the patient's functioning improves, his or her transfer to outpatient status is possible and desirable. Such a course of action is a reasonable use of resources; if the patient were not transferred, he or she would have had to remain at a higher level of care for a longer period of time.

THE PULMONARY REHABILITATION TEAM

Pulmonary rehabilitation programs integrate medical management with training, the teaching of coping skills, and exercise; such integrated programs require a wide spectrum of medical and paramedical disciplines.[1-3, 5] Ideally, a team of medical and paramedical professionals—each of whom represents a specific function, perspective, or skill—conducts the program in an organized fashion. The composition of the pulmonary rehabilitation team can vary. Even the roles of specific members or disciplines can differ. However, in a complete rehabilitation team, the major players include a medical director, a nurse coordinator, a respiratory therapist, an occupational therapist, a physical therapist, a social worker, and a dietitian. Additional support can be obtained from the clinical pharmacist, psychologist, case manager, and exercise physiologist.

In most instances, the medical director is a pulmonologist who serves as the medical and physiologic consultant to the team. He or she is usually not the patient's primary physician. Typically, he or she conducts the team's rounds or leads the conference at which the course of a patient's rehabilitation is established. The medical director can assess the patient's medication regimen, determine if he or she has other health problems that might complicate the rehabilitative process, and interact with the patient's primary physician. In an inpatient program, the medical director may temporarily assume responsibility for the patient's care and subsequently relinquish that role to the patient's primary physician at the end of the program. He or she also provides the primary physician with a report and recommendations for the patient's continued care. The medical director is the program's medical advocate in the hospital, among the medical staff, and in the community.

The other allied health professionals on the team practice their specialties. Each member of the team has a specific teaching role. A nurse who is trained in respiratory care or a respiratory therapist is chosen to coordinate the day-to-day activities of the team. The nurse is involved in the clinical aspects of the program and is the team member most often in contact with the medical director. The nurse also teaches the self-medication program. The respiratory therapist teaches the self-administration of respiratory medications, oxygen therapy, and chest physiotherapy. He or she also arranges for home oxygen supplies and other respiratory equipment.

The physical therapist conducts exercise programs that are designed to improve endurance and strength, teaches stretching exercises, and provides support to patients with back problems that are caused by osteoporosis and spinal compressions commonly associated with steroid therapy. The occupational therapist often administers the upper extremity exercises and teaches ADL techniques for self-care and management of the home. Included among the ADL techniques are problem-solving methods, pacing and motion economy disciplines, relaxation training, and stress management. The social worker teaches the patients how to manage within their home or work environments and secures community resources as necessary. Sometimes the social worker provides psychologic support services to the patient and rehabilitation team. The dietitian helps the patients to meet their nutritional needs, to lose or gain weight, and to reduce their sodium intake.

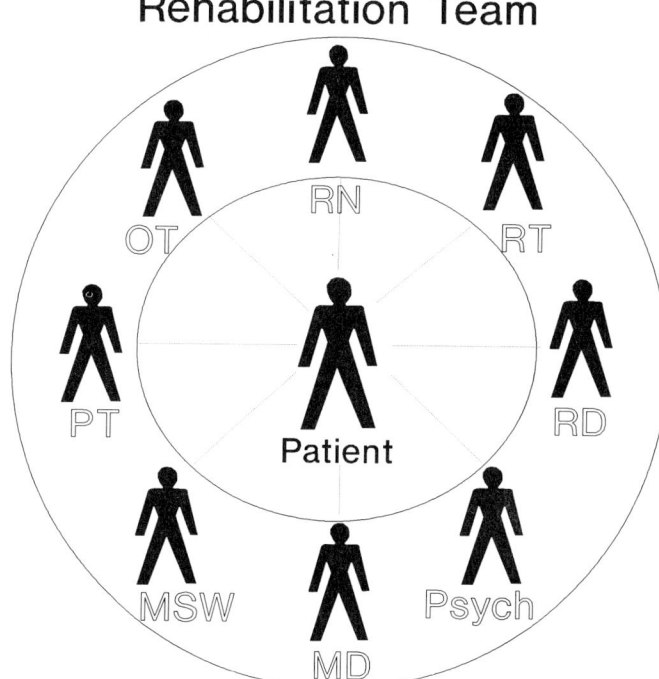

FIGURE 22-1. The rehabilitation team. (RN: registered nurse; RT: registered technician; RD: registered dietitian; Psych: psychiatrist; MD: medical doctor; MSW: medical social worker; PT: physical therapist; OT: occupational therapist.) (Courtesy of Casa Colina Hospital for Rehabilitation Medicine, Pomona, CA.)

There are several areas that are addressed by several disciplines. For example, stress management might be conducted by the psychologist, social worker, or the occupational therapist within different contexts. Both the nurse and respiratory therapist train patients in the effective use of metered-dose inhalers.

Because self-management is a major goal, the patient is also considered to be the central member of the team with respect to his or her program (Fig. 22-1).

In many or perhaps most instances, a team of participants such as that described may not be available, particularly in this era of cost restraints. Very effective rehabilitation can be administered by fewer therapists who are well trained in the areas crucial to the patient's rehabilitation. It is not unusual for a nurse, respiratory therapist, or physical therapist to conduct the vast majority of the program and call on other health care professionals as necessary.

The Team Concept

The pulmonary rehabilitation team is an interdisciplinary, interactive, and coordinated group of health care

TABLE 22-3. THE CHARACTERISTICS OF THE PULMONARY REHABILITATION TEAM

Interdisciplinary with a common purpose
Interactive and collaborative
Overlapping roles
Authority at the lowest levels
Trust
Knowledge of specialized area
A philosophic leader and coordinator (may or may not be same person)

professionals whose common goal is to restore function to patients with pulmonary disability and handicap.[9-11] Since each health care team member is a professional and a specialist, each contributes to decision-making and is regarded as a colleague by the physician. Consistency and continuity are important; therefore, most team members should be regular rather than rotating-shift therapists. Problems are identified and managed early.[9,10] This improves efficiency and prevents myriad greater problems. A key nurse or therapist coordinates the team's daily operations.[10] Each team member contributes to major decisions in regard to the direction of or a change in the patient's care. There is significant authority at the lowest levels.

The function of the team is truly collaborative. Members have autonomy, and yet their roles overlap.[10,11] Team members have shared knowledge, mutual trust, and a common purpose. Most important, the team takes on the personality of its individual members as it forms its own collective personality. The team usually has a philosophic leader who devotes more time and energy to supporting the team than to actually directing it. Previous studies have demonstrated that a well-functioning team is a major factor contributing to successful clinical outcome in both the acute and chronic settings.[9] A summary of the characteristics of an effective rehabilitation team is presented in Table 22-3.

PROGRAM COORDINATION

Patients with chronic lung disease are usually clinically stable during the pulmonary rehabilitation program. However, chronic lung disease can sometimes become acute very suddenly. Since many chronic lung disease patients come to pulmonary rehabilitation programs after they have experienced multiple exacerbations that require hospitalization, rapid change in patient health status during rehabilitation is common. During the course of the program, patients are observed for signs and symptoms that indicate the need for prompt intervention. Thus, the team should include a coordinator who is aware of all aspects of the patient's condition and who is prepared to react appropriately to changes in the patient's physical and emotional states. Also, a physician should be available at all times.

CONFERENCES AND ROUNDS

One of the features of the rehabilitation team is that the patient and the team mutually participate in conferences and rounds.[10,11] The utility of this function is manifold: goals are planned, progress is evaluated, problems are identified, and treatment directions are determined. Patients have the opportunity to function within the team, and family members can understand and participate in the rehabilitative process. Also, this form of patient-team participation provides an excellent opportunity for case managers and newly initiated health professionals to observe how a health care team functions.

CONTRACT

A pulmonary rehabilitation program is a unique experience in health care. It requires patient and family involvement in the treatment process. Participation in it requires hard work, and yet it is designed to be enjoyable. Most of all, a pulmonary rehabilitation program demands the patient's lifetime commitment. A contract that describes the program and the commitment it involves is an excellent introduction for the patient. The contract immediately initiates the patient in the rehabilitation process, and his or her signature is the first sign of commitment.[4]

The contract can take one of several forms, but in general it describes the program, specifies the commitment required of the patient, and appears somewhat legal. The contract should have a title such as "Pulmonary Rehabilitation Therapeutic Contract," and it should be printed on paper that is official in appearance. There should be specific places on the document for both the patient's and team coordinator's signatures.

PATIENT GUIDEBOOK

Patients undergoing a rehabilitation program receive a large amount of information that they must process and incorporate into their daily lives. A manual or guidebook can help to put this information into perspective.[12,13] Also, the patient will require a reference listing of resources after completion of the program. The guidebook should be short and concise and have a clear table of contents as well as large, readable type, and the information it contains should be relevant and consistent with the program.

The guidebook may list emergency information and important telephone numbers on the inside of the front cover. A one-page summary of the program might appear on the first page of the guidebook. The table of contents should be consistent with the summary page. Each section should be clearly labeled.

An introduction that describes the philosophy of the program and tells how to use the guidebook can set the stage for better patient understanding. Also, the daily instructions and descriptions as to how to maintain the

TABLE 22–4. SUMMARY OF THE CHARACTERISTICS OF A PULMONARY REHABILITATION GUIDEBOOK

Format
  Simple and clear
  Large readable type
  No crowding of pages
  Simple illustrations
  Upbeat and encouraging
  Some repetition for emphasis
  Section tabs

Table of Contents
  Reveals important points of the program
  Simplifies location of subjects in guidebook

Summary of Program
  Conveniently located and interrelated with the table of contents
  Gives rehabilitation information at a glance

Introduction
  Describes the philosophy of rehabilitation
  Explains goals and expectations

Descriptions
  Short description of the heart and lungs and of their role in the body
  COPD, asthma, and fibrosis

Relevance
  Information provided is related to the program and relevant to the patient

Important Emergency Information Page
  Emergency telephone numbers, including 911 and the numbers of the hospital, the patient's physician, and the local pharmacies

Glossary
  Explanation of common terms

---

daily record should be conveniently located. Also, there should be a description of the lungs and of how COPD and other lung diseases affect the lungs. All of the program's components should be simply and clearly presented. A glossary and an index at the end of the guidebook can add to the ease of its use and to its effectiveness. A summary of the recommended features of a pulmonary rehabilitation guidebook is presented in Table 22–4.

PROGRAM COMPONENTS

Attitudes and Motivation

Patients with chronic lung disease are disabled largely as a result of their adaptive response to progressive impairment rather than of the impairment itself. As their lungs have deteriorated, they have become progressively inactive. They conceive of themselves as sedentary onlookers to life rather than as active participants. Thus, the major tasks of the pulmonary rehabilitation program are not only to change how patients are able to function but also to improve their self-images. Changes in function and self-image come from the experience of being active that is gained in the program. Through the encouragement of the rehabilitation team, this experience translates into increased confidence. The encouragement of the team should be designed into the structure of the program.

Acceptance of the Disease

For the pulmonary rehabilitation intervention to be successful, the patient must accept the problem against which the intervention is directed.[14, 15] Denial is common in chronic lung disease patients and is firmly based in the disease's slow progression. Patients do not accept oxygen or any other medication or therapy if they do not accept their disease. This is one area in which a program's educational component must be individualized if a patient is to recognize that the description of the pathology directly applies to him or her. It is especially helpful to relate physiologic findings to symptoms. Finally, each patient should have pulmonary function studies and their significance explained to him or her.

Active Lifestyle

Patients are taught that the development and maintenance of an active lifestyle are basic to successful rehabilitation. In the program, the patients retake charge of their own lives.[15, 16] Not only is it necessary for them to perform the daily essentials, such as self-care, home maintenance, and self-management of their disease, but also for them to do something enjoyable. Patients are taught to be good to themselves as a part of maintaining physical and mental health.

Critical Knowledge

"Critical knowledge" includes an understanding of the lungs and of how illness affects them. This understanding must be functional so that the patient's self-management of his or her illness takes on a logical meaning.[7, 8] Patients learn to recognize early warning signs of an exacerbation and the importance of seeking prompt medical attention. They come to understand and adhere to a no-smoking policy that includes the avoidance of both personal and second-hand smoke. They learn self-assessment skills and how to report their symptoms to their physicians. Finally, they learn how to keep a daily record and how to use that record when reporting to their doctors and their teams.

Smoking

The "great common denominator" of most patients entering pulmonary rehabilitation programs is a history of smoking. Typically, patients quit smoking before entering a rehabilitation program. Those patients who still smoke have two options: (1) they must first become nonsmokers as a prerequisite to entry into the program, or (2) they enter the program while undergoing parallel smoking cessation therapy. Both approaches are workable, but their success depends on the philosophy of the team.

Another role of the program is to help the patients and their families to understand the importance of maintaining a smoke-free environment. In order to accomplish this, family members and patients must learn to appreciate the damaging nature of second-hand smoke.

Medicines

Accurate and reliable self-administration of medicines by patients is critical to their maintaining independence.[17] The primary concern in the development of any self-medication program is patient compliance. Without compliance, there is no basis for patient self-management. It is generally assumed that if the patient really understands the value of a particular medication, he or she is more likely to take it as prescribed. As more medications are prescribed and as their administration schedules become more complex, life itself becomes complicated, and patients are less likely to remain compliant. Patients should keep a list of their medications with them at all times (Fig. 22–2).

Most patients consider pills, elixirs, and "shots" as medicines, but some patients do not regard inhaled medications as such. Patients in pulmonary rehabilitation programs learn that medications administered using metered-dose inhalers and motor-driven nebulizers are an important part of their medication program.

In self-medication programs, patients are taught how to chart their use of medicines in a simple and straightforward fashion. The lettering on the chart should be large because some patients are visually impaired. All charts should be helpful tools for the patient rather than a burden. Medication charts should include the names of the medicines, their doses, what they are for, their administration schedules, and check-off boxes (Fig. 22–3).

Exercise Rationale

In pulmonary rehabilitation programs, patients start exercise regimens that they must continue for the rest of their lives.[18–20] They learn to fully understand that the benefits of exercise include not only improvement in endurance and strength but also the relief of dyspnea, anxiety, and depression as well as the mobilization of secretions. For the exercise program to be effective, the patient must intellectually and emotionally understand that it must be performed almost daily.

Nutrition

Some patients are markedly underweight, whereas others are grossly overweight. Thus, many patients need specific nutritional counseling. Underweight patients require measures to improve their overall nourishment, and thus their strength and stamina, whereas overweight patients need to lose weight in order to lower the workload on their heart and ventilatory muscles.[21] The dietitian can be helpful in this regard. Nutritional intervention is difficult, requires continuous attention, and often yields disappointing long-term results.

Skills and Techniques

Daily Instructions

A summary of the rehabilitation program is very useful to the patient and should be included in their rehabilitation guidebook. This summary can include a brief description of the goals of rehabilitation, a general description of daily requirements, and instructions for how to react when signs of an exacerbation are recognized or in the event of an emergency. The summary is essentially a one-page "refresher" on the nature of pulmonary rehabilitation (Fig. 22–4). A patient who has strayed from the program can use the summary as the first step in returning to his or her daily regimen.

Patient Daily Charting

Daily charting is a tool for patients to understand and communicate their health status. Recordkeeping should be neither cumbersome nor intrusive. It should be simple, straightforward, convenient, and meaningful to both the patients and their physicians (Fig. 22–5). A considerable amount of information can be recorded in less than 1 minute, particularly if the patient is only required to check off or circle a number or entry. If each circled entry is connected by a line to the previous day's circled entry, then a graph is created. This procedure is similar to peak flow rate monitoring by asthmatic patients. When a downturn in patient status occurs, it can be easily detected on the graph, making it possible to quell an exacerbation more rapidly.

The chart shown in Figure 22–5 assesses exercise status, dyspnea, cough, sputum production, and general status. These indicators are compared from day to day as better than ($+$), the same as ($=$), or worse ($-$) than on the previous days.

Breathing Retraining

Patients are taught pursed-lip breathing and diaphragmatic breathing techniques to reduce dyspnea and improve gas exchange.[22–27] These techniques, which are useful in controlling anxiety and panic, should become second nature to the patient if they are to be of lasting benefit. The patient's breathing technique is observed and corrected by all members of the team throughout the program.

Biofeedback

There are several forms of biofeedback that are useful to patients with chronic lung disease. The most common are electromyographic data, galvanic skin resistance, and skin temperature, knowledge of which can be useful in relaxation. Other biofeedback modalities that are more specific to the needs of pulmonary patients reduce

Casa Colina Pulmonary Rehabilitation
MEDICATIONS

Drug dose	Purpose	Morning	Afternoon	Evening	Bedtime	Xtra
Theophylline 300 mg	Breathing	1		1		
Prednisone 5 mg	Breathing	3				
Lasix 40 mg	Water	1				
Potassium 10 mEq	Potassium replacement	1		1		
Atrovent MDI	Open Airways	3	3	3	3	PRN
Albuterol MDI	Open Airways	2	2	2	2	PRN
Azmacort MDI	Open Airways	4			4	

Patient:_____ Patient #:_____

FIGURE 22-2. Medication list. (MDI: metered dose inhaler; PRN: as needed.) (Courtesy of Casa Colina Hospital for Rehabilitation Medicine, Pomona, CA.)

the work of breathing, relax bronchospasm, and improve gas exchange.[28] Pulse oximetry feedback has been used in conjunction with pursed-lip breathing training to increase oxygen saturation.[25] Some patients who require supplemental oxygen only during exertion are able to maintain adequate oxygen saturation during exercise by using such biofeedback-guided pursed-lip breathing.

Clearing Secretions

While in the program, patients learn methods of coughing and clearing secretions. They learn the importance of being well hydrated and of avoiding salt to reduce fluid retention. They learn to associate their metered-dose inhaled medication and nebulized medication with secretion clearance.

Chest Physiotherapy

Not all patients require chest physiotherapy. Those who do are taught self-administration so that physiotherapy can become a part of their daily ritual.[29-30] Chest physiotherapy is particularly important early in the morning when secretions are copious and difficult to expel.[31]

Oxygen

Patients who are hypoxemic require oxygen supplementation.[32, 33] Many patients find it difficult to accept their need for oxygen as oxygen use implies the presence of severe disease and impending death.[34] The patients are taught the rationale for oxygen prescription. They must also learn that they cannot use dyspnea as an indicator of oxygen deficiency, but rather that they must base their oxygen therapy on the results of blood gas testing. Patients learn the special importance of using supplemental oxygen both when exerting themselves and during sleep.

If patients are learning to be active, oxygen therapy should focus on the use of portable oxygen systems. These systems should be lightweight, easy to transfill or

CASA COLINA HOSPITAL FOR REHABILITATIVE MEDICINE   PULMONARY ACTIVATION PROGRAM

MEDICATION CHART

MEDICATION INHALERS: MDIs	MONDAY M N E N Xtra	TUESDAY M N E N Xtra	WEDNESDAY M N E N Xtra	THURSDAY M N E N Xtra	FRIDAY M N E N Xtra	SATURDAY M N E N Xtra	SUNDAY M N E N Xtra
Atrovent 3pf							
Albuterol 2pf							
Azmacort 4pf							

ORAL MEDICINE	M N E N Xtra	M N E N Xtra	M N E N Xtra	M N E N Xtra	M N E N Xtra	M N E N Xtra	M N E N Xtra
TheoSlo 300mg							
Prednisone 5mg							
Lasix 40mg							
KCl 10 mEq							

FIGURE 22-3. Medication charts, such as the one shown here, should be simple check-off forms that include the names of the medicines administered to the patient, their dosages, and the times they are to be administered. (M: morning; N: noon; E: evening; N: night.) (Courtesy of Casa Colina Hospital for Rehabilitation Medicine, Pomona, CA.)

PULMONARY REHABILITATION ENCAPSULATED

CONCEPTS:

Be active and in control of your life. Try to enjoy life every day. Don't let anxiety, panic, or depression take over.
Use your breathing techniques for good control.
Exercise daily for strength, stamina, and confidence.
Maintain good nutrition for strength and energy. Avoid salt.
Recognize your health status. Know your medicines. Carry your medication list with you at all times! Clear your secretions, get help early if you are getting worse, communicate well with your doctor.

DAILY INSTRUCTIONS:

Know your body, your lungs, and your illness. Recognize early warning signs that you need medical help and seek rapid attention. NO SMOKING—yours or anyone else's!
How are you doing compared to yesterday? Better, the same, or worse? Keep your daily record so that you can see any change in your condition!

Medicines
   Inhalers: Use every 4 hours or more often as needed.
   Oral Medications: Know your medicines and instructions.

Breathing Control
   Use your breathing techniques: Inhale through your nose and exhale slowly through pursed lips.

Exercise
   Walk daily!
   Perform arm exercises every other day.
   Perform other prescribed exercise as directed.

Clear Your Secretions
   Drink some fluids throughout the day, take your inhalers, cough effectively, and exercise.

Nutrition
   Maintain a proper diet for strength and stamina, as prescribed. Avoid salt.

On Oxygen?
   Take as prescribed (determined by your blood gases).

Feelings
   Control anxiety and depression via your exercise, good nutrition, and your breathing techniques. Avoid panic! Be in control.

Insomnia
   Avoid sleeping pills, stimulants near bedtime, and daytime sleeping. Use your relaxation methods; reading, TV, or radio are good distractions. If you awaken at night short of breath, get up, take your inhalers, drink some water, and cough clear secretions.

Active Lifestyle
   Be good to yourself. Be active and in control, and do something nice every day.

Your Doctor
   Go to your doctor prepared to communicate any change in your symptoms. Take your daily record, medication list, and list of questions.

IN THE EVENT OF AN EMERGENCY:

Don't panic. Call 911, use pursed-lip breathing, use metered-dose inhalers or nebulizers continuously, and have your medication list close by.

FIGURE 22–4. Daily patient instructions, consisting of a one-page summary of the patient's pulmonary rehabilitation program. (Courtesy of Casa Colina Hospital for Rehabilitation Medicine, Pomona CA.)

exchange, and acceptable to the patient and family. Oxygen-conserving devices can greatly improve the portability and range of ambulatory oxygen systems from the home.[35] A good working relationship should exist among the rehabilitation team, the patient, and the home oxygen supplier so that the transition to home oxygen therapy is smooth and nonthreatening to the patient. The rehabilitation team should understand the rules and regulations regarding reimbursement for home oxygen therapy so that patients can be provided with the most appropriate systems.

Activities of Daily Living

Training in ADL is key to all successful rehabilitation.[36] ADL comprise all of the methods and techniques for independent living and include self-care, home management, and work and leisure activities. ADL training helps patients to learn to perform life's activities more efficiently and comfortably. The patient in Figure 22–6 is being taught energy conservation methods while cooking in an ADL kitchen. Patients learn economy of work, pacing, and how to prioritize daily chores. All of the other aspects of pulmonary rehabilitation contribute to ADL training. Arm exercises lend strength and endurance to upper body activity, particularly grooming activity. Walking programs build generalized strength and endurance, whereas the reduction of dyspnea and breathing retraining directly control dyspnea and improve gas exchange.

Psychosocial Factors

Inherent in pulmonary rehabilitation programs are methods for addressing the psychosocial component of chronic lung disease.[37] Physiologic impairment is only one component of the pulmonary patient's progressive disability.[15, 16] A patient's progressive inactivity and dependence on others have an impact on the psychosocial make-up of the patient and his or her family. Thus, the program that addresses psychosocial factors is able to manage these areas. Often, patients with chronic lung disease have other psychosocial and family-centered impairments that require special attention. If such is the case, a psychologist or marriage and family counselor should be requested. Also, many patients become depressed and anxious. The general rehabilitation program

COMPONENTS OF THE PULMONARY REHABILITATION PROGRAM

CASA COLINA HOSPITAL		PULMONARY ACTIVATION PROGRAM											DAILY RECORD
INSTRUCTIONS:	**Monday**		**Tuesday**		**Wednesday**		**Thursday**		**Friday**		**Saturday**		**Sunday**
SOB:	SOB		SOB		SOB		SOB		SOB		SOB		SOB
(+) less SOB	+		+		+		+		+		+		+
(=) no change	=		=		=		=		=		=		=
(−) more SOB	−		−		−		−		−		−		−
COUGH:	COUGH		COUGH		COUGH		COUGH		COUGH		COUGH		COUGH
(+) more cough	+		+		+		+		+		+		+
(=) no change	=		=		=		=		=		=		=
(−) less cough	−		−		−		−		−		−		−
SPUTUM:	SPUTM		SPUTM		SPUTM		SPUTM		SPUTM		SPUTM		SPUTM
(+) thin, light	+		+		+		+		+		+		+
(=) no change	=		=		=		=		=		=		=
(−) thick, dark	−		−		−		−		−		−		−
WALK:	WALK		WALK		WALK		WALK		WALK		WALK		WALK
Minutes of	60		60		60		60		60		60		60
continuous	50		50		50		50		50		50		50
walking.	40		40		40		40		40		40		40
	30		30		30		30		30		30		30
	20		20		20		20		20		20		20
	10		10		10		10		10		10		10
	5		5		5		5		5		5		5
	0		0		0		0		0		0		0
SOB:	SOB		SOB		SOB		SOB		SOB		SOB		SOB
After walking,	1		1		1		1		1		1		1
count to 20. Circle	2		2		2		2		2		2		2
the no. of breaths	3		3		3		3		3		3		3
required.	4		4		4		4		4		4		4
ARM EXERCISES:	ARM		ARM		ARM		ARM		ARM		ARM		ARM
(+) easier	+		+		+		+		+		+		+
(=) no change	=		=		=		=		=		=		=
(−) harder	−		−		−		−		−		−		−
SOB:	SOB		SOB		SOB		SOB		SOB		SOB		SOB
Count to 20.	1		1		1		1		1		1		1
Circle the no. of	2		2		2		2		2		2		2
breaths required.	3		3		3		3		3		3		3
	4		4		4		4		4		4		4
Since yesterday do you feel:	GENRL		GENRL		GENRL		GENRL		GENRL		GENRL		GENRL
(+) better?	+		+		+		+		+		+		+
(=) no change?	=		=		=		=		=		=		=
(−) worse?	−		−		−		−		−		−		−
WEIGHT:		XXX		XX		XX		XX		XX		XX		

FIGURE 22–5. Patient's daily record. (SOB: shortness of breath; GENRL: general.) (Courtesy of Casa Colina Hospital for Rehabilitation Medicine, Pomona, CA.)

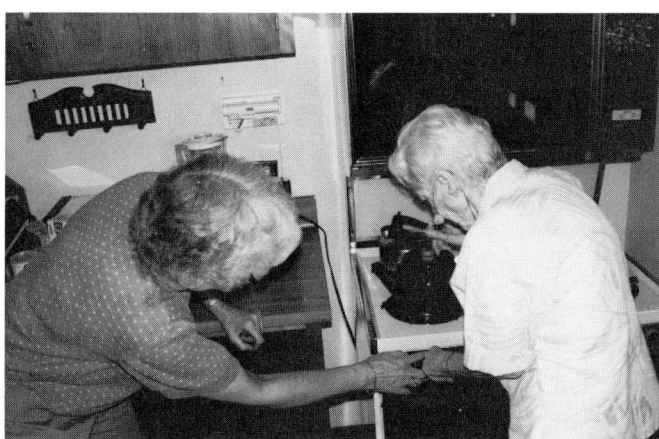

FIGURE 22-6. A patient in an activities of daily living kitchen learning energy conservation methods during cooking and other common household tasks.

may relieve the causes of depression and anxiety for some patients, but others require individual or group counseling.

Feelings

Patients learn that anxiety and depression are common among people with lung disease.[14, 16] They also learn that these potentially disabling emotions are controllable, often without medications. Patients are provided with relaxation training as well as with psychologic means for directly controlling their uncomfortable feelings. Exercise programs often bolster self-confidence and afford a "time out" (rest) period from depressing and anxiety-provoking thoughts. Thus, the general process of a rehabilitation program can help in this important area. Occasionally, a patient might require medication, psychologic support, or both.

Insomnia

Chronic lung disease patients often suffer from insomnia that is the result of a variety of causes.[14] In the rehabilitation program, they learn that a lack of sleep is not itself dangerous. This removes a major source of anxiety and can mitigate sleeplessness. Patients are taught to avoid taking sleeping pills. They should not take stimulants, nor should they exercise near their bedtime. They are taught relaxation methods that include progressive muscle relaxation (Fig. 22–7) and biofeedback. More commonly, they are taught that reading, listening to the radio, or watching television can induce somnolence in some people.[38] If the cause of insomnia is dyspnea, then the cause of the dyspnea is addressed. The patients learn to accept middle-of-the-night awakenings to open their airways and to clear their secretions. They get up, use their inhalers, drink some water, cough, and clear their secretions before resuming sleep.

Sexuality

Sexuality is part of human existence. It includes not only the physical sex act, but also how a person perceives himself or herself. As long as we are alive, we are sexual beings, even if we have not had physical sex in years.[39] Many rehabilitation programs address sexuality as a regular part of the program, whereas others offer assistance in this area to patients who request it. In any case, patients should be helped to feel comfortable when discussing sex, and specific help should be made available to those who require it.

The Patient and the Physician

Patients are taught that a visit to the physician is not simply a passive experience. The patient must take an active role, and communication must flow in both directions.[40] The patients become extensions of their physicians and are thus trained to prepare for the visit; specifically, they are taught to be able to report any change in their condition. If an exacerbation occurs, the patient must report it early or an emergency situation might result. Patients are taught to bring their daily records (see Fig. 22–5) when they visit their physicians. The records provide an instant history of their progress since the previous visit. In addition, patients are instructed to bring their list of medications and a written list of any questions they may have. The program teaches patients how to communicate accurately and efficiently with their physicians. The visit to the physician should be a pleasant and productive experience.

Endurance and Strength

Upper and Lower Extremity Exercise Program

Therapeutically, the most essential ingredient of pulmonary rehabilitation is the exercise program.[18, 19] Walking is the most practical exercise for most patients as it improves both mobility and independence. It is a sub-

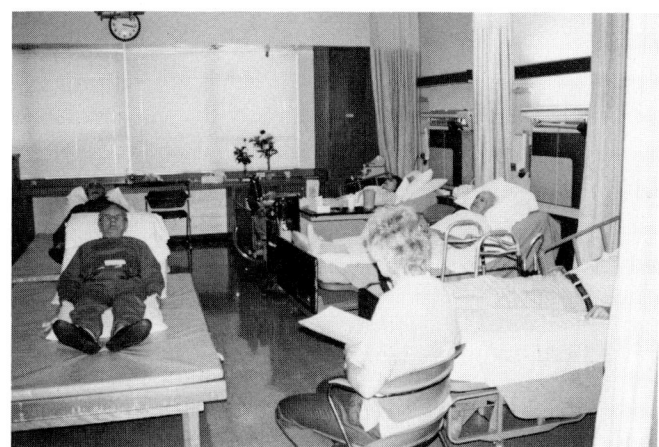

FIGURE 22-7. Patients learning progressive muscle relaxation to facilitate sleep and to control anxiety and panic.

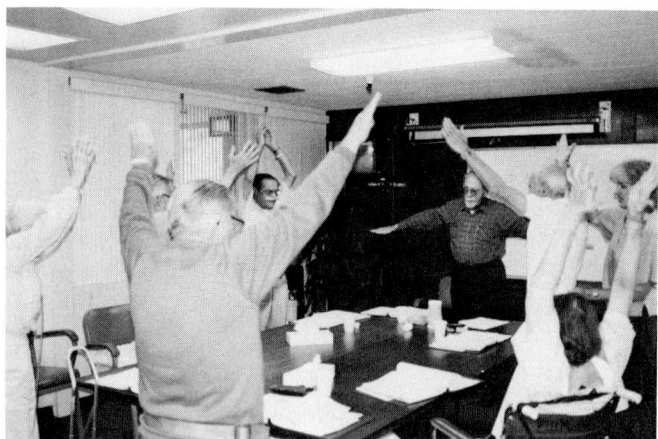

FIGURE 22–8. Gravity-resistive exercises; unsupported arm exercises are shown here.

maximal exercise for persons without lung disease, but it can be a major effort for the patient with cardiopulmonary impairment. Bicycle ergometry is not an ideal alternative to walking because it exercises a different set of muscles than walking and does not require weight-bearing. The obvious advantage of bicycle ergometry is its utility during inclement weather.

Upper extremity exercise builds strength and endurance in the muscle groups most involved in self-care.[41] Patients with chronic lung disease typically become dyspneic from any activity that requires the arms to work at shoulder level or above.[42] Arm bicycle ergometry (cranking) training is effective, although the arms must be supported by the hands on the pedal-cranks.[43] However, gravity-resistive exercises require the arms to work unsupported against the force of gravity.[42, 44] In such exercise, the patient performs repetitive exercises with the arms in various positions (usually at shoulder level or above; Fig. 22–8).

Before starting any exercise program, the patient should undergo exercise testing to determine the safety of program participation as well as the need for oxygen prescription.[45, 46] This testing is often performed on a treadmill or stationary bicycle, although it can consist of a hallway walking test. At a minimum, vital signs, dyspnea, the electrocardiogram, and pulse oximetry should be monitored.

Ventilatory Muscle Training

As a relative newcomer to rehabilitation, ventilatory muscle training has been shown to increase strength and endurance in the ventilatory muscles. There are three forms of such training: (1) isocapneic hyperpnea, which selectively builds endurance[47, 48]; (2) inspiratory resistance training, which builds strength in the inspiratory muscles[49]; and (3) inspiratory threshold training, which trains both endurance and strength, the proportions of which depend on the training protocol.[50] The benefits of ventilatory muscle training seem to be specific to the ventilatory muscle groups; its role in the general pulmonary rehabilitation program is discussed in Chapter 17.

Family Training

Ideally, the patient lives within a supportive family environment. Even if this is true, dynamics within the home are addressed by the rehabilitation team. The family plays an extremely important role in the rehabilitation of the chronic lung disease patient, and thus family members are urged to participate in the rehabilitative process.[15, 51] The relationship of the family to the patient can range from too supportive (i.e., family members do not allow the patient to do anything for himself or herself) to disinterested or even hostile. Family members are taught how to create a balance between being supportive and understanding and allowing the patient reasonable independence and dignity.[51]

Patients and families are encouraged to interact in a manner that allows the patient to participate in the home environment and that permits him or her to be less of a patient and more of a contributing family member.

Family members often participate in the program so that they are better able to assist their loved ones in hard times. They are taught the signs and symptoms of an impending exacerbation and how to manage the patient while seeking medical assistance. They learn problem-solving techniques, how to avoid panicking, and how to report to the physician.

The family is taught the value of maintaining a smoke-free environment. Even if other members of the family smoke, they must spare the patient from breathing the harmful chemical-laden air that results from their tobacco use. Also, if the patient has just quit smoking, exposure to the second-hand smoke of a family member can often produce irresistible urges to return to smoking.

Home Program

In preparing patients with chronic lung disease to return home, the health care team must provide them and their families with the tools and skills to live at home safely.[38] This is the overall task of the rehabilitation program. Going home is not a natural transition. Patients are discharged from a program that is both intense and supportive. Many patients become fearful of the outside environment because they have become dependent on their skilled and trusted therapists. In addition, patients leaving the program are often in an accelerated stage of improvement and have not yet reached their peak function levels. Thus, they are provided with a home program to continue their rehabilitation independently. Their progress is assessed during follow-up clinical visits. It is useful to provide the home patient with a call-in support system through which he or she can contact the rehabilitation team and sometimes other patients. The team or, ideally, the medical director, communicates the patient's progress to his or her private physician.

Team Follow-up

Naturally, a follow-up program is highly recommended. If possible, patients should be seen in a rehabilitation follow-up clinic to monitor and strengthen their rehabilitation disciplines. If the program is directed by a physician, then the follow-up evaluation may be performed by that physician. More commonly, it is conducted by other team members.

Physician Follow-up

The most important follow-up is performed by the patient's personal physician.[2, 4] For this follow-up to be successful, the patient's physician should understand the value and rationale of the rehabilitative approach. Good communication between the program physician and the patient's physician is essential.

Immediately after the conclusion of the pulmonary rehabilitation program, the patient should make an appointment to see his or her personal physician. In so doing, the personal physician can see the patient at his or her best; this gives the physician a frame of reference should the patient suffer an exacerbation. Also, physicians unaware of the value of rehabilitation will have a better perception of the overall benefits of these programs. In turn, this improves physician support of rehabilitation's goals and methods. Greater physician support of rehabilitation makes it available to other patients who need it.

The rehabilitation physician should not assume the general care of the patient unless requested to do so by the patient's physician. This policy helps to ensure the continuation of referrals.

Patient Support Groups

Patient support groups, such as Better Breather Clubs, can provide important help and encouragement. These support groups help patients to relate to other patients who have many of the same problems and concerns as they do.[7, 12] Also, patient support groups provide continuing education that brings hope to the demoralized patient. Patient support groups that participate in some of life's most enjoyable events bolster the morale of these patients and give them a reason to fight to survive.[52-54]

SUMMARY

Pulmonary rehabilitation is an interdisciplinary approach to the treatment of patients with chronic lung disease. The rehabilitation program is administered by an interactive team of medical and health care paraprofessionals whose members represent specific functions, perspectives, and skills. The team typically comprises a pulmonologist, a nurse, a respiratory therapist, an occupational therapist, a physical therapist, a social worker, a dietitian, and a psychologist.

The goals of pulmonary rehabilitation are to improve the patient's comfort, mobility, and ability to function independently in daily life. In rehabilitation, patients learn to employ a wide variety of skills and disciplines in their lives. The programs are structured in a manner that nurtures the training and practicing of these techniques by patients while they learn the rationale for incorporating them into daily life. Patients learn bronchial hygiene, upper and lower extremity exercises, stress and panic control techniques, and breathing skills. The entire process helps to reduce dyspnea, to promote an active lifestyle, and to improve quality of life.

Family training is critical to the overall success of rehabilitation. It is sometimes beneficial to train the family right along with the patient. After the patients complete the rehabilitation program, they are provided with a home program to continue their rehabilitation independently.

Follow-up is necessary to solidify and maintain life pattern changes. During follow-up sessions, the rehabilitation team reinforces what the patients learned during the program. Patients are also instructed to visit their personal physicians. The team sends a summary of the program to the private physician; this summary describes the patient's progress and includes recommendations for his or her long-term management. During the program, patients have learned to recognize signs and symptoms of exacerbation and how to report them to their physicians. These skills can be used in the home program as well. In addition, support groups provide hope and encouragement through opportunities for interaction with other patients. They also serve as forums for discussion of the latest advances in the treatment of lung disease.

Pulmonary rehabilitation is comprehensive in its approach as well as in its impact on patients and their families. The human drama of struggle and achievement unfolds with each new patient who enters a program. Those team members who participate in this drama are rewarded with the joys of accomplishment and of knowing that they have contributed to making the lives of their patients more livable.

REFERENCES

1. Hodgkin JE, Petty TL (eds). Chronic Obstructive Lung Disease: Current Concepts. Philadelphia: W.B. Saunders Co., 1987.
2. Hodgkin JE, Zorn EG, Connors Gl (eds). Pulmonary Rehabilitation: Guidelines to Success. Stoneham, MA: Butterworth's, 1984.
3. Petty TL, Nett LM, Finigan MM. A comprehensive care program for chronic airway obstruction: Methods and a preliminary evaluation of symptomatic and function improvement. Ann Intern Med 1969; 70:1109–1120.
4. Hodgkin JE. Organization of a pulmonary rehabilitation program. Clin Chest Med 1986; 7:541–550.
5. Holden DA, Stelmach KD, Curtis PS, et al. The impact of a rehabilitation program on functional status of patients with chronic lung disease. Respir Care 1990; 35:322–341.
6. Mahler DA. Dyspnea. Mt. Kisco, NY: Futura Publishing Co., 1990.
7. Burns M. Outpatient pulmonary rehabilitation. Postgrad Med 1989; 86:129–140
8. Tiep BL. Inpatient pulmonary rehabilitation: A team approach to the more fragile patient. Postgrad Med 1989; 86:141–150.
9. Knaus WA, Draper EA, Wagner DP, Zimmerman JE. An evalu-

ation of outcome from intensive care in major medical centers. Ann Intern Med 1986; 104:410–418.
10. Blake R, Mouton J, Allen R. Spectacular Teamwork: How to Develop the Leadership Skills for Team Success. New York: John Wiley & Sons, Inc., 1987.
11. Axelrod R. The Evaluation of Cooperation. New York: Basic Books, 1984.
12. Petty TL, Tiep BL, Burns M. Essentials of Pulmonary Rehabilitation: A "Do It Yourself" Program. Pulmonary Education and Research Foundation. Lomita, CA, 1991.
13. Tiep BL, Chow M. Pulmonary Activation Program: Rehabilitation Guidebook 1991. Pomona, CA, 1991.
14. Kinsman RA, Yaroush RA, Fernandez E, et al. Symptoms and experiences in chronic bronchitis and emphysema. Chest 1983; 83:755–761.
15. Williams SJ. Chronic respiratory illness and disability: A critical review of the psychosocial literature. Soc Sci Med 1989; 28:791–803.
16. Agle DP, Baum GL, Chester EH, Wendt M. Multidiscipline treatment of chronic pulmonary insufficiency: 1. Psychologic aspects of rehabilitation. Psychosom Med 1973; 35:41–49.
17. Theodore AC, Beer DJ. Pharmacotherapy of chronic obstructive pulmonary disease. Clin Chest Med 1986; 7:657–672.
18. Belman MJ. Exercise in chronic obstructive pulmonary disease. Clin Chest Med 1986; 7:585–598.
19. Casaburi R, Patessio A, Ioli F, et al. Reductions in exercise lactic acidosis and ventilation as a result of exercise training in patients with obstructive lung disease. Am Rev Respir Dis 1991; 143:9–18.
20. Daly J, Cooper C, Casaburi R, et al. Exercise training as a mediator of increased exercise performance in COPD patients undergoing rehabilitation. Am Rev Respir Dis 1989; 139:A330.
21. Wilson DO, Rogers RM, Openbrier D. Nutritional aspects of chronic obstructive pulmonary disease. Clin Chest Med 1986; 7:643–656.
22. Mueller RE, Petty TL, Filley GF. Ventilation and arterial blood gas changes induced by pursed lips breathing. J Appl Physiol 1970; 28:784–789.
23. Ingram RH, Schilder DP. Effect of pursed lips expiration on the pulmonary pressure-flow relationship in obstructive lung disease. Am Rev Respir Dis 1967; 96:381–388.
24. Schmidt RW, Wasserman K, Lillington FA. The effect of air flow and oral pressure on the mechanics of breathing in patients with asthma and emphysema. Am Rev Respir Dis 1964; 93:564–571.
25. Tiep BL, Burns M, Kao D, et al. Pursed lips breathing using ear oximetry. Chest 1986; 90:218–221.
26. Tiep BL, Burns M, Chow M, et al. Pursed lips breathing increases oxygen saturation in restrictive lung disease patients. Chest 1989; 96:205s.
27. Tiep BL, Burns M, Branum N. Pursed lips breathing and gas exchange. Chest 1990; 98:31s.
28. Tiep BL. Biofeedback and ventilatory muscle training. In: Hodgkin JE, Zorn EG, Connors GL (eds). Pulmonary Rehabilitation: Guidelines to Success. Philadelphia: J.B. Lippincott Co. (in press).
29. Bateman JRM, Newman SP, Daunt KM, et al. Regional lung clearance of excessive bronchial secretions during chest physiotherapy in patients with stable chronic airways obstruction. Lancet 1979; 1:294–297.
30. Bateman JRM, Newman SP, Daunt KM, et al. Is cough as effective as chest physiotherapy in removal of excessive tracheobronchial secretions? Thorax 1981; 36:683–687.
31. Faling LJ. Pulmonary rehabilitation: Physical modalities. Clin Chest Med 1986; 7:599–618.
32. Long term domiciliary oxygen therapy in chronic hypoxic cor pulmonale complicating chronic bronchitis and emphysema: Report of the Medical Research Council Working Party. Lancet 1981; 1:681–686.
33. Continuous or nocturnal oxygen therapy in hypoxemic chronic obstructive lung disease: A clinical trial, Nocturnal Oxygen Therapy Trial Group. Ann Intern Med 1980; 93:391–398.
34. Tiep BL. Long term oxygen therapy. In: Hodgkin JE (ed). Chronic obstructive pulmonary disease. Clin Chest Med 1990; 11:505–521.
35. Tiep BL. Portable oxygen therapy: Including oxygen conserving methodology. Mt Kisco, NY: Futura Publishing Co, 1991.
36. Walsh RL. Occupational therapy as part of a pulmonary rehabilitation program. Occup Ther Health Care 1986; 3:65–77.
37. Sandhu HS. Psychosocial issues in chronic obstructive pulmonary disease. Clin Chest Med 1986; 7:629–642.
38. Tiep BL, Lewis Y, Branum N, et al. Respiratory management at home. In: Portnow J (ed). Physical Medicine and Rehabilitation: State of the Art Reviews 1988; 2:385–403.
39. Selecky PA. Sexuality and the COPD patient. In: Hodgkin JE, Petty TL (eds). Chronic Obstructive Lung Disease: Current Concepts. Philadelphia: W.B. Saunders Co., 1987.
40. Powers JS. Patient-physician communication and interaction: A unifying approach to the difficult patient. South Med J 1985; 78:445–447.
41. Celli BR, Rassulo J, Make B. Dyssynchronous breathing during arm but not leg exercise in patients with chronic airflow obstruction. N Engl J Med 1986; 314:1485–1490.
42. Celli B, Criner G, Rassulo J. Ventilatory muscle recruitment during unsupported arm exercise in normal subjects. J Appl Physiol 1988; 64:1936–1941.
43. Ries AL, Ellis B, Hawkins RW. Upper extremity exercise training in chronic obstructive pulmonary disease. Chest 1988; 93:688–692.
44. Banzett RB, Topulos GP, Leith DE, Nations CS. Bracing arms increases the capacity for sustained hyperpnea. Am Rev Respir Dis 1988; 138:106–109.
45. Belman MJ, Wasserman K. Exercise training and testing in patients with chronic obstructive pulmonary disease. Basics of RD 1981; 10:1–6.
46. Wasserman K, Hansen J, Sue DY, Whipp BJ. Principles of Exercise Testing and Interpretation. Philadelphia: Lea & Febiger, 1987, pp 3–26.
47. Leith DE, Bradley M. Ventilatory muscle strength and endurance training. J Appl Physiol 1976; 41:508–516.
48. Belman MJ, Mittman C. Ventilatory muscle training improves exercise capacity in chronic obstructive pulmonary disease patients. Am Rev Respir Dis 1980; 121:273–280.
49. Sonne LJ, Davis JA. Increased exercise performance in patients with severe COPD following inspiratory resistive training. Chest 1982; 81:436–439.
50. Larson JL, Kim MJ, Sharp JT, Larson DA. Inspiratory muscle training with a pressure threshold breathing device in patients with chronic obstructive pulmonary disease. Am Rev Respir Dis 1988; 138:689–696.
51. Gilmartin M. Patient and family education. Clin Chest Med 1986; 7:619–628.
52. Burns M. Travel hints for the persons with COPD. In: Petty T, Nett L (eds). Enjoying Life with Emphysema. 2nd ed. Philadelphia: Lea & Febiger, 1987, pp 103–107.
53. Burns M. Travel and the COPD patient: Planning for problems. Respir Times 1988; 4:10–11.
54. Gong H. Guidelines for travel with oxygen in advanced COPD. Respir Times 1986; 1:22–23.

Chapter 23

Candidate Evaluation

ROGER S. GOLDSTEIN, M.B. Ch.B.,
F.R.C.P.(UK), F.R.C.P.(C), F.C.C.P.
MONICA A. AVENDANO, M.D., F.R.C.P.(C)

In this chapter, we address the process of candidate selection for pulmonary rehabilitation programs. Our approach has been developed based on practical experience with a 52-patient (26 inpatients and 26 outpatients) rehabilitation program at West Park Hospital in Toronto, Canada, and on numerous conversations with colleagues who have interests similar to our own. Our inpatient program is of 6 to 8 weeks' duration and consists of morning and afternoon activities conducted from Monday to Friday. On weekends, most patients return home. Our outpatient program is of 10 to 12 weeks' duration; patients attend on average 2 days per week and continue the program at home on the other days. In order to quantify some of our remarks, we reviewed all admissions to our program in 1990 and 1991. We believe that the proper selection of candidates is an important determinant of a successful rehabilitation program. It must be remembered, however, that respiratory rehabilitation is a treatment modality, and as such, it should always be medically indicated.

SOURCES OF REFERRAL

All patients are referred by physicians who are either family practitioners or internists with a respiratory subspecialty. Referrals are written and include either a brief medical history or a photocopy of a recent consultation note. Most patients live or have been hospitalized within 20 miles of our center (139 out of 182 admissions), but a substantial number of them live farther away. The patient's location is less important than is his or her clinical condition as a determinant of whether hospitalization or an outpatient program is required.

REASONS FOR REFERRAL

Many patients are referred to rehabilitation programs because a decrease in function has been documented or is suspected as being consequent to respiratory impairment. Common reasons for referral include the following:

1. Dyspnea experienced during rest or exertion. Rehabilitation is usually suggested when dyspnea begins to interfere with the patient's lifestyle.
2. Oxygen evaluation. Monitoring of blood oxygen saturation that results in either the initiation of or an adjustment to supplemental oxygen therapy.
3. Reduced exercise tolerance or a reduction in the ability to perform activities of daily living.
4. An unexpected deterioration. This includes worsening symptoms that occur against a background of longstanding dyspnea and a reduced but stable exercise tolerance level.
5. Preoperative rehabilitation in order to maximize medical status prior to the resection of a lung nodule or lung transplantation.
6. Evaluation of respiratory failure and the elective initiation of mechanical ventilation.

REASONS FOR ADMISSION

A large percentage of patients are admitted to a conventional, multidisciplinary, supervised exercise program of the type described elsewhere in this book. Some patients, however, are admitted for the investigation, management, or re-evaluation of hypoxemia, hypercapnia, or both. Depending on their underlying diagnosis,

TABLE 23-1. DIAGNOSTIC GROUPINGS AND REASONS FOR ADMISSION TO RESPIRATORY REHABILITATION*

Disease	No. of Admissions	(% of Total)	No. of Patients in Rehabilitation Program	No. of Other Patients (Reason for Admission)
Obstructive disease	146	(80)	124	22 (Oxygen evaluation)
Restrictive disease	35	(20)		
Thoracic restrictive and neuromuscular disease	31		11	20 (Ventilatory assessment)
Parenchymal disease	4		4	
Total	182	(100)		

*Data from West Park Hospital, Toronto, Ontario, Canada, for 1990 and 1991.

such patients may require supplemental oxygen or mechanical ventilation as part of their rehabilitation program (Table 23–1).

SYMPTOMS

Most patients complain of dyspnea on exertion (85%), of decreased exercise tolerance (67%), or both. Other symptoms commonly noted include difficulties during activities of daily living (53%), mood changes (36%), hypoxemia (35%), weight changes (23%), and soft tissue pain (47%).

SELECTION OF CANDIDATES

Important patient characteristics that determine the effectiveness of the rehabilitation program should be sought during the initial candidate evaluation.

Preprogram Motivation[1]

Good motivation is essential for a successful outcome. A well-motivated candidate has recognized the existence of his or her progressive physical limitation and the need for assistance. Establishing a patient's motivation for self-improvement and commitment to the necessary lifestyle changes brings together the patient and the health care team to the best effect.

Realistic Expectations

Even well-motivated patients should have realistic expectations both as to what is expected from them and as to what they are likely to achieve from participation in the program. If these expectations are unrealistic, the apparent lack of progress can be disruptive and detrimental to the patient, the health care team, and other individuals currently participating in the rehabilitation program. The patient and the health care team should agree on realistic goals at the time of the initial evaluation and candidate selection.

Adequate Comprehension

This is another essential component contributing to a successful outcome. Language problems might be dealt with by locating an interpreter from among the health care professionals. Simple hearing problems can also often be effectively addressed. Organic brain syndromes, however, preclude a successful rehabilitation program.

Adequate Home Situation

It must be established at the outset that there is a home for the patient to go to and that reasonable facilities for sleeping, cleaning, and washing exist there. Environmental considerations (e.g., possible exposure to smoke and pollution) are important, as are the physical facilities available in the home (e.g., an elevator for an upstairs apartment). Candidates with supportive families or other caregivers tend to do better than those who are socially isolated. For those patients who may require elective mechanical ventilatory support, special considerations (both social and financial) may apply, and for such individuals an inadequate home situation precludes this modality of treatment.

Clinical Factors[2,3]

Cessation of Smoking. Our policy has been to accept only nonsmokers for respiratory rehabilitation. Cessation of smoking reflects the patient's motivation and active commitment to a lifestyle change. Our past experience of accepting those patients who vowed to quit on the first day of their program is that they frequently start smoking soon after program completion. Moreover, supplemental oxygen therapy is unsafe and probably ineffective for those patients who continue to smoke. Other patients in the program may be sensitive to and antagonized by the smell of smoke. Therefore, our approach is to direct smokers to a smoking cessation program and to request that they contact us for reassessment 2 months after they have quit completely.

Patient Age. The age of the patients does not determine whether they are accepted for rehabilitation. Patients range from ages 20 years to 80 years or more. The mean age of 182 patients (94 men and 88 women) accepted to our program last year was 62 ± 13 years.

Respiratory Stability. Of 126 chronic obstructive pulmonary disease (COPD) patients admitted for rehabilitation, 110 came from home and 16 were transferred from an acute care hospital. Of those requiring home ventilation, 24 patients came from home and 7 were transferred from an acute care hospital. Although rehabilitation is easier for patients who are clinically stable, it may be introduced (if medically indicated) during the recovery phase of an exacerbation provided that the acute component has been fully treated. Thus, rehabilitation may become part of a patient's convalescence provided that the intensity of the program is modified. It is important, however, that a referral for rehabilitation not be used as a substitute for convalescence; if such is the case, then a confusing and frustrating situation can arise in which the referring physician, the patient, and the rehabilitation team all have quite different expectations. In our experience, the severity of a patient's exacerbation does not influence the outcome of the rehabilitation unless complications (e.g., intractable heart failure or anoxic brain damage) have occurred. A severe exacerbation may prolong a patient's length of stay in the inpatient program (the mean length of stay in our program for patients with a diagnosis of COPD was 52 ± 18 days). Ventilation administered prior to the patient's entry into a rehabilitation program does not contraindicate rehabilitation whether or not the patient has been weaned. Patients transferred from hospitals often have the sequelae of prolonged illness and are sometimes completely bedridden at the start of their program. Such patients may experience a dramatic improvement in functional status during rehabilitation. However, some patients who appear to be ideal candidates become unstable. If candidates are carefully selected, this is not a common occurrence; in the last year, only 4 of 182 patients who were admitted to our service had to be transferred to an acute care facility.

Maximum Pharmacologic Therapy. The full approach to pharmacologic management of pulmonary disease is discussed elsewhere in this text. It is important, however, that pharmacologic therapy be maximized at the time of the initial evaluation. In the presence of airflow limitation, we usually test for reversibility and attempt to address this component with appropriate sympathomimetic or anticholinergic medications or with a trial of oral steroids, as indicated.

Associated Medical Conditions. Active associated medical conditions influence a patient's progress unless they are treated prior to admission to the program. Time allocated to the identification and management of such conditions often reduces the overall length of a patient's stay. This is especially the case when a cardiovascular disease—such as symptomatic ischemia, arrhythmias, or heart failure—is present. Similarly, active joint disease or claudication can militate against achieving benefits from an exercise program unless it is first treated. Malnutrition can be addressed at the time of the initial evaluation by implementing appropriate dietary changes.

CANDIDATE ASSESSMENT

The objectives of the medical evaluation for respiratory rehabilitation include (1) confirming the diagnosis, (2) establishing and characterizing the severity of the main symptoms, and (3) identifying the impact of the disease on the patient's lifestyle. One can separate the components of a baseline medical assessment into those that are essential and those that are optional.

Essential Investigations

Medical History. Candidate assessment begins with a medical evaluation that includes a medical history with a special focus on respiratory problems. In the history, the main limiting symptom of the patient is usually shortness of breath on exertion, but a reduced exercise tolerance that results from muscle weakness, pain, or generalized fatigue can also influence the initial approach to rehabilitation. Other symptoms that might denote cardiorespiratory failure (e.g., morning headaches, ankle edema, recent memory loss, and changes in weight) are important because they might indicate the need to consider ventilation as part of the rehabilitation process.[4, 5] The duration of the respiratory impairment is important as is its progression; when assessed in conjunction with physiologic measurements of pulmonary function, these factors may give some indications as to the patient's prognosis. A history of recurrent respiratory exacerbations, hospital admissions, and intensive care management may reflect the patient's respiratory stability and reserve.

A history of smoking is important for obvious reasons. The patient should be asked about any exposure to smoke he or she might have at the workplace or in the home or about other factors that trigger the patient's symptoms. The physician should know whether the patient drives, as important decisions relating to mobility and, thus, quality of life may need to be made. All current medications, including oxygen, are noted as is the frequency of antibiotic and steroid prescription.

A more thorough impression of the patient may be obtained if the medical assessment is carried out in the presence of a spouse or close caregiver. First, the physician might gain a sense of the motivation and support at home, factors that influence the patient's long-term compliance with the rehabilitation program. Second, the patient might be too dyspneic to give a good history. Third, the spouse might sometimes indicate whether an individual who has previously been stable is now experiencing an unexpected decline. This may be especially important if associated medical conditions such as anemia, malignancy, or heart failure are to be diagnosed or if a stressful social circumstance such as marriage, divorce, or a recent bereavement has occurred. We try to establish the patient's premorbid personality and to gain a sense of how he or she copes with other stresses in life. We are especially interested in learning about the presence of anxiety or depression as a usual response to dealing with stress as it might focus the health care team on the possibility of a similar response to the present stress.[6]

Physical Examination. The physical examination follows usual principles. Special attention is given to signs that may reflect respiratory distress or cardiorespiratory failure.

Hematologic and Biochemical Investigations. These investigations are limited to standard measurements (e.g., a blood count) that might reflect the presence of anemia or polycythemia; determinations of serum electrolytes, urea, creatinine, and blood glucose levels are also made. When appropriate, we usually measure serum levels of commonly used drugs such as theophylline and digoxin. The initial radiologic evaluation is usually restricted to a posteroanterior and lateral radiograph; other radiologic tests are performed as indicated.

Pulmonary Function Tests. Standard measurements of lung volumes, maximum forced expiratory flow rates, and diffusion are important in quantifying the disease and in establishing the relationship among the disease, the disability, and the handicap. This is not a predictable relationship and therefore needs to be established for each patient at the outset. We usually include measurements of respiratory muscle strength (maximum inspiratory pressure and maximum expiratory pressure), especially if muscle weakness is thought to be a contributing factor to the patient's level of functioning. Arterial blood gas parameters are measured while the patient breathes room air in a standardized body position.

The widespread use of oximetry has made it possible to make a more detailed assessment of arterial oxygen saturation (SaO_2) at rest, during exercise, during activities of daily living, and during sleep. All patients undergo this assessment before receiving an individualized oxygen prescription. We always include a simple measurement of global endurance such as a 6- or 12-minute walking test.[7,8] This test allows exercise tolerance to be assessed using the familiar activity of walking in a nonlaboratory setting. The distance covered during the test has been found to be significantly related to the patient's forced vital capacity, symptom-limited maximum oxygen uptake, and symptom-limited maximum ventilation.

Allied Health Clinical Assessments. Medically directed questions are sharply focused and make it difficult to explore the wider impact of the disease on the patient's life. Therefore, the allied health multidisciplinary clinical assessment is considered an essential preprogram step in candidate selection and evaluation. Rehabilitation must address not only the medical aspects of a disease, but also its broad impact on the life of the patient and on his or her family. Although the composition of a rehabilitation team varies depending on the specific requirements of the patient, in addition to the physician, core members consistently include nurses, physical therapists, occupational therapists, respiratory therapists, and social workers.

Nursing Evaluation. The nursing evaluation begins with a record of the standard patient characteristics and physical signs. Language and the ability to communicate are recorded as is any sensory impairment (e.g., hearing or vision impairment). The nursing history explores the patients' impressions as to the reasons for their admission to the rehabilitation program as well as their expectations of it. Details of previous admissions to the hospital often expand on the information obtained by the physician. The need for assistive devices, prostheses, and appliances is documented. When the patient has been transferred directly from an acute care hospital, risk factors for pressure sores are defined. Any obvious behavioral problems are noted. The nurses administer a questionnaire to assess the patient's baseline knowledge of his or her respiratory condition and general health habits. The results of this test guide the educational aspects of the program. The test is readministered midway through the program as a guide to the patient's progress.

Physical Therapy. The physical therapist determines the patient's baseline functional activity level based on his or her history and examination. It may range from being bedridden to being able to participate in outdoor activities. Dyspnea is assessed both by using standardized grading scales and by recording its impact on the patient's awareness of the need to breathe and the ability to converse. The general examination focuses on the patient's posture and flexibility, range of motion, and strength and endurance of the upper extremities. The more specific examination of the respiratory system focuses on breathing pattern, accessory muscle use, pursed-lip breathing, and any indications of respiratory muscle dysfunction. Cough effectiveness is tested. Finally, the physical therapist usually conducts the 6-minute walking test.

Occupational Therapy. The occupational therapist records the interaction between the patient's environment and his or her disease. The living situation is explored with respect to the number of individuals residing in the patient's home, the presence of stairs, the location of the home within the community, and the accessibility of transportation to shops and municipal facilities. Activities of daily living, which include self-care and household duties such as meal preparation, cleaning, clothes laundering, and grocery shopping, are discussed in detail. The patient's vocational and leisure activities are explored, as is his or her driving history. A description of a typical day can be most helpful in providing a more comprehensive assessment of the impact of disease on the patient's lifestyle.

Respiratory Therapy. The respiratory therapist measures resting SaO_2 and obtains arterial blood samples for blood gas analysis. If the patient is hypoxemic ($SaO_2 < 85\%$), the respiratory therapist measures the flow of supplemental oxygen (administered by nasal prongs) that is needed to maintain resting SaO_2 between 85 and 90%. The respiratory therapist assesses tracheostomy care and the effectiveness of mechanical ventilation if it has been established prior to admission to the respiratory rehabilitation program.

Social Work. The social worker's assessment expands the information available in several areas that are not fully addressed by other members of the team. For example, the patient's family history includes an assessment of family dynamics and of cultural and religious influences that might affect the patient's receptiveness to the rehabilitation program. The adequacy of the housing situation is recorded. The impact of the disease on the patient's work environment is noted, as is the presence of appropriate community support networks. The social worker completes the psychosocial assessment by establishing the patient's and the family's perceptions of and reactions to the illness. Important social risk indicators that have an impact on the candidate's selection and management are noted. These include not only financial circumstances, employment concerns, and placement problems but also possible social isolation, change-of-role pressures, and loss of control on the part of the patient.

Optional Investigations

Although several investigations can be considered as optional (i.e., they are helpful but not strictly essential for patient management), it should be emphasized that any categorization of this type is arbitrary. Under certain circumstances, optional tests are essential, and so-called essential tests are optional. This is especially the case if patients are involved in clinical trials in which detailed measurements are needed to clarify our understanding of physiologic mechanisms and treatment protocols.

Formal exercise testing is addressed in detail elsewhere in this book. A properly conducted test provides an objective assessment of symptoms, identifies an abnormal exercise response, and measures a patient's physiologic reserve. However, not all patients can complete a formal exercise evaluation. Severely obstructed, restricted, or malnourished patients may be unable to exercise sufficiently for meaningful measurements to be made. For some patients, such as those with poorly controlled left ventricular dysfunction, exercise may actually be contraindicated. For others who have little self-confidence or limited previous laboratory experience, a great deal of coaching is required, and the test being performed may have to be modified considerably. Detailed measurement of central and peripheral chemoresponsiveness can be useful if primary or secondary alterations in respiratory control are thought to contribute to the patient's disability. Full respiratory polysomnographic measurements have their place in the diagnosis and management of sleep-disordered breathing. Examples include central or obstructive apnea and nocturnal hypoventilation. Whereas positive changes in laboratory or clinical measurements may be relevant to clinicians, patients are ultimately concerned with the prospect of functioning at an optimal level. The impact of disease on their physical, social, and emotional functions is difficult to quantify; however, in an attempt to measure such changes, sophisticated quality of life instruments that are valid, reliable, and sensitive have been devised.[9] General health profiles with well-established reliability and validity allow for a comparison among interventions or conditions. An example of such a profile is the Sickness Impact Profile,[10] which requires approximately 15 minutes to administer and can be scored at several levels of aggregation to provide individual category scores, two-dimensional scores (physical and pyschosocial), and an overall score. Disease-specific instruments are clinically sensitive and more responsive than general health profiles but may be limited in their application in the making of such comparisons. An example of such an instrument is the Chronic Respiratory Questionnaire,[11] which is an interviewer-administered instrument that describes a patient's dyspnea, fatigue, emotional function, and mastery. Utility instruments, such as the Standard Gamble,[12] address the preference of an individual for a particular health status. The Standard Gamble is a test designed to determine how a patient actually feels about his or her present state of health. We have found that the inclusion of such questionnaires during the initial assessment broadens our evaluation and allows us to better define the impact of the disease on the patient's life.

CONCLUSION

Careful patient selection identifies those patients most likely to benefit from respiratory rehabilitation. Medical considerations that influence the effectiveness of respiratory rehabilitation include confirmation of the diagnosis, maximization of therapy, and the identification and management of associated medical conditions. Other important influences include patient motivation, an adequate home situation, and realistic goals and expectations. The initial assessment of referred candidates should include measurements of pulmonary function and an evaluation of the impact of the disease on both the lifestyle of the patient and that of his or her family.

REFERENCES

1. Goldstein RS, McCullough C, Contreras MA. Approaches to rehabilitation of patients with ventilatory insufficiency. Eur Respir J 1989; 2:655s–660s.
2. Hass A, Cardon H. Rehabilitation in chronic obstructive pulmonary disease. A 5-year study of 252 male patients. Med Clin North Am 1969; 53:593–606.
3. Petty TL, Nett LM, Finigan MM, et al. A comprehensive care program for chronic airway obstruction: Methods and preliminary evaluation of symptomatic and functional improvement. Ann Intern Med 1969; 70:1109–1120.
4. Goldstein RS, Molotiu N, Skrastins R, et al. Assisting ventilation in respiratory failure by negative pressure ventilation and by rocking bed. Chest 1987; 92:470–474.
5. Goldstein RS, Molotiu N, Skrastins R, et al. Reversal of sleep-induced hypoventilation and chronic respiratory failure by nocturnal negative pressure ventilation in patients with restrictive ventilatory impairment. Am Rev Respir Dis 1987; 135:1049–1055.
6. Agle DP, Baum GL. Psychological aspects of chronic obstructive pulmonary disease. Med Clin North Am 1977; 61:749–758.
7. McGavin CR, Gupta SP, McHardy GJR. Twelve-minute walking test for assessing disability in chronic bronchitis. Br Med J 1976; 1:822–823.
8. Crockcroft AE, Saunders MJ, Berry G. Randomized controlled trial of rehabilitation in chronic respiratory disability. Thorax 1981; 36:200–203.
9. Guyatt GM, Valdhuyzen Van Zanten SJO, Feeny DH, Patrick DL. Measuring quality of life in clinic trials: A taxonomy and review. Can Med Assoc J 1989; 40:1441–1448.
10. Bergner M, Bobbitt RA, Carter WB, Gilson, BS. The Sickness Impact Profile: Development and final revision of a health status measure. Med Care 1981; 19:787–805.
11. Guyatt G, Berman LB, Townsend M, et al. A measure of quality of life for clinical trials in chronic lung disease. Thorax 1987; 42:773–778.
12. Torrance GW, Feeny D. Utilities and quality-assisted life years. Int J Technol Assess Health Care 1989; 5:559–575.

Chapter 24

Exercise Prescription

ANTONIO PATESSIO, M.D.
FRANCESCO IOLI, M.D.
CLAUDIO FERDINANDO DONNER, M.D.,
F.C.C.P.

Patients with chronic obstructive pulmonary disease (COPD) are generally limited in the performance of exercise to inappropriately low work rates. This decrease in exercise capacity is well documented to be a result of a decrease in maximum oxygen consumption.[1,2] The mechanism of reduced exercise capacity is multifactorial, but it can be conceptualized as an imbalance between an increased ventilatory requirement, which is caused by worsened gas exchange,[3] and a decrease in ventilatory capacity, which is the result of altered pulmonary mechanics.[4,5] Dyspnea is the end-point symptom responsible for the limitation of physical activity: patients enter a vicious circle of increasing inactivity, deconditioning, increased dyspnea for a lower level of activity, and further deconditioning (Fig. 24–1). This spiral also has a negative impact on social and emotional functions. In many patients, the loss of physical abilities induces anger, frustration, and depression,[6,7] which need to be recognized and treated as independent clinical entities if a positive outcome is to be achieved in exercise training programs. The widespread use of such programs is justified by the improvement in exercise tolerance that participants achieve.[8–11] Although the mechanism of this improvement is controversial and not completely elucidated, exercise therapy has become a cornerstone of almost all rehabilitative programs and should be prescribed with the aim of increasing the performance or the autonomy of COPD patients. A major problem in formulating an exercise prescription is that COPD patients do not form a homogeneous population. A wide range of pulmonary functional impairment interacts with factors such as duration of illness, cardiac function, lean body mass, and bronchoreactivity to determine the potential to achieve a training response, and few studies of the responses of COPD patients to exercise programs have acknowledged these factors in their experimental designs. Designing for each individual patient the program that is most likely to improve his or her exercise

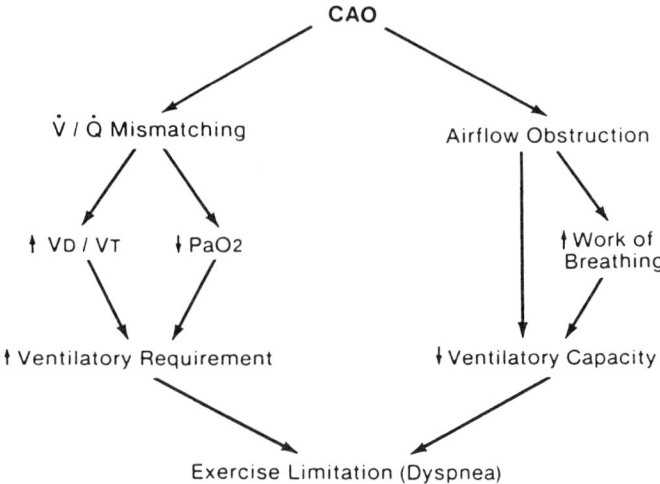

FIGURE 24–1. The pathologic derangements due to COPD impair both gas exchange and the mechanics of breathing. Much work must be performed by a less capable system, which leads to functional impairment and eventually dyspnea. (From Brown HV, Wasserman K. Exercise performance in chronic obstructive pulmonary disease. Med Clin North Am 1981; 65:525–547.)

tolerance should be the goal of the pulmonary specialist. Although this is not always possible, a complete evaluation of each patient who is to be admitted to a program of exercise reconditioning is important.

SELECTION CRITERIA

Since almost all patients with chronic airflow obstruction have limited exercise tolerance, it can be affirmed that there is a general indication for programs of exercise therapy in COPD. In practice, many factors should be taken into consideration before a patient is included in such programs. The basic requirement for prescribing exercise therapy is that the patient should be stable and not likely to experience disease exacerbation, and that he or she should be receiving appropriate pharmacologic therapy. As far as associated diseases are concerned, it is our practice to exclude patients with a history of recent myocardial infarction, unstable or frequent angina, serious arrhythmias, orthopedic problems, and uncompensated metabolic disorders. Beyond these considerations, whether a patient should or should not be admitted to an exercise training program depends on factors such as (1) motivation, (2) lung function, (3) age, and (4) exercise evaluation.

Motivation

Before exercise is prescribed, the attitudes of individual patients should be investigated and the most suitable and widely accepted mode of exercise should be sought. It is not surprising that many pulmonary disease patients have to be motivated and convinced to exercise regularly. Some of them fear the breathlessness that exercise induces. In many instances, the dyspnea experienced at levels of exercise near their maximum oxygen consumption ($\dot{V}O_2$max) is further aggravated by the fear of the sensation, which in turn amplifies the breathlessness. The role of personnel in reassuring and encouraging these patients in the early stages of the program is a key component for a successful outcome of exercise therapy. There is not much information in the literature about patient compliance in programs of exercise therapy. In one study, 12 of 130 patients did not complete their program because of a lack of motivation[12]; in another study, 16 of 68 patients dropped out for reasons other than a lack of motivation (e.g., exacerbations of their disease, transportation difficulties, and severe coronary artery disease).[11] In our experience, compliance with an exercise program depends on the length of time the patient has to spend in the hospital once he or she has recovered from acute episodes of bronchospasm or infection, on the facilities he or she has available for an outpatient program, on the support of the patient's family, on the opportunity to exercise regularly at home, and on the degree of recovery from exertional dyspnea.[13] Under the most favorable conditions, it is still expected that 15% of patients "will not want" to continue. In our opinion, it is worthwhile to enroll in exercise therapy programs all participants in formal rehabilitation programs who are physically able; outpatient programs should be recommended only for those patients who do not have psychosocial factors that are likely to interfere with exercise therapy.

Lung Function

Resting lung function can be easily measured, and thus there have been many attempts to find a correlation between it and factors that characterize exercise limitation. Equations have been developed that allow the prediction of the maximum ventilation achievable during exercise; these equations are based on spirometric measures taken at rest.[14–16] If the difference between the predicted maximum ventilation and the observed maximum ventilation ($\dot{V}$Emax) during exercise is small, the patient is presumed to be ventilatorily limited. However, the relation between measures such as forced expiratory volume in 1 second (FEV_1) or 12-second maximum voluntary ventilation (MVV) and observed $\dot{V}$Emax during exercise in patients who are presumed to be ventilatorily limited shows considerable scatter. The 4-minute maximum sustained ventilatory capacity may be a somewhat superior index,[17] but it is more difficult to measure. However, it is questionable whether any of these resting measures are of use in determining if an individual patient is ventilatorily limited. Furthermore, exercise induces a variable amount of bronchodilation[18] and a variable increase in functional residual capacity (FRC),[19, 20] both of which would tend to induce a variable increase in a patient's ability to ventilate during exercise in excess of the levels predicted based on resting measurements. Defining whether a patient is ventilatorily limited is important, since it might be argued that only those who are ventilatorily limited are able to gain from exercise therapy. It is generally true that patients with an FEV_1 greater than 50% of that predicted (or roughly above 1.5 L) are probably not limited in performing common daily activities. However, it should be considered that most of these subjects are employed; if they are engaged in a physically demanding occupation, they will be strongly motivated to improve their physical performance in order to retain their ability to work. We think that it is valuable to include these patients in programs of exercise therapy because it is often possible to restore them to an almost fully functional lifestyle. At the other extreme, it has been suggested that patients with very severe obstruction are unable to obtain physiologic benefits because their ventilatory limitation makes them unable to exercise above a critical training intensity (see Chapter 16). However, it has been demonstrated that even patients with hypercapnia ($PaCO_2 > 54$ mm Hg) are still able to derive benefit from exercise therapy[21] (e.g., to increase their exercise tolerance in terms of distance walked).

Moreover, resting spirometric values do not correlate well with $\dot{V}O_2$max because other factors are important in limiting exercise performance. It has been contended that $\dot{V}O_2$max can be predicted using an equation that

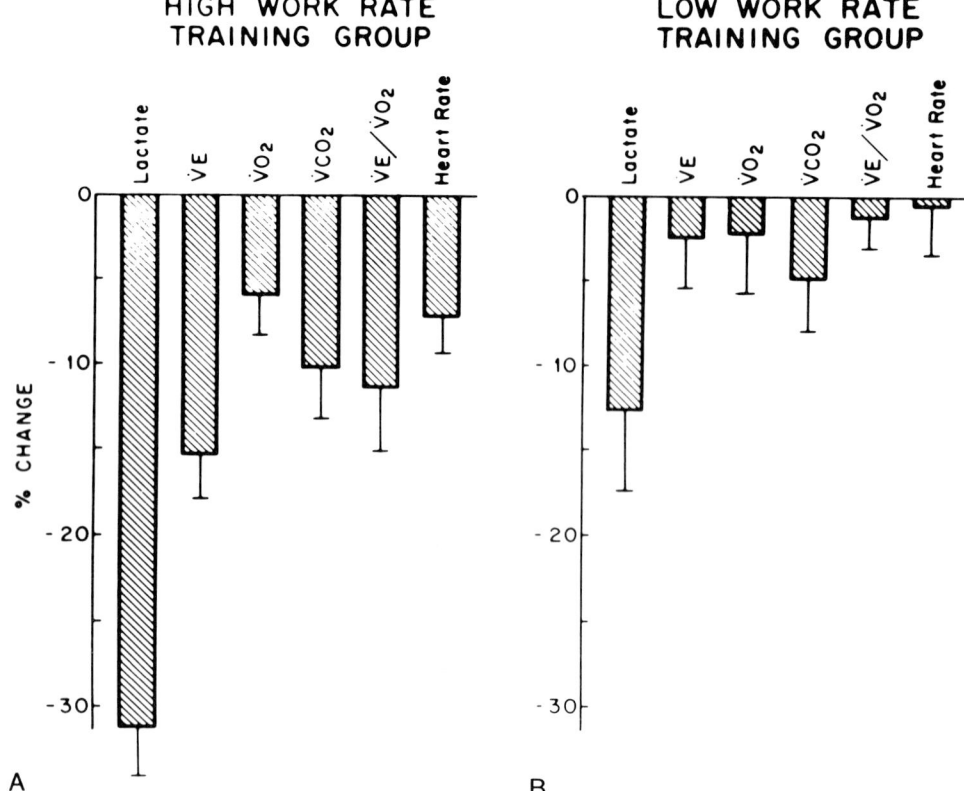

FIGURE 24–2. Changes in physiologic variables in response to an identical exercise task (high constant work rate) after two exercise training programs in 19 COPD patients. A, Average per cent change in 11 patients trained at work rates engendering high levels of lactic acidosis. B, Average per cent change in eight patients trained at work rates engendering low levels of lactic acidosis. The group trained at higher work rates had a significantly greater physiologic response. The total amount of work performed by the two groups of patients was the same. (The low-work-rate training group had a longer work duration.) (From Casaburi R, Patessio A, Ioli F, et al. Reductions in exercise lactic acidosis and ventilation after exercise training in obstructive lung disease patients. Am Rev Respir Dis 1991; 143:9–18.)

includes FEV_1, diffusing capacity, and peak inspiratory pressure to reflect the physiologic effects of expiratory airflow, the gas transfer factor, and inspiratory muscle strength on exercise capacity.[22] Even if it were possible to predict $\dot{V}O_2$max, so far there are no resting lung function parameters that can serve as accurate predictors of which patients are likely to derive physiologic benefits from exercise training. It has been suggested that one of the requirements for patients to experience physiologic improvement is the ability to develop metabolic acidosis during exercise[10]; this ability cannot be predicted from resting lung function data.[10–23]

Exercise Evaluation

Important information can be obtained from formal exercise testing. A recent study has shown that training at a work rate associated with lactic acidosis is more effective in inducing a training effect in COPD patients than is a work rate not associated with lactic acidosis (Fig. 24–2).[10] The concept that early onset of lactic acidosis may be an important contributor to exercise limitation in COPD patients has only recently been emphasized.[24, 25] In fact, it had been contended that ventilatory fatigue occurs well before the anaerobic threshold is reached (the work rate at which blood lactate levels increase appreciably) in most patients with moderate to severe disease. However, recent studies document that the anaerobic threshold is reached by most patients, even those with severe disease.[10, 11, 23] Thus, exercise testing is necessary because the work rate at which the anaerobic threshold occurs does not correlate well with resting spirometric measures (such as FEV_1 or carbon monoxide diffusing capacity; Fig. 24–3). This is likely in part because the degree of impairment of the pulmonary vasculature is not determined by the same pathologic changes that lead to airways obstruction. The ability of COPD patients to develop metabolic acidosis at lower work rates than do normal subjects[26] can be the result of different causes such as the abnormal response of the pulmonary vasculature to exercise (which limits the oxygen supply to exercising muscle) or the very sedentary lifestyle typical of these patients. Disuse makes the muscles more prone to anaerobiosis.[27] An earlier onset of lactic acidosis is explained by the decrease in the level of phosphocreatine in underused muscles.[28] The fact that many COPD patients who undergo incremental exercise testing are able to generate a substantial level of lactic acidosis demonstrates that the exercising muscles are being stressed.

Age

A great part of the population of COPD patients are over 55 years of age, and this should be considered in evaluating realistic goals in terms of improvement of exercise performance. A progressive decline in all physiologic functions is evident in all individuals as they get older (even though most of our information comes from cross-sectional rather than longitudinal studies). There is a distinct decrease in $\dot{V}O_2$max that is associated with

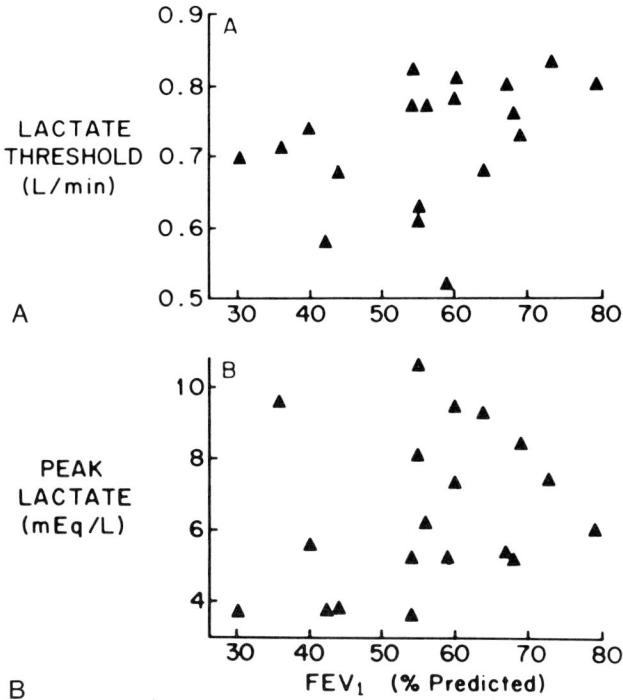

FIGURE 24–3. Relationship between the severity of airways obstruction (expressed as a percentage of predicted forced expiratory volume in 1 second [FEV_1]) and lactate threshold (A), as well as peak lactate level at the highest tolerated work rate (B) during an incremental exercise test in 19 COPD patients. Neither correlation is statistically significant. (Modified from Casaburi R, Patessio A, Ioli F, et al. Reductions in exercise lactic acidosis and ventilation after exercise training in obstructive lung disease patients. Am Rev Respir Dis 1991; 143:9–18.)

aging; thus, any absolute work rate represents a higher stress for the older individual.[29, 30] Most information regarding the effects of physical training comes from studies carried out in young people, but it has been demonstrated that such effects (e.g., a decrease in blood lactate concentration, heart rate, and ventilation at the same submaximum work rates and an increase in $\dot{V}O_2$max and the maximum work output) can also be obtained in healthy older men and women (over 60 yrs of age) after prolonged programs of physical activity.[31, 32] It has been shown that older sedentary subjects are able to tolerate exercise training at an intensity of 70% of their $\dot{V}O_2$max for 1 hour per day without any unfavorable metabolic or physiologic effects, so that in some ways they do better than younger sedentary patients. Equations have been recently developed for predicting $\dot{V}O_2$max in healthy older people.[33, 34] They provide useful values for the evaluation of the degree of impairment of patients with lung disease. In particular, it was observed that this population had values of $\dot{V}O_2$max that were 17.5 ± 22% higher than predicted values based on subjects of all ages. Thus, if aging itself does not preclude normal older subjects from participating in programs of exercise training and from obtaining the positive effects usually reported for younger subjects,[35] exercise programs should also be applicable to older COPD patients once other coexisting contraindications can be eliminated.

EVALUATION

The basic requirement for prescribing exercise is the performance of a preliminary exercise test by the patient. Much important information can be obtained from such a test, such as initial exercise tolerance, whether lactic acidosis is present, and whether hyopoxemia, hypercapnia, arrhythmias, or hypertension has developed. Exercise testing should be carried out in a good environment (e.g., one with controlled relative humidity and temperature) that is not too noisy. The patient should be instructed to wear comfortable clothes and to have a light meal at least 2 hours before the test.

Testing Modalities

In one sense, it is preferable that the preliminary exercise test be performed using the same kind of exercise that the patient will undergo during the training program because it is easier to discern the effectiveness of a program of training when testing modalities are similar to the predominant training modality. However, this is sometimes problematic, since certain kinds of exercise tests reveal physiologic effects of training more reliably than do others; also, there are differences in the reproducibility of test methods. We normally use the bicycle ergometer for preliminary evaluation because it allows a more accurate quantitation of external work that is easily reproducible and readily measured.[36] The mechanical efficiency of pedaling varies little among subjects (4–5%), and the $\dot{V}O_2$max obtained is also very reproducible in COPD patients.[1] In contrast, the oxygen uptake requirement for a given treadmill speed and grade varies substantially among subjects and is clearly a function of body weight, and the familiarization (improvement of pacing strategy) with treadmill exercise can lead to the accomplishment of a given task with lower oxygen uptake and ventilatory responses[37] for the same speed and inclination of the belt. This can be confusing when one evaluates the results of an exercise program: less ventilation for the same workload can be regarded as a physiologic benefit, and we might not be sure how much of this benefit is attributable to training and how much to the improvement of the skill in performing the exercise. However, a method for translating exercise performance from incremental bicycle ergometry testing to steady-state treadmill walking speed has been described for patients with COPD.[38] This method provides very useful and practical information because it combines the advantages of an incremental test on a bicycle ergometer (during which a complete assessment can be easily carried out) and the advantages of training patients with walking (which is simpler and in many instances better accepted than bicycle ergometry).

Testing Protocols

We normally use an incremental symptom-limited maximum test because it is likely to provide the greatest information on factors that limit exercise performance and on possible unfavorable effects that are induced by exercise. We choose to increment the work rate each minute by 5 to 15 watts, according to the characteristics of the individual patient (e.g., age, sex, height, lung function, and the presence of concomitant heart disease), so that the test lasts about 8 to 10 minutes. A shorter test does not yield enough data, and a longer one is at risk to be terminated for reasons not related to exercise intolerance, such as boredom and seat discomfort.

Patients with very advanced disease might find exercise on a bicycle ergometer is very stressful because their $\dot{V}O_2$max is often equal to that necessary for pedaling at 0 watts. In addition, treadmill exercise testing requires many attempts to find a suitable speed, and a significant amount of time is required to familiarize the patients with the treadmill. In this case, we use a "walking test" for the preliminary assessment because walking is a natural mode of exercise and because all patients in stable condition are able to perform it. Moreover, this test can be carried out even in those laboratories that cannot provide a complete assessment of exercise performance. It can be considered a simple, practical, and objective measurement of the disability of COPD patients in performing everyday physical efforts. In comparison with questionnaires, this test is objective and allows patients to be placed on a continuous scale of performance rather than in arbitrary grades of disability. However, one must consider the walking test to be a submaximal test, as it is unable to stress patients to their limits and to diagnose the causes of exercise limitation. Performance depends on many other factors, such as patient attitude and motivation.[39] The "12-minute walking test" was originally described by Cooper,[40] who showed in healthy subjects that the distance covered in the 12-minute field performance test (which allows subjects to run or walk) correlated fairly well ($r = .897$) with the $\dot{V}O_2$max assessed during an incremental treadmill test. The 12-minute walking test for the evaluation of COPD patients was introduced in 1976 by McGavin.[41] The test was performed in a hospital corridor, and an attempt was also made to standardize the verbal instructions. The walked distance correlated weakly with forced vital capacity ($r = .406$), maximum oxygen uptake ($r = .52$), and minute ventilation ($r = .53$), which were measured during an incremental test on a bicycle ergometer, whereas no significant correlation was found with FEV_1. A learning effect occurred between the first test and the second test, whereas no difference was found between the second test and the third test.[41] In another study[42] comparing serial 12-minute walking distances, the improvement in the distance walked attributable to the learning effect reached its maximum at the third test of a series carried out on different days, and the variability of the 12-minute test was less than that of the other common respiratory function tests (provided that the first two assessments were discarded).

A comparison[43] of the 12-minute walking test with an incremental bicycle ergometer test and with a fixed-rate paced-step test in patients with a high degree of lung function impairment showed that there is a progressive and significant increase in performance in all the tests up to the fourth run. This demonstrates how the comparison between the maximum performance before and after a treatment might be misleading. The tests performed were symptom-limited, and it was not surprising that increasing familiarity with the tests may have led to an increase in confidence and motivation. A further investigation[44] on the learning effect showed that over either a short or long period there is an increase in the walked distance from the first to the last of 12 walks (33% over 3 days and 8.5% over 4 wk). In the first instance, most of the increase was observed in the first three walks, whereas for the longer period, the increase occurred between the third and the twelfth walks. Figure 24-4 summarizes the different percentages of improvement in the distances walked that are only a result of the learning effect in these previous studies. The need to repeat the tests before comparable results can be obtained and the long duration of testing required to do so represent the major disadvantages of the 12-minute walking test.

The "6-minute" walking test is now most commonly used, since it has been demonstrated[45] that the distances walked in 6 and 12 minutes correlate well ($r = .955$), and even if the 12-minute test is more discriminating in assessing exercise tolerance, the 6-minute test represents a good compromise. It is also useful to emphasize the need for the careful standardization of instructions given by test supervisors to encourage patients, since the nature of these instructions can possibly have a great impact on the distance walked ($+30.5$ m on average).[46] In studies aimed at evaluating the effect of drugs or rehabilitation techniques, it has been found that different kinds of encouragement may bias walking test results. Nevertheless, since this test reflects the ability to perform everyday activities, it is a useful tool in successive evaluations of patients in rehabilitation programs if the procedure is accurately standardized and if at least four initial practice attempts are made to minimize the learning effect.

Measurements

During the preliminary test, a minimal assessment should consist of the monitoring of arterial blood pressure, electrocardiographic study with 12 leads, and an analysis of arterial oxygen saturation (SaO_2). The most common method for SaO_2 monitoring[47, 48] is the use of pulse oximeters because these devices are portable, easy to use, do not require calibration, are noninvasive, and have a high level of reliability[47] at SaO_2 levels greater than 90%. However, at SaO_2 levels below 90%, their reliability progressively worsens; at levels of 65% and lower, they have been found to be substantially inaccurate.[47] The differences among the various instruments for measuring SaO_2 and discrepancies between them and oximetry have been described.[48, 49] In fact, some studies show that oximetry has major limitations in detecting

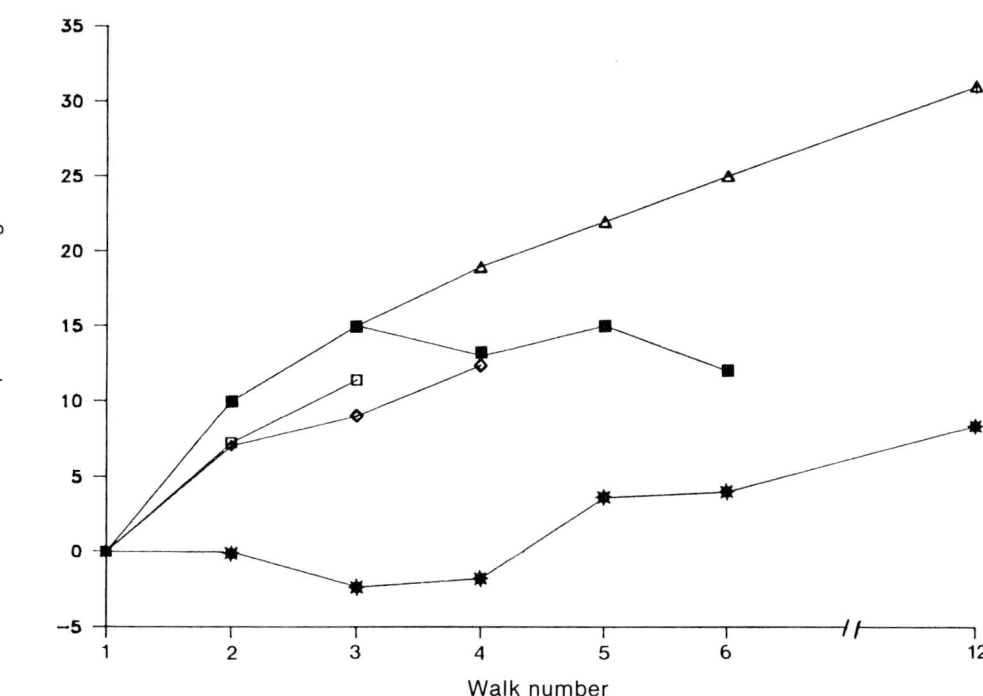

FIGURE 24–4. Mean per cent change in the distance walked in the 12-minute walking test. (Data from McGavin CR, Gupta SP, McHardy GJR. Twelve-minute walking test for assessing disability in chronic bronchitis. BMJ 1976; 1: 822–823; Mungall IPF, Hainsworth R. Assessment of respiratory function in patients with chronic obstructive airways disease. Thorax 1979; 34:254–258; Swinburn CR, Wakefield JM, Jones PW. Performances, ventilation, and oxygen consumption in three different types of exercise test in patients with chronic obstructive lung disease. Thorax 1985; 40:581–586; and Knox AJ, Morrison JF, Muers MF. Reproducibility of walking test results in chronic obstructive pulmonary disease. Thorax 1988; 43:388–392.)

exercise hypoxemia, particularly when SaO_2 is less than 85%.[47] Some other studies demonstrated that oximetry is reliable in detecting desaturation, both in pulmonary patients and in normal subjects.[48–50] However, these studies did not explore low SaO_2, which occasionally is observed during light exercise in COPD patients. It may be reasonable to simply use these devices to detect desaturation episodes and eliminate any concern about their reliability in detecting the lowest SaO_2 levels, since from the clinical point of view, a desaturation episode may be corrected by supplemental oxygen without taking into account the precise degree of the desaturation. However, some authors have shown that in some patients hypoxemia detected in the analysis of arterial blood samples was not detected by pulse oximetry, and in other patients oximeter readings were falsely depressed, perhaps due to local hypoperfusion.[51] Thus, pulse oximetry cannot be considered the equivalent of arterial blood sampling; however, it is often used in the clinical setting for detecting desaturation between rest and exercise, although false positive and false negative results should be expected.

If a more complete assessment is necessary, recording of the time courses of oxygen uptake, carbon dioxide output, and ventilation should be made. When possible, periodic arterial blood samples should be taken for measurement of Po_2, Pco_2, pH, and lactate concentration, preferably through an indwelling arterial catheter (brachial or radial). It should be particularly stressed that arterial puncture performed immediately after the cessation of exercise may give results that do not accurately represent end-exercise values, particularly those for PaO_2.[52]

Breathlessness during exercise is an almost universal complaint of patients with COPD. The cause of dyspnea has been thoroughly investigated; different factors have been claimed to play a role in it, including the quantitative disturbance of the sense of respiratory loads,[53] respiratory muscle fatigue,[54] and excessive ventilation in relation to maximum breathing capacity.[55] Irrespective of its etiology, dyspnea can be a very useful index for evaluating the results of exercise programs. Psychophysical methods using both categorical and continuous scales have been validated and are considered to be reproducible (although with a great intersubject variability).[56,57] However, there is also a report of the very variable perception of breathlessness using the Borg scale during exercise, whereas the physiologic indices are quite reproducible.[58] It seems reasonable to include measures of breathlessness with the other physiologic data, since breathlessness changes independently of ventilation following exercise programs.

Questioning the patient about the intensity of dyspnea also suggests (particularly in very disabled patients) those work rates or modalities of exercise that will allow him or her to perform programs with greater motivation and better acceptance.

EXERCISE THERAPY PROGRAMS

If no major contraindications emerge from the baseline assessment, exercise training should be initiated under the supervision of a trained therapist (e.g., a physical therapist) and overseen by a physician.

Training Modalities

Three general training modalities are used: (1) walking (or running), (2) treadmill exercise, and (3) bicycle ergometer exercise. These modalities are directed at training the legs. Training of the arms may be an important goal, since the arms are used for many daily activities such as combing hair, brushing teeth, lifting, bathing, and dressing. It has been demonstrated that patients with COPD tolerate arm exercise particularly poorly, since the muscles of the shoulders and chest participate both in breathing and in moving the arms.[59] In fact, the endurance of unsupported arm exercise is dramatically lower than that of leg exercise in the same subject; severe dyspnea has been reported as the main limiting factor of arm exercise. Dyssynchronous breathing has a higher incidence with arm than with leg exercise in the more severely obstructed patients. The concomitant observation that electromyographic signs of diaphragmatic fatigue develop in the same way during both arm and leg exercise suggests that other factors may contribute to severe dyspnea and uncoordinated breathing, such as the extra demand placed on the accessory muscles of inspiration, which also participate in positioning the torso and the arms. An improvement in upper-extremity performance has been observed after a specific program of arm training.[60] A controlled study on the effect of arm and leg training was carried out in 28 severe but stable COPD patients; the study showed specific and useful improvement of exercise performance after a program of training. It is interesting that the quality of life improved only as a result of a combined program of arm and leg exercise, but not when only arm exercise was performed.[61]

Training Characteristics

It must be acknowledged that the prescription of exercise programs for COPD patients with the goal of inducing a physiologic training effect is not yet a developed science. It is important to decide whether physiologically based improvement in exercise tolerance is an achievable goal for a given COPD patient. If so, it seems clear that exercise rehabilitation programs must be designed with consideration of the principles used to train healthy individuals. The physiologic responses to exercise training have been well studied and are widely applied in the field of competition athletics, where increase in endurance of a given task is the desired result (see Chapter 16).

It seems appropriate to suppose that duration and frequency characteristics appropriate for healthy subjects are likely to be appropriate for patients with COPD. However, exercise intensity considerations are different. COPD patients are likely to require training work rates that are a higher fraction of their maximum heart rate or $\dot{V}O_2$max to achieve a physiologic training effect. It has been suggested that they are unable to gain these physiologic benefits because they are unable to exercise above a "critical training intensity."[62-65] It has been demonstrated that three of the most important enzymes of the skeletal muscle responsible for producing the adenosine triphosphate necessary for muscle contraction are not increased by exercise training in COPD patients because they are not able to exercise above the critical intensity.[65] However, it is unclear even in normal subjects whether a "critical level" exists because the biochemical mediators of the changes in the exercising muscles are unknown.[66] Thus, a supervised program involving 30 to 45 minutes of exercise per day and 3 to 5 days per week for 5 to 8 weeks at a work rate involving lactic acidosis seems a reasonable strategy for patients who are able to increase blood lactate concentrations during exercise. To date, we are unable to provide a physiologic rationale for training patients who do not develop lactic acidosis during exercise and who are generally the most compromised and the oldest. However, since increased endurance and better exercise performance have also been demonstrated in this group, exercise training is surely worthwhile. We use walking as the mode of exercise at a speed chosen by the patient, which usually ranges between 1 and 3 km/h, for 20 minutes per day at the beginning of the training program. Later, we try to increase the duration of the walking rather than the speed. We apprise the patient of increases in 6-minute walking distance that he or she achieves; we find that this encourages the patient to perform further training.

PRACTICAL STEPS IN PRESCRIBING EXERCISE THERAPY

Easing Patients into Exercise

The first important step is to use the preliminary exercise testing to show the patient that maximum exercise does not cause injury, even though he or she may feel highly dyspneic. During this test, the presence of the physician is important also from a psychologic point of view because he or she becomes the patient's reference point during the training program. We attend the first sessions of training with the physiotherapist; these sessions are carried out in the hospital. We try to reassure the patient that he or she is able to tolerate dyspnea on exercise. After several sessions, we have always noted a decrease in this sensation at the same work rate. Another advantage of starting training in the hospital environment is that patients can talk to each other and are encouraged by seeing those who have already obtained some benefits from the training program.

Training Session

We usually start with a 5-minute warm-up period performed on a bicycle ergometer at 0 watts or on a treadmill at 0% inclination and at a speed chosen by the patient. The patient is encouraged to exercise at the chosen work rate (see Training Characteristics, discussed previously) for as long as he or she is able (5–10 min on average in the first sessions). After 5 to 10 minutes of rest, the patient starts again and continues to take as many breaks as he or she needs to complete the working session.

During these sessions, the rehabilitation therapist checks the patient's heart rate and rhythm and blood pressure while he or she is exercising. The therapist teaches the patient to monitor his or her own heart rate in order to have a useful guide to quantify physical activities performed outside the hospital.

Maintenance Programs

It is well known that the physiologic benefits of exercise training disappear over a 1- to 2-month period if regular exercise is not continued.[67] Moreover, even patients who do not show physiologic improvements are likely to lose their increased exercise tolerance if they return to a sedentary lifestyle. Therefore, a maintenance program of exercise must be part of the rehabilitation process. We instruct the patients to continue with the same form of exercise that was started in the hospital and recommend regular exercise for 1 hour per day. One of the major difficulties in maintaining a regular exercise activity in the long term is the occurrence of exacerbations of disease. The deterioration in lung function, even though it is only transient, acts to increase dyspnea for a work rate lower than that previously tolerated. This sometimes leads patients to believe that all the benefits of exercise have been lost and that it is not worth spending time and effort in continuing exercise therapy. We usually see our patients with COPD after exacerbations, and on those occasions we encourage them to resume an active lifestyle.

Realistic Goals

As illustrated in Table 24–1, a preliminary lung function assessment and exercise testing provide as much information as is needed to design a program of exercise therapy in terms of the mode of exercise, its duration, and its intensity aimed at obtaining an overall improvement in the quality of life of the patient. Within these general indications, the prescription should be tailored to the individual patient and should incorporate a knowledge of his or her actual needs.

POTENTIAL RISKS

Cardiac Arrhythmias

Cardiac arrhythmias can constitute an important problem. They have been reported to be common in COPD patients (20–86%[68–70]) at rest, and exercise is known to be a potential arrhythmogenic stimulus because it increases the oxygen consumption of the heart and sympathetic tone. In many COPD patients, exercise is associated with additional factors such as hypoxemia and metabolic acidosis, which can provoke arrhythmias. However, it is still unclear whether these arrhythmias play a role in the rate of mortality of COPD patients[71] and whether they should be treated with antiarrhythmic drugs. There is also a large variability in the prevalence of arrhythmias reported by different investigators that can be attributed to the severity of the disease, to the methods of monitoring cardiac rhythm, and to the concomitant use of drugs such as theophylline and beta$_2$ stimulants.[72]

The prevalence of serious arrhythmias (e.g., ventricular premature beats at a rate greater than 6/min, bigeminy, and multiform, couplet, and nonsustained ventricular tachycardia) is not well correlated with the severity of lung disease, oxyhemoglobin desaturation, or drug use (i.e., use of theophylline or beta$_2$ stimulants); they are more related to coexisting coronary artery disease.[73] Based on our present knowledge, it seems that only a few COPD patients develop severe arrhythmias during exercise if they are not already present at rest and if these patients have no significant history of coronary artery disease. Our personal experience is that we have not observed cardiac arrhythmias to develop during a training program if the baseline incremental exercise test did not elicit such a problem.

Arterial Desaturation

Patients with COPD, particularly those in whom the disease is severe, often develop hypoxemia during light exercise. This has been ascribed by some investigators to the worsening of ventilation/perfusion inequality[74, 75] and by others to the decrease in the mixed venous PO_2 that results from a greater increase in oxygen uptake than in cardiac output.[76, 77] Hypoxemia constitutes an important problem, since it provokes high grades of dyspnea and contributes to an increase in pulmonary artery pressure. There are conflicting data about the possibility of detecting exercise desaturation from resting lung function (carbon monoxide diffusing capacity, PaO_2, and FEV_1).[78–80] The correct detection of oxygen desaturation is important because supplemental oxygen given to patients who desaturate during exercise is able to improve exercise tolerance,[81, 82] relieve exercise dyspnea, and increase the capacity to perform useful daytime activities. These effects are achieved through different physiologic mechanisms. First, the oxygen delivery to tissues can be increased, allowing the cardiovascular and the respiratory systems to work more efficiently (i.e., to cause a decrease in heart and respiratory rates).[81, 83, 84] Second, the greater availability of oxygen to the tissues shifts the anaerobic threshold to a higher workload, reducing the necessity of hyperventilation to compensate for the metabolic acidosis.[81] Third, the raised PaO_2 may reduce the ventilatory requirement by removing the hypoxemic drive on the carotid bodies (although a greater carbon dioxide retention may follow oxygen administration, which worsens the acidemia that occurs during the exercise).[82–85] Finally, the threshold of impending diaphragmatic fatigue is delayed, probably as a result of the reduction of ventilatory requirement.[82–85]

With respect to the level of desaturation that should be corrected, it seems reasonable to correct desaturation if it leads to a substantial improvement in exercise

330 COMPONENTS OF THE PULMONARY REHABILITATION PROGRAM

TABLE 24–1. DECISION-MAKING FLOW CHART AND EXPECTED RESULTS OF EXERCISE TRAINING IN COPD PATIENTS

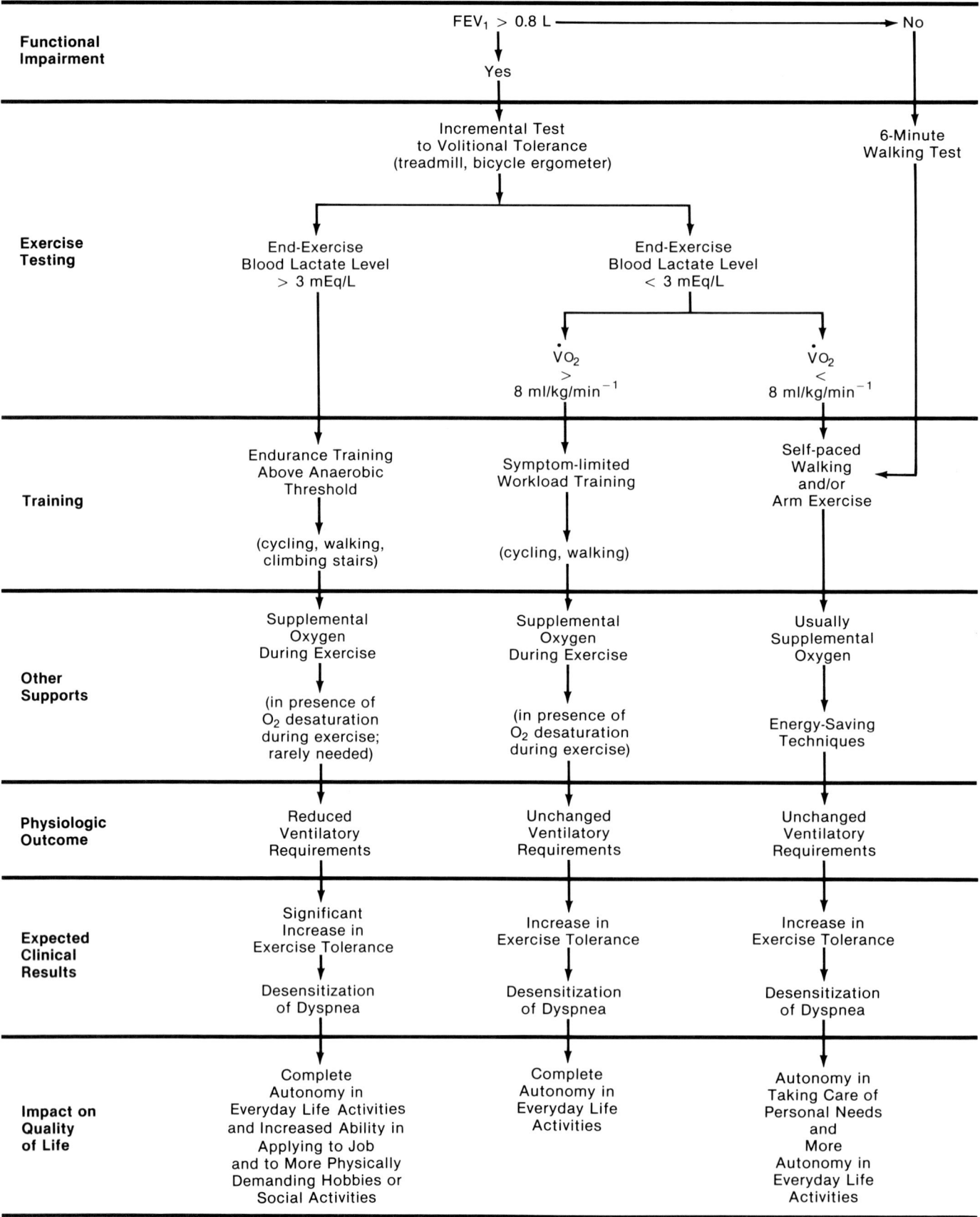

tolerance. Two populations can be identified: (1) patients with resting PaO_2 greater than 60 mm Hg who desaturate during exercise, and (2) patients receiving long-term oxygen therapy who desaturate during exercise while breathing oxygen at resting flow rates. Although it seems adequate to increase the oxygen flow rate for the latter group during exercise, the prescription of oxygen for patients who need it only during effort is more debatable. In practice, the oxygen flow that is capable of preventing desaturation during exercise and of restoring an SaO_2 of greater than 90% is usually prescribed to induce a significant increase in exercise tolerance.[86, 87] In patients receiving long-term oxygen therapy at rest, the increment of 1 L/min over the resting flow rate is widely used.[86] However, this strategy does not always correct desaturation; supplemental oxygen during exercise should be prescribed only after appropriate testing. Such testing might consist of the 12- or 6-minute walking test, an incremental bicycle ergometer test, or a treadmill test. Comparison can be made between the results obtained while a patient breathed air and those recorded while he or she breathed supplemental oxygen (the patient being unaware of the inhaled mixture).[86] A portable source is usually employed to afford the patient the greatest possible independence.[86-87] The difficulties associated with the refilling of portable cylinders and their limited period of use usually lead to the favoring of liquid oxygen supplies. The reliability of the supplied flow is usually acceptable, even if there is an occasional underflowing immediately after refilling. Also, after a long-term continuous use, the internal serpentine can freeze, which can decrease the precision of the system. The need for the possible use of these sources by those who lead active lifestyles fostered the development of oxygen-conserving devices that allow increased autonomy. A reservoir nasal cannula can reduce the amount of wasted oxygen by one half in COPD patients and is less expensive than a pulse-demand valve.[88, 89] This device delivers oxygen only at the beginning of the inspiratory phase, triggered by negative pressure.[90] In patients needing 24-hour oxygen therapy, the transtracheal catheter is presently experiencing increased popularity. The fraction of inspired oxygen is independent of the pattern of breathing, which is often of crucial importance during exercise. It causes little interference with daily activities and makes possible 24-hour administration. Because virtually all of the oxygen administered via the transtracheal catheter reaches the lung, patients who require higher oxygen flow rates than those that can be easily accommodated by conventional means are good candidates for this modality.[87]

The administration of supplemental oxygen during exercise improves exercise tolerance, but the pathophysiologic mechanisms underlying this benefit have not been completely elucidated. A more comprehensive knowledge of these aspects could lead to the more correct prescription of supplemental oxygen for use during exercise and to a better understanding of the role played by the correction of exercise desaturation in modifying the prognosis of COPD patients. There are many difficulties in carrying out studies in this area, since most patients spend little time exercising. Also, there is evidence of psychologic reticence in the use of portable sources by some patients. So far, supplemental oxygen therapy during exercise has been used more as a means to manage the "dyspnea symptom" and to correct PaO_2 if it decreases below an essentially arbitrary level rather than as a pivotal component of a comprehensive strategy for the long-term management of severe chronic airway obstruction.

Other Problems

Mild to moderate carbon dioxide retention during exercise is common in COPD patients and is largely dependent on the degree of airway obstruction at rest.[10] The normal respiratory alkalosis that occurs in response to the metabolic acidosis of exercise is rarely seen. This causes a more profound decrease in pH during exercise. Whether the exercise-induced hypercarbia and acidosis have a long-term adverse effect on the survival of these patients is unknown.

Hypoglycemia and muscle cramps that have been described after prolonged exercise in normal subjects are not reported in COPD patients. Also, exercise-induced bronchoconstriction is rarely observed.

Exercise puts an additional stress on the respiratory muscles, which work in unfavorable conditions in COPD patients owing to the deranged lung mechanics. This increases the oxygen consumption necessary to sustain respiration. At rest, respiratory muscle work is roughly 12 times greater in the COPD patient than in the healthy subject,[91] and the work of breathing accelerates rapidly with exercise.[91, 92] However, it is very unlikely that exercise can precipitate acute respiratory failure; whether whole-body exercise can train the respiratory muscles is currently being studied.

The hypothesis that exercise training can improve pulmonary hemodynamics is still very controversial (an inappropriate increase in pulmonary vascular pressure is often seen in COPD patients during exercise). The results of pulmonary artery catheterization during exercise are difficult to interpret. Although studies performed to date have shown no clear change in pulmonary artery pressure and although no consistent change in arteriovenous PO_2 difference has been observed,[93, 94] these studies have featured small numbers of patients or exercise programs that were unlikely to achieve a physiologic training effect. Furthermore, the measurement of pulmonary artery pressure in these patients is difficult because of profound swings in this parameter resulting from respiratory fluctuations in intrapleural pressure. A related question is whether exercise training sessions can predispose patients to right-sided heart failure by raising pulmonary artery pressure. Although this is a theoretical possibility, to our knowledge no reports of this problem occur in the literature.

ADDITIONAL CONSIDERATIONS

Drugs and Exercise

The classic therapeutic medications for COPD patients, including bronchodilators, corticosteroids, and antibiotics, are well known. There is, however, an increasing interest in investigating the possible effects of other drugs on breathlessness during exercise.

Carbimazole, an agent inducing the reduction of thyroid hormone levels, was studied in COPD patients with severe dyspnea,[95] but no significant symptomatic or objective improvement in exercise tolerance was found.

Many studies have shown that exogenous opioids decrease exertional dyspnea and increase the maximum external work of COPD patients. The mechanism responsible for the improved exercise tolerance is unknown. It has been suggested that the primary factor is a decreased metabolic requirement at a given workload. It has been demonstrated that after the ingestion of morphine, the maximum workload and the $\dot{V}O_2$max increased significantly.[96] Other investigators studied naloxone, an opioid antagonist, to uncover possible opioid influences in specific situations. They speculated that naloxone would block the endogenous endorphins and decrease the exercise capacity of COPD patients.[97] They did not find any difference in exercise performance between patients who took naloxone and those who took a placebo. These results do not support the hypothesis that endogenous opioids play a significant role in dampening dyspnea on exercise and in improving exercise tolerance.

Many studies suggest that inhaled beta agonists may improve exercise performance. The effect of inhaled metaproterenol on exercise performance was studied in patients with moderate to severe irreversible COPD.[98] The walked distance after metaproterenol administration improved significantly, but individual improvements in exercise performance did not correlate with corresponding changes in FEV_1 or forced vital capacity or with the baseline measurement of carbon monoxide diffusing capacity.

Pentoxifylline is a xanthine derivative with rheologic and vasomotor effects. The net effect of its pharmacologic properties seems to result in an improvement of gas exchange, possibly by increasing cardiac output, raising mixed venous PO_2, or improving blood flow to underperfused alveoli, or a combination of these effects.[99]

Nutrition

Malnutrition has been estimated to occur in as many as 40 to 50% of hospitalized patients with severe COPD. The consequent decrease in respiratory muscle strength contributes to reduced exercise capacity and to increased dyspnea on exertion. Reduced activity in turn leads to muscle atrophy, which may contribute to further weight loss.

Increasing caloric intake may be beneficial, but attention should be paid to paradoxical potential impairment of exercise capacity. Brown and coworkers[100] have found that a large liquid carbohydrate load adversely affects walking performance in patients with COPD. However, it is theoretically possible to influence the ventilatory requirement by manipulating the diet (e.g., if more fat is to be metabolized, a lower $\dot{V}CO_2$ is produced, resulting in a lower ventilatory requirement for the same work rate), but results in normal subjects have not been very encouraging.[101] In conclusion, the pharmacologic and nutritional approaches to reduce dyspnea during exercise have not yet been established in clinical practice.

CONCLUSION

Exercise therapy increases the exercise tolerance of patients with obstructive lung disease and should be regarded as a mainstay of pulmonary rehabilitation. Although it has been generally accepted and demonstrated that baseline pulmonary function (as determined by the measure of lung volumes, airway resistance, diffusing capacity, and blood gas indices at rest) does not change as a result of exercise training, such training has been shown to result in improved aerobic capacity, desensitization to the sensation of dyspnea, improved mechanical skill in performance, and greater confidence in the performance of everyday activities. Controversy exists as to whether improvements in exercise tolerance are based on physiologic changes in performing work or whether psychologic factors play the major role. A definite answer should come from future studies that might acknowledge in their selection factors the total amount of work performed, lung function, and the ability to develop exercise lactic acidosis. It seems possible that some subsets of patients can achieve a training response, whereas others cannot. The characterization of patients may be determined by a particular combination of characteristics derived from resting and exercise studies.

Psychologic factors do play a role in exercise training. For example, an almost constant finding of exercise therapy is an improved sense of well-being. Agle and associates reported decreased excessive body preoccupation, anxiety, and depression in most patients undergoing programs of exercise training.[102] The reassuring role of the medical personnel and possible desensitization of the fear of dyspnea encourages patients to tolerate higher levels of activity, particularly when they exercise under the supervision of the medical care team. It seems, however, that psychologic and physiologic benefits should go hand in hand because it is difficult to explain those benefits derived from a program of exercise training solely on a psychologic basis. Thus, the exercise program needs to be designed with consideration of the physiologic impairment of the pulmonary and cardiovascular systems. It seems unlikely that the degree of airways obstruction in itself should be a major selection criterion for entry into a program of exercise training. However, in the patient with severe COPD, coexisting factors, such as the presence of severe arrhythmias, may rule out exercise training. The need for supplemental oxygen during the training process needs to be considered. It seems prudent to supply oxygen to those patients with substantial arterial desaturation during exercise, but whether patients with only mild desaturation are more likely to obtain a training effect if oxygen is supplied requires study. A final question whose answer it is hoped is forthcoming is whether exercise training improves survival.

REFERENCES

1. Brown SE, Fischer CE, Stansbury DW, Light RW. Reproducibility of $\dot{V}O_2$max in patients with chronic airflow obstruction. Am Rev Respir Dis 1985; 131:435–438.
2. Servera E, Gimenez M. $\dot{V}O_2$max during progressive and constant bicycle exercise in patients with chronic obstructive lung disease. Respiration 1984; 45:197–206.
3. Jones NL. Pulmonary gas exchange during exercise in patients with chronic airway obstruction. Clin Sci 1966; 31:39–50.
4. Clark TJH, Freedman S, Campbell EJM. The ventilatory capacity of patients with chronic airways obstruction. Clin Sci 1969; 36:307–316.
5. Patessio A, Casaburi R, Ioli F, Donner CF. Mechanisms of exercise limitations. In: Donner CF Howard P (eds). SEPCR Guidelines and Recommendations for Pulmonary Rehabilitation (with Particular Regard to COPD Patients). Eur Respir Rev 1991; 1:482–485.
6. Salata PA, Berman LB. Variables which distinguish good and poor outcome following a respiratory rehabilitation program. Am Rev Respir Dis 1981; 123:A117.
7. Dudley DL, Glaser EM, Jorgenson BN, Logan DL. Psychosocial concomitants to rehabilitation in chronic obstructive pulmonary disease. Chest 1980; 77:677–684.
8. Cockcroft AE, Sanders MJ, Berry G. Randomized controlled trial of rehabilitation in chronic respiratory disability. Thorax 1981; 36:200–203.
9. Sinclair DJM, Ingram CG. Controlled trial of supervised exercise training in chronic bronchitis. BMJ 1980; 1:519–521.
10. Casaburi R, Patessio A, Ioli F, et al. Reductions in exercise lactic acidosis and ventilation after exercise training in obstructive lung disease patients. Am Rev Respir Dis 1991; 143:9–18.
11. Holle RHO, Williams DV, Vandree JC, et al. Increased muscle efficiency and sustained benefits in an outpatient community hospital-based pulmonary rehabilitation program. Chest 1988; 94:1161–1168.
12. Mall RW, Medeiros M. Objective evaluation of results of a pulmonary rehabilitation program in a community hospital. Chest 1988; 94:1156–1160.
13. Donner CF, Braghiroli A, Lusuardi M. Selection criteria. In: Donner CF, Howard P (eds) SEPCR Guidelines and Recommendations for Pulmonary Rehabilitation (with Particular Regard to COPD Patients). Eur Respir Rev 1991; 1:472–474.
14. Dillard TA, Piantadosi S, Rajagopal KR. Prediction of ventilation at maximal exercise in chronic airflow obstruction. Am Rev Respir Dis 1985; 132:230–235.
15. Spiro SG. Exercise testing in clinical medicine. Br J Dis Chest 1977; 71:145–172.
16. Carter R, Pevler M, Zinkgraf S, et al. Predicting maximal exercise ventilation in patients with chronic obstructive pulmonary disease. Chest 1987; 92:253–259.
17. Clark TJH, Freedman S, Campbell EJM. The ventilatory capacity of patients with chronic airways obstruction. Clin Sci 1969; 36:307–316.
18. Sean NC, Stulbarg MS, Doherty JJ, et al. Exercise-induced bronchodilatation in patients with severe COPD. Am Rev Respir Dis 1989; 139:(Suppl)A85.
19. Sergysels R, Degré S, Garcia Herreros P, et al. The ventilatory pattern during exercise in chronic obstructive pulmonary disease. Bull Eur Pathophysiol Respir 1979; 15:57–70.
20. Jones NL, Berman LB. Gas exchange in chronic airflow obstruction. Am Rev Respir Dis 1984; 129:(Suppl)581–583.
21. Foster S, Lopez D, Thomas III HM. Pulmonary rehabilitation in COPD patients with elevated PCO_2. Am Rev Respir Dis 1988; 138:1519–1523.
22. Dillard TA, Piantadosi S, Rajagopal KR. Determinants of maximum exercise capacity in patients with chronic airflow obstruction. Chest 1989, 96:267–271.
23. Sue DY, Wasserman K, Moricca R, Casaburi R. Metabolic acidosis during exercise in patients with chronic obstructive pulmonary disease. Chest 1988; 94:931–938.
24. Casaburi R, Wasserman K. Exercise training in pulmonary rehabilitation. N Eng J Med 1986; 314:1509–1511.
25. Casaburi R, Wasserman K, Patessio A, et al. A new perspective in pulmonary rehabilitation: Anaerobic threshold as a discriminant in training. Eur Respir J Suppl 1989; 7:618S–623S.
26. Shuey CD Jr, Pierce AK, Johnson RL Jr. An evaluation of exercise tests in chronic obstructive lung disease. J Appl Physiol 1969; 27:256–261.
27. Hainaut K, Duchateau J. Muscle fatigue, effects of training and disuse. Muscle Nerve 1989; 12:660–669.
28. McDougall JD, Ward BR, Sale DG, Sutton JR. Biochemical adaptation of human skeletal muscle to heavy resistance training and immobilization. J Appl Physiol 1977; 43:700–703.
29. Astrand I. Aerobic work capacity in men and women with special reference to age. Acta Physiol Scand 1960; 169:(Suppl)1–92.
30. Heath GW, Hagberg JM, Ehsani AA, Holloszy JO. A physiological comparison of young and older endurance athletes. J Appl Physiol 1981; 51:634–640.
31. Seals DR, Hagberg JM, Hurley BF, et al. Endurance training in older men and women: I. Cardiovascular responses to exercise. J Appl Physiol 1984; 57:1024–1029.
32. Seals DR, Hurley BF, Schultz J, Hagberg JM. Endurance training in older men and women: II. Blood lactate response to submaximal exercise. J Appl Physiol 1984; 57:1030–1033.
33. Blackie SP, Fairbarn MS, McElvaney GN, et al. Prediction of maximal oxygen uptake and power during cycle ergometry in subjects older than 55 years of age. Am Rev Respir Dis 1989; 139:1424–1429.
34. Jones NL, Summers E, Killian KJ. Influence of age and stature on exercise capacity during incremental cycle ergometry in men and women. Am Rev Respir Dis 1989; 140:1373–1380.
35. Hagberg JM, Seals DR, Yerg JE, et al. Metabolic responses to exercise in young and older athletes and sedentary men. J Appl Physiol 1988; 65:900–908.
36. Hansen JE, Casaburi R, Cooper DM, Wasserman K. Oxygen uptake as related to work rate increment during cycle ergometer exercise. Eur J Appl Physiol 1988; 57:140–145.
37. Nicholas JJ, Gilbert R, Gabe R, Auchincloss JH. Evaluation of an exercise therapy program for chronic obstructive pulmonary disease. Am Rev Respir Dis 1970; 102:1–9.
38. Ries AL, Moser KM. Predicting treadmill/walking speed from cycle ergometry exercise in chronic obstructive pulmonary disease. Am Rev Respir Dis 1982; 126:924–927.
39. Donner CF, Patessio A. Performance indicators in chronic obstructive lung disease: Walking test. Eur Respir J 1989; 2:670–673.
40. Cooper KH. A means of assessing maximal oxygen intake. JAMA 1968; 203–138.
41. McGavin CR, Gupta SP, McHardy GJR. Twelve-minute walking test for assessing disability in chronic bronchitis. BMJ 1976; 1:822–823.
42. Mungall IPF, Hainsworth R. Assessment of respiratory function in patients with chronic obstructive airways disease. Thorax 1979; 34:254–258.
43. Swinburn CR, Wakefield JM, Jones PW. Performances, ventilation, and oxygen consumption in three different types of exercise test in patients with chronic obstructive lung disease. Thorax 1985; 40:581–586.
44. Knox AJ, Morrison JF, Muers MF. Reproducibility of walking test results in chronic obstructive airways disease. Thorax 1988; 43:388–392.
45. Butland JA, Pang J, Gross BR, et al. Two-, six-, and 12-minute walking tests in respiratory disease. BMJ 1982; 284:1607–1608.

46. Guyatt GH, Pugsley SO, Sullivan MJ, et al. Effect of encouragement on walking test performance. Thorax 1984; 39:818–822.
47. Nickerson BG, Sarkisian C, Tremper K. Bias and precision of pulse oximeters and arterial oximeters. Chest 1988; 93:515–517.
48. Ries AL, Farrow JT, Clausen JL. Accuracy of two ear oximeters at rest and during exercise in pulmonary patients. Am Rev Respir Dis 1985; 132:685–689.
49. Carlin BW, Clausen JL, Ries AL. The use of cutaneous oximetry in the prescription of long-term oxygen therapy. Chest 1988; 94:239–241.
50. Escourrou PJL, Delaperche MF, Visseaux A. Reliability of pulse oximetry during exercise in pulmonary patients. Chest 1990; 97:635–638.
51. Hansen JE, Casaburi R. Validity of ear oximetry in clinical exercise testing. Chest 1987; 91:333–337.
52. Ries AL, Fedullo PF, Clausen JL. Rapid changes in arterial blood gas levels after exercise in pulmonary patients. Chest 1983; 83:454–456.
53. Killian KJ, Campbell EJM. Dyspnea and exercise. Annu Rev Physiol 1983; 45:465–479.
54. Gandevia SC, Killian KJ, Campbell EJM. The effect of respiratory muscle fatigue on respiratory sensations. Clin Sci 1981; 60:463–466.
55. Jones NL, Jones G, Edwards RHT. Exercise tolerance in chronic airway obstruction. Am Rev Respir Dis 1971; 103:477–491.
56. Adams L, Chronos N, Lane R, Guz A. The measurement of breathlessness induced in normal subjects: Validity of 2 scaling techniques. Clin Sci 1985; 69:7–16.
57. Mahler DA, Rosiello RA, Harver A, et al. Comparison of clinical dyspnea ratings and psychophysical measurements of respiratory sensation in obstructive airway disease. Am Rev Respir Dis 1987; 135:1229–1233.
58. Brooks LR, Ross DJ, Mohsenifar Z, Belman MJ. Comparison of clinical dyspnea ratings and psychophysical measurements of respiratory sensation in obstructive airway disease. Am Rev Respir Dis 1989; 138:A13.
59. Celli BR, Rassulo J, Make BJ. Dyssynchronous breathing during arm but not leg exercise in patients with chronic airflow obstruction. N Engl J Med 1986; 314:1485–1490.
60. Ries AL, Ellis B, Hawkins RW. Upper extremity exercise training in chronic obstructive pulmonary disease. Chest 1988; 93:688–692.
61. Lake FR, Henderson K, Briffa T, et al. Upper-limb and lower-limb exercise training in patients with chronic airflow obstruction. Chest 1990; 97:1077–1082.
62. Belman MJ, Kendregan BA. Exercise training fails to increase skeletal muscle enzymes in patients with chronic obstructive pulmonary disease. Am Rev Respir Dis 1981; 123:256–261.
63. Weg JG. Therapeutic exercise in patients with chronic obstructive pulmonary disease. In: Wenger NK (ed) Cardiovascular Clinics: Exercise and the Heart. 2nd ed. Philadelphia: F. A. Davis Co., 1985, pp 261–275.
64. Hughes RL, Davison R. Limitations of exercise reconditioning in COLD. Chest 1983; 83:241–249.
65. Belman MJ, Kendregan BA. Exercise training fails to increase skeletal muscle enzymes in patients with chronic obstructive pulmonary disease (letters). Am Rev Respir Dis 1981; 124:347–348.
66. Casaburi R, Storer T, Sullivan C, et al. Influence of training intensity on the physiologic responses to heavy exercise. FASEB J 1990; 4:A1073.
67. Coyle EF, Martin WH, Sinacore DR, et al. Time course of loss of adaptations after stopping prolonged intense endurance training. J Appl Physiol 1984; 57:1857–1864.
68. Brasher RE. Arrhythmias in patients with chronic obstructive pulmonary disease. Med Clin North Am 1984; 68–981.
69. Shih HT, Webb CR, Conway WA, et al. Frequency and significance of cardiac arrhythmias in chronic obstructive pulmonary disease. Am Rev Respir Dis 1988; 94:44–48.
70. Holford FD, Mithoefer JC. Cardiac arrhythmais in hospitalized patients with chronic obstructive pulmonary disease. Am Rev Respir Dis 1973; 108:879–885.
71. Pratt CM. Asymptomatic ventricular arrhythmias in patients with obstructive lung disease: Should they be treated? Chest 1988; 94:2–4.
72. Edelman DH, Sami MH, McGregor M, Cosio MG. Combination of theophylline and salbutamol for arrythmias in severe COPD. Chest 1987; 91:808–812.
73. Cheong TH, Magder S, Shapiro S, et al. Cardiac arrhythmias during exercise in severe chronic obstructive pulmonary disease. Chest 1990; 97:793–797.
74. Cutillo A, Bigler AH, Perondi R, et al. Exercise and distribution of inspired gas in patients with obstructive pulmonary disease. Bull Eur Physiopathol Respir 1981; 17:891–901.
75. Minh V, Lee HA, Dolan GF, et al. Hypoxemia during exercise in patients with chronic ostructive pulmonary disease. Am Rev Respir Dis 1979; 120:787–794.
76. Wagner PD, Dantzker DR, Dueck R, et al. Ventilation-perfusion inequality in chronic obstructive pulmonary disease. J Clin Invest 1977; 59:203–216.
77. Dantzker DR, D'Alonzo GE. The effect of exercise on pulmonary gas exchange in patients with severe chronic obstructive pulmonary disease. Am Rev Respir Dis 1986; 134:1135–1139.
78. D'Urzo AD, Mateika J, Bradley DT, et al. Correlates of arterial oxygenation during exercise in severe chronic obstructive pulmonary disease. Chest 1989; 95:13–17.
79. Ries AL, Farrow JT, Clausen JL. Pulmonary function tests cannot predict exercise-induced hypoxemia in chronic obstructive lung disease. Chest 1988; 93:454–459.
80. Sue DY, Oren A, Hansen JE, Wasserman K. Diffusing capacity for carbon monoxide as a predictor of gas exchange during exercise. N Engl J Med 1987; 316:1301–1306.
81. Stein DA, Bradley BL, Miller WC. Mechanisms of oxygen effects on exercise in patients with chronic obstructive pulmonary disease. Chest 1982; 81:6–10.
82. Bye PTP, Esau SA, Levy RD, et al. Ventilatory muscle function during exercise in air and oxygen in patients with chronic airflow limitation. Am Rev Respir Dis 1985; 132:236–240.
83. Vyas MN, Banister EW, Morton JW, Grzybowski S. Response to exercise in patients with chronic airway obstruction: II. Effects of breathing 40% oxygen. Am Rev Respir Dis 1971; 103:401–412.
84. Cotes JE, Pisa Z, Thomas AJ. Effect of breathing oxygen upon cardiac output, heart rate, ventilation, systemic and pulmonary blood pressure in patients with chronic lung disease. Clin Sci 1963; 25:305–321.
85. Bye PTP, Esau SA, Walley KR, et al. Ventilatory muscles during exercise in air and oxygen in normal men. J Appl Physiol 1984; 56:464–471.
86. American Thoracic Society. Standards for the diagnosis and care of patients with chronic obstructive pulmonary disease (COPD) and asthma. Am Rev Respir Dis 1987; 136:225–244.
87. SEP Task Group. Recommendations for long term oxygen. Eur Respir J 1989; 2:160–164.
88. Soffer M, Tashkin DP, Shapiro BJ, et al. Conservation of oxygen supply using a reservoir nasal cannula in hypoxemic patients at rest and during exercise. Chest 1985; 88:663–668.
89. Wesmiller SW, Hoffman LA, Sciurba FC, et al. Exercise tolerance during nasal cannula and transtracheal oxygen delivery. Am Rev Respir Dis 1990; 141:789–791.
90. Winter RJD, Moore-Gillon JC, George RJD, Geddes DM. Inspiration-phased oxygen delivery. Lancet 1984; ii:1371–1372.
91. McGregor M, Becklake, MR. The relationship of oxygen cost of breathing to respiratory mechanical work and respiratory force. J Clin Invest 1961; 40:971–980.
92. Levison H, Cherniack RM. Ventilatory cost of exercise in chronic obstructive pulmonary disease. J Appl Physiol 1968; 25:21–27.
93. Alpert JS, Bass H, Szucs MM, et al. Effects of physical training on hemodynamics and pulmonary function at rest and during exercise in patients with chronic obstructive pulmonary disease. Chest 1974; 66:647–651.
94. Degré S, Sergysels R, Mesin R, et al. Hemodynamic responses to physical training in patients with chronic lung disease. Am Rev Respir Dis 1974; 110:395–402.
95. Butland RJA, Pang JA, Geddes DM. Carbimazole and exercise tolerance in chronic airflow obstruction. Thorax 1982; 37:64–67.
96. Light RW, Muro JR, Sato RI, et al. Effects of oral morphine on breathlessness and exercise tolerance in patients with chronic

obstructive pulmonary disease. Am Rev Respir Dis 1989; 139:126–133.
97. Kirsch JL, Muro JR, Stansbury DW, et al. Effect of naloxone on maximal exercise performance and control of ventilation in COPD. Chest 1989; 96:761–766.
98. Berger R, Smith D. Effect of inhaled metaproterenol on exercise performance in patients with stable "fixed" airway obstruction. Am Rev Respir Dis 1988; 138:624–629.
99. Haas F, Bevelaqua F, Levin N, et al. Pentoxifylline improves pulmonary gas exchange. Chest 1990; 97:621–627.
100. Brown SE, Nagendran RC, McHugh JW, et al. Effect of a large carbohydrate load on walking performance in chronic airflow obstruction. Am Rev Respir Dis 1985; 132:960–962.
101. Sue DY, Chung MM, Grosvenor M, Wasserman K. Effect of altering the proportion of dietary fat and carbohydrate on gas exchange in normal subjects. Am Rev Respir Dis 1989; 139:1430–1434.
102. Agle DP, Baum GL, Chester EH, Wendt M. Multidiscipline treatment of chronic pulmonary insufficiency: 1. Psychological aspects of rehabilitation. Psychosom Med 1973; 35:41–49.
103. Brown HV, Wasserman K. Exercise performance in chronic obstructive pulmonary diseases. Med Clin North Am 1981; 65:525–547.

Chapter 25

Nutritional Assessment and Therapy

JULIET M. MANCINO, M.S., R.D.
MICHAEL DONAHOE, M.D.
ROBERT M. ROGERS, M.D.

Nutrition intervention in pulmonary rehabilitation lacks a research-based rationale. Interactions of nutritional status and lung disease have been the focus of research interest only in the recent past. The focus of this chapter is nutritional intervention for malnourished chronic obstructive pulmonary disease (COPD) and cystic fibrosis (CF) patients.

The problem of obesity and its implications for respiratory muscle function have been greatly overlooked. The role of nutrition in lung transplantation, pulmonary fibrosis, and bronchiectasis remains minimally addressed. In pulmonary rehabilitation literature, the nutrition component of the multidisciplinary approach is often oversimplified or ignored, despite the general impression that the goals of rehabilitation are more readily attained with optimal nutritional status. Therefore, practical clinical approaches based on sound scientific inquiry should be elicited. Pulmonary rehabilitation has been shown to be successful in improving outcome, quality of life, and exercise capacity.[1] More attention and skill applied to nutritional intervention in this setting should help to further improve these parameters. Optimal nutritional status should help to maximize the patient's state of health, respiratory muscle function, and overall sense of well-being and could possibly improve disease outcome.

In this chapter, nutritional intervention in the context of comprehensive pulmonary rehabilitation is explored by first examining techniques of nutritional assessment. Second, a review of interventions that should be incorporated into pulmonary rehabilitation programs to allow for optimal nutritional status and muscle function is presented. Both research and clinical applications of assessment and intervention tools are discussed so as to provide a comprehensive picture of what is available and appropriate for practitioners' use at present. The needs of patients with COPD (including those who are under- and overweight) and with CF are addressed; some lung diseases whose nutritional implications have received little attention, such as bronchiectasis and interstitial lung disease as well as the needs of lung transplantation candidates, are also discussed. In this manner, practitioners can utilize forms of nutritional intervention in the treatment of lung disease patients as effectively as they do in the management of other diseases and thus advance this aspect of the multidisciplinary rehabilitation program.

NUTRITIONAL ASSESSMENT

The detection of chronic nutrient excesses or deficits that result in compromised nutritional status has been a developing science over the past 20 years. In the 1970s, Bistrian and coworkers focused attention on the importance of nutritional status with their reports of malnutrition and surgical outcome.[2] Their program of nutritional assessment has been the model for this field[3] and forms the basis for concepts of nutritional assessment in all disease states. The protocol can be altered for use in pulmonary rehabilitation by applying data from lung disease populations. We have recently reviewed nutritional assessment and support for COPD patients.[4] The tools discussed are applicable for use in the COPD patient population as well as for patients with other lung diseases. Suggestions for utilization of these tools for nutritional assessment and planning of care for patients in the pulmonary rehabilitation setting follow.

Anthropometric Assessment

Physical measurements of the body allow assessment of bodily stores of nutrients. Anthropometry uses common quantitative measures to assess nutritional status by recording body weight, height, skin fold thickness, and skeletal measurements. Total body weight is accepted as a gross indicator of total body stores of visceral and somatic protein, intracellular and extracellular fluid, adipose tissue stores, and skeletal mass. In the clinical setting, body weight is obtained ideally on a calibrated beam balance scale, with the patient in light clothing and after voiding. Serial readings have greater validity if patients are weighed at the same time each day. All patients, regardless of weight status, should be screened upon entry into a pulmonary rehabilitation program. Although the problems of the underweight patient or the obese patient obviously necessitate nutritional intervention, the patient of normal body weight in the rehabilitation setting also must have his or her body weight documented to assure that it is maintained over time. Early detection of a consistent change in body weight may allow early intervention.

The calculation of percentage of *ideal body weight* by comparing measured body weight to a standard or group norm has been a traditional method. Two commonly used standards are the Metropolitan Life Insurance Tables and the Dietary Guidelines for Americans.[5,6] The use of weight standards to assess nutritional status has significant limitations. Existing standards utilize populations with limited demographics and often exclude the elderly and minorities. The Metropolitan Tables are based on a sample of 19- to 59-year-old, mostly white, middle class, insured individuals. An effort is ongoing to establish a database in the third National Health and Nutrition Examination Survey of nutritional indices for the United States population. Unlike the other resources, this survey utilizes a more diverse population base. When complete, the database will allow for a more appropriate comparison of body weight by utilizing a broad demographic population.

Weight standards are an incomplete assessment of nutritional status because they do not detail variations in specific body components, most notably lean body mass (LBM). Standards also fail to assess weight appropriateness on an individual level and do not take into consideration individual and family history of body weight, clinical measures of blood pressure, lipid levels, and other factors. To compensate for these deficiencies, the assessment of percentage of ideal body weight is usually combined with measures of body composition to provide a more complete assessment of nutritional status.

Serial measurements (or the obtaining of a weight history) to determine per cent of usual body weight are useful to reference the individual to himself or herself. They make possible the identification of trends or abrupt changes in body weight and the need for early intervention. Our data of 153 patient interviews conducted in an outpatient pulmonary clinic suggest that patients can recall their weight accurately within the past year (recalled weight versus actual weight, $r = .96$, $P < .05$).[7]

Body Composition

Although body weight is a useful parameter to monitor overall changes in nutritional status, clinicians in pulmonary rehabilitation can avail themselves of additional methods to assess body tissue compartments. As the primary goal of nutrition intervention is the maintenance or repletion of LBM, measurement of this compartment would be a useful outcome parameter. LBM, which includes the muscles of respiration, can be measured at a one-time assessment or serially to monitor ongoing changes.

One approach to the determination of LBM involves the use of anthropometric measurements. Anthropometric measurements assess the size of skin fold, skeletal breadth, and circumference at various body sites. It should be noted that anthropometric measurements need to be performed by a skilled technician using standardized techniques[8] to lessen observer error. Anthropometric measurements are limited by at least two assumptions fundamental to their use: first, that the thickness of subcutaneous fat is evenly distributed throughout the body; and second, that the measurement sites represent the average thickness of the body fat. Despite the obvious potential error in these assumptions, anthropometry can be utilized in a variety of ways in nutritional assessment.

One use is to compare (as a one-time or serial assessment) individual measurement sites with a group norm, utilizing traditional measurement sites such as the triceps skin fold and midarm circumference.[8] Second, measurement sites can be monitored serially, that is, successive values can be compared to original values to monitor therapeutic effect over the course of an intervention. Third, anthropometry can be used to determine body composition or estimate LBM and fat mass. The use of skin fold measurements to calculate body composition assumes a uniform distribution of total body fat. This assumption may be false, particularly for the elderly, who may centralize and internalize adipose tissue in the trunk.[9] Various investigators have developed regression equations utilizing assorted measurement sites to predict body density that can be used to calculate body composition.[10,11] The populations selected to develop these regression equations varied more technically precise methods for measuring body composition are too expensive for large populations or impractical for ill populations. Recent work by Schols and colleagues suggests that despite its limitations, BIA is preferable to anthropometry for use in the elderly with COPD. Anthropometry was found to overpredict LBM when compared with BIA and the measurement of total body water using deuterium isotopes.[13] Preliminary data from our laboratory confirm an overestimation of LBM by anthropometry compared with BIA.[14] Further work in the area of body composition measurement for the elderly COPD population will help to clarify these issues.

For pulmonary rehabilitation programs, regular screening of body weight is indicated. The use of anthropometry or BIA to measure body composition is suggested to detect individuals with specific depletion of LBM and to monitor the adequacy and effects of intervention.

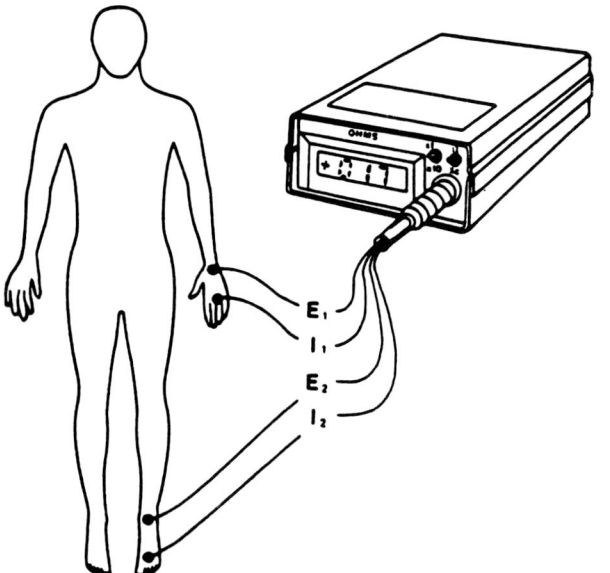

FIGURE 25–1. Diagrammatic representation of bioelectric impedance analysis electrode placement. (E_1: Medial surface between the two distal prominences of the radius and the ulna; I_1: Midline dorsal surface of the hand proximal to the metacarpal-phalangeal joint; E_2: Distal surface between the medial and lateral malleoli at the ankle; I_2: Midline dorsal surface of the foot proximal to the metacarpal-phalangeal joint.) (From Lukaski HC, Johnson PE, Bolonchuk WW. Assessment of fat-free mass using bioelectrical impedance measurements of the human body. Am J Clin Nutr 1985; 41:812.)

demographically but did not include patients with lung disease.

An alternative approach to estimating LBM is bioelectrical impedance analysis (BIA, RJL Systems, Inc.). It can be applied clinically because of its ease of use, noninvasive method of measurement, and relatively low cost. BIA measures body impedance to a nondetectable current. Electrodes are placed at a unilateral hand and foot (Fig. 25–1). Briefly summarized, the theoretical basis of BIA for the determination of body composition lies in the assumption that the human body is a series of connected cylinders; impedance is related to the length and area of these cylinders. In humans, the current is conducted by body water and electrolytes. Because the body's water and electrolytes are concentrated in the LBM, a mathematic relationship exists between the length (or height) of a person, the resistance to current flow, and the size of the LBM.

BIA has been well validated in normal populations but suffers from lack of substantiation in ill, obese, or malnourished individuals. In addition, although the relationship of body fluid and electrolytes to impedance is accepted, the constant relationship of fluid and electrolytes to LBM is not. Subjects with alterations in total body water and electrolytes may appear to have changes in lean tissue that may not exist. In the pulmonary patient, edema, malnutrition, or the use of steroids may influence fluid status, which is unrelated to LBM change. It has been suggested that BIA overestimates LBM in obese populations,[12] which might include those with lung disease. Additionally, the validation of this measurement against a gold standard has been difficult, since

Biochemical Parameters

Biochemical assessment of various body fluids has been advocated as a marker of nutritional status. Proteins, which circulate in the plasma and include the hepatic secretory proteins, are strongly influenced by dietary intake and therefore have been used to assess the adequacy of protein and calorie intake. They include albumin, prealbumin, transferrin, and retinol-binding protein. Although it has been suggested that albumin correlates highly with arm muscle circumference,[15] malnourished COPD patients generally do not present with decrements in this parameter. A number of clinical trials of nutritional support in malnourished COPD patients report depleted body weight and anthropometric indices with normal serum albumin or transferrin in the studied patients.[16–19] The influence of other diseases, infection, and steroid therapy also complicates the use of these indices. Thus, these tools do not appear to be reliable indicators of an inadequately nourished state and therefore cannot be used alone in assessing nutritional status. The use of these parameters in the nutritional assessment of patients with other lung diseases, such as interstitial lung disease, has not been explored.

A major goal of nutritional rehabilitation is the achievement of an optimal immune response in the infection-prone COPD population. A blood parameter that provides evidence concerning nutritional status and that is related to immunocompetence is the *total lymphocyte count*. This value is usually depressed in malnutrition and responds to patient refeeding. In COPD patients, low lymphocyte levels have been reported, particularly in respiratory failure patients[20,21]; however, reports of hospitalized patients[22] and stable malnourished outpatients have revealed normal lymphocyte counts.[18,19,21] Fuenzalida and coworkers reported significant increases in total lymphocyte count in COPD in patients with recent weight loss who were given supplemental feeding.[23] It appears that this measure is influenced by dietary intake, but multiple additional regulators may complicate the interpretation of this parameter. As with the visceral proteins, this parameter may serve an adjunct role as an additional marker of protein and calorie malnutrition.

Creatinine and 3-methyl histidine are urine metabolites degraded from skeletal muscle that have been used in comprehensive nutritional assessments in hospital and research settings. Urinary excretion of creatinine or 3-methyl histidine is representative of total skeletal muscle mass; excretion data can be compared with standards for height and sex to determine skeletal muscle depletion.[24] Measurement of both of these metabolites requires precise 24-hour urine collections and is most valid in the presence of controlled dietary protein intake. Other influential factors limiting its usefulness are stress, renal disease, and age.[24] Few studies have reported data based on urine collections in the nutritional assessment of malnourished COPD patients because of these details. Practically speaking, other measures of LBM are more appropriate for the rehabilitation setting.

A third measurement of urine metabolites is utilized in nitrogen balance studies. These studies are performed not for the assessment of tissue stores but rather to make a determination of how the current dietary intake is meeting the body's protein needs. Nitrogen output is determined by measurement of urinary urea nitrogen from a 24-hour urine collection. A constant of 3 g is often added to account for fecal and integumentary losses. Nitrogen intake is determined from dietary protein intake over the same time period. Subtraction of output from intake yields the nitrogen balance, with positive levels interpreted as nitrogen retention and anabolism and negative values indicating catabolism. Again, the detail and cost of urine collections make these tools impractical for use in pulmonary rehabilitation. As an alternative, serial measures of LBM, weight, or muscle function can be used to assess the effects of interventions.

In addition to the examination of the body compartments and fluids, there are additional methods of assessing nutritional status. Delayed cutaneous hypersensitivity responses are decreased or completely suppressed in malnutrition. A response of less than 10 mm of induration following intradermal injection of Candida or tuberculin or other antigens is indicative of compromised immune status. Although abnormal measures have been reported in malnourished COPD inpatients,[22] this method is limited by the influence of steroids, infection, and other disease.

Muscle Function Testing

Nutritional status can also be explored indirectly by measures of muscle function. Measurement of handgrip strength has been utilized in surgical populations to predict outcome more precisely than other nutritional parameters such as triceps skin fold thickness or albumin level.[25] This measure provides an inexpensive and simple means of assessing muscle function and is easily obtained in the outpatient setting. Several investigators report improvement in handgrip strength with weight gain after administration of oral nutritional support in the COPD patient population.[16, 26, 27] Although the use of this tool in the pulmonary rehabilitation population has not been defined, handgrip strength can be incorporated into an initial assessment with little difficulty and can be used serially to confirm strength changes stimulated by nutrition and exercise.

Respiratory pressures, although not traditionally nutritional parameters, have value in the monitoring of the function of the respiratory muscles. It has been suggested that respiratory muscle function is diminished in malnourished patients, including those with COPD.[28, 29] Several investigators report improvement in respiratory pressures with weight gain in this same population.[16, 26, 27, 30, 31] A logical goal of pulmonary rehabilitation is improved respiratory muscle function; to this end, the provision of an adequate substrate with restoration of muscle mass should produce measurable changes in muscle function. Serial measurement of inspiratory and expiratory pressures can be used to monitor nutritional progress in pulmonary rehabilitation.

Micronutrients play a role in the muscle function and nutritional status of patients with lung disease, and thus the monitoring of these parameters is essential. Electrolytes, including potassium, calcium, magnesium, and phosphates, are important contributors to overall respiratory muscle strength. Multiple factors, including poor dietary intake and diuretic use, can combine in COPD patients to produce marked depletion of these electrolytes. Fisher and associates have suggested that 28% of patients admitted to a chest ward with pulmonary infection are hypophosphatemic.[32] The issue of micronutrient deficiency is further complicated by evidence that suggests that malnourished COPD patients may experience intracellular electrolyte depletion when serum electrolyte levels are within normal limits. Monitoring of electrolyte status is a key component of the nutritional assessment program.[33]

Diet History

There are nonphysiologic aspects of nutritional assessment that need to be addressed in the pulmonary rehabilitation setting. A diet history compiled by a dietitian includes an assessment of nutritional, medical, and socioeconomic factors as well as other pertinent details that affect adequate nutrient intake. Diet intake can be assessed using a number of methods, including verbal recall techniques (e.g., a 24-hour recall by the patient regarding his or her diet) or a usual food history. Food frequency questionnaires (usually of a checklist format) require the patient to describe which foods he or she most frequently consumes and their quantities per unit of time (i.e., in days, weeks, or months). In the research setting, 24-hour recalls (verbal) or written food records are frequently used, with patients instructed in the accurate reporting of food intake. These methods suffer in varying degrees from measurement biases and inaccuracies in reporting. It is important that a dietitian be consulted to most accurately assess the patient's nutrient intake.

The summary of all physiologic and historical findings is then used to identify the specific nutritional problems of the individual patient and to develop a comprehensive care plan. Then, forms of nutritional intervention appropriate and beneficial to each patient can be implemented, and their outcome can be evaluated.

Although the scope of this chapter includes discussion of nutritional issues directly related to lung disease, it should be noted that in the clinical setting a patient is often afflicted with other medical conditions that warrant alternate diet therapy. These include cardiac disease, diabetes, and hypertension. It is expected that conflicting diet therapies may be indicated, such as sodium restriction and calorie supplementation in an underweight COPD patient with hypertension. In this instance, the skills of a dietitian and the leadership of a physician are required to prioritize the goals of nutritional intervention for the patient.

In summary, the nutritional assessment of the COPD patient is complicated by the imprecision of measurement tools. Body weight and serum electrolytes should be the basic parameters studied prior to the admission of a patient to any pulmonary rehabilitation program. Additional assessment tools, including anthropometry, BIA, visceral protein measurement, and total lymphocyte counts, may be indicated based on the patient's characteristics and the overall goal of the treatment protocol. The remainder of this chapter addresses the condition-specific nutritional implications for pulmonary disease patients.

CONDITION-SPECIFIC NUTRITIONAL CONCERNS

Malnutrition in Chronic Obstructive Pulmonary Disease

The malnourished patient with COPD has received the most attention with respect to the study of chronic lung disease and nutrition. The occurrence of weight loss in obstructive lung disease is well documented. Descriptive studies of this phenomenon were performed in the mid-1960s.[34–36] Later, Hunter and colleagues reported a near 50% incidence of protein and calorie malnutrition in hospitalized COPD patients.[22] Other investigators reported evidence of malnutrition predominantly in emphysema patients as opposed to in those with chronic bronchitis.[37] Braun and coworkers examined the predictive nature of nutritional parameters and found that triceps skin fold thickness was a significant predictor of hospitalization in the following year.[38] More recently, it was shown that COPD patients who required hospitalization and mechanical ventilation exhibited the most severe nutritional decrements of a group of 90 patients who received varying levels of health care.[21]

These investigations of malnutrition and outcome have resulted in the theorization of mechanisms for weight loss in COPD. These mechanisms have been reviewed by Wilson and associates.[39] The exact mechanism of weight loss has not been identified. Openbrier and colleagues and others reported a relationship between decreased diffusing capacity and alterations in nutritional status.[37, 40] This suggests that the pathologic type of airflow obstruction may play a part in the weight loss mechanism. Others have discussed the increased calorie needs of the COPD population. Some metabolic measurement data indicate that malnourished COPD patients have resting energy expenditures that are 15 to 19% above those predicted by the Harris-Benedict equation.[41–43]

What is the appropriate and effective nutritional intervention for the malnourished COPD patient that will have an impact on important outcomes, including but not limited to morbidity, mortality, and quality of life? A number of investigations of standard oral nutritional support for malnourished COPD outpatients have attempted to answer this question.[16–18, 31, 44] Although study design and outcomes varied, the results of these investigations indicated that standard intervention can result in weight gain, but returning patients to their ideal or usual body weight is not readily achieved. The weight gain in such patients appears to be associated with physiologic improvements.

Clinical Guidelines for Intervention

Rogers and associates[26] established, and others have repeated the finding, that the adequate provision of calories causes malnourished COPD patients to gain weight. Metabolic and nutritional studies of underweight COPD patients in our institution have suggested that calorie provision at 1.7 times the resting energy expenditure results in weight gain in this population.[27, 44] If indirect calorimetric measurements are not feasible, data reported in the literature suggest that malnourished COPD patients' resting energy expenditures are approximately 15 to 19% above those predicted by the traditional Harris-Benedict equation.[41–43] However, wide variation in this average value was noted in individual patients. If available, the use of indirect calorimetry to assess energy expenditure is preferred. The challenge that still faces investigators is to identify the combination of parameters and constants that predicts calorie needs on an individual basis without the use of indirect calorimetry. To determine the calorie requirements for weight gain, the resting energy expenditures that are obtained must be multiplied by a factor to account for the calorie needs of diet-induced thermogenesis, activity, and weight gain. A standard approach for the repletion of nonstressed surgical populations is to provide energy in an amount that is 1.7 times the resting energy expenditure.

Another concern in lean tissue repletion is the provision of adequate nitrogen. Nitrogen from amino acid sources needs to be supplied to maintain body stores, replete tissue mass, and spare calories for energy. In the hospital setting, stressed patients are commonly provided protein in a 150:1 nonprotein-calorie to nitrogen ratio. Although COPD is not a traditional stress, such as trauma or burns, the amount of protein necessary for the accretion of LBM in malnourished COPD patients has not been clearly established. This is in part owing to the lack of long-term repletion data. Based on two of the more successful trials aimed at inducing weight gain and physiologic improvements, it appears that protein supplementation of at least 1.7 g/kg of body weight is associated with nitrogen retention and physiologic improvement.[16, 44]

Another issue of nutrition intervention that is still not entirely clear is carbohydrate and fat composition. It has been suggested that the manipulation of enteral and parenteral feedings to increase the percentage of fat calories reduces carbon dioxide production. This concept has been reported to accelerate the weaning of patients from ventilators.[45] The application of this hypothesis to patients on oral diets who are not ventilator-dependent has not been thoroughly investigated, despite its common acceptance in the clinical setting. Whether this technique can alter respiratory function on a clinical level has not been clearly demonstrated.

For malnourished patients, this issue may be precluded by the difficulty of inducing patients to consume a diet that is adequately high in calories to cause weight gain, as has been evidenced in multiple clinical trials.[17–19] Some patients may only be able to tolerate a high-calorie diet of a traditional composition (e.g., one consisting of 50% carbohydrates). Attempts to manipulate a diet's fat content may be deferred to meet individual food preferences and tolerance. Early satiety and bloating, for example, may require consumption of fewer fat-dense foods. The use of an altered diet composition is not contraindicated, but patient acceptance on the clinical level is a priority.

Nutrition counseling to address the planning and preparation of a nutritionally adequate meal plan, the adequacy of the food supply in the home, the use of nutritional supplements, and other details is essential to the success of any intervention program. Frequently, this involves the inclusion of family members or the development of social support systems when patients lack familial support. Patients may suffer from the limitation of activity, including of their ability to obtain and prepare meals. The possible use of convenience food, social support, and meal providers is an important consideration for these individuals. Some pulmonary patients suffer from a number of disease-related symptoms that appear to limit their food intake, including dyspnea, fatigue, early satiety, and bloating.[46] Management strategies have been suggested to counteract the effect of these symptoms on food intake (Table 25–1).[47] Additionally, the accurate use of metered-dose inhalers, nebulizer treatments, chest physical therapy, or other modalities should help to control symptoms and further facilitate the patient's ability to maintain food intake. Patients should demonstrate their ability to appropriately administer these treatments in the course of pulmonary rehabilitation to show that they have been adequately taught by the pulmonary nurse or respiratory professional. A summary of the decision-making process in the nutritional care of malnourished individuals appears in Figure 25–2.

What improvements can be expected from the provision of standard oral nutrition support? Existing data suggest patients gain weight more readily in an inpatient setting,[26, 31, 44] whereas weight gain in an outpatient setting is difficult to achieve. If weight gain is achieved, it should result in improvements in respiratory pressures, handgrip strength, and walking distance.[16, 26, 44] There are no reports of mortality in those for whom compromised nutritional status has been effectively addressed, presumably owing to the requirement of a large sample of patients in whom significant weight change has been achieved. However, future research may address this question. More aggressive approaches have been suggested, including exploration of the use of enteral support.[31] The results of this work promise to give insight into the refeeding of this population as well as into the delivery and outcome of nutritional support for other malnourished populations. Additionally, approaches utilizing nutrition support, anabolic hormones, and specific exercise should be investigated and may yield more effective protocols and outcomes in the future.

In view of the limitations of standard oral intervention to facilitate weight gain and LBM repletion, the prevention of weight loss is key. Ideally, intervention in those patients who are at high risk of losing weight would maximize the efficiency of clinical efforts. However, preliminary data suggest that there are no clinical variables that can predict the onset of weight loss in COPD patients up to 1 year in the future.[7] The excessive financial and temporal drain on the health care system that is required to intervene in patients in whom risk is uncertain makes treatment of all patients unreasonable.

Therefore, efficient nutritional screening and continued medical and nutritional management appears essential to maintain nutritional status during high-risk periods, such as disease exacerbations. Patient education in weight maintenance techniques and the importance of the preservation of muscle mass and tissue stores need to be emphasized as do other instructions for managing their disease, particularly for those who have lost or will lose weight.

In summary, health care professionals have been stymied by or have ignored the problem of malnutrition in the 20 to 40% of COPD patients in whom it occurs. There is fairly clear evidence that the onset of weight loss is a poor prognostic indicator[48] and that modest weight gain facilitates improved muscle function. Interventions that target the mechanisms of weight loss and that have greater impact on nutritional status and muscle function show promise as an important part of disease management. Future research needs to clarify the role of aggressive nutritional support and the role of health care providers in the prevention of weight loss.

Obesity in Chronic Obstructive Pulmonary Disease

Obesity, which is defined as body weight that is 20% greater than ideal body weight, has been established as a risk factor in epidemiologic studies of a number of

TABLE 25–1. SUMMARY OF SYMPTOMS AND COUNSELING STRATEGIES FOR NUTRITIONAL THERAPY IN CHRONIC OBSTRUCTIVE PULMONARY DISEASE*

Complaint	Estimated Frequency (%)	Recommendations
Anorexia	73	Eat high-calorie food first Have favorite foods available Try more frequent meals and snacks throughout the day Push yourself to eat Add margarine, butter, mayonnaise, sauces, and gravies to diet to add calories
Early satiety	87	Eat high-calorie foods first Limit liquid consumption during meal; sip liquids 1 h after meals Eat cold foods first, as they can give less of a sense of fullness than hot foods
Dyspnea	73	Rest before meals Use bronchodilators before meals Use secretion clearance strategies if indicated Eat more slowly Use pursed-lip breathing between bites Use tripod position for meals Have readily prepared meals available for periods of increased shortness of breath Physician should evaluate for meal desaturation; refer patient for oxygen evaluation if necessary
Fatigue	60	Rest before meals Have readily prepared meals available for periods of increased fatigue or illness Try to eat larger meals in periods of less fatigue
Bloating	80	Treat shortness of breath early to prevent the swallowing of air Eat smaller, more frequent meals Avoid rushed meals Avoid gas-forming foods (individual to patient)
Constipation	50	Incorporate exercise as tolerated Eat high-fiber foods and drink adequate quantities of fluids Physician should determine the need for a stool softener
Dental problems	30	Eat soft, high-calorie foods Facilitate use of dental services as appropriate

*From Donahoe M, Rogers RM. Nutritional assessment and support in chronic obstructive pulmonary disease. Clin Chest Med 1990; 11:499.

diseases, including hypertension, noninsulin-dependent diabetes, and certain cancers.[49] Although obese COPD patients may be at increased risk for such diseases, the detrimental effect of obesity on respiratory function has been assumed but has not generated the same degree of attention as has malnutrition in COPD. The implications of obesity for the COPD patient are related to the limitations of function, but the approach to the treatment of this diagnostic group remains unexplored. It is logical to assume that metabolically inactive added fat mass increases the work of the compromised respiratory system, particularly during weight-bearing activities. Therefore, one could assume that reductions in body fat mass would be beneficial to this patient population.

However, obesity is notoriously resistant to treatment, and current recommendations for its treatment are comprehensive in scope, including careful assessment and long-term, multidisciplinary intervention. Although a variety of commercial weight loss programs and traditional nutritional counseling are available as interventions, the use of these options in pulmonary rehabilitation has not been explored. Investigation in this area requires consideration of a number of aspects, including the individualized evaluation of long-term predictors of weight reduction outcome, the goals of pulmonary rehabilitation, and the commitment of the personal and professional resources that are needed for successful weight reduction.

First, the indication for treatment involves the identification of suboptimal status that is the result of excess body weight. The identification of obesity is made difficult by a lack of precision similar to that seen in the detection of malnutrition. Although morbid obesity (200% of ideal body weight, or a body weight 100% greater than ideal body weight) is visually obvious, there is less distinction as to what defines moderate obesity by various weight standards and what risk this represents for the individual (see the use of weight standards discussed earlier). Some research has suggested that the anatomic localization of body fat determines health risk more than does overall body fat. Upper-body, centrally located excess body fat is associated with a high risk of coronary heart disease, hypertension, and certain cancers.[50] One could theorize that fat localized in this region may impede pulmonary function to a greater degree than that in other areas because of its impairment of the ventilatory apparatus. Lower-body obesity (e.g., at the hips or femoral region) is relatively insignificant with respect to disease risks. Recognition of this can be used

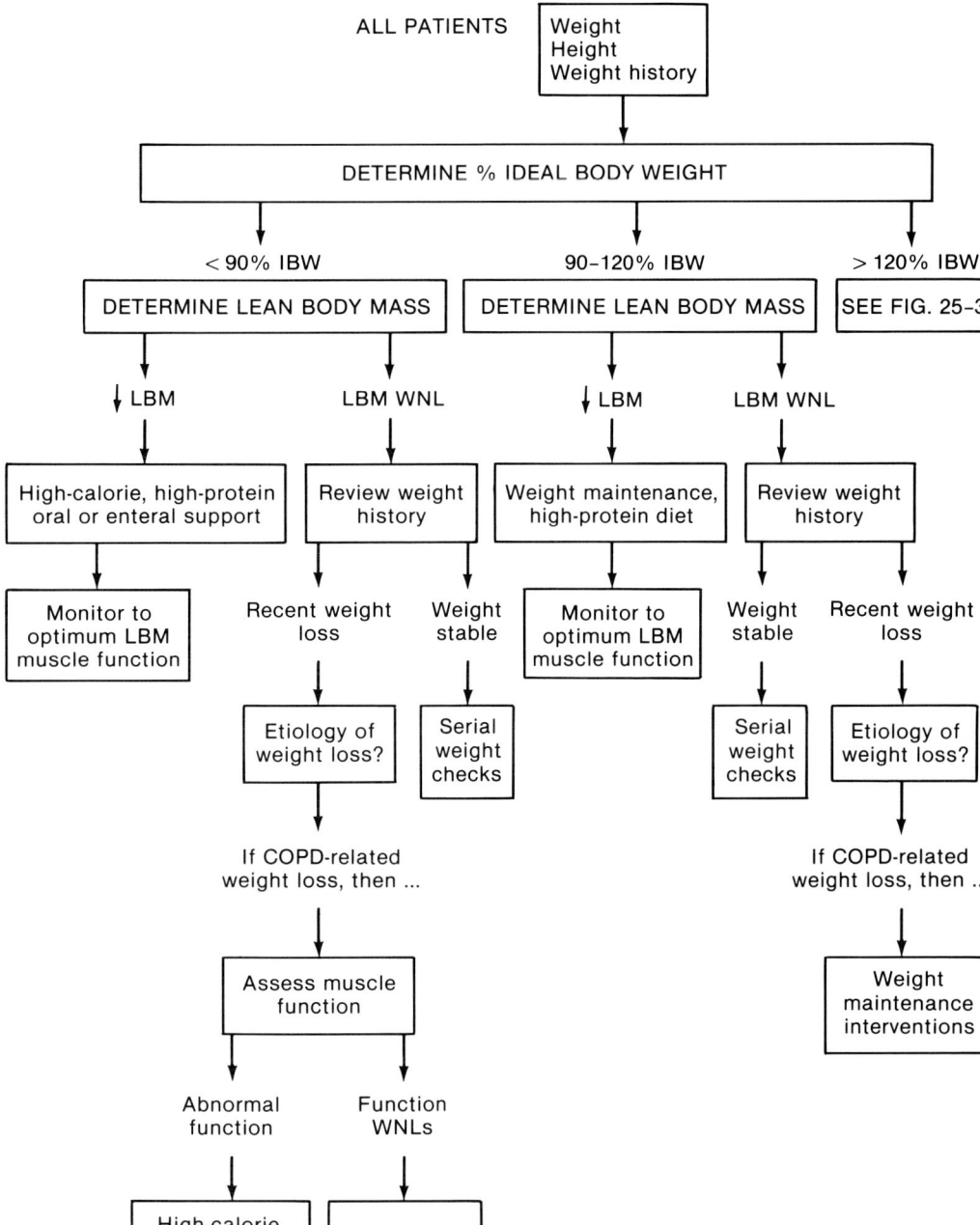

FIGURE 25–2. Suggested guidelines for the decision-making process in the nutritional care of normal and underweight patients. (IBW: ideal body weight; LBM: lean body mass; WNL: within normal limits; COPD: chronic obstructive pulmonary disease.)

in clinical decision-making in combination with knowledge of blood lipid levels, the presence of hypertension, family history, the presence of smoking, and other factors that may elucidate whether a person is a candidate for weight reduction therapy.

Although the treatment of obesity has diversified and continues to be the subject of extensive research, obesity still has a poor long-term prognosis for many individuals. Studies of identical twins suggest a genetic component of obesity that may explain the refractory nature of weight loss efforts for some individuals.[51] Adult-onset obesity without familial precedent may be more amenable to treatment. It appears that clinicians must evaluate the detriment of the added weight on pulmonary function and other medical problems and compare it with the potential for long-term weight reduction and risks of recidivism. At present, this is clearly a subjective judgment made by the clinician. Weight cycling (repeated weight loss and gain) may contribute to a loss of lean mass, lead to an increased body weight, and make long-term weight maintenance more difficult.[52] This would not serve the goals of pulmonary rehabilitation well.

Additionally, older or chronically obese patients who are to undergo pulmonary rehabilitation may be resistant to behavioral change. Although it has been suggested that the increased health risks of severe obesity warrant higher-risk treatments (e.g., very low-calorie diets or surgical procedures),[53] a more conservative, realistic approach may be to prevent continued weight gain. Preliminary evidence suggests that this in itself may be a challenge. Data on 153 COPD patients in a Veterans Affairs Medical Center pulmonary clinic revealed a high incidence (37.2%) of obesity (greater than 120% of the midpoint body weight provided by the Metropolitan Life Insurance Tables).[7] Of these obese patients, two thirds had maintained or gained weight in the previous year.

The population of patients who are greater than 140% of ideal body weight presents a difficult management question for pulmonary rehabilitation. The immediate response when encountering such patients in clinical settings is often automatic weight reduction efforts. The high risk of heart disease, hypertension, and other problems suggests that this is imperative. However, all patients should be evaluated individually to develop the intervention that will give the greatest long-term benefit. There is a subset of individuals with COPD for whom weight loss may be contraindicated. A number of investigations yield evidence that may lead to this conclusion. For example, it is well established that weight loss to subnormal status in COPD is associated with earlier mortality. The population of COPD patients at risk for such weight loss has not been defined. In an unpublished report, Openbrier compared nutritional patterns of normal-weight and underweight COPD patients and found that the 70% of the normal-weight patients (90–110% of ideal body weight) were losing weight. In preliminary data, we found that 22% of obese patients and 34% of normal-weight patients in a Veterans Administration clinic population had a documented weight loss of 5% or greater in the previous year.[7] These findings suggest that a careful review of weight history is indicated for patients before a weight reduction program is initiated. For patients who are of borderline status, further weight reduction may be contraindicated. Factors such as weight or appetite fluctuations, weight loss during disease exacerbations, or weight gain associated with prolonged steroid use must be examined when selecting a treatment plan. Weight reduction may exacerbate an existing risk for weight loss associated with disease and lead to a decrease in pulmonary function.

Weight Gain Prevention

Although some patients are motivated and show potential for success in a weight reduction program, others may utilize alternative interactions. These patients should receive treatments aimed at preventing further weight gain, such as instruction in how to maintain a prudent diet that is low in fat and has a normal calorie content as well as how to adhere to an exercise program. Nutrition intervention for these individuals should concentrate on modifications in the current diet to control total fat and calories as well as on behavioral techniques to deter overeating. The role of exercise is vital in preventing weight gain and maximizing the function of lean tissue, which may have become deconditioned because of the limitation of activity that resulted from the increased body weight.

Information can be utilized to assess patients who are moderately obese (120–140% of ideal body weight) for the appropriate intervention. The clinical parameters previously discussed should be assessed. Candidates can be screened for predictors of success in obesity treatment; the most important of these—participation in regular exercise—complements pulmonary rehabilitation. Three other factors are described as essential for success: (1) a shift in motivation from external to internal reasons (e.g., losing weight for health reasons as opposed to for an event), (2) the ability to attend to positive health changes (e.g., decreased dyspnea in the pulmonary patient), and (3) social support.[50] Of course, these factors are dependent on the patient's recognition of and willingness to address his or her weight problem. The detection of the existence of these factors depends on the skill of the clinician and calls for specific expertise within the weight loss program. Conservative treatment includes behavior modification techniques, exercise, modest calorie restriction, and slow weight loss (1/2–1 lb/wk). The inclusion of social support and relapse prevention training can help to optimize success for moderately overweight individuals.[50] The availability of skilled clinicians who can implement these elements in pulmonary rehabilitation or refer patients to programs that provide such services is vital. Interventions should be monitored so that patients lose weight at a slow rate and minimize lean tissue losses. The use of nutritional assessment tools to monitor muscle strength during periods of weight loss is suggested so that clinicians can intervene if there is evidence of a change in muscle function that is caused by electrolyte abnormalities or LBM catabolism.

If the patient and clinician agree that a weight reduction regimen is imperative and appropriate, the most current diet therapies utilize low-fat, calorie-controlled regimens or very low-calorie diets that emphasize relapse prevention and weight maintenance. As stated earlier, one of the keys to the maintenance of weight loss is regular exercise, which is probably limited in severely obese individuals with lung disease. Thus, the issue of weight maintenance is still problematic.[50] Suggested guidelines for decision-making concerning the obese patient in pulmonary rehabilitation are summarized in Figure 25–3.

Smoking and Weight Management

An important aspect related to the nutrition of pulmonary patients concerns smoking cessation. The event of weight gain (average of 6 lb) after smoking cessation has been documented.[54] The mechanism of this weight gain appears to be an increase in the total dietary intake of calories and, although it has not been shown conclusively, a decrease in metabolism.[54] Activity levels appear to be unrelated to smoking cessation and changes in body weight.[54]

Interventions for this problem are being addressed. Continuance of smoking cessation despite weight gain must remain a priority because the health risks of smoking are relatively greater than those of added

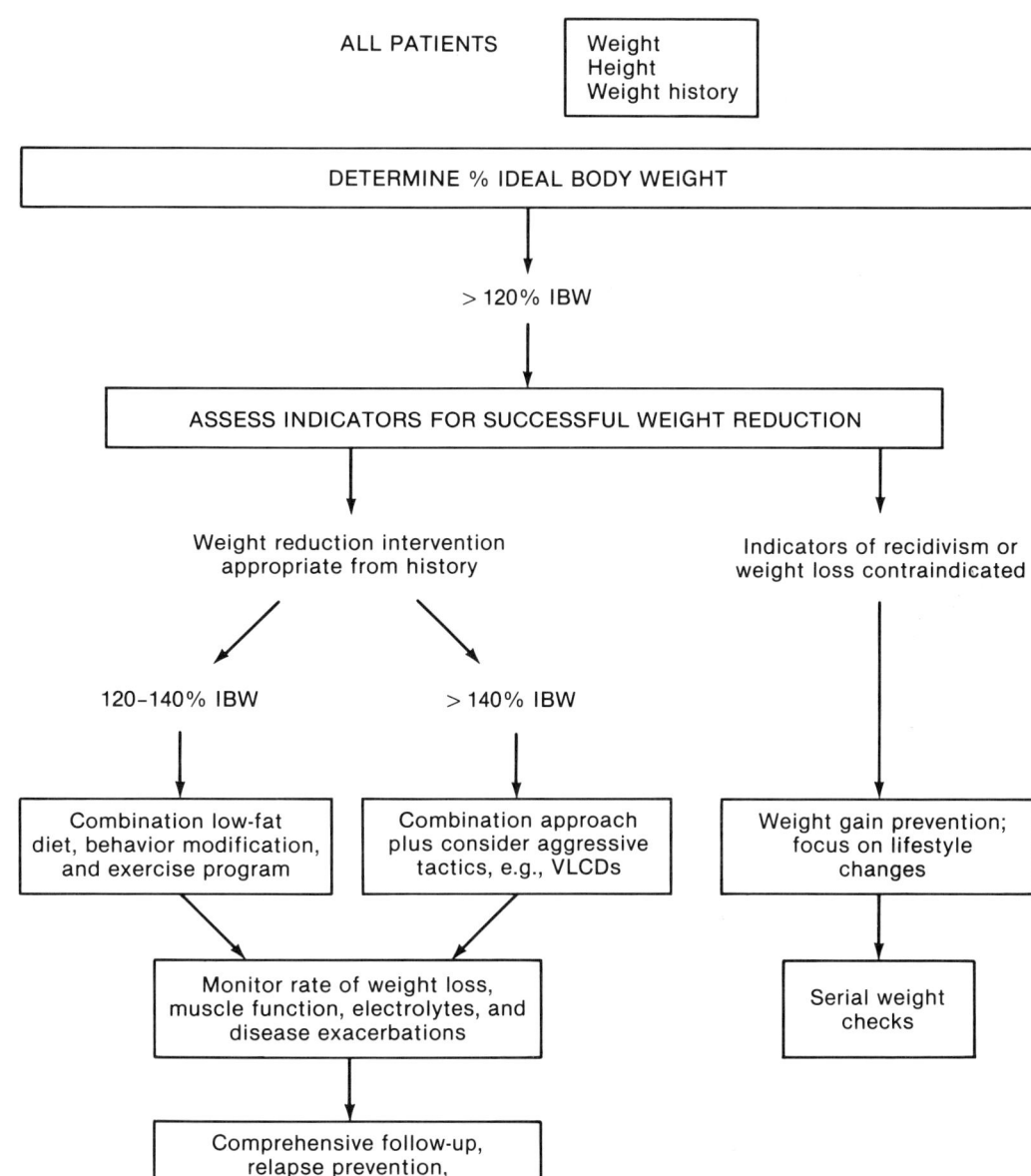

FIGURE 25–3. Suggested guidelines for the decision-making process in the nutritional care of obese patients. (VLCD: very low-calorie diet.)

weight. Patients report fear of weight gain as a reason for their inability to quit smoking, although only one third of them express concern about weight gain in a smoking cessation program.[54] It is unclear in which patient populations intervention strategies should be targeted and what effect such interventions have on the smoking cessation effort. However, the same intervention strategies that are currently advocated for weight reduction are utilized in smoking cessation (e.g., cognitive and behavioral techniques, exercise, nutritional modifications, and the use of social support). The use of nicotine gum may play a role in weight gain prevention strategies.[54] Research into the relationship between smoking cessation and body weight is relatively recent but is warranted owing to the importance of smoking abstinence in the rehabilitation of patients with chronic lung disease.

Cystic Fibrosis and Bronchiectasis

Nutritional intervention for CF patients has been suggested to prevent infection and slow the rate of pulmonary decline in patients with successful weight gain.[55] In contrast, the population of adult bronchiectasis patients is relatively smaller, and, unfortunately, few data have been published on the nutritional implications of this disease. However, the pulmonary complications of recurrent infections, sputum production, and worsening obstructive lung disease are similar to those of the patient with CF. Nutritional intervention for patients with these diseases can be similarly addressed, with the emphasis being on the rehabilitation of the malnourished patient. However, it should be noted that the malabsorption component of CF does not apply to the bronchiectasis patient. Ideally, nutritional intervention is ongoing throughout the CF patient's life span and helps to facilitate patient survival to almost 30 years, as is now reported.[56] However, nutritional compromise continues to be a result of the many complicating nutritional factors of CF; as a result, presentation of the patient in need of nutritional rehabilitation is not uncommon.

The dramatic effect of nutritional intervention in CF was reported in a comparison of survival rates at two CF clinics, one in Boston, Massachusetts, and the other in Toronto, Canada.[57] The Toronto patients were noted to have a survival time approximately 9 years longer than that of the patients in the Boston clinic. The only outstanding difference was that the Toronto patients were counseled to maintain a *high-fat*, high-calorie diet and were taller and heavier than the Boston patients, who were counseled to maintain a *low-fat*, high-calorie diet regimen. The longer survival of the Toronto patients could be attributed to diet composition or caloric level; the clinical evidence of enhanced growth suggests that the caloric contribution was a significant component. Recent recognition of the role dietary lipids have in immune system function[58] may suggest an additional mechanism of benefit.

Clinical Investigations of Nutrition Intervention in Cystic Fibrosis

The effects of nutrition intervention have been reported in a number of projects utilizing a variety of forms of nutritional support but most commonly in those using nighttime enteral feeding.[59-65] Although these were uncontrolled investigations, they all reported weight gain, growth, and clinical benefits. This is in contrast to the COPD patient population, in which attempts at weight gain have proved difficult despite comprehensive oral diet intervention. It has been our experience that COPD patients have a limited ability to maintain an increased oral intake beyond a certain point in time after intervention.[44] The CF patient's ability to maintain oral intake while receiving supplementation over an extended time period[60, 62, 65] to enhance total caloric intake suggests a difference in the mechanism that limits adequate intake in these two populations. It could also be speculated that the metabolic presence of growth hormone in the younger CF patient may favorably alter the tissue composition of the weight gain achieved. LBM accretion would then most effectively contribute to improvement in physiologic and, consequently, clinical and quality-of-life parameters.

The genetic potential for growth is normal in CF; abnormalities are related to inadequate energy balance, not a catabolic disease process.[56] Several investigations document the influence of nutrition counseling to augment oral intake in CF patients.[56, 66] Furthermore, progressive weight loss contributes to pulmonary decline, and therefore attempts to halt and reverse this process are vital and appear to have an impact on survival. Thus, nutritional intervention in the CF patient has several aims and includes the maintenance of optimal nutritional status within the context of the disease through normal growth and development, the minimization of alterations in growth rate, and the fulfillment of energy, macronutrient, and micronutrient needs (including the increased needs caused by sweat, sputum, and malabsorption losses).

Issues in Nutritional Assessment of Cystic Fibrosis Patients

As in COPD, initial nutritional care for the CF patient begins with a thorough assessment of objective and subjective factors. Important objective medical information includes knowledge of the presence of infection, the degree of malabsorption, and the need for pancreatic enzyme replacement as well as of the presence of anemia, gastroesophageal reflux, diabetes, liver disease, or cor pulmonale.[67] Serial nutritional assessment is useful to monitor adequate growth and the maintenance of tissues. Anthropometric assessment should include the measurement of height, weight, growth velocity or chronologic progress (e.g., on growth charts), and triceps skin fold thickness and midarm circumference. Utilizing serial weight measurements or a weight history is important in the close monitoring of CF and bronchiectasis patients at risk of weight loss associated with their lung diseases. Shepherd and Cleghorn have also suggested the use of the creatinine height index to assess LBM, although this may not be appropriate in the pulmonary rehabilitation setting.[55] Biochemical assessment can include measurement of hepatic secretory proteins; for example, measurement of albumin level is useful, although this common index may be altered artificially by elevated globulin levels or hemodilution.[55] An alternative is the measurement of retinol-binding protein, which may respond more rapidly to changes in protein stores; however, the use of this measure in the rehabilitation of CF and bronchiectasis patients has not been reported.

Subjective information obtained during compilation of a diet history may include usual food intake, which can be obtained from food records or verbal recall by the patient or the patient's family. The clinician needs to ascertain the usage pattern of pancreatic enzyme replacements and the frequency of steatorrhea. Pancreatic enzymes need to be administered with all meals and snacks, and a regimen individualized for each patient that is dependent on tolerance and the degree of steatorrhea is suggested.[66] Although it can be a source of pain, mild steatorrhea is not harmful. As with the malnourished COPD patient, a variety of disease-related symptoms can limit food intake, and coping strategies are important for the patient. Chest physical therapy—an important treatment regimen for CF and bronchiectasis patients—can contribute to decreased appetite and fatigue and needs to be considered when planning meals and snacks. Additional chest therapy sessions may be needed as disease worsens, and therefore food intake may be decreased when chest therapy needs are increased.[66] Current prudent (low-fat and low-salt) diet recommendations espoused for the general public are contraindicated in CF, and this needs to be communicated to the patient and his or her family.

Nutritional Needs in Cystic Fibrosis

CF patients have unique elevated nutrient needs of several types. Calorie needs are characterized by increased resting energy expenditure and other disease factors. The increased resting energy expenditure (which can be up to 153% of that predicted[60] appears to result from two sources. The first is increased work of breathing caused by the obstructive process in the lungs similar to that demonstrated in the COPD and interstitial lung disease populations.[41–43, 68] The second is the suggestion of an increase in cellular metabolism associated with the genetic defect in CF, but this possibility has not been investigated thoroughly and remains speculative at this point.[55, 56, 69]

The calorie needs of CF patients are also influenced by nutrient losses associated with malabsorption and the presence of low-grade fevers and infection. These factors, along with generally suboptimal food intake,[66] create the need for a high-calorie diet.[56] In trials in which successful weight gain has been achieved, calories have been provided in quantities ranging from 109 to 137% of the Recommended Daily Allowance (Table 25–2).[59–65] Hubbard and Mangrum suggest a calorie intake that is 150% of the Recommended Daily Allowance; this level appears to be the standard recommendation at present. It could also be theorized that the bronchiectasis patient would have elevated calorie needs because of the obstructive process and the presence of infections. Metabolic measurement data on the bronchiectasis population have not been reported.

CF patients have specific nutrient requirements related to diet composition. A low-fat diet has been demonstrated to be contraindicated in these patients because of their need for a calorie-dense diet and because CF is characterized by fat malabsorption. It is generally recommended that CF patients obtain between 35 and 50% of their calories from fat, including 5% from essential fatty acid sources. CF patients may have abnormal essential fatty acid profiles owing to their maldigestion and malabsorption of linoleate; they therefore require adequate fatty acid sources in their diet.[70]

Protein requirements are increased by the need for nutritional repletion and by nitrogen losses in sputum. Various standards for protein intake have been suggested, including 1.5 times the Recommended Daily Allowance, 15 to 20% of calorie needs, or 1.5 to 2.0 g/kg of body weight.[56, 67] Any of these three methods is adequate to achieve a higher than normal amount of protein in the diet.

In addition to protein and calorie needs, CF patients have increased micronutrient needs. Primarily as a result of fat malabsorption, higher requirements exist for the fat-soluble vitamins A, D, E, and K. Shepherd and Cleghorn report supplementation of the water-soluble vitamins (twice the Recommended Daily Allowance of B-complex and C vitamins), although no evidence of need has been identified.[55] The loss of nutrients in sweat, especially in warm weather, requires that salt consumption remain unrestricted and that salty foods and table salt be consumed. The role of exercise is being explored in the treatment of CF patients; sodium chloride lost in the sweat of exercising patients needs to be recovered. A summary of CF patient nutrient needs appears in Table 25–3.

It is essential, therefore, to address the nutritional status of CF patients throughout their life span and not only in the rehabilitation setting. Measures to maintain an oral diet adequate to sustain growth are an integral part of treatment. With respect to those patients who become malnourished (despite efforts to the contrary) or who are unable to consume an adequate diet in advanced lung disease, more aggressive forms of intervention have been explored and have shown reasonable success in maintaining or repleting the nutritional status of some patients.

Other Lung Disease

Other patients for whom nutritional intervention might facilitate improved clinical outcomes include the lung transplant candidate and the patient with interstitial lung disease. Data on the incidence or implications of altered nutritional status and the results of intervention are sparse. Nutritional problems and interventions are intuitive or anecdotal at present.

Lung Transplant Patients

The patient who is to undergo lung transplantation could be expected to have an indication for nutritional intervention. Transplant candidates are often end-stage COPD and CF patients, in whom the incidence of malnutrition is well documented. Additionally, the application of nutritional support to end-stage CF patients can be complicated by the complete absence of pancreatic enzyme function, diabetes mellitus, or carbohydrate load–induced hypercapnia.[71] Alternatively, patients who are obese are poor surgical risks and, like malnourished patients, have impaired postoperative mobility, which is associated with decreased survival.[72] Morrison and colleagues suggested that transplant candidates maintain weight within 10 to 15 kg of their ideal body weight.[72] For patients who are not within this range, the appropriate intervention to achieve optimal nutritional status for transplantation involves the same problematic issues as for underweight and obese COPD patients (discussed previously). Clinical work regarding the documentation of nutritional status and surgical outcome to identify predictors needs to be refined for pulmonary transplant patients as it has been for other disease populations. This is complicated by the limited size of this population and by the many factors affecting the success of lung transplantation. More specific data regarding the surgical risks associated with deficits in a variety of nutritional parameters (e.g., lean and fat mass, immune system function, and hematopoietic status) may be helpful in determining the indications for and the aggressiveness of intervention efforts.

The development of aggressive nutritional support regimens or other forms of intervention that contribute to a more favorable outcome for potential transplant

TABLE 25–2. REPORTS OF NUTRITIONAL SUPPORT IN CYSTIC FIBROSIS PATIENTS

Investigator	Year	No. of Patients	Study Type	Form of Nutrient Delivery	Nutrients Provided	Improvements Seen Clinically in:
Shepherd et al.[59]	1980	12	Pilot	TPN	>130% RDA, 20% protein	Weight, growth, rate of infection, well-being, and p.o. intake post-TPN
Levy et al.[60]	1985	14	NR, NC, historical comparison	h.s. g-tube	30% of REE in formula	Weight, LBM, growth, and rate of PFT decline
Boland et al.[63]	1986	10	Pilot	h.s. j-tube	Details not given	Weight, growth, and rate of FVC decline
Shepherd et al.[62]	1986	10	NR, NC, comparison group	h.s. ng-tube	120% RDA of calories and protein	Weight, growth, infection rate, and rate of PFT decline
O'Loughlin et al.[61]	1986	13	NR, NC	h.s. ng-tube	150% RDA in formula	Weight, LBM, infection rate, and well-being
Soutter et al.[64]	1986	15	Pilot	h.s. g-tube	Up to 137% RDA	Weight, growth, and well-being
Luder et al.[65]	1989	37	NR, NC	p.o. high-calorie diet	Up to 126% RDA	Weight, rate of PFT decline

Key: TPN: total parenteral nutrition; RDA: Recommended Daily Allowance; NR: nonrandomized; NC: noncontrolled; REE: resting energy expenditures; PFT: pulmonary function test; FVC: forced ventilatory capacity; h.s.: at night; p.o.: by mouth; g-tube: gastric tube; j-tube: jejunal tube; ng-tube: nasogastric tube.

candidates or make transplantation a possibility has not been reported. Nutritional support in CF and COPD patients has already been discussed. Weight reduction in the COPD patient was also discussed and may present the challenging problem of how to maintain optimal nutritional status preoperatively while depleting only body fat. Weight loss through exercise may not be realistic for the patient with a degree of pathology that necessitates transplantation.

It has been suggested that there are unique nutritional problems facing the postoperative lung transplant patient. Anecdotes of postoperative hypercholesterolemia and excessive weight gain have been reported by Maurer after unilateral and bilateral lung transplants.[71] The mechanisms of each of these sequelae may be related to steroid use, pretransplant eating behavior, or other factors. The role of post-transplantation nutrition intervention has yet to be defined. Clearly, individualized assessment and treatment goals are necessary.

Interstitial Lung Disease

Interstitial lung disease affects a relatively small population of individuals. The nutritional implications of the disease have been the subject of minimal investigation. Hypermetabolic calorie needs in interstitial lung disease patients have been hypothesized because of these patients' increased work of breathing that is similar to that of COPD patients. However, owing to the lung inflammatory processes in this disease, an actual increase in lung metabolism was proposed.[68] In COPD hypermetabolism, it is theorized that the diaphragm operates at a mechanical disadvantage. In interstitial lung disease patients, resting energy expenditure measurements were a mean of 17% above those predicted. The sample of 12 patients included 8 who had recent weight loss, although it was not noted if the presence of certain other diseases with nutritional implications was a criterion for exclusion. This early report suggests nutritional implications for interstitial lung disease patients. Further investigation may provide insight into the scope of the nutritional problems of interstitial lung disease patients and the implications for treatment and outcome.

CONCLUSION

The application of nutrition therapy has developed rapidly over the past two decades and has paralleled an increasing focus on cost efficiency in health care. Indeed, nutrition has gained importance as the significance of adequate nutritional status in recovery from disease and its impact on the need for and length of hospitalization have been recognized. Malnutrition is no longer viewed as an inevitable consequence of disease. Research efforts verify that clinicians must continue to investigate the

TABLE 25–3. NUTRITIONAL NEEDS OF THE OLDER CYSTIC FIBROSIS PATIENT*

Nutrient	Daily Requirement
Energy	RDA × 1.5
Protein	RDA × 1.5
Fat	40% of energy
Essential fatty acids	5% of total energy
Fat-soluble vitamins	
A	5–1000 I.U./day in water-miscible form
D	4–80 I.U./day
E	1–300 I.U./day of alpha-tocopherol acetate
K	5 mg twice daily
Water-soluble vitamins	
B group	RDA × 2
C	RDA × 2
B_{12}	RDA unless ileal resection present
Sodium chloride	4–6 g/day in hot weather
Zinc	RDA
Iron	RDA unless anemia present

*From Shepherd RW, Cleghorn GJ. Nutritional management. In: Shepherd RW (ed.). Cystic Fibrosis: Nutritional and Intestinal Disorders. Boca Raton, FL: CRC Press, Inc., 1989, p 58.

role of nutrition intervention in treating the pulmonary disease patient. Pharmacologic effects of nutrients on immune function and hormonal influence on body composition are promising new tools that, after investigation, may allow clinicians to alter disease outcome in the future. The continued use and investigation of these tools in pulmonary rehabilitation only serves to better refine and enhance the comprehensive treatment of the pulmonary disease patient.

REFERENCES

1. Hodgkin JE. Pulmonary rehabilitation. Chest 1990; 11:447–454.
2. Bistrian BR, Blackburn GL, Hallowell E. Protein status of general surgical patients. JAMA 1974; 230:858.
3. Blackburn GL, Bistrian BR, Maini BS, et al. Nutritional and metabolic assessment of the hospitalized patient. J Parenter Enter Nutr 1977; 1:11–22.
4. Donahoe M, Roger RM. Nutritional assessment and support in chronic obstructive pulmonary disease. Clin Chest Med 1990; 11:487–504.
5. Metropolitan Life Insurance Company. New weight standards for men and women. New York: Metropolitan Life Insurance Company, 1983.
6. Nutrition and your health: Dietary guidelines for Americans, 3rd ed. Washington, D.C.: U.S. Department of Agriculture and Department of Health and Human Services; 1990. Home and Garden Bulletin No. 232.
7. Donahoe M, Rogers RM, Mancino JM, et al. Clinical variables do not predict weight loss in patients with chronic obstructive pulmonary disease. Am Rev Respir Dis 1991; 143:A453.
8. Lohman TG. Anthropometry and body composition. In: Lohman TG (ed). Anthropometric Standardization Reference Manual. Champaign, IL: Human Kinetics Books, 1988, pp 39–55.
9. Seidell JC, Oosteriee A, Thyssen MAO, et al. Assessment of intraabdominal and subcutaneous fat: Relation between anthropometry and computed tomography. Am J Clin Nutr 1987; 12:217–225.
10. Durnin JVGA, Womersley J. Body fat assessment from total body density and its estimation from skinfold thickness: Measurements on 481 men and women aged from 16–72 years. Br J Nutr 1974; 32:77–97.
11. Lohman TG. Skinfolds and body density and their relation to body fatness: A review. Hum Biol 1981; 53:181–225.
12. Segal KR, Van Loan M, Fitzgerald PI, et al. Lean body mass estimation by bioelectrical impedance analysis: A four-site cross-validation study. Am J Clin Nutr 1988; 47:7–14.
13. Schols AM, Wouters EF, Soeters PB, et al. Body composition by bioelectrical impedance analysis compared with deuterium dilution and skinfold anthropometry in patients with chronic obstructive pulmonary disease. Am J Clin Nutr 1991; 53:421–424.
14. Mancino JM, Donahoe M, Rogers RM, et al. Determination of lean body mass in patients with chronic obstructive pulmonary disease. Am Rev Respir Dis 1990; 141:A34.
15. Grant A, DeHoog S. Biochemical assessment. In: Nutritional Assessment and Support. Seattle: Grant-DeHoog, 1985, p 36.
16. Efthimiou J, Fleming J, Gomes C, et al. The effect of supplementary oral nutrition in poorly nourished patients with chronic obstructive pulmonary disease. Am Rev Respir Dis 1988; 137:1075–1082.
17. Lewis MI, Belman MJ, Dorr-Uyemura L. Nutritional supplementation of ambulatory patients with chronic obstructive pulmonary disease. Am Rev Respir Dis 1989; 135:1062–1068.
18. Otte KE, Ahlburg P, D'Amore F, et al. Nutritional repletion in malnourished patients with emphysema. J Parenter Enter Nutr 1984; 13:152–156.
19. Knowles JB, Fairbarn MS, Wiggs DJ, et al. Dietary supplementation in respiratory muscle performance in patients with COPD. Chest 1988; 93:977–983.
20. Driver AG, McAlevy MT, Smith JL. Nutritional assessment of patients with chronic obstructive pulmonary disease and acute respiratory failure. Chest 1982; 82:568–571.
21. Fiaccadori E, Del Canale SD, Coffrini E, et al. Hypercapnic-hypoxemic chronic obstructive pulmonary disease (COPD): Influence of severity of COPD on nutritional status. Am J Clin Nutr 1988; 48:680–685.
22. Hunter AMB, Carey MA, Larsh HW. The nutritional status of patients with chronic obstructive pulmonary disease. Am Rev Respir Dis 1981; 124:376–381.
23. Fuenzalida CE, Petty TL, Jones ML, et al. The immune response in short-term nutritional intervention in advanced chronic obstructive pulmonary disease. Am Rev Respir Dis 1990; 142:49–56.
24. Heymsfeld SB, Arteaga C, McManus C, et al. Measurement of muscle mass in humans: Validity of the 24-hour urinary creatinine method. Am J Clin Nutr 1983; 37:478–494.
25. Hunt DR, Rowlands BJ, Johnston D. Hand grip strength: A simple prognostic indicator in surgical patients. J Parenter Enter Nutr 1985; 36:680–690.
26. Wilson DO, Rogers RM, Sanders MH, et al. Nutritional intervention in malnourished patients with emphysema. Am Rev Respir Dis 1986; 134:672–677.
27. Donahoe M, Rogers RM, Openbrier DR, et al. Effect of calorie intake on muscle strength and walking distance in malnourished COPD. Am Rev Respir Dis 1989; 139:A334.
28. Arora NR, Rochester DF. Respiratory muscle strength and maximal voluntary ventilation in undernourished patients. Am Rev Respir Dis 1982; 126:5–8.
29. Rochester DF, Braun NMT. Determinants of maximal inspiratory pressure in chronic obstructive pulmonary disease. Am Rev Respir Dis 1985; 132:42–47.
30. Goldstein SA, Thomashow B, Askanazi J. Functional changes during nutritional repletion in patients with lung disease. Chest 1986; 7:141–155.
31. Whittaker JS, Ryan CF, Buckley PA, et al. The effects of refeeding in peripheral and respiratory muscle function in malnourished chronic obstructive pulmonary disease patients. Am Rev Respir Dis 1990; 142:283–288.
32. Fisher J, Magid N, Kallman C, et al. Respiratory illness and hypophosphatemia. Chest 1983; 83:504–508.
33. Fiaccadori E, Del Canale S, Coffrini E, et al. Muscle and serum magnesium in pulmonary intensive care unit patients. Crit Care Med 1988; 16:751–760.
34. Sukumalchantra Y, Williams MH. Serial studies of pulmonary function in patients with chronic obstructive pulmonary disease. Am J Med 1965; 39:941–945.
35. Renzetti AD, McClement JH, Litt BD. The Veterans Administration cooperative study of pulmonary function: Mortality in relation to respiratory function in chronic obstructive pulmonary disease. Am J Med 1966; 41:115–129.
36. Vandenbergh E, Woestijne KP, Gyselen A. Weight changes in the terminal stages of chronic obstructive pulmonary disease. Am Rev Respir Dis 1967; 96:556–565.
37. Openbrier DR, Irwin MM, Rogers RM, et al. Nutritional status and lung function in patients with emphysema and chronic bronchitis. Chest 1983; 83:17–22.
38. Braun SR, Dixon RM, Keim NL, et al. Predictive clinical value of nutritional assessment factors in COPD. Chest 1984; 85:353–357.
39. Wilson DO, Rogers RM, Hoffman RM. Nutrition and chronic lung disease. Am Rev Respir Dis 1985; 132:1347–1365.
40. Braun SR, Keim NL, Dixon RM, et al. The prevalence and determinants of nutritional changes in chronic obstructive pulmonary disease. Chest 1984; 86:558–563.
41. Donahoe M, Rogers RM, Wilson DO, et al. Oxygen consumption of the respiratory muscles in normal and malnourished patients with chronic obstructive pulmonary disease. Am Rev Respir Dis 1989; 140:385–391.
42. Wilson DO, Donahoe M, Rogers RM, et al. Metabolic rate and weight loss in chronic obstructive lung disease. J Parenter Enter Nutr 1990; 14:7–11.
43. Goldstein SA, Askanazi J, Weissman C, et al. Energy expenditure in patients with chronic obstructive pulmonary disease. Chest 1987; 91:222–224.
44. Rogers RM, Donahoe M, Costantino JP. Physiologic effects of

oral supplemental feeding on malnourished COPD patients: A randomized control study. Am Rev Respir Dis 1992 (in press).
45. Askanazi J, Rosenbaum SHH, Hyman AI, et al. Respiratory changes induced by the large glucose loads of total parenteral nutrition. JAMA 1980; 243:1444–1447.
46. Openbrier DR, Donahoe M, Rogers RM. Eating patterns and factors associated with weight loss in patients with COPD. Am Rev Respir Dis 1989; 139:A134.
47. Openbrier DR, Covey M. Ineffective breathing pattern related to malnutrition. Nurs Clin North Am 1987; 22:225–247.
48. Wilson DO, Rogers RM, Wright EC, et al. Body weight in chronic obstructive pulmonary disease: The National Institutes of Health intermittent positive pressure breathing trial. Am Rev Respir Dis 1989; 139:1435–1438.
49. Centers for Disease Control. Prevalence of overweight—Behavioral risk factor surveillance system, 1987. MMWR 1989; 38:421–423.
50. Foreyt JP. Issues in the assessment and treatment of obesity. J Consult Clin Psychol 1987; 55:677–684.
51. Stunkard AJ, Foch TT, Hrubec Z. A twin study of human obesity. JAMA 1986; 356:51–54.
52. Buckmaster L, Brownell KD. Behavior modification: The state of the art. In: Frankle RT, Yang M (eds). Obesity and Weight Control: The Health Professional's Guide to Understanding and Treatment. Rockville, MD: Aspen Publishers, Inc., 1988, p 228.
53. Owen OE. Obesity. In: Kinney JM, Jeejeebhoy KN, Hill GL, Owen OE (eds). Nutrition and Metabolism in Patient Care. Philadelphia: W.B. Saunders Co., 1988, pp 185–188.
54. Klesges RC. Area review: Smoking and body weight. Ann Behav Med 1989; 11:123–157.
55. Shepherd RW, Cleghorn GJ. Nutritional management. In: Shepherd RW (ed.). Cystic Fibrosis: Nutritional and Intestinal Disorders. Boca Raton, FL: CRC Press, 1989, pp 53–65.
56. Luder E. Nutritional care of patients with cystic fibrosis. Top Clin Nutr 1991; 6:39–50.
57. Corey M, McLaughlin FJ, Williams M, et al. A comparison of survival, growth and pulmonary function in patients with cystic fibrosis in Boston and Toronto. J Clin Epidemiol 1988; 41:583–591.
58. Kinsella JE, Lokesh B. Dietary lipids, eicosanoids, and the immune system. Crit Care Med 1989; 18:S94–S113.
59. Shepherd R, Cooksley WGE, Cooke WDD. Improved growth and clinical, nutritional, and respiratory changes in response to nutritional therapy in cystic fibrosis. J Pediatr 1980; 97:351–357.
60. Levy LD, Durie PR, Pencharz PB, et al. Effects of long-term nutritional rehabilitation on body composition and clinical status in malnourished children and adolescents with cystic fibrosis. J Pediatr 1985; 107: 225–230.
61. O'Loughlin E, Forbes D, Parsons H, et al. Nutritional rehabilitation of malnourished patients with cystic fibrosis. Am J Clin Nutr 1986; 43:732–737.
62. Shepherd RW, Holt TL, Thomas BJ, et al. Nutritional rehabilitation in cystic fibrosis: Controlled studies of effects on nutritional growth retardation, body protein turnover, and course of pulmonary disease. J Pediatr 1986; 109:788–794.
63. Boland MP, Stoski DS, MacDonald NE, et al. Chronic jejunostomy feeding with non-elemental formula in undernourished patients with cystic fibrosis. Lancet 1986; 1:232–234.
64. Soutter VL, Kristidis P, Gruca MA. Chronic undernutrition/growth retardation in CF. Clin Gastroenterol 1986; 15:138–155.
65. Luder E, Kattan M, Thornton JC, et al. Efficacy of a nonrestricted fat diet in patients with cystic fibrosis. Am J Dis Child 1989; 143:458–464.
66. Hubbard VS, Mangrum PJ. Energy intake and nutrition counseling in cystic fibrosis. J Am Diet Assoc 1982; 80:127–131.
67. Daniels LA, Davidson GP. Current issues in the nutritional management of children with cystic fibrosis. Aust Paediatr J 1989; 25:261–266.
68. Fitting J, Frascarolo P, Jequier E, et al. Resting energy expenditure in interstitial lung disease. Am Rev Respir Dis 1990; 142:631–635.
69. Heymans HSA. Gastrointestinal dysfunction and its effects on nutrition in CF. Acta Paediatr Scand Suppl 1989; 363:74–79.
70. Farrell PM. Nutrition in cystic fibrosis. Contemp Nutr 1989; 8:1–2.
71. Maurer JR. Therapeutic challenges following lung transplantation. Clin Chest Med 1990; 11:285–286.
72. Morrison DL, Maurer JR, Grossman RF. Preoperative assessment for lung transplantation. Clin Chest Med 1990; 11:213.

Chapter 26

Psychosocial Issues in the Rehabilitation of Patients with Chronic Obstructive Pulmonary Disease

ROBERT M. KAPLAN, Ph.D.
ELIZABETH G. EAKIN, B.A.
ANDREW L. RIES, M.D.

Patients with chronic obstructive pulmonary disease (COPD) confront significant limitations in the performance of daily activities. These limitations may be associated with important psychosocial problems, including depression and anxiety. Furthermore, the complex regimen suggested by most physicians is sometimes confusing and difficult for patients to follow. In this chapter, some of the psychosocial issues faced by patients with COPD are reviewed, and some suggestions for intervention are offered. All of the psychosocial issues confronting patients with COPD cannot be covered within this chapter. Therefore, problems related to depression and anxiety, issues in social support, and adherence to regimens are emphasized. Some of the methodologic issues relevant to the evaluation of psychosocial interventions for patients with COPD are also described.

Comprehensive pulmonary rehabilitation programs have been developed to provide a multidisciplinary therapeutic program tailored to the needs of the individual patient. As suggested in this volume and elsewhere,[1-3] rehabilitation efforts are well justified. Such programs may comprise several components, including individual assessment, education, instruction in respiratory and chest physiotherapy techniques, elements of psychosocial support that are designed to address the difficult psychologic and emotional problems of COPD patients, and supervised exercise training. The primary goal of pulmonary rehabilitation is to restore the patient to the highest possible level of independent function. Successful programs can help patients to become better educated and more involved in their own care. In addition, patients may experience reduced physical and psychologic symptoms,[4] improved exercise tolerance,[5] fewer hospitalizations and physician visits, and more gainful employment.[6] Pulmonary rehabilitation programs have expanded substantially in the last two decades and are now an accepted form of comprehensive therapy for many patients with COPD. In 1981, the American Thoracic Society recommended standards for pulmonary rehabilitation programs.[7] The scientific basis for pulmonary rehabilitation has recently been reviewed.[8]

The development of an effective rehabilitation program must consider psychosocial issues. Some of these common issues are reviewed in the next section.

COMMON PSYCHOSOCIAL ISSUES AMONG PATIENTS WITH CHRONIC OBSTRUCTIVE PULMONARY DISEASE

Depression

Depression is a common problem for patients with chronic pulmonary disease as well as other chronic diseases. Substantial evidence suggests that individuals with physical disabilities or chronic diseases experience more depression and psychologic distress than do nondisabled populations.[9–11] In a recent meta-analysis of 101 studies, depression was more commonly observed in various disease groups than was any other personality variable.[12] Several studies indicate that the prevalence of depression is higher in patients with COPD than in patients with other medical conditions.[13–17] Both McSweeny and coworkers[15] and Light and associates[16] reported prevalence rates of depression of approximately 42% in patients with moderate to severe COPD.

One explanation for the high levels of depression in patients with COPD is that depression is a psychologic response to the limitation of activities that is common for patients. The gradually deteriorating course of COPD often results in numerous lifestyle changes, including the loss of many activities. Many patients with COPD find themselves avoiding active jobs or discontinuing work altogether. Social activities are curtailed, the ability to walk comfortably with others of the same age is greatly diminished, and in later stages of the disease, even self-care may become too taxing. As a result of disability, patients are no longer able to obtain the reinforcers that make daily life enjoyable.

If this theory is correct, then pulmonary rehabilitation programs that increase functional performance should reduce depression. Unfortunately, few studies of pulmonary rehabilitation have evaluated the effects of increased functioning on depression. Toshima and colleagues[17] randomly assigned 119 patients with COPD to a rehabilitation program or an education control group. The rehabilitation program was designed to enhance physical functioning and the performance of activities of daily living. The education control group received only information without specific instruction in physical activity training. Following the 2-month treatment, there was no significant reduction in depression in either group. Patients were then categorized according to whether they had increased or decreased depression between the initial and post-treatment evaluations. Within the rehabilitation group, those who had a decrease in depression increased their exercise endurance. Within the education group, increase or decrease in depression was unrelated to change in exercise endurance.

In an uncontrolled trial of rehabilitation in COPD, Agle and coworkers[13] reported that those patients who showed significant increases in physical function over the course of the study experienced significant reductions in both depression and anxiety. These two studies can be viewed as partially supporting the theory that depression results from decreased functional ability in patients with COPD.

Because of the high prevalence of depression in COPD, assessment of depression should be a standard part of the patient assessment protocol. Severe levels of depression may interfere with the ability to adhere to complex medical or rehabilitative regimens. Difficulty in concentrating, fatigue, and lack of motivation—all common symptoms of depression—may also make it difficult for patients to benefit from pulmonary rehabilitation programs. In the case of severe depression, it may be necessary to refer the patient to a mental health practitioner prior to beginning pulmonary rehabilitation. The treatment of depression is discussed in Chapter 19.

Anxiety and Dyspnea

Over the past two decades, a number of investigators have reported a high prevalence of anxiety in patients with COPD.[10, 13, 17–20] However, a number of recent studies have reported mixed results. In a sample of 50 outpatients with stable COPD, Karajgi and associates[19] found that 16% had an anxiety disorder. Yellowlees and colleagues[20] reported that of their sample of 50 patients with COPD who were admitted to a respiratory unit, 34% had an anxiety disorder. In contrast, Light and coworkers[16] found that of 45 outpatients with COPD, only 2% had significantly elevated levels of anxiety.

Although the true prevalence of anxiety disorders in COPD is unclear, numerous investigators have described the anxiety and distress that accompany the symptom of breathlessness in COPD. In fact, dyspnea has been described as one of the most common and distressing symptoms of COPD.[10, 21–24] By the time patients seek medical attention, they are frequently caught in a dyspnea-panic cycle.[25, 26] The experience of breathlessness can be extremely distressing and is often accompanied by panic or anxiety. Panic leads to increased dyspnea. Patients begin to give up many activities of daily living for fear of becoming short of breath. Inactivity leads to deconditioning, which increases the likelihood of dyspnea during exertion. This dyspnea-panic cycle often perpetuates to the point where patients are greatly limited in their daily functioning or even completely housebound. Teaching patients to cope with dyspnea and ensuing anxiety is an important focus of pulmonary rehabilitation and is discussed in Chapter 9.

Behavioral interventions may be valuable for helping patients to cope with dyspnea and depression. In addition to depression and anxiety, other behavioral issues may interfere with the achievement of outcomes for patients with COPD. Perhaps the most common behavioral problem concerns adherence to the medical and rehabilitative regimen. Adherence is reviewed in the next section.

ADHERENCE IN THE PATIENT WITH PULMONARY DISEASE

Most medical encounters result in a physician or other health care professional advising a patient to follow a specific regimen. Patients are told to take medication on a specific schedule, to exercise, or to engage in some other routine. Nonadherence occurs when this advice is not followed. It is widely believed that many patients fail to get the optimal benefits of therapy because of nonadherence. In this section, the issue of nonadherence for patients with pulmonary diseases is explored. Some authors prefer the terms "noncompliance," "noncooperation," and "patient resistance." Others prefer the terms "adherence" and "cooperation" to "compliance" because they give more emphasis to the patient's active role in the encounter. In this chapter, the terms "adherence" and "compliance" are used interchangeably.

Most authors agree that patient nonadherence is a common problem. Nonadherence rates vary between 15 and 93%, depending on patient population and the definition of nonadherence.[27, 28] Most estimates suggest that about one third of patients fail to comply with any particular medical regimen.[29, 30] Nonadherence for patients with chronic lung diseases may be higher. Studies that examine nonadherence rates by disease state have consistently shown that chronically ill individuals comply less than do those with acute illnesses.[31, 32]

In considering the adherence problem, it is important to recognize that many factors influence adherence behavior. Some regimens are easy to follow, such as taking only one pill per day. Other treatments may be more complex if, for instance, they involve side effects or frequent dosing schedules (for medications) or lifestyle changes that can be time-consuming and painful. Thus, adherence rates need to be estimated for specific regimens. Although most physicians believe that their patients satisfactorily comply with prescribed treatments, the evidence does not support these beliefs.[33] Physicians typically overestimate the extent to which their patients comply and overstate the extent to which patient behaviors correspond with their orders.[34]

Drugs may be used to relieve airflow obstruction that is caused by inflammation, secretions, and smooth muscle spasm, to treat chronic and acute infections, or to control fluid retention. It is not uncommon for patients with COPD to simultaneously use several types of medications, including bronchodilators, corticosteroids, antibiotics, and diuretics. Dosing schedules are typically complex. In addition, patients with more severe hypoxemia often use supplemental oxygen. Thus, the medical regimen for patients with COPD is often complex and involves a variety of different medications and behavioral changes. Ultimately, the determinants of adherence may be different for each of these varied regimens.

In the next sections, adherence in the areas of exercise and medicine taking is considered.

Adherence to an Exercise Program

An important component of most pulmonary rehabilitation programs is the establishment of a regular exercise regimen. Specific physical conditioning exercises, such as walking, can be undertaken by the patient to help to maintain physical functioning.[6, 35] Improvements in patients with COPD following exercise training have been documented in several studies.[36–41] Specifically, appropriate physical conditioning exercises can improve maximum exercise tolerance and endurance and improve ventilatory and mechanical efficiency for exercise.[6]

There have been few controlled studies evaluating COPD rehabilitation programs or their components. Reports from nonrandomized studies typically suggest that the objectives can be achieved.[36–38] Recently, several controlled trials documented the benefits of exercise programs for patients with COPD. Cockcroft and colleagues[42] randomly assigned 39 patients to a 6-week exercise training program or to a control group that received no treatment. In comparison with the control group, patients in the exercise group experienced subjective benefits and increased the distance they could walk in 12 minutes. However, the length of follow-up was only 2 months. McGavin and coworkers[43] randomly allocated 24 patients with COPD to a 3-month unsupervised stair-climbing home exercise program or to a nonexercise control group. The 12 patients in the exercise group noted subjective improvements, an increased sense of well-being, and decreased breathlessness. They also reported an objective increase in the 12-minute walking distance and maximum level of exercise on a bicycle ergometer. These changes did not occur in the control group. However, the length of follow-up was limited to 3 months. Ambrosino and associates[44] randomly assigned 23 patients to a 1-month medical and rehabilitative therapy group and 28 patients to medical therapy alone (without exercise training). The experimental group improved in exercise tolerance and ventilatory pattern (as evidenced by a decrease in respiratory rate and an increase in tidal volume). Again, these changes were not present in the control group.

Developing exercise programs for patients with COPD is difficult for several reasons. First, principles of training that have been well studied for normal individuals or for cardiac patients do not necessarily apply to patients with COPD.[45] Adherence is often a major problem for the patient with COPD. Some studies suggest that the degree of benefit is related to compliance with the exercise regimen.[46] Although patients can benefit from exercise, the exercise routine is typically not comfortable for them. Many participants in rehabilitation programs have become physically deconditioned over a long period of time. Exertion may be uncomfortable and commonly leads to the frightening symptom of breathlessness (dyspnea). Because of these problems, discontinuation of the exercise regimen is common.

Remarkably few studies have evaluated methods to improve adherence to an exercise regimen. In one experimental trial, patients with COPD underwent exercise testing and were given an exercise prescription.[47] They were then randomly assigned to one of five experimental or control groups. The experimental groups were based on the principles of behavior modification or a variant of behavior modification known as "cognitive behavior modification." These principles involve setting goals, analyzing the reinforcers for walking, and using behavioral contracts. The experimental programs included six weekly sessions in the patient's home. One control group received attention through regular meetings with the staff but did not have the behaviorally based sessions, whereas the other control group received no treatment. After 3 months, greater compliance with the exercise program was observed among the experimental groups in comparison with the two control groups. These changes were reflected in changes in exercise tolerance that were measured 1 month after the treatment. However, there were no significant changes in spirometric parameters.[47]

Adherence to Medical Regimens

Although some aspects of COPD are treatable, the medical regimen is extremely complex. Traditional medical management of patients with COPD relies heavily on pharmacologic intervention. However, treatment regimens may also include additional modalities, such as chest physiotherapy, exercise, and smoking cessation. Most patients are confronted with complex combinations of treatment options.

Despite a large amount of literature on adherence to medical regimens, surprisingly little has been written about adherence in patients with chronic pulmonary disease. We recently reviewed the literature and found only a handful of published studies of this subject.[48] Two comprehensive reviews of the literature published prior to 1980[49, 50] did not identify studies on adherence to medical regimens for patients with COPD. For example, the exhaustive annotated bibliography by Haynes and colleagues[50] does not include a single reference to a study limited to patients with COPD. In order to summarize the literature following the comprehensive 1979 review by Haynes and colleagues,[50] we conducted a computerized literature review dating back to 1980. The search revealed few studies that have directly addressed the issue of adherence with traditional medical regimens for patients with COPD. The studies considered different treatments in diverse samples and employed various definitions and measurements for adherence.

The traditional view of adherence and nonadherence in the literature, in which the patient either strictly follows or fails to follow a treatment recommendation, may no longer be optimal for adherence research in the future. The degree of adherence required for the desired outcome—whether it is adherence to a prescribed regimen or the maximization of the quality of life—varies from treatment to treatment and should be considered. To date, few studies have systematically evaluated adherence to medical treatments for the patient with COPD, and in these few cases, the focus has been on drug and oxygen therapy. In the United Kingdom, for example, James and coworkers[51] reported that only one half of their patients took medicines regularly. We found only one study evaluating interventions to improve adherence for patients with COPD. This report suggested that simple counseling interventions by pharmacists might increase adherence to prescriptions commonly used by patients with COPD.[52]

Patients with COPD with significant hypoxemia may be treated with oxygen. Two important clinical trials demonstrated the benefits of oxygen therapy. In the multicenter Nocturnal Oxygen Therapy Trial sponsored by the National Institutes of Health, hypoxemic patients with COPD were randomly assigned to receive oxygen therapy for either 12 or 24 hours.[53] In the British Medical Research Council study, hypoxemic patients with COPD received either no oxygen or 15 hours of oxygen therapy.[54] Both studies demonstrated a significant reduction in mortality associated with the use of oxygen. Patients receiving continuous oxygen therapy had significantly reduced mortality compared with patients receiving intermittent oxygen therapy (12 or 15 h). The highest mortality rate was seen in patients who received no oxygen. In addition, the group receiving 24-hour oxygen therapy experienced higher scores on general quality of life measures[15] and, after 1 year, on selected tests of cognitive function.[55]

Oxygen is expensive and inconvenient for patients to use. Several types of oxygen therapy systems are now available, including portable units that allow continuous therapy for ambulatory patients. Thus, by using oxygen systems, hypoxemic patients with COPD can remain active and engage in a variety of physical activities and beneficial exercises. Despite these advances, adherence rates remain low. Estimated or measured adherence values do not appear to converge on a specific rate or even a specific pattern.

Alternative methods for oxygen delivery may be useful for increasing compliance with therapy. For example, Heimlich and Carr[56] demonstrated that transtracheal oxygen therapy can increase the number of patients who use therapy 24 hours per day. Using the results of the Nocturnal Oxygen Therapy Trial to estimate the impact of improved adherence on life expectancy suggests that transtracheal oxygen therapy can improve life expectancy because it improves adherence.

Overadherence

Most of the literature on adherence behaviors focuses on the extent to which patients underuse medications. A less common but perhaps equally important problem involves the overuse of medications. Overadherence is a more common problem in those patients who use medications that provide prompt symptomatic relief. In the study by Chryssidis and coworkers,[57] for example, the use of high doses of aerosol therapy often exceeded prescription rates. The mean percentage of prescribed dose actually used was 98.5% at the 1-month follow-up and 110.8% at the 2-month follow-up. Since there was variability for each of these estimates, it appears that some portion of the patients took considerably more medication than was prescribed. It is not surprising that patients suffering from COPD, a highly symptomatic disorder, would overuse a medication that provides rapid symptomatic relief.

Some of the evidence for patient overcompliance comes from innovative studies on the assessment of adherence. For example, in one clinical trial on antihypertensive medications, patients were asked to bring their medications with them to follow-up visits. Adherence rates were remarkably high, sometimes approaching 100%. However, there was considerable variability among subjects, with those at higher adherence levels obtaining better clinical results. Using innovative methods that attach microprocessors to pill blister packs or to the caps of standard pill bottles,[58] it was possible to estimate not only how many of the pills were removed from the packages but also specifically when they were removed. These studies suggested that patients often had lapses in adherence in periods between visits or that medicine taking was erratic. Also, they may have overused medication or engaged in "pill dumping" just prior to a clinic visit. These findings imply that medications may not be used as prescribed. Often, patients overuse medication prior to a clinic visit. This may substantially bias estimates of dose-response in clinical trials as well as provide an inaccurate measure of treatment side effects.[59, 60]

Rational Nonadherence

There are several competing theories about why patients fail to comply with medical regimens (see Becker[28] for review). Explanations for why patients fail to adhere might be divided into three categories: (1) those that focus on the patient, (2) those that focus on the patient's environment, and (3) those that focus on the interaction between the patient and the provider. Patient-oriented explanations suggest that certain personalities fail to adhere to medical treatments or that patients intentionally reject therapy because of some flaw in their personality.[61] These explanations have failed to gain empiric support. There is some evidence that patients misunderstand instructions,[62] but there is relatively little evidence that patients intentionally try to harm themselves by ignoring advice.

Environmental explanations suggest that elements in the patient's environment, such as family variables, reminders, or other environmental stimuli, influence adherence behavior.[63] Evidence for this view of adherence is suggested by studies demonstrating that reminders and simple environmental cues increase adherence.[64] These simple reminders might be notes attached to a refrigerator or electronic devices that beep when a dose of medication is indicated. In one study, it was shown that individual rather than block appointments and simple appointment reminders significantly improved adherence.[66]

The third view of adherence emphasizes the role of the patient-provider relationship. Although the evidence cannot be reviewed in detail here, a substantial amount of literature demonstrates that information exchanged between patients and providers is often poor.[67, 68] This view of adherence suggests that the remedy to the problem is to improve communication between patients and their health care providers.

In considering the three views of noncompliant behavior, we find little evidence that patient personality variables explain much of the variability in nonadherence.[69] The environmental view is valuable in identifying simple manipulations that may enhance adherence behavior in some settings. However, the environmental view is not a comprehensive explanation that considers the patient's role in the choice to use or not use medications. The patient-provider interaction view comes closest to dealing with the realities of the problem. Substantial evidence suggests that patients often do not comprehend instructions offered to them by their providers.[68] Conversely, providers often have an inadequate picture of the responses their patients have to treatment recommendations. In the following sections, this issue is explored in more detail.

In a 1989 paper, Liang[70] offered reasons why his chronically ill patients failed to take their medications. Common explanations were "I forgot" and that the medications were "too expensive," that they made them feel "dopey" or "constipated," and that they "didn't work." Patients often have poor responses to medications, find that the medications are not providing the expected benefit, or cannot afford to purchase the medications. These patients are taking several factors into consideration in their decision to use or not use a product. Although the provider may describe the patient as irrational, the patient may be making what he or she considers to be an informed choice. Kaplan and Simon[69] suggested that patients are more likely to comply with treatment when they perceive a net health benefit from it. Nonadherence occurs when the perceived negative consequences outweigh expected benefits. In this decision process, patients may discount future benefits because of current side effects. A corollary of the theory is that treatments that produce a short-term benefit may evoke better adherence than those that produce a delayed benefit. For example, treatments that provide immediate symptomatic relief, such as inhalers, may be associated with higher adherence than those such as antihypertensive therapies that exchange current inconvenience for future benefit.

One major reason for nonadherence is that patients experience treatment side effects, and, thus, increased medicine use results in increased discomfort.[70, 71] In one study, 36% of patients in a large tertiary care hospital had some iatrogenic disease.[72] Older individuals may experience a seven-fold increase in adverse reactions in comparison to those aged 20 to 29 years.[73] Evidence from the United Kingdom indicates that as many as 10% of admissions to geriatric units result from adverse reactions attributable to drug interactions.[74] Observed nonadherence might reflect patient feedback about bad experiences with the regimen. Although patients may be less direct about their decision not to adhere, observations of nonadherence may be a stimulus for discussion of treatment side effects.

Several authors have argued that nonadherence can be rational.[28] Patients may adhere to a regimen but fail to obtain the desired benefit. If the probability of an expected benefit is low and if there are undesirable side effects, nonadherence may be rational. For example, a patient with streptococcal pharyngitis who discontinues the use of an antibiotic on the 8th day of a 10-day course might be regarded as a noncomplier. However, if the patient decides that the inconvenience and side effects associated with the medication are a greater concern than is the low probability of developing rheumatic fever, the decision may be regarded as rational. Nonadherence might also be regarded as rational when the patient achieves the desired result despite nonadherence. Indeed, studies in many areas do not show a systematic relationship between adherence and health outcome.[64] Many studies in the adherence literature fail to take health outcomes into consideration.

Problems such as poor adherence often benefit from behavioral interventions. Behavior therapy programs may help address depression and anxiety. In the next section, behavioral intervention methods are discussed, and strategies that may be useful in modifying several behaviors for patients with COPD are presented.

BEHAVIORAL INTERVENTIONS

The goal of pulmonary rehabilitation is to return the patient to the highest possible level of independent functioning.[75] Because there is no known cure for COPD, improvement in function depends largely on the patient's taking an active role in his or her rehabilitation. Patients with COPD are asked to make numerous changes in behavior and lifestyle, including the cessation of smoking, the initiation and maintenance of regular exercise, adherence to complex medical regimens, and the use of various techniques to manage the sensation of dyspnea.

This section addresses the many issues involved in assisting patients in making these behavioral changes and describes the application of behavior modification techniques to pulmonary rehabilitation. Behavioral techniques have been successfully applied in the areas of smoking cessation, diet, exercise, medication compliance, and stress reduction. Given that similar behavior changes are required in pulmonary rehabilitation, it seems reasonable to incorporate what we know from each of these areas into the comprehensive care of patients with COPD.

Behavioral techniques—such as clearly defining the target behavior, setting realistic goals, evaluating obstacles, self-monitoring, making use of social support, and self-reward—are discussed in relation to pulmonary rehabilitation. These issues are often not addressed in the traditional approach to working with patients with COPD. Few physicians have been trained in the theory and techniques of behavior change, and many do not have time to address these issues with their patients. The result is that patients are given advice to make numerous changes in behavior without being trained in the skills necessary to follow through on the physicians' advice. What follows is a description of some techniques that can be used to assist patients in making behavior changes.

Defining the Target Behavior

The behavior or behaviors expected of the patient must be clearly defined. The patient should be provided with a detailed plan of action and a list of exactly what it is that he or she is expected to do. This avoids the miscommunication that can occur when patients are given general instructions that they do not know how to follow. For example, it is not sufficient to tell the patient that he or she needs to exercise. The specific exercises need to be defined. The physician must consider many questions. Is the patient to walk? How often? What distance? At what pace? Is there a target heart rate? Should he or she start out slowly and gradually increase the frequency or intensity? If so, how should he or she judge when to increase the pace or distance? Like a prescription, the target behavior or plan of action should be written out for the patient to take home so that he or she can use it as a prompt to engage in the necessary behaviors.

Providing a Rationale for the Behavior Change

It is important for the patient to understand why he or she is being asked to engage in new behaviors (e.g., to take medications, exercise, and practice relaxation). If the patient does not understand why these behaviors are necessary and does not believe that engaging in the behaviors will be beneficial, he or she is unlikely to follow through with them. After providing a rationale, assessing the patient's understanding can be as simple as asking if he or she can explain how engaging in such behaviors is beneficial. Many patients nod their heads in agreement even when they do not understand the rationale for treatment. Having the patient repeat back his or her understanding of the rationale is a means of ensuring that the patient does indeed understand why the treatment is necessary and provides an opportunity to clear up any confusion.

Evaluating Obstacles

This is a crucial step that is often overlooked. It is rare that patients are asked directly if they can foresee problems or obstacles to changing their behavior. This step is critical; if patients are not asked directly, they will not often volunteer that they think they will be unable to follow through with the prescribed changes. Yet, when asked, they can usually identify the things that will make it difficult for them to adhere to the target behaviors.

Medication adherence provides an excellent example, particularly with the COPD population for whom medication schedules are time-consuming and complex. A large body of research has identified astoundingly low rates of medication compliance among these patients (discussed earlier in this chapter). The likelihood of some level of noncompliance combined with patients' ability to identify obstacles to compliance suggests that

TABLE 26–1. SUGGESTIONS FOR HELPING PATIENTS ADHERE TO TREATMENT

Clearly define the target behavior and write it for the patient in "prescription" form.
Provide a rationale for the prescribed regimen and assess the patient's understanding of the rationale.
Evaluate obstacles. Ask the patient if he or she can foresee obstacles that will interfere with adherence and help the patient work around these obstacles.
Evaluate the patient's self-efficacy and provide the necessary referral if he or she lacks the skills necessary to follow the prescribed regimen (e.g., referral to a smoking cessation program, nutritionist, or exercise physiologist).

physicians should work with patients to develop medication schedules to which patients believe they can adhere rather than prescribe a medically optimal schedule with which patients are unlikely to comply.

Common obstacles are confusion due to the complexity of the medication schedules (e.g., when are what medications taken, and how are bronchodilators used), forgetfulness, and unpleasant side effects. Helping the patient to work out and write down a daily schedule of medications (or exercise) and suggesting that he or she wear a watch with an alarm that can be set according to that schedule are simple strategies that can increase the likelihood of adherence. As suggested previously, patient nonadherence may be a stimulus for a discussion of treatment side effects. Taking a few minutes to assist the patient in finding ways to work around obstacles can have a significant effect on the likelihood that the patient will follow through with the prescribed behaviors. Table 26–1 provides a summary of suggestions for helping patients adhere to treatment.

Evaluating Self-Efficacy

Self-efficacy refers to the belief that one has the ability to successfully perform a given behavior. Self-efficacy is an important factor in behavior change because people who feel confident in their ability to change their behaviors are much more likely to be successful in doing so. Patients with COPD are instructed to engage in numerous behaviors (e.g., to stop smoking, start exercising, take daily medications, and relax as a means of reducing the anxiety associated with dyspnea). Yet, they are rarely asked whether they feel they have the ability or skills to successfully follow through with these changes in behavior. The next section delineates four simple skills that can assist patients in making the recommended changes in behavior.

Behavior Change

Changing old behaviors or initiating new ones involves more than a decision to change. Following through with a complex pulmonary rehabilitation regimen is not always a matter of will power. There are a number of specific skills that patients can use to assist them in making the desired behavioral changes. Presented in this way, behavior change revolves around learning and practicing new skills rather than relying on will power. Will power is an amorphous construct over which many people feel they have little control. Changing behaviors via learning, practicing, and perfecting skills implies that the patient can be in control. The following four techniques can be presented to patients as skills that they can use to assist them in making the necessary changes in behavior that are a part of pulmonary rehabilitation.

Goal Setting. When initiating a new and complex behavior, such as an exercise program, it can be helpful to break the behavior into *small*, *realistic*, and *attainable* goals. Being overwhelmed by a goal that seems unattainable may make it difficult for some people to take any steps toward the goal. For example, the goal of walking for 30 minutes twice per day may seem impossible for someone who currently walks 3 minutes at a time. Setting small, attainable goals allows the person to gain confidence (increase self-efficacy) and have a number of experiences with success, thus making it more likely that he or she will continue to work toward the larger goal.

Self-Monitoring. Self-monitoring means having the patient keep track of the number of times that he or she engages in the target behavior. This can be done using a calendar or diary and is a way for the patient to monitor his or her progress. When initiating a new behavior, it is helpful to have the patient keep track not only of the frequency but also of the time and situation in which the behavior was performed. If the patient is having trouble achieving his or her daily goals, the diary or calendar can be used to assess whether there are particular times or situations in which the patient is having difficulty engaging in the behavior.

Self-Reward. One of the most basic principles of behavior theory states that behaviors followed by reinforcement are likely to be repeated. Patients should be encouraged to reward themselves for engaging in the target behaviors. This may be as simple as postponing their morning coffee until after they have completed their walk. For someone who is trying to quit smoking, the reward could be buying something at the end of each week with the money saved by not buying cigarettes. Following a comprehensive program of pulmonary rehabilitation takes a great deal of effort, and patients should be encouraged to feel good about their accomplishments, and reward themselves for them.

Social Support. Social support is an important contributor to patients' ability to cope with chronic illness. Social support entails having a person or network of people to whom the patient can turn for support. Often, this is a spouse who reminds the patient to take his or her medications or encourages the patient to exercise daily or to seek regular medical attention rather than use the emergency room for acute exacerbations. Better Breathers Clubs of the American Lung Association may also provide a source of support for the patient. Patients should be encouraged to find a person or group of people who can support them in coping with their illness and in following through with their pulmonary rehabilitation program. In the next section, we will explore the potential of social support in greater detail.

SOCIAL SUPPORT

A growing body of data suggests that social support may be an important determinant of health outcomes for adults with chronic illnesses. In this section, the relationship between social support and health outcomes in COPD is considered. The epidemiologic data linking social support to mortality are also briefly reviewed.

Most epidemiologic studies were started some years before formal measures of social support had been developed. Nevertheless, simple measures of social network appeared to be predictive of health outcomes in a variety of studies. The Alameda County Population Monitoring Study demonstrated that a simple measure of social network was a significant predictor of longevity. The measure included marital status, the number of close family members and friends, church membership, and group affiliation. Men with weak social networks were nearly 2.5 times as likely to die within a defined time period than were men with extensive networks. Women benefited even more from established social networks.[76]

Similar results were obtained in Tecumseh, Michigan, where 2754 men and women were studied. In this investigation, men who were married, attended church, and participated in voluntary organizations and community activities were significantly less likely to die within a 10-year period than were men who were without such social connections. The Tecumseh Study did not show similar relationships for women.[77] In contrast to the findings of Berkman and Breslow[77] and of the Durham County (North Carolina) Study,[78] no consistent pattern of increased mortality rates was associated with a progressive decrease in social support. Rather, there appears to be a threshold effect in which only those individuals, either male or female, who were at the extreme end of the continuum in terms of the least amount of social support had increased mortality rates. In the Evans County (Georgia) Study,[79] similar findings to those of the Durham County Study were reported. The relationship between social support and mortality did not suggest a gradient of risk. Rather, those individuals with the fewest ties were at increased risk for mortality. The findings reported were significant for older white males only, and the trends for black individuals and for white females, although in the expected direction, were weak and nonsignificant. In the Honolulu Heart Study, social support was not related to mortality or the incidence of cardiovascular disease.[80]

The Functional Effects of Social Support

It is typically assumed that social support has positive effects for chronically ill patients. However, social relationships may have different functions for the chronically ill than they have for other members of the population. This may occur when a support-giver, out of empathy or concern, reinforces a behavior that is incompatible with optimal health outcomes. For example, patients with COPD need to comply with regimens that are difficult, painful, or burdensome. A caring and empathetic support-giver may reinforce comfortable but noncompliant behaviors. Immediate comfort may be emphasized over the long-term consequences of noncompliance. This is most likely to occur when the support-giver believes that any suffering should be avoided. For example, if the spouse of a male COPD patient believes that exercise is harmful, she may discourage activity. This may occur because of inadequate information about the condition or as a result of enduring beliefs. We conceptualize these as functional effects of social support. Functional effects may have a positive influence on health outcomes if the support-giver reinforces appropriate health behaviors. In cases in which support-givers reinforce maladaptive health behaviors, functional effects may have a negative influence. We feel it is important to make the distinction between a "positive-functional-effects" model and a "negative-functional-effects" model. Although there are few studies of social support and health outcomes in COPD, studies of patients with chronic heart disease are instructive.

Negative Functional Effects. Several studies have provided support for the negative-functional-effects model, which suggests that the involvement of supportive but overconcerned family members may lead to poorer health outcomes. In one study, congestive heart failure patients who were not working 3, 6, or 9 months after hospitalization were reported to have more overprotective families than those patients who resumed work during the same time periods.[81] Garrity[82] studied first-time myocardial infarction patients and found that the more concerned the patient's family, the fewer hours the patient worked at his or her job, regardless of the severity of the heart attack. These findings suggest that the patients' families, although concerned, interfered with the recovery. Furthermore, the actions of family members may actually harm patients by not allowing them to exercise and strengthen their cardiac muscle tissue. Presumably, the family members are supportive and want to see recovery. However, their personal beliefs about the frailty of the patient may lead to the reinforcement of sedentary behaviors.

Positive Functional Effects. Positive social influences have also been documented. Significant others in the support environment may encourage adherence to the medical regimen and the adoption of appropriate health behaviors. A related positive functional effect is achieved through modeling. Members of the support environment may model appropriate coping skills as well as health behaviors.[83] Thus, if a network member makes these changes at the same time, outcomes may be enhanced through mutual encouragement, mutual modeling, and a reduction in the perceived difficulty of making changes. Another mechanism accounting for the benefits of social support is the *stress buffering channel*. That is, adaptation may be facilitated by having network members absorb some of the stress.

TABLE 26-2. SUGGESTIONS FOR USING SOCIAL SUPPORT

Discuss with the patient the importance of social support in coping with COPD.
Assess whether the patient feels that he or she has adequate social support and whether the support is positive or negative.
Refer the patient to a local chronic illness support group or a Better Breathers Club (American Lung Association).

Some studies have confirmed the positive-functional-effects model of a social support network. An intervention study with hypertensive patients[84] found that lectures alone did little to help patients control blood pressure. However, lectures in conjunction with social support and encouragement were significantly more effective. Social support has also been found to aid in the maintenance of desirable health behaviors (e.g., weight loss) in post–myocardial-infarction patients.[85] In addition, dropout rates from coronary heart disease rehabilitation and intervention programs were also shown to be correlated with the amount of perceived social support in female hypertensive patients.[86] Thus, perceived social support may prevent or reduce attrition in such programs.

Miller and coworkers[87] examined specific prescriptive factors (diet, medication, exercise, smoking cessation, and other lifestyle changes) that lead to optimal health functioning in post–myocardial-infarction patients. They found that adherence to medical regimens after recovery from an initial myocardial infarction is generally low but varies according to the prescription component. Those behaviors requiring minimal lifestyle changes, such as taking medication, were more readily adopted. Conversely, there was poorer compliance with prescriptions involving more intense lifestyle alterations, such as a challenging regular exercise program. Of particular interest was the finding that attitudes and perceived beliefs of significant others toward the prescriptive components were strong correlates of actual regimen adherence. These findings parallel those found in the diabetes compliance literature.

In summary, social support may be an important variable in adaptation to chronic disease.[85, 88] However, to date, few empiric studies have addressed the contribution of overconcerned spouses and family members in the reinforcement of maladaptive or inappropriate behaviors that ultimately lead to decreased health outcomes. Furthermore, there have been very few studies of social support interventions for patients with COPD. Although social support is a part of many established rehabilitation programs, there is little current evidence to suggest that this component of the program is helpful. Future evaluations of social interventions in COPD are encouraged. Table 26-2 provides a summary of suggestions for using social support to help patients with COPD.

METHODOLOGIC ISSUES IN THE EVALUATION OF PSYCHOSOCIAL INTERVENTIONS

Although this chapter focuses on psychosocial interventions, we also need to consider methods for evaluating outcomes in intervention studies. Since rehabilitation programs are designed to enhance functioning and quality of life, the definition and quantification of these outcomes become an important focus. A wide variety of measures has been used to evaluate health-related quality of life for patients with COPD or related pulmonary diseases. We conducted a Medline search and requested papers on quality of life and COPD published between 1983 and 1991. The search identified 18 papers. Among these papers, two were literature reviews that did not include original data. Three papers did not specifically identify the quality of life measure that they used. In one case, the paper simply said that quality of life is commonly measured and that there is a growing interest in this field. The methods section of this paper noted that a questionnaire including nine quality of life items was administered.[89] Another paper measured quality of life using linear analog scales. Nine of the scales concerned performance problems, whereas two assessed the side effects of chemotherapy.[90] A third paper suggested that corticosteroids may improve quality of life for patients with COPD; however, no quality of life measure was used.

Outcome Measures

The measure that has been used most frequently for patients with chronic respiratory diseases is the Chronic Respiratory Questionnaire (CRQ) developed by Guyatt and colleagues.[91] This questionnaire evaluates four aspects of quality of life for patients with lung diseases: dyspnea, fatigue, emotional function, and mastery. The final version of the questionnaire includes 20 items and can be administered in between 15 and 25 minutes. In one study, it was demonstrated that the questionnaire was responsive to change for 13 patients participating in a drug treatment protocol and 28 patients participating in a respiratory rehabilitation program. In both of these studies, changes on the questionnaire correlated with changes in spirometric values, exercise performance, and subjective ratings of improvement of both the patients and physicians.[91] In another study, the questionnaire was demonstrated to be sensitive to bronchodilator treatment.[92] Guyatt and colleagues[93] also administered the CRQ in a pretest/post-test study on the effects of bronchodilators. At the time of the post-test, one half of the patients were shown their previous responses. When patients were given information about their previous responses, changes in CRQ scores for dyspnea and fatigue were more strongly correlated with changes in spirometry, exercise performance, and subjective ratings of improvement than they were for patients who had not been given the information. Guyatt and colleagues believe this finding supports giving patients feedback on their previous responses. In a fourth study, Jaeschke and associates[94] evaluated changes in CRQ scores against changes in global ratings of change. Using global rating change as the criterion, they attempted to establish a clinically important difference.

Although the CRQ has attracted attention, we also

have some concerns about its application. For example, the CRQ is a point-in-time measure. It does not measure change. Instead, it depends on subjective judgments of change, which are highly susceptible to expectancy effects. The second issue is the meaning of CRQ scores. The CRQ is not scaled against a meaningful unit that places scores into perspective. The study of Jaeschke and associates[94] did attempt to define minimal clinically important differences, but these differences were unrelated to other clinical outcome assessments. The CRQ cannot be used in cost utility studies, nor can it be used for comparisons across these conditions.

Another commonly used health-related quality of life measure is the Sickness Impact Profile (SIP).[95] The SIP is a measure that describes physical and psychosocial impacts of illness. It has been used in at least four studies involving COPD patients. In the Nocturnal Oxygen Therapy Trial, the SIP was administered to 203 patients with COPD and to 73 healthy controls. In comparison with the controls, COPD patients were significantly more impaired on every scale except that for employment.[15] In another study of 985 patients with mild hypoxemia and COPD, most SIP scores indicated significant impairment with the exception of body movement and eating.[96] A British version of the SIP, the Functional Limitation Profile, was used in an evaluation by Williams and Bury.[97]

Considering the studies on functional outcomes, we observed several common themes. First, several studies have observed low correlations between measures of health outcome and measures of lung functioning. For example, Williams and Bury[97] reported that only 14% of the variance in patient functioning could be explained by lung function. However, the correlation between functioning and dypsnea was substantial. Schrier and colleagues[98] found no correlation between lung function tests and SIP scores. However, they did observe substantial correlations between the symptoms of wheezing and dyspnea and SIP scores. These findings are important because they help clarify the appropriate outcomes for behavioral intervention studies. Medical interventions work through physiologic mediators to improve patient functioning and quality of life. However, a treatment might be considered a failure if it improved lung functioning but had no effect on patient functioning and quality of life. Conversely, psychosocial intervention might have little direct impact on physical measures, such as forced expiratory volume in 1 second, but may be successful in directly improving patient health status as measured by quality of life and functional assessments. In the next section, an approach to the measurement of patient outcomes that quantifies the impact of any treatment (medical, surgical, or psychosocial) in a common unit is considered. In addition, the measure can be used for cost effectiveness comparisons among psychosocial and other interventions.

Evaluating Cost-Effectiveness

Within the last few years, there has been growing interest in using quality of life data to help evaluate the cost-utility or cost-effectiveness of health care programs. Cost studies have gained in popularity because health care costs have grown rapidly. Not all health care interventions are equally efficient in returning benefit for the expended dollar. Objective cost studies might guide policymakers toward an optimal and equitable distribution of scarce resources. Cost-effectiveness analysis typically quantifies the benefits of a health care intervention in terms of years of life or Quality-Adjusted Life Years (QALYs). Cost-utility is a special use of cost effectiveness that weights observable health states by preferences or utility judgments of quality.[99] In cost-utility analysis, the benefits of medical care, behavioral interventions, or preventive programs are expressed in terms of "well-years." These outcomes have also been described as QALYs,[100] discounted life years,[101] or healthy years of life.[102] Since measurement in terms of QALYs has become most popular, it is used in this chapter. QALYs integrate mortality and morbidity to express health status in terms of equivalents of well-years of life.

If an adult dies of COPD at age 60 years, but it was expected that he or she would live to age 75 years, it might be concluded that the disease was associated with 15 lost life years. If 100 adults died at age 60 years (and they also had a life expectancy of 75 years), we might conclude that 1500 (100 adults × 15 yr) life years had been lost. Yet, death is rarely the outcome of concern in COPD. Many adults may suffer from conditions like COPD that leave them somewhat disabled over long periods of time. Because of respiratory problems, the quality of their lives has diminished. QALYs take into consideration the quality of life consequences of these illnesses. For example, a disease that reduces quality of life by one half takes away 0.5 QALY over the course of each year. If it affects two people, it will take away 1.0 years (equal to 2 × 0.5) over each year period. A medical treatment that improves quality of life by 0.2 for each of five individuals results in the equivalent of 1 QALY if the benefit is maintained over a 1-year period. This system has the advantage of considering both benefits and side effects of programs in terms of the common QALY units. One of the major issues in the proposed studies is the assessment of toxic effects of new treatments for COPD. The general measurement system is capable of quantifying the side effects. Furthermore, it can be used to evaluate the relative importance of side effects so that a net assessment of the treatment can subtract the side effects from the benefits.

Although there are several different approaches for obtaining quality-adjusted life years, most of them are similar.[103] The approach that our group prefers involves several steps. First, patients are classified according to objective levels of functioning. These levels are represented by scales of mobility, physical activity, and social activity. The dimensions and steps for these levels of functioning are shown in Table 26–3. The reader is cautioned that these steps are not actually the scale, but rather only listings of labels representing the scale's steps. Standardized questionnaires have been developed to classify individuals into one of each of these scale

TABLE 26–3. QUALITY OF WELL-BEING/GENERAL HEALTH POLICY MODEL: ELEMENTS AND FORMULAS (FUNCTION SCALES, STEP DEFINITIONS, AND CALCULATING WEIGHTS)

Step No.	Step Definition	Weight
	Mobility Scale (MOB)	
5	No limitations for health reasons	−.000
4	Did not drive a car, health-related; did not ride in a car as usual for age (younger than 15 yr), health-related, *and/or* did not use public transportation, health-related; *or* had or would have used more help than usual for age to use public transportation, health-related	−.062
2	In hospital, health-related	−.090
	Physical Activity Scale (PAC)	
4	No limitations for health reasons	−.000
3	In wheelchair, moved or controlled movement of wheelchair without help from someone else; *or* had trouble or did not try to lift, stoop, bend over, or use stairs or inclines, health-related; *and/or* limped, used a cane, crutches, or walker, health-related; *and/or* had any other physical limitations in walking, or did not try to walk as far as or as fast as others the same age are able, health-related	−.060
1	In wheelchair, did not move or control the movement of wheelchair without help from someone else, *or* in bed, chair, or couch for most or all of the day, health-related	−.077
	Social Activity Scale (SAC)	
5	No limitations for health reasons	−.000
4	Limited in other (e.g., recreational) role activity, health-related	−.061
3	Limited in major (primary) role activity, health-related	−.061
2	Performed no major role activity, health-related, but did perform self-care activities	−.106
1	Performed no major role activity, health-related, *and* did not perform or had more help than usual in performance of one or more self-care activities, health-related	−.106

Calculating Formulas

Formula 1. Point-in-time well-being score for an individual (W):
$$W = 1 + (CPXwt) + (MOBwt) + (PACwt) + (SACwt)$$
where "wt" is the preference-weighted measure for each factor, and CPX is the Symptom/Problem complex. For example, the W score for a person with the following description profile may be calculated for 1 day as:

CPX = 11	Cough, wheezing, or shortness of breath, with or without fever, chills, or aching all over body	−.257
MOB = 5	No limitations	−.000
PAC = 1	In bed, chair, or couch for most or all of the day, health-related	−.077
SAC = 2	Performed no major role activity, health-related, but did perform self-care	−.061

$$W = 1 + (-.257) + (-.000) + (-.077) + (-.061) = .605$$

Formula 2. Well-years (WY) as an output measure:
$$WY = \text{No. of persons} \times (CPXwt + MOBwt + PACwt + SACwt) \times Time$$

---

steps.[104, 105] In addition to classification into these observable levels of function, individuals are also classified by the one symptom or problem that bothered them most (see Table 26–2). About one half of the population reports at least one symptom on any day. Symptoms may be severe (e.g., serious chest pain) or minor (e.g., the inconvenience of taking medication or a prescribed diet for health reasons). The functional classification (see Table 26–3) and the accompanying list of symptoms or problems (Table 26–4) were created after extensive reviews of the medical and public health literature.[99] Over the last decade, the function classification system and symptom list were repeatedly shortened until we arrived at the current versions. Various methodologic studies on the questionnaire have been conducted.[105–107] With structured questionnaires, an interviewer can obtain classifications on these dimensions in 11 to 16 minutes.

When observable behavioral levels of functioning have been classified, a second step is required to place each individual on the 0 to 1.0 scale of wellness. To accomplish this, the observable health states are weighted by "quality" ratings of their desirability. Human value studies have been conducted to place the observable states onto a preference continuum that has an anchor of 0 for death and a rating of 1.0 for completely well. In several studies, random samples of citizens from a metropolitan community evaluated the desirability of over 400 case descriptions. Using their ratings, a preference structure that assigned the weights to each combination of an observable state and a symptom or problem has been developed.[108] Cross-validation studies have shown that the model can be used to assign weights to other states of functioning with a high degree of accuracy ($R^2 = .96$). The regression weights obtained in these studies are given in Tables 26–1 and 26–2. Studies have shown that the weights are highly stable over a 1-year period and that they are consistent across diverse groups of raters.[108] Finally, it is necessary to consider the duration of stay in various health states.

TABLE 26–4. QUALITY OF WELL-BEING/GENERAL HEALTH POLICY MODEL: SYMPTOM/PROBLEM COMPLEXES (CPX) WITH CALCULATING WEIGHTS

CPX No.	CPX Description	Weight
1	Death (not on respondent's card)	−.727
2	Loss of consciousness such as seizure (fits), fainting, or coma (out cold or knocked out)	−.407
3	Burn over large areas of face, body, arms, or legs	−.387
4	Pain, bleeding, itching, or discharge (drainage) from sexual organs (does not include normal menstrual [monthly] bleeding)	−.349
5	Trouble learning, remembering, or thinking clearly	−.340
6	Any combination of one or more hands, feet, arms, or legs either missing, deformed (crooked), paralyzed (unable to move), or broken (includes wearing artificial limbs or braces)	−.333
7	Pain, stiffness, weakness, numbness, or other discomfort in chest, stomach (including hernia or rupture), side, neck, back, hips, or any joints or hands, feet, arms, or legs	−.299
8	Pain, burning, bleeding, itching, or other difficulty with rectum, bowel movements, or urination (passing water)	−.292
9	Sick or upset stomach, vomiting, or loose bowel movement, with or without chills, or aching all over	−.290
10	General tiredness, weakness, or weight loss	−.259
11	Cough, wheezing, or shortness of breath, with or without fever, chills, or aching all over	−.257
12	Spells of feeling upset, depression, or crying	−.257
13	Headache, dizziness, or ringing in ears, or spells of feeling hot, nervous, or shaky	−.244
14	Burning or itching rash on large areas of face, body, arms, or legs	−.240
15	Trouble talking, such as lisp, stuttering, hoarseness, or being unable to speak	−.237
16	Pain or discomfort in one or both eyes (such as burning or itching) or any trouble seeing after correction	−.230
17	Overweight for age and height or skin defect of face, body, arms, or legs, such as scars, pimples, warts, bruises, or change in color	−.188
18	Pain in ear, tooth, jaw, throat, lips, tongue; several missing or crooked permanent teeth (includes wearing bridges or false teeth); stuffy, runny nose; or any trouble hearing (includes wearing a hearing aid)	−.170
19	Taking medication or staying on a prescribed diet for health reasons	−.144
20	Wearing eyeglasses or contact lenses	−.101
21	Breathing smog or unpleasant air	−.101
22	No symptoms or problems (not on respondent's card)	−.000
23	Standard symptom/problem	−.257
X24	Trouble sleeping	−.257
X25	Intoxication	−.257
X26	Problems with sexual interest or performance	−.257
X27	Excessive worry or anxiety	−.257

For example, 1 year in a state that has been assigned the weight of 0.5 is equivalent to 0.5 QALY. Table 26–1 provides an illustrative example of a calculation. Both reliability[107, 108] and validity studies[109] have been published.

The *well-life expectancy* is the current life expectancy adjusted for diminished quality of life that is associated with dysfunctional states and the duration of stay in each state. Using the system, it is possible to simultaneously consider mortality, morbidity, and the preference weights for these observable behavioral states of function. When the proper steps have been followed, the model quantifies the health activity or treatment program in terms of the QALYs that it produces or saves. A QALY is defined conceptually as the equivalent of a completely well year of life or a year of life free of any symptoms, problems, or health-related disabilities.

The Quality of Well-being (QWB) system is currently in use in several multisite clinical trials. It was demonstrated to be sensitive to minor changes in health status in the multicenter clinical trial of auranofin (oral gold) for patients with rheumatoid arthritis.[110] Among many clinical trials currently using the QWB system are the 15-center Modification of Diet in Renal Disease (MDRD), trials evaluating the benefits of exercise in patients with noninsulin-dependent diabetes mellitus,[111] and a trial of exercise in cystic fibrosis.[112, 113] The measure has also been used in clinical trials evaluating azidothymidine for men infected with the human immunodeficiency virus,[114] and specific validity data are available for infected patients with this virus. The National Center for Health Statistics is currently analyzing QWB scores for several years of the National Health Interview Survey and the Health and Nutrition Examination Survey (HANES).[115] These data will allow the comparison of representative samples.

Studies using the QWB system suggest that psychosocial interventions may produce benefits for COPD patients at a cost comparable to that of many widely advocated programs.[116] We encourage the performance of more cost-utility studies in the future.

SUMMARY

Psychosocial problems—including anxiety, depression, and limitations in functioning—are common for patients with COPD. One goal of rehabilitation is to provide remedies for these psychosocial problems. Some aspects of dysfunction for COPD patients may be remediated through participation in exercise and greater compliance with medications. Evidence suggests that behavioral intervention programs may be useful for increasing adherence to an exercise protocol and for facilitating appropriate medication use.

A review of the literature suggests that there are very few systematic studies evaluating behavioral interventions for patients with COPD. Furthermore, problems such as adherence to the COPD regimen may be poorly understood. For example, many patients may fail to adhere because they are experiencing undesirable side effects of their medications. Patient resistance may be regarded as rational from the patient's perspective. Other studies suggest that patients with COPD may overadhere to certain medical regimens.

The behavioral intervention components of rehabilitation programs may help remediate the problems of anxiety and depression. Social support may also be an essential ingredient of a successful rehabilitation program. Substantial evidence relates social support to health outcomes for patients with other chronic diseases. However, we know very little about the role of social relationships for patients with COPD. More research is needed to clarify this issue.

Finally, it is important to emphasize that psychosocial interventions can be evaluated using general health outcome measures. The ultimate goal of medical, surgical, and psychosocial interventions is to permit patients to live longer and to improve their health-related quality of life. Methods to quantify these outcomes are currently available. These methods can also be used to compare the cost-effectiveness of rehabilitation with that of other health care services.

REFERENCES

1. American Thoracic Society. Standards for the diagnosis and care of patients with chronic obstructive pulmonary disease (COPD) and asthma. Am Rev Respir Dis 1987; 136:225.
2. Hodgkin JE. Pulmonary rehabilitation: Structure, components, and benefits. J Cardiopulmon Rehabil 1988; 11:423.
3. Hodgkin JE, Zorn EG, Connors GL (eds). Pulmonary Rehabilitation: Guidelines to Success. Boston: Butterworth's, 1984.
4. Guyatt GH, Berman LB, Townsend M. Long-term outcome after respiratory rehabilitation. Can Med Assoc J 1987; 137:1089.
5. Petty TL, Nett LM, Finigan MM, et al. A comprehensive care program for chronic airway obstruction: Methods and preliminary evaluation of symptomatic and functional improvement. Ann Intern Med 1969; 70:1109.
6. Belman MJ. Exercise in chronic obstructive pulmonary disease. Clin Chest Med 1986; 7:585.
7. American Thoracic Society. Pulmonary rehabilitation. Am Rev Respir Dis 1981; 124:663.
8. Ries AL. Position paper of the American Association of Cardiovascular and Pulmonary Rehabilitation: Scientific basis of pulmonary rehabilitation. J Cardiopulmon Rehabil 1990; 10:418–441.
9. Murrell SA, Himmelfarb S, Wright K. Prevalence of depression and its correlates in older adults. Am J Epidemiol 1983; 117:173–185.
10. Gift AG, Plaut SM, Jacox A. Psychologic and physiologic factors related to dyspnea in subjects with chronic obstructive pulmonary disease. Heart Lung 1986; 15:595–601.
11. Schwab JJ, Traven ND, Warheit GJ. Relationships between physical and mental illness. Psychosomatics 1978; 19:458–463.
12. Friedman HS, Booth-Kewley S. The "disease-prone personality": A meta-analytic view of the construct. Am Psychol 1987; 42:539–555.
13. Agle DP, Baum GL, Chester EH, Wendt M. Multidiscipline treatment of chronic pulmonary insufficiency: 1. Psychologic aspects of rehabilitation. Psychosom Med 1973; 35:41–49.
14. Dudley DL, Glaser EM, Jorgenson BN, Logan DL. Psychosocial concomitants to rehabilitation in chronic obstructive pulmonary disease. Part I: Psychosocial and psychological considerations. Chest 1980; 77:413–420.
15. McSweeny AJ, Grant I, Heaton RK, et al. Life quality of patients with chronic obstructive pulmonary disease. Arch Intern Med 1982; 142:473–478.
16. Light RW, Merrill EJ, Despars JA, et al. Prevalence of depression and anxiety in patients with COPD: Relationship to functional capacity. Chest 1985; 87:35–38.
17. Toshima MT, Kaplan RM, Ries AL. Experimental evaluation of rehabilitation in chronic obstructive pulmonary disease. Health Psychol 1990; 9:237–252.
18. Hodgkin JE. Prognosis in chronic obstructive pulmonary disease. Clin Chest Med 1990; 11:555–569.
19. Karajgi B, Rifkin A, Doddi S, Kolli R. The prevalence of anxiety disorders in patients with chronic obstructive pulmonary disease. Am J Psychiatry 1990; 147:200–201.
20. Yellowlees PM, Alpers JH, Bowden JJ, et al. Psychiatric morbidity in patients with chronic airflow obstruction. Med J Aust 1987; 146:305–307.
21. Dudley DL, Martin CJ, Holmes TH. Dyspnea: Psychologic and physiologic observations. J Psychosom Med 1968; 11:325–339.
22. Kinsman RA, Yaroush RA, Fernandez RA, et al. Symptoms and experiences in chronic bronchitis and emphysema. Chest 1983; 5:755–761.
23. Rosser R, Denford J, Heslop A, et al. Breathlessness and psychiatric morbidity in chronic bronchitis and emphysema: A study of psychotherapeutic management. Psychol Med 1983; 13:93–110.
24. Renfroe KL. Effect of progressive relaxation on dyspnea and state anxiety in patients with chronic obstructive pulmonary disease. Heart Lung 1988; 17:408–413.
25. Hoffman LA, Berg J, Rogers RM. Daily living with COPD: Self-help skills to improve functional ability. Postgrad Med 1989; 86:153–166.
26. Kaplan RM, Atkins CJ. Behavioral interventions for patients with COPD. In: McSweeny AJ, Grant I (eds). Chronic Obstructive Pulmonary Disease: A Behavioral Perspective. New York: Marcel Dekker, Inc., 1985.
27. Becker MH, Maiman LA. Strategies for enhancing patient compliance. J Community Health 1980; 6:113.
28. Becker MH. Patient adherence to prescribed therapies. Med Care 1985; 23:539.
29. Blackwell B. Patient compliance. N Engl J Med 1973; 289:249.
30. Gates SJ, Colborn DK. Lowering appointment failures in a neighborhood health center. Med Care 1976; 14:263.
31. Sackett DL. A compliance practicum for the busy practitioner. In: Haynes RB, Taylor DW, Sackett DL (eds). Compliance in Health Care. Baltimore: The Johns Hopkins Press, 1979.
32. Sackett DL, Snow JC. The magnitude and measurement of compliance. In: Haynes RB, Taylor DW, Sackett DL (eds). Compliance in Health Care. Baltimore: The Johns Hopkins Press, 1979.
33. Caron HS, Roth HP. Objective assessment of cooperation with an ulcer diet: Relation to antacid intake and to assigned physician. Am J Med Sci 1971; 261:61.
34. Norell SE. Accuracy of patient interviews and estimates by clinical staff determining medication compliance. Soc Sci Med 1981; 15:57.
35. Bell CW, Jensen RH. Physical conditioning. In: Jensen RH, Kass I (eds). Pulmonary Rehabilitation Home Programs. Omaha: University of Nebraska Medical Center, 1977.
36. Unger K, Moser K, Hansen P. Selection of an exercise program for patients with chronic obstructive pulmonary disease. Heart Lung 1980; 9:68.
37. Moser KM, Bokinsky GE, Savage RT, et al. Results of a comprehensive rehabilitation program: Physiologic and func-

tional effects on patients with chronic obstructive pulmonary disease. Arch Intern Med 1980; 140:1596.
38. Bass H, Whitcomb JF, Forman R. Exercise training: Therapy for patients with chronic obstructive pulmonary disease. Chest 1970; 57:116.
39. Fishmen DB, Petty TL. Physical, symptomatic and psychological improvement in patients receiving comprehensive care for chronic airway obstruction. J Chron Dis 1971; 24:775.
40. Pierce AK, Paez PN, Miller WF. Exercise training with the aid of a portable oxygen supply in patients with emphysema. Am Rev Respir Dis 1965; 91:653.
41. Shephard RJ. On the design and effectiveness of training regimens in chronic obstructive lung disease. Bull Eur Physiopathol Respir 1977; 13:457.
42. Cockcroft AE, Saunders MT, Berry G. Randomized controlled trial of rehabilitation in chronic respiratory disability. Thorax 1981; 36:200.
43. McGavin CR, Gupta SP, Lloyd EL, McHardy JR. Physical rehabilitation of chronic bronchitis: Results of a controlled trial of exercises in the home. Thorax 1977; 32:307.
44. Ambrosino N, Paggiaro PL, Macchi M, et al. A study of short-term effect of rehabilitative therapy in chronic obstructive pulmonary disease. Respiration 1981; 41:40.
45. Belman MJ, Wasserman K. Exercise training and testing in patients with chronic obstructive pulmonary disease. Basics RD 1981; 10:1.
46. Mertens DJ, Shephard RJ, Kavanagh T. Long-term exercise therapy for chronic obstructive lung disease. Respiration 1978; 35:96.
47. Atkins CJ, Kaplan RM, Timms RM, et al. Behavioral programs for exercise compliance in COPD. J Consult Clin Psychol 1984; 52:591.
48. Kaplan RM, Toshima MT, Atkins CJ, Ries AL. Adherence to prescribed regimens for patients with chronic obstructive pulmonary disease. In: Shumaker SA, Schron EB, Ockene JK (eds). The Handbook of Health Behavior Change. New York: Springer Publishing Co., Inc., 1990, pp 126–143.
49. Atkins CJ. A randomized clinical trial comparing cognitive and behavioral strategies for exercise compliance among chronic obstructive pulmonary disease patients. Riverside, CA: University of California, 1981; Doctoral dissertation.
50. Haynes RB, Taylor DW, Sackett DL. Compliance in Health Care. Baltimore: The Johns Hopkins Press, 1979.
51. James PNE, Anderson JB, Priar JG, et al. Patterns of drug taking in patients with chronic airflow obstruction. Postgrad Med J 1985; 61:7.
52. DeTullio PL, Kirkling DM, Arslanian C, Olson DE. Compliance measure development and assessment of theophylline therapy in ambulatory patients. J Clin Pharm Ther 1987; 12:19.
53. Nocturnal Oxygen Therapy Trial Group. Continuous or nocturnal oxygen therapy in hypoxemic chronic obstructive lung disease: A clinical trial. Ann Intern Med 1980; 93:391.
54. Medical Research Council Working Party. Long term domiciliary oxygen therapy in chronic hypoxic cor pulmonale complicating chronic bronchitis and emphysema. Lancet 1981; 1:681–686.
55. Heaton RK, Grant I, McSweeney AJ, et al. Psychologic effects of continuous and nocturnal oxygen therapy in hypoxemic chronic obstructive pulmonary disease. Arch Intern Med 1983; 143:1941.
56. Heimlich HJ, Carr GC. The micro-trach: A seven-year experience with transtracheal oxygen therapy. Chest 1989; 95:1008.
57. Chryssidis E, Frewin DB, Frith PA, Dawes ER. Compliance with aerosol therapy in chronic obstructive lung disease. N Z Med J 1981; 94:375.
58. Cramer JA, Mattson RH, Prevey ML, et al. How often is medication taken as prescribed? A novel assessment technique. JAMA 1989; 261:3273.
59. Rudd P, Byyny RL, Zachary V, et al. Pill count measures of compliance in a drug trial: Variability and suitability. Am J Hypertens 1988; 3:309.
60. Rudd P, Byyny RL, Zachary V, et al. The natural history of medication compliance in a drug trial: Limitations of pill counts. J Clin Pharm Ther 1989; 46:176.
61. Appelbaum SA. The refusal to take one's medicine. Bull Menninger Clin 1977; 41:511.
62. Stone GC. Patient compliance and the role of the expert. J Soc Issues 1979; 35:34.
63. Corish CD, Richard B, Brown S. Missed medication doses in rheumatoid arthritis patients: Intentional and unintentional reasons. Arthritis Care Res 1989; 2:3.
64. Agras WS. Understanding compliance with the medical regimen: The scope of the problem and a theoretical perspective. Arthritis Care Res 1989; 2:S2
65. Stamler R, Stamler J, Civinelli J, et al. Adherence and blood pressure response to hypertension treatment. Lancet 1975; 2:1227.
66. Finnegan DL, Suler JR. Psychological factors associated with maintenance of improved health behaviors in postcoronary patients. J Psychol 1984; 119:87–94.
67. Inui TS, Carter WB. Problems and prospects for health services research on provider-patient communication. Med Care 1985; 23:521.
68. DiMatteo MR, DiNicola D. Achieving Patient Compliance. New York: Pergamon Press, Inc., 1982.
69. Kaplan RM, Simon HJ. Compliance in medical care: Reconsideration of self-prediction. Ann Behav Med 1990; 12:66–71.
70. Liang MH. Compliance and quality of life: Confessions of a difficult patient. Arthritis Care Res 1989; 2:S71.
71. Green LW, Mullen PD, Stainbrook GL. Programs to reduce drug errors in the elderly: Direct and indirect evidence from patient education. In: Improving Medication Compliance. Reston, VA: National Pharmaceutical Council, 1984, p 59.
72. Steel K, Gertman P, Crescenzi C, Anderson J. Iatrogenic illness on a general medicine service at a university hospital. N Engl J Med 1981; 304:638.
73. Williamson J, Chapin JM. Adverse reactions to prescribed drugs in the elderly: A multicare investigation. Age Ageing 1980; 9:73.
74. Hurwitz N. Predisposing factors in adverse reactions to drugs. BMJ 1969; 1:536.
75. Dudley DL, Glaser EM, Jorgenson BN, Logan DL. Psychosocial concomitants to rehabilitation in chronic obstructive pulmonary disease: Part 2. Psychosocial treatment. Chest 1980; 77:544–551.
76. Berkman LF, Breslow L. Health and Ways of Living: Findings from the Alameda County Study. New York: Oxford University Press, Inc., 1983.
77. House JS, Robbins C, Metzner HL. The association of social relationships and activities with mortality. Prospective evidence from the Tecumseh community health study. Am J Epiemiol 1982; 116:123–140.
78. Blazer DG. Social support and mortality in an elderly community population. Am J Epidemiol 1982; 115:684–694.
79. Boadhead WE, Kaplan BH, James SA, et al. The epidemiologic evidence for a relationship between social support and health. Am J Epidemiol 1983; 117:521–537.
80. Reed D, McGee D, Yano K, Feinleib M. Social networks and CHD among Japanese men in Hawaii. Am J Epidemiol 1983; 117:384–396.
81. Lewis CE. Factors influencing the return to work of men with congestive heart failure. J Chron Dis 1966; 19:1193–2013.
82. Garrity TF. Vocational adjustment after first myocardial infarction: Comparative assessment of several variables suggested in the literature. Soc Sci Med 1973; 7:705–717.
83. Pearlin LI, Aneshensel CS. Coping and social supports: Their functions and applications. In: Aiken L, Mechanic B (eds). Applications of Social Science to Clinical Medicine and Health Policy. New Brunswick, NJ: Rutgers University Press, 1986.
84. Caplan R, Robinson EAR, French JR, et al. Adhering to Medical Regimens. Lecture presented at the Institute for Social Research, Ann Arbor, MI, 1976.
85. Atkins CJ, Kaplan RM, Toshima MT. Close relationships in the epidemiology of heart disease. In: Pearlman D (ed). Advances in Interpersonal Relationships. Vol 3. London: Jessica Kingsley Press, 1992, pp 207–231.
86. Williams CA, Beresford SAA, James SA, et al. The Edgecome County high blood pressure control program: III. Social support, social stressors, and treatment dropout. Am J Public Health 1985; 75:483–486.
87. Miller P, Wikoff RL, McMahon M, et al. Indicators of medical

regimen adherence for myocardial infarction patients. Nurs Res 1985; 34:268–272.
88. Davidson TN, Bowden L, Tholen D. Social support as a moderator of burn rehabilitation. Arch Phys Med Rehab 1979; 60:556.
89. Osby E, Reizenstein P. Quality of life and care in leukemia, myeloma and non-malignant disease: Opinions of patients and relatives, and effects of geography and time. Med Oncol Tumor Pharmacother 1989; 6:133–141.
90. Maasilta PK, Rautonen JK, Mattson MT, Mattson KV. Quality of life assessment during chemotherapy for non-small cell lung cancer. Eur Cancer 1990; 26:706–708.
91. Guyatt GH, Berman LB, Townsend M, et al. A measure of quality of life for clinical trials in chronic lung disease. Thorax 1987; 42:773–778.
92. Guyatt GH, Townsend M, Pugsley SO, et al. Bronchodilators in chronic air-flow limitation: Effects on airway function, exercise capacity and quality of life. Am Rev Respir Dis 1987; 135:1069–1074.
93. Guyatt GH, Townsend M, Keller JL, Singer J. Should study subjects see their previous responses: Data from a randomized control trial. J Clin Epidemiol 1989; 42:913–920.
94. Jaeschke R, Singer J, Guyatt GH. Measurement of health status: Ascertaining the minimal clinically important difference. Controlled Clin Trials 1989; 10:407–415.
95. Bergner M, Bobbitt RA, Carter WB, Gilson BS. The sickness impact profile: Development and final revision of a health status measure. Med Care 1981; 19:787–805.
96. Prigatano GP, Parsons O, Wright E, et al. Neuropsychological test performance in mildly hypoxemic patients with chronic obstructive pulmonary disease. J Consult Clin Psychol 1983; 51:108–116.
97. Williams SJ, Bury MR. Impairment, disability and handicap in chronic respiratory illness. Soc Sci Med 1989; 29:609–616.
98. Schrier AC, Dekker FW, Kaptein AA, Dijkman JH. Quality of life in elderly patients with chronic nonspecific lung disease seen in family practice. Chest 1990; 98:894–899.
99. Kaplan RM, Bush JW. Health related quality of life measurement for evaluation research and policy analysis. Health Psychol 1982; 1:61–80.
100. Weinstein MC, Stason WB. Foundations of cost/effectiveness analysis for health and medical practice. N Engl J Med 1977; 296:716–721.
101. Kaplan RM, Bush JW, Berry CC. Health status: types of validity for an index of well-being. Health Serv Res 1976; 11:478–507.
102. Russell L. Is Prevention Better Than Cure? Washington, D.C.: The Brookings Institution, 1986.
103. Kaplan RM, Anderson JP. The quality of well-being scale: Rationale for a single quality of life index. In: Walker SR, Rosser RR (eds). Quality of Life: Assessment and Application. London: MTP Press, 1988, pp 51–77.
104. Anderson JP, Bush JW, Berry CC. Classifying function for health outcome and quality-of-life evaluation: Self-versus interviewer modes. Med Care 1986; 24:454.
105. Anderson JP, Bush JW, Berry CC. Internal consistency analysis: A method for studying the accuracy of function assessment for health outcome and quality-of-life evaluation. J Epidemiol 1988; 41:127.
106. Anderson JP, Kaplan RM, DeBon M. Comparison of responses to similar questions in health surveys. In: Fowler F (ed). Health Survey Research Methods. Washington, D.C.: National Center for Health Statistics, US Department of Health and Human Services, pp 13–21.
107. Anderson JP, Kaplan RM, Berry CC, et al. Interday reliability of function assessment for a health status measure: The quality of well-being scale. Med Care 1989; 27:1076–1084.
108. Kaplan RM, Bush JW, Berry CC. The reliability, stability and generalizability of a health status index. Proc Soc Stat Sec 1978; 26:415–418.
109. Kaplan RM, Atkins CJ, Timms R. Validity of a quality of well-being scale as an outcome measure in chronic obstructive pulmonary disease. J Chron Dis 1984; 37:85–95.
110. Bombardier C, Ware J, Russell IJ, et al. Auranofin therapy and quality of life for patients with rheumatoid arthritis: Results of a multi-center trial. Am J Med 1986; 81:565–578.
111. Kaplan RM, Hartwell SL, Wilson DK, Wallace JP. Effects of diet and exercise interventions on control and quality of life in non-insulin-dependent diabetes mellitus. J Gen Intern Med 1987; 2:220–228.
112. Orenstein DM, Nixon PA, Ross EA, Kaplan RM. The quality of well-being in cystic fibrosis. Chest 1989; 95:344–347.
113. Orenstein DM, Pattishall EN, Ross EA, Kaplan RM. Quality of well-being before and after antibiotic treatment of pulmonary exacerbation in cystic fibrosis. Chest 1990; 98:1081–1084.
114. Kaplan RM, Anderson JP, Wu AW, et al. The quality of well-being scale: Applications in AIDS, cystic fibrosis, and arthritis. Med Care 1989; 27:S27–S43.
115. Kaplan RM, Anderson JP, Erickson P. Estimating well-years of life for a new public health indicator. In: Proceedings of the 1989 Public Health Conference on Records and Statistics. Washington, DC: National Center for Health Statistics; 1989. US Department of Health and Human Services publication (PHS) 90–1214, pp 298–303.
116. Toevs CD, Kaplan RM, Atkins CJ. The costs and effects of behavioral programs in chronic obstructive pulmonary disease. Med Care 1984; 22:1088–1100.

Chapter 27

Relaxation and Biofeedback: Coping Skills Training

ANNE JERMAN, R.N., M.S.
MARGARET CAMPBELL HAGGERTY,
R.N.C., M.S.N.

THE CHALLENGE OF CHRONIC LUNG DISEASE

As the average age of the population in the United States has shifted to middle age and older, the incidence of chronic illness has increased. The aging process in the United States requires learning to live with a chronic illness or disability for an increasing number of our patients. This presents new challenges not only to the patient suffering from the condition but to the health care provider as well. We are called upon to provide the medical treatments required to control the illness, which in itself is a stimulating challenge. More important to our patients, we are often called upon to help them cope with the many changes that are caused by the chronic illness: changes in lifestyle, goal setting, career, recreational activities, and roles inside and outside the home.

People with chronic lung disease encounter several challenges that are brought about by their condition. Shortness of breath and fear of shortness of breath may limit activity, may lead to chronic deconditioning, and may cause panic. Increased work of breathing, problems with oxygenation, ineffective secretion clearance, increased risk of infection, respiratory failure, and the time requirements of a prescribed therapeutic regimen often cause drastic changes in lifestyle and self-concept. Patients can feel conspicuous and embarrassed when their illness is made evident to others by the equipment they must carry or the outward symptoms they display.

Patients may feel stigmatized or may suffer from overwhelming guilt because of an illness that they may have brought on themselves with poor health habits.

Adequate treatment of chronic lung disease requires a comprehensive, biopsychosocial approach. Pharmacologic therapy, smoking cessation, breathing retraining, exercise reconditioning, and nutrition are among the therapeutic modalities used to help the patient meet the challenge of chronic lung disease. An additional challenge to patients and health care providers is the development of strategies to reduce the impact of the disease on the patient, the family, and support systems and not simply to focus on the illness alone. Providing patients with an opportunity to learn new coping skills is an effective way to decrease the disease's negative impact. New coping skills can improve the functional ability of the patient and enhance self-esteem by helping the patient take some control of the disease process.

This chapter focuses on relaxation methods, biofeedback interventions, and cognitive techniques to help the patient develop some coping strategies, decrease symptoms, and enhance functioning.

STRESS RESPONSE

In order to understand how coping skills training can be helpful, the patient requires a rationale for training. Although most patients have some understanding of what stress is, few understand the stress response and its function in the body. Until they become ill, most patients have understood stress to be the transient annoyances of life that are often dealt with and then forgotten. With the onset of chronic illness, stress becomes a part of life, but few patients actually understand what is happening to their bodies or why they feel and react in the many ways that they do.

Stress may refer to a stimulus, a response, or a combination of the two. A stressor is usually referred to as a stimulus that a person perceives as a threat. A stressor may be physical, psychologic, or psychosocial.[1] The physical stressors that challenge a COPD patient include dyspnea-inducing physical activities, environmental pollutants, changes in temperature, exposure to disease, and the medications used to modify some of these experiences. Psychologic stressors are the thoughts, feelings, and concerns that the patient has about perceived threats. Psychologic stressors are subjective and involve the patient's interpretation of the situation. Often these interpretations are distorted. Psychosocial stressors occur in the context of the patient's interpersonal relationships. These may be problems that occur in very intimate relationships, such as with a parent or a spouse, or in less intimate relationships, such as with friends or acquaintances; they may occur because of social isolation.

Potentially, everything is stressful, but the same stressors do not stress each person equally. In order for an event to be stressful, it must be recognized and acknowledged by the person as a stressor. Situations and events become decreasingly stressful to individuals as the perceived ability to cope with the stressor increases. Therefore, the more coping skills we can provide for our patients, the more likely it is that they will be able to maintain control and cope effectively with the stressful event.

It is not the intent of this chapter to review the physiology of the stress response. Readers interested in a full and up-to-date description are referred to Asterita.[1] The message the health care provider should give the patient is that the stress response has cognitive, behavioral, and physiologic components and that a trigger of any one component can and will trigger the other two components.

In the early 1900s, Cannon[2] described the emergency reaction displayed by an organism when it is threatened or in danger. This reaction, called the "fight or flight" reaction, is intended as a self-protection mechanism to prepare the organism to fight the threat or to avoid it. It was Cannon's belief that arousal of the autonomic nervous system was a basic response to stress. The most noticeable effects of autonomic nervous system arousal are summarized in Figure 27–1. Although many of the changes are obvious, patients often are not aware of them because of the triggering of this stress response.

In 1956, Selye[3] used Cannon's ideas in a more complex description of the stress response that he called the "General Adaptation Syndrome" (Fig. 27–2). Selye expanded on the "all-or-nothing concept" of Cannon to describe a process that enables the body to deal with stress in an effective manner.

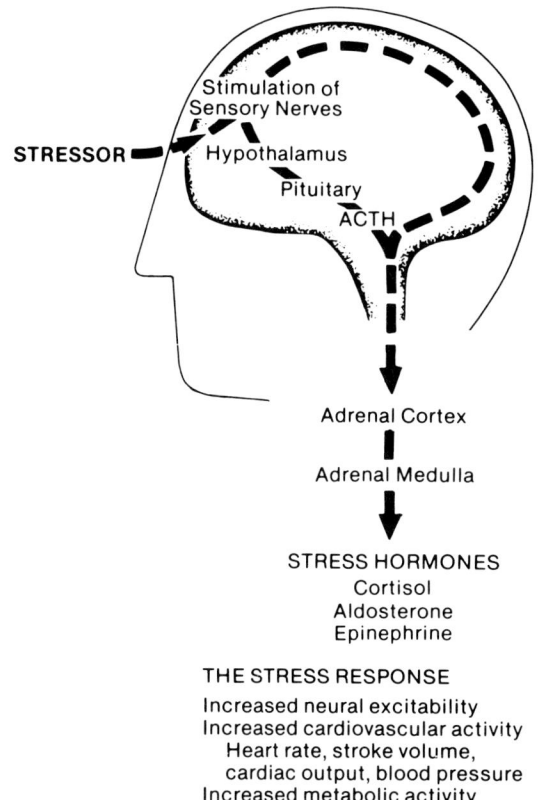

FIGURE 27–1. The stress response pathway. (From Girdano DA, Everly GS, Dusek DE. Controlling Stress and Tension. Englewood Cliffs, NJ: Prentice-Hall, Inc., 1990, p 35.)

The General Adapatation Syndrome has three phases. The *alarm phase* is the initial response of the body's defense mechanisms. Sympathetic arousal occurs, and the body prepares to defend itself against the threat or to flee from it. The second phase, the *stage of resistance*, is the stage at which coping and adaptation occur. Most of the changes that have occurred at the *alarm stage* have been reversed. The body provides maximum resistance to the threat through increased metabolism and increased muscle strength. However, the body is at risk from other stressors secondary to decreased inflammatory responses, decreased immunity, and depleted body resources. Unless the stress is resolved, the body's defense mechanisms will weaken. The *stage of exhaustion* is the third phase. Adaptation no longer occurs, and shock and lowered resistance to infection become apparent.

During the alarm stage, little thought is required. Cognitive function tends to be disorganized during fight or flight because energy is being directed to the survival of the body. However, if the stress continues to the second stage, a chronically stressed person may dem-

GENERAL ADAPTATION SYNDROME

Stage I: Alarm reaction	Stage II: Stage of resistance	Stage III: Stage of exhaustion
Mobilization of the body's defensive forces and activation of the "fight or flight" mechanism	Optimal adaptation to stress within the person's capabilities	Loss of ability to resist stress because of depletion of body resources

Physical Change

Release of norepinephrine and epinephrine, causing vasoconstriction, increased blood pressure, and increased rate and force of cardiac contraction	Hormone levels readjust	Decreased immune response with suppression of T cells and atrophy of thymus
Increased hormone levels	Reduction in activity and size of cortex	Depletion of adrenal glands and hormone production
Enlargement of adrenal cortex	Lymph nodes return to normal size	Weight loss
Marked loss of body weight	Weight returns to normal	Enlargement of lymph nodes and dysfunction of lymphatic system
Shrinkage of thymus, spleen, and lymph nodes		If exposure to the stressor continues, cardiac failure, renal failure, or death may occur
Irritation of the gastric mucosa		

Psychosocial Changes

Increased level of alertness	Increased and intensified use of coping mechanisms	Defense-oriented behaviors become exaggerated
Increased level of anxiety	Tendency to rely on defense-oriented behavior	Disorganization of thinking
Task-oriented, defense-oriented, inefficient or maladaptive behavior may occur		Disorganization of personality
		Sensory stimuli may be misperceived with appearance of illusion
		Reality contact may be reduced with appearance of delusions or hallucinations
		If exposure to the stressor continues, stupor or violence may occur

FIGURE 27–2. General adaptation syndrome. (From Kneisl CR, Ames SW. Adult Health Nursing: A Biopsychosocial Approach. Menlo Park, CA: Addison-Wesley Publishing Co., Inc., 1987, p 20.)

onstrate increased difficulty in solving problems, misinterpret situations, demonstrate difficulty making decisions, and worry excessively. Often these individuals begin to demonstrate some mental status impairments, including irritability, easy frustration, lack of energy, loss of interests, a focus on the negative, and verbalization of guilt and anger.

Behaviorally, a person under increased stress may become more aggressive or more passive. The aggressive person may complain about the care that he or she has received and become more demanding, argumentative, confrontational, and stubborn. As the distress continues, potentially stressful situations are increasingly avoided. The passive individual demonstrates difficulty making decisions, becomes increasingly isolated, and generally waits to be taken care of. As isolation increases, the focus of attention is drawn inward and worries about present performance and anticipation of a negative outcome for the future increase.

When the stress response is triggered, people may fear a loss of control. For example, a person may fear going insane, having a heart attack, suffocating, or at best, embarrassing himself or herself in front of others. Each person responds uniquely to a stressor. Understanding the stress response can provide the patient with an understanding of the experience and with a model to increase awareness of the physiologic, cognitive, and behavioral cues of the stress response. He or she can become aware of situations that are likely to trigger the stress response and of how to slow down the process and regain a sense of control.

RELAXATION THERAPY

The useful properties of relaxation training in the alleviation of the symptoms of stress have been well documented, especially over the past 20 to 30 years. The relaxation techniques on which there is the greatest amount of empirical data are progressive muscle relaxation,[4] autogenic relaxation,[5,6] electromyographic feedback,[7,8] meditation,[9] and modified meditation.[10]

Goals of Treatment

The goals of relaxation training include gaining mastery over the physiologic effects of the stress response in the body, increasing awareness of early physiologic distress, and developing techniques to reduce the effects of anxiety and distress on the body. Patients can feel helpless to control the effects of illness on their lifestyle. Teaching relaxation is one way to empower the patient and give him or her a degree of responsibility and control over the illness experience.

Through relaxation techniques, the patient redirects energy from what cannot be controlled to what can be controlled. During the process, the patient redefines what is controllable. As stress levels begin to rise, the patient begins to feel increasingly out of control. When attempts are made to regain control by controlling the environment, frustration increases. When energies are directed toward changing and controlling the individual's response to the situation instead of the environment, frustration and distress decrease.

Identifying the Appropriate Patients

The relaxation response is a learned response, and almost anyone can learn it. However, it should not be used with patients who are psychotic. Relaxation techniques with these patients can intensify symptoms such as delusions and hallucinations. This includes not only patients with a known history of mental illness but also patients who are experiencing delusions or hallucinations as a side effect of medications or of the withdrawal of medications.

Preparing the Patient

Relaxation is a skill, and learning it requires practice and work. Disappointment occurs when quick results are expected, and motivation to continue rapidly decreases. Assessing one's own as well as the patient's expectations is an important part of the learning process. Frequent reminders of the importance of practice and patience are necessary. Research evidence indicates that home practice of relaxation plays a critical role in the persistence of positive results gained from biofeedback and relaxation training.[11]

There are many ways to trigger a relaxation response. Relaxation techniques should be adapted to the patient according to his or her own individual needs. The technique should be tailored to the individual, not to the disease. There is no one technique that is best for a specific diagnosis. There may be one or two specific techniques that are best for the individual, and it is the job of the health care provider to help the patient find the techniques that work best. Children as well as adults can benefit from relaxation training. However, children can become bored with relaxation, and the challenge to the health care provider is often how to keep the child's interest. Relaxation and mental imagery exercises have been taught at the Minneapolis Children's Medical Center. Forty children were followed from 6 months to 2 years. Evaluation of the results showed that most of the children had experienced a greater than 50% improvement in symptoms. Improvements included a reduction in the number of visits to emergency rooms, decreased symptom severity, and reduced medication use.[12] Once an appropriate relaxation technique has been identified and the relaxation response has been learned, the techniques are simple to use.

Prior to teaching relaxation techniques, it can be very helpful for the health care provider to practice the relaxation techniques so as to become acquainted with the sensations associated with a relaxation response and the problems that can be encountered as practice procedes and will identify some possible solutions to those problems. There can be a positive influence on the patient when the health care provider demonstrates the ability to maintain a relaxed manner or looks like a relaxed person. A tense practitioner can elicit tension in the patient. Patients are often aware of whether the health care provider is using the health promoting techniques that the patient is being encouraged to use. Motivation and receptiveness to learning can increase when the patient knows the health care provider is following the same prescription.

Positioning

In practicing a relaxation technique, body positioning is important. Thus, care should be taken to ensure that the patient is as comfortable as possible. Often, the most comfortable position is lying in bed, with the head of the bed elevated, the knees bent, and a pillow placed beneath the knees. Lying back in a reclining chair can achieve the same effect. Patients who become drowsy during relaxation or fear reclining because of possible dyspnea should perhaps sit up with the head and neck supported. If the patient tends to get cold, a light blanket to retain warmth may be helpful. Removing glasses, loosening tight clothing, and taking off shoes is helpful. If seated, the patient should not cross his or her legs, since this interferes with circulation, can become uncomfortable, and may require movement in less than the time needed to complete the relaxation technique.

Expected Sensations

The sensations of relaxation are described in many different ways. Descriptions are individual and can include a feeling of heaviness (as if one were "sinking down" and getting very comfortable), a feeling of pleasant warmth, a feeling of lightness (as if there were a thin layer of air between the patient and the chair), a feeling of a pleasant coolness, or a pleasant tingling sensation. Some people may even describe a combination of these sensations.

Patients can be frightened by their initial experience with relaxation. Patients are afraid of losing control and may experience these relaxed feelings as a loss of control. Because the sensations frighten them, they cannot relax. Reassurance that the mind is alert and can respond to any sudden emergency in the environment even when the patient is deeply relaxed can significantly reduce anxiety.

Intrusive Thoughts

When using any relaxation technique, it is to be expected that the mind will wander and that these intrusive thoughts can become a barrier to triggering a relaxation response. Patients can become frustrated with their inability to control their thoughts; if they become frustrated enough, they might give up their attempt to learn. During the initial training period, it is helpful to anticipate with the patient if this will be a problem. Relaxation requires passive concentration, whereas most tasks require active concentration. Most people are more accustomed to active concentration. Directions to the patient to refocus each time an intruding thought occurs eventually minimize this problem. Although intruding thoughts continue to occur, the patient learns to experience the intrusive thoughts in a more passive way.

After a relaxation sequence has been completed, the patient should be encouraged to remain seated or lying down and to change position slowly. Triggering of the relaxation response slows heart rate, slows respiration, and reduces blood pressure slightly. Moving too quickly causes orthostatic blood pressure changes, and moving slowly minimizes any dizziness.

Relaxation Tapes

Relaxation training takes time, not only in the office but at home as well. Relaxation is a skill that must be practiced if any benefit is to be derived from it. Anxiety about learning something new, doing it well, and doing it right can interfere with concentration and with the learning process. Training can be easiest if the patient has a taped relaxation sequence to listen to at home. Making the tape with the patient in the office during the first trial is an easy and practical way to provide the patient with a tape. Making the tape with the patient also allows for individual adjustments to be made if the patient requires some changes in the standard instruction routine.

When recording a relaxation tape or using relaxation during a session with the patient, it is important to use a tone of voice that is slow, quiet, calming, and relaxing. Maintaining this tone of voice may require some practice before it is used with a patient. Making a tape of one's own voice and then using it to relax can help the practitioner make the necessary adjustments and ensure that the right atmosphere is created for optimal relaxation.

Just as the health care provider creates the right atmosphere to begin relaxation training in the office, the patient must work to create the right atmosphere at home. The slightest noise can be very distracting when trying to practice the relaxation techniques. Anticipating together what interruptions may occur at home can help minimize them before they begin. Temporarily disconnecting the telephone during this brief period and speaking with family members about minimizing noise are helpful. Family pets can interfere when the relaxation techniques are practiced. Helping the patient anticipate problems can help decrease frustration later and improve compliance. To improve a patient's motivation and compliance, the practitioner should ask him or her about home practice at each visit. Inquiries about home practice communicate to the patient that home practice is important and that he or she is accountable for it. Inquiries about home practice may help identify problems early and allow for easier solutions.

Relaxation Techniques

There are many useful techniques that can trigger a relaxation response, and no one technique is best for a specific problem. Some studies seem to indicate that one form of relaxation may be of greater benefit than another. Maher-Loughman and associates[13] reported encouraging results using hypnotherapy to reduce wheezing and drug use in 62 patients. Similar results have been obtained since that time.[14, 15] Edmundston[16] has suggested that hypnotherapy and relaxation therapy are essentially the same. It can be concluded that it is more important to find the technique or techniques that work best for the individual. The more individualized the treatment program, the more likely it is that the patient will be compliant.

Progressive Muscle Relaxation

Perhaps the easiest technique to use is progressive muscle relaxation. First employed by Jacobson,[4] it requires that the patient be actively involved in the relaxation process. Patients often find that it is easier to concentrate using this technique because it is an active technique.

Reductions in dyspnea, anxiety, and respiratory rate have been reported in patients with COPD who are undergoing progressive muscle relaxation training.[17] Patients with chronic debilitating illnesses often are unable to attend to the subtle physical cues from their bodies. They have become experts at using denial as a coping skill to ignore the pain and discomfort of their illnesses. Denial is a useful and appropriate coping technique to a certain degree, but the consequence of overuse is insufficient awareness of rising levels of discomfort. Patients are often unaware of a problem until the sensations are much stronger and more difficult to cope with. The sensations of relaxation are initially quite subtle. A patient who uses distraction from or denial of a physical sensation may have difficulty recognizing the changes as they occur. If the patient is actively involved, such as with progressive muscle relaxation, the changes are more likely to be observed by the patient.

Many patients have a limited understanding of how the mind influences the body and how the body influences the mind. They can be very skeptical of imagery techniques, self-hypnosis techniques, or meditation. This skepticism can interfere with participation in the treatment. Progressive muscle relaxation can be less threatening for patients because it is an active technique. Patients perceive that they are doing something for themselves and not that something is being done for them. A sequence for progressive muscle relaxation is described in Table 27–1.

Autogenic Techniques

Autogenic or autosuggestion relaxation trains the patient to use passive attention to trigger a relaxation response. Training with this technique can follow quite naturally after the patient has gained some competence

TABLE 27-1. PROGRESSIVE MUSCLE RELAXATION

- Begin by closing your eyes and settling back comfortably with your arms and legs uncrossed.
- Take a deep breath and let it out slowly.
- Focus on your right arm and hand. When I say the word "now," place a lot of tension in your right arm and hand by making a fist, pushing down with your forearm into the arm of the chair or the mattress of the bed. Create just enough pressure to feel it up to your shoulder. Ready, NOW (hold for 5 sec).
- Now relax, allowing all the tension to flow out of your right arm and hand.
- When I say the word "now," again tense up your right arm and hand. Ready, NOW (hold for 5 sec).
- And relax, allowing all the tension to flow down your arm, out your finger tips.
- Now turn your focus to your left arm and hand, thinking about how your left arm feels compared with your right arm.
- When I say the word "now," tense up your left arm and hand by making a fist and by pushing down into the arm of the chair or the mattress of the bed, creating just enough pressure to feel it up to your left shoulder. Ready, NOW (hold for 5 sec).
- Now relax, allowing all the tension to flow out of your left arm and hand.
- When I say the word "now," again, tense up your left arm and hand. Ready, NOW (hold for 5 sec).
- Relax, allowing all the tension to flow down your arm and out your finger tips.
- Think about both arms and hands sinking comfortably into the chair or bed.
- Each time you lose your concentration, take a deep breath, let it out slowly, and refocus on the tension/relaxation contrasts, noticing the difference between the tension and the relaxation you are beginning to feel.
- Turn your focus to your neck and shoulder muscles. Think about how high or low your shoulders seem and how the back of your neck feels.
- When I say the word "now," tense your neck and shoulders by shrugging your shoulders up and by tilting your head forward, chin toward your breast bone. Ready, NOW (hold for 5 sec).
- Relax, allowing your shoulders to drop down and your neck to become loose and limp.
- When I say the word "now," again tense up your neck and shoulders. Ready, NOW (hold for 5 sec).
- Relax, allowing your shoulders to sink down and all the tension to flow down your neck, across your shoulders, down your arms, and out your finger tips. Feel the tension drain right out.
- Turn your focus to your facial muscles. When I say the word "now," tense up your facial muscles by wrinkling your brow, closing your eyes even more tightly, and clenching your teeth. Ready, NOW (hold for 5 sec).
- Relax by smoothing out your brow, relaxing your mouth, and allowing your tongue to lie still in your mouth.
- When I say the word "now," again, tense up your facial muscles. Ready, NOW (hold for 5 sec).
- Relax, allowing all the muscles of your face to relax, your jaw to loosen, and your teeth to move slightly apart. Think about how different it feels compared with the tension.
- Now focus on your chest, back, and abdomen. When I say the word "Now," tense up your chest, back, and abdomen by arching your back very slightly away from the bed or the chair, tightening your abdominal muscles, and holding your breath *(note: Eliminate breathholding if the patient is very anxious)*. Ready, NOW (hold for 5 sec).
- Relax, allowing your abdomen to relax, your breathing to return to normal, and your back to sink back comfortably into the chair.
- When I say the word "now," again, tighten up your check, back, and abdomen. Ready, NOW (hold for 5 sec).
- And relax, allowing all the tension to flow out of your chest, back, and abdomen.
- Each time you lose your concentration, take in a deep breath and let it out slowly and focus on the tension/relaxation contrast.
- Focus now on your right leg and foot, having no other thoughts except how your right leg and foot feel. When I say the word "now," tighten up your right leg and foot by lifting your leg very slightly off the bed or chair, and pointing your toes up toward your head *(note: If the patient has difficulty picking up the leg, simply have him or her point the toes of the appropriate foot)*. Ready, NOW (hold for 5 sec).
- Relax, allowing your leg to sink back comfortably onto the chair or bed.
- Once again, tense up your right leg and foot. Ready, NOW (hold for 5 sec).
- Relax, allowing all the muscles to relax, to feel loose and limp, and to sink down comfortably into the chair or bed.
- Focus now on your left leg and foot, thinking about how your left side feels compared with your right. When I say the word "now," tense up your left leg and foot by lifting the leg very slightly off the bed or the chair and pointing your toes up toward your head. Ready, NOW (hold for 5 sec).
- Relax, allowing your leg to sink back down and lie limp and loose against the chair or bed.
- Once again, tense up your left leg and foot. Ready, NOW (hold for 5 sec).
- Relax, allowing your leg to sink back comfortably.
- Think about all the muscles in your legs lying loosely and limply against the chair or the bed.
- Take a moment now to think about all the muscles of your body and about where there is remaining tension.
- Take a deep breath, and as you breathe out, allow the tension to flow out, replacing it with a deeply relaxed feeling.
- I am going to count backwards now from 10 to 1. At the count of five, you may open your eyes, and at the count of one you may stretch out if you want to.
  10...9...8...7...6...5...4...3...2...1

with progressive muscle relaxation. Training with progressive muscle relaxation helps the patient become more aware of bodily sensations and of how the body feels when a relaxation response has been triggered.

After several weeks or months of using progressive muscle relaxation, the patient becomes conditioned to the response. When beginning autogenic training, it is helpful to use this conditioned response by making a taped sequence that is similar to the sequence used in progressive muscle relaxation. The taped sequence is at once familiar and different to the patient, and learning is enhanced because of this conditioned effect. A sequence for autogenic relaxation is described in Table 27-2.

Abdominal Breathing

Abdominal breathing or diaphragmatic breathing can be a quick and easy way to trigger a relaxation response. It can be done anywhere with a minimum of self-consciousness because others are not aware of any change. It can be used in combination with other relax-

TABLE 27-2. AUTOGENIC RELAXATION

- Begin by closing your eyes and settling back comfortably.
- Start off by focusing on your breathing; try to make it a little deeper and slower than usual.
- Remember, if you lose your concentration, take a deep breath, let it out slowly, and refocus on the sensations of relaxation.
- Think of breathing in relaxation and breathing out the tension.
- Now focus on your right arm and hand, having no other thoughts except how your right arm and hand feel.
- As you release the tension, allow your right arm and hand to go limp and become deeply relaxed.
- Try saying to yourself, "My right arm and hand are heavy and warm; warmth is flowing into my right arm and hand."
- Allow the tension to drain from your shoulder, down your arm, and out your fingertips.
- Turn your focus now on your left arm and hand and think about how your left arm feels compared with your right.
- As you release the tension, allow your left arm and hand to go limp, to become deeply relaxed.
- Try saying to yourself, "My left arm and hand are heavy and warm; warmth is flowing into my left arm and hand."
- Imagine a wave of warmth and heaviness flowing down your arm, into your hand, and out your fingertips.
- Think about a warm, relaxed feeling in both arms and hands, and concentrate on how they feel against the chair or bed.
- They may feel heavy or light. Think about the pleasant feeling.
- Turn your focus now to your neck and shoulder muscles. Think about how your neck and shoulders feel as you allow your shoulders to drop down.
- Think about the back of your neck being more flexible and loose as you say to yourself, "My neck and shoulders are heavy and warm; warmth is flowing into my neck and shoulders."
- Think about the tension draining out of your neck, through your shoulders, down your arms, and out your fingertips.
- Turn your focus now to your facial muscles.
- Try to relax all the muscles in your face, allowing them to become more smooth, more relaxed.
- Think about your brow unwinding and your eyelids becoming more calm, your face smooth, your jaw more slack.
- Think about a comfortable, smooth feeling across your face.
- Turn your attention to your chest, back, and abdomen. Think about a relaxed feeling spreading down now into your back muscles, chest, and abdomen.
- As you allow your back to sink more comfortably into the chair or bed, think about your abdomen becoming very calm and smooth, not tight.
- Try to imagine the whole upper part of your body being deeply relaxed, lying limply against the chair or bed.
- Turn your attention now to your legs and feet. Think about both legs and feet, and as you allow the relaxation to replace the tension, say to yourself, "My legs and feet are heavy and warm; warmth is flowing into my legs and feet."
- Imagine a wave of warmth and heaviness moving down your thighs, down your calves, down into your feet and into your toes.
- Take a moment now to think about your whole body and how the muscles feel. Notice where there is remaining tension and tightness.
- Each time you breathe out, imagine a little bit more of the tension leaving with each breath. Think about what you might do the next time to loosen up even a little bit more.
- I am going to count backwards from 10 to 1. At the count of five, you may open your eyes, and at the count of one you may stretch. 10...9...8...7...6...5...4...3...2...1

ation techniques to promote rapid relaxation of the autonomic nervous system. The breathing centers of the brain are closely related to the reticular activating system; thus, relaxed, steady breathing promotes relaxation in general. Diaphragmatic breathing helps to relax the striated and smooth muscles, saves mechanical energy, and promotes ventilation of the lower lobes of the lungs.

Many patients can be taught the basics of diaphragmatic breathing in a short period of time. The patient should be seated in a comfortable chair or be lying in a comfortable position in a way that increases awareness of the relaxation of the abdominal muscles. The patient should place his or her hands on the abdomen to feel the diaphragm working to displace abdominal organs and inflate the lungs. The patient takes a deep breath that is sufficient to cause the shoulders to rise. As the patient exhales completely, the shoulders return to a more relaxed position. With the next inhalation, the patient should breathe without moving the shoulders from the relaxed position to avoid use of the accessory muscles. As with pursed-lip breathing that is used in breathing retraining, the expiratory phase should be at least twice as long as the inspiratory phase to relieve dyspnea and hyperventilation. The patient must relax the abdominal muscles to breathe comfortably. It can be helpful to cue the patient to relax the shoulders first when diaphragmatic breathing is attempted. Relaxing the shoulders first can help some patients expand the diaphragm more easily.

Initially, the patient will feel uncomfortable with this slower, more efficient breathing. Discomfort decreases with practice. Encourage the patient to use this technique in times of distress as well as in times of less stress. Patients can begin to condition themselves to use this technique by using selected cues in the environment as a reminder to practice. Such reminders might include each time the car stops at a red light or a stop sign, each time a commercial appears on the television, or each time the telephone rings. Encourage the patient to begin to look for opportunities to relax; such opportunities might include events that have been irritating in the past, such as waiting on line at a supermarket, waiting in a clinic waiting room, waiting for an elevator, or sitting in a dentist's chair.

Abdominal breathing may produce asynchronous and paradoxical rib cage motion and therefore may not be useful for some patients.[18] Careful observation of the patient can help determine if this technique is contraindicated.

Imagination

Visualization and guided imagery are two ways to stimulate the imagination. They reduce distress by helping one to imagine a different feeling in the body or to imagine the self in a more comfortable or safe place. Imagery can be particularly useful when working to help reduce symptoms in children.

Visualization

Visualization can help minimize distressing thoughts and emotions or physical distress by refocusing awareness. Tape recording a visualization sequence can help minimize the distracting nature of intruding thoughts.

Many visualization sequences use the concept of giving the tension or the focus of the distress (e.g., pain, dyspnea, tension in one part of the body, and a distress-

TABLE 27-3. VISUALIZATION

- Close your eyes and settle back comfortably.
- Take a deep breath and let it out slowly.
- Each time you breathe out, allow the tension to flow out of your body.
- As you breathe in and out, slowly and evenly, think about your (whatever the patient has identified as the problem).
- Give this problem you are struggling with a symbol.
- Now give your concept of relaxation a symbol.
- Think about these symbols interacting in such a way that the tension is replaced by the relaxation.

ing emotion such as fear) a symbol or a color. As the visualization progresses, the patient gradually imagines the changing of the symbol. It becomes softer, quieter, less threatening, or easier to manage. For example:

"Imagine the tight, hard knot of muscles between the shoulders becoming softer, looser, more flexible, smooth, and pliant. Imagine a hard, jagged rock changing to a soft, pliant clay, and then imagine the shape of that clay reforming, changing into a smoother shape. Give the problem a color such as red. Gradually change the color from a hot, painful red to a cool, soothing blue. Visualize a tight, closed fist clamping down on the areas of tension or distress, such as your dyspnea, and then gradually allow the fist to open and turn with palm up. Allow the problem to 'sit quietly' in the palm of the hand or even to float away from the hand."

Whatever the image, it should be one that is meaningful or useful to the patient. Patients very often have very vivid, graphic ways of describing what it is they are struggling and trying to cope with. The patient should try this technique several times. After the patient has described a symbol or symbols, the practitioner should make a tape that the patient can use at home. A visualization sequence format is described in Table 27-3.

Guided Imagery

Guided imagery uses the concept of imagining a safe, quiet, comfortable place to slow the stress response. Although almost any image of a quiet, restful place can be useful, perhaps one of the most helpful ways to use imagery is to have the patient describe his or her own place. It might be a quiet place in a park, garden, or wooded area. It may be a pleasant day on a deserted beach or even the description of a favorite painting. Ask the patient about the details of the image, and then use them during the recording of a tape of the guided imagery. A description of a guided imagery format is described in Table 27-4.

Music

Many therapists trained in relaxation techniques include music in their relaxation strategies.[19-21] Auditory nerve impulses trigger a thalamic response that influences the limbic system. The response can be either sympathetic or parasympathetic and can have an effect on sleep/wakefulness cycles, hormone release, heart rate, blood pressure, and other physiologic parameters. Altshuler[22] theorized that music alters moods unconsciously through the stimulation of an autonomic response at the thalamic level. Brody[23] explained that music appears to influence right-sided brain activity, causing the pituitary gland to release endorphins (the body's natural opiates) and generate a soothing, calming effect. But, as McClelland[24] has noted, there is still no well-defined scientific explanation for why we respond to music.

Music works well with other relaxation strategies and can enhance their effects. The challenging task in teaching diaphragmatic breathing is to achieve full exhalation. Hyperventilators usually cannot relax the diaphragm fully and thus experience shallow respirations. Asthmatics appear to hold some air in reserve; this results in poor air exchange. The use of music during diaphragmatic breathing training is a simple, pleasant, and relaxing way to teach full exhalation. The cadence of soothing music gives the patient something other than counting on which to focus. Relaxing with music also has the additional benefit of conditioning. Once the patient has been trained to relax with music, simply recalling the music during a stressful time can help trigger a relaxation response. Fried[25] has done considerable work in teaching his clients deep, diaphragmatic breathing with music. He reported that he and his clients prefer several pieces in particular during breathing relaxation, including:

1. "Pachelbel Canon" from Daniel Kobialka's *Timeless Motion* (Li-Sem Enterprises).
2. "Oxygene" by Jean Michel Jarre (Polygram Records).
3. "Minuet" from Boccherini's *String Quintet in E*, Opus 13, No. 5. (Phillips compact disk No. 410-606-2).
4. "Infini" (Pan Communications Compact Disk No. 9001).

TABLE 27-4. GUIDED IMAGERY

- Close your eyes and settle back comfortably.
- Take a deep breath and let it out slowly.
- Each time you breathe out, allow the tension to flow out of your body.
- Imagine yourself leaving the place where you are now.
- Take a short break from your daily problems, leave them behind for this brief time out.
- Imagine yourself gradually approaching your quiet place (use the details the patient has described to you).
- What is the first thing that you notice here?
- Think about the colors in this place (adding details from the patient's description).
- Think about how the air feels here.
- What is the weather like in your place?
- What do you hear in this place?
- Select a spot to sit down, settle in, and allow yourself to gradually relax.
- Allow yourself to feel totally relaxed in this place, totally calm, peaceful, and relaxed.
- Allow yourself to spend a few minutes here, and remind yourself that you can return to this place any time you choose.

In 1975, Bonny recognized the value of music to enhance, prolong, and experience mood.[26] Meditative music is one of two types that can affect the mind. Meditative music affects the mind and the body and creates an atmosphere of calm and inner reflection. It is quiet and slow. Its purpose is to slow and deepen breathing.

In the United States, the music most commonly used as an adjunct to relaxation is contemporary American meditative music.[27] It uses three to seven tones, its melodies progress by steps, and its durations of phase equal one breath. It is moderately soft, smooth, and flowing and has no rapid rhythmic changes. It is simple music with little emotion. Well-known music pieces include the various "Environments" as well as compositions by Steven Halpern and Kitaro.

Systematic Desensitization

In 1958, Wolpe proposed the idea of reciprocal inhibition as a way to reduce fear.[28] He theorized that an anxiety response and a state of relaxation are physiologically incompatible and that the relaxation response could be used to reciprocally inhibit an anxious response. Wolpe combined a modified form of Jacobson's progressive muscle relaxation technique with systematic desensitization. Systematic desensitization is probably the most common behavior therapy technique used in the past 20 years.[29] Using progressive muscle relaxation, it has been shown to be an effective treatment for phobias and some psychosomatic symptoms.[29-31] The notion of desensitization is well known to most physicians and other health care providers in the treatment of allergic asthmatics. The patient gradually develops a tolerance for greater and greater amounts of a specific allergen by being exposed systematically to increasing amounts of the allergen. Desensitization to increasing levels of dyspnea has also been suggested as a way to encourage anxious patients with COPD to exercise. The patient is asked to exercise at levels that produce dyspnea and is then instructed to use breathing techniques to regain comfortable or controlled breathing.[32] Wolpe's desensitization works much the same way to control the toxic effects of anxiety and the stress response.

The patient and the clinician construct a hierarchy of stressful stimuli or events. The hierarchy is prioritized from the lowest threat to the highest threat. After the patient has learned relaxation, the patient is instructed to relax and imagine a series of scenes involving a stressful stimulus or event. The patient continues to practice the relaxation for a number of sessions until he or she can maintain relaxation while imagining the stressful stimulus. When the image is mastered, the patient moves on to the next image in the hierarchy.

Systematic desensitization has been used effectively with some asthmatic patients.[33-36] Patients create a hierarchy involving a series of events associated with an asthma attack. They work their way up the hierarchy by using the relaxation techniques, imagining encounters with the stressful stimuli, and remaining relaxed. Creer[33] claimed 100% improvement in a sample group of 30 asthmatic patients. He evaluated the success of the desensitization in this group by measuring changes in pulmonary function (peak expiratory flow rate).

Systematic desensitization is a useful treatment technique for other patients with COPD. Anxiety is frequently a concomitant feature of COPD. Anxiety is often related to fear of suffocation and of those activities that might upset what seems to the patient to be an already marginal balance. Many patients begin to live increasingly restricted lives in response to their fears about their inability to cope with outside stressors. The avoidance behavior of the COPD patient is analogous to the development of agoraphobia, in which the fear of an anxiety attack—not the anxiety attack itself—results in increasingly limited behavior. Although many of these fears are quite premature, the fear of loss of control and embarrassment in front of others is a powerful deterrent.

Patients with COPD are often afraid of changes in routine brought about by special events, visits of friends or relatives, or proposed travel. Fear of dyspnea, fatigue, or contagion from others may cause patients to restrict themselves to a hermit-like existence. Breathing retraining, exercise reconditioning, and other therapeutic modalities may help patients maximize their ability to cope with changes in routine. Systematic desensitization is an additional technique that may help patients cope with their fears and may assist them in resuming many previously enjoyed activities. For example, a patient who is afraid to travel may construct a hierarchy involving travel by airplane, he or she might imagine organizing luggage, traveling to and in the airport, and exposure to potentially adverse environmental conditions. Visualization of these stressful events while relaxing can help the patient feel more in control and thus more likely to tackle the travel experience. In this way, systematic desensitization with the anxiety-provoking stimuli can help patients broaden the scope of their world.

Anticipatory Rehearsal

Anticipatory rehearsal is similar to systematic desensitization. Although the patient feels very anxious in many situations, he or she does not develop avoidance behavior. The patient may complain of an increase in symptoms in certain situations. High levels of anxiety can restrict pleasure or a sense of accomplishment or success that might have been derived from the experience. As in systematic desensitization, once a relaxed state is achieved, the patient visualizes himself or herself doing well in the anxiety-provoking anticipated situation. While relaxed, the patient can anticipate problems that may occur and seek possible solutions. This can decrease anxiety once the patient is actually in the anticipated event. Imagining oneself maintaining breath control while negotiating stairs or rehearsing calmly the setting up of a portable fan to minimize the effect of unexpected humidity are two possible ways to use this technique. Creer[37] found anticipatory rehearsal to be an important part of strategy development in the self-management system entitled *Living with Asthma* developed at the National Asthma Center in Denver, Colorado. Patients were found to be better prepared to deal with stressful events. Using anticipatory rehearsal, patients recalled instructions that they had been taught, imagined how they would perform these instructions, and later wrote down their responses.

Anticipatory rehearsal may also be used with severely dyspneic patients who are entering an exercise program. For example, one of our patients reported severe anticipatory dyspnea each time she prepared for her exercise walk. She was taught to apply anticipatory rehearsal, using her previously learned relaxation technique, and to visualize herself maintaining relaxed and controlled breathing during her walk. This was followed by the performance of paced walking. The patient was able to walk for longer periods of time with less severe dyspnea when she used this technique.

BIOFEEDBACK

Biofeedback is "the technique of using equipment (usually electronic) to reveal to human beings some of their internal physiologic events, normal and abnormal, in the form of visual and auditory signals, in order to teach them to manipulate these otherwise involuntary or unfelt events by manipulating the displayed signals."[38] In clinical practice, biofeedback most often refers to electromyographic feedback. Using electromyographic feedback, the patient learns to decrease or increase muscle tension in a chosen area of the body. Other commonly used biofeedback methods include thermal or skin temperature feedback, galvanic skin response feedback, and alpha brain wave (or electroencephalogram) feedback. Other types of biofeedback have been used with asthmatics but have not proved efficacious. Mussell and Hartley[39] proposed that asthmatics would be able to consciously reverse bronchospasm using trachea-noise biofeedback, but concluded that conscious reversal of a full asthma attack was limited. Erskine-Milliss and Cleary[40] conducted two studies to evaluate feedback of total respiratory resistance of the airways as a treatment for adults with moderate to severe chronic bronchial asthma. Biofeedback failed to produce any significant improvements, and any improvements that were demonstrated could not be attributed to the biofeedback.

The somatic measurements from any of these techniques are converted instantly to audio or visual displays. It is from this information that the patient learns to enhance the relaxation training. Audio feedback most frequently involves tones, buzzes, or clicks that change as the patient increases or decreases muscle tension, skin potential, or temperature. Visual feedback is usually displayed using lights, oscilloscopic tracings, or a video display. It is not known if any one form of feedback has merit over any other. The type of display chosen is based on options offered by the manufacturer and the preference of the purchaser.

There is considerable controversy about whether biofeedback is a useful or necessary addition to relaxation training. In 1985, Roberts reviewed biofeedback research findings and concluded that there is "little relationship between research findings in the area of biofeedback and the clinical practice of biofeedback."[41] He found that many studies were poorly controlled and that results were not generalizable and conflicted from laboratory to laboratory. However, he did believe that biofeedback is a useful addition to treatment when used as part of a multimodal approach. Green and Shellenberger[42] agree that conclusions cannot be drawn about the efficacy of biofeedback because of research methodology problems. Biofeedback alone probably cannot be considered an appropriate or useful treatment modality, but it does have its place in treatment when used in a comprehensive multimodal treatment plan.[43-46] In a related study, Kotses and associates[47] concluded that biofeedback was not adequate to treat childhood asthma and that the long-term improvements they noted were probably dependent on both the biofeedback training and home practice.

Biofeedback is not a relaxation technique, but rather a tool that can be used to enhance the learning of relaxation techniques. Although biofeedback can be used without training in the use of relaxation techniques, it is rarely used in this way in the clinical setting. Most clinical strategies involve training the patient in at least one relaxation technique before using biofeedback.

Biofeedback can be useful to help legitimize the relaxation experience. Because the experience of relaxation is an internal one in which patients appear to others to be simply lying down and resting, patients sometime complain that they "feel like" they are doing nothing. Some patients label this outwardly appearing nonproductive task as laziness and experience a resultant decrease in motivation. Biofeedback demonstrates to patients that they in fact are accomplishing something. This change in perception can improve compliance. Measurement of physiologic parameters provides the patients with evidence that they are learning something. Patients are frequently learning more than they are aware. This knowledge can be encouraging for patients and may decrease dropout rates. Stoyva[48] reports a 15% dropout rate in his clinic. He believes the encouragement that patients get from the biofeedback information helps keep the dropout rate low.

Patients can feel out of control when they experience the symptoms of stress. Often, in attempting to control their stress response, they actually intensify the distressing symptoms. Biofeedback training can enhance the understanding of how to stop trying to control the stress response and how to start controlling the relaxation response. During initial sessions with biofeedback, the patient can focus on the feedback itself and attempt to control the sound or the visual image change. Focusing on the feedback can actually cause the tension to intensify; this is a paradoxical effect. When the patient makes the shift to a focus on the feelings of relaxation, a sense of control and a sense of success are achieved.

Using biofeedback presents some disadvantages. Patients can develop a sense of reliance on the feedback machines. Some patients enter into biofeedback training with the understanding that the machines are controlling the relaxation. Conversely, they believe they cannot relax without the machines. The emphasis in training must be placed on the learning that occurs away from the machines. Clinicians might give the patient the message that the machine is more important than it actually is by focusing on the instrumentation, measurement, and recording of data too much. The focus must remain on the patient and on the patient's perception of the process.

Before beginning biofeedback training, the patient must be prepared. For the training to be of any benefit, the patient must be cooperative. To derive benefit from the biofeedback sessions in the office, the patient must practice the relaxation response daily at home.

Patients are prepared for biofeedback the same way they are prepared for the relaxation techniques. The rationale for using the relaxation is the same rationale as that for using the biofeedback training: to reduce the physiologic effects of distress by gaining some control over their physiologic responses. The patient should be seated in a comfortable chair or lying down on a couch or reclining chair. Restrictive clothing should be loosened. A pillow under the head and under the knees can improve comfort, as can a light blanket if the patient complains of feeling cold.

Once the patient is comfortable, baseline data are recorded. This baseline data can be compared from session to session to assess if the patient is learning anything. The patient is instructed to observe when there is either an audio or visual change in the feedback that indicates a reduction in tension and an increase in relaxation. The patient is asked to notice what physical changes occur (e.g., changes in symptoms or sensations) that can be correlated with the change indicated by the biofeedback. It is this information that is most useful to the patient because it is the information that will be used at home during practice.

A typical session lasts 15 to 20 minutes. It is important to ask the patient what the session was like for him or her, what went well, and what needs more attention. This can be a very important part of the training. The patient talks about and clarifies those strategies that trigger relaxation and what his or her perceptions are about the biofeedback; the patient also helps to pinpoint specific problems that may be occurring during and outside the session.

There are many biofeedback units available on the market. When selecting equipment, it is most important to find units that are easy to use and easily understood by the patient and that will withstand frequent use over time. Thermography units measure and feed back temperature changes in the skin, usually using the tip of a finger. Galvanic skin response units measure skin conductance or electrical potential. Most commercial machines are simple hand-held units. Electromyography measures the electrical discharges of motor neurons and is the most complex type of biofeedback unit of the three types. Electromyographic feedback involves the placement of sensors on the muscle to be monitored, which is often the frontalis muscle of the face.

ANTICIPATING PROBLEMS

One of the most common problems encountered by patients and clinicians is finding that a task is too difficult. This can occur whether the focus is the relaxation response or the use of the biofeedback. If the patient finds the task at hand to be too demanding, then the clinician should choose an easier task. Switching to a simpler, slower, or shorter relaxation sequence may be helpful. The time of day at which sessions occur may be a problem, thus finding a less stressful time of day to practice might also help. Some patients initially have difficulty in practicing a technique every day. Helping the patient structure his or her day can improve compliance or provide more information about the nature of the problem.

The challenge for the clinician is to help the patient feel successful. Often patients with chronic illnesses have a sense of failure because they have not been able to control the course of their illness or its impact on their lives. This sense of failure can generalize to other areas of their lives. Helping patients achieve success with relaxation practice or successfully attain the goal of that particular session can provide an energy boost and improve compliance.

Some patients become frustrated with their inability to stop the frequent intrusion of thoughts. The problem is magnified when attempts are made to force these thoughts out of conscious awareness. The same effect results when a patient tries to control the symptoms of stress that are experienced rather than to control the relaxation response. Encouragement to merely notice the intruding thoughts and to "drift along with them" for a moment or so is a useful way to stop attempts to control these thoughts and to decrease their intrusiveness. Occasionally, changing to a more active relaxation technique, such as progressive muscle relaxation, can be a way to decrease the intrusions. The patient focuses on the action in the activity and shifts attention away from the thoughts.

Poor compliance with home practice can be a problem. Taking time to understand the problem may be frustrating but is worth the effort. Does the patient understand or believe the rationale? By focusing on the learning of coping skills, does the patient think the health care provider is minimizing the importance or the severity of the problem? Is the problem with other family members? Are they unconsciously sabotaging the training because they do not understand the rationale? Do they have unresolved feelings about the illness of the patient or the lifestyle changes that have occurred because of the illness? Problem-solving cannot begin until the nature of the problem is clarified. Compliance is more likely when the experience is easy and fun.

GENERALIZING AND MAINTAINING THE ABILITY TO RELAX

During skill development, the patient is asked to use a relaxation tape at least once per day. Although patients frequently believe that using the tape is no longer necessary once it is memorized, relaxation does not occur as easily or as deeply when the patient simply relies on memory. Skill development requires 4 to 6 weeks, depending on the patient and the situation. Once a skill has been developed, daily use of the tape is not required to maintain the skill, but home practice remains important to continuing the success of this coping skill. Patients should be encouraged to use the tape two to three times per week to maintain the relaxation skill as well as to continue to look for daily opportunities to relax. Any time spent waiting is an opportunity to relax. Waiting for the bus, waiting in the clinic waiting room, waiting at a stop light, waiting on line, or waiting for a friend are all good opportunities to relax. Periodically throughout the day, noticing muscle tension and releasing it is an opportunity to relax. Routine practice several times per day—for example, before the beginning of each meal—is useful. The patient should be encouraged to notice the development of unnecessary tension in the course of an activity such as walking, cooking, cleaning, writing, or driving and then to allow that tension to be released.

COGNITIVE-BEHAVIORAL TREATMENT: A MULTIMODAL APPROACH

In addition to physical problems, patients with COPD suffer from the consequences of negative emotions. Emotional discomfort is experienced as fear, depression, anger, or guilt that is elicited by threats to self-concept, uncertainty, fears about the future, changes in family roles and responsibilities, changes in social and vocational roles, increased dependence, and decreased autonomy.[49, 50] The stressors associated with physical disability require significant coping. The way in which an individual copes with a stressful situation may determine how disabling the problem becomes. How patients respond depends on several factors, including emotional strength and support systems that were available to them before the onset of the illness. Strong emotions can challenge the respiratory system, and respiratory symptoms can elicit strong emotions. Dyspnea and anxiety are frequent problems for patients with COPD. Emotional stress may even precipitate some symptoms (e.g., bronchospasm). Dekker and Groen selected stressful emotional stimuli from the records of patients and then used the stimuli to trigger asthma attacks.[51] However, this was not a simple cause-and-effect phenomenon, that is, it was difficult to distinguish whether the emotions were the cause or the effect of respiratory symptoms.

Patients with COPD frequently do not complain of emotional distress but often "transfer" their complaints and concerns to somatic complaints.[52] Beneath the physical complaints often lie fears of the same symptoms they are complaining of as well as fears concerning the future.

Patients with COPD have been described as living in "emotional straitjackets."[53] Feelings evoked by dyspnea may trigger greater dyspnea and more intense emotions. Action-related reactions, such as anxiety or anger, or nonaction reactions, such as depression and withdrawal, can trigger more dyspnea and exacerbate the patient's feelings; this can result in respiratory insufficiency combined with hypoxia or hypercapnia.[54] This constriction of emotions is an adaptive reaction and requires slow change. Relaxation and coping skills training is a way to help patients avoid or emerge from the emotional straitjacket.

Adaptation to changing events, changes in function, and change in ability is constant. The amount of stress that is experienced by the individual depends on how the individual interprets the stressor or the change. If the individual believes that there are adequate resources to deal with the stressor, the level of distress is relatively low. As the number of perceived resources decreases, distress increases. The resources may be external or internal. How an individual perceives and interprets the resources is determined in part by his or her past experience. This perception-interpretation process is called "self-talk."

Problem Clarification

Through relaxation training, the patient has learned a skill to decrease physiologic arousal. At the same time, the patient has begun to identify the prodromal signs that herald an intensification of a symptom or the signal that a problem has not been addressed and requires attention. Relaxation provides a basis with which to maintain control while engaging in problem clarification and problem-solving. Mandel and Keller[55] found that patients experienced a significant reduction in anxiety and somatization following completion of a stress management program, suggesting that they had a lesser preoccupation with physical symptoms.

Using a relaxation skill, the individual has a means of decreasing the anxiety or the distressing symptoms of the stress response. He or she might have enough clarification of what the source of a problem is or the ability to identify what the contributing stressors to a given situation may be. Once the source of the stress is clarified, the patient can begin problem-solving. Problem-solving might include changing the stressor or its source or altering the reaction to the stressor.

Stressors may be environmental (e.g., smoke or cold), physical (e.g., an upper respiratory infection or inadequate sleep), social (e.g., a disagreement with a spouse), organizational (e.g., difficulty getting an appointment with a physician when desired because of scheduling conflicts, or difficulties in dealing with insurance companies), or internal (e.g., thinking "I am a burden to my family" or "I must not leave the house because I will catch a cold and die from complications").

The patient can learn to control some of the events that precipitate anxiety or dyspnea. Control can be attained by avoiding, altering, or accepting a situation. The pattern of behavior might be to underutilize or overutilize any of these options. Overexposure has its obvious consequences; underexposure leads to withdrawal and avoidance behaviors that contribute to the "emotional straitjacket." The goal is to avoid relying too heavily on either of the two extremes and to work toward a more balanced response.

Problem Solving

Altering the situation could mean invoking other coping skills, such as communication skills or problem-solving skills. Patients frequently communicate in a passive way; they believe that the health care provider should know what they mean when they speak or know what they need without having to ask for it. This can lead to feelings of frustration, anger, fear, hopelessness, and helplessness. By validating the patient's feelings and encouraging the patient to verbalize his or her needs, an increased sense of self-control and control of the situation can occur.

Some situations cannot be controlled. Patients with COPD experience many losses that occur gradually over time. Patients lose their health, independence, careers, responsibilities at home, and ability to participate in activities that they previously enjoyed. Relationships with others are changed, often permanently. For these reasons, patients with COPD can become depressed. In order to accept these losses, the losses must be grieved for. These feelings are often confusing for the patient. Validating and encouraging expression of sadness can help the patient begin to accept losses. Acceptance also involves choice. Patients often feel as if they have no choice. Helping patients to learn to choose, even between the lesser of two negatives, aids them in achieving some control over situations.

Self-Talk

People almost continually engage in self-talk. Self-talk is the way in which people describe and interpret themselves, others, and their world. When the self-talk is accurate and reasonable, negative emotions are well controlled. When the self-talk is distorted, negative emotions become increasingly distressing. Using the model described by Beck and associates,[56] cognitive therapists have described 10 ways in which people misinterpret information. This faulty interpretation includes arbitrary inference (drawing a specific conclusion in the absence of evidence to support the conclusion), selective abstraction (focusing on a detail out of context and ignoring other, more salient features of the situation), overgeneralization (drawing a general conclusion and then applying it to all situations), magnification and minimization (errors in evaluating the significance or magnitude of an event), personalization (blaming oneself for events or problems when there is no basis for such a connection), and dichotomous thinking (the tendency to categorize all experiences into one of two opposite categories).[56]

TABLE 27–5. DISPUTING AND REDUCING COGNITIVE DISTORTIONS

Situation
- I was out with my family at a restaurant.

Physical/Emotional State
- I started to cough and had difficulty catching my breath. I felt uncomfortable, as if everyone was watching me. I started to feel short of breath, and I became afraid that I would not be able to catch my breath. I felt guilty that I was ruining my family's meal. My dyspnea worsened. I felt sad, lonely, isolated, and scared.

Thoughts
- Everyone's watching me; they feel sorry for me.
- I am not going to be able to clear my airway; I'll choke to death.
- I am ruining their meal; they probably wish that I had not come.
- They would have more fun without me here.
- Next time I'll send them off without me and I'll stay home alone.

Changing the Self-Talk
- Some people might be looking at me, but everyone isn't. Even if they are looking at me it isn't because they think I shouldn't be here; they might be concerned about my welfare. There are other people here who probably have chronic illnesses as well.
- I can clear my airway; it will take a minute. I can breathe more slowly and evenly, and that will help me catch my breath.
- I am not ruining my family's meal. They have told me that they want me to be here and that it is more fun when I am here, even if I do have a coughing spell.
- If I stay home, I won't be happy and they won't be happy.

Substituting a More Empowering Message
- It takes courage to come out to a restaurant. I have courage.

Altering Negative Thinking

Patients can be taught to dispute and reduce cognitive distortions, reduce the intensity of negative emotions, and feel more in control. The following five steps are helpful:

- Identify the situation that generated the negative emotions or the physical symptoms
- Write down how the physical and emotional feelings increased as the situation occurred
- Write down the thoughts and feelings as they occurred
- Dispute and change the distorted self-talk, often by asking oneself, "Would my friend see this the same way that I do?" or "What would I tell my friend in this situation?"
- Substitute a more balanced, empowering message

An example of how to use this technique is described in Table 27–5.

SLEEP DISTURBANCES

Many patients complain of difficulty in falling asleep, remaining asleep, or of excessive sleepiness during the day. Accurate diagnosis is important because specific treatments exist for some sleep disorders. Often these complaints are a symptom of depression, which itself must be treated. Sleep disturbances can be medical, psychiatric, or behavioral in origin, and can be a combination of the three. Whatever the origin, the principles of sleep hygiene should be considered.[57] They include (1) sleeping as much as needed to feel refreshed during the day; (2) understanding that the sleep requirement is completely individual and tends to be reduced somewhat with age; (3) maintaining a regular rising time in the morning tends to strengthen the sleep/wakefulness cycle and leads to a regular sleep-onset time; (4) knowing that regular daily exercise probably helps to deepen sleep; (5) insulating against noise, as occasional loud noises interfere with sleep; (6) understanding that an excessively warm room disrupts sleep; (7) understanding that hunger may disrupt sleep; (8) occasionally using sleeping medication, especially during periods of acute stress (but understanding that chronic use of sedative hypnotics is ineffectual for some patients and may be harmful to others); (9) knowing that caffeine in the evening disturbs sleep; (10) understanding that alcohol can hasten sleep onset but disrupts rapid eye movement sleep, making sleep less restful; and (11) understanding that tension disrupts sleep.

After other causes of sleep disturbance have been eliminated or after diagnosis has been made and treatment initiated, behavioral interventions using the principles of sleep hygiene can be employed. The patient should be encouraged to go to bed only when sleepy and not to take naps during the day. If the patient is able to exercise, he or she should not exercise after 4 PM. A small snack before bedtime decreases hunger. Patients having difficulty with sleep should be cautioned about consuming any caffeine after breakfast. If difficulty falling asleep is the complaint, a relaxation technique can be used to decrease muscle tension as well as provide distraction. Any of the relaxation techniques, including progressive muscle relaxation, is appropriate. If midcycle awakening is the complaint, a relaxation technique can also be useful.

Patients must have some experience and skill with relaxation before attempting to use it for a sleep disturbance. Most patients are very frustrated with their inability to sleep in a satisfactory way. If they have the expectation that the relaxation will induce sleep and it actually does not, frustration will increase, making it even less likely that sleep will occur. A patient experienced with relaxation knows that using the technique can make it more likely that sleep will occur, but even if sleep does not occur, frustration is less likely because the patient has a reasonable expectation.

WHEN THE PATIENT IS OVERWHELMED

Many patients approach coping skills training already believing that they have failed. They may feel they have failed to keep themselves healthy, to stay in their jobs, to provide for their families, to take care of their responsibilities at home, and to control the progress of their illness. Now, they fear that they will fail at their coping skills training. They feel helpless to make any changes and hopeless that the changes will help. The more intensely the feelings are felt, the less energy is available to devote to skills training. The challenge to the health care provider is to help the patient attain some success.

Some patients have the expectation that the new intervention will work perfectly, will work the first time, and will work under the most difficult circumstances. When this expectation is not met, the new intervention is discounted by the patient as being totally worthless. The patient needs help to identify which aspects of the intervention have worked well and then to build on that success. For example, the patient might have anticipated that he or she would have trouble finding the time to relax. The patient may, in fact, have practiced 3 of 7 days. Congratulating the patient for finding the time, reviewing how the time was set aside, and making suggestions for improvement reinforce the patient's success. The patient may have noticed the circumstances and the emotions that precipitated an episode of dyspnea. The experience may have been discounted because he or she did not remember to use relaxation and became overwhelmed; alternatively, he or she may have tried to use some relaxation but employed it too late in the cycle, thereby minimizing the effect. The awareness of the circumstances and the emotions that predisposed the patient to the dyspneic episode were discounted. Previously, the patient may have believed that an episode of dyspnea occurred with little or no warning. Noticing the prodromal factors is a successful change. Reinforcing the awareness of these factors can help maintain motivation.

Family Support

Enlisting the support and assistance of family members can help identify some of the patterns of behavior that contribute to the feeling of being overwhelmed. Patients can have difficulty prioritizing; they place their own needs last and attempt to meet those of the family first. Family members are often aware of this but are confused as to what to do to help change the maladaptive behavior and support new, more adaptive behavior. Families frequently offer very creative solutions to these problems when they are encouraged to do so.

WHEN TO REFER

When the patient continues to feel overwhelmed and is having difficulty with compliance, when family intervention has not helped, or when the family is unsupportive, a referral for further evaluation should be considered. The patient may be developing a major depressive episode, may have an underlying anxiety disorder, or may have long-standing psychologic problems that interfere with compliance and contribute to feelings of hopelessness and helplessness. Depression and anxiety not only influence already compromised respiration but also influence a patient's ability to participate in treatment programs. When a patient suffers from a major depressive episode or an anxiety disorder, he or she is less likely to participate in self-care activities. Anxiety and depression place the patient at risk for self-destructive behaviors, such as smoking and alcoholism. A referral to a behavioral medicine service would be appropriate; at such a service, an understanding of the interaction of body and mind is well understood. Depending on the resources in the area of practice of the health care provider, a referral to a therapist specializing in cognitive behavioral psychotherapy or to a psychotherapist specializing in medical psychotherapy would also be appropriate. In more rural areas, these services may not be available. In such a case, referral to a psychiatrist or mental health clinic should be considered so that the patient's depression and anxiety can be evaluated. If treatment is indicated, close collaboration among medical and psychiatric disciplines is needed to avoid treatment recommendations that might be confusing for the patient.

CONCLUSION

As the incidence of chronic illness increases, the challenge to treat the illness and to help patients cope increases as well. Relaxation training offers effective ways to modify the symptoms of anxiety, dyspnea, muscle tension, and general distress. In addition to physical symptoms, patients with chronic illness can suffer from the effects of guilt, unexpressed anger, embarrassment, and shame. Relaxation techniques in combination with other behavioral and cognitive techniques can help patients cope with the many changes that result from living with a chronic illness. In the past, patients with COPD have coped by narrowing the scope of activity in their lives. Providing patients with adequate coping skills can help them broaden that scope and live not only longer but also fuller, more complete lives.

REFERENCES

1. Asterita MF. The Physiology of Stress. New York: Human Sciences Press, Inc., 1985.
2. Cannon WB. Bodily Changes in Pain, Hunger, Fear and Rage. New York: Appleton-Century-Crofts, 1920.
3. Selye H. The Stress of Life. New York: McGraw-Hill Book Co., 1956.
4. Jacobson E. Progressive Relaxation. 2nd ed. Chicago: University of Chicago Press, 1938.
5. Luthe W. (ed). Autogenic Therapy. Vol 1–4. New York: Grune & Stratton, Inc., 1969.
6. Schultz JH. Das Autogene Training: Konzentrative Selbstentspannung. Georg Thieme Verlag, Stuttgart, 1932.
7. Budzynski RH, Stoyva JM, Peffer KE. Biofeedback Techniques in Psychosomatic Disorders. In: Foa E, Goldstein A (eds). Handbook of Behavioral Interventions. New York: John Wiley & Sons, Inc., 1980, pp 186–265.
8. Budzynski RH, Stoyva JM. Biofeedback Techniques in Behavioral Therapy. In: Birbaumer N (ed) Neuropsychologie der Angst: Reihe Fortschritte der Klinischen Psychologie. Vol 3. Munich: Urban & Schwarzenberg, 1973, pp 248–270.
9. Hirai R. Psychophysiology of Zen. Tokyo: Igaku-Shoin Medical Publishers, 1974.
10. Benson H. The Relaxation Response. New York: William Morrow & Co., 1975.
11. Tarler-Benlolo L. The role of relaxation in biofeedback training: A critical review of the literature. Psychol Bull 1978; 85:727–755.
12. Kohen D. A biobehavioral approach to managing childhood asthma. Child Today 1987; 16:6–10.
13. Maher-Loughman G, MacDonald N, Mason A, Fry L. Controlled trial of hypnosis in the symptomatic treatment of asthma. BMJ 1962; 2:371–376.
14. Morrison JB. Chronic asthma and improvement with relaxation induced by hypnotherapy. J R Soc Med 1988; 81:701–704.
15. Nagarathna R, Magendra HR. Yoga for bronchial asthma: A Controlled Study. BMJ 1985; 291:1077–1079.
16. Edmundston WE. Hypnosis and Relaxation: Modern Verification of an Old Equation. New York: John Wiley & Sons, Inc., 1981.
17. Renfroe KL. Effect of progressive relaxation on dyspnea and state anxiety in patients with chronic obstructive pulmonary disease. Heart Lung 1988; 17:408–413.
18. Lareau S, Larson JL. Ineffective breathing pattern related to airflow limitation. Nurs Clin North Am 1987; 22:179–191.
19. Hanser SB. Music therapy and stress reduction research. J Music Ther 1985; 22:193–206.
20. Hanser SB. Controversy in music listening/stress reduction research. Arts Psychother 1988; 15:211–217.
21. Standley JM. Music research in medical/dental treatment: Meta-analysis and clinical applications. J Music Ther 1986; 23:56–122.
22. Altshuler J. A psychiatrist's experiences with music as a therapeutic agent. In: Schullian M, Schoen M (eds). Music and Medicine. New York: Henry Schulman, Inc., 1948.
23. Brody R. Music medicine. Omni 1984; 6:24, 110.
24. McClelland R. The Healing Forces of Music. New York: Amity House, 1988.
25. Fried R. Integrating music in breathing training and relaxation: I. Background, rationale, and relevant elements. Biofeedback Self Regul 1990; 15:161–169.
26. Bonny H, Savary L. Music and Your Mind: Listening with a New Consciousness. New York: Harper & Row Publishers, Inc., 1975.
27. Fried R. Integrating Music in Breathing Training and Relaxation: II. Applications. Biofeedback Self Regul 1990; 15:171–177.
28. Wolpe J. Psychotherapy by Reciprocal Inhibition. Stanford, California: Stanford University Press, 1958.
29. Wolpe J. Behavior therapy for psychosomatic disorders. Psychosomatics 1980; 21:379–385.
30. Davison GC. Systematic desensitization as a counterconditioning process. J Abnorm Psychol 1968; 73:91–99.
31. Wolpe J, Lazurus AA. Behavior Therapy Techniques. New York: Pergamon Press, Inc., 1966.
32. Kohlman-Carrieri V, Janson-Bjerklie S. Coping and Self-Care Strategies. In: Mahler D (ed). Dyspnea. Kisco, New York: Futura Publishing Co., 1990.
33. Creer T. Biofeedback and asthma. Adv Asthma Allergy 1974; 1:7–12.
34. Renne C, Creer TL. The effects of training on the use of inhalation therapy equipment by children with asthma. J Appl Behav Anal 1976; 9:1–11.
35. Moore N. Behavior Therapy in Bronchial Asthma: A controlled Study. J Psychosom Res 1965; 9:257–276.
36. Walton D. The application of learning theory to the treatment of a case of bronchial asthma. In: Eyesenck (ed). Behavior Therapy and the Neuroses. New York: Pergamon Press, Inc., 1960.
37. Creer TL. Living with asthma: Replications and extensions. Health Educ Q 1987; 14:319–331.
38. Basmajian JV. Biofeedback: Principles and Practice for Clinicians. Baltimore: Williams & Wilkins, 1979.
39. Mussell MJ, Hartley JPR. Trachea-noise biofeedback in asthma: A comparison of the effect of trachea-noise biofeedback, a bronchodilator, and no treatment on the rate of recovery from exercise- and eucapnic hyperventilation-induced asthma. Biofeedback Self Regul 1988; 13:219–234.
40. Erskin-Milliss JM, Cleary PJ. Respiratory resistance feedback in the treatment of bronchial asthma in adults. J Psychosom Res 1987; 31:765–775.
41. Roberts A. Biofeedback: Research, training, and clinical roles. Am Psychol 1985; 40:938–941.
42. Green J, Shellenberger R. Biofeedback research and the ghost in the box: A reply to Roberts. Am Psychol 1986; 41:1003–1005.
43. McGovern H. Comment on Roberts's criticism of biofeedback. Am Psychol 1986; 41:1007.
44. Smith JC. Meditation, biofeedback, and the relaxation contro-

versy: A cognitive behavioral perspective. Am Psychol 1986; 41:1007–1009.
45. White S, Tursky B. Commentary on Roberts. Am Psychol 1986; 41:1005–1007.
46. Norris R. On the status of biofeedback and clinical practice. Am Psychol 1986; 41:1009–1010.
47. Kotses H, Harver A, Segreto J, et al. Long-Term effects of biofeedback-induced facial relaxation on measures of asthma severity in children. Biofeedback Self Regul 1991; 16:1–21.
48. Stoyva J. Autogenic training and biofeedback combined: A reliable method for the induction of general relaxation. In: Basmajian JV (ed). Biofeedback: Principles and Practice for Clinicians. Baltimore: Williams & Wilkins, 1979.
49. Cohen F, Lazarus R. Coping with stresses of illness. In: Stone GC, Adler NE (eds). Health Psychology. San Francisco: Jossey-Bass, 1979; pp 217–254.
50. Gruen W. Effects of brief psychotherapy during hospitalization period on recovery process in heart attack. J Consult Clin Psychol 1975; 43:223–232.
51. Dekker E, Groen J. Reproducible psychogenic attacks of asthma. J Psychosom Res 1957; 2:97–108.
52. Zitter RE, Dent T. How to help release COPD patients from "emotional lock-in" lifestyles. Behav Med 1981; Jan.:12–16.
53. Dudley DL, Glaser EM, Jorgenson B, et al. Psychosocial concomitants to rehabilitation in chronic obstructive pulmonary disease: Part I. Psychosocial and psychological considerations. Chest 1980; 77:413–420.
54. Dudley DL, Martin CJ, Holmes TH. Dyspnea: Psychological and physiologic observations. J Psychosom Res 1968; 11:325–339.
55. Mandel AR, Keller SM. Stress management in rehabilitation. Arch Phys Med Rehab 1986; 67:375–379.
56. Beck A, Rush JA, Shaw BF, Emery G. Cognitive Therapy of Depression. New York: Guilford Press, 1979.
57. Hauri P. The sleep disorders. In: Current Concepts. A Scope Publication. Kalamazoo, Michigan: The Upjohn Company, 1977.
58. Girdano DA, Everly GS, Dusek DE. Controlling Stress and Tension. Englewood Cliffs, New Jersey: Prentice-Hall, Inc., 1990.
59. Kneisl CR, Ames SW. Adult Health Nursing: A Biopsychosocial Approach. Menlo Park, California: Addison-Wesley Publishing Co., Inc., 1987.

Chapter 28

Sexuality and the Patient with Lung Disease

PAUL A. SELECKY, M.D.

Somewhere in the rehabilitative process of the lung disease patient, after medical and physical needs have been successfully addressed, the issue of sexuality may arise.[1] The primary basis for pulmonary rehabilitation is to help the patient understand and cope with his or her lung disease and to attempt to help the patient achieve the "highest possible functional capacity allowed by his pulmonary handicap and overall life situation."[2] We are therefore interacting with the patient as a person, including his or her sexuality. Our patients are men and women of various ages who have differing sexual roles as husbands or wives or as single adults who are involved in a variety of relationships. Caregivers are sexual beings as well. Our sexuality impacts on our interpersonal relationships, including the interactions with our patients.

It is evident, therefore, that sexuality is a far-reaching subject. Addressing sexuality clearly comes within the scope of our responsibilities as members of a pulmonary rehabilitation team. It is our job to help our patients cope with the impact of the disease process on their lives and all its intricacies, including their lives as sexual beings, and to help them better understand this impact as a part of the rehabilitative process.[3]

SEX VERSUS SEXUALITY

A discussion of sex within the context of a pulmonary rehabilitation program most often begins with a focus on the physical aspects of sex—namely, sexual intercourse and other physical expressions of sexual functioning. This is understandably an area of great interest, but it is important that we paint a broader picture for ourselves and our patients. The word "sex" triggers many different images in each individual, depending on his or her experiences and expectations as well as on the context in which the word is being used. "Sexuality" is a more complex term, as it involves the total personality of an individual—how he or she thinks, how he or she acts and feels; in essence, who he or she *is*. It has been said that sex is something we do, but that sexuality is something we are. Both are important and unique in each of us.

As described in Table 28–1, sex is a biologic term; sexuality addresses the total person. Our sex is our gender; it also establishes our role as male or female with a varying combination of masculine and feminine traits. Our sexuality colors our emotions, our understanding of ourselves, and our interactions with others. Together, sex and sexuality encompass the whole individual. Men and women respond differently to many situations in life because they are men or women, and

TABLE 28–1. SEX VERSUS SEXUALITY

Sex (Biology)	Sexuality (Total Person)
Facts	Attitudes
Male/female	Maleness/femaleness
Genitality	Personality
Physical pleasure	Intimacy
Doing	Being
Self-oriented	Relational

"never the twain shall meet."[4] It is our responsibility as health care workers to better understand those differences if we are to be useful to our patients.

SEXUAL HEALTH CARE

The World Health Organization defines sexual health as "the integration of the somatic, emotional, intellectual, and social aspects in ways that are positively enriching and will enhance personality, communication, and love."[5] Health care workers must attempt to achieve this objective through *sexual health care*, a concept that may seem a bit foreign to our roles as respiratory care professionals. It requires our focusing on the impact of chronic lung disease and its attendant symptoms on the sexual health of the patient. It is not sufficient for us to inquire about physical sexual dysfunctions, such as impotence, decreased libido, or ejaculatory problems; we must gain an understanding of the impact of the chronic lung disease on the sexuality of our patient as a total person.

A *sexual problem* has been appropriately defined by Calderone as "the malfunction of any part of an individual's organism or life in such a way as to cause his sexual life to appear to him unrewarding or inadequate, or to be potentially harmful to another individual and therefore to himself."[6] In the context of these definitions, the delivery of sexual health care is a responsibility of the entire pulmonary rehabilitation team, which should integrate discussions of sexuality into the entire rehabilitative process. This is in contrast to assigning the rehabilitation coordinator to elicit responses to specific questions about sexual functioning and then to refer the patient for specialty evaluation determined by the specific dysfunction. Schover and Jensen describe this as a kind of "relay race," in which one health care worker passes the "baton" to the next. Instead, a more appropriate integrative approach should be applied that involves the entire rehabilitation team in the process and that ideally includes the patient's sexual partner in the evaluation and treatment plan.[7]

SEXUALITY LASTS A LIFETIME

The delivery of sexual health care is based on the thesis that sexuality lasts a lifetime, in contrast to the popular view expressed by the media that sexuality is relegated to the young. As Munjack and Oziel have pointed out, ". . . there is no time when one abruptly becomes old; there is no cut-off point for sexual desire, response, or ability."[8] The significance of sexuality in later life is merely an extension of an individual's past life experiences, with the addition of (1) the normal expected aging process, (2) the availability of a partner, and (3) one's general health.

In simple analysis, a person who is sexually active during younger years is expected to become less active in later years, and the younger person who is sexually less active is expected, therefore, to become inactive.

Thienhaus states that a reasonable attitude to assume concerning sexual activity in later life is that "some do, some don't, and there is nothing wrong with either."[9]

The patient with lung disease fits well into this concept of a lifetime of sexuality, as he or she is most often an older individual who is facing the impact of aging on sexuality and sexual functioning, may be lacking a sexual partner, and is trying to cope with progressive breathing problems. It is important that the rehabilitation team be knowledgeable of these factors if it is to minister to the patient's concerns about sexuality.

"LOVE, SEX, AND AGING"

Consumers Union conducted a comprehensive study of the sexual attitudes and activities of over 4000 men and women from 1978 to 1979 entitled "Love, Sex, and Aging."[10] The study revealed a significant interest in sex in both men and women that was affected only slightly by increasing age. For example, the data reproduced in Table 28–2 are in response to the question, "How would you describe your present interest in sex?" They indicate that many seniors have a strong interest in sex.[11] In addition, 79% of men and 65% of women between 70 and 80 years of age stated that they were sexually active; of these, one half or more reported having intercourse at least once per week.[12]

The level of sexual activity is obviously impacted by the availability of a partner. The 1985 census revealed that approximately 39% of women aged 65 to 74 years were widowed; this figure increased to 68% by the age of 75 years or older.[13] The loss of a marital partner may not be an obstacle to sexual activity for all of our patients. Consumers Union reported that 50% of unmarried women and 75% of unmarried men aged 70 years and older were sexually active.[12]

SEXUALITY AND CHRONIC ILLNESS

Sexual functioning can be affected by chronic illness in a variety of ways. Sometimes the effect is related to the specific disease (e.g., impotence in diabetic men).[14] Dyspnea is the major symptom of the patient with lung disease, but studies reveal that this does not appear to be a major obstacle to successful sexual intercourse, except perhaps for those with severe impairment who are dyspneic at rest.[15-17] Although the scientific data are somewhat contradictory, the impact of the disease on sexual functioning is not to be measured by pulmonary function tests; rather, it is found in an understanding of the psychosocial impact of the disease on the patient, as depicted in Table 28–3.[18-19] Regardless of these factors, some patients have good coping skills and stand out as model patients because they are able to maintain an active lifestyle despite their chronic illness. This ability generally flows over into their sexual functioning.

Wise organizes the obstacles to sexual functioning into three categories.[20] The lung disease patient has to struggle with *impersonal* factors, such as limited exercise

TABLE 28-2. "HOW WOULD YOU DESCRIBE YOUR PRESENT INTEREST IN SEX?"*

	Age		
	50–59 Yr	60–69 Yr	≥ 70 Yr
Women (No.)	783	658	260
Interest in sex that is strong or moderate (%)	75	67	59
Weak (%)	20	23	23
Absent (%)	4	10	18
Total (%)	99	100	100
Men (No.)	820	963	567
Interest in sex that is strong or moderate (%)	94	88	75
Weak (%)	5	10	18
Absent (%)	1	2	8
Total (%)	100	100	101

*From Love, Sex, and Aging by Edward Brecher and The Editors of Consumer Reports Books. pp. 318–336. Copyright © 1984 by Consumers Union of the United States, Inc. By permission of Little, Brown, and Company.

tolerance, chronic cough, sputum production, and the potential side effects of medications. He or she also often struggles with *intrapersonal* obstacles, such as a decreased self-esteem and an altered view of his or her masculine or feminine role and the attendant anxiety. These then lead to *interpersonal* obstacles with a spouse or intimate other, including the fear of sexual failure and ultimately a suppression of sexual desire. It is important to realize, however, that this is not a universal finding linked only to chronic illness. A significant number of healthy couples also complain of sexual problems.[21] Moreover, many patients do continue to live full and very satisfying sexual lives.

WHAT CAN A HEALTH PROVIDER DO?

Our primary role as health care professionals is to attend to our patient's needs. In the field of sexual health care, this must begin with a self-examination of our knowledge and attitudes about sexuality. Any deficits in sexual information can be corrected by further study of a number of published resources,[22, 23] but the *facts* we know are not nearly as important to our patients as our *attitudes* concerning sex and sexuality. Ideally, we want our attitude to be "sex-positive" and accepting of others' points of view and lifestyles, and we want to avoid making value judgments. Our lack of sexual knowledge can be an obstacle in communicating with our patients; this obstacle is worsened by their perceiving negative nonverbal messages or negative attitudes concerning their sexual interests and behavior.

Before embarking on the subject of sexuality in a

TABLE 28-3. PSYCHOSOCIAL COMPOSITE OF THE PATIENT WITH CHRONIC OBSTRUCTIVE PULMONARY DISEASE

Social, family, and/or sexual roles altered
Activities of daily living limited
Recreation limited
Body preoccupation
Increased anxiety
Decreased self-esteem
Depressed
Overdependent

rehabilitation program, it is important that the rehabilitation team conduct an introspective evaluation of their sexual attitudes. This can be accomplished by conducting discussions of sexuality at team conferences. Team members might respond to such probing questions as: What are your attitudes about sexual activity in the elderly, masturbation, homosexuality, oral sex, and a wide variety of sexual subjects and practices? How comfortable are you with talking about sex? Ideally, training in the diagnosis and treatment of sexual dysfunctions should be sought. A model for a 1-day training session is described by Schover and Jensen.[24] At the very least, we need to be good listeners; we must respond to our patients' needs and concerns and not shut them out or turn them away.

SEXUAL COUNSELING

Many health care workers feel unprepared to become involved in sexual counseling and feel more comfortable with almost every other subject in the field of pulmonary rehabilitation. Regardless of our hesitancy in discussing sexuality with our patients, we may have no choice other than to become involved when our patients ask questions. It is a subject for which the entire team should be prepared; the team should not relegate the responsibility to just one member, such as the coordinator. Although the responsibility is often placed on the coordinator, the patient may feel more comfortable discussing questions concerning sexuality with some other member of the team. It is likely to be someone who appears to the patient to be most comfortable with the subject, someone who is approachable, and someone who appears able to discuss such intimate subjects in a relaxed and nonjudgmental manner. The coordinator may be the one to introduce the subject, but all members of the team should be open to continuing that discussion in their interactions with the patient.[25]

Most questions can be addressed from the resource of our own life experiences without the need for specialized training. Francoeur offers three cautions in this regard: (1) be aware of your limitations; (2) be sensitive to your position within the health care team so as not to interfere with the role of others, such as that of the primary physician; and (3) making a detailed recommendation to a patient may go beyond the team's limitations.[26]

A model for sexual counseling that many have found useful has been described by Annon as the PLISSIT model, a four-step process progressing from simple to complex counseling.[27] The caregiver proceeds through the four steps guided by the patient's needs and his or her own professional knowledge and personal comfort. The steps are described in Table 28–4. Kravetz has aptly applied this model to the counseling of the patient with lung disease and has developed accompanying professional and patient education materials.[28-30] Other guides to sexual counseling are available as well.[7, 8, 31, 32]

Permission-giving

The steps of the first level of counseling are listed in Table 28–5.[28] They begin by merely introducing the subject to the pulmonary rehabilitation patient. This can be done by asking a few open-ended questions on the entry questionnaire and by allowing time for the patient to elaborate on the responses during the intake interview. It is best to avoid questions that require a yes or no answer and to use instead questions such as (1) How does your breathing problem affect your sexual activity? (2) You mentioned you were limited by your shortness of breath; how has it affected your sexual functioning? (3) Many people have sexual concerns; what concerns you about your sexual functioning? What concerns your partner?

It is important that the interviewer asks such questions in a relaxed and comfortable manner and expects the patient to respond. We must be cautious of body language that may be telling the patient that we really do not want to hear about his or her sexual problems because they embarrass us. The look on our face is more important than the words we use.

Ideally, such an interview should be conducted in privacy to maintain patient confidentiality. The interviewer should allow sufficient time for discussion, pointing out to the patient that there will be other opportunities for addressing his or her concerns during the rehabilitation program. The patient's sexual partner should be involved in these discussions at some point, although initially it may be more comfortable for the patient to address the subject alone with the interviewer. Schover and Jensen point out that couple therapy is more productive than addressing the patient alone.[33] The interviewer is often able to assess the potential benefit of involving the patient's sexual partner in the discussion by assessing the role that the partner is

TABLE 28–4. PLISSIT MODEL FOR SEXUAL COUNSELING

P = Permission-giving
LI = Limited information
SS = Specific suggestions
IT = Intensive therapy

TABLE 28–5. GIVING PERMISSION TO BE SEXUAL

Introduce the subject of sex and sexuality
Communicate acceptance by your words and behavior
Provide educational materials
Use open-ended questions in the interview
Do not categorize or stereotype the patient's behavior
Use terms that are comfortable to you and the patient
Be "sex positive"
Be a good listener
Encourage and support the patient

already playing in the patient's illness. These authors point out that "general coping skills and sexual function are linked in the chronically ill," and advise the clinician that the best way to treat any sexual concerns is by fostering the strengths of the couple's relationship.[34] They identify a strong relationship as one in which the couple has developed four important marital skills: (1) they are comfortable and flexible in allocating their individual marital roles, (2) they respect each other's boundaries and allow these boundaries to change over time, (3) they have achieved good communication, and (4) they have reached agreement on the rules of their relationship that govern its daily functioning.[35] The same four skills apply to their sexual relationship as well.

This first step of permission-giving may generate no response from the patient. It should be remembered that "some do, some don't, and there is nothing wrong with either."[9] Nonetheless, sexual concerns are common. Giving permission to discuss them is likely to bring results. A study in a general medicine practice of adults of all ages, both sexes, different marital statuses, and different education levels revealed that over 50% reported sexual problems or concerns (e.g., related to the frequency of intercourse, a lack of sexual desire, marital or relationship problems, painful intercourse, and difficulties achieving an erection).[36] We should be prepared to address these concerns.

The solution to many patients' sexual concerns lies in education. Various institutions have produced materials that can be offered to patients or placed in the packet of educational materials that they receive as a part of the rehabilitation program.[37-39] Some teams utilize the slide-tape programs developed by Kravetz, including them among the various audiovisual programs that are presented to the patient.[29, 30] Such efforts introduce the subject of sexuality but are of only limited usefulness unless the patient is given an opportunity to discuss individual concerns. Some programs introduce the topic of sexuality to discussions in patient support groups, but this requires the presence of an experienced facilitator in order to make the discussion productive.[40]

Limited Information

Introducing the topic of sexuality may open the door to further discussion. If such is the case, the clinician should be prepared to offer at least limited information of a general nature, such as that listed in Table 28–6. The first step is to broaden the patients' focus from

TABLE 28–6. PROVIDING LIMITED INFORMATION ABOUT SEXUAL HEALTH

Sexuality involves the total person
Aging has predictable effects on sexual functioning
Many fears and myths about sex exist
Physiologic stress of sexual functioning is limited
Some medications can impair sexual functioning
Describe common sexual dysfunctions
Encourage discussion with sexual partner

TABLE 28–8. SOME CLASSES OF MEDICATIONS THAT CAN AFFECT SEXUAL FUNCTIONING

Impotence	Decreased Libido
Diuretics	Antihypertensive drugs
Antihypertensive drugs	Antihistamines
Anticholinergic drugs	Antipsychotic drugs
Antipsychotic drugs	Antidepressant drugs
Antihistamines	Sedatives
Antidepressants	Alcohol
Anorectic drugs	
Sedatives	
Alcohol	

genital functioning to the impact of sexuality on their total being, explaining that sexuality also includes how a person thinks and feels and not just what he or she does. This is particularly important for the patient with lung disease who has often developed a negative sexual self-image and who chooses to focus on his or her own frailties and limitations. This negative attitude often springs from society's image of the sexually active person as being young and attractive. Many patients unfortunately succumb to these myths, feeling that they are too old, too unattractive, or too sickly to have sexual feelings, let alone to consider being sexually active.

It is important that patients also understand the impact of normal aging on sexual functioning; this is described in Table 28–7.[41, 42] Although this knowledge does not resolve patients' concerns entirely, it often alleviates their belief that they are not normal. Patient education materials are available on this subject as well.[43, 44]

Some medications can be the source or an aggravating factor for sexual dysfunction. Most notably, they can contribute to impotence in the male. Antihypertensive medications are commonly the culprit.[45] Patients should be made aware of these interactions and advised to discuss them further with their prescribing physician. Other medications may result in decreased libido in both sexes (Table 28–8).[46, 47] Sexual impotence has also been linked to obstructive sleep apnea.[48] A history of loud interrupted snoring and excessive daytime sleepiness is strongly suggestive of this sleep disorder and may warrant further evaluation in a sleep disorders center.

Patients and their sexual partners may limit their sexual activity because they fear that the physical exertion and associated increase in breathing may trigger an attack of coughing or dyspnea. They need to be reassured that although the breathing rate increases, the physical stress of sexual intercourse is limited and is comparable with that of climbing only one or two flights of stairs.[49] The value of making such comparisons is limited, however, as individual styles of lovemaking are quite varied, and the stress is often limited to only a few minutes in most circumstances.[50]

Specific Suggestions

As we progress through this model of progressive counseling in sexual health, patients may ask for specific suggestions to address their problems or concerns. These may also be presented in a general way as part of the lecture series attended by patients in the pulmonary rehabilitation program or to patient support groups or more general patient education forums, such as the Better Breathers Clubs of the American Lung Association. A list of such suggestions that focus on ways to enhance sexual performance is found in Table 28–9. Many of the suggestions are based on common sense but are worth reiterating for the patient and his or her sexual partner. Making these suggestions often reassures both partners and may encourage their discussing the subject further in private. The rehabilitation team can advise patients to schedule their lovemaking for their "best breathing time," usually in the late morning or early afternoon after their daily morning bronchial hygiene has been completed and before late afternoon fatigue has begun to set in. Advise them to be creative and romantic in their sexual encounters and urge them to avoid the "touchdown" mentality that has often been the driving force for many couples (i.e., attempting to achieve orgasm or "score" on every sexual encounter). They need to be reminded of the sexual benefits of cuddling, caressing, and just spending some sexual time

TABLE 28–7. IMPACT OF AGING ON SEXUAL RESPONSE

Female
Vagina decreases in length and width
Vagina is less elastic
Vagina takes longer to become lubricated
Less vaginal lubrication
Decrease in frequency of orgasm

Male
Erections take longer to achieve
Erections not as firm
Takes longer to ejaculate
Less ejaculate volume
Longer recovery time

TABLE 28–9. SPECIFIC SUGGESTIONS FOR LOVEMAKING

Be physically and emotionally rested
Start and progress slowly
Choose the "best breathing" time
Avoid a "touchdown" mentality
Avoid alcohol and heavy meals
Use medications and/or oxygen to your advantage
Choose less stressful positions
Be creative and romantic

together. They should be encouraged to explore a wide range of sexual behaviors "from smiling to orgasm."[51] Specific variations on body position can be offered as alternatives to their usual habits of lovemaking.[18, 38–40, 52] For the male patient, the female-on-top position may be less stressful. Such a suggestion is less important if the change in position appears too unnatural to the couple. Our role is simply to offer the suggestions in an attempt to give them permission to change their habits, if they so desire, and to point out the wide variety of ways in which couples conduct their lovemaking.

The team can remind patients to avoid lovemaking after a heavy meal or the use of alcohol because of the tendency for both to generate fatigue. Alcohol can also be a risk factor for male impotence—even Shakespeare pointed out in *Macbeth* that "drink . . . provokes the desire, but it takes away the performance." Cigarette smoking is also a risk factor for male impotence because the vasoconstrictive effects of nicotine alter the complex vascular mechanism associated with erection of the penis. More often than not, most physicians have already convinced their male patients to stop smoking because of its impact on their lung disease.

Intensive Therapy

If our suggestions have not resolved the patient's concerns up to this point or if we detect problems that need specialty care, appropriate referrals should be made. Care options are described in Table 28–10. Referral requires our having knowledge of appropriate resources that are available in the community.

Impotence can be a problem for the aging male. Estimates indicate that as many as 55% of men report problems with impotence by the age of 75 years.[53] It is not an all-or-nothing symptom. Impotence is defined as the failure to achieve an erection that is adequate for intercourse in 25% or more of all attempts. Regardless of the expected increase in incidence with age, impotence in an elderly man should not be accepted as a normal course of events. Many patients can be successfully treated. An erection is the result of a complex physiologic process that can go awry in a number of ways; this emphasizes the importance of an appropriate diagnosis and treatment. Diagnosis and treatment usually begin with the primary care physician, who refers the patient for specialty evaluations as needed. Evaluations are performed by such specialists as an endocrinologist, urologist, vascular surgeon, or sex therapist. Studies identifying the various causes are influenced by the population being studied, but most indicate that the majority of patients have an organic cause (fewer than one in five causes are psychogenic in origin).[53, 54] Possible organic causes include medication effects, endocrine abnormalities (e.g., hypogonadism and diabetes), neurologic diseases, and vascular dysfunction. The effects of alcohol and nicotine have already been mentioned. The complex nature of impotence therefore requires the physician to perform physical examination and compile a thorough history that includes a detailed discussion of the sexual dysfunction. This should be supplemented by appropriate laboratory studies. Sleep disorders that may impair nocturnal penile tumescence should be excluded, if possible.[55] A variety of treatment modalities that can be guided by the evaluation are available. They include such therapies as testosterone supplementation, intracavernous injections of medications to produce or enhance erections, vascular surgery, vacuum tumescent devices, and the placement of a penile prosthesis. Sexual counseling is an important part of all these therapies.[56, 57]

Review of Table 28–11 indicates that there are also many nonorganic causes of sexual problems that can occur at any age and that may be corrected by ongoing counseling. The patient, his or her sexual partner, or both may focus on the problems they are having in their sexual interactions, but these problems may just be a symptom of a more general problem with their relationship. Couples need to be reminded that their lovemaking at night is an extension of their daytime interactions. They may be suffering from monotony and boredom in their daily life together; this flows over into their love life. Both partners need to be reminded that each needs to continue to work on their relationship on an ongoing basis and to continue to romance each other. Patients with lung disease are often so involved in the management of their illness that they neglect their personal relationships. They may need to be reminded that they must work at being feminine or masculine and focus on expressing their sexuality in the way they dress, in their general attitude, and in how they interact with others. Most individuals enjoy being attractive and gaining the attention of others. We may need to remind patients how they pursued those goals in the past.

SEXUALITY AND THE CAREGIVER–PATIENT RELATIONSHIP

To a certain extent, our own sexuality has an effect on the relationships we have with our patients. On the

TABLE 28–10. MODES OF INTENSIVE THERAPY FOR SEXUAL PROBLEMS

Training in communication techniques
Marriage counseling
Urologic/gynecologic consultation
Psychologic counseling
Psychiatric consultation
Sex therapy

TABLE 28–11. NONORGANIC CAUSES OF SEXUAL PROBLEMS

Lack of a partner
Monotonous sexual interactions
Marital disharmony
Unreasonable sexual expectations
Fear of failure in sexual performance

other hand, sometimes this effect is insignificant (e.g., when the healthcare professional administers a therapy). It may be ongoing over a period of time, such as in a pulmonary rehabilitation program or in the delivery of home care on a recurring basis to a lung disease patient. As mentioned above, we are sexual beings as males or females, and thus cannot divorce sexuality from our interpersonal relationships. Male and female caregivers may act differently with male patients than with female patients. The difference in these interactions is not necessarily good or bad, but it is important that the caregiver be aware of how sexuality can have a negative impact on these relationships from time to time.

It is quite natural that a caregiver might be sexually attracted to a patient. There are many people in the world who are beautiful in mind, body, and soul, and it is natural that we might be sexually attracted to them. These feelings are neither right nor wrong; they simply exist. However, we must recognize our sexual feelings and deal with them if they interfere with the professional nature of our relationship. We are told to be loving and caring individuals, and at the same time we are expected to be scientifically objective. This combination is difficult. We must compromise each of these goals in some way. If we are to be successful caregivers, we must be loving and caring, but we must also be aware of our sexual feelings, needs, and desires and guard against their interfering with our roles as loving and caring health care professionals.

The relationship with our patient is unique. It has been described as a *fiduciary* relationship, that is, the patient has the trust and confidence that the caregiver will act in his or her best interest.[58] By its very nature, therefore, this relationship is asymmetric, with the patient being in a dependent and vulnerable position. The patient entrusts us with many personal and sometimes intimate aspects of his or her life, and we are obliged to preserve the patient's dignity and privacy. This ranges from how we initially address the patient to how we physically touch the patient and maintain an ongoing relationship.

As professionals, we have developed a sensitivity to calling the patient by his or her proper name and avoid the use of familiar and often insulting labels. We have also learned about respecting the patient's "personal space" and about assessing when and how it is appropriate to touch the patient, either in the process of physical examination or in social touching. Touch is an important part of healing in many instances, but limits and boundaries to touching do exist, and they may vary from patient to patient.[59] It may seem appropriate at times to hold the hand of a depressed patient to offer comfort and support; other patients may consider this gesture an intrusion. Our actions are generally guided by our own good sense and by the awareness of our own personal level of comfort, but the asymmetric and fiduciary nature of the relationship must be kept in mind, particularly when we may sense sexual feelings rising to the surface, either in ourselves or in our patients.

ETHICAL ISSUES IN SEXUAL HEALTH CARE

Acknowledging the impact of sexuality on our professional relationships (described earlier) brings the realization that sexual feelings by either the caregiver or the patient can disrupt and alter the goals of the professional relationship. This leads to a number of concerns regarding medical ethics. The caregiver may inadvertently or sometimes consciously become involved in circumstances with a patient that might be termed "boundary violations," which implies that the professional nature of the relationship has been breached. The "violations" by either the caregiver or the patient may be at times seemingly innocent and perhaps trivial—such as an inappropriate word or unwelcome familiarity—and simply be excused as a brief intrusion into the privacy of either the caregiver or the patient. On the other hand, more significant violations can occur; if not corrected, they can lead to complete disruption of the relationship and sometimes become associated with charges of impropriety or ethical misconduct.

Most health care professionals have had little or no training on how to identify and avoid or correct sexually oriented disruptions in the professional relationship. Those in the field of psychiatry and related professions who become involved in long-term counseling have been the most vocal in addressing these issues. We can learn from their experiences as they apply to the field of pulmonary rehabilitation and respiratory care.

Seductive Behavior

The caregiver may sometimes find that a patient exhibits behavior that is sexually seductive and he or she may be at a loss as to how to respond, except for the instinctual urge to turn and run. Such seductive behavior may be subtle and may actually be innocent, such as a wink of the eye, a touch on the hand, or other behavior of the patient that makes the caregiver feel that the patient is crossing the professional boundary, causing the caregiver to feel uncomfortable. On the other hand, the behavior may be rather obvious, such as the male patient exposing his genitals to the female caregiver who enters the hospital room or the female patient whose manner of dress becomes progressively seductive while interacting over time with a male caregiver. Regardless of the intent of the behavior, its sexual content is disruptive to the relationship and needs to be recognized and perhaps addressed, depending on the nature of the behavior.[58]

At times, the caregiver may sense a sexual attraction to the patient, which by itself is neither right nor wrong but which clearly must be recognized by the caregiver and suppressed. Sexual feelings are natural and spontaneous in each of us and should be recognized for what they are, that is, simply feelings. Acting on those feelings, on the other hand, is inappropriate and unethical. Seductive behavior by a patient to a vulnerable caregiver is understandably a formula for disaster for both individuals.

The caregiver should try to analyze and interpret the motivation for the patient's behavior. Is it expressing a truly sexual need or physical urge, or is the patient lonely and depressed and craving personal attention? Is the patient utilizing this inappropriate behavior in an attempt to fulfill those needs? Perhaps the behavior is merely representative of the patient's personality, that is, he or she might be flirtatious or a sexual "tease" by nature. On the other hand, the behavior may represent the patient's attempt to control the relationship by manipulating the caregiver's feelings. Under these circumstances, the caregiver should suppress the urge to "play along," however tantalizing it might appear. It is important to realize that the patient is responding to the relationship with the caregiver, not to the caregiver as an individual. It is at this point that the caregiver should identify what it is in his or her own behavior that may be generating sexual attraction in the patient.

If possible, the caregiver should try to preserve the relationship unless the behavior is totally disruptive. Suggestions for this are listed in Table 28-12.[58] It is important to reaffirm the professional nature of the relationship. Words or touches by the patient that are blatantly sexual must be addressed, and it must be pointed out to the patient that such liberties are not acceptable. The male patient who exposes his genitals during the female caregiver's visit to his hospital room should be told to cover up and that such actions are not welcomed and make the caregiver uncomfortable. More subtle behavior by the patient may be more difficult to address. The situation may be resolved simply by refocusing the relationship and pointing out to the patient that the behavior suggests that his or her feelings for the caregiver may be other than professional.

It is important to preserve the patient's self-esteem by acknowledging and affirming his or her sexuality. The patient may feel sickly and unattractive and fear that the caregiver looks on him or her with pity or disgust. A negative response by the caregiver would then confirm the patient's sense of low self-worth. The caregiver should try not to focus on the actual behavior but rather on the reason for the behavior. At times, unfortunately, the professional nature of the relationship is beyond repair and this relationship must be severed. In such a case, the caregiver transfers the patient to the care of another, if possible. It is wise that the caregiver discuss this problem with the rehabilitation team or an appropriate supervisor.

TABLE 28-12. POTENTIAL RESPONSES TO A SEDUCTIVE PATIENT

Do not play along
Identify motive (tease versus hysteric versus control)
Indicate your discomfort
Reaffirm professional nature of relationship
Preserve patient's self-esteem
Acknowledge patient's sexuality
Address patient's emotional needs
Transfer patient to other caregiver, if necessary

Sexual Bias

Another sexual issue that may impact negatively on the caregiver-patient relationship is a pre-existing sexual bias. As discussions concerning sexuality ensue in a pulmonary rehabilitation program, the caregiver may learn of sexual behavior or sexual preferences of the patient that the caregiver finds personally unacceptable (e.g., the patient is "different from me"). Learning about a patient's homosexual preference, for example, may activate a sexual bias in the caregiver who feels that homosexual behavior is morally wrong or somehow abnormal. As has been stated many times, feelings about sexuality are an integral part of our personality. The rightness or wrongness of a sexual bias is not the subject of this discussion. Rather, it is important that the caregiver recognize a personal sexual bias and take precautions that it does not interfere with the professional relationship.

This re-emphasizes the importance of preparing for patient encounters by examining one's feelings and attitudes about sexuality and sexual behavior and by coming to grips with one's own sexual values and levels of comfort. It is not our place to make value judgments about the sexual preferences or behavior of our patients unless we feel that the behavior is harmful to the patient or to others. Even though we may avoid making any comments to the patient, we must also guard against sending nonverbal messages of disapproval, such as through the look on our face or our body language, or by how we choose to continue the discussion. We may not agree with the patient's choices, but we must accept them and work to accept the patient unconditionally as a person.

Sexual Abuse

Our interactions with patients may reveal evidence or generate suspicion of sexual abuse of the patient. This most commonly involves individuals who are dependent on others for their care and support (e.g., children and the elderly). All health care professionals are legally required in most states to report suspected incidents of abuse and neglect, and legal immunity is provided for those making such reports. Victims of such abuse would seem to be unlikely participants in a pulmonary rehabilitation program, but this depends on the age and nature of the population that the program is serving.

The sexual abuse of children is a major problem in the United States, and we must be knowledgeable of the behavioral and physical signs that may indicate that such abuse is taking place.[61] This is particularly important in caregivers who serve children and young adults. Although we often think of sexual abuse as occurring mainly in children, the caregiver must also consider whether elderly patients have been abused sexually. Most commonly, the patient who has been abused will be an elderly woman who has lost her spouse and who is physically or mentally dependent on another person for care. Often the abused person will be unwilling to talk about the abusive incidents because he or she is afraid that the abuser will find out and that the abuse will worsen. The caregiver is obliged to protect the patient from injury and thus should be familiar with the necessary steps to obtain protection or to seek appropriate professional resources.

Sexual Interactions

It is difficult for a caregiver to know how to respond when a patient expresses attraction or "makes a pass" at him or her. The initial reaction is often one of flattery, the caregiver feeling pleased that the patient has found him or her to be attractive. However, it is important to focus on the nature of the relationship. The patient's response may appear genuine, but it is more commonly an expression of *transference*.[58] This is a behavioral phenomenon first identified by Freud, who noted that patients displace previous experiences, behavior, and emotions onto the caregiver. This can be a source of confusion for both the patient and the caregiver. Transference is not necessarily pathologic or sexual, but it can be either or both. Regardless of its nature, it must be recognized and understood by the caregiver and be addressed when the behavior oversteps the boundary limitations of the relationship.

It is understandable that patients may confuse their feelings toward the caregiver with feelings that may have been expressed to others in intimate relationships in the past. The patient may feel lonely and unloved and sense that the caregiver is beginning to fill those needs. After all, our professional behavior is to focus on the patient as a person, giving him or her our attention and addressing his or her needs and desires. Our actions tell the patient that we think that he or she is a special person and worthy of our attention; the patient may feel the desire to respond to that attention, even though that desire is misguided.

Countertransference is the caregiver's return response to the patient. Again, such interaction is not necessarily bad and can sometimes act to cement the relationship (e.g., talking about things the caregiver and patient may have in common, such as love of movies, theater, and books). Such discussions make the patient and caregiver feel more familiar and thus more comfortable with each other. On the other hand, sexual transference and countertransference are generally disruptive. In these circumstances, the caregiver must be reminded of the asymmetric nature of the relationship and of the fact that the patient is vulnerable and at risk for exploitation. Any encouragement that the caregiver gives to the patient's expression of sexual interest is a violation of the trust that the patient has placed in the relationship, with the patient suffering the consequences of the breach of that trust. Even if the patient continues to pursue the caregiver and appears to consent to an ongoing sexual relationship, many would argue that the initial fiduciary basis for the relationship prevents any true consent from occurring.[63] As a result, sexual interactions between caregiver and patient, particularly sexual intercourse, are unethical.[64]

SUMMARY

Sexuality is an integral and, at times, an important part of the human experience. It contributes to our understanding of ourselves as individuals and colors our interactions with others. Chronic illness has an impact on persons and thus impacts on their sexuality. As health care professionals, we must come to know and understand how chronic lung diseases can influence our patient's self-image as a man or woman and how it might influence and possibly impair their sexual interactions with others. In order to fulfill these responsibilities, we must assess our knowledge of sexuality and sexual functioning and examine our own attitudes about this intimate and often emotion-laden subject. If we are to minister to our patient's needs, we must first come to grips with any negative attitudes we have about sexuality, as they are likely to influence our interactions with our patients.

Within the context of a pulmonary rehabilitation program, creating opportunities for discussions about sexuality is likely to bring positive results. At the very least, the patient will be better informed. This is likely to result in decreased fear and anxiety concerning sexual matters and lead to a more accepting and permissive attitude about sexuality and the potential impact of a breathing disorder. This can lead to an improved self-esteem, which opens the door to improved communication within relationships. The end result may be increased sexual activity, if that is the patient's desire.[65]

It is clear that our role is not to preach about sex and sexuality but to support and encourage those who are struggling with their feelings. Our concerns are not necessarily the concerns of the patient, and we must be cautious of being too zealous. It is best to create the opportunity and then follow the patient's lead. In brief, as health care professionals, we must be prepared, be available, be responsive, and, whenever possible, be useful.

REFERENCES

1. Petty TL. Health, sex and better quality of life for your COPD patient. Med Aspects Human Sex 1986; August:70–85.
2. Petty TL. Pulmonary Rehabilitation: Basics of RD. Vol 4. New York: American Thoracic Society, 1975, pp 1–6.
3. Hanson EI. Effects of chronic lung disease on life in general and on sexuality. Heart Lung 1982; 11:435–441.
4. Kipling R. The Ballad of East and West. 1889. In: Bartlett J. Familiar Quotations. Boston: Little, Brown & Co., Inc., 1968, p 872b.
5. World Health Organization. Education and treatment in human sexuality: The training of health professionals. Geneva: World Health Organization Technical Reports, Series 572, 1975.
6. Calderone MS. Sexual problems in medical practice. J Am Med Wom Assoc 1968; 23:140–146.

7. Schover LR, Jensen SB. Sexuality and chronic illness: An integrative model. In: Schover LR, Jensen SB (eds). Sexuality and Chronic Illness. New York: The Guilford Press, 1988, pp 3–13.
8. Munjack DJ, Oziel LJ. Sexual Medicine and Counseling in Office Practice: A Comprehensive Treatment Guide. Boston: Little, Brown & Co., Inc., 1980, p 203.
9. Thienhaus OJ. Practical overview of sexual function and advancing age. Geriatrics 1988; 43:63–67.
10. Brecher EM. Love, Sex, and Aging. Boston: Little, Brown & Co., Inc., 1984.
11. Brecher EM. Love, Sex, and Aging. Boston: Little, Brown & Co., Inc., 1984, pp 330–331.
12. Brecher EM. Love, Sex, and Aging. Boston: Little, Brown & Co., Inc., 1984, pp 313–315.
13. U.S. Bureau of the Census. Statistical Abstract of the United States: 1987. 107th ed., Washington, DC: 1986, p 39.
14. Conine TA, Evans JH. Sexual reactivation of chronically ill and disabled adults. J Allied Health 1982; 11:261–270.
15. Fox LS, Light R. Physiological correlates of sexual performance capacity in the male pulmonary patient. Annual Meeting, American Thoracic Society. New York: American Lung Association, 1982.
16. Fletcher EC, Martin RJ. Sexual dysfunction and erectile impotence in chronic obstructive pulmonary disease. Chest 1982; 81:413–421.
17. Levine SB, Stern RC. Sexual function in cystic fibrosis. Chest 1982; 81:422–428.
18. Thompson WL. Sexual problems in chronic respiratory disease. Postgrad Med 1986; 17:41–52.
19. McSweeny AJ, Grant I, Heaton RK, et al. Life quality of patients with chronic obstructive pulmonary disease. Arch Intern Med 1982; 142:473–478.
20. Wise TN. Sexual dysfunction in the medically ill. Psychosomatics 1983; 24:787–805.
21. Frank E, Anderson C, Rubinstein D. Frequency of sexual dysfunction in "normal" couples. N Engl J Med 1978; 299:111–115.
22. Kolodny RC, Masters WH, Johnson VE. Textbook of Sexual Medicine. Boston: Little, Brown & Co., Inc., 1979.
23. Lief HI (ed). Sexual Problems in Medical Practice. Monroe, Wisconsin: American Medical Association, 1981.
24. Schover LR, Jensen SB. Sexuality and chronic illness: An integrative model. In: Schover LR, Jensen SB (eds). Sexuality and Chronic Illness. New York: The Guilford Press, 1988, pp 293–306.
25. Conine TA, Evans JH. Sexual adjustment in chronic obstructive pulmonary disease. Respir Care 1981; 26:871–874.
26. Francoeur RT. Sexual components in respiratory care. Respir Management 1988; March-April:35–39.
27. Annon JS. Brief therapy. In: Annon JS (ed). The Behavioral Treatment of Sexual Problems. Vol 1. Honolulu: Enabling Systems, 1974.
28. Kravetz HM, Weiss M, Meadows R. Sexual counseling for the male pulmonary patient (slide-tape program). Prescott AZ, Kravetz HM (eds), 1980.
29. Kravetz HM. A visit with Harry (slide-tape program). Prescott AZ, Kravetz HM (eds), 1981.
30. Kravetz HM. A visit with Helen (slide-tape program). Prescott AZ, Kravetz HM (eds), 1982.
31. Kennedy E. Sexual Counseling: A Practical Guide for Those Who Help Others. New York: Continuum Publishing Co., 1989.
32. Croft LH. Sexuality in Later Life: A Counseling Guide for Physicians. Boston: John Wright, 1982.
33. Schover LR, Jensen SB. Couple therapy and the integrative model. In: Schover LR, Jensen SB (eds). Sexuality and Chronic Illness. New York: Guilford Press, 1988, pp 14–35.
34. Schover LR, Jensen SB. Couple therapy and the integrative model. In: Schover LR, Jensen SB (eds). Sexuality and Chronic Illness. New York: Guilford Press, 1988, p 18.
35. Schover LR, Jensen SB. Couple therapy and the integrative model. In: Schover LR, Jensen SB (eds). Sexuality and Chronic Illness. New York: Guilford Press, 1988, pp 18–32.
36. Ende J, Rockwell S, Glasgow M. The sexual history in general medicine practice. Arch Intern Med 1984; 144:558–561.
37. Selecky PA. Sexuality and Chronic Breathing Problems. Santa Ana, California: American Lung Association of Orange County, 1989.
38. Eckert RC, Bartsch K, Dowell D, et al. Being Close. Denver: National Jewish Hospital/National Asthma Center, 1984.
39. Hossler CJ, Cole SS. Intimacy and Chronic Lung Disease. Ann Arbor: University of Michigan, 1983.
40. Hahn K. Sexuality and COPD. Rehabil Nurs 1989; 14:191–195.
41. Brecher EM. Love, Sex, and Aging. Boston: Little, Brown & Co., Inc., 1984, pp 318–336.
42. Mooradian AD, Greiff V. Sexuality in older women. Arch Intern Med 1990; 150:1033–1038.
43. Butler RN, Lewis MI. Love and Sex After Sixty: A Guide for Men and Women for Their Later Years. New York: Perennial Publications, 1976.
44. Nebraska Projects, University of Nebraska—Lincoln. Sexuality and aging (videotape). Lincoln, Nebraska: Great Plains National, 1987.
45. Croag SH, Levine S, Sudilovsky A, et al. Sexual symptoms in hypertensive patients. Arch Intern Med 1988; 148:788–794.
46. The Medical Letter. Drugs that cause sexual dysfunction. Med Lett 1980; 22:108–110.
47. Arsdalen KN, Wein AJ. Drug-induced sexual dysfunction in older men. Geriatrics 1984; 39:63–70.
48. Guillemenault C. Clinical features and evaluation of obstructive sleep apnea. In: Kryger MH, Roth T, Dement WC (eds). Principles and Practice of Sleep Medicine. Philadelphia: W. B. Saunders Co., 1989, pp 552–558.
49. Kolman PBR. Sexual dysfunction and the post-myocardial infarction patient. J Cardiac Rehabil 1984; 4:335–340.
50. Bohlen JG, Held JP, Sanderson MO, Patterson RP. Heart rate, rate-pressure product, and oxygen uptake during four sexual activities. Arch Intern Med 1984; 144:1745–1748.
51. Romano MD. Sexuality and the disabled female. Accent Living 1973; 18:28–29.
52. Della Bella L. Sexuality and the pulmonary patient. In: Hodgkin JE, Zorn EG, Connors GL (eds). Pulmonary Rehabilitation. Boston: Butterworth's, 1984, pp 239–262.
53. Cooke M. Evaluation of impotence. West J Med 1986; 145:106–110.
54. Slag MF, Morley JE, Elson MK, et al. Impotence in medical clinic outpatients. JAMA 1983; 249:1736–1740.
55. Pressman MR, DiPhillipo MA, Kendrick JI, et al. Problems in the interpretation of nocturnal penile tumescence studies: Disruption of sleep by occult sleep disorders. J Urol 1986; 136:595–598.
56. Kaiser FE. Sexuality and impotence in the aging man. Clin Geriatr Med 1991; 7:63–72.
57. Morley JE. Impotence. Am J Med 1986; 80:897–905.
58. Selecky PA. Sexuality in respiratory care. In: Pierson DJ, Kacmarek R (eds). Foundations of Respiratory Care. New York: Churchill Livingstone, Inc., 1992, pp 1237–1246.
59. Ebersole P, Hess P. Touch, intimacy, and sexuality. In: Toward Healthy Aging. St. Louis: C. V. Mosby Co., 1985, pp 481–497.
60. Kennedy E. Sexual Counseling: A Practical Guide for Those Who Help Others. New York: Continuum Publishing Co., 1989, pp 34–39.
61. Council on Scientific Affairs. AMA diagnostic and treatment guidelines concerning child abuse and neglect. JAMA 1985; 254:796–800.
62. Kallman H. Detecting abuse in the elderly. Med Aspects Human Sex 1987; March:89–99.
63. Kennedy E. Sexual Counseling: A Practical Guide for Those Who Help Others. New York: Continuum, 1989, pp 63–72.
64. American Psychiatric Association. The Principles of Medical Ethics with Annotations Especially Applicable to Psychiatry. Washington, DC: American Psychiatric Association Press, 1985.
65. White CB, Catania JA. Psychoeducational intervention for sexuality with the aged, family members of the aged, and people who work with the aged. Int J Aging Hum Dev 1982; 15:121–138.

Chapter 29

Chronic Obstructive Pulmonary Disease: Treatment of Advanced Stages of Disease

THOMAS L. PETTY, M.D.

The course and prognosis of chronic obstructive pulmonary disease (COPD) have changed during the past 25 years. Several important advances in respiratory care technologies and their application have led to improved survival and a better quality of life, even in the setting of chronic and irreversible airflow obstruction. Ventilatory management of acute respiratory failure can lead to recovery in as many as 80% of selected patients.[1] However, the long-term survival of such individuals is not very good. Figure 29–1 presents survival data on 48 consecutive patients who were managed with mechanical ventilation for the first episode of acute respiratory failure in our Denver, Colorado, pulmonary care unit.[2] These data have been previously reported.[2] More contemporary data on outcomes with mechanical ventilation in COPD are not available. In addition, the so-called conservative management of acute respiratory failure that consists of the controlled administration of low-flow oxygen[3,4] and the use of antibiotics (because of the high likelihood of a bacterial component for exacerbations of COPD), methylxanthines (to improve respiratory muscle function), and corticosteroids (to improve airflow) results in an excellent hospital survival (94%)[5] and posthospital survival at 2 years (76%).[6] Thus, the occurrence of acute respiratory failure in COPD does not necessarily mean that further outcome will be dismal.

In addition, both the Nocturnal Oxygen Therapy Trial[7] and the British Medical Research Council Study[8] have shown that oxygen can improve survival in chronic stable patients with hypoxemia. It was shown that some oxygen delivered from a stationary source, including during the hours of sleep, was better than no oxygen at all. However, the best survival rates occurred in patients who received almost continuous ambulatory oxygen therapy using a portable system (see Chapter 15, Fig. 15–1). Accordingly, there is no question that the late and life-threatening course of COPD can be improved by mechanical ventilation and long-term home oxygen therapy.

ADVANCED CHRONIC OBSTRUCTIVE PULMONARY DISEASE DEFINED

The severity of COPD is gauged by simple measures of airflow, most notably the forced expiratory volume in 1 second (FEV_1). Most patients become symptomatic with an FEV_1 of 1.5 L or less, depending on their age and activity level. On average, patients older than 60 years of age with an FEV_1 of approximately 1.0 to 1.2 L/sec have a 5-year survival rate of 50 to 60%. Patients with carbon dioxide retention and those requiring home oxygen are often considered to have advanced disease. However, the prognosis for both longevity and an excellent quality of life is much better for patients in this category than has been previously thought. Much of the improvement in length and quality of life can be attrib-

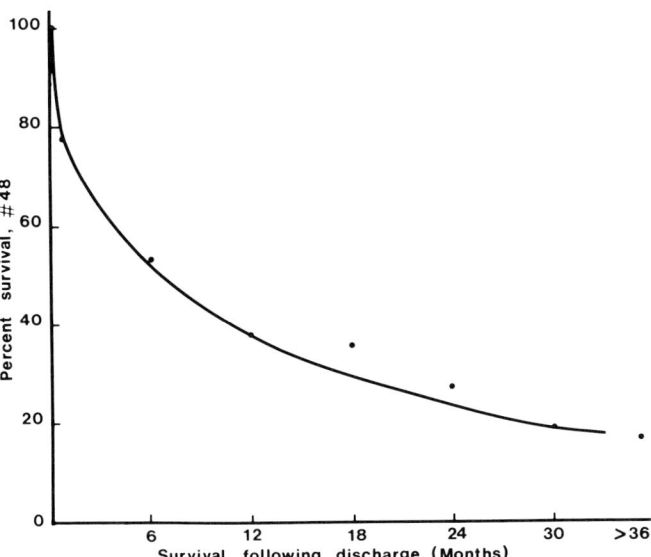

FIGURE 29–1. Survival rate (in per cent) for 48 consecutive patients managed with intubation and mechanical ventilation for the first episode of acute respiratory failure at University Hospital, Denver, CO. (From Petty TL. Acute respiratory failure in chronic obstructive pulmonary disease. In: Shoemaker WC, Ayres S, Grenvik A, et al. (eds). Textbook of Critical Care. 2nd ed. Philadelphia: W. B. Saunders Co., 1989, p 565.)

uted to pulmonary rehabilitation programs and their support groups, the continued dedication of physicians, respiratory therapists, and nurses, and the home health care industry; together they have helped patients cope successfully with advanced stages of COPD.

PHARMACOLOGIC THERAPY

Beta Agonists

Virtually all patients with advanced pulmonary disease continue to benefit from the use of inhaled beta agonists. Often, these individuals use their metered dose inhalers 20 or more times per day. This is appropriate because it is the peak effect rather than duration of the pharmacologic response that provides relief. Since the peak effect of inhaled beta agonists lasts only 1 to 2 hours, it is quite reasonable for patients to use their metered dose inhalers once or twice every 1 to 2 hours. Most of these individuals have learned this on their own.

Anticholinergics

Anticholinergics appear to be even more effective bronchodilators than inhaled beta agonists in patients with advanced stages of pulmonary disease.[9, 10] However, their onset of action is somewhat more delayed. In contrast, the duration of action of the inhaled anticholinergics is somewhat longer. Many patients use both an inhaled beta agonist and an anticholinergic (e.g., ipratropium [Atrovent]) to provide a small but clinically significant improvement in airflow throughout the day.

Theophyllines

Theophyllines remain useful in some patients probably because of their beneficial effect on respiratory muscle function.[11] Thus, if theophyllines are tolerated in terms of the gastrointestinal symptoms and the cardiac arrhythmias they can produce, they should continue to be used at a modest dose to achieve a blood level of approximately 8 to 12 µg/ml. Once-per-day theophyllines are most practical when used at bedtime. Patients are taught to keep their nighttime dose of 24-hour theophylline with their toothbrush so that they can remember to take it once per day.

Corticosteroids

Corticosteroids also continue to remain the mainstay of management for patients with advanced COPD. For some reason, whatever inflammatory processes are still operative in very advanced stages of disease can be at least partly reversed or controlled with corticosteroids. Inhaled corticosteroids seem to be less effective than oral preparations. Single maintenance doses of 10 to 20 mg of prednisone administered on a morning dosing schedule are most practical. It is recognized that long-term side effects of steroids occur in many patients, particularly in women. However, the global benefit of corticosteroids in terms of improved airflow, which results in a better quality of life, commonly outweighs the long-term side effects of osteopenia, eye complications, atrophic skin changes, and other less common manifestations of long-term steroid toxicity. Whether corticosteroids can slow the rate of decline in pulmonary function in advanced stages of disease and help prevent the progression of moderately advanced to advanced disease has been questioned. Some uncontrolled studies suggest that this may be the case.[12, 13]

BLUNTING DYSPNEA

Dyspnea with almost any activity occurs in the most advanced stages of pulmonary disease. Breathing training and physical conditioning (described in other chapters of this book) are useful in dealing with dyspnea. Many patients can be "trained through" their dyspnea with graded exercises and continued daily activity. It is important for daily walks to take place once or twice per day. Walks can be taken both inside and outside the home. During cold weather, exercising within heated shopping malls has become a popular morning routine for many patients. Pharmacologic agents can also be used to blunt dyspnea. Low doses of narcotics in the form of codeine have been shown to improve dyspnea in selected patients with advanced COPD.[14] Benzodiazepine tranquilizers may have a similar effect.[15] One review presents information about other pharmacologic agents that have been used to reduce the impact of dyspnea in chronic respiratory insufficiency.[16] One should not be concerned about creating slow carbon dioxide retention by blunting respiratory drives. In fact, it is this mechanism that the "wisdom of the body" employs in some patients. Chronic compensation carbon dioxide retention occurs in some individuals who are receiving home oxygen therapy. The appropriate generation and reclamation of bicarbonate can result in a normal pH in states of hypercarbia in the range of 80 to 100 mm Hg. The long-term survival of such patients has been reported.[17] Living for 1 to 2 years with a chronic compensated carbon dioxide pressure greater than 80 mm Hg is well documented.[17] When chronic compensation carbon dioxide retention can be achieved, pH and carbon dioxide homeostasis occurs at a very low level of minute ventilation. Often, this can be translated into a reduced work of breathing and, thus, less dyspnea.

Higher flows of oxygen are often required in advanced stages of disease. This should not be of concern to physicians, suppliers, or those who control reimbursement. The correct dose of any drug is that which provides the desired pharmacologic effect without undue side effects.

COUNSELING

The frustrations, anxieties, and concerns about dealing with advanced COPD are innumerable. In this respect, the caring physician, therapist, or nurse can play the most important role in dealing with the human aspects of illness. Frequent clinic visits are required to deal with the numerous frustrations, anxieties, and concerns of patients and their families. A "laid-back" and relaxed atmosphere appears to be salutary for many patients and their families. The use of the telephone is also helpful. Encouraging patients to call at a specific time (i.e., during "telephone hours") often minimizes abuses of the physician's time. Answering patients' letters is another valuable technique. Often, patients feel that physicians have not had enough time to listen to their concerns. It is wise for physicians to encourage patients to come to office visits with lists of questions or to ask them to write a letter when they feel that their questions have not been answered adequately during the clinic visit. Patients appreciate the time it takes for physicians to respond to their letter requests. It only takes a few minutes to answer questions that have been accumulated and set to paper over weeks, months, or years. In today's modern society of high-technology communication, we often forget the impact of the personal letter or note.

Counseling is also important in order to identify patients' expectations of the health care system in times of emergency and to determine whether or not heroic measures are expected whenever an inevitable respiratory failure appears to threaten an end to life. Our job as physicians is to prevent or forestall premature morbidity and mortality. But it is not and never will be our job to extend suffering and death. Accordingly, when a patient's life is at best miserable, and further attempts at the use of high-technology care are futile, it is this author's opinion that it is ethically, morally, and legally inappropriate to intervene. The President's Commission has clearly stated that there is no difference between withdrawing or withholding therapy when this decision is made jointly between mentally competent patients and physicians.[18] The right to refuse medical therapy is established by the United States Constitution and by common law.

Problems arise when there is not a clear understanding of a patient's wishes and expectations. Many physicians feel uncomfortable about discussing the inevitability of death and how it will occur and be managed. The physician should learn to be comfortable about "discussing the future." This is an acceptable concept to most patients and their families, since virtually all patients with advanced stages of COPD know that they will die of it. They often do not focus on this inevitability but they are very concerned about how they will die. Patients frequently imagine horrible scenarios about suffocating, climbing the walls, or being trapped and tethered to a mechanical ventilator. It is wise for the physician to liken the transition out of life and to death as a long, pleasant sleep. We recognize sleep as natural, peaceful, and refreshing. Fear of going to sleep should be discussed and dealt with. Some patients may sleep for many hours or even days while breathing oxygen, only to awaken feeling refreshed. In these instances, there is a "détente" with death.

At times, this period of détente may last for up to 2 years of meaningful life. The détente, of course, is followed by what I call "the long sleep." Indeed, sleep and death have been equated in literature:

"O sleep, thou ape of death, lie full upon her and be her sense but as a monument . . ."
William Shakespeare, *Cymbeline*

and

"How wonderful is death, Death and his brother, Sleep . . ."
Percy Bysshe Shelley, *Queen Mab*

When patients understand death, they often cease to have any further anxiety about the dying process. They recognize the tranquil nature of carbon dioxide-induced unconsciousness, which is probably mediated by endorphins. If nature can be so kind to our patients, why can't we?

Thus, in the final days and hours of illness, I believe that it is quite appropriate to offer narcotic relief, which includes the use of intravenous morphine. If patients rally to achieve another period of conscious life, their temporary recovery can be applauded and accepted; however, the inevitability of death is not in doubt.

It would be easy to offer numerous case examples to illustrate the important points of this chapter. However, only two are presented. The first will also appear in another publication,[19] but it is published in this book as well because of its impact on me and on the caregivers involved in the patient's final care. The other case example is also unique. It is best to recount these two examples from a personal point of view.

CASE HISTORIES

Case No. 1. RK first came to me at age 48 because of worsening cough, wheeze, and dyspnea. He had smoked extremely heavily throughout his life and had consumed the equivalent of 37 pack-years at the time he was first examined. He expressed a desire to be able to live to the age of 60 years, which would be about the time that all of his children would be grown. He followed every detail of my medical advice and counseling, including my recommendation to stop smoking and to systematically use bronchodilating agents. Since he was responsive to corticosteroids and had marked improvement during their use, he frequently took these drugs on my advice and, at times, on his own with my permission. At age 60 years, the patient had deteriorated to the point that he was nearly housebound. At this time, he began to receive continuous oxygen therapy from a portable source via nasal cannulas. He had extremely high respiratory drives and often would use pursed-lip breathing to the extent that he could not achieve the degree of hypoxemia required for reimbursement under Medicare. That is, he would often maintain an oxygen saturation higher than 88%, but he still experienced extreme dyspnea while using pursed-lip breathing. On other occasions, while he sat quietly, his oxygen saturation would fall to 78%. The patient did improve when he received oxygen during physical reconditioning training as part of a pulmonary rehabilitation program. Later, however, dyspnea became intolerable. At this point, I prescribed codeine, 32 mg to be taken every 4 hours, and also as needed to help blunt dyspnea. This was only modestly effective. The patient freely used inhaled beta agonists and anticholinergics and required increasingly high doses of corticosteroids. Two compression fractures occurred during the patient's last year of life. In an attempt to extend the patient's oxygen use and because of nasal complications, he received a transtracheal oxygen catheter,[20] which he believed helped relieve his dyspnea. Full pharmacologic management and oxygen therapy via transtracheal catheter were maintained until dyspnea became overwhelming. At this point, he requested a prescription of 40 100-mg secobarbital (Seconal) tablets, which he had read would be a lethal dose should he ever decide to take the entire prescription. He wanted a method of "getting out" if he wished, as well as control of this decision. I gave him the prescription after full discussions with his wife. At the time that a living will was signed, his wife was given durable power of attorney to help carry out the patient's wishes in the event that he would become incompetent and thus unable to express his wishes about further treatment. However, he never did take the entire secobarbital prescription at once; on occasion, he did take individual capsules when overwhelming nocturnal anxiety and insomnia were present. He reported that it was a great comfort to have the medication available in case he wanted or needed it. Finally, the patient deteriorated to the point where he could not leave his house. Still later, he could not leave his room or even get dressed without involuntarily urinating. He was miserable. Accordingly, he called me and asked to be admitted to the hospital to receive intravenous morphine and to discontinue his oxygen therapy. He felt his wife could not deal with his dying at home. It was agreed that he would be admitted to the hospital unit that cares for terminal cancer patients. In this setting, it is commonplace to give sufficient morphine by intravenous administration to provide comfort. The patient's family was in general agreement, but a son-in-law struggled with anxiety about what he viewed as euthanasia. It was clearly explained that relieving patients' suffering is something quite different from euthanasia.

The patient became hungry on his last day of life. He had an abundant breakfast consisting of scrambled eggs, bacon, and hash browns, all with salt (which had previously been restricted in his diet because of right-sided heart failure). Later that day, he wanted to watch a professional football game one more time. During the game, he ordered a prime rib of beef with plenty of salt. He was jovial because he was surrounded by his family and me. He was receiving intravenous morphine at this time. He and his family also enjoyed a bottle of excellent wine with their meal. Casual observers could not believe that he was a dying man. After the meal and following the advice of the family, the patient stopped his oxygen flow and went to sleep. However, there was much anxiety on the part of the nursing support staff, who felt that stopping oxygen therapy was inappropriate. Indeed, they almost always used oxygen for the care and comfort of terminal cancer patients. Finally, I had to write an order to discontinue oxygen, and the patient died quietly while receiving morphine. This case was discussed before the hospital's ethics committee; all members were in unanimous agreement that his care was proper.

This case illustrates many of the problems faced by those who care for terminally ill patients. The patient died at age 63.5 years, which was longer than predicted or expected when I first saw him. His quality of life was excellent at first and at least tolerable until his last year. Even his last few days of life were meaningful because of the discussions he could have with his family, the saying of goodbyes, and the offering of forgiveness for past transgressions.

Medical care is designed to relieve suffering as well as to promote health, happiness, and longevity. These principles must always be kept in mind as we strive to serve our patients' best interests.

Case No. 2. IK is an extremely successful businessman. He originally came to me at the age of 70 years because he wanted to have a second opinion about his care and prognosis. This patient had seen an excellent pulmonologist 2 years earlier. The pulmonologist had provided state-of-the-art treatment and, on request, offered his opinion that the patient's survival would only

TABLE 29-1. SERIAL PULMONARY FUNCTION TESTS: CASE HISTORY NO. 2*

	Age 70		Age 71		Age 72				Age 73		Age 75+	
	Before BD	After BD	Before BD†	After BD†	Before BD‡	After BD‡	Before BD‡	After Beta Agonists and Ipratropium‡	Before BD‡	After Beta Agonists‡	After Beta Agonists‡	After Ipratropium‡
FVC (L)	1.52	1.99	2.18	2.22	1.35	1.41	2.08	2.59	2.01	2.78	2.45	2.16
FEV₁ (L)	0.54	0.70	0.63	0.75	0.43	0.55	0.70	0.86	0.62	0.71	0.76	0.35
DLCO (ml/min/mm Hg)	9.5		11									

*Performed using a hand-held spirometer, which underestimates low flows.
†After steroid use.
‡Steroid use continued.
Key: BD: bronchodilators; FVC: forced vital capacity; FEV₁: forced expiratory volume in 1 second; DLCO: carbon monoxide diffusing capacity.

be approximately 2 years. "The two years are up," the patient said at the time of his initial consultation with me. On this occasion, he was accompanied by his son and wife. It was obvious that an excellent family support system was present. History revealed a lifetime of smoking that had ended 8 years before following an acute myocardial infarction. He also had long-standing diabetes, which was partly controlled by oral hypoglycemic agents. Physical examination revealed a highly intelligent man in a good state of nutritional health. He had mild hypertension, a blood pressure of 140/90 mm Hg, marked hyperinflation with decreased breath sounds, and no signs of pulmonary hypertension. Serum parameters were normal except for a randomly obtained blood glucose level of 180 mg%. Serial spirometric pulmonary functions are cited in Table 29–1. Recent blood gas determinations obtained by his internist at my request are listed in Table 29–2. Severe airflow with minimum response to bronchodilators was evident. An abnormal diffusion test indicated emphysema. The patient was given a trial of corticosteroids, 40 mg per day each morning for 2 weeks. During this time, in spite of the mild hypertension and worsening chemical diabetes, the patient experienced significant clinical improvement. When he returned for follow-up, there was objective evidence of a small response to the corticosteroids. Accordingly, their use was continued in varying doses to the present time (usually 15–20 mg prednisone each morning). In addition, he was taught to use a metered dose inhaler on every occasion of dyspnea. His worsened chemical diabetes, aggravated by the use of corticosteroids, was managed with increasing doses of oral hypoglycemic agents. Within 1 year, it was necessary for the patient to begin oxygen use at night to manage nocturnal dyspnea and insomnia. Nocturnal oxygen was helpful at first. After 2 years, it was necessary for the patient to receive continuous ambulatory oxygen therapy in order to be able to function in his job. It also became difficult for the patient to come to Denver because of the high altitude. Accordingly, I began to provide management by telephone and mail in conjunction with the patient's local internist. At approximately 3- to 4-month intervals, it was possible for me to see the patient near sea level during my various travels. Examinations and consultations took place in a hotel room near an airport. On one occasion, I visited the patient's home upon the request of both the patient and his family. All were concerned that the end of his life was near. This visit was almost 2 years before the time of this writing. In the meantime, the patient achieved his 77th birthday and welcomed his first grandson into the world. He continues to be a successful executive despite extremely severe physiologic impairment. He is able to get from his house to his place of business with the assistance of a wheelchair and aided by his wife. The social support system provided by his family is outstanding and unusual. Equally outstanding and somewhat unusual is this patient's "keep on keepin' on" attitude. Intelligence and social support become the final driving forces for long-term survival in many patients with extreme degrees of disease.

I have personally cared for many such individuals who live into their late 70s and early 80s with relative comfort and with the feeling of accomplishment that success brings.

TABLE 29-2. ARTERIAL BLOOD GAS VALUES

	Age		
	74 Yr	75 Yr	75.5 Yr
Po₂ (mm Hg)	58*	50*	55†
Pco₂ (mm Hg)	51	62	89
pH	7.43	7.41	7.33
HCO₃ level (mEq/L)	34	39	40

*Breathing O₂ at 3 L.
†Breathing O₂ at 3.5 L.

REFERENCES

1. Petty TL, Lakshminarayan S, Sahn S, et al. Intensive respiratory care unit: Review of ten years' experience. JAMA 1975; 233:34–37.
2. Petty TL. Chronic airflow limitation. In: Petty TL (ed). Intensive and Rehabilitative Respiratory Care. 3rd ed. Philadelphia: Lea & Febiger, 1982, 222–245.
3. Cherniack RM, Hakimpour K. The rational uses of oxygen in respiratory insufficiency. JAMA 1967; 199:178–182.
4. Bigelow DB, Petty TL, Levine BE, et al. The effect of oxygen breathing on arterial blood gases in patients with chronic airway obstruction living at 5,200 feet. Am Rev Respir Dis 1967; 96:28–34.
5. Albert RK, Martin TR, Lewis SW. Controlled clinical trial of methylprednisolone in patients with chronic bronchitis and acute respiratory insufficiency. Ann Intern Med 1980; 92:753–758.
6. Martin TR, Lewis SW, Albert RK. The prognosis of patients with

chronic obstructive pulmonary disease after hospitalization for acute respiratory failure. Chest 1982; 82:310–314.
7. Nocturnal Oxygen Therapy Trial Group. Continuous or nocturnal oxygen therapy in hypoxemic chronic obstructive lung disease: A Clinical Trial. Ann Intern Med 1980; 93:391–398.
8. Report of the Medical Research Council Working Party. Long term domiciliary oxygen therapy in chronic hypoxic cor pulmonale complicating chronic bronchitis and emphysema. Lancet 1981; 1:681–686.
9. Gross NJ. Ipratropium bromide. N Engl J Med 1988; 319:486–494.
10. Braun SR, McKenzie WN, Copeland C, et al. A comparison of the effect of ipratropium and albuterol in the treatment of chronic obstructive airway disease. Arch Intern Med 1989; 149:544–547.
11. Murciano D, Aubier MH, Pariente R, et al. A randomized, controlled trial of theophylline in patients with severe chronic obstructive pulmonary disease. N Engl J Med 1989; 320:1521–1525.
12. Postma DS, Steenhuis EJ, van der Weele LH, et al. Severe chronic airflow obstruction: Can corticosteroids slow down progression? Eur J Respir Dis 1985; 67:56–64.
13. Postma DS, Peters I, Steenhuis EJ, et al. Moderately severe chronic airflow obstruction. Can corticosteroids slow down obstruction? Eur Respir J 1988; 1:22–26.
14. Woodcock AA, Gross ER, Gellert A, et al. Effects of dihydrocodeine, alcohol, and caffeine on breathlessness and exercise tolerance in patients with chronic obstructive lung disease and normal blood gases. N Engl J Med 1981; 305:1611–1616.
15. Mitchell-Heggs P, Murphy K, Minty K, et al. Diazepam in the treatment of dyspnoea in "Pink Puffer" Syndrome. Q J Med 1980; 49:9–20.
16. Stark RD. Dyspnea: Assessment and pharmacologic manipulation. Eur Respir J 1988; 1:280–287.
17. Neff TA, Petty TL. Tolerance and survival in severe chronic hypercapnia. Arch Intern Med 1972; 129:591–596.
18. President's Commission for the Study of Ethical Problems in Medicine and Biomedical and Behavioral Research: Making Health Care Decisions. Vol 1. Washington, DC. US Government Printing Office; 1982:1–196.
19. Petty TL. Ethical considerations in the case of advanced and final stages of COPD. In: Hodgkin JE, Zorn EG, Connors GL (eds). Pulmonary Rehabilitation: Guidelines to Success. Philadelphia: J.B. Lippincott Co., 1993 (in press).
20. Christopher KL, Spofford BT, Petrun MD, et al. A program for transtracheal oxygen delivery. Ann Intern Med 1987; 107:802–808.

Chapter 30

Continuing Care Programs

MARY BURNS, R.N., B.S.

Dramatic improvements can occur in the respiratory patient during the few short weeks that he or she undergoes intensive pulmonary rehabilitation (PR). Maintaining these improvements in the months and years that follow, however, is a challenge to everyone concerned with the patient's care. Some form of continuing care and encouragement is usually required for the patient to maintain an exercise program, to maintain and update his or her knowledge of the disease, and to provide for psychosocial needs.

EXERCISE

Maintaining a regular exercise regimen is often difficult for the most physically fit individuals. For the respiratorily impaired, it is even more of a struggle, but it is essential to the maintenance or improvement of these patients' physical well-being.

Ideally, after PR the patient should continue to come to maintenance exercise sessions with the same staff and in the same location as the original sessions several times per week. Since the staff already knows the patient, only minimal supervision is usually required. Good exercise regimens are maintained, reinforced, and improved. Unfortunately, PR programs often have budgetary constraints that limit the space and personnel available for continuing programs. Sometimes arrangements can be made for rehabilitation programs to share facilities with a cardiac treatment center or a wellness center. Medicare and insurance carriers usually do not reimburse for maintenance programs, so it is a challenge to price these sessions attractively. Since many patients are on fixed incomes, PR departments are also constrained by cost containment measures that are necessary in today's medical community.

If group exercise facilities are not available in the hospital setting or if the patient population is too financially limited to participate in regular maintenance programs, group walks may be a solution.

Group Walks

Patients can meet at a regular time and place and walk with or without medical supervision. Walks can take place on the hospital grounds or at a local park, if weather permits. However, air-conditioned malls are ideal for respiratory patients in all seasons. They are level and have seating areas and rest rooms.

When forming a walking group, interest and enthusiasm can be generated by making an "event" of the initial day. Even if medical staff cannot be present at all times, having them participate in the initial walk helps motivate some of the less enthusiastic patients to join in.

If you have access to a mall, the mall management is often pleased to assist by providing prizes and publicity. One of the malls in our area even marked the corridors in tenths of a mile and provided banners and a sign dedicating the specially named walking area to our respiratory patient group, the PEP Pioneers.*

Patients should be provided with exercise logs or diaries to keep track of the amount of time they walk (Fig. 30–1). The practitioner should plan to give out prizes for as many things as possible (e.g., to anyone who walks daily, to the patient who walks the longest time, and to the one who shows the most improvement). Having separate prizes for each sex makes it possible to

---

*The PEP Pioneers are graduates of the Pulmonary Education Program of Little Company of Mary Hospital in Torrance, California.

WALKING DIARY OF _____

DATE	HOUR	HEART RATE	MINUTES WALKED	HEART RATE	COMMENTS

FIGURE 30–1. An example of an exercise diary in which a patient might record the amount of time he or she walks. (From Petty T, Tiep B, Burns M, Essentials of Pulmonary Rehabilitation: A "Do It Yourself" Program. Pulmonary Education and Research Foundation. Lomita, CA, 1991, pp 6–7.)

give out two awards in each category. Another possibility is to give an award to each person who brings someone new to join the group.

Prizes can be simple, such as a gold star, or much more elaborate if the budget permits. Patients recognize that that the staff is trying to motivate them and thus get into the spirit of the walks. The names of the monthly winners should be posted in a prominent place, and annual awards should be presented.

For several years, our group engaged in a "Walk to New York" and then a "Walk Up the Coast." The rules of the walks were simple. Each month, participants turned in a record of the amount of time they walked. One half hour of walking and 15 minutes of riding a bicycle were each considered the equivalent of 1 mile. We had a large map on which we charted our patients' combined progress across the country. Each month, one of the patients researched a town we "stopped at" and wrote about it in our newsletter. He really got into the spirit of things and managed to get Mayor Ed Koch of New York to send a letter welcoming the PEP Pioneers to the "Big Apple." Getting Mayor Clint Eastwood to do the same when we symbolically reached Carmel, California, created so much excitement that even the most reluctant joined in the fun and exercise. The grand climax occurred when we finally ended our symbolic walk. We arranged for all of our hospital's senior administrators as well as the mayor of our city to welcome our group of walkers "back home" and present to them an official document that proclaimed April 17th "Welcome Back Home—PEP Walkers' Day." These proclamations are framed and hang on the walls of the rehabilitation department to inspire future participants in the PR program. It is interesting to note that of the three proclamations, it is the one from Mayor Clint Eastwood that continues to generate the most excitement.

Other Exercise Options

Another possibility for patients looking for inexpensive places to exercise in groups may be found at community colleges. In addition to access to exercise facilities, patients may be fortunate enough to receive some supervision from future physical education teachers or exercise physiologists.

Local YMCAs may be willing to offer specialized exercise classes. The YMCA in our area has reserved the outside lane of its pool for patients on oxygen. By switching to a 25- or 50-ft supply tube that attaches to their cannulas and by putting their strollers at the pool's side at the midpoint of the lane, patients on oxygen can swim as freely as anyone else and certainly float more easily.

Adult education programs offer another option. Some patients in our group and their spouses have been taking dance lessons for years, and another local patient group is forming a special dance class just for the respiratorily impaired.

PATIENT CLUBS

Maintaining and updating the patient's knowledge of his or her medications and disease process and providing psychosocial support are much easier if patients have a support group. If one is not already available for your patients, the benefits of forming such a group should be seriously considered. In addition to the benefits already mentioned, a group that meets on a regular basis can be very beneficial to the public relations of a hospital and to the physicians involved with the group as speakers. Local lung associations are pleased to be cosponsors and to send out flyers about the meetings. Some newspapers also print announcements at no charge. By forming a support group, your hospital will maintain better ties with patients, and your PR program will potentially recruit more patients. Monthly meetings are also a good way of following patients who have graduated from your rehabilitation program.

Starting a Patient Club

Some factors need to be taken into account before holding a first meeting. An easily accessible location with nearby parking is most important. If your hospital can provide valet parking on the meeting day, its effort will be more than repaid by the good will of grateful patients. If it cannot manage to provide valet parking, parking spaces should be reserved in the closest location that can be found.

Daytime meetings are much better than evening ones. Most members of respiratory patient clubs tend to be retired, but those patients who still work can occasionally come during their lunch breaks. Many of those who will attend no longer drive at night; for some, mornings can also be difficult. Mid-day or early afternoon seems to be a good time to have the group meet, especially if the guest speaker is allowed to conclude by 2:00 PM in time for afternoon office hours.

Some patient clubs meet once per month, whereas others meet weekly. A buffet lunch that is catered at cost by the hospital cafeteria may be feasible, but many groups simply provide beverages and have club members supply cookies or a cake.

Other than payment for meals or beverages, there should be no dues for belonging to a patient club. Many of the people who attend are on very restricted budgets, and any additional costs, no matter how small, may prevent their participation.

Money for the group can be raised by holding a raffle each month. Prizes can include white elephants, baked goods, homegrown fruits and vegetables, or a few dollars that are returned from the money collected. An annual holiday bazaar held in November or December can be another fund raiser. These activities, in addition to an occasional donation, can provide a treasury with a healthy balance.

Topics for monthly meetings should be subjects specifically of interest to those with respiratory problems. Asthma and prednisone are good subjects, and any meeting title that includes the word "new" guarantees full attendance. Discussions of emotional stresses that are exacerbated by respiratory disease are also always of interest. These problems can be addressed by psychologists or just discussed in open dialogue in small groups, with or without a group facilitator. In the newly formed patient club, speakers can be recruited from the PR staff. When other physicians see that a reasonably sized audience can be attracted, they are more willing to donate their time. Pharmacists, psychologists, and, on occasion, paramedics, members of police departments, or Medicare representatives are others who might be asked to speak.

Improving Established Groups

Perhaps you already have a patient club but need to stimulate more active participation. A telephone committee is invaluable in this respect for several reasons. Even the most inactive and shy patient feels able to handle a few phone calls each month. Speaking on the phone is a good way for the patient to gain confidence in the ability to help and makes him or her more willing to take on bigger tasks in the future. It also helps the patient to develop closer relationships with some of the other club members.

Limiting each person on the committee to calling 10 members on the phone list is recommended. In this way, more people become involved in assisting without the work becoming a burden for anyone. The committee phones patients the week before a meeting not only to remind them about the upcoming meeting but also to learn if they are having any health problems. The patient who is homebound or ill is usually grateful to know that someone cares. If your group is large, have each telephone committee member report to the chairperson rather than make individual calls to the PR office. The chairperson coordinates all the information; with one phone call to the PR staff, he or she can give a head count for the patient club luncheon and provide an update on any problems in the group. This is an easy way to follow patients without spending inordinate amounts of staff time.

Another easy way to get patients to be more active in your group is to ask them to sit with a new member and help make him or her feel welcome. Someone new to the group can be uncomfortable about walking into a crowd of strangers. Having someone act as a host or hostess, introduce new members to others at a table, and answer questions about rehabilitation or the patient club is very effective in ensuring the return of the first-time visitor. The member who makes the newcomer welcome in turn enjoys being able to make a contribution. If your group is large and staff time is limited, several official hosts and hostesses can be in charge of greeting the new members and seating them with someone in the group.

Getting patients to volunteer for anything is almost impossible, since almost all are afraid that they will not be physically capable of completing an assignment. The more easy tasks you can find for patients to do, the easier it is to develop in them the confidence needed to eventually accept more complicated projects.

Some of the other easy things your patients can do are help sell raffle tickets or just pick out the winning numbers. Getting someone to read out the winning numbers and the names of the patients who win can be more difficult, but it is wonderful to watch the growing self-confidence and willingness to take charge that are achieved by patients with time.

PATIENT CLUB BOARD OF DIRECTORS

As your group becomes larger, it may wish to form a board of directors to help plan future activities. Again, the spoken or unspoken fear of many patients is whether they will get sick and let everyone down. One way to overcome this reasonable concern is to have co-officers for each position. Allowing a patient's spouse to be a co-officer helps in that it includes nonrespiratory patient members on your board and encourages the family closeness that is so helpful to many patients. In theory, this means that there can be four people for each position on the board; in practice, however, this rarely occurs. Only the sickest patients feel overwhelmed by the duties of such a board. Board meetings become fun gatherings, and members rarely decline re-election. Board members also become the strongest advocates of your group and often begin to display a previously hidden talent of leadership as soon as they realize how important their contributions are.

Bylaws of the group can be as simple or as complex as desired, and many groups can function quite well without any. *Robert's Rules of Order* are probably unknown to the majority of members and are certainly not necessary to achieve an enthusiastic, functioning board.

One caveat worth mentioning is the care that must be taken in choosing the cotreasurers. Based on our past experience, it is strongly recommended that selection for that office be biased in favor of the healthier asthmatics or of those with spouses who can play a strong role.

COMMITTEES

Committees can be established according to the needs of the group. As previously discussed, a telephone committee is extremely valuable.

An historian can be in charge of a committee that keeps scrapbooks and photo albums of club events. These mementos can "get out of hand" if such a group is not started early in the club's organization, the result being the accumulation of boxes of pictures and slides that no one can identify.

A librarian might be chosen to record all guest lecturers on audio or video cassette. The cassettes can then be mailed to members who are unable to attend club meetings. A lending library of books on respiratory disease and diet is good to establish, as is a collection of joke books for members who are hospitalized.

There is usually at least one person in the group who enjoys organizing holiday bazaars and making the decorations and favors to be used in celebrating the various holidays. A "sunshine" committee also can have an important impact. This committee sends get-well cards and birthday cards to club members. Sometimes, these cards are the only ones that patients receive, as witnessed by the touching thank-you letters occasionally sent in acknowledgment.

If club members are homebound, arrangements can be made to visit them if they want company. Sometimes, a daily or weekly phone call can be made to let such members know that they are not forgotten and that friends still care. This type of caring spreads far beyond the committee and spills over into the very essence of your group. A pervasive atmosphere of continuing mutual care develops that achieves what no individual medical caregiver, no matter how dedicated, could ever attain alone. Besides displaying care and concern for members it has grown to know, the group as a whole can be counted on to help the stranger who enters the group skeptical that rehabilitation can help overcome some of the limitations imposed by respiratory disease.

On the first day of a PR program, graduates of previous programs are honored to be asked to come in and encourage new students. Their stories of life before and after PR inspire the staff and new class members alike to aim for even greater achievements.

Patients who live alone or who have unsupportive spouses find support or companionship in the clubs if they wish to take advantage of them. Sometimes, close friendships develop among members of the class who encourage each other. At other times, graduates can assist by coming to classes on a regular basis to motivate students; graduates might invite students to walk with a group in the mall or park when their exercise capacity allows it. In the meantime, graduates can assure new students of the value of pacing and of continuing to increase the duration of their exercise sessions by telling stories about how short of breath they used to be. It is very difficult for even the most withdrawn and shy patients not to respond to the caring atmosphere around them.

Our continuing care program has been quite successful. In order to maintain interpatient bonds after rehabilitation, new graduates of our program and their significant others automatically become members of the PEP Pioneers. On graduation day, they are officially made members by one of the board and given a PEP badge with their name on it, a copy of the bylaws, a roster of other members, and a complimentary pass to the first luncheon attended after graduation. At this first club meeting, they have reserved, front-row seats. After being warmly applauded as new Pioneers, a board member gives a brief biographic sketch of each, so that each new member is seen as someone special who may share unique interests with other Pioneers.

As the treasury of our patient club grew larger, members began making donations in memory of deceased members or their families. Christmas lunch for each Pioneer and his or her significant other is paid for by the club. At Christmas, the club provides a gift certificate for a year of free meals to six members whose names are selected at random. Three of these "random" selections are earmarked for needier members. In a similar manner, during the year, an anonymous member (supposedly one who is unable to attend an event) provides a free ticket for a bus trip to someone who might otherwise have been unable to go on a group excursion. In order to protect the pride of the recipient, his or her name is known only to a few of the members.

NEWSLETTERS

A newsletter can be a good marketing tool and method of maintaining the cohesiveness of a group. It can be as simple as a one-page flyer or as elaborate as *Second Wind*, which is published by the PEP Pioneers.* Since the preparation of newsletters can be very time-consuming, depending on staffing and writing skills, arrangements can sometimes be made to reprint parts of other newsletters, such as Dr. Petty's monthly letter in *Second Wind*; such a reprint might then be supplemented by local news.

Folding, taping, labeling, and sorting *Second Wind*

---

*A complimentary copy of *Second Wind* may be obtained by writing to Pulmonary Rehabilitation, Little Company of Mary Hospital, 4101 Torrance Blvd., Torrance, California 90503.

issues in preparation for mailing is one of the most popular monthly events of the PEP Pioneers. The chairperson in charge of organizing the volunteers must be sure to phone everyone on his or her list; someone who is not called to participate may feel hurt. Since it is never known when the newsletter will arrive from the printer, these phone calls are often made at the last minute; nevertheless, up to 12 people usually are able to attend, eager for the camaraderie of the paper party.

RESPIRATORY RALLY

A popular annual event in our organization is the Respiratory Rally at which patients, families, and medical staff from around southern California gather for a day of education, fun, and fellowship. Although the Rally's format has changed over the years, it usually consists of a pace race, exhibits, and entertainment and is addressed by a well-known keynote speaker who is usually flanked by a panel of other well-recognized physicians. This format has been successfully implemented in various locations such as Texas, Washington D.C., and even Belgium.

The Pace Race

"What is a 'pace race,' and how can respiratory patients possibly be part of a race?" is a question that is frequently heard. Winning the pace race is more dependent on pacing skills than on speed; thus our respiratory patients not only can take part but also usually do better than the medical personnel who compete with them. The object of the race is to estimate the time it will take to complete a very short course without shortness of breath. "Guesstimate" might be a better word than "estimate," since time is measured in hundredths of a minute. Official race timers are borrowed from the local high school track team. Eight participants compete at one time and are cheered on by respiratory therapy students and the surrounding crowd. First, second, and third place winners have their names put on a plaque, receive a certificate, and are awarded a prize.

Door prizes for the rally can be solicited from local restaurants and hotels. Pharmaceutical and durable medical equipment companies are often willing to sponsor guest speakers or to pay for a bus that is used to bring groups from a distance.

Although there may be educational benefits to be gained by listening to your keynote speaker, the emphasis of the day should be on making the rally enjoyable for everyone who attends.

TRAVEL

Often, the first goal of patients who complete a PR program is to attempt vacation plans that have been long postponed because of their physical limitations.

Guidelines for successful trips are provided to the patient during PR, and the PR staff remains a good resource for questions that may arise.

The patient who receives oxygen should also be able to rely on the expertise and guidance of his or her oxygen supplier. Detailed information on traveling with portable oxygen can be obtained in other books and articles.[1–4]

However, the physician often is the first medical caregiver to be asked for advice. Answers depend on the patient's destination, the altitude of the destination, and the length of stay in addition to the obvious concerns about the physical limitations of the patient.

A summary of the patient's history and physical examination results, including arterial blood gas and pulmonary function test results, along with the name of a physician to contact in the event of an emergency, are usually requested, as are extra prescriptions for current medications. Antibiotics and steroids for acute exacerbations of illness may also be prescribed, depending on the patient and type of trip being undertaken. Stool softeners are also good for the patient to have available. An oximetry walk for exercise evaluation may reassure the physician and patient that oxygen prescriptions are current, especially if higher altitudes are to be encountered during travel.[1]

Patients who receive oxygen need extra oxygen prescriptions and should be advised to discuss their itinerary in detail with their oxygen supplier; the oxygen supplier should make arrangements for refills in other areas. Patients need to be prepared to pay for their oxygen refills with cash or credit card rather than count on insurance. Private insurance refunds can be obtained later, but billing Medicare correctly can sometimes be a problem. Advise your patients to keep their invoices until they have been correctly reimbursed.

Although the patient's oxygen supplier should be able to handle the problems of traveling with oxygen, capability and reliability may vary from one company to another. The physician might remind the patient that liquid oxygen is not available in all areas, and when arranging for refills, it is necessary for the physician to specify the manufacturer of the oxygen supply system. It is important to note that *there are no universal adapters for oxygen systems on the market.* Our local durable medical equipment supplier, Pioneer Home Care, has developed such refill adapters for our patients to use when traveling; other suppliers in different areas may do the same. Your patient needs to find out if such a device can be taken on his or her trip.

Air travel can be complicated, since each airline has different regulations and forms for physicians to complete (often in triplicate) about patient oxygen needs at 8000 ft. Although many airlines say they require only 1 to 3 days' notice before the patient's departure, it is best to complete these forms earlier, if possible.[5,6]

Many airlines still provide oxygen via face-mask, but they do allow patients to use their own cannulas. Airline personnel are often not knowledgeable about oxygen equipment. Patients should come prepared with scissors and adapters to switch from the masks to their cannulas.

Government regulations do not allow patients to bring their own oxygen supplies on board airplanes. Because of this, those requiring continuous oxygen therapy need to make arrangements to be met by an oxygen supplier at their destination.

Group Travel

Because of the problems of traveling mentioned earlier, especially those associated with oxygen supplies, respiratory patients find group trips attractive. There are now various travel agencies and hospitals throughout the country that sponsor trips for respiratory patients at regular intervals. If this is not being done in your area, you might consider organizing your own group trips. If your patient support group is not large enough, networking with other groups in the area can be beneficial.

Bus Trips

The easiest way for patients to start traveling is by taking a 1-day bus trip. The bus should be air-conditioned and have a bathroom and a step stool to help patients when boarding. Sometimes, a signed consent form from a physician is also required. We always bring a stationary oxygen supply (donated by our local durable medical equipment supplier) for oxygen refills.

Before planning a trip, altitude changes as well as the amount and type of walking required at the final destination should be taken into consideration.

Popular trip destinations include dinner theaters and the racetrack. Although trips such as these serve as an incentive for patients to maintain their exercise capacity (we discourage the use of wheelchairs), occasional assistance is required if some patients are to accompany the group. An example of a trip during which such assistance may be needed is an outing to a racetrack. The distance from the bus to center field can be so great that it is necessary to have wheelchairs ready for some of the patients. Sometimes, a physically able spouse can assist the staff; youth volunteers might also be recruited to help. The extra work is more than worth the effort when the laughter and enjoyment shared by the group are seen and heard.

Cruises

In 1985, our group of patients went on a cruise, marking the first time that oxygen-dependent patients were allowed on board a cruise line.[7] It was such a successful event that since then, with the help of the Coast Guard,[8] many other cruises have been arranged at regular intervals.

The best way to ensure a safe and enjoyable trip for all is to plan ahead.[9] Although travel agents are becoming more knowledgeable about the problems associated with traveling with oxygen, it is essential that the staff planning the cruise verify all details and work closely with the oxygen supplier.

Consent forms must be obtained from the hospital legal department, and permission for the patient to go on the cruise must be requested from the referring physician. Obtaining a referral, however, does not necessarily mean that the patient is a good candidate for a cruise. Each patient should be individually interviewed and evaluated after his or her history and physical examination record are received and the latest arterial blood gas and pulmonary function test results are obtained. One patient who had received a referral to participate in our original cruise seemed irritable and slow. When we insisted on the performance of blood gas testing—the first such testing he had ever undergone—we discovered a Po_2 of 40 mm Hg and a Pco_2 of 70 mm Hg. Enrolling this man in a PR program after initiation of continuous oxygen therapy improved his status so much that he was able to accompany the group not only on that cruise but also on many other trips in subsequent years.

Practitioners should be aware that some respiratory patients may exhibit confusion with the excitement of travel and that sometimes a patient's traveling companion who has not been evaluated can have a problem that is more serious than those of the patient. The other major problem that may be encountered during a cruise is fluid retention due to high sodium intake. Not only are many foods that are served on cruises high in sodium, but the amounts of them that are consumed may be much greater than those usually eaten at home.

In general, however, cruising is the ideal vacation for respiratory patients. The sea air is free of pollens, the decks encourage walking, and the many activities tempt even the most inactive patient. These many factors combine to make for a wonderful trip.

SUMMARY

PR provides the tools that can make a positive change in the lives of most patients. Continuing care is needed, however, to maintain or even increase the improvement begun in a formal rehabilitation program. This care includes assisting patients to find ways to continue exercising, to maintain a current understanding of respiratory disease, to keep socially involved, and to expand the horizons of their life through travel.

REFERENCES

1. Burns M. Travel with oxygen. In: Tiep BL (ed). Portable Oxygen: Including Oxygen Conserving Devices. Spring Valley, NY: Futura Press, 1991, pp 421–436.
2. Burns M. Travel hints for the person with COPD. In: Petty T, Nett L (eds). Enjoying Life with Emphysema. 2nd ed. 1987, pp 103–107.
3. Smeets F. Eurolung Assistance Guide. Centre Hospitalier de Saint-Ode, Saint-Ode, Belgium.
4. Maguire J, Randazzo J, Lundstedt D, Bobeck J. Requirements for traveling with oxygen. AARC Times 1988; 4:31–35.
5. Gong H. Flying with oxygen. In: Tiep BL (ed). Portable Oxygen: Including Oxygen Conserving Devices. New York: Futura Press, 1991, pp 437–465.
6. Gong H, Tashkin D, Lee EY, Simmons D. Hypoxia-altitude simulation test. Am Rev Respir Dis 1984; 130:980–986.
7. Burns MR. Cruising with COPD. Am J Nurs 1987; 87:479–482.
8. Olenik P. Planning a cruise? AARC Times 1988; 4:24–29.
9. Burns M. Travel and the COPD patient: Planning for problems. Respir Times 1988; 4:10–11.

Chapter 31

Evaluating the Results of Pulmonary Rehabilitation Treatment

CHRISTOPHER J. CLARK, M.D., F.R.C.P.

The paradigm of pulmonary rehabilitation treatment has been succinctly defined by Petty as the "art of medical practice where an individually tailored, multidisciplinary program is formulated which through accurate diagnosis, therapy, emotional support and education, stabilizes or reverses both the physio- and psycho-pathology of pulmonary diseases and attempts to return the patient to the highest possible functional capacity allowed by his pulmonary handicap and overall life situation."[1] The global concept of treatment in this definition and also the recognition of involvement of "art" as well as science in the application of treatment give some indication of the potential difficulties involved in the evaluation of rehabilitation treatment.

Consider the resources involved in evaluating drug treatment as compared with those for assessing rehabilitation programs. In the case of the former, the mode of administration of a drug, the frequency of its administration, and its dosage are predetermined, and the clinician's resource commitment is solely directed toward evaluation of drug efficacy. Rehabilitation treatment requires an additional major resource commitment that includes staff and facilities. For logistic reasons, it is often not feasible to test and retest hypotheses on rehabilitation treatment without having a major impact on the daily function of the rehabilitation unit. The difficulty in conducting research on rehabilitation is further complicated by the fact that patients with broadly similar resting lung function levels not only have marked variability in exercise capacity[2] but also in disability, that is, "the total effect of impairment on the patient's life" is very much influenced by psychosocial factors.[3] Wide *intersubject* variability with respect to all parameters measured is not the only factor involved; an illness such as chronic obstructive pulmonary disease (COPD) is dynamic, and as a result it is subject to intercurrent exacerbations—this produces *intrasubject* variability. In rehabilitation, the therapeutic program should therefore differ from one patient to the next, depending on the needs of each.[4] However, this makes it extremely difficult to evaluate pulmonary rehabilitation in a standardized fashion. Even when procedures have apparently been standardized, the teacher's or trainer's relationship with the patient has a major influence on therapeutic outcome.[5] Table 31–1 summarizes areas for consideration in the evaluation of rehabilitation treatment.

ASPECTS OF STUDY DESIGN

A number of studies have now established that there are potential benefits to be gained from pulmonary rehabilitation; however, speculation remains as to how benefits are derived.[6] Major difficulties arise in comparing the results of different rehabilitation centers because of variations in study design with respect to the duration of rehabilitation programs, patient selection, the type of exercise chosen, and the methodology for testing.[7] In

TABLE 31–1. ASPECTS OF EVALUATION OF REHABILITATION TREATMENT

1. Study design, including methodology for data analysis
2. Resting lung function assessment (e.g., spirometry and arterial blood gas testing)
3. Exercise evaluation, including determination of exercise tolerance
4. Outcome analysis, including longevity, quality of life, analysis of failure to achieve physiologic goals, and cost-benefit analysis

view of the wide variation in patient impairment within the definition of COPD, the large number of factors independently affecting improvements in exercise performance, and the plethora of possible treatment approaches, it is not surprising that implementation of an appropriate study design remains one of the most difficult aspects of assessing the results of rehabilitation. A large number of research contributions suffer because of their lack of adequate control groups.[3] This is not the result of carelessness or oversight but simply of the logistic difficulties in including control groups in such research. Even in studies in which a control group is identified, the subsequent statistical analysis may be inadequate. In a recent study using univariate analysis, cardiorespiratory performance variables were not significantly different among patient and control groups. However, multiple regression analysis revealed highly significant differences among the groups.[8] Therefore, there are a number of key issues that must be considered when creating an appropriate study design, including the methodology for data analysis.

Patient Numbers

The comment ". . . one of the most serious ethical problems in clinical research is that of placing subjects at risk of injury, discomfort, or inconvenience in experiments where there are too few subjects for valid results . . ."[9] is particularly pertinent to pulmonary rehabilitation treatment, in which there may be a number of confounding variables occurring during prolonged observation of each patient and in which highly subjective data such as "quality of life" scores are collated. If the sample size is too small, there is an increased risk of false-negative findings. This can be prevented by estimating the statistical power of the sample size necessary to predict a clinically important effect and to ensure that a negative finding provides strong grounds for concluding that no important effect has occurred.[10] Thus, before embarking on a study, it would be helpful to calculate the appropriate sample size and to indicate this in the subsequent report.

Patient Selection

It is important to minimize heterogeneity within the study group. If two patients with similar lung function have a major difference in exercise capability, an additional variable influencing outcome is introduced. Similarly, patients with pure emphysema cannot be considered identical to those with chronic bronchitis, carbon dioxide retention, and incipient cor pulmonale. The best approach is to restrict entry to the study to well-defined patient subgroups. The advantage of this approach is that study results are less likely to be undermined by the inclusion of patients with varying degrees of disability; however, the disadvantage is that the results can only be considered applicable to the particular subgroup chosen. We have recently combined rating scales for mild, moderate, and severe impairment of lung function,[11] the presence or absence of impairment in diffusing capacity, arterial oxygen desaturation during exercise, or both, and the assessment of daily activity as expressed using a four-point scale reflecting inactivity to full participation in sports. This facilitates the recruitment of patients to appropriate programs and reduces heterogeneity with respect to disability. An interesting paper has recently confirmed that exercise tolerance can be predicted reasonably well from measurements of lung function and gas exchange in patients with COPD[12]; the inclusion of an index of daily activity in our assessment reduces some of the residual variability in exercise tolerance. A more detailed assessment of disability in COPD is the subject of continuing debate.[13,14]

Control Groups

Since the usual question to be evaluated is whether the particular pulmonary rehabilitation treatment protocol does or does not have a beneficial effect on outcome measures (e.g., exercise tolerance) in COPD, an appropriate control group consists of patients with similar respiratory impairment and disability who are undergoing sequential evaluations of exercise tolerance and analysis identical to those of the treatment group. The appropriate statistical analysis is then of the significance of any difference in *changing* outcome measures between the two groups on sequential testing throughout the study period. A pitfall in studies of this kind is analyzing the significance of a change (e.g., in exercise tolerance) after training the control and treatment groups separately and then commenting on the presence or absence of "significant" changes in the treatment group that were not seen in the control group. Another problem results from choosing normal subjects without COPD to serve as the control group. This allows a comparison of the effects of a rehabilitation program on patients with COPD with those on normal subjects, but it does not take into account aspects such as placebo effects or improvement due to familiarization with training that may be common to both groups. The potential problems that arise from the absence of control data are particularly relevant in the evaluation of rehabilitation treatment. The methods of assessment are subject to the major influence of learning or familiarization, and the treatment itself involves important, potentially confounding factors, such as improved medication and increased well-being that result from increased supervision. For example, one study[15] showed a significant improvement in psychologic variables in the treatment group of a controlled trial of exercise training; however, a similar magnitude of improvement was seen in the control subjects, indicating the potential confounding effect of even minimal management intervention. A recent study serves as a useful example of how clinically important information can be obtained relatively easily by using an appropriate study design that includes control data.[16] A particular error to be avoided is the use of a run-in period for "control" measurements. The consecutive design automatically introduces bias owing to its lack of randomization. In addition, since patients have a tendency to improve with familiarization, an analysis relying on within-patient change (e.g., paired statistical analysis) will likely be a source of error.

If any doubt remains regarding the heterogeneity of disability in the patient group after the patients have been stratified into well-defined subgroups and if a large enough patient group has been studied, the independent contribution of rehabilitation treatment versus control status to outcome measures can be identified by moving from univariate analysis to multiple regression analysis, which allows the influence of variables affecting performance (e.g., prestudy respiratory impairment and exercise capacity) to be taken into account.

If for any reason a control group is not considered feasible, then a different question has to be answered for a study of rehabilitation treatment to be meaningful: accepting that this treatment can be anticipated to have measurable effects on exercise tolerance, what factors within the program or patient best predict outcome, that is, the magnitude of improvement in exercise tolerance? An approach with this focus cannot distinguish placebo effects within the overall outcome measures but can provide insight into the quantitative changes that are likely to result from rehabilitation. An example of this can be seen in a recent study[17] that examined multiple physiologic and psychologic variables in order to produce a model explaining improvements in exercise performance in asthmatics following rehabilitation treatment. The important predictors were the initial level of disability or fitness, the variability of asthma severity, its coincidence with fixed training sessions, and, finally, the prestudy motivational assessment. There was no correlation of these factors with indices of lung function. This is a finding similar to that reported for 33 patients with COPD who completed a rehabilitation program; the program resulted in significant improvements in endurance measurements and 12-minute walking distance that did not correlate with lung function data.[18] Another recent study of 50 ambulatory outpatients who completed a 6-week rehabilitation program used stepwise regression analysis to identify predictors of improvement in 12-minute walking distance. The more disabled the patients were at the outset—that is, the lower the initial peak oxygen consumption, the shorter the initial 12-minute walking distance, and the higher the baseline lung volumes—the greater the improvement in exercise tolerance gained.[19]

One of the problems in using multiple regression analysis is that there are often many independent and dependent measures to select in evaluating outcome. The selection of single measures, however, may fail to identify significant relationships. An interesting approach reported recently[20] used factor analysis to consolidate multiple outcome measures into a smaller number of reliable composites. This approach has the advantage of reducing the number of variables and, therefore, the likelihood of type I statistical errors (the detection of spurious significant differences). The disadvantage of this approach is that it transforms variables that have clinical meaning into multivariate composites that may not provide specific diagnostic information. Factor analysis appears to be a promising statistical tool for evaluation of the outcome of pulmonary rehabilitation when there are many potentially confounding variables.

Randomization

The most essential component of study design is the inclusion of patient randomization to minimize bias. Randomization can create particular problems with regard to the organization and implementation of rehabilitation treatment programs. There are major economic and even ethical issues that are involved in running a parallel, nonintervention group that requires a considerable commitment of investigative time. The high "dropout" rate within the intervention group compounds the waste of resources. It is often not appreciated that *randomization need not be equal*. Thus, if the approximate rate of failure of completion can be anticipated (e.g., 30%), then a 3:1 randomized allocation of patients to treatment and control groups can help to ensure adequate patient recruitment for a realistic length of time.

Longevity of Benefits

For rehabilitation programs to have validity, the longevity of the benefits needs to be assessed. Short studies (e.g., of 6 weeks' duration) fail to present a complete picture. Quarterly or semiannual assessment is recommended.

RESTING LUNG FUNCTION ASSESSMENT

Most studies show little average change in routine lung function data following rehabilitation treatment.[6] However, sequential evaluation routinely includes such data in order to characterize the patients in terms of severity and variability of illness during the study period. These measurements also serve as variables in the analysis of outcome.

TABLE 31-2. AREAS OF POSSIBLE EXERCISE EVALUATION

1. Maximum exercise performance (direct [progressive incremental exercise] and indirect [timed walking tests])*
2. Endurance of submaximum exercise (bicycle ergometer or treadmill)*
3. Respiratory muscle function (strength* and endurance testing)
4. Skeletal muscle function (isokinetic testing)

*Feasible in a community hospital setting.

EXERCISE EVALUATION

The rationale in pulmonary rehabilitation for the emphasis on improving exercise capacity is justified by the aphorism that the "condition of exercise is not a mere variant of the condition of rest, it is the essence of the machine."[21] In the evaluation of exercise rehabilitation in COPD, the various questions to be asked can be reduced to only two: (1) Does the treatment improve exercise tolerance in some measurable way? and (2) What is the most likely physiologic basis for the effects of the treatment?

We know from the experimental approaches to understanding exercise physiology in normal subjects[22] that we are most likely to find a basis for the effects of the treatment in (1) central cardiorespiratory adaptations, (2) peripheral mechanisms within the exercising muscle, or (3) psychosocial factors that have an impact on performance.

An increasing number of methods are available for evaluating pulmonary rehabilitation, ranging from simple, noninvasive techniques for care in community hospitals to comprehensive methods of exercise evaluation that use computerized data collection and are suitable for larger-scale studies in specialized centers. Table 31-2 identifies areas of possible measurement that relate to exercise performance.

Maximum Exercise Performance

Progressive incremental exercise testing provides objective measurement of work capacity either directly (as maximum oxygen uptake determined using a gas exchange system) or indirectly (based on the power output during treadmill or bicycle ergometer exercise). The short-duration protocols[23] should use 1-minute time increments that employ work rates modified according to disease severity to give an optimal total test duration of approximately 12 minutes. This requires a reduction of work increments in COPD patients to as low as 10 watts in men and 6 watts in women,[11] although considerably higher work rates can be used in patients with mild disease. A variety of treadmill protocols are available; for example, in patients with COPD, a treadmill speed of 3 kph with an increasing grade of 2.5% per minute is usually very suitable and well tolerated. A uniform protocol is not necessary for all patients, but the protocol should be standardized for each patient so that a longitudinal assessment of treatment benefits can be made. Progressive incremental exercise testing provides further physiologic data on changes in cardiorespiratory parameters following rehabilitation, including anaerobic threshold, oxygen pulse, ventilatory equivalent for oxygen, and the "dyspnea index" (the ratio of maximum minute ventilation to maximum voluntary ventilation [$\dot{V}_{E}max/MVV$])—all of which may show beneficial adaptive changes following rehabilitation.[17, 24, 25] Anaerobic threshold should be measured based on the slope of the carbon dioxide output/oxygen uptake relationship ($\dot{V}_{CO_2}/\dot{V}_{O_2}$) using the method of Wasserman.[26] Although anaerobic threshold is often not attained in severely disabled patients, when it is identified, it is a useful monitor of cardiovascular adaptive changes, particularly when the reliability of the progressive incremental exercise endpoint is uncertain. The interpretation of submaximum data obtained from progressive incremental exercise testing suffers from the large confidence limits for normal values.

Wide interpatient variability is less relevant in longitudinal studies of rehabilitation treatment, but it does require adequate statistical analysis in such studies.[8, 17] Measurement of the perception of breathlessness is also recommended during progressive incremental exercise using psychophysical methods that rely on either a visual analog score or the categorical (modified Borg) scale. Both are characterized by validity and reproducibility, but both also result in wide intersubject variability.[27] Measurement of the effects of rehabilitation treatment on the perception of breathlessness requires the same data processing and statistical analysis as do other measurements taken during progressive incremental exercise.[17]

A number of reports have used maximum exercise performance as a principal outcome measure of the benefits of rehabilitation. Although many of these reports did not include control data, virtually all showed patient improvement of a clinically relevant magnitude in either peak work rate or maximum oxygen consumption ($\dot{V}_{O_2}max$).[28–39] Controlled studies that include adequate patient populations confirm the impression that rehabilitation using a wide range of programs results in considerable improvement in maximum exercise tolerance.[40–47] In one study, for example,[45] regular stair climbing at home for 3 months led to a 16% increase in $\dot{V}_{O_2}max$ and a 23% increase in maximum workload in the treatment group (as compared with a 12% and 4% decrease in the same measures, respectively, in the control group). Another study[44] showed that attention to rehabilitation techniques, such as breathing control without exercise training, improved maximum exercise tolerance during bicycle ergometry. Important subjective improvements reported in these controlled studies included an increase in the performance of activities of daily living[41, 43, 45, 47] and a reduction in symptoms, such as breathlessness during exercise[40, 41]; this confirms the clinical relevance of the changes seen in laboratory exercise testing. Additional measurements—such as improvements in stride length during walking and the relationship of $\dot{V}_{O_2}max$ to work rate—have shown that changes in maximum exercise tolerance may be due to increased mechanical efficiency, increased physiologic work capacity, or both.[32, 33, 45] However, regardless of the underlying mechanism, improved exercise tolerance is a worthy goal for disabled patients and one that studies have shown to be achievable. A useful table was provided by one author to compare the magnitude of improvements in peak work rate that was observed in his study with that found in a number of other reports. Results ranged from no change to 143% improvement, with an average increase in tolerance of 33%.[28]

Timed Walking Tests

Timed walking tests can be used to indirectly measure exercise capacity following rehabilitation treatment, particularly when limited resources are available.[48] The main advantages of walking tests are simplicity, minimal resource requirements (i.e., a corridor and a supervisor), and general applicability.

For patients with moderate to severe disease, the 6-minute walk is preferable to the 12-minute walk. The main disadvantages of these tests are patient and supervisor susceptibility to motivation,[49] their nonstandardized nature, and their dependence on a single quantitative measure of distance achieved. Although walking tests are capable of meeting stringent test-retest criteria,[50] the plethora of circumstances in which testing takes place limits comparison of the magnitude of various rehabilitation treatment results from different centers.[51] Where facilities are limited, the timed walking test remains a simple method of assessing exercise capacity in individual patients provided that reproducibility of the measurement is demonstrated. The effects of learning on initial walks need to be taken into account.

Those studies that have used timed walking tests to evaluate the benefits of rehabilitation treatment[34, 43, 45–47] have virtually all shown a clinically relevant improvement in the distance walked after treatment. For example, a 42% increase was observed in one uncontrolled study of 24 patients undergoing supervised exercise for 3 months,[46] a 51% increase was reported in another study of 63 patients,[34] and a 6% increase was noted in a controlled study of 28 patients compared with a 2% decrease in control subjects.[45] These changes parallel other measures of exercise tolerance (although the magnitude of the changes can be markedly different). Therefore, timed walking tests have validity in showing "responsiveness" to change in exercise performance following pulmonary rehabilitation.

Effects of Treatment on the Endurance of Submaximum Exercise

In addition to determination of maximum work capacity, it is useful to measure tolerance of submaximum steady-state exercise as an index of the effects of rehabilitation treatment on the tolerance of daily activities. A number of studies show improvements in the endurance time for steady-state exercise at between 50 and 60% of predetermined $\dot{V}O_2$max following rehabilitation treatment.[40, 52] Treadmill and bicycle ergometer exercise

TABLE 31–3. COMPARISON OF TREADMILL AND CYCLE ERGOMETERS FOR EXERCISE TESTING*

Feature	Treadmill	Cycle
Higher maximum $\dot{V}O_2$ and maximum O_2 pulse	+	
Similar maximum heart rate and maximum $\dot{V}E$	+	+
Familiarity of exercise	+ +	+
Quantitation of external work	– –	+ +
Freedom from artifacts in electrocardiography, gas flow, and pressure tracing	– –	+ +
Ease of obtaining arterial blood specimens	– –	+ +
Safe (fewer musculoskeletal injuries)		+
Useful in supine position		+
Less vertical and horizontal laboratory space		+
Less noise		+
Less expensive		+
Portable	–	+
Greater experience in United States	+	
Greater experience in Europe		+

*From Wasserman K, Hansen JE, Sue DY, Whipp BJ. Principles of Exercise Testing and Interpretation. Philadelphia: Lea & Febiger, 1987.
Key: $\dot{V}E$: minute ventilation; + +: more important advantage; – –: more important disadvantage; +: less important advantage; –: less important disadvantage.

can be used, and each has advantages and disadvantages. The most important advantage of the treadmill is patient familiarity with the form of exercise, whereas the bicycle ergometer's primary asset is the ease with which it can be used to quantitate work. These points are summarized in Table 31–3.[26] The improvements in endurance time may be of a magnitude greater than that anticipated from improvements in maximum exercise level. For example, one study of 63 patients[34] showed no improvement in peak work rate or $\dot{V}O_2$ max but did demonstrate a 57% increase in endurance time. Another study[35] evaluating 15 patients for 6 weeks showed a doubling of endurance time with no increase in peak work rate. Endurance evaluation may therefore reveal other components that strongly affect training outcome; these include an improved strategy for the performance of steady-state work and skeletal muscle conditioning in addition to central cardiorespiratory adaptations to rehabilitation. Steady-state submaximum exercise also affords the possibility of performing the additional gas exchange measurements recommended in the Stage 3 exercise test protocols of Jones.[53] However, these measurements are not specifically indicated for the evaluation of rehabilitation treatment, since studies that have measured gas exchange at rest and during exercise[39, 40] have shown no change in these parameters despite the presence of improved exercise tolerance.

The Effects of Treatment on Respiratory Muscle Function

Some indication of the difficulties in understanding the exact role of respiratory muscle in exercise tolerance in COPD can be seen in the recent shift in research emphasis from attempts to train respiratory muscle using overload techniques (i.e., performance of work beyond a critical level[54]) to the potential role of periodic rest in the reduction of incipient muscle fatigue.[55] Despite a major emphasis on the possible benefits of respiratory muscle training,[56] its failure to consistently produce favorable results is disappointing[57] and is probably related to multiple factors such as patient selection and specific methods of respiratory muscle training. Clearly, there is a need for further longitudinal controlled studies of the effects of this form of treatment in selected patients with COPD. In the meantime, since rehabilitation treatment of many kinds may induce a component of respiratory muscle training,[56] it is logical to include simple measurements of respiratory muscle function such as determination of maximum inspiratory pressure.[58] More complex and invasive assessment of respiratory muscle function is not warranted for the routine evaluation of rehabilitation treatment unless respiratory muscle training is specifically being investigated. In such a case, detailed evidence of improved respiratory muscle strength and endurance is to be included with general measures of exercise tolerance. One particular study illustrates this approach.[59] The effects of additional target flow in inspiratory muscle training on the performance of the respiratory muscles, general exercise capacity, and psychologic parameters during a 10-week pulmonary rehabilitation program were measured. A significant improvement in respiratory muscle function and the 12-minute walking distance (but not in peak work rate or psychologic symptoms) was observed in the treatment group compared with control patients (i.e., those undergoing exercise rehabilitation alone). The clarity of the study's design allowed not only an investigation of the physiologic changes introduced by the specific treatment but also the estimation of the likely clinical importance of the improvement seen. The authors rightly concluded that respiratory muscle training had an "extra beneficial effect on . . . exercise performance."[59] However, the data allowed for a more conservative interpretation. The mean increase in exercise tolerance—although significantly greater in the respiratory muscle training group than in control patients—was not of a magnitude sufficient to suggest a clinically important benefit. Further studies of respiratory muscle training using this methodology are required.

The Effects of Treatment on Skeletal Muscle Function

An important component of perceived exertion is the sense of discomfort and fatigue in exercising muscle[60] that causes enforced periods of inactivity in any patient with chronic illness. Suboptimal conditioning of skeletal muscle is likely to be present. The adaptations resulting from chronic dynamic exercise can be divided into those affecting the cardiorespiratory system and those affecting peripheral muscle; the distinction between the two types is made operationally by examining the effects of dynamic exercise on trained and untrained limbs. By increasing peripheral oxygen extraction through muscle fiber hypertrophy, increased muscle mitochondrial volume and increased capillary blood volume, and by shunting blood from inactive muscle to exercising muscle,[61] an increase in work capacity may occur. The evidence of skeletal muscle deconditioning cycles as a contributory factor limiting exercise tolerance in COPD is circumstantial but convincing. Jones and coworkers[62] showed that the intensity of leg discomfort in COPD patients at maximum exercise was on average twice that expected for normal subjects at the same exercise intensity. Although breathlessness was a major limiting factor, it seems reasonable to conclude from this study that the symptoms attributable to the exercising peripheral muscles were excessive and thus an additional factor adding to disability. There is also some evidence that muscle fatigue can be demonstrated at maximum exercise levels in patients with COPD.[63] This evidence was presented in a study that measured quadriceps electromyographic fatigue criteria during progressive incremental exercise. The study demonstrated that 50% of the patients had evidence of fatigue at peak exercise levels. It is likely that a cycle of deconditioning occurs, particularly after periods of enforced inactivity that cause negative reinforcement of the patient's association of exercise with discomfort. In a further study,[64] the static strength of peripheral skeletal muscle was significantly lower in patients with airflow limitation than in normal control subjects, confirming the likelihood of deconditioning cycles. These data suggest that conditioning of skeletal muscle may contribute to improvements in exercise tolerance following pulmonary rehabilitation. The specificity of the muscle groups trained and the preponderance of strength-versus-endurance benefits depend critically on the type of program used. Monitoring such responses using techniques such as isokinetic exercise evaluation[65] is possible but not routinely available. Such techniques make possible not only measurement of the impact of the treatment program on isolated muscle groups but also assessment (using multiple regression analysis) of the contribution of skeletal muscle adaptation to overall improvements in exercise performance following pulmonary rehabilitation.

OUTCOME ANALYSES

Longevity

The rationale for rehabilitation treatment is not dependent on demonstration of improved patient survival. Nevertheless, there is important evidence that the comprehensive approach involved, which concentrates medical expertise longitudinally on patient care, may improve life expectancy[66] by identifying problems and initiating treatment early. Examples include the identification of oxygen desaturation during exercise and appropriate prescription of supplemental oxygen, the improvement of nutritional status, and the cessation of smoking, all of which are of very obvious immediate prognostic significance. In early COPD, in which rehabilitation may mobilize a proportion of patients from an unnecessarily sedentary lifestyle, there may be a reduced risk of cardiac events relating to ischemic heart disease. Although this is speculative, there remains encouraging evidence that pulmonary rehabilitation does improve survival. In one study,[67] the 5-year survival rate for 252 patients who had undergone comprehensive rehabilitation was 20% greater than that of a comparison group of outpatients with COPD. Another study of 182 patients[68] revealed a 17% greater survival rate than expected from the mortality figures for comparable patients with COPD. There are other similar reports of improved survival compared with life expectancy data.[69–71] Consideration of aspects such as which component of therapy was responsible for improved survival and in which patients is not possible from studies of this kind. The requirements to produce such information would include large patient groups, evaluation over a number of years, and adequate contrast groups. It would necessitate the multicenter evaluation of a comprehensive standardized rehabilitation program, which is logistically not feasible. However, such an approach has been used to demonstrate improved life expectancy with a single treatment (long-term oxygen therapy) and to show which patients are most likely to benefit from such treatment.[72]

The Effects of Treatment on "Quality of Life" Measures

There is increasing interest in the development of instruments for the measurement of "quality of life" that have adequate validity and are sufficiently practical to be of use in monitoring the effects of pulmonary rehabilitation. The requirements for such instruments have recently been reviewed by Guyatt.[73] Considerable controversy remains even as to the perspective from which quality of life is defined. McSweeny[3] has recently stressed that the patient's viewpoint is different from that of the health care provider. This researcher gives a definition of quality of life that encompasses (1) emotional functioning, (2) social role functioning, (3) the ability to perform daily living activities, and (4) the ability to participate in enjoyable activities.

In many studies, difficulties in analysis arise from a lack of proven validity and from limitations in the psychometric methods applied. However, recent studies have managed to produce quantitative information regarding the contribution of psychologic factors to disability in COPD.[74, 75] The main pitfalls for any prospective treatment evaluation lie in the sample size, which, if too small, limits not only the statistical validity but also the applicability of conclusions to other patients and settings. There have been several approaches to the question of analysis of quality of life improvements following treatment in the context of a specific disease such as COPD. The first is a separate analysis of "quality of life" measurements that assesses patient responses to rehabilitation treatment. Measurements are most conveniently summarized when quality of life questionnaires are health profiles (i.e., they produce a single aggregate score or small numbers of scores that can be used to monitor treatment response).[76] A second approach is to use multiple regression analysis to identify interrelationships among patient responses to treatment with respect to psychosocial variables. Yet another, more complex multivariate analysis technique integrates physiologic and social factors to produce a model that explains the improvements that are observed and the various linkages involved.[77] The complexity of such analyses can be seen in the changing importance of the predictor variables that occur with changing disease severity.

For most proposed studies to evaluate the benefits of rehabilitation treatment, a less complex approach using a separate analysis of responses to treatment with respect to specific psychologic and "quality of life" factors is adequate. Several studies using this methodology have shown significant improvements in symptom scores, the performance of activities of daily living, psychologic factors (e.g., mood), and general well-being.[33, 47, 70, 78] These benefits of rehabilitation may be measurable several years after the completion of rehabilitation. Guyatt and associates[79] demonstrated a marked improvement in quality of life measures during the long-term follow-up of 31 patients who completed a comprehensive rehabilitation program. More important, virtually all of the patients showed some degree of improvement. Cockroft and colleagues[47] reported improvements in psychologic variables in a treatment group following exercise training; they also found beneficial changes in the control group, which illustrates the potential for measured psychologic and subjective status to change with even minimal attention from the health care professional. Several reports have demonstrated long-term benefits in terms of reduced symptoms, increased activity, and greater self-confidence several years after the conclusion of a comprehensive pulmonary rehabilitation program.[33, 70, 79]

Studies using the techniques discussed previously have now also shown the importance of both psychologic and "quality of life" factors not only as outcome measures but also as predictors of physiologic outcome following rehabilitation.[70, 80, 81] The emphasis on such measurements is likely to increase with the development of psychosocial interventions that are incorporated into multimodal pulmonary rehabilitation treatment.[82] One carefully designed, randomized controlled study[78] has shown highly beneficial changes in quality of life measurements when a behavioral intervention program is used in addition to regular exercise.

Analysis of Failure of Treatment to Achieve Physiologic Goals

It is important to include an analysis of failure to achieve physiologic goals as a distinct strategy component because without it the overall *effectiveness* of the treatment and its applicability in a general clinical setting cannot be established. Factors influencing adherence (i.e., the extent to which individuals follow treatment recommendations) include motivation, the extent of disability, intercurrent exacerbations of disease, external socioeconomic factors, work commitments, and travel requirements, among others. By devolving responsibility for compliance, a community-based treatment program may suffer from these problems to a greater extent than a hospital-based program. In addition, the potential discrepancy between the physician's knowledge of treatment compliance and the patient's actual compliance may radically reduce the reliability of a study. Not only are noncompliance rates higher among patients with chronic conditions, they are also higher in patients whose therapy involves lifestyle modification and exercise (as do rehabilitation programs).[83, 84] There is very little information regarding patient compliance as an *outcome variable* in studies of rehabilitation in COPD.[85] Reasons for failure to achieve physiologic goals, including lack of compliance, should be carefully documented to give some indication of the likely success of rehabilitation treatment (e.g., acceptability to the patient) that might otherwise be overlooked.

Cost-Benefit Analysis

Although it is not possible to compare the health costs that result from COPD across Europe, it is likely that the magnitude of impact of the disease on health care systems in Europe is similar to that in the United States, where an age-adjusted COPD mortality of 1.4% per year is rising with a correspondingly increased economic impact from the use of health care resources (e.g., 4.55 billion dollars in the 1970s). There have been reports of reduced hospitalization, more gainful employment, and the slowing of disease progression when comprehensive rehabilitation programs are used, and it is assumed that an important benefit will accrue from reduced health care costs overall.[86] This has been investigated in more detail by Toevs and coworkers[87] in a comparison of the effects of different pulmonary rehabilitation programs. Using a "health policy model," improvements were seen in experimental subjects with respect to cost-utility figures that were very comparable to those of other types of health care programs, such as those for hypertension screening and hospital renal dialysis. This kind of analysis is likely to be an increasing component of medical audit and is therefore worth considering within the overall evaluation of rehabilitation treatment. However, it does require the expertise of a health economist from the onset of program planning.

A simpler form of cost-utility analysis that has been used by a number of investigators provides strong evidence that comprehensive rehabilitation programs can be a cost-effective method of providing treatment for patients with COPD. These various authors have estimated the financial savings likely to have resulted from a reduction in the number of days spent in the hospital following pulmonary rehabilitation. Their findings are very encouraging. Petty and associates[88] reported a decrease in hospital days from 868 to 542 (38%) for 85 patients 1 year after the conclusion of pulmonary rehabilitation. Johnson and colleagues[89] similarly reported a 55% decrease in days of hospitalization for 96 patients over a similar period. Another study[90] has shown a marked reduction in the number of repeat admissions in a group of 24 patients in the year after pulmonary rehabilitation (5 admissions compared with 30 in the previous year). Several reports indicate that comprehensive rehabilitation programs are also cost-effective on a long-term basis. For example, two studies[39, 89] reported a similar average decrease in hospital stay per year of 20 and 21 days, respectively. The latter included the cost of the pulmonary rehabilitation program in the cost-benefit analysis and concluded that there had been highly significant net cost savings. Another study[91] has shown that a reduction in the hospital stays of 64 patients after rehabilitation was maintained over a 4-year period (73% reduction in the first year and 61% in the fourth for the 44 patients who survived). Persistent reductions in hospitalization have been shown over periods as long as 5 years[67, 69] and 8 years.[92] In the case of the latter, only 8% of the rehabilitation group required sheltered care (nursing home) compared with 17% of the comparison group. A number of factors might have influenced these reported outcomes, including the active participation of the investigators in the decision-making regarding outpatient versus inpatient care. Bias in patient selection also cannot be excluded. Nevertheless, all of the information supports the conclusion that pulmonary rehabilitation can be not only a highly beneficial treatment for individual patients but also cost-effective therapy for COPD in general. A note of caution must be sounded, however. Not all aspects of rehabilitation are likely to be cost-effective; for example, a recent study[93] has found that no measurable cost benefit in terms of reduced morbidity was gained from the outpatient intervention of a respiratory health worker (nurse specialist). Paradoxically, this may be because a beneficial treatment outcome that reduces mortality in such frail patients may increase health care costs. Therefore, cost should not be the predominant factor in determining the effectiveness of pulmonary rehabilitation programs.

In conclusion, there is an increasing requirement to comprehensively evaluate the benefits and problems of pulmonary rehabilitation, and there is now a wide range of methods available for use in such evaluation in a variety of clinical settings. Prior consideration of the requirements for evaluation will improve the outcome, both in the management of the individual patient and in the processing of group data.

REFERENCES

1. Petty TL. Pulmonary rehabilitation. Respir Care 1977; 22:68–77.
2. Wasserman K, Whipp BJ. Exercise physiology in health and disease. Am Rev Respir Dis 1975; 112:219–249.
3. McSweeny J. Quality of life in COPD. In: McSweeny J, Grant I (eds). Chronic Obstructive Pulmonary Disease: A Behavioural

Perspective. Lung Biology in Health and Disease. Vol 36. New York: Marcel Dekker, Inc., 1988.
4. Make BJ. Pulmonary rehabilitation: Myth or reality? Clin Chest Med 1986; 74:519–540.
5. Dimatteo MR. A social-psychological analysis of physician-patient rapport: Towards a science of the art of medicine. J Soc Issues 1979; 35:12–33.
6. Hughes RL, Davison R. Limitations of exercise reconditioning in COLD. Chest 1983; 83:241–249.
7. Gimenez M. Exercise training in patients with chronic airways obstruction. Eur Respir J Suppl 1989; 2:611s–617s.
8. Clark CJ, Cochrane LM. Assessment of work performance in asthma for determination of cardiorespiratory fitness and training capacity. Thorax 1988; 43:745–749.
9. May WW. The composition and function of ethical committees. J Med Ethics 1975; 1:23–29.
10. Freiman JA, Chalmers TC, Smith H, Kuebler RR. The importance of beta, the type II error and sample size in the design and interpretation of the randomized control trial. N Engl J Med 1978; 299:690–694.
11. American Thoracic Society: Standards for the diagnosis and care of patients with chronic obstructive pulmonary disease (COPD) and asthma. Am Rev Respir Dis 1987; 136:225–244.
12. Carlson DJ, Ries AL, Kaplan RM. Prediction of maximum exercise tolerance in patients with COPD. Chest 1991; 100:307–311.
13. Jones PW, Baveystock CM, Littlejohns P. Relationships between general health measured with the sickness impact profile and respiratory symptoms, physiological measures and mood in patients with chronic airflow limitation. Am Rev Respir Dis 1989; 140:1538–1543.
14. Cotes JE, Bishop JM, Capel LH, et al. Disabling chest disease; prevention and care: A report of the Royal College of Physicians by the College Committee on Thoracic Medicine. JR Coll Physicians Lond 1981; 15:69–87.
15. Cockroft AE, Saunders MT, Berry G. Randomised controlled trial of rehabilitation in chronic respiratory disability. Thorax 1981; 36:200–203.
16. Lake FR, Henderson K, Briffa T, et al. Upper-limb and lower-limb exercise training in patients with chronic airflow obstruction. Chest 1990; 97:1077–1082.
17. Cochrane LM, Clark CJ. Benefits and problems of a physical training programme designed for asthmatic patients. Thorax 1990; 45:345–351.
18. Neiderman MS, Clemente PH, Fein AM, et al. Benefits of a multidisciplinary pulmonary rehabilitation programme: Improvements are independent of lung function. Chest 1991; 99:798–804.
19. Zu Wallak RL, Patel K, Reardon JZ, et al. Predictors of improvement in the 12 minute walking distance following a six week outpatient pulmonary rehabilitation programme. Chest 1991; 99:805–808.
20. Ries AL, Kaplan RM, Blumberg E. Use of factor analysis to consolidate multiple outcome measures in chronic obstructive pulmonary disease. J Clin Epidemiol 1991; 44:497–503.
21. Barcroft J. Features in the Architecture of Physiological Function. Cambridge, England: Cambridge University Press, 1934.
22. Astrand PO, Rodahl K. Textbook of Work Physiology. 2nd ed. New York: McGraw-Hill Book Co., 1977.
23. Whipp BJ, Davis JA, Torres F, Wasserman K. A test to determine parameters of aerobic function during exercise. J Appl Physiol 1981; 50:217–221.
24. Casaburi R, Wasserman K, Patessio A, et al. A new perspective in pulmonary rehabilitation: Anaerobic threshold as a discriminant in training. Eur Respir J Suppl 1989; 2:618s–623s.
25. Casaburi R, Patessio A, Ioli F, et al. Reductions in exercise lactic acidosis and ventilation as a result of exercise training in patients with obstructive lung disease. Am Rev Respir Dis 1991; 143:9–18.
26. Wasserman K, Hansen JE, Sue DY, Whipp BJ. Principles of Exercise Testing and Interpretation. Philadelphia: Lea & Febiger, 1987.
27. Wilson RC, Jones PW. A comparison of the visual analogue scale and modified Borg scale for the measurement of dyspnoea during exercise. Clin Sci 1989; 76:277–282.
28. Holle RHO, Williams DV, Vandree JC, et al. Increased muscle efficiency and sustained benefits in an outpatient community hospital-based pulmonary rehabilitation programme. Chest 1988; 94:1161–1168.
29. Carter R, Nicotra B, Clark L, et al. Exercise conditioning in the rehabilitation of patients with chronic obstructive pulmonary disease. Arch Phys Med Rehabil 1988; 69:118–222.
30. Vyas MN, Banister EW, Morton JW, Grzybowski S. Responses to exercise in patients with chronic airway obstruction: Effects of exercise training. Am Rev Respir Dis 1971; 103:390–400.
31. Pierce AK, Taylor HF, Archer RK, Miller WF. Responses to exercise training in patients with emphysema. Arch Intern Med 1964; 113:28–36.
32. Paez PN, Phillipson EA, Masangkay M, Sproule BJ. The physiologic basis of training patients with emphysema. Am Rev Respir Dis 1967; 95:944–953.
33. Mall RW, Medeiros M. Objective evaluation of results of a pulmonary rehabilitation programme in a community hospital. Chest 1989; 94:1156–1160.
34. Zack MB, Palange AV. Oxygen supplemented exercise of ventilatory and nonventilatory muscles in pulmonary rehabilitation. Chest 1985; 88:669–675.
35. Mohsenifar Z, Horak D, Brown HV, Koerner SK. Sensitive indices of improvement in a pulmonary rehabilitation programme. Chest 1983; 83:189–192.
36. Christie D. Physical training in chronic obstructive lung disease. BJ 1968; 2:150–151.
37. Bass H, Whitcomb JF, Forman R. Exercise training: Therapy for patients with chronic obstructive pulmonary disease. Chest 1970; 57:116–121.
38. Woolf CR, Suero JT. Alterations in lung mechanics and gas exchange following training in chronic obstructive lung disease. Dis Chest 1969; 55:37–44.
39. Alpert JS, Bass H, Szucs MM, et al. Effects of physical training on hemodynamics and pulmonary function at rest and during exercise in patients with chronic obstructive pulmonary disease. Chest 1975; 66:647–651.
40. Chester EH, Belman MJ, Bahler RC, et al. Multidisciplinary treatment of chronic pulmonary insufficiency: 3. The effect of physical training on cardiopulmonary performance in patients with chronic obstructive pulmonary disease. Chest 1977; 72:695–702.
41. Booker HA. Exercise training and breathing control in patients with chronic airflow limitation. Physiotherapy 1984; 70:258–260.
42. Busch AJ, McClements JD. Effects of a supervised home exercise programme on patients with severe chronic obstructive pulmonary disease. Phys Ther 1988; 68:469–474.
43. Sinclair DJM, Ingram CG. Controlled trial of supervised exercise training in chronic bronchitis. BMJ 1980; 280:519–521.
44. Ambrosino N, Paggiaro PL, Macchi M, et al. A study of short-term effect of rehabilitative therapy in chronic obstructive pulmonary disease. Respiration 1981; 41:40–44.
45. McGavin CR, Gupta SP, Lloyd EL, McHardy JR. Physical rehabilitation of chronic bronchitis: Results of a controlled trial of exercises in the home. Thorax 1977; 32:307–311.
46. Tydeman DE, Chandler AR, Graveling BM, et al. An investigation into the effects of exercise tolerance training on patients with chronic airways obstruction. Physiotherapy 1984; 70:261–264.
47. Cockroft A, Bagnall P, Heslop A, et al. Controlled trial of respiratory health worker visiting patients with chronic respiratory disability. BMJ 1987; 294:225–228.
48. McGavin CR, Gupta SP, McHardy GJR. 12 minute walking test for assessing disability in chronic bronchitis. BMJ 1976; 1:822–823.
49. Guyatt GH, Pugsley SO, Sullivan MJ, et al. Effect of encouragement on walking test performance. Thorax 1984; 39:818–822.
50. Knox AJ, Morrison JF, Muers MF. Reproducibility of walking test results in chronic obstructive airways disease. Thorax 1988; 43:388–392.
51. Donner CF, Patessio A. Performance indicators in chronic obstructive lung disease: Walking test. Eur Respir J Suppl 1989; 2:670s–673s.
52. O'Donnell DE, Sanii R, Younas M. Improvement in exercise endurance in patients with chronic airflow limitation using continuous positive airway pressure. Am Rev Respir Dis 1988; 138:1510–1514.

53. Jones NL. Clinical exercise testing. 3rd ed. Philadelphia: W.B. Saunders Co., 1988.
54. Pardy RL, Reid DW, Belman MJ. Respiratory muscle training. Clin Chest Med 1988; 9:287–296.
55. Rochester DF. Does respiratory muscle rest relieve fatigue or incipient failure? Am Rev Respir Dis 1988; 138:516–517.
56. Grassino A. Inspiratory muscle training in COPD patients. Eur Respir J Suppl 1989; 2:581s–586s.
57. Belman MJ. Respiratory muscle training should be instituted in COPD patients: ATS highlights. Am Rev Respir Dis 1988; 138:1072.
58. Black LF, Hyatt RE. Maximal respiratory pressures: Normal values and relationship to age and sex. Am Rev Respir Dis 1969; 99:696–702.
59. Dekhuijzen PN, Folgering HT, van Herwaarden CL. Target-flow inspiratory muscle training during pulmonary rehabilitation in patients with COPD. Chest 1991; 99:128–133.
60. Clausen JP. Circulatory adjustments to dynamic exercise and effect of physical training in normal subjects and patients with coronary artery disease. Prog Cardiovasc Dis 1976; 18:459–495.
61. Holloszy JO. Adaptations of muscular tissue to training. Prog Cardiovasc Dis 1976; 18:445–458.
62. Jones NL, Kearon MC, Leblanc P, et al. Symptoms limiting activity in chronic airflow limitation. Am Rev Respir Dis 1989; 139:A319.
63. Guell R, Gimenez M, Marchand M. Dyspnoea, pain in the legs and quadriceps electro-myographic fatigue at maximal exercise in patients with chronic airway obstruction. Eur Respir J Suppl 1989; 2:385s.
64. Allard C, Jones NL, Killian KJ. Static peripheral skeletal muscle strength and exercise capacity in patients with chronic airflow limitation. Am Rev Respir Dis 1989; 138:A90.
65. Clarke DH. Adaptations in strength and muscular endurance resulting from exercise: Part 5. Exerc Sports Sci Rev 1973; 1:83–84.
66. Petty TL. Pulmonary rehabilitation. Am Rev Respir Dis 1980; 122:159–161.
67. Haas A, Cardon H. Rehabilitation in chronic obstructive pulmonary disease: A 5 year study of 252 male patients. Med Clin North Am 1969; 53:593–606.
68. Sahn SA, Nett LM, Petty TL. Ten year follow-up of a comprehensive rehabilitation programme for severe COPD. Chest 1980; 77:311–314.
69. Sneider R, O'Malley JA, Kahn M. Trends in pulmonary rehabilitation at Eisenhower Medical Center: An 11 years' experience (1976–1987). Cardiopulmon Rehabil 1988; 11:453–461.
70. Bebout DE, Hodgkin JE, Zorn EG, et al. Clinical and physiological outcomes of a university-hospital pulmonary rehabilitation programme. Respir Care 1983; 28:1468–1473.
71. Anthonisen NR, Wright EC, Hodgkin JE. Prognosis in chronic obstructive pulmonary disease. Am Rev Respir Dis 1986; 133:14–20.
72. Nocturnal oxygen therapy trial group. Continuous or nocturnal oxygen therapy in hypoxaemic chronic obstructive lung disease. Ann Intern Med 1980; 93:391–398.
73. Guyatt G. Measuring health status in chronic airflow limitation. Eur Respir J 1988; 1:560–564.
74. Rutter BM. The prognostic significance of psychological factors in the management of chronic bronchitis. Psychol Med 1979; 9:63–70.
75. Morgan AD, Peck DF, Buchanan DR, McHardy GJR. Psychological factors contributing to disproportionate disability in chronic bronchitis. J Psychosom Res 1983; 27:259–261.
76. Jones PW, Baveystock CM, Littlejohns P. Relationship between general health measured with the Sickness Impact Profile and respiratory symptoms, physiological measures and mood in patients with chronic airflow limitation. Am Rev Respir Dis 1989; 140:1538–1543.
77. Asher HB. Causal Modeling. Beverly Hills, CA: Sage, 1976.
78. Atkins CJ, Kaplan RM, Timms RM, et al. Behavioral exercise programmes in the management of chronic obstructive pulmonary disease. J Consult Clin Psychol 1984; 52:591–603.
79. Guyatt GH, Berman LB, Townsend M. Long-term outcome after respiratory rehabilitation. Can Med Assoc J 1987; 137:1089–1095.
80. Kass I, Dyksterhuis JE, Rubin H, Patil KD. Correlation of psychophysiological variables with vocational rehabilitation outcome in patients with chronic obstructive pulmonary disease. Chest 1975; 67:433–440.
81. Jensen PS. Risk, protective factors, and supportive interventions in chronic airway obstruction. Arch Gen Psychiatry 1983; 40:1203–1207.
82. Dudley DL, Glaser EM, Jorgenson BN, Logan DL. Psychosocial concomitants to rehabilitation in chronic obstructive pulmonary disease: Part 2: Psychosocial treatment. Chest 1980; 77:544–684.
83. Sackett DL. The magnitude of compliance and noncompliance. In: Sackett DL, Haynes RB (eds). Compliance with Therapeutic Regimens. Baltimore: The Johns Hopkins Press, 1976.
84. Carmody T, Senner J, Malineau M, Matarazzo G. Physical exercise rehabilitation: Long term dropout rate in cardiac patients. J Behav Med 1980; 3:163–168.
85. Mertens DJ, Shepherd RJ, Kavanagh T. Long term exercise therapy for chronic obstructive lung disease. Respiration 1978; 35:96–107.
86. Petty T, Cherniak RM. Comprehensive care of COPD. Clin Notes Respir Care 1981; 20:3–13.
87. Toevs CD, Kaplan RM, Atkins CJ. The costs and effects of behavioural programs in chronic obstructive pulmonary disease. Med Care 1984; 22:1088–1100.
88. Petty TL, Nett LM, Finigan MM, et al. A comprehensive care programme for chronic airway obstruction: Methods and preliminary evaluation of symptomatic and functional improvement. Ann Intern Med 1969; 70:1109–1120.
89. Johnson HR, Tanzi F, Balchum OJ, et al. Inpatient comprehensive pulmonary rehabilitation in severe COPD. Respir Ther 1980; 3:15–19.
90. Agle DP, Baum GL, Chester EH, Wendt M. Multidiscipline treatment of chronic pulmonary insufficiency: 1. Psychologic aspects of rehabilitation. Psychosom Med 1973; 35:41–49.
91. Hudson LD, Tyler ML, Petty TL. Hospitalisation needs during an outpatient rehabilitation programme for severe chronic airway obstruction. Chest 1976; 70:606–610.
92. Nicol J, Hodgkin JE, Connors G, et al. Strategies for developing a cost-effective pulmonary rehabilitation programme. Respir Care 1983; 28:1451–1455.
93. Littlejohns P, Baveystock CM, Parnell H, Jones PW. Randomised controlled trial of the effectiveness of a respiratory health worker in reducing impairment, disability, and handicap due to chronic airflow limitation. Thorax 1991; 46:559–564.

4

Special Considerations in Pulmonary Rehabilitation

Chapter 32

Rehabilitation of Patients with Chronic Ventilatory Limitation from Nonobstructive Lung Diseases

RICHARD S. NOVITCH, M.D.
HENRY M. THOMAS III, M.D.

The availability of multidisciplinary rehabilitation programs for patients with chronic obstructive pulmonary disease (COPD) has led to the admission of patients with ventilatory limitation resulting from other causes to these programs. As the scope and breadth of pulmonary medical practice expand, it would seem inevitable that there will be a need to expand the spectrum of indications for pulmonary rehabilitation. The restoration of function in those patients with impaired exercise capability due to lung disease that is nonobstructive in nature is the focus of a relatively small but expanding field. One source of the growth in the number of such patients comes from progress in critical care medicine. The widespread availability of sophisticated intensive care units and the success of physicians in salvaging patients with severe lung injury and pneumonia have provided a new pool of severely disabled patients. Extended periods of enforced bed rest as well as poor caloric intake combined with increased metabolic demands may leave cardiovascular and muscle function depressed despite the resolution of respiratory failure. Once depleted, cardiovascular reserve, muscle mass, and strength are difficult to regain, in particular in the presence of the ventilatory limitation that these patients experience during exercise.

In our inpatient multidisciplinary pulmonary rehabilitation program, we find that approximately 10% of those admitted are patients with nonobstructive diseases. The range of diagnoses is broad, and a partial list of these diagnoses can be found in Table 32–1. The large majority of these patients have severe restrictive ventilatory defects as indicated by pulmonary function testing. Although the causes of their disease vary widely, we have designated all such patients as *nonobstructive lung disease patients* for the purpose of discussing rehabilitation. The application of pulmonary rehabilitation techniques to these non–COPD lung disease patients has not been extensively studied.[1, 2]

In many respects, the clinical sequelae of nonobstructive chronic lung disease are similar to those of COPD. Patients' major complaint is dyspnea, which is provoked by exertion. There is a marked diminution in exercise tolerance as measured by timed ambulation distance.[3] Others have shown that oxygen consumption during exercise is reduced as well.[4] The patients may have significant malnutrition and weight loss. Reduction in weight by itself, independent of airflow limitation, is negatively correlated with exercise capacity and timed ambulation distance.[5, 6] There may be weakness of the respiratory muscles (especially the diaphragm) and use of the accessory muscles. Resting levels of ventilation are elevated in both groups of patients.[7] Patients may have resting or exercise-induced hypoxemia and associated cor pulmonale that require oxygen therapy.[8] The

TABLE 32-1. SUMMARY OF DIAGNOSES OF NON-COPD PATIENTS ADMITTED FOR PULMONARY REHABILITATION

Fibrothorax
Bronchiectasis
Neuromuscular disease
Interstitial lung disease
    Sarcoidosis
    Idiopathic pulmonary fibrosis
    Radiation fibrosis
    Scleroderma
Chest wall deformity
    Kyphoscoliosis
    Postpolio syndrome
    Thoracoplasty
Diaphragmatic paralysis
    Post coronary artery bypass graft
    Post thoracotomy
Post lung resection
    Lobectomy
    Pneumonectomy
    Bronchopleural (cutaneous) fistula
Post respiratory failure
    Pneumonia
    Adult respiratory distress syndrome

ability to perform the activities of daily living may be impaired, as chest wall mechanics can be adversely affected when shoulder girdles that optimize the length-tension relationships of the accessory muscles are not anchored.[9] Patients may also be receiving corticosteroid medications and can suffer proximal myopathies and mood alterations associated with this class of drugs. As a general rule, both COPD and non-COPD patients have a poor understanding of pulmonary function and of the way in which it relates to the symptoms they are experiencing. Both groups usually have undergone extended or recurrent hospitalizations with prolonged periods of bed rest that have led to loss of muscle mass and deconditioning of skeletal and cardiac muscle. One distinct difference between the two groups is that the anger and self-recrimination with regard to smoking that many patients with COPD experience are not usually present in patients with non-COPD lung diseases.

The presence of a diverse patient population in a group pulmonary rehabilitation program is stimulating but also challenging for the staff that must individualize programs for non-COPD patients, especially in regard to education. One of the major objectives of pulmonary rehabilitation is education. However, many of the visual and printed materials that are available are addressed to COPD patients only. Therefore, not only do nonobstructive lung disease patients have to be instructed as to the differences between their lung disease and COPD, but ongoing in-service training of staff about different pulmonary conditions must be conducted as well. Most of the nonmedical staff on the pulmonary rehabilitation unit are well versed in the pathophysiology of COPD; however, their knowledge does not extend to the restrictive lung diseases. The task of individualizing the educational component of the program for the patient as well as the staff is the responsibility of the physician.

Thus, the entry of patients with chronic ventilatory limitation arising from non-COPD lung disease to rehabilitation programs is both of interest and of increasing importance for those involved with pulmonary rehabilitation in the 1990s.

CHRONIC OBSTRUCTIVE PULMONARY DISEASE REHABILITATION AS THE BASIS FOR THE REHABILITATION OF PATIENTS WITH NONOBSTRUCTIVE LUNG DISEASE

The Burke Experience

COPD is the most common chronic lung disease; in 1986, an estimated 11.4 million Americans had chronic bronchitis, and another 2 million had emphysema.[10] The desire for pulmonary rehabilitation is an outgrowth of the insidiously progressive nature of COPD and of the disability that ensues. Advanced age and smoking-accelerated declines in vital capacity result in the reduction of airflows below the level necessary to maintain a constant level of activity.[11,12] The physiologic derangements, resultant dyspnea, cycling of exacerbations, and the unrelenting nature of the disease have led to the development of a multidisciplinary treatment approach.[13]

A review of 317 patients admitted to our multidisciplinary rehabilitation program over a 5-year period revealed that exercise capacity (measured based on 6-minute ambulation distance) was significantly correlated with airway obstruction (measured based on forced expiratory capacity in 1 second [FEV_1]) but accounted for only 9% of its variance (Fig. 32–1).[14] This suggests that the generation of disability in chronic lung disease is a multifactorial process. Identification and treatment of cofactors may be important to the rehabilitation process. One area of substantial interest is the role of behavioral processes (e.g., depression) in the generation of disability.[15]

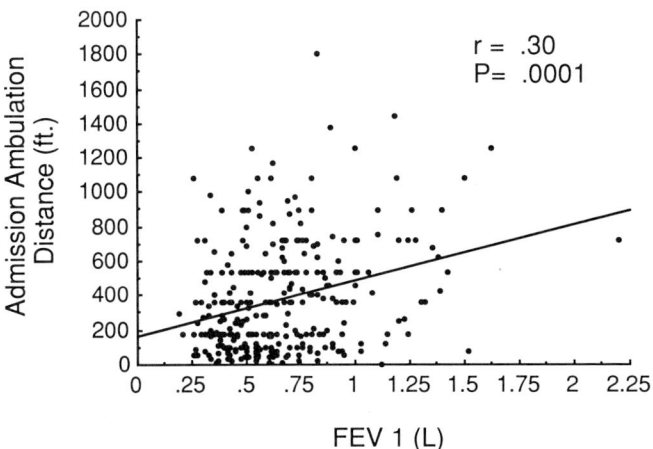

FIGURE 32-1. In this study, FEV_1 accounted for only 9% of the variance in exercise capacity (6-minute ambulation distance) at the time of patient admission to the hospital. (From Foster S, Lopez D, Thomas HM III. Pulmonary rehabilitation in COPD patients with elevated P_{CO_2}. Am Rev Respir Dis 1988; 138:1519–1523.)

The cornerstone of therapy in pulmonary rehabilitation is the reduction of ventilatory requirements for activity through exercise training. The phenomena of reduced heart rate and blood lactate production for a given level of oxygen consumption have been demonstrated in normal subjects after maximum oxygen consumption ($\dot{V}O_2$max) has been increased by an exercise training program.[16] The value of exercise training in patients with lung disease has always been questioned because ventilatory limitation renders achieving this physiologic phenomenon difficult, if not impossible. Recently, Casaburi and coworkers[17] found that certain patients with COPD also achieved reductions in lactic acidosis and ventilation after an exercise program that increased $\dot{V}O_2$max. Their data seem to be in conflict with those of earlier studies by Belman and colleagues,[18] who found no improvement in muscle mitochondrial enzymes in COPD patients after rehabilitation. Studies by several authors have attempted to determine physiologic discriminants for identifying candidates for exercise training.[19, 20] They have demonstrated that there is no correlation between the degree of airway obstruction and the ability to generate blood lactate in selected groups of COPD patients. Therefore, the ability to cross the anaerobic threshold may be an independent variable in predicting which candidates can develop a true training effect from an exercise program, and it might possibly assist in identifying those candidates who have the greatest potential for improvement after an exercise program. However, the fact that activity beyond the anaerobic threshold is most effective in increasing maximum exercise capacity in stable COPD patients[21] does not preclude the other aspects of the rehabilitation process (e.g., education, relaxation, nonaerobic activity, and repetition) from having an effect on the improvement of exercise capacity. Clearly, there seem to be aerobic and nonaerobic mechanisms for increases in $\dot{V}O_2$max after rehabilitation.

Our experience with COPD patients in an inpatient rehabilitation setting has generally been a positive one. Figure 32–2 shows a frequency histogram of the admission 6-minute ambulation distances of the 317 patients whom we studied. The mean admission ambulation distance was 380 ft ± 313 ft (SD), with 29% of the patients unable to walk 180 ft (one-half lap of the 360-ft walking circuit) in 6 minutes. An improvement of at least 100 ft was demonstrated by 80.1% of the patients in their 6-minute walking test by the time of discharge—this is a clinically significant improvement. A review of this data at first glance suggests that patients with end-stage COPD are quite disabled and can make only small improvements even after undergoing rehabilitation. Other investigators have come to similar conclusions, including Moser and associates,[22] who suggested that pulmonary rehabilitation may be of little value in caring for the most severely impaired COPD patients. Most of the homebound patients of these investigators tended to remain homebound, and only a fraction of the most impaired patients improved in functional classification.

In our clinical experience, however, there are great differences in functional levels even among homebound patients. For example, being at home is a more attractive alternative than living in an institutional setting, using a bathroom is preferable to using a commode, and ambulating inside an apartment is more satisfactory than being bedridden. Figure 32–3 is a frequency histogram of the discharge ambulation distances for the patients in our study. Although the discharge ambulation distances were generally short, only 8 patients were unable to ambulate 150 ft in 6 minutes. This is quite an important number because it represents the minimum ambulation distance necessary to maintain independent living in an apartment setting.[24]

Conclusions Based on Chronic Obstructive Pulmonary Disease Data

It has been our experience that there is a benefit to pulmonary rehabilitation across the spectrum of severity of both pulmonary function and level of disability in patients with COPD. In patients with severe impairment of ventilation and daily function, the goals of rehabilitation are small in an absolute sense but significant for the disabled individual.

The observation that small increases in function can make a significant impact on the quality of life of patients with severe disability has not been lost on the rehabilitation community in general. It has been noted that the use of pulmonary rehabilitation is not as widespread as the use of rehabilitation in other types of disabling conditions. The small incremental gains and short life expectancy of most patients with chronic ventilatory limitation seem to have created a nihilistic approach toward the rehabilitation of COPD patients in general.[24]

Comparison of Rehabilitation Results of Patients With and Without Chronic Obstructive Pulmonary Disease

An analysis of the outcome of multidisciplinary pulmonary rehabilitation in nonobstructive lung diseases was performed by Foster and Thomas.[1] Improvement of non-COPD patients was compared with that of COPD patients undergoing the same 4-week inpatient rehabilitation program. Table 32–2 shows the pulmonary function test results, respiratory muscle strength, and blood gas analysis results of the patients with restrictive lung disease undergoing the program as compared with those of their COPD counterparts. Improvement was assessed by comparing the 6-minute ambulation distances performed on admission with those attained at discharge. The 6-minute walking test revealed that the 32 non-COPD patients had initial ambulation distances of 276 ± 219 ft (SD). At the completion of the program, the ambulation distances were 574 ± 267 ft. The increase in ambulation distance was 298 ± 290 ft. The results of these patients were compared with those of the patients with COPD undergoing the same rehabilitation program (Table 32–3) and were quite similar to them.

In our experience, patients with non-COPD lung

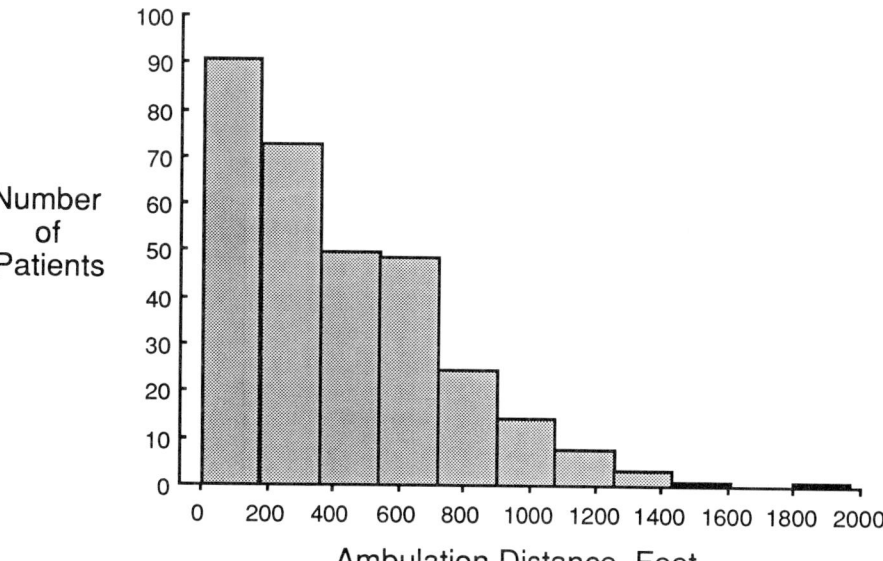

FIGURE 32-2. Patient 6-minute ambulation distance at the time of hospital admission. (From Foster S, Lopez D, Thomas HM III. Pulmonary rehabilitation in COPD patients with elevated P_{CO_2}. Am Rev Respir Dis 1988; 138:1521.)

diseases who are referred for inpatient multidisciplinary rehabilitation have essentially the same level of disability as do patients with COPD and thus have similar potential benefits. The mechanism by which patients with non-COPD lung disease improve $\dot{V}O_2$max, mobility, and daily functioning has yet to be investigated.

Clinical Presentation of non-COPD Lung Diseases for Rehabilitation

The hallmark of exercise limitation in non-COPD lung diseases is similar to that found in COPD: ventilatory limitation. The overwhelming prevalence of COPD dictates that only a fraction of all of our patients have nonobstructive diagnoses. Even so, of those patients with restrictive diseases, few seem to be chronic stable patients admitted from home.

The majority of patient referrals for non-COPD lung disease are from acute care hospitals. The referred patients have generally had complicated hospital courses that involved prolonged episodes of respiratory failure, and as a result they have required mechanical ventilation. The cause of respiratory failure has usually been pneumonia or the syndrome of diffuse alveolar damage.

Patients who have had pulmonary resections, lobectomies, or pneumonectomies are among those frequently referred. In addition to the early complications of adult respiratory distress syndrome and pneumonia, late complications may include bronchopleural (cutaneous) fistulas. Patients with a breakdown of the bronchial stump are especially dyspneic because of the diversion of large amounts of ventilation to dead space. Lung resections to treat bronchogenic carcinoma are typically performed in cigarette smokers who may have concurrent diffuse lung pathology, which may further reduce lung volumes and impair gas exchange.

Patients with diaphragmatic paralysis as a result of phrenic nerve injury constitute another group of individuals referred for rehabilitation. The injuries are usually iatrogenic and transient (6 wk to 18 mo in duration) and occur after extensive thoracotomy with mediastinal manipulation. Hypothesized origins of phrenic nerve palsy include the use of cardioplegic agents at low temperatures in cardiac surgery, the manipulation of the phrenic nerve itself, and the interruption of the blood supply to the nerve (which may be more frequent after left internal mammary artery grafting). The paralysis may be unilateral or bilateral, and patients with this condition may need assisted ventilation when they are in the supine position. This is accomplished using positive-pressure ventilation through a tight-fitting mask, a cuirass, or a rocking bed.[25]

Patients with deformities of the chest wall constitute

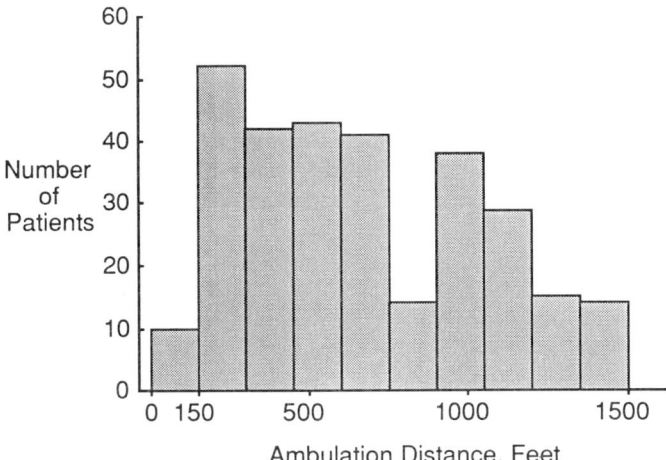

FIGURE 32-3. Patient 6-minute ambulation distance at the time of discharge from the hospital. Note that only eight patients were able to walk less than the 150-ft distance necessary to maintain independent living at the time of discharge. See text for additional details. (From Foster S, Lopez D, Thomas HM III. Pulmonary rehabilitation in COPD patients with elevated P_{CO_2}. Am Rev Respir Dis 1988; 138:1521–1523.)

TABLE 32-2. ADMISSION PULMONARY FUNCTION TESTS FOR COPD AND NON-COPD PATIENTS*†

	COPD	(% Pred)	Non-COPD	(% Pred)
No. of Patients	317		32	
FVC(L)	1.58 ± 0.62	(47 ± 16)	1.20 ± 0.45	(39 ± 16)
FEV_1 (L)	0.65 ± 0.28	(29 ± 12)	0.88 ± 0.35	(41 ± 22)
FEV_1/FVC (%)	42 ± 10		75 ± 14	
P_{Imax} (cm H_2O)	38 ± 17	(44 ± 18)	39 ± 22	(41 ± 24)
P_{Emax} (cm H_2O)	51 ± 28	(31 ± 15)	43 ± 23	(27 ± 13)
pH	7.42 ± 0.04		7.41 ± 0.03	
P_{CO_2} (mm Hg)	44 ± 8		43 ± 8	
P_{O_2} (mm Hg)	63 ± 14		67 ± 12	

*Adapted from Foster S, Thomas HM III. Pulmonary rehabilitation in lung disease other than chronic obstructive pulmonary disease. Am Rev Respir Dis 1990; 141:602–603.
†Values are means ± SD.
Key: VC: vital capacity; P_{Imax}: maximum inspiratory pressure; P_{Emax}: maximum expiratory pressure; % Pred: per cent of that predicted.

another subgroup that we admit to our program with some frequency. Patients with thoracoplasty, kyphoscoliosis, and postpolio syndrome have a variable combination of decreased chest wall compliance and respiratory muscle weakness; as a result, carbon dioxide retention and cor pulmonale may ensue. Many of these patients receive nighttime positive-pressure ventilation in order to rest fatigued muscles and to correct daytime hypercapnia.[26]

One group of patients that has not done well in our program is that with interstitial pulmonary fibrosis. These patients are generally referred late in the course of their disease when they are severely debilitated; they frequently show little improvement after therapy.

CASE HISTORIES IN THE REHABILITATION OF LUNG DISEASE OTHER THAN CHRONIC OBSTRUCTIVE PULMONARY DISEASE

Case No. 1. A 55-year-old woman with a 9-year history of a scleroderma and SLE overlap syndrome was admitted to pulmonary rehabilitation from an acute care hospital. The patient had chronic systemic scleroderma involving the lungs that had been diagnosed approximately 7 years earlier, digital infarctions that caused severe deformity in both hands, massive esophageal dilatation with recurrent vomiting and aspiration, and episodes of pericarditis and pleurisy. She developed peptic ulcers, osteoporosis, and spinal compression fractures as a result of corticosteroid use; this drug therapy had no impact on her lung disease. The patient had been suffering from malabsorption and malnutrition and was admitted to the hospital for total parenteral nutrition. She began to gain weight when steroid use was tapered. During her hospitalization, she experienced cardiac arrest. The patient was resuscitated successfully and remained on mechanical ventilation for 3 days.

Upon the patient's transfer to Burke Rehabilitation Hospital, a physical examination was performed and showed a respiratory rate of 24 breaths per minute with nasal flaring. The patient was anxious and somewhat depressed. There were rales at the lung bases bilaterally. The patient had shallow respiratory movements and poor lower rib cage excursions, but there was no evidence of abdominal paradox. There was an accentuated second pulmonic heart sound. The examination also revealed the presence of severe digital deformities.

The patient's blood gas analysis on admission revealed a pH of 7.41, a P_{CO_2} of 40 mm Hg, and a P_{O_2} of 89 mm Hg. No desaturation was observed during exercise oximetry. Pulmonary function testing showed a forced vital capacity (FVC) of 0.86 L (26% of that predicted); an FEV_1 of 0.80 L; and an FEV_1/FVC of 93%. The maximum voluntary ventilation was 37 L/min (39% of that predicted), the maximum inspiratory pressure was 29 cm H_2O (37% of that predicted), and the maximum expiratory pressure was 74 cm H_2O (51% of that predicted). The chest radiograph revealed fibrotic infiltration scattered throughout both lung fields, more prominently at the left base, but showed no acute infiltrates. The electrocardiogram showed sinus tachycardia, right atrial enlargement, and a nonspecific intraventricular conduction delay.

The initial 6-minute ambulation distance was 180 ft, with the patient walking behind a wheelchair. No thoracoabdominal paradox was noted after exercise. The

TABLE 32-3. AMBULATION DISTANCES ON A 6-MINUTE WALKING TEST IN COPD AND NON-COPD PATIENTS*†

		Ambulation Distance		
	No. of Patients	At Admission	At Discharge	Increase
COPD	317	380 ± 313	751 ± 562	371 ± 419
Non-COPD	32	276 ± 219	574 ± 367	298 ± 290
Non-COPD versus COPD		$P = .06$	$P = .08$	$P = .3$

*From Foster S, Thomas HM III. Pulmonary rehabilitation in lung disease other than chronic obstructive pulmonary disease. Am Rev Respir Dis 1990; 141:603.
†Values are means ± SD. All distances measured in feet.

patient rode a stationary bicycle without resistance for 15 minutes and was unable to perform any other activities. During occupational therapy it was noted that although the patient was independent in dressing, she only had fair endurance for activities of daily living, demonstrated fair incorporation of labor-saving techniques, and showed weakened strength proximally.

After undergoing the rehabilitation program for 25 days, the patient was able to ambulate 1080 ft without the aid of walking devices. She performed upper body exercise for 10 minutes at 120 rpm using an arm ergometer and rode a stationary bicycle for 20 minutes at 55 rpm, both without resistance. The patient was able to climb up and down 33 6-in steps.

In summary, this patient had multiple and complicated medical problems. She had been admitted to the hospital for hyperalimentation, had experienced cardiac arrest, was put on a ventilator for 3 days, and had bed rest for 6 weeks. She had steroid-induced compression fractures of the lumbosacral spine and possibly mild proximal steroid myopathy. Both her lung volumes and her muscle mass were markedly decreased. The patient had a good response to therapy with improvement in strength (as evidenced by stair climbing) and in stamina (as evidenced by substantial increases in walking distance and independence from supportive devices, such as a walker or wheelchair). After discharge, she was able to live independently.

Case No. 2. A 49-year-old woman was transferred to the Burke Rehabilitation Hospital after a 5-month stay at an acute care hospital. The patient had been admitted for abdominal pain and vomiting. She became somnolent, vomited and aspirated, and experienced respiratory arrest; following respiratory arrest, she was intubated and developed adult respiratory distress syndrome. The patient required high concentrations of oxygen and large amounts of positive end-expiratory pressure. The course was complicated by bilateral pneumothoraces and fungal pneumonia. Three weeks prior to transfer to the Burke Rehabilitation Hospital, the patient had been weaned from the ventilator. A transtracheal oxygen catheter was placed in the previous tracheostomy site.

Upon admission for rehabilitation, this anxious patient's physical examination revealed cachexia, severe muscle wasting in both upper and lower extremities, and muscle weakness in the shoulder and hip girdles. There was an accentuated second pulmonic heart sound and a soft S3 gallop rhythm. The breath sounds were decreased throughout, and good bilateral lower rib cage excursions were noted. There were coarse rales at both lung bases.

A room air arterial blood gas analysis on admission showed a pH of 7.37, a P_{CO_2} of 49 mm Hg, and a P_{O_2} of 57 mm Hg. The chest radiograph revealed substantial dense fibrosis with a honeycomb pattern throughout both lung fields. The heart appeared normal.

The initial physical therapy evaluation revealed that the patient could tolerate stationary bicycling for 4 minutes and upper body exercise for 7 minutes; she performed a 6-minute walking test of 360 ft without the aid of walking devices. Occupational therapy evaluation revealed that the patient needed minimal assistance for transfers and became markedly dyspneic during any routine activities.

The patient did well during a 28-day rehabilitation program. At the time of discharge, her arterial blood gas parameters had improved and showed a pH of 7.40, a P_{CO_2} of 40 mm Hg, and a P_{O_2} of 63 mm Hg. With exercise, oximetry revealed that oxygen saturation decreased from 92% to 69%. The patient was discharged with a prescription for supplemental oxygen via nasal cannula for her exercise program. At the time of discharge, the patient was able to ambulate 600 ft in 6 minutes without walking devices and to climb up and down 12 stairs. She could perform upper body exercise with an arm ergometer for 13 minutes and ride on a stationary bicycle for 6 minutes with minimal resistance. The patient was independent in her activities of daily living and was able to perform light household tasks. She was able to transfer independently without the aid of walking devices and performed light resistive exercise of the upper extremities with good coordination of her breathing patterns. Three months after discharge, her FVC was 1.17 L (34% of that predicted), FEV_1 was 1.17 L, and FVC/FEV_1 was 99%; maximum voluntary ventilation (MVV) was 66 L/min (65% of that predicted) and diffusing capacity was 9.6 ml/min/mm Hg (36% of that predicted). These results indicated a severe restrictive ventilatory defect with impaired diffusing capacity. Approximately 1 year after discharge, the patient was reported to be able to walk approximately 1 mile daily uninterrupted; however, she remained short of breath on exertion and had severe residual restrictive disease.

This patient was in good health prior to an episode of adult respiratory distress syndrome. Subsequent to an extended stay in an intensive care unit, she was malnourished and deconditioned and had residual pulmonary dysfunction and hypercapnia. The emotional support, nutrition, and muscle conditioning that she received enabled her to return to a normal lifestyle.

Together, these two patients illustrate the effects of rehabilitation in patients with non-COPD lung disease. Following either a chronic (Case No. 1) or acute (Case No. 2) illness, the patients are severely restricted in the performance of activities of daily living. Their disability is multifaceted and frequently medically complex, but pulmonary impairment is the central feature. Multidisciplinary pulmonary rehabilitation is not only "treadmills" but also an approach to the disabled patient with chronic lung disease that is directed toward improving mobility and coping skills in order to foster independent living and maintain as active a life as possible.

Physiology of Exercise Limitation in Restrictive Lung Disease

From the standpoint of the respiratory system, the key to performing muscular work of any type is the ability to maintain gas exchange in the face of increased metabolic demands. In the presence of lung disease, the impairment of gas exchange is severe enough to demand increased ventilation and energy expenditure even at basal levels.[7, 27] Increases in the resting level of ventilation and in the work of breathing can therefore be demonstrated in both restrictive and obstructive lung diseases.

The ability of patients with restrictive lung diseases to maintain high levels of ventilation despite increases in static recoil was noted by Austrian and coworkers.[28] The strategy these patients employ to minimize the work of breathing during exercise is to increase minute ventilation solely by increasing respiratory frequency while maintaining a constant tidal volume.[29] The maximum work output, however, is limited and correlates with the decline in vital capacity.[30]

In exercise testing, exercise limitation can be ascribed to ventilatory impairment in those patients whose minute ventilation during maximum exercise is greater than 70% of their MVV.[31] Maximum sustainable levels of exercise ventilation are often expressed as a percentage of the MVV in 12 seconds. The maximum sustainable ventilation is a relatively constant fraction of MVV in both normal and disease states.[32] MVV correlates with respiratory muscle strength in normal individuals and in patients with restrictive lung disease, whereas it correlates with airway resistance in COPD.[33-35] De Troyer and Yernault[36] found that respiratory muscle strength is normal when corrected for vital capacity in interstitial lung diseases. Therefore, both reductions in vital capacity and in respiratory muscle strength contribute to reductions in MVV and in maximum sustainable ventilation during exercise in patients with restrictive lung disease.

Gallagher and associates[37] found that maximum levels of sustained ventilation during exercise were 71%, 76%, and 111% of MVV in normal subjects, patients with restrictive lung disease, and patients with COPD, respectively. The tendency of patients with restrictive lung disease to exercise at a lower percentage of MVV may postpone the onset of respiratory muscle fatigue. This situation is profoundly different from that in the physiology of COPD, in which hyperinflation places respiratory muscles on a disadvantageous portion of their length-tension curve. In restrictive lung diseases, lung shrinkage tends to maximize inspiratory muscle strength based on Laplace's relationships.[38] In COPD, the activation of inspiratory muscles throughout the respiratory cycle may predispose patients with the disease to the early onset of muscle fatigue.[39] On the other hand, in restrictive lung diseases, increases in static recoil passively facilitate the return of the lung to end-expiratory volume.

Relatively few patients with restrictive lung diseases are referred for rehabilitation for a variety of reasons that relate to the epidemiology, physiology, and natural history of restrictive lung diseases. All of the conditions listed in Table 32–1 occur less frequently than does COPD. From a physiologic standpoint, there may be a greater ability to maintain higher levels of exercise ventilation in restrictive lung diseases than in COPD for a comparable reduction in vital capacity.

The Rehabilitation Program for Patients with Lung Diseases Other Than Chronic Obstructive Pulmonary Disease

As a general rule, the patients with non-COPD lung diseases participate in the same multidisciplinary rehabilitation programs as do their counterparts with COPD. They undergo an intensive inpatient program that has an average length of stay of 4 weeks. Those patients with hypoxemia are given supplemental oxygen according to the guidelines of the American College of Chest Physicians and the National Heart, Lung and Blood Institute.[8] The program uses a multidisciplinary approach[13] that involves multiple daily therapy sessions to achieve its goals.

Most of the improvement seen in muscular and cardiac conditioning occurs during physical therapy. Patients start with one daily session of individual physical therapy; after 1 week, this is extended to a second session of group therapy. The 45-minute physical therapy sessions emphasize strength and conditioning through repetitive work against resistance. Included are floor walking, treadmill walking, stationary bicycle riding, and work on an upper body cycle ergometer; each of these exercises is performed repetitively to the patient's tolerance. Breathing retraining attempts to develop a slow, deep diaphragmatic (abdominal) respiratory pattern and desensitization to dyspnea. Each day, a 45-minute occupational therapy session is conducted; it emphasizes upper extremity resistive exercise to tolerance, improvement in the performance of activities of daily living, and incorporation of breathing techniques into the activities of daily living. Training in surface-to-surface transfers, labor-saving techniques, and safety is also given. Patients participate in either an education or relaxation class for 1 hour daily. Respiratory therapy provides the patient with chest physiotherapy and instruction in the use of nebulizers and inhalers. Patients are seen at least four times per week by the physician for medical management. Instruction given in the classroom and gym is reinforced in the patient unit by the nursing staff. Progress is assessed at a weekly multidisciplinary conference. The 6-minute walking test is performed at both admission and discharge.

SUMMARY

Patients with non-COPD lung diseases admitted for multidisciplinary pulmonary rehabilitation are characterized by a broad spectrum of diagnoses. However, the disability of these patients may have similar origins to that of COPD patients. Dyspnea is a prominent factor in the limitation of exercise. Fatigue, enforced periods of bed rest, and muscular deconditioning may also contribute to the overall debility in these patients. The patients may have behavioral and cognitive dysfunction, which often causes a withdrawn and depressed state coupled with a sense of hopelessness. Participating in a rehabilitation program that provides a structured and supportive environment in addition to extensive exercise training tends to maximize the level of physical functioning that these patients' ventilatory limitation allows.

REFERENCES

1. Foster S, Thomas HM III. Pulmonary rehabilitation in lung disease other than chronic obstructive pulmonary disease. Am Rev Respir Dis 1990; 141:601–604.
2. Cherniak RM, Handford RG, Svanhill E. Home care of chronic respiratory disease. JAMA 1969; 208:821–824.
3. Butland RJA, Pang J, Gross ER, et al. Two, six and 12 minute walking tests in respiratory disease. BMJ 1982; 284:1607–1608.
4. Belman MJ. Exercise in chronic obstructive pulmonary disease. Clin Chest Med 1986; 7:585–597.
5. Donahoe M, Rogers RM, Wilson DO, et al. Oxygen consumption of the respiratory muscles in normal and in malnourished patients with chronic obstructive pulmonary disease. Am Rev Respir Dis 1989; 140:385–391.
6. Wilson DO, Rogers RM, Wright EC, et al. Body weight in chronic obstructive pulmonary disease. Am Rev Respir Dis 1989; 139:1435–1438.
7. Lourenco RV, Turino GM, Davidson LAG, et al. The regulation of ventilation in diffuse pulmonary fibrosis. Am J Med 1965; 38:199–216.
8. Fulmer JD, Snider GL. American College of Chest Physicians (ACCP): National Heart, Lung and Blood Institute (NLHBI) Conference on Oxygen Therapy. Arch Intern Med 1984; 144:1645–1655.
9. Martinez FJ, Courser JI, Celli BR. Respiratory response to arm elevation in patients with chronic airflow obstruction. Am Rev Respir Dis 1991; 143:476–480.
10. Current Estimates from the National Health Interview Survey, United States, 1986: Vital and Health Statistics. Hyattsville, MD: National Center for Health Statistics; 1987. US Department of Health and Human Services publication (PHS) 897-1592, Series 10.
11. Tager IB, Segal MR, Speizer FE, et al. The natural history of forced expiratory volumes: Effect of cigarette smoking in respiratory symtoms. Am Rev Respir Dis 1988; 138:837–849.
12. Sorlie PD, Kannel WB, O'Connor G. Mortality associated with respiratory function and symptoms in advanced age: The Framingham Study. Am Rev Respir Dis 1989; 140:379–384.
13. Fishman DB, Petty TL. Physical, symptomatic and psychological improvement in patients receiving comprehensive care for chronic airways obstruction. J Chron Dis 1971; 24:775–785.
14. Foster S, Lopez D, Thomas HM III. Pulmonary rehabilitation in COPD patients with elevated PCO2. Am Rev Respir Dis 1988; 138:1519–1523.
15. Daughton DM, Fix AJ, Kass I, et al. Physiological-intellectual components of vocational rehabilitation success in patients with chronic obstructive pulmonary disease (COPD). J Chron Dis 1979; 32:405–409.
16. Casaburi R, Storer TW, Ben-Dov I, et al. Effect of endurance training on possible determinants of $\dot{V}O_2$ during heavy exercise. J Appl Physiol 1987; 62:199–207.
17. Casaburi R, Patessio A, Ioli F, et al. Reductions in exercise lactic acidosis and ventilation as a result of exercise training in patients with obstructive lung disease. Am Rev Respir Dis 1991; 143:9–18.
18. Belman MJ, Kendregan BA. Exercise training fails to increase skeletal muscle enzymes in patients with chronic obstructive pulmonary disease. Am Rev Respir Dis 1981; 123:256–261.
19. Mohsenifar Z, Horak D, Brown HV, et al. Sensitive indices of improvement in a pulmonary rehabilitation program. Chest 1983; 83:189–192.
20. Wasserman K, Sue DY, Casaburi R, Moricca RB. Selection criteria for exercise training in pulmonary rehabilitation. Eur Respir J Suppl 1989; 7:604–610.
21. Casaburi R, Wasserman K, Patessio A, et al. A new perspective in pulmonary rehabilitation: Anaerobic threshold as a discriminant in training. Eur Respir J Suppl 1989; 7:618–623.
22. Moser KM, Bokinsky GE, Savage RT, et al. Results of a comprehensive rehabilitation program: Physiologic and functional effects on patients with chronic obstructive pulmonary disease. Arch Intern Med 1980; 140:1596–1601.
23. Donaldson SW, Wagner CC, Gresham GE. A unified ADL evaluation form. Arch Phys Med Rehabil 1973; 54:175–179.
24. Make BJ. Pulmonary rehabilitation: Myth or reality? Clin Chest Med 1986; 7:519–540.
25. Abd AG, Braun NMT, Baskin MI, et al. Diaphragmatic dysfunction after open heart surgery: Treatment with a rocking bed. Ann Intern Med 1989; 111:881–886.
26. Goldstein RS, Avendano MA, De Rosie J, et al. Intermittent positive-pressure ventilation via a nasal mask in patients with restrictive ventilatory failure. Chest 1990; 97:80s.
27. Fitting JW, Frascarolo P, Jequier E, et al. Resting energy expenditure in interstitial lung disease. Am Rev Respir Dis 1990; 142:631–635.
28. Austrian R, McClement JH, Renzetti AD, et al. Clinical and physiologic features of some types of pulmonary diseases with impairment of alveolar-capillary diffusion. Am J Med 1951; 11:667–684.
29. Bradley GW, Crawford R. Regulation of breathing during exercise in normal subjects and in chronic lung disease. Clin Sci Mol Med 1976; 51:575–582.
30. Burdon JGW, Killian KJ, Jones NL. Pattern of breathing during exercise in patients with interstitial lung disease. Thorax 1983; 38:778–784.
31. Wasserman K, Hansen JE, Sue DY, Whipp BJ. Principles of Exercise Testing and Interpretation. Philadelphia: Lea & Febiger, 1987.
32. Rochester DF, Arora NS, Braun NMT, et al. The respiratory muscles in chronic obstructive pulmonary disease (COPD). Bull Eur Physiopathol Respir 1979; 15:951–975.
33. Aldrich TK, Arora NS, Rochester DF. The influence of airway obstruction and respiratory muscle strength on maximal voluntary ventilation in lung disease. Am Rev Respir Dis 1982; 126:195–199.
34. Ringqvist T. Ventilatory capacity in normal subjects: Analysis of causal factors with special reference to the respiratory forces. Scand J Clin Lab Invest Suppl 1966; 88:1–179.
35. Lavietes MH, Clifford E, Silverstein D, et al. Relationship of static respiratory muscle pressure and maximum voluntary ventilation in normal subjects. Respiration 1979; 38:121–126.
36. De Troyer A, Yernault J-C. Inspiratory muscle force in normal subjects and patients with interstitial lung disease. Thorax 1980; 35:92–100.
37. Gallagher CG, Im Hof V, Younes M. Effect of inspiratory muscle fatigue on breathing pattern. J Appl Physiol 1985; 59:1152–1158.
38. Gibson GJ, Pride NB. Pulmonary mechanics in fibrosing of alveolitis. The effects of lung shrinkage. Am Rev Respir Dis 1977; 116:637–647.
39. Campbell EJM, Agostoni E, Davis JN. The Respiratory Muscles: Mechanics and Neural Control. Philadelphia: W.B. Saunders Co., 1970.

Chapter 33

The Role of Physical Training in Asthma

CHRISTOPHER J. CLARK, M.D., F.R.C.P.

THE RELATIONSHIP BETWEEN ASTHMA AND EXERCISE

It can be seen from the broad definition of bronchial asthma as a "clinical syndrome characterized by reversible obstruction to airflow and increased bronchial responsiveness to a variety of stimuli both allergic and environmental"[1] that there are two important implications for rehabilitation management of the resulting disability. First, there is a wide *interpatient* variability in disease severity that ranges from very mild asthma, which allows participation in athletic competition at the highest level,[2, 3] to severe disease, which is characterized by irreversible airways obstruction despite optimal medication. Second, there is often a significant *intrapatient* variability in disease severity either in the form of illness exacerbations or background lability of airways obstruction. The issue is also complicated by the fact that the resultant disability, that is, "the total effect of impairment on the patient's life,"[4] is influenced by additional psychosocial variables, including attitude toward exercise, education, social circumstances, and the patient personality. Strategies for the management of these variables have recently been the subject of a good review,[5] and in this chapter I concentrate on exercise rehabilitation programs in particular. Because asthma is a chronic illness that arises during early childhood, many long-standing misconceptions about the effect of exercise on the illness exist. There are few analogous conditions—for example, angina and osteoarthritis—in which exercise has such a potentially deleterious effect on the patient, not only by limiting exercise capability but also by acting as a direct stimulus to the underlying pathophysiologic process. Whether the mechanism is respiratory heat loss,[6] increased osmolarity due to respiratory water loss,[7] or other postulated vascular events,[8] increasing minute ventilation during exercise is a potent stimulus to exercise-induced asthma. It is not surprising that asthmatic patients often have a negative attitude toward exercise, and this attitude is compounded by the personal problems that they experience in safely and effectively participating in athletic activities.[9] The unnecessary restriction of sporting activities for certain children with asthma has been recognized for some time,[10] and an attempt has been made to remedy this problem through better education and by advising the use of a beta-selective agonist before exercise[11] as well as the avoidance of conditions that are apt to produce exercise-induced asthma. Certain activities, such as swimming, are often encouraged because of the favorable conditions of humidity and temperature in which they are performed.[12] However, the routine management of physical exercise in schoolchildren remains difficult. The results of a questionnaire recently given to physical education teachers[13] suggested that their knowledge was insufficient to offer sporting activities to individual children in a satisfactory manner and that they were in favor of receiving more education on this topic. There is an increasing requirement to provide more specific exercise prescription for individual patients of all ages based on objective criteria of exercise capability, and there is evidence to suggest that this approach can improve fitness.[14, 15]

Many patients are between the two extremes of

asthma severity, that is, they have moderate airflow limitation. The pursuit of exercise as a recreational activity or as part of the widely advertised promotion of a "healthy lifestyle"[16] raises a difficult question for these patients that is paradoxically not faced by severely disabled patients, namely, How much exercise can and should be undertaken? A previously sedentary nonasthmatic adult who attends a training session of vigorous intensity may experience considerable breathlessness and chest discomfort (or "tightness") while exercising but will, depending on his motivation level, respond to the encouragement (or harrassment!) of the trainer and attempt to continue training at an intensity that is likely to improve fitness. In this case, breathlessness is physiologic and occurs for a variety of reasons, including a heightened awareness of unfamiliar increasing hyperpnea.[17] The asthmatic patient faces a dilemma when experiencing the same symptoms; he or she must ask if the discomfort and breathlessness are normal or abnormal. At one extreme, the patient may attribute breathlessness to lack of fitness when the illness is the limiting factor, and at the other extreme, the patient may attribute exercise limitation to asthma despite good residual capacity for exercise participation. In the former case, objective exercise evaluation would allow the patient to be counseled, and exercise could be directed toward a realistic program that works within the limitations of the underlying condition; however, in the latter case, management should be directed toward encouragement of confidence to participate in more vigorous exercise programs. Such objective information is not routinely available to the asthmatic patient, whose decision is heavily weighted against continuing to exercise whenever breathlessness is a significant component of the perceived exertion, regardless of its etiology, because exercise in these circumstances may be viewed as potentially dangerous. In a recent study,[18] experimentally induced "harmful anticipation" significantly intensified the perception of visceral changes, including the subjective cost of exercise, and even had some influence on specific asthma-related responses, such as airways resistance. Several papers highlight the complexity of the relationships between breathlessness, exercise tolerance, and resting lung function in asthma. In one,[19] a regression model using nine independent physiologic variables could explain only 63% of the variance in breathlessness rating of asthmatics during progressive incremental exercise. Although the relationship of breathlessness to work intensity showed responsiveness to change induced by bronchoconstriction with methacholine, wide intrapatient and interpatient variabilities were seen. There is similar evidence of a wide variability between exercise tolerance and measures of airways obstruction[20] as well as between the severity of breathlessness and measures of lung function in asthma.[21]

This complexity can even obscure the diagnosis of exercise-induced asthma. By way of illustration, a physician in our unit underwent exercise evaluation to determine her fitness level. She had attributed the breathlessness that occurred frequently during exercise to a lack of fitness. In fact, she developed a 30% decrease in forced expiratory volume in 1 second (FEV_1) after progressive incremental exercise testing in the laboratory without overt wheezing. Retrospectively, she could not identify any features of the breathlessness that were suggestive of a pathologic cause such as asthma. This is perhaps a more common problem than is often appreciated. For example, a screening test of 503 children[22] recently revealed that an average of one child in every classroom had previously undiagnosed exercise-induced asthma, the symptoms of which were often absent or attributed to other causes.

In summary, there is a potential for misinterpretation of exercise capability in the absence of objective measurement of cardiorespiratory responses to exercise. Formal exercise evaluation is the keystone to success in rehabilitation of the asthmatic patient.

CARDIORESPIRATORY PERFORMANCE CHARACTERISTICS OF ASTHMATICS

When considering cardiorespiratory performance characteristics of asthmatics in the context of pulmonary rehabilitation, three aspects may act as conflicting variables. First, intrasubject variability of airways obstruction at the time of measurement may be associated with a corresponding variability in exercise performance. There is no current evidence to suggest a fundamentally different cardiorespiratory response to exercise in the asthmatic patient when he or she is free from airways obstruction compared with normal subjects.[23] However, there are predictable alterations in ventilatory patterns associated with airways obstruction[24] that may confound accurate measurement of true performance capability. For example, ventilatory limitation may produce a variable respiratory endpoint rather than a true cardiovascular endpoint during evaluation of work capacity. The importance of this in the asthmatic patient is that this respiratory endpoint is determined mainly by the relationship of minute ventilation to maximum voluntary ventilation ($\dot{V}E/MVV$) during exercise, and since MVV has a close relationship to FEV_1,[25] mild variability in asthma severity at the time of testing has a very significant influence on measured work capacity. This makes it difficult not only to compare patients' performance but also can confound longitudinal measurement in individual patients of the impact of rehabilitation programs on cardiorespiratory variables that may be responsive to change in underlying disease severity.

Second, the presence or absence of exercise-induced asthma has an important implication in determining performance capability. Exercise-induced asthma should be viewed as a specific entity about which there remains debate not only concerning the initial stimulus to the development of airflow limitation but also about the circulatory and metabolic changes that result. This is of limited relevance to pulmonary rehabilitation in asthmatics, as medication prior to training can usually prevent exercise-induced asthma and the related physiologic sequelae. Pulmonary rehabilitation involves exercise under optimal conditions, and thus prevention of exercise-induced asthma with appropriate therapy is a prerequisite. Anderson and coworkers[26] have shown that treadmill exercise without prior treatment produces an increase in ventilation/perfusion inequality, alveoloarterial oxygen tension, physiologic dead space, and arterial blood lactate levels. If exercise-induced asthma is prevented by premedication with beta$_2$-agonist therapy, then drug effects on the cardiovascular responses to exercise cannot be completely excluded,[27] although these effects appear to be small if standard therapeutic doses via the inhaled route are used.[28]

Third, there is conflicting evidence on impaired metabolic responses to exercise in asthmatics that could also influence cardiorespiratory performance in individual patients. Two studies[29, 30] have suggested a "blunted" sympathoadrenal response to exercise in asthmatic subjects, implying that a failure of the usual increase in plasma adrenaline and noradrenaline concentrations during submaximum exercise may be a contributing factor to exercise-induced asthma. However, other studies[31, 32] have failed to confirm these findings; furthermore, the postulated abnormalities have not been associated with abnormal cardiorespiratory responses to exercise (provided that appropriate premedication was given). There are other studies that suggest altered metabolic responses, including conflicting reports of potassium homeostasis during exercise in asthmatics as compared with normal subjects (i.e., a prolongation of the normal exercise-provoked elevation in serum potassium level).[32, 33] Impairment of free fatty acid metabolism[34] and excessive growth hormone secretion after exercise (regardless of inspired air conditions or the development of exercise-induced asthma)[35] have been reported. Finally, a recent study of asthmatic patients suggested the presence of an impaired plasma cortisol response to exercise in 10 asthmatic subjects, none of whom were being treated with systemic corticosteroids.[36] It is important to stress that there is no direct evidence to suggest that these abnormalities, if present, directly impinge on exercise performance, and thus they are of limited relevance in the specific context of asthma rehabilitation.

A number of studies have investigated fitness levels in asthmatic subjects. As illustrated in Table 33–1, published data largely refer to childhood asthma. There are considerable differences in the size of sample populations, the type of control subjects, measurements, and the use of bronchodilators prior to testing. Instruments chosen for the measurement of work performance included maximum oxygen consumption ($\dot{V}O_2$max), maximum work rate measured externally (e.g., from bicycle ergometry settings), and peak work capacity at a heart rate of 170 beats/min. These differences in study design, including the illness severity of the asthmatic subjects chosen, may explain the conflicting performance data in these studies. Work capacity is likely to have been underestimated in those studies in which exercise-induced bronchoconstriction was not prevented by premedication with bronchodilators. Inadequate patient sample size in most of the studies limits the general applicability of the conclusions, and in a number of studies, a control group was either absent or inappropriate, that is, there had been no attempt to match for age, sex, and habitual activity. However, it is clear from these studies that exercise evaluation of asthmatic patients very frequently reveals suboptimal fitness levels. Three studies of childhood asthma[37–39] and one of adult asthma,[23] in which subjects exercised to exhaustion after premedication with bronchodilators to prevent exercised-induced asthma, present particularly compelling evidence that asthmatic subjects tend to be less fit than their peers. One study of 65 children with moderate to severe asthma revealed that 60% were unfit and that 50% were "severely" deconditioned.[37] This was not simply a function of the severity of airways obstruction, as fitness level could not be predicted from asthma history alone. Another study of 39 children with milder asthma revealed a marked reduction in maximum oxygen consumption when compared with that of normal children.[38] The third recent large-scale study, again in children and using validated "field" testing of fitness by a 9-minute run, showed poor conditioning (i.e., a score below the 25th percentile for values obtained from screening over 12,000 normal children) in 74% of subjects that was not attributable to anthropometric differences.[39] Recently,[23] we used progressive incremental exercise testing not only to determine work performance but also to assess the contribution of respiratory factors to exercise limitation and to determine the likely capacity for endurance training in a group of patients with well-controlled asthma of moderate severity. This form of exercise evaluation is particularly suitable for a variety of reasons. The use of short-step increments (i.e., 25 watts at 1-minute intervals to a symptom-limited maximum) provides the necessary data over a practical time scale (on average 12 minutes). The physiologic variables measured include heart rate, $\dot{V}E$, tidal volume, oxygen consumption, and carbon dioxide production; "cardiovascular fitness" variables include anaerobic threshold, oxygen pulse, and $\dot{V}O_2$max. Simultaneous measurement of $\dot{V}E$ and heart rate allows an analysis of the interrelation of the ventilatory and the cardiovascular responses to exercise at submaximum workloads.

The 44 asthmatic subjects with chronic stable asthma of moderate severity all required regular prophylactic treatment and had reproducible airways obstruction when treatment was withheld. In all cases, the provocative concentration of histamine causing a 20% decrease in FEV_1 (PC_{20}) was less than 8 mg/ml, according to the method described by Hargreave and associates,[40] and 39 of the 44 patients fulfilled criteria for exercise-induced asthma. The 64 control subjects had no concomitant illness, past history of respiratory disease, or family history of asthma. All had a sedentary lifestyle and did not participate in any form of regular exercise or training.

Because some of the measurements made during exercise are dependent on several variables, including age, sex, weight, and height, multiple regression analysis was used to compare the two groups after adjustment for these factors. Asthma accounted for a mean reduction in $\dot{V}O_2$max of 199 ml/min ($P < .001$). The relation-

TABLE 33-1. REVIEW OF STUDIES REPORTING FITNESS LEVELS IN ASTHMATIC SUBJECTS

Reference	Asthma Patients	Healthy Control Subjects	Fitness Measurement	Pre-exercise Medication	Conclusion
Nickerson et al.[67] (1983)	15 C	No data	Work rate	NO*	Less fit
Mallinson et al.[69] (1981)	5 C	No data	No measurement	N/S	Less fit
Fitch et al.[71] (1976)	46 C	10 C	PWC 170	NO*	Less fit
Ludwick et al.[37] (1986)	65 C	ref 1980	Work rate	YES	Less fit
Vavra et al.[66] (1971)	16 C	No data	$\dot{V}O_2$max	N/S	Less fit
Freeman et al.[28] (1989)	9 A	6 A	$\dot{V}O_2$max	YES	Less fit
Orenstein et al.[38] (1985)	23 C	No data	Work/$\dot{V}O_2$	YES	Less fit
Bevegaard et al.[89] (1976)	20 C	ref 1950	$\dot{V}O_2$max	NO	No difference
Cropp and Tanakawa[87] (1977)	21 C	13 C	$\dot{V}O_2$max	NO	No difference
Kivilog et al.[88] (1975)	86 A	ref 1969 (L)	Work rate	NO*	No difference
Ingemann-Hansen et al.[90] (1980)	5 A	ref 1970 (L)	$\dot{V}O_2$max	NO	No difference

Key: C: children; A: adults; (L): local population; N/S: no statement regarding pre-exercise medication; *: studies documenting exercise-induced asthma; PWC 170: peak work capacity at a heart rate of 170 beats/min. "Ref" followed by date indicates that a historical comparison group was used. "Less fit" is with respect to the control/comparison population.
Further details can be found in references 37, 38, and 66 to 90.

ship between $\dot{V}O_2$ and the diagnosis of asthma is described in the following equation:

$$\dot{V}O_2\text{max (ml/min)} = 1906.3 + 13.33 \times \text{WT} - 723.8 \times \text{SEX} - 14.19 \times \text{AGE} - 199.23 \times \text{ASTHMA}$$
$$(\text{SEE} = 27.03, r = 0.88)$$

where ASTHMA equals 1 for asthmatics and 0 for control subjects, SEX equals 1 for females and 0 for males, AGE is in years, WT is weight in kilograms, and SEE is standard error of the estimate.

The anaerobic threshold was 125 ml/min lower ($P < .001$) and maximum oxygen pulse was 0.805 ml/beat lower ($P < .001$) in asthmatic than in nonasthmatic subjects.

The dyspnea index ($\dot{V}_E$max/MVV%) was significantly higher in the asthmatic subjects during maximum exercise (61 ± 19 versus 49 ± 10, $P < .001$) and also at the submaximum workload that produced 75% of the predicted maximum heart rate (34 ± 15 versus 25 ± 6, $P < .001$).

Within the asthmatic group, there was no linear correlation between FEV_1 before or after bronchodilator use and the "cardiovascular fitness" variables ($\dot{V}O_2$max, anaerobic threshold, and oxygen pulse), whether FEV_1 was expressed in absolute terms or as percentages of predicted values. Once age, weight, and sex had been taken into account, there was no separate contribution from FEV_1 to these variables. A relatively poor correlation was found between postbronchodilator FEV_1 and the dyspnea index at peak exercise (Fig. 33-1).

This study highlights several important aspects of exercise performance in patients with moderate asthma. Contrary to the subjects' expectation that their condition would not permit exercise of high intensity, they achieved a maximum heart rate that was similar to that of control subjects and therefore had a cardiovascular rather than respiratory endpoint to exercise. Furthermore, the absence of correlation of airways obstruction with the measures of fitness in the asthmatic subjects revealed that factors other than the severity of asthma were likely to be responsible for their lack of fitness. The subjects were young adults. In early adolescence, it is possible that their asthma had been much worse so that they were less able to carry out exercise; thus, they developed a sedentary lifestyle. Alternatively, they may have a more fundamental and continuing aversion to exercise as a result of long-standing asthma.[41] This is supported by a recent study of 90 asthmatic children that identified the interrelationships between cardiorespiratory fitness, asthma severity, and psychologic functioning.[42] Disease severity variables (e.g., FEV_1) accounted for only 8% of the variability in fitness within the group, whereas a psychologic assessment (using the Child Global Assessment Scale) correlated with fitness

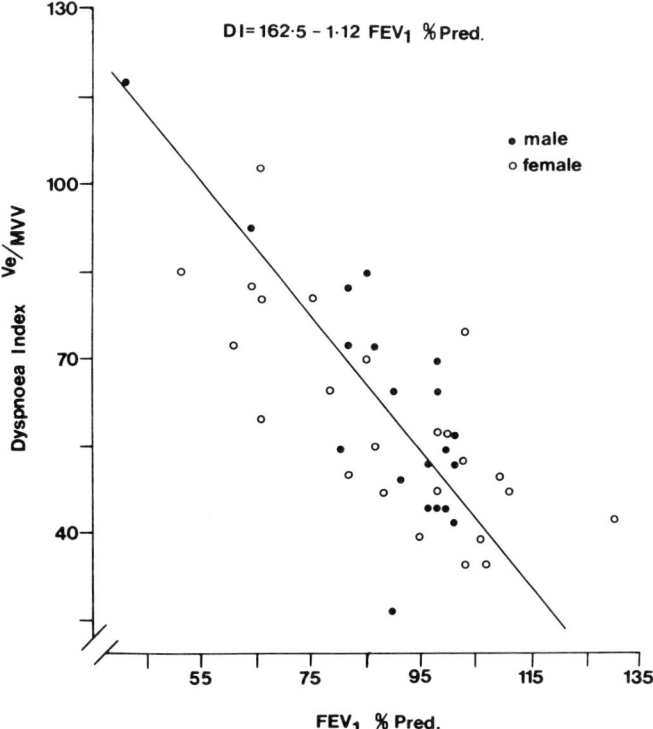

FIGURE 33-1. Relationship between the dyspnea index ($\dot{V}_E$/MVV, in per cent) at maximum exercise and FEV_1 per cent predicted in 44 asthmatic patients. (DI: dyspnea index; $r = -.533$; $P < .001$). (From Clark CJ, Cochrane LM. Assessment of work performance in asthma for determination of cardiorespiratory fitness and training capacity. Thorax 1988; 43:745-749.)

better than all the medical variables combined. The authors concluded that adjustment to disease was at least as important as disease severity in determining fitness in asthmatic children. Another study examining attitudes about physical activity and asthma in 408 children[43] showed that, although they enjoyed exercise and were generally active, they were more anxious prior to exercise than were normal children. Perhaps these problems in attitude are compounded in young adult asthmatics by the absence of medical advice and ongoing flexible exercise prescription. Even for the normal, healthy individual, exercise will improve aerobic fitness only if certain criteria for intensity, frequency, and duration are consistently fulfilled over several months. The recommended guidelines[14] suggest a workload that produces about 75% of the predicted maximum heart rate for 20 minutes at least three times per week. In those with asthma, the underlying obstruction may limit exercise tolerance if there is inadequate ventilatory reserve. It is not clear how individuals should determine the extent of their ventilatory reserve and how the recommended guidelines should be adapted to their own circumstances. These uncertainties may deter even well-motivated individuals from participating in exercise. High levels of $\dot{V}E$ close to the MVV can only be tolerated for a short time because of breathlessness. This principle is used routinely in progressive incremental exercise testing, where the relationship $\dot{V}Emax/MVV$ during maximum exercise is used to identify "respiratory limitation."[24] The potential contribution of reduced ventilatory reserve to intolerance of the submaximum exercise level necessary for endurance training has been shown in a study that measured the endurance time for various levels of $\dot{V}E$ in relation to the MVV by using voluntary isocapnic hyperventilation.[44] As $\dot{V}E$ decreased to 60% of MVV, endurance time increased to about 15 minutes. At this point in the relationship, the "asymptote"—that is, the tangent to the curve of $\dot{V}E$ versus endurance time—"extended to infinity." Lower levels of ventilation were comfortable and could be sustained continuously. The importance of this for endurance training in the person with asthma is that for a given frequency and intensity of exercise, the ventilatory reserve determines the duration of exercise and, therefore, the potential for achieving a training effect. This is illustrated schematically in Figure 33–2. Sector A represents the case where exercise intensity (maximum heart rate is less than 75% of that predicted) is inadequate for achieving a training effect. Because they misinterpret the perceived severity of more strenuous exertion as being caused by their underlying condition, patients who choose this pattern of performance fail to improve their level of fitness, despite adequate ventilatory reserve and regardless of the duration of exercise sessions. Sector B represents the case where the patients choose an adequate exercise intensity and have sufficient ventilatory reserve (low $\dot{V}E/MVV\%$) to allow the necessary duration of exercise to achieve a training effect. (This was the pattern seen in the subjects of the previously mentioned study, as the dyspnea index—although higher at each stage of exercise than in the control subjects—decreased below 60% in all the asthmatic subjects at a submaximum workload that produced 75% of the predicted maximum heart rate.) In Sector C, the duration of exercise at high workloads is impaired by inadequate ventilatory reserve. In Sector D, inadequate ventilatory reserve at low workloads makes even mild exercise difficult and precludes a training effect.

In Figure 33–3, the progressive incremental exercise data for four asthma patients are superimposed on the four-quadrant diagram. Although they have a very similar extent of obstruction (FEV_1 60–70% of the predicted norm), each has a markedly different ventilatory response during exercise. Since such patients may have difficulty in interpreting the appropriateness of their subjective response to various levels of exercise and since resting lung function does not predict their exercise ventilation accurately, objective exercise testing with emphasis on measurements of heart rate and $\dot{V}E$ has a valuable practical application in allowing individual exercise prescription. This is considered further later in this chapter in the discussion of the rehabilitation management of asthmatic patients.

PHYSIOLOGIC OUTCOME OF MEDICALLY SUPERVISED PHYSICAL TRAINING

A number of studies have reported beneficial changes in cardiorespiratory performance indicators in asthmatic subjects following physical training. Table 33–2 summarizes these studies and indicates the categories of patients chosen, the control groups selected, and the physiologic measurements used to examine the effects of physical training. It is important to identify methodologic difficulties that the various authors have experienced. Before doing so, however, it is equally important to stress that almost universally these exhaustive clinical studies have shown a major improvement in exercise performance occurred in patients after participation in rehabilitation programs.

There have been few studies of adult asthmatic patients. Most of the publications cite no control groups for comparison, and those that did have control groups mainly used young, fit adults already participating in regular physical activity, thus introducing bias into the analysis. Randomization to training and nontraining asthmatic groups is essential to rule out the possibility that any change in performance indicators resulted not from the rehabilitation program but rather from the normal variability in illness severity with time or from changes in medication that occur as a result of increased access to medical advice. Table 33–3 summarizes the variety of training schedules that have been used as well as the frequency, duration, intensity, and time scale of the programs. Most of the studies do not identify whether premedication with inhaled bronchodilators was given before exercise participation. Table 33–4 summarizes the reported effects on lung function and asthma severity following physical training. Virtually all of the studies showed no change in spirometric indices of airways obstruction. In two of the studies that reported

FIGURE 33-2. Interrelation between exercise intensity and the resulting ventilatory response in determining training effect in an individual with asthma. The heart rate, expressed as a percentage of predicted maximum, represents the intensity of work undertaken. The minute ventilation (VE) produced by that level of exercise is expressed as a percentage of maximum voluntary ventilation (MVV). The thick horizontal line represents the work intensity below which a training effect is unlikely. The thick vertical line represents the VE/MVV above which exercise is unlikely to be tolerated for long enough to achieve a training effect. (See also reference 65.) (From Cochrane LM, Clark CJ. Benefits and problems of a physical training programme for asthmatic patients. Thorax 1990; 45:345–351.)

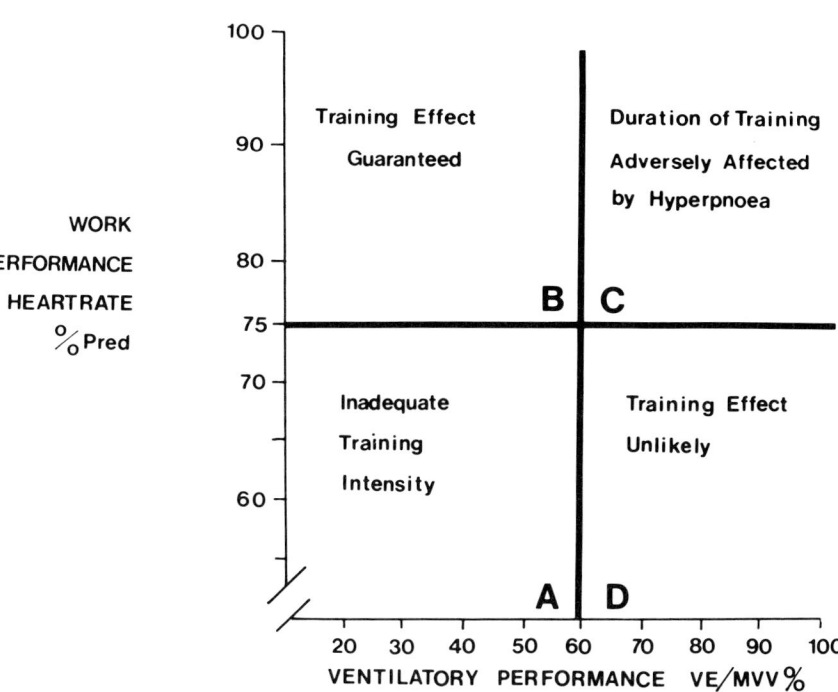

an increase in peak flow rate, no actual data were given. Assessment of exercise-induced asthma produced conflicting results (of the nine reports, only three showed a decrease in exercise-induced asthma; furthermore, no physiologic rationale for the apparent improvement was provided in these three studies). We have recently piloted a carefully controlled program of exercise training under medical supervision in a group of patients with asthma of moderate severity in order to evaluate the benefits not only in terms of cardiorespiratory fitness

FIGURE 33-3. Progressive incremental exercise data for the heart rate and ventilatory responses of four patients with similar airways obstruction. The data are superimposed on the four-quadrant diagram.

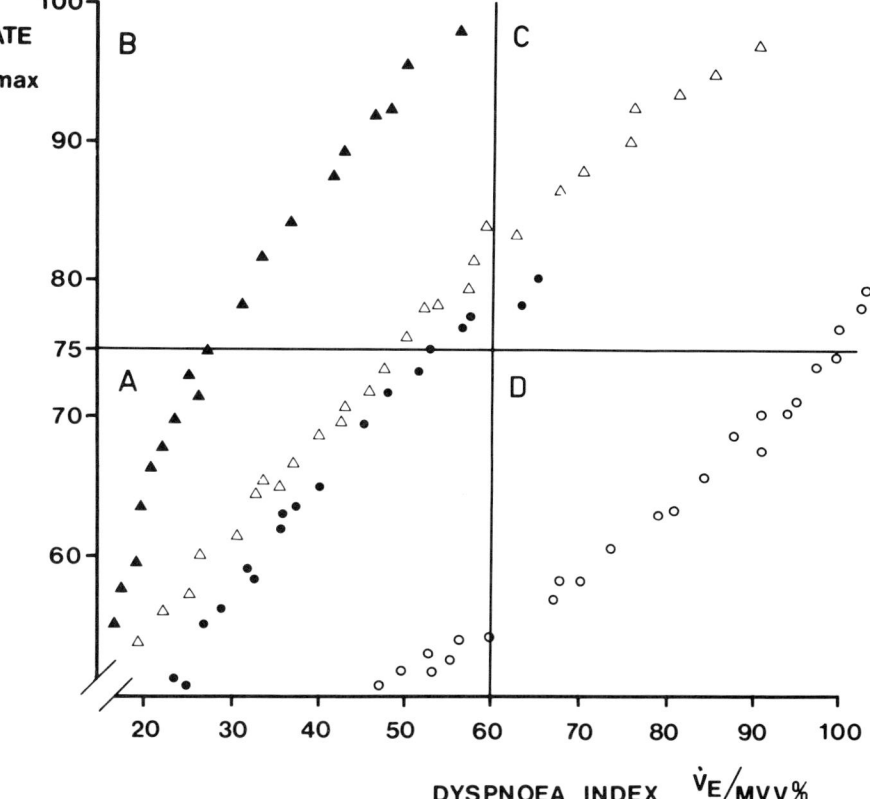

TABLE 33–2. A REVIEW OF THE PHYSIOLOGIC CHANGES OBSERVED IN STUDIES THAT EXAMINED THE EFFECTS OF PHYSICAL TRAINING IN ASTHMA

Reference	Asthma Patients	Control Subjects	Fitness Measurement			Other Physiologic Measurements	
Vavra et al.[66] (1971)	16 C	None	$\dot{V}O_2$	→			
Nickerson et al.[67] (1983)	15 C	None	Work	↑	: 12-min run ↑		
Green and Coggings[68] (1982)	6 C	None	No data				
Mallinson et al.[69] (1981)	5 C	None	No data				
Sly et al.[70] (1972)	26 C	None	"Fitness"	↑			
Fitch et al.[71] (1976)	46 C	Healthy	PWC 170	↑	: swim distance ↑		
Itkin and Nacman[72] (1966)	29 YA	10 YA	$\dot{V}O_2$	↑		Heart rate response	→
Ludwick et al.[37] (1986)	65 C	None	$\dot{V}O_2$	↑	(only in 5 subjects)		
Orenstein et al.[38] (1985)	23 C	13 C	$\dot{V}O_2$	↑	: PWC ↑	Heart rate, submaximum	↓
Sevonius et al.[73] (1983)	50 C	C	PWC	↑		Heart rate, submaximum	↓
Henriksen and Nielsen[74] (1983)	42 C	C	No data			Heart rate and lactate level	↓
Graff-Lonevig et al.[75] (1980)	11 C	9 C	$\dot{V}O_2$	→			
Guebelle et al.[76] (1971)	11 C	None	PWC 170	→			
Scherr and Frankel[77] (1958)	25 C	None	No data				
Hyde and Swarts[78] (1968)	36 C	None	No data				
Peterson and McElhenny[79] (1965)	18 C	None	"Gym tests"	↑			
Bundgaard et al.[80] (1982)	27 A	11 A	$\dot{V}O_2$	↑			
Chai et al.[81] (1967)	80 C	10 C	"Fitness"	↑			
Hirt[82] (1964)	23 YA	40 YA	$\dot{V}O_2$	↑	: Work ↑	$\dot{V}E$	
Leisti et al.[83] (1979)	16 C	None	PWC 180	↑	: Lactate level, submaximum →		
Millman et al.[84] (1965)	9 C	None	"Step test"	↑			
Seligman et al.[85] (1970)	18 C	None	"Treadmill test"	↑			
Freeman and Williams[86] (1989)	9 YA	Healthy	$\dot{V}O_2$	↑			

Key: YA: young adults; WC: work capacity; ↑: increased; ↓: decreased; →: unchanged.
Further details can be found in references 37, 38, and 66 to 90.

(which has been shown to improve in normal individuals following a similar regimen[14]) but also with respect to the ventilatory and metabolic adaptations during submaximum exercise, the effects on breathlessness during exercise, and the changes in disease severity, including nonspecific bronchial responsiveness to inhaled histamine.[44] We also tried to identify which factors determine whether an individual is successful in achieving the training goals. The 3-month indoor training program was carefully defined in terms of frequency, duration, intensity, progression, and mode of physical activity. The optimum duration and frequency of exercise were set at 30 minutes 3 times per week, during which the subjects had a target heart rate of 75% of the predicted

TABLE 33–3. DETAILS OF TRAINING SCHEDULES USED IN STUDIES EXAMINING THE EFFECTS OF PHYSICAL TRAINING IN ASTHMA*

Reference	Mode of Exercise	Frequency (per wk)	Duration	Intensity	Time (wk)	Bronchodilator Used Before Exercise?
Vavra et al.[66] (1971)	Gym/games	3	1 h	Gradual	12	Not stated
Nickerson et al.[67] (1983)	Distance running	4	Distance	Distance	6	No
Green and Coggings[68] (1982)	Gym/breathing	1	Not stated	Hard	8	Not stated
Mallison et al.[69] (1981)	Interval/ball games/strength	2	Gradual	Gradual	24–32	Yes
Sly et al.[70] (1972)	Physical conditioning/breathing	3	2 h	Not stated	12	Not stated
Fitch et al.[71] (1976)	Swimming	3–5	1 h	Increased	20	Not stated
Itkin and Nacman[72] (1966)	Sports activity/calisthenics	5	2 h	Not stated	12	Not stated
Ludwick et al.[37] (1986)	Cycling	5	1 h	60–75%	6	Yes
Orenstein et al.[38] (1985)	Exercises/ball games/jogging	3	1 h	Heart rate	16	Not stated
Sevonius et al.[73] (1983)	Interval/swimming	—	1 h	Not stated	12–16	Yes
Henriksen and Nielsen[74] (1983)	Ball games/circuits/team games	2	1½ h	Gradual	6	Yes
Graff-Lonevig et al.[75] (1980)	Interval/circuits/ball games/breathing	2	1 h	Gradual	80	No
Guebelle et al.[76] (1971)	Altitude training/hill climbing	7	4 h	Heavy	12	No
Scherr and Frankel[77] (1958)	General exercises/games/breathing	2	Not stated	Not exhausting	Not stated	Not stated
Hyde and Swarts[78] (1968)	Light endurance/strength/breathing	1	1 h	Tolerable	25	Not stated
Peterson and McElhenny[79] (1965)	Calisthenics/tumbling/games	3	1 h	Required effort	32	Not stated
Bundgaard et al.[80] (1982)	Interval/gymnastics	2	1 h	Heavy	8	Not stated
Chai et al.[81] (1967)	Physical exercise/breathing	7	2 × 20 min	Not stated	40	Not stated
Hirt[82] (1964)	Games/weights	5	2 h	Vigorous	12	Not stated
Leisti et al.[83] (1979)	Interval/gymnastics	2	1 h	Short burst	16	No
Millman et al.[84] (1965)	Interval/gymnastics	3	45 min	Tolerable pace	16	Not stated
Seligman et al.[85] (1970)	Interval/games/swimming/breathing	1	1½ h	Not stated	8	Not stated
Freeman and Williams[86] (1989)	Treadmill running	3	Not stated	Self-selected	6	Yes

*Further details can be found in references 37, 38, and 66 to 90.

TABLE 33-4. REPORTED EFFECTS ON LUNG FUNCTION AND ASTHMA SEVERITY FOLLOWING PHYSICAL TRAINING

Reference	FEV_1	Peak Flow	Exercise-induced Asthma	Other Effects
Vavra et al.[66] (1971)				Increased PaO_2
Nickerson et al.[67] (1983)	No change	No change	No change	No change in sGaw or RV
Green and Coggings[68] (1982)	No change			Increased FVC
Mallison et al.[69] (1981)		Increased		"Clinical improvement"
Sly et al.[70] (1972)	No change		No change	Decreased "wheeze"
Fitch et al.[71] (1976)			No change	
Itkin and Nacman[72] (1966)	No change			
Ludwick et al.[37] (1986)	No change			
Orenstein et al.[38] (1985)	No change	No change	No change	
Sevonius et al.[73] (1983)	No change		Decreased	"Subjective improvement"
Henriksen and Nielsen[74] (1983)	No change		Decreased	
Graff-Lonevig et al.[75] (1980)	No change			
Scherr and Frankel[77] (1958)		Increased (no data given)		
Hyde and Swarts[78] (1968)	No change			Increased MVV
Peterson and McElhenny[79] (1965)				Increased VC
Bundgaard et al.[80] (1982)			No change	
Chai et al.[81] (1967)		Increased (no data given)		
Leisti et al.[83] (1979)			No change	
Millman et al.[84] (1965)	No change			Increased MBC
Seligman et al.[85] (1970)	No change			
Freeman and Williams[86] (1989)			9 patients showed no change; 7 patients experienced a decrease	

Key: sGaw: specific airways conductance; RV: residual volume; FVC: forced vital capacity; VC: slow vital capacity; MBC: maximum breathing capacity. Further details can be found in references 37, 38, and 66 to 90.

maximum heart rate. Medical supervision was provided during all hospital training sessions. Each session consisted of a warm-up period followed by 30 minutes of continuous but varied aerobic exercise, including cycling, jogging, and "aerobic" dance movements. Patients then cooled down with a mixture of light calisthenics and stretching exercises designed to improve muscle strength and joint flexibility. A training log detailed the number of hospital and home sessions attended and the time spent exercising. A symptom score for each particular training day was also recorded. For this, subjects were asked to consult their daily diary cards and give an approximate aggregate score that ranged from 0 (no symptoms) to 4 (severe symptoms).

Cardiovascular Responses

After training, there were significant increases in mean maximum oxygen uptake (ml/kg/min) from 23 ± 5 to 28 ± 6, oxygen pulse (ml/beat) from 8.8 ± 2.3 to 10.8 ± 2.4, and anaerobic threshold (L/min) from 1.11 ± 0.27 to 1.38 ± 0.33. No significant changes were seen in the nontraining asthmatic control group.

Respiratory and Metabolic Responses

$\dot{V}_{Emax}$ (L/min) increased in the training group from 58.8 ± 14.8 to 66.1 ± 15.5 ($P < .001$), with an increase in tidal volume at peak exercise from 1.93 ± 0.69 L to 2.12 ± 0.67 L ($P < .01$). The respiratory rate was unchanged. The ventilatory equivalent for oxygen was reduced from 38 ± 4 to 34 ± 4 ($P < .01$) in the training group but not in the control group. There was no change in $\dot{V}_{Emax}/MVV$ in either group. Submaximum exercise performance data are shown in Figure 33-4. There were significant changes in blood lactate level, carbon dioxide production, and $\dot{V}_E$ at the higher levels of exercise in the training group but no corresponding changes in the control group. The latter data are useful not only as a contrast to the changes seen in the training group; they also demonstrate the reliability of this methodology in the longitudinal assessment of cardiorespiratory performance in asthmatic patients who might be expected to have considerable random variability in the parameters measured. The changes in the training group demonstrate that altered ventilatory responses are linked to underlying metabolic changes that would be anticipated in normal nonasthmatic subjects following endurance training.

Subjective (Perceived Exertion) Responses

During progressive incremental exercise, the subjects were instructed to estimate their sense of breathlessness according to a Borg scale.[45] This is essentially a category scale in which simple verbal expressions that describe increasing degrees of effort expenditure in exercise are

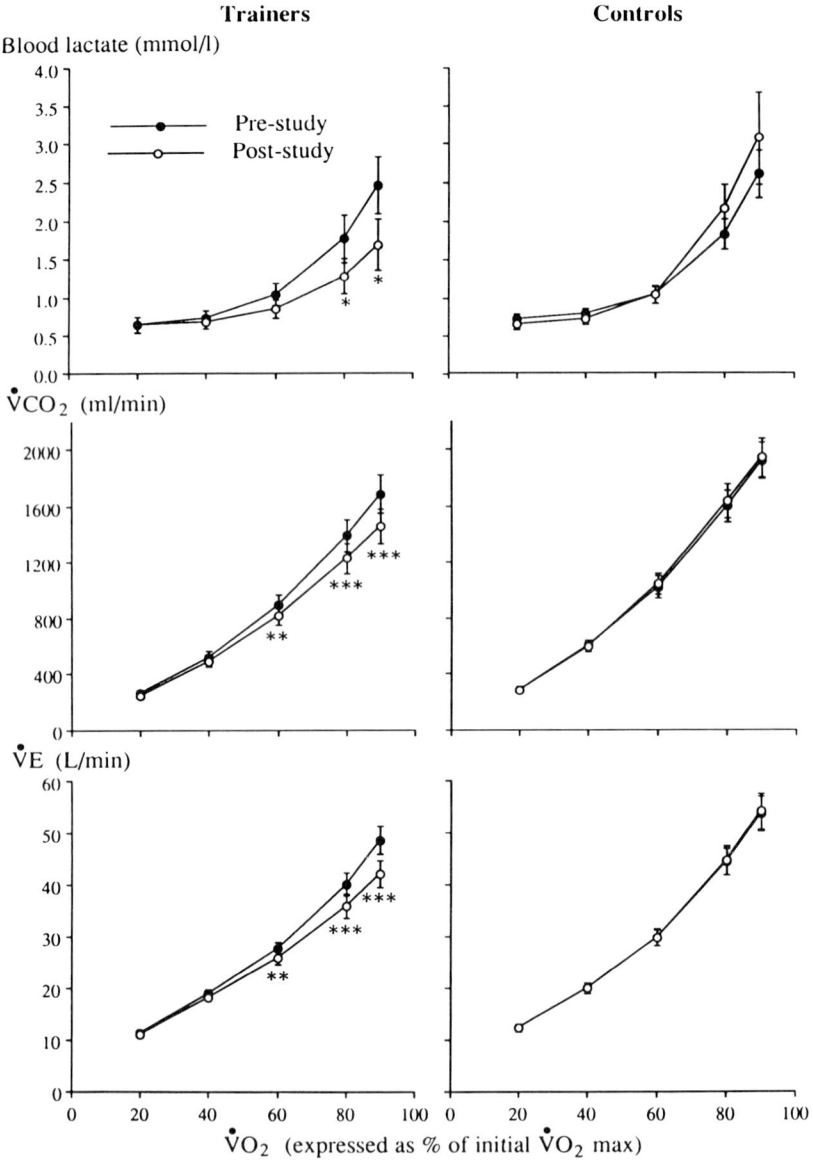

FIGURE 33-4. Relationship among blood lactate level (mean ± SEM, mmol/L), carbon dioxide production ($\dot{V}CO_2$, ml/min), and minute ventilation ($\dot{V}E$, L/min) to oxygen consumption ($\dot{V}O_2$ expressed as a percentage of initial $\dot{V}O_2$max) before and after the study period for the training and control groups. (*$P < .05$; **$P < .01$; ***$P < .001$ [before versus after the study].) (From Cochrane LM, Clark CJ. Benefits and problems of a physical training programme for asthmatic patients. Thorax 1990; 45:345–351.)

linked to numbers. After training, breathlessness was found to be reduced at workloads equivalent to those required by a wide range of daily activities (Fig. 33–5). This confirms the general observation that patients with asthma may notice a diminution in symptoms (including breathlessness) after participating in an exercise program.[46] Although a decrease in ventilation at submaximum workloads is likely to contribute to a reduction in breathlessness during exercise,[47] physical training may have a central desensitizing effect on the sensation of breathlessness. Rhythmic, repetitive exercise can produce improvements in electroencephalographic synchronicity[48] and can increase endorphin levels without reducing ventilatory chemosensitivity.[49] An analogy can be drawn between this and the type II effects of drugs, such as chlorpromazine, that reduce breathlessness by a central effect that is independent of changes in ventilation.[50]

Disease Severity

There was a slight improvement in mean FEV_1 (before and after bronchodilator use) in both groups after the study period. However, no significant difference between the mean change in FEV_1 of 0.38 ± 0.48 L in the training group and 0.19 ± 0.53 L in the control group was observed. There was also no difference when the change in FEV_1 was expressed as a percentage of the predicted normal value. Histamine PC_{20} was unchanged for the two groups. The absence of significant change in nonspecific bronchial responsiveness suggests that reported improvements in exercise-induced asthma after training (see Table 33–4) are probably due to the reduction in $\dot{V}E$ at equivalent high-intensity workloads; this results in a decrease in the stimulus for exercise-induced asthma rather than any change in the underlying

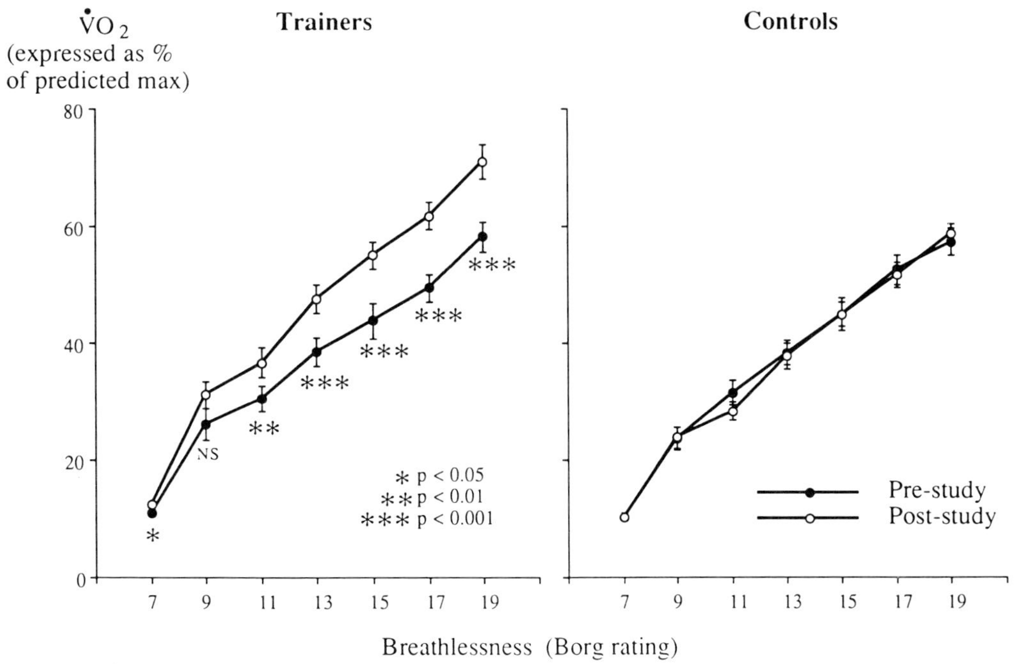

FIGURE 33-5. Relationship between perceived breathlessness (Borg scale rating) and oxygen consumption ($\dot{V}O_2$, mean ± SEM) expressed as a percentage of predicted $\dot{V}O_2$max before and after the study period for the training and the control groups. (*$P < .05$; **$P < .01$; ***$P < .001$ [before versus after the study].) (From Cochrane LM, Clark CJ. Benefits and problems of a physical training programme for asthmatic patients. Thorax 1990; 45:345–351.)

pathophysiologic process involved. The mild improvements in airflow obstruction seen in individual patients in both groups was probably caused by the optimization of treatment that arose as an indirect benefit of the continuous medical supervision provided during the program. Furthermore, optimal treatment was likely to have enhanced the ability of patients to comply with training requirements. This experience highlights the importance of having clinical expertise available during physical training programs.

This study suggests that reported differences in expiratory airflow between fit and unfit asthmatics[46] are likely to reflect underlying illness severity and that improvement in lung volumes is therefore not a primary objective of physical training in asthma. Recently, however, the authors of the latter study have suggested an additional hypothesis: that training enhances the mechanisms causing exercise-induced bronchodilation.[51] This enhancement might partially counterbalance any reduction in airflow that occurs during exercise under unfavorable conditions in which exercise-induced asthma is not completely prevented by premedication. This is unlikely to be of additional benefit during physical training under optimal conditions in which premedication is adequately prescribed.

Factors Influencing Physiologic Outcome

The effects of motivation, initial level of fitness, training attendance, and asthma severity and variability on the change in the $\dot{V}O_2$max within the training group were analyzed by multiple regression analysis.[44] The best model for predicting training improvement (i.e., the percentage change in $\dot{V}O_2$max) was described by the following equation:

Per cent change in $\dot{V}O_2$max = 46.9 − 1.01 × SYMP + 6.23 × MOT − 0.56 × INFIT
($R^2 = .80$, SEE = 6.66)

where SYMP is the average symptom score for all the training days, MOT is subject motivation, and INFIT is the initial level of fitness expressed as prestudy $\dot{V}O_2$max (per cent of predicted maximum). Those who were least fit at the outset of the training gained most in terms of a training effect, as has been reported in healthy subjects.[52] The motivation score taken early in the introductory period was also highly predictive, despite subsequent education, discussion, and access to medical advice. An initial motivational assessment may therefore save limited resources by identifying potential noncompliers early. The symptom score at the time of training was the third important factor determining training outcome; it reflected not only the severity and variability of asthma but also the inevitable asynchrony between the optimal training condition of the patient and the availability of supervised exercise sessions. A practical solution would be to supplement scheduled sessions with home exercise once the patients have been familiarized with all aspects of exercise with particular reference to their asthma. Exacerbations may still result in enforced periods of reduced activity with consequent detraining. The exercise supervisor should be aware that these periods are likely to present asthmatic patients with a particularly difficult challenge in terms of their motivation.

Clearly, exercise rehabilitation can bring many improvements in cardiorespiratory performance to asthmatic patients—including a reduction in breathlessness—across a range of workloads equivalent to widely varying daily activities.[53]

The challenge is to identify those patients who can benefit from rehabilitation programs, to maximize outcome in individual patients, and to develop alternative approaches to rehabilitation for those who are less able to participate.

RECOMMENDATIONS FOR PULMONARY REHABILITATION OF ASTHMATIC PATIENTS

The objective of pulmonary rehabilitation in asthma should be viewed as twofold: (1) to provide specific exercise prescription and advice for individual patients based on objective criteria of exercise capability and (2) to implement adequate programs for the various groups of asthmatic patients. This latter goal requires an integrated approach to rehabilitation across the spectrum of asthma that interfaces rehabilitation programs for asthmatics with those already in existence for patients with chronic obstructive airways disease. The two main issues for consideration are the category of patients to be selected and the choice of rehabilitation programs.

Patient Selection

Asthmatic patients can be categorized into three broad groups. Within this approximate categorization, the extent of diurnal peak flow variation and intermittent illness exacerbations must be taken into account to determine the individual patient's suitability for rehabilitation treatment. The choice of program varies for each of the three patient groups. Those patients with mild disability are normally free of airways obstruction with the exception of occasional asthma exacerbations. Patients with pure exercise-induced asthma that is relieved by beta$_2$ agonists would also be included in this category. The patient with mild disability primarily requires objective evaluation and education regarding exercise. After evaluation and exercise education, the responsibility for regular physical training lies with the patient, who mainly uses local gymnasium facilities rather than hospital resources. The program for improving fitness in this group would be no different than that used in healthy subjects to improve aerobic fitness.[14] Hospital facilities would be used by mild asthmatics for periodic medical and fitness assessment to monitor progress and promote motivation. The potential benefits in terms of work capacity (in addition to the health benefits of improved lifestyle) for a limited commitment of resources justify the inclusion of this group of patients under the "umbrella" of rehabilitation treatment. Patients with moderate disability have variable airways obstruction despite prophylactic treatment but have preserved reasonable mobility and exercise tolerance. These patients have a "therapeutic window" of opportunity to improve exercise tolerance that is not readily available to chronically disabled patients with severe asthma. The devotion of pulmonary rehabilitation resources solely to the latter category of patients would disenfranchise those patients for whom this form of therapy is most likely to be beneficial. Thus, if selection is limited by the resources available, in our view patients with moderate disability are the optimal group to consider for exercise rehabilitation. Furthermore, prior implementation of programs with this group of patients provides invaluable experience to assist in constructing modified rehabilitation programs for asthmatic patients with severe disability (i.e., significant chronic airflow obstruction that causes a major limitation in exercise tolerance despite optimal medical treatment).

It is important to note that since the content of programs for these three groups of patients differs substantially, it can be counterproductive to mix patient groups. Those with very mild disease may feel they are not being challenged (i.e., trained at an adequate intensity); likewise, severely disabled patients may become extremely disillusioned by the greater exercise tolerance of less disabled program participants. It is also worth noting that patients with asthma should not be treated together with those who have other pulmonary diseases, not only for the reasons already mentioned but also because each specific disease group requires very different educational components. Mixed programs have the effect of diluting the educational message and can create some confusion as to the objectives of the different groups of patients.

Choice of Program

Broadly considered, there are two basic strategies that rehabilitation programs can follow, either (1) to improve aerobic capacity and cardiorespiratory fitness or (2) to focus on improving muscle strength and endurance in order to increase general mobility and work performance without producing central physiologic adaptive effects, particularly on the cardiovascular system. Programs for the aerobic training of mild and moderate asthmatics do not need to meet any specific requirements and are generally the same as those for normal individuals. However, in view of the variability of the disease, important additional features that these programs should have are ongoing access to medical supervision and a flexible programmed response to exacerbations of asthma. The "flexibility" component should be designed to motivate and encourage continued participation in the program on a long-term basis. The principles used in our program for aerobic exercise rely on established criteria for intensity, frequency, and duration[14] and include a slightly extended warm-up period combined with beta$_2$ agonist therapy to reduce the likelihood of exercise-induced asthma.[11] Regardless of the specific exercises used, these criteria can be reliably implemented using heart rate monitors to control for exercise intensity. In the gymnasium, we alleviate the potential boredom of repetitious exercises by continuously presenting music with a standardized rhythm. Individual schedules are based on initial evaluation of exercise capability and fitness requirements. Patients are divided into small groups; at the various work stations, we use a mixture of floor exercises, including dance movement, circuit training, bicycle ergometry, treadmill exercise, rowing, and isokinetic weight training. Provided that exercise intensity is monitored, the actual mode of aerobic training can be varied to best take advantage of the facilities available within a community setting. Several programs with an emphasis on childhood asthma have been recently reviewed.[54] For example, one program has arranged special reduced rates for entry to local sporting facilities to encourage participation. Three studies report marked improvement in cardiorespiratory fitness following swimming programs of different intensity and duration. Thirty-six children between 10 and 16 years of age showed improved work tolerance after exercising for 10 swimming units of 30 minutes' duration each every week for 3 months.[55] Forty-five asthmatic children in Baltimore, Maryland, showed a similar marked improvement in clinical variables and an increase in school attendance after a 2-month program of swimming as compared with age-matched controls.[56] In a third study,[56] 12 children participated in a 3-month program of weekly swimming lessons, each of which was preceded by an appropriate warm-up period and interspersed with rest. Premedication was given via aerosol bronchodilator, and a significant improvement in cardiorespiratory status was found to be associated with a slight increase in lung volumes. Bronchial lability remained the same. For adults, an aerobic dance program[57] that incorporated pulse rate monitoring during exercise sessions conducted three times per week and an approach similar to our own proved successful. Specialized centers for the residential care and rehabilitation of asthmatic patients are rare. However, two studies report that favorable benefits arise from such intensive therapy centers. In one,[58] a 5-day residential course of rehabilitation for asthmatic children produced improvements in asthma symptoms, peak flow, and exercise tolerance that were not seen in a similar group of control subjects. This led the authors of the study to conclude that a short intensive course of inpatient rehabilitation is of benefit physically, socially, and psychologically to children with asthma, at least in the short term. In a controlled study at another residential center,[55] improvements could be identified specifically as a result of physical activity. Other nonspecific benefits, such as improved general well-being, were a result of the increased medical supervision that was a part of the residential care. In practice, however, it is likely that the general trend will be a continuation of community-based programs for asthma rehabilitation rather than the implementation of such residential care programs.

Respiratory muscle training has not been used in our rehabilitation programs for asthmatic patients, nor have there been any published reports of its use in this context. There is also no current evidence to suggest that respiratory muscle deconditioning or fatigue is a feature of asthma, either in acute exacerbations of the disease[59] or in its stable state.[60] Furthermore, any respiratory muscle deconditioning that might conceivably be present should be responsive to the general physical training program undertaken, and reduction of airflow limitation with bronchodilators is likely to be the best method of optimizing the strength and efficiency of the respiratory muscles in the asthmatic patient.[61]

After a 6-week period of intensive assessment and supervision of training, in our rehabilitation program individual patients attend a single supervised weekly exercise session and complete the remaining schedules using a training log either at home or at local health clubs; this maximizes overall patient access to the limited hospital gymnasium facilities. The hospital session allows an opportunity for the patient's log to be reviewed; problems that occur at the home sessions can be identified by the trainer. Patients who experience exacerbations of their illness that prevent them from participating in aerobic training are allocated to a less strenuous "holding program" for the period of the exacerbation and for a 2- or 3-week period of convalescence thereafter. The holding program concentrates on nonaerobic muscle conditioning by combining isotonic and isokinetic exercise with low-intensity aerobic exercise, such as gentle walking and bicycle ergometry at low workloads. The objective is clearly not to improve cardiorespiratory fitness but rather to maintain mobility, work capacity, and exercise tolerance until the more strenuous program can be resumed. For all our rehabilitation programs for patients with lung disease, including those for asthmatics, we are increasingly using the progressive incremental exercise test as the basis for individual program prescription (an approximate schema of this is illustrated in Figure 33–6). This test has been particularly useful in our experience with the treatment of patients with marked variability of airways obstruction and moderate to severe disability. Nonaerobic muscle conditioning from the outset is the exercise of choice for severely disabled asthmatics. The principles of this form of training are well known.[62] Our program concentrates on the training of the large muscle groups of both the lower limbs and the upper limb girdles, with the understanding that strengthening of the accessory muscles of respiration translates into benefits in performing activities of daily living.*

We have also considered the additional therapeutic option of oxygen prescription during exercise for all patients assessed for rehabilitation (see Fig. 33–6). Although oxygen desaturation is more frequently encountered in patients with other lung diseases, it is occasionally precipitated or exacerbated by exercise in asthmatic patients presumably because of pre-existing gas exchange abnormalities.[63, 64] It is therefore checked routinely during progressive incremental exercise testing using pulse oximetry or transcutaneous oxygen tension measurement.

SUMMARY

Bearing in mind the wide range of disability among asthmatic patients, the objectives of rehabilitation management in asthma are (1) to determine the exercise capacity of the individual patient and provide appropriate advice, (2) to prescribe specific exercise rehabilitation according to illness severity, and (3) to provide supervised hospital-based programs that cater as much

---

*The specific program descriptions for both types of training are available from the author on request. Please write to the Department of Respiratory Medicine, Hairmyres Hospital, East Kilbride, Glasgow, UK.

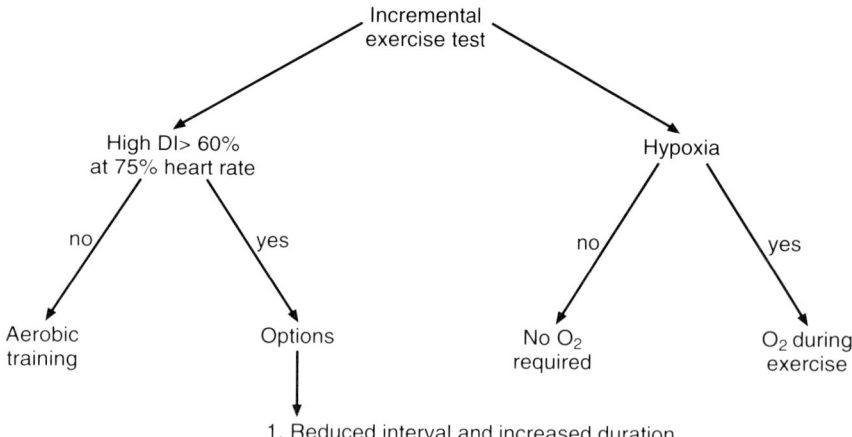

FIGURE 33-6. Exercise testing protocol for rehabilitation programs for patients with lung diseases, including asthma. The first option involves low-intensity work (e.g., relaxed walking or bicycle exercise at low workloads), with the duration of exercise prolonged at each consecutive session. The second option involves repeated periods of high-intensity exercise for short duration and with longer recovery periods between exercises. The third option is interval training, which refers to isotonic and isokinetic circuit training usually consisting of repetitions of exercises 30 seconds in duration (DI: dyspnea index). (Department of Respiratory Medicine, Hairmyres Hospital, East Kilbride, Glasgow, UK.)

as possible to the broadest spectrum of patient disability. The therapy of this group of patients, for whom pulmonary rehabilitation is an eminently suitable but previously neglected adjunct to other forms of treatment, can be both challenging and rewarding.

ACKNOWLEDGMENTS

I gratefully acknowledge the contributions of my colleague Dr. Lorna Cochrane to the rehabilitation program of our unit, the technical staff of the Department of Respiratory Medicine, and my secretary Mrs. Ann Glen, whose administrative skills have been essential in the preparation of this chapter.

REFERENCES

1. American Thoracic Society. Standards for the diagnosis and care of patients with chronic obstructive pulmonary disease (COPD) and asthma. Am Rev Respir Dis 1987; 136:225–243.
2. Katz RM. Exercise-induced asthma/other allergic reactions in the athlete. Allergy Proc 1989; 10:203–208.
3. Freeman W, Williams C, Nute MG. Endurance running performance in athletes with asthma. J Sports Sci 1990; 8:103–117.
4. American Thoracic Society. Evaluation of impairment/disability secondary to respiratory disease. Am Rev Respir Dis 1981; 124:663–666.
5. Guidelines for the diagnosis and management of asthma. J Allergy Clin Immunol 1991; 883:424–534.
6. Deal EC, McFadden ER Jr, Ingram RH, et al. Role of respiratory heat exchange in the production of exercise-induced asthma. J Appl Physiol 1979; 46:467–475.
7. Sheppard D, Eschenbacher WL. Respiratory water loss as a stimulus to exercise-induced bronchoconstriction. J Allergy Clin Immunol 1984; 73:640–642.
8. McFadden ER Jr. Hypothesis: Exercise-induced asthma as a vascular phenomenon. Lancet 1990; 335:880–883.
9. Anonymous. Exercise training, fitness and asthma (editorial). Lancet 1989; i:763–764.
10. Anonymous. The asthmatic child's participation in sports and physical recreation. Pediatrics 1984; 74:155–156.
11. Sly RM. Beta-adrenergic drugs in the management of asthma in athletes. J Allergy Clin Immunol 1984; 73:680–685.
12. Fitch KD, Morton AR. Specificity of exercise-induced asthma. BMJ 1971; 4:577–581.
13. Menardo-Mazeran G, Michel FB, Menardo JL. Childhood asthma and sports in school: A survey of teachers of sports and physical education. Rev Mal Respir 1990; 7:45–49.
14. American College of Sports Medicine. Guidelines for Graded Exercise Testing and Exercise Prescription. 2nd ed. Philadelphia: Lea & Febiger, 1980.
15. Varray AL, Mercier JG, Terral CM, Prefaut CG. Individualised aerobic and high intensity training for asthmatic children in an exercise readaptation program: Is training always helpful for better adaptation to exercise? Chest 1991; 99:579–586.
16. Bannister R. Sport, physical recreation and the national health. BMJ 1972; 4:711–715.
17. Cockroft A, Adams L. Measurement and mechanisms of breathlessness. Bull Eur Physiopathol Respir 1986; 22:85–92.
18. Meyer R, Kroner-Herwig B, Sporkel H. The effect of exercise and induced expectations on visceral perception in asthmatic patients. J Psychosom Res 1990; 34:455–460.
19. Mahler DA, Faryniarz K, Lentine T, et al. Measurement of breathlessness during exercise in asthmatics: Predictor variables, reliability and responsiveness. Am Rev Respir Dis 1991; 144:39–44.
20. Peel ET, Soutar CA, Seaton A. Assessment of variability of exercise tolerance limited by breathlessness. Thorax 1988; 43:960–964.
21. Burdon JGW, Juniper EF, Killian KJ, et al. The perception of breathlessness in asthma. Am Rev Respir Dis 1982; 126:825–828.
22. Tsanakas JN, Milner RD, Bannister OM, Boon AW. Free running asthma screening test. Arch Dis Child 1988; 63:261–265.
23. Clark CJ, Cochrane LM. Assessment of work performance in asthma for determination of cardiorespiratory fitness and training capacity. Thorax 1988; 43:745–749.
24. Wasserman K, Hansen JE, Sue DY, Whipp BJ. Principles of Exercise Testing and Interpretation. Philadelphia: Lea & Febiger, 1987.
25. Jones NL, Campbell EJM. Clinical Exercise Testing. 2nd ed. Philadelphia: W.B. Saunders Co., 1981.
26. Anderson SD, Silverman M, Walker SR. Metabolic and ventilatory changes in asthmatic patients during and after exercise. Thorax 1972; 27:718–725.
27. Smith SR, Ryder C, Kendall MJ, Holder R. Cardiovascular and biochemical responses to nebulised salbutamol in normal subjects. Br J Clin Pharmacol 1984; 18:641–644.
28. Freeman W, Packe GE, Cayton RM. Effect of nebulised salbutamol on maximal exercise performance in men with mild asthma. Thorax 1989; 44:942–947.
29. Warren JB, Keynes RJ, Brown MJ, et al. Blunted sympathoadrenal response to exercise in asthmatic subjects. Br J Dis Chest 1982; 76:147–150.
30. Barnes PJ, Brown MJ, Silverman M, Dollery CT. Circulating catecholamines in exercise and hyperventilation-induced asthma. Thorax 1981; 36:435–440.

31. Berkin KE, Walker G, Inglis GC, et al. Circulating adrenalin and noradrenalin concentrations during exercise in patients with exercise-induced asthma and normal subjects. Thorax 1988; 43:295–299.
32. Gugger M. Changes in serum potassium concentration in asthmatic and normal subjects during exercise. Thorax 1989; 44:605–606.
33. Haas F, Levine N, Ackson K, et al. Changes in serum K^+ in healthy and in asthmatic subjects during exercise. Am Rev Respir Dis 1988; 137:833–836.
34. Barboriak JJ, Sosman AJ, Fink JN, et al. Metabolic changes in exercise-induced asthma. Clin Allergy 1973; 3:83–89.
35. Amirav I, Dowdeswell RJ, Plit M, et al. Growth hormone response to exercise in asthmatic and normal children. Eur J Pediatr 1990; 149:443–446.
36. Kallenbach JM, Panz V, Girson MS, et al. The hormonal response to exercise in asthma. Eur Respir J 1990; 3:171–175.
37. Ludwick SK, Jones JW, Jones TK, et al. Normalisation of cardiopulmonary endurance in severely asthmatic children after bicycle ergometry therapy. J Pediatr 1986; 109:446–451.
38. Orenstein DM, Reed ME, Grogan FT Jr, Crawford LV. Exercise conditioning in children with asthma. J Pediatr 1985; 106:556–559.
39. Strunk RC, Rubin D, Kelly L, et al. Determination of fitness in children with asthma: Use of standardized tests for functional endurance, body fat composition, flexibility and abdominal strength. Am J Dis Child 1988; 142:940–944.
40. Hargreave FE, Ryan G, Thomson NC, et al. Bronchial responsiveness to histamine or methacholine in asthma: Measurement and clinical significance. J Allergy Clin Immunol 1981; 68:347–355.
41. Limitation of Activity Due to Chronic Conditions, United States, 1969 and 1970, Vital Health Statistics 1973. Rockville, MD: Public Health Service; 1973. US Department of Health, Education and Welfare publication (PHS) 8010, Series 10.
42. Strunk RC, Mrazek DA, Fukuhara JT, et al. Cardiovascular fitness in children with asthma correlates with psychological functioning of the child. Pediatrics 1989; 84:460–464.
43. Weston AR, Macfarlane DJ, Hopkins WG. Physical activity of asthmatic and nonasthmatic children. J Asthma 1989; 26:279–286.
44. Cochrane LM, Clark CJ. Benefits and problems of a physical training programme for asthmatic patients. Thorax 1990; 45:345–351.
45. Borg G. Perceived exertion as an indicator of somatic stress. Scand J Rehabil Med 1970; 2:92–98.
46. Haas FH, Pineda K, Axen D, et al. Effects of physical fitness on expiratory airflow in exercising asthmatic people. Med Sci Sports Exerc 1985; 17:585–592.
47. Cockcroft A, Adams L. Measurement and mechanisms of breathlessness. Bull Eur Physiopathol Respir 1986; 22:85–92.
48. Fernal B, Daniels FS. Electroencephalographic changes after a prolonged running period: Evidence for a relaxation response (abstract). Med Sci Sports Exerc 1984; 16:181.
49. Mahler DA, Cunningham LN, Skrinar GS, et al. Activity and hypercapnic ventilatory responsiveness after marathon running. J Appl Physiol 1989; 66:2431–2437.
50. Stark RD. Dyspnea: Assessment and pharmacologic manipulation. Eur Respir J 1988; 1:280–287.
51. Haas F, Pasierski S, Levine N, et al. Effect of aerobic training on forced expiratory airflow in exercising asthmatic humans. J Appl Physiol 1987; 63:1230–1235.
52. Wenger HA, Bell GJ. The interaction of intensity, frequency and duration of exercise training in altering cardiorespiratory fitness. Sports Med 1986; 3:346–356.
53. Astrand PO, Rodahl H. Physical training. In: Textbook of Work Physiology. 2nd ed. New York: McGraw-Hill Book Co., 1977.
54. Strunk RC, Mascia AV, Lipkowitz MA, Wolf SI. Rehabilitation of a patient with asthma in the outpatient setting. J Allergy Clin Immunol 1991; 87:601–611.
55. Rothe T, Kohl C, Mansfield HJ. Controlled study of the effect of sports training on cardiopulmonary functions in asthmatic children and adolescents. Pneumologie 1990; 44:1110–1114.
56. Huang SW, Veiga R, Sila U, et al. The effect of swimming in asthmatic children: Participants in a swimming programme in the city of Baltimore. J Asthma 1989; 26:117–121.
57. Wolf SI, Lampl KL. Pulmonary rehabilitation: The use of aerobic dance as a therapeutic exercise for asthmatic patients. Ann Allergy 1988; 61:357–360.
58. Dean M, Bell E, Kershaw CR, et al. A short exercise and living course for asthmatics. Br J Dis Chest 1988; 82:155–161.
59. Lavietes MH, Grocela JA, Maniatis T, et al. Inspiratory muscle strength in asthma. Chest 1988; 93:1043–1048.
60. Picado C, Fiz JA, Montserrat JM, et al. Respiratory and skeletal muscle function in steroid-dependent bronchial asthma. Am Rev Respir Dis 1990; 141:14–20.
61. Weiner P, Suo J, Fernandez E, Cherniack RM. The effect of hyperinflation on respiratory muscle strength and efficiency in health subjects and patients with asthma. Am Rev Respir Dis 1990; 141:1501–1505.
62. Clausen JK, Klaussen K, Rasmussen B. Central and peripheral circulatory changes after training of the arms and legs. Am J Physiol 1973; 225:675–682.
63. Levine G, Hounsley F, Macleod P, Macklem PT. Gas exchange abnormalities in mild bronchitis and asymptomatic asthma. N Engl J Med 1970; 282:1277–1282.
64. Packe GE, Freeman W, Cayton RM. Effects of exercise on gas exchange in patients recovering from acute severe asthma. Thorax 1990; 45:262–266.
65. Leith DE, Bradley M. Ventilatory muscle strength and endurance training. J Appl Physiol 1976; 41:508–516.
66. Vavra J, Macek M, Mrzena B, Spicak V. Intensive physical training in children with bronchial asthma. Acta Paediatr Scand Suppl 1971; 217:90–92.
67. Nickerson BG, Bautista DB, Namey MA, et al. Distance running improves fitness in asthmatic children without pulmonary complications or changes in exercise-induced bronchospasm. Pediatrics 1983; 71:147–152.
68. Green JM, Coggings D. A movement and exercise group for asthmatics. Practitioner 1982; 226:961–964.
69. Mallinson BM, Cockcroft C, Burgess DA, David TJ. Exercise training for children with asthma. Physiotherapy 1981; 67:106–108.
70. Sly RM, Harper RT, Rosselot I. The effect of physical conditioning on asthmatic children. Ann Allergy 1972; 30:86–94.
71. Fitch KD, Morton AR, Blanksby BA. Effects of swimming training on children with asthma. Arch Dis Child 1976; 51:190–194.
72. Itkin IH, Nacman M. The effect of exercise on the hospitalized asthmatic patient. J Allergy Clin Immunol 1966; 37:251–263.
73. Sevonius E, Kautto R, Arborelius M. Improvement after training of children with exercise-induced asthma. Acta Paediatr Scand 1983; 72:23–30.
74. Henriksen JM, Nielsen TT. Effects of physical training on exercise-induced broncho-constriction. Acta Paediatr Scand 1983; 72:131–136.
75. Graff-Lonevig V, Bevegard S, Erikson BO, Kraepelien S, Saltin B. Two years follow-up of asthmatic boys participating in a physical activity programme. Acta Paediatr Scand 1980; 69:347–352.
76. Guebelle F, Ernould C, Jovanovic M. Working capacity and physical training in asthmatic children at 1800m altitude. Acta Paediatr Scand Suppl 1971; 217:93–98.
77. Scherr MS, Frankel L. Physical conditioning programme for asthmatic children. JAMA 1958; 168:1996–2000.
78. Hyde JS, Swarts CL. Effect of an exercise programme on the perennially asthmatic child. Am J Dis Child 1968; 116:383–396.
79. Peterson JH, McElhenny TR. Effects of a physical fitness program upon asthmatic boys. Pediatrics 1965; 32:295–299.
80. Bundgaard A, Ingemann-Hansen T, Schmidt A, Kristensen JH. Effect of physical training on peak oxygen consumption rate and exercise-induced asthma in adult asthmatics. Scand J Clin Lab Invest 1982; 42:9–13.
81. Chai H, Falliers CH, Dietiker F, Franz B. Long term investigation into the effects of physical therapy in chronically asthmatic children. J Allergy 1967; 39:109.
82. Hirt M. Physical conditioning in asthma. Ann Allergy 1964; 22:229–237.
83. Leisti S, Finnila MJ, Kiuru E. Effects of physical training on

hormonal responses to exercise in asthmatic children. Arch Dis Child 1979; 54:524–528.
84. Millman M, Grundon WG, Kasch F, et al. Controlled exercise in asthmatic children. Ann Allergy 1965; 23:220–225.
85. Seligman T, Randel HO, Stevens JJ. Conditioning program for children with asthma. Phys Ther 1970; 50:641–648.
86. Freeman W, Williams C. The effect of endurance running training on asthmatic adults. Br J Sports Med 1989; 23:115–122.
87. Cropp GJA, Tanakawa N. Cardiorespiratory adaptations of normal and asthmatic children to exercise. In: Dempsey JA, Reed CE (eds). Muscular Exercise and the Lung. Madison, WI: University of Wisconsin Press, 1977, pp 265–278.
88. Kivilog J, Irnell L, Gunnar E. Ventilatory capacity, work capacity and exercise-induced bronchoconstriction in a population sample of subjects with bronchial asthma or chronic bronchitis. Scand J Respir Dis 1975; 56:73–83.
89. Bevegaard S, Eriksson BO, Graff-Lonevig V, et al. Respiratory function, cardiovascular dimensions and work capacity in boys with bronchial asthma. Acta Paediatr Scand 1976; 65:289–296.
90. Ingemann-Hansen T, Bundgaard A, Halkjaer-Kristensen J, et al. Maximal oxygen consumption rate in patients with bronchial asthma: The effect of beta$_2$-adrenoreceptor stimulation. Scand J Clin Lab Invest 1980; 40:99–104.

Chapter 34

Cystic Fibrosis

DAVID M. ORENSTEIN, M.D.
BLAKESLEE E. NOYES, M.D.

OVERVIEW OF CYSTIC FIBROSIS

Cystic fibrosis (CF) is the most common lethal genetic disease among white populations.[1] Although the complex of signs and symptoms that characterize this syndrome has been recognized since 1938,[2] its basic biochemical defect has only recently begun to come to light.[3] CF affects virtually every organ system that has epithelial surfaces—most important, the lungs, pancreas, intestinal mucous glands, and sweat glands. A common pathogenetic mechanism underlying the involvement of the major target systems is an alteration of ion transport across epithelial surfaces. Faulty functioning of the chloride channel and excessive sodium reabsorption through these epithelial cells lead to relative dehydration of luminal secretions.[3] These abnormally viscous secretions cause the blockage of ducts and air passages.

Genetics and Prevalence

CF is a hereditary autosomal recessive disorder that occurs in approximately 1 in every 2500 live births in white American and northern European populations and in about 1 in every 17,000 births in the American black population; it is virtually unheard of in Asian populations.[4] There are an estimated 30,000 patients with CF in the United States, and since more than 5% of the white population are presumed to be heterozygous for CF, there are likely to be about 10 million asymptomatic carriers. The gene for CF is located on the long arm of chromosome 7. The most common mutation is a deletion of phenylalanine at position 508 ("ΔF508").

This mutation apparently alters a protein product, referred to as CFTR (cystic fibrosis transmembrane conductance regulator), which accounts for the basic defect in ion transport.[5] Recent evidence suggests that this protein may actually be the epithelial chloride channel itself.[6] The ΔF508 mutation accounts for 70 to 80% of cases of CF.[7] More than 120 other mutations at the CF locus—most of them very uncommon or even unique to a given family—have been discovered, raising the proportion of CF cases identifiable with genetic analysis to about 85%.[8] The influence of genotype on phenotype among the 120 or so specific CF mutations is not yet clear.[9]

Clinical Manifestations

Gastrointestinal Tract and Nutrition

Exocrine pancreatic insufficiency is present at birth in about 50% of CF patients[9a] and develops in others, so that by a few years of age it is present in approximately 90% of CF patients. It is manifested by maldigestion of fats and protein with consequent malabsorption, steatorrhea, and failure to thrive.[10] Malnutrition in CF may be a problem at any age and is attributable to malabsorption, poor dietary intake, excessive caloric expenditure associated with increased work of breathing and cough, or any combination of these factors. Patients may come to the physician with evidence of deficiencies in fat-soluble vitamins.[10] Bowel obstruction—a result of thickened intestinal mucus and pancreatic insufficiency—may be present at birth (meconium ileus) in 10% of patients or later in life (meconium ileus equivalent, now referred to as *distal intestinal obstruction syndrome*) in 20 to 25% of patients.[10] Rectal prolapse, which is caused by the same factors (and perhaps by malnutrition with loss of musculature), is seen in 20% of CF patients in the first years of life.[11] Intussusception is much less common, but CF patients account for a significant portion of the patients with intussusception after 1 year of age.[12] Liver pathology, including nonspecific steatosis and a specific lesion *(focal biliary fibrosis)*, is commonly seen histologically[13]; however, cirrhosis with clinically important manifestations such as hepatic failure or portal hypertension with hypersplenism, bleeding esophageal varices, or both, is fortunately rare.[13] Children or adults with clinically intact pancreatic function may develop acute pancreatitis.

The absence of gastrointestinal manifestations often delays the diagnosis of CF.

Sweat Glands

The chloride transport defect seen in all epithelia in CF is expressed clearly in the sweat glands. It results in the characteristic high-salt content of CF sweat and provides the basis for the sweat test (discussed later). CF patients lose more salt during exercise in the heat than do normal persons,[14] and they may experience heat prostration. In hot weather, infants with CF may require medical care for hyponatremia and hypochloremia.[15]

Respiratory Tract

The upper respiratory tract is involved in CF in most patients, with radiographic evidence of pansinusitis. Such involvement is seldom clinically bothersome to the patient but occasionally is helpful diagnostically. Nasal polyps may be found in as many as 25% of these patients.[16]

Lower respiratory tract involvement accounts for over 90% of the morbidity and mortality in CF.[1] Although the lungs are histologically normal at birth, obstructive pulmonary disease, which begins in the small airways, is eventually present in almost all patients. Recurrent cough, wheeze, or both—which may lead to diagnoses such as recurrent bronchiolitis, asthma, or pneumonia—are often the first indications of pulmonary involvement. As the disease progresses, hyperinflation, crackles, and rhonchi become apparent. The rate and intensity of the progression of the lung disease vary tremendously among patients; some infants have severe disease, whereas some 30-year-old patients have normal or nearly normal pulmonary function.

The older child (6–7 yr of age and older) who is able to cooperate in the pulmonary function laboratory and who has had respiratory involvement generally has test results that indicate a pattern of obstructive airways disease (decreased vital capacity, decreased forced expiratory volume in 1 second [FEV_1], decreased peak expiratory flow, and increased residual volume [RV], which is indicative of air trapping).[17] These obstructive changes show varying responses to bronchodilator inhalation: some patients apparently improve, many do not change, and others actually worsen. The response to bronchodilators is not consistent over time.[18] Exercise testing (discussed more fully later) typically shows reduced exercise tolerance and fitness, with a comparatively large minute volume for the oxygen consumed, presumably because of greater than normal dead space ventilation. Typically, a higher than normal proportion of the ventilatory capacity is required at peak workloads.

The pulmonary function and exercise tests are relatively sensitive tools for following progression of disease in the older cooperative child, the adolescent, and the adult.

Chronic pulmonary infection with acute exacerbations is characteristic of CF patients. *Staphylococcus aureus*, *Haemophilus influenzae*, and a variety of gram-negative organisms may be involved in the early stages, but eventually the lungs of the vast majority of patients become colonized by *Pseudomonas aeruginosa*.[19] Many patients have *Pseudomonas* at diagnosis. There seems to be a unique relationship between CF patients and *Pseudomonas*; at least one half of all CF patients are colonized by a peculiar mucoid strain of this organism that is seldom seen in other human disease states.[19, 20] Recently, other organisms, such as *Aspergillus fumigatus* and *Pseudomonas cepacia*, have become increasingly important as pulmonary pathogens.[19] Despite the universal finding of chronic pulmonary colonization and infection, extrapulmonary infection is unusual and indicates that any defect in defense mechanisms is limited to the lungs. Pulmonary defenses are almost certainly inhibited by viscid mucus. Mucociliary transport rates are dramatically reduced in CF patients.[21] There may be circulating toxins, locally secreted toxins, or both that inhibit the phagocytosis and killing of *Pseudomonas* by pulmonary alveolar macrophages and neutrophils.[22, 23]

The chain of events caused by chronic infection with acute disease exacerbations begins with bronchiolitis and progresses to bronchitis, bronchiectasis, peribronchial fibrosis, and progressive loss of pulmonary function. Figure 34–1 illustrates the cascade of events that lead to and result from airways infection.

The progression of pulmonary dysfunction leads to hypoxemia. Hypoxemia appears during sleep before it becomes evident during the day.[24] Oxyhemoglobin desaturation also occurs during exercise in some of the most severely affected patients,[25] but there is no clear correlation between sleep-related and exercise-related desaturation.[26]

Pulmonary complications include pneumothorax, hemoptysis, segmental and lobar atelectasis, and pulmonary hypertension that leads to cor pulmonale.

Other Organ Systems

The reproductive tract is involved in most male patients, with atresia of the vas deferens and consequent obstructive azoospermia and sterility.[27] In female patients, thick cervical mucus often results in decreased fertility.[27a] Delayed puberty may be seen in either sex as a consequence of chronic illness and poor nutrition. Some adolescents and adults have a unique pattern of

CASCADE OF PROBLEMS IN CYSTIC FIBROSIS

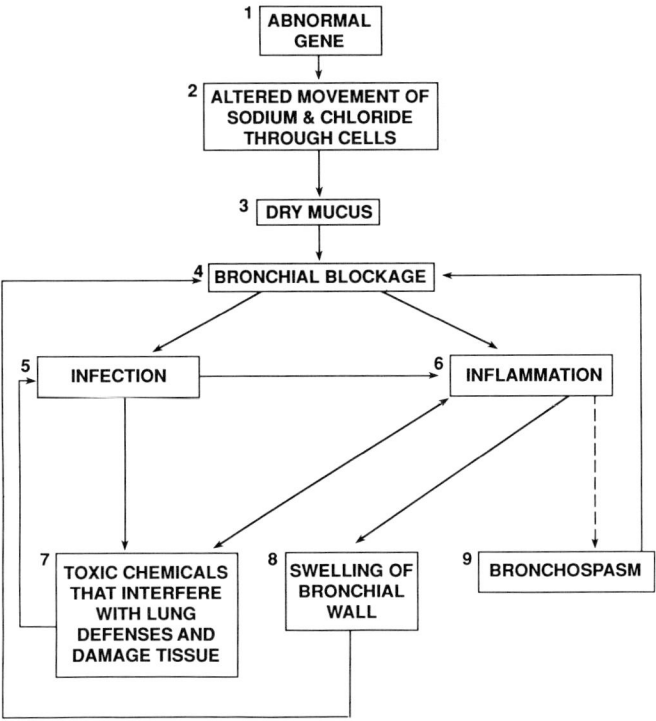

FIGURE 34–1. The cascade of factors leading to bronchial obstruction and destruction in cystic fibrosis. The abnormal gene (1) encodes an abnormal protein that alters the movement of sodium ions and chloride ions through epithelial cell membranes (2), leading to the production of dry mucus (3) that blocks bronchioles and bronchi (4). With bronchial blockage, infection (5) and inflammation (6) occur. Both infection and inflammation can cause the release of toxic chemicals (7) that interfere with lung defenses and damage tissues, thus worsening the infection and inflammation. Inflammation also causes swelling of the bronchial wall (8), which worsens bronchial blockage. Finally, in some individuals, inflammation may lead to bronchospasm (9). (Adapted from Orenstein D. Cystic fibrosis. Respir Care 1991; 36:746–754.)

hyperglycemia and abnormal glucose tolerance test results, but they almost never have ketoacidosis.

Hypertrophic pulmonary osteoarthropathy may be present in the long bones and adjacent joints. Digital clubbing is a nearly universal finding in patients with even mildly abnormal lung function.

Diagnosis

Diagnosis usually must be based on the clinical features of the disease.[28] Currently, the accepted criteria for the diagnosis of CF are (1) a positive sweat test—that is, a sweat chloride concentration greater than 60 mEq/L in a sample of at least 100 mg obtained after maximum stimulation by pilocarpine iontophoresis, (2) the presence of chronic obstructive pulmonary disease (COPD), (3) the presence of exocrine pancreatic insufficiency, and (4) a family history of the disease.[28] Most experts require the satisfaction of at least two of these criteria for establishing a diagnosis of CF, and the diagnosis is almost never made without a positive sweat test. Theoretically, the sweat test is simple, but false-positive and false-negative results are very common in tests performed outside established CF centers.[29] It must be stressed that the key to making the diagnosis is a high index of suspicion in the presence of any of the manifestations. Table 34–1 lists the indications for a sweat test. Most physicians are sufficiently aware of the disease, and few children with the symptom triad of growth failure, steatorrhea, and COPD escape diagnosis. However, atypical patients, especially those who have no clinically apparent pancreatic involvement (as many as 10% of all CF patients[10]) or who have normal growth, may escape accurate diagnosis for years. There is no such thing as a child, adolescent, or even adult who "looks too good" to have CF. Molecular genetic techniques may help establish the diagnosis in some cases. Identification of the most common CF mutation (ΔF508) along with about one-half dozen other CF mutations has now become routine through the use of polymerase chain reaction technology in some genetics laboratories.[30] The absence of these mutations does not rule out the possibility of CF, and dozens of less common mutations are not detectable in any but a few research laboratories.

Newborn Screening

An elevation of blood immunoreactive trypsin (IRT) is found in most newborns with CF.[31] The assay for IRT can be carried out on the dried blood spots obtained from newborns for routine screening (e.g., for phenylketonuria and hypothyroidism). This test has been used in a number of states and countries, and its use is likely to continue. There appear to be very few false-negative results but many false-positive results with this screening technique.[31] Repeat analyses for IRT are required after one positive test result is obtained. If the second test (usually at several weeks of age) still shows elevated IRT, definitive testing (sweat test or DNA analysis) must be carried out.

Finally, it must be emphasized that CF is a disease in which early diagnosis and institution of an aggressive treatment program may make a difference in quality and length of life.[32] Efforts at pursuing diagnosis are rewarded by the family's peace of mind in the case of a negative result and by the knowledge of an improved outlook for the patient in the event of a positive result.

Standard Treatment

CF is a complex disease, and CF patients require a comprehensive care program. This is usually best carried out in (or at least coordinated from) a specialized CF center at which many different specialists are available.[33] Therapy has three primary components: a pulmonary component, a gastrointestinal component, and a psychologic component.

TABLE 34–1. INDICATIONS FOR SWEAT TESTING*

Pulmonary Indications	Gastrointestinal Indications	Other Indications
Chronic cough	Meconium ileus, steatorrhea, malabsorption	Family history of cystic fibrosis
Digital clubbing	Rectal prolapse	Failure to thrive
Recurrent or chronic pneumonia	Cirrhosis (portal hypertension; esophageal varices)	Salty sweat; salty taste when kissed
Recurrent bronchiolitis	Prolonged neonatal jaundice	Low serum sodium or chloride; heat prostration
Mucoid *Pseudomonas*	Hypoprothrombinemia beyond newborn period	Two positive IRT blood spot tests in newborn period
Hemoptysis	Pancreatitis	Nasal polyps
Atelectasis	Intussusception (in patients >2 yr of age)	Pansinusitis
		Obstructive azoospermia

*Modified from Orenstein DM. Cystic Fibrosis. Respir Care 1991; 36:746–754.

Pulmonary Therapy

The goal of pulmonary therapy is to prevent or delay progression of the pulmonary lesion. This goal is also the foundation for a rehabilitation program and is accomplished through the relief of airway obstruction and inflammation and through the control of infection.

Therapy for Obstruction. Chest physiotherapy with percussion and postural drainage is the mainstay of most treatment programs and is effective[34] despite the lack of definitive studies indicating the ideal time for instituting this treatment or the benefits of various techniques. It is recommended that most patients undergo chest physiotherapy to all pulmonary segments at least once and up to four times daily, with increased frequency at the time of clinical pulmonary disease exacerbation.[34] Many patients have found that mechanical percussors ease this arduous task.

Aerosol Therapy. Continuous aerosol therapy came into and went out of vogue in the past 20 years without undergoing adequate evaluation.[1] Intermittent aerosols are much more widely used but are also somewhat controversial.[1] Aerosols for intermittent use have been employed to deliver various types of medication. Bronchodilators clearly increase airflow acutely in some patients, but they make no difference in many others, and in a few they actually reduce airflow (perhaps because of a reduction in bronchomotor tone in airways that are kept patent only by abnormally high tone).[35] One 4-week study[36] suggested benefit from regular beta agonist inhalation in those CF patients who had clear evidence of bronchial hyperreactivity on methacholine challenge. Whether long-term use of beta agonists is helpful to any or all CF patients is unclear. Possible benefits in addition to bronchodilatation include increased mucociliary transport rates, improved ventilatory muscle endurance, and decreased dyspnea.[37] Possible harm could result from mucous gland hyperplasia, dynamic collapse of airways, worsened epithelial ion transport, or any combination of these.[37] Mucolytic agents (e.g., *N*-acetylcysteine) are favored by some experts and are effective in vitro, but they may cause irritation, bronchoconstriction, and bronchorrhea in vivo.[38] Vasoconstrictors (e.g., phenylephrine) are commonly used to reduce mucosal edema, although their efficacy has yet to be established. Antibiotics (especially aminoglycosides and the anti-*Pseudomonas* penicillin derivatives[19]) have been delivered by aerosols, apparently with favorable results.

Several experimental aerosol therapies have been introduced and await definitive study to confirm their safety and efficacy. These include amiloride,[39] which may improve epithelial chloride and sodium transport and thus make airway luminal contents less viscous; DNase, which can degrade neutrophil-derived DNA and therefore decrease the viscosity of airway secretions[40]; and alpha$_1$-antitrypsin, which may diminish the inflammatory effects of neutrophil-derived proteases.[41]

Therapy for Inflammation. Several approaches have been suggested to diminish airways inflammation in CF, including the use of systemic steroids (alternate-day prednisone[42]) and ibuprofen.[43] Early studies, particularly with alternate-day prednisone, have had mixed results, with apparent benefits in some patients[42] but unacceptable side effects in others.[44] A definitive statement about the efficacy and toxicity of such anti-inflammatory therapy must await the results of several collaborative studies that are currently under way.

Therapy for Infection. There is general agreement that antibiotic treatment has probably been the single most important factor in the greatly improved prognosis in CF. Colonization and infection with *Staphylococcus* and, later, *Pseudomonas* are nearly universal, and clinical exacerbations of pulmonary disease have been convincingly linked to worsening infection. *Staphylococcus* and *Haemophilus* may occasionally be eliminated from the bronchial tree in CF, but once *Pseudomonas* colonization is established, it is almost never eradicated. It may, however, be controlled.

Antibiotic Strategies. Some CF centers advocate continuous "prophylactic" antibiotic treatment. There is some concern that this approach might lead to the early emergence of drug-resistant flora.[19] Another approach is to restrict the use of antibiotics to times of exacerbation of pulmonary disease, as evidenced by increased symptoms or signs (e.g., cough or sputum production[19]) or by worsening chest radiograph or pulmonary function test results. Because some patients (especially those with advanced disease) experience disease exacerbations whenever they are not being treated with antibiotics, virtually continuous treatment is occasionally indicated.[19] A third approach is to treat patients with full-dose drugs for 2 to 3 weeks every 1 or 2 months if there is any evidence of pulmonary disease based on culture results.[19] A Danish group has adopted a more aggressive antibiotic policy of elective hospitalization for 2 weeks of intravenous anti-*Pseudomonas* antibiotic therapy every 3 months for all patients, regardless of their clinical condition.[44a] Although it cannot be said that this policy alone is responsible, survival statistics for CF patients in Denmark have become among the best in the world since the institution of this policy. It is not clear at present which of the many antibiotic strategies is most successful.

A cornerstone of most successful treatment programs is the frequent evaluation of patients by physicians. Evaluation should include bacterial examination of respiratory tract flora.[19] Oral antibiotics (e.g., dicloxacillin, cephalosporins, amoxicillin, trimethroprim with sulfamethoxazole, tetracyclines, and chloramphenicol) are often adequate when the offending organism is *Staphylococcus* or *Haemophilus,* and even on occasion when *Pseudomonas* is the only organism isolated in culture.[19]

The quinolones (e.g., ciprofloxacin and norfloxacin) are a relatively new class of oral antibiotics with impressive activity against *Pseudomonas* in the lung. Because most studies have suggested that there is a rapid emergence of resistant organisms during treatment with quinolones, many experts recommend reserving their use in CF to severe exacerbations of pulmonary disease that otherwise would have prompted initiation of intravenous therapy.[45]

Intravenous antibiotics are indicated when the patient does not respond to outpatient oral administration of antibiotics.[19] The important consideration in the decision to hospitalize a patient and begin parenteral therapy is whether the patient is sicker than his or her own baseline, and not whether he or she seems very ill. It is clear that a tremendous amount of lung can be lost irreversibly while a child still looks reasonably well. Because *Pseudomonas aeruginosa* is usually the offending organism, intravenous therapy is commonly carried out with an aminoglycoside and an anti-*Pseudomonas* penicillin or a third-generation cephalosporin.[19] Intravenous antibiotics have traditionally been administered during hospitalization, but in recent years they have increasingly been used successfully at home.[19]

Aerosolized antibiotics may be effective in many patients whose lungs are colonized with *Pseudomonas.*[19] In those who have severe airways obstruction, aerosol penetration into the lung may be limited, rendering this form of treatment less valuable. Patients who cannot tolerate the intravenous administration of certain drugs (e.g., colistin) may do well with the same drugs delivered by aerosol.

Lung Transplantation. Heart-lung or bilateral lung transplantation has been successful in a limited number of CF patients with end-stage disease.[46] One-year survival ranges from 50 to 75%. Donor organ availability is a limiting factor for most North American lung transplant programs, and pretransplant mortality is very high among those on many transplant waiting lists. After transplantation, problems with organ rejection, immunosuppression, infection, finances, and psychologic adjustment require constant attention.[46] Nonetheless, some patients have had excellent results and have returned to work or school full time.[46]

Gastrointestinal Therapy

The main goal of gastrointestinal therapy is to establish good nutrition. Since pancreatic enzyme replacement preparations and especially enteric-coated preparations became available, the once insurmountable problem of poor nutrition has become quite manageable.[10] The correct dose of enzyme is determined through trial and error by titrating against the symptoms and signs of maldigestion and malabsorption (steatorrhea, abdominal discomfort, excessive hunger, and poor weight gain). Supplemental vitamins, especially fat-soluble A and E vitamins, should be administered at twice their recommended daily doses.[10] Diet need not be specially tailored for the well-grown CF patient as long as adequate calories are supplied. In the poorly nourished patient, however, it may be necessary to go to some lengths to assure adequate caloric intake.

Gastrointestinal Complications. Meconium ileus and distal intestinal obstruction can usually be treated with careful administration of meglumine diatrizoate (Gastrografin) enemas.[10] Distal intestinal obstruction in its early stages may respond to large volumes of oral or nasogastric GoLytely bowel prep, obviating the need for enemas.[47] Rectal prolapse is treated by gentle manual pressure on the protruding rectum and is prevented by adjustment of diet and enzyme activity to reduce bulky stools.[11] There is no treatment yet for the uncommon cirrhosis, but endoscopic sclerotherapy may be lifesaving and obviate the need for portocaval shunting in the uncommon cases of symptomatic esophageal varices.[48] Liver transplantation has been carried out in a number of patients with CF, with results similar to those in non-CF liver recipients.[49] Surprisingly, pulmonary function did not worsen and may even have improved in these CF patients after transplantation.[49]

Psychologic Considerations

The emotional burdens of a genetic, incurable, progressive, life-shortening, financially draining, and activity-limiting disease on patient and family are great. It is remarkable how well the large majority of patients and families adjust; a very low incidence of depression has been observed.[50] Issues that patients must face include education and vocation, marriage, reproduction, medical expenses, independent living, and anticipation of disability and death. Establishing and maintaining a positive and optimistic yet realistic attitude are extremely important. These goals are attainable, especially if the primary physician shares this attitude and maintains a close, supportive relationship with the patient and family. Knowledge of the tremendously improved prognosis in CF over the past decades facilitates such an attitude.

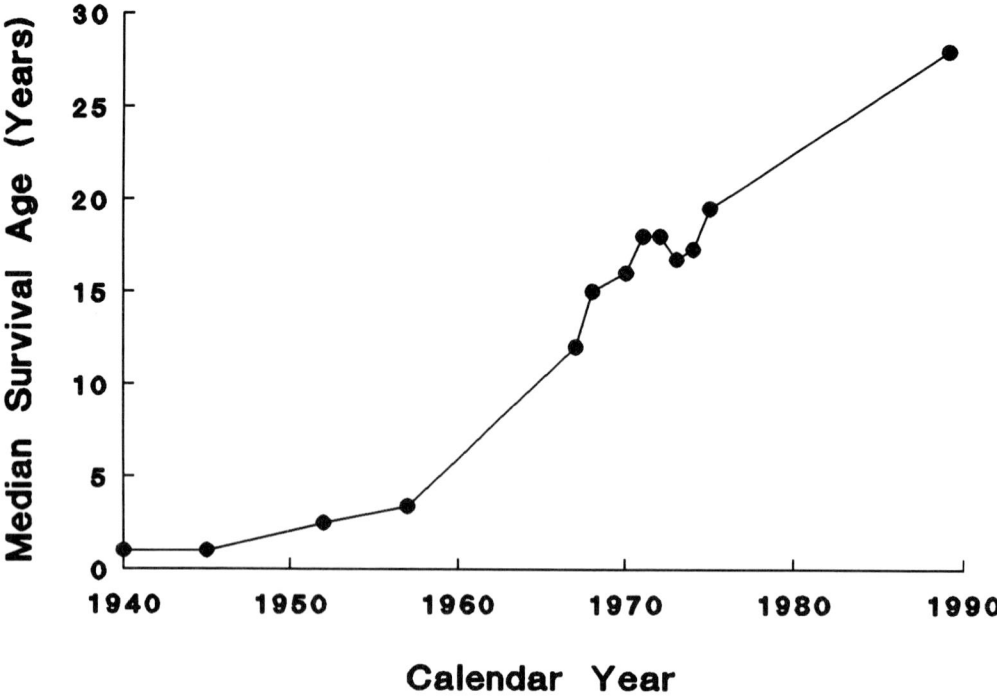

FIGURE 34–2. The change in prognosis for patients with cystic fibrosis over the decades since the disease was recognized. Change in prognosis is plotted as median survival for the given years. (Data from the Cystic Fibrosis Foundation, Bethesda, MD.)

Miscellaneous Treatment Considerations

Hyperglycemia occurs in a small but important group of CF patients and may necessitate insulin therapy.[51] Salt loss may be excessive, especially during exertion in warm weather.[14] Infants may require small amounts of supplemental salt in warm weather, but older children and adults regulate their salt intake quite adequately if given free access to the salt shaker. Salt tablets are not necessary and may be harmful.

Prognosis

When CF was first recognized in the late 1930s, almost all children with it died before school age. Institution of specialized CF centers and comprehensive, aggressive treatment programs beginning in the 1950s has improved the prognosis tremendously. National median survival was 10.6 years in 1966, 20 years in 1981, and 28 years in 1989 (Fig. 34–2). There are currently many patients over 20 and even 30 years of age with excellent lung function and, at the end of 1990, 32.7% of CF patients in the United States were 18 years of age or older.[52] Survival probably depends on several factors, including inherent severity of the disease, which is perhaps influenced by genotype[53]; aggressiveness of the treatment program as prescribed by the physician and carried out by the patient and family; and some degree of chance, especially concerning contact with various bacterial and viral pathogens. Perhaps most important, long-term prognosis may depend on the timing of the diagnosis and institution of treatment. Factors shown to be associated with good prognosis have included care in a CF center,[33] male sex,[54] a good chest radiograph score,[55] good nutrition,[56] high cardiopulmonary fitness,[57] and the absence of colonization of the respiratory tract by *P. cepacia*.[58] Several studies indicate that those CF patients who are diagnosed and who begin an aggressive treatment program before the onset of irreversible pulmonary damage have significantly better pulmonary function and survival than those discovered and treated only after considerable pulmonary tissue has been lost.[55] The recent discovery of the gene for CF,[7] the uncovering of the basic defect,[5] and the very exciting research breakthrough of using gene-transfer techniques to cure the basic defect in CF cells in the test tube[59] have all raised hopes for improved treatments and even the possibility of a cure within the foreseeable future.

REHABILITATION IN CYSTIC FIBROSIS

Rehabilitation is an idea and a process long applied to patients with CF, yet it is one that has not been explicitly acknowledged until quite recently. It has been said that "rehabilitation is a therapeutic program designed to minimize the consequences of a permanent or protracted disability"[60] and that rehabilitative efforts differ from standard medical care in that standard medical care attempts to reverse the primary disease process, whereas rehabilitation "concentrates on restoring function."[60] Yet, in CF, the primary disease process has not been amenable to reversal, and thus the thrust of therapy has not been cure but the restoration and preservation of function. Therefore, more than in many other clinical settings, the boundaries between standard medical care and rehabilitative efforts have been unclear. The primary thrust of standard care has been to preserve function. The remainder of this chapter focuses on the role of exercise and nutrition in CF, two areas

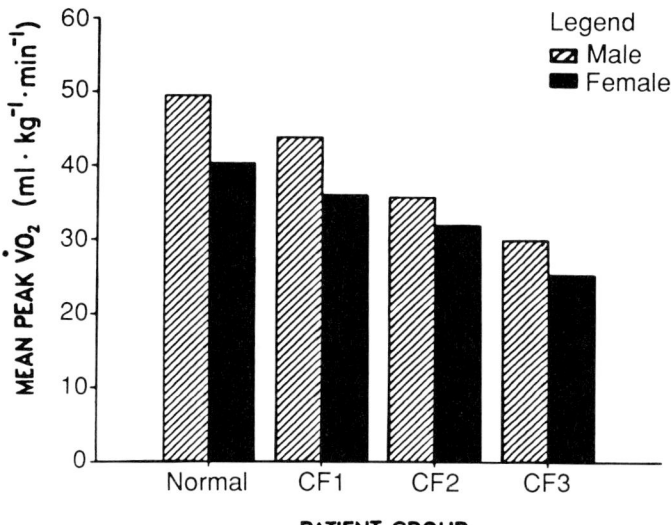

FIGURE 34-3. Overall correlation of exercise tolerance (expressed as peak oxygen consumption [$\dot{V}O_2$] in ml/kg/min) with pulmonary function. The "normal" group comprised 56 male and 51 female healthy subjects. The graph reflects data recorded on 57 male and 52 female cystic fibrosis patients categorized in 3 groups: CF1, where forced expiratory volume in 1 second (FEV_1) ≥ 70% of forced vital capacity (FVC); CF2, where FEV_1 = 50–69% FVC; and CF3, where FEV_1 < 50% FVC. (From Orenstein DM, Nixon PA. Patients with cystic fibrosis. In: Franklin BA, Gordon S, Timms GC (eds). Exercise in Modern Medicine. Baltimore: Williams & Wilkins, 1989, pp 204–214.)

that are generally associated with rehabilitation medicine. It will be clear that successful rehabilitative efforts in CF are impossible without strong and continuing standard care.

Exercise in Cystic Fibrosis

Responses to Single Bouts of Exercise

Just as the severity of airways obstruction varies tremendously among patients with CF, so too does the response to exercise. Some patients are nearly bedridden, whereas others have completed marathons[61] and "Ironman" distance triathlons (i.e., they consecutively swam 2.4 miles, biked 112 miles, and ran 26.2 miles). In general, studies have shown that exercise tolerance in patients with CF is related to the severity of the underlying lung disease[62-64] (Fig. 34–3) and have suggested that ventilatory mechanics may limit exercise tolerance in these patients; this is in contrast to healthy populations, in which the lungs seldom limit exercise.

Amount of Work Tolerated. In study after study, most CF patients perform less well on exercise tests than do their normal peers, whether the tests employed are cycle ergometer tests,[62-67] time to exhaustion on a run test,[65] distance walked in 2 minutes,[68] or minimum time required to complete a sprint obstacle course.[65] Patients with normal or nearly normal lung function at rest tend to have normal or nearly normal exercise tolerance, whereas those with more severe pulmonary function abnormalities fare less well on exercise challenge.[63] In fact, the correlation between disease severity (as indicated by FEV_1) and exercise tolerance (as indicated by peak oxygen consumption) is strong and statistically significant.[69] Exercise tolerance also correlates significantly with an overall life-quality measure, the Quality of Well-being Scale.[70]

Among patients with comparable disease severity, female patients have a lower exercise tolerance than do males.[69] Despite the high group correlation between pulmonary function and exercise tolerance, there is tremendous individual variation, making the resting pulmonary function test a poor predictor of exercise tolerance. Figure 34–4 shows peak oxygen consumption plotted against the ratio of RV to total lung capacity. The correlation is highly significant statistically but nearly useless as a guide to predicting exercise tolerance from the resting pulmonary function. This is not to imply that pulmonary function does not influence exercise tolerance in the individual, but rather that the exact relationship between pulmonary function test results and exercise tolerance differs from patient to patient. An important study demonstrated what most patients report, namely, that a change in pulmonary function alters exercise tolerance in individual patients.[71] Seventeen patients with CF were studied at the beginning and end of a 2-week hospitalization for intensive treatment of pulmonary disease exacerbation. The patients achieved much higher work rates, markedly improved peak oxygen consumption, and a lower perception of exertion when their pulmonary function improved (Fig. 34–5).[71]

Cardiovascular Responses. Except in the most se-

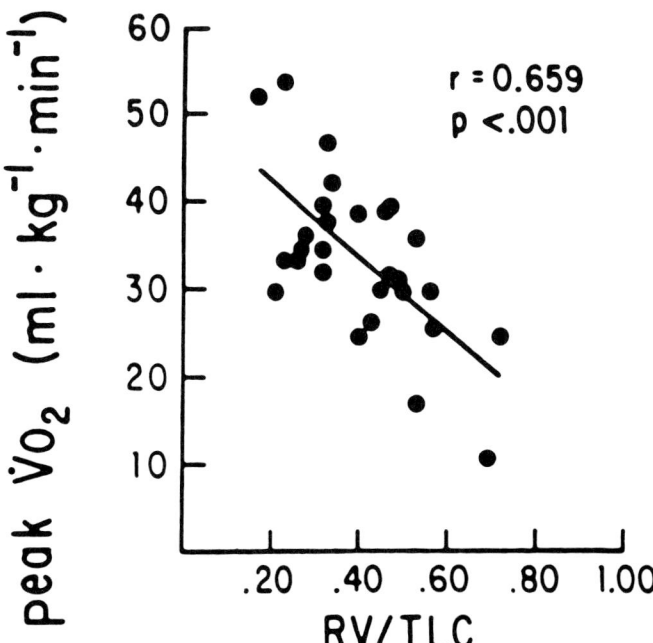

FIGURE 34-4. Correlation between the ratio of residual volume to total lung capacity (RV/TLC, a sensitive measure of air trapping) and exercise tolerance (expressed as peak $\dot{V}O_2$). The worse the air trapping, the higher the value of RV/TLC. The correlation is highly significant, but the tremendous scatter makes the resting pulmonary function value meaningless in predicting exercise tolerance in the individual patient. (From Orenstein DM, Nixon PA. Patients with cystic fibrosis. In: Franklin BA, Gordon S, Timms GC (eds). Exercise in Modern Medicine. Baltimore: Williams & Wilkins, 1989, pp 204–214.)

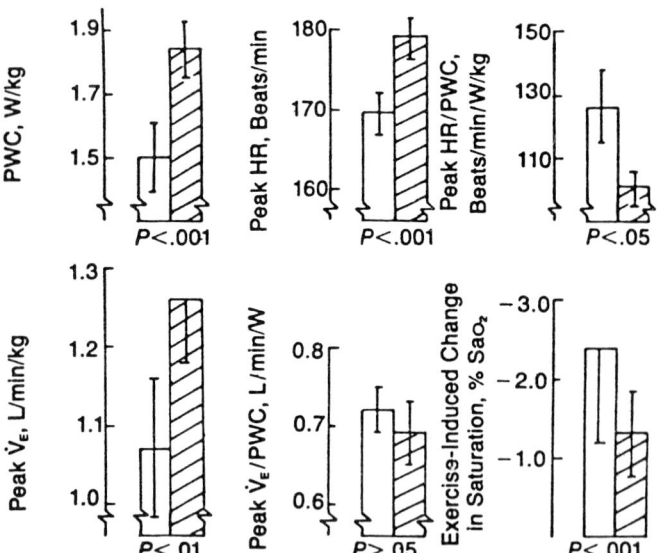

FIGURE 34–5. Exercise tolerance at the beginning of hospitalization for treatment of pulmonary exacerbation (open bars) and at the end of hospitalization (lined bars) after pulmonary function had improved. Thus, improved pulmonary function is correlated with improved exercise tolerance. (PWC: peak work capacity; $\dot{V}_E$: expired volume; HR: heart rate; Sao_2: arterial blood oxygen saturation). (From Cerny FJ, Cropp GJ, Bye MR. Hospital therapy improves exercise tolerance and lung function in cystic fibrosis. Am J Dis Child 1984; 138:261–265. Copyright 1984, American Medical Association.)

verely affected patients, heart rate tends to be normal at rest and increases normally with increasing workloads.[72] Maximum heart rates, however, do not reach normal levels (except in those patients with the mildest lung disease[63]) almost certainly because other noncardiac factors limit exercise before the heart is pushed to the maximum rates of which it is capable.[73] Cardiac output is also normal for workload.[62, 74, 75] In 11 patients from Montreal with relatively severe airways obstruction, cardiac stroke volume as a per cent predicted correlated with resting PaO_2 and even more strikingly with FEV_1 and the respiratory duty cycle,[76] suggesting a mechanical element of cardiopulmonary interdependence. Another Canadian study suggested that nutrition has an important influence on cardiac function, at least in CF patients with low resting PaO_2.[75] In 22 patients with severe resting oxyhemoglobin desaturation, stroke volume during submaximum exercise was reduced in 13 poorly nourished patients compared with a normal stroke volume in the 9 well-nourished patients, an effect that was independent of resting pulmonary function.[75] Radionuclide angiographic studies have shown some CF patients to have impaired right or left ventricular function, or both, without relation to resting pulmonary function.[77]

Ventilatory Responses. Ventilation increases with increasing work rate, and at peak exercise, minute ventilation is greatest for those with the best pulmonary function and least for those with the most compromised resting pulmonary function (consistent with the amount of work accomplished).[69] The components of ventilation—namely, tidal volume and breathing frequency—do not correlate with pulmonary function.[69] However, the sickest patients show a trend toward using a greater proportion of their VC for each breath than do the healthiest patients.[69] Breathing frequency seems to be more closely related to age (i.e., younger patients breathe faster than older patients) than to disease severity (Table 34–2).

Despite the fact that peak minute ventilation is highest for the healthiest patients (because of the greater work rates achieved), when ventilation is examined in relation to work rates achieved or units of oxygen consumed, patients require a larger minute ventilation than do subjects without lung disease[72]; this is almost certainly to compensate for a larger than normal dead space.[62] It is interesting to note that this increased ventilatory requirement during exercise is most pronounced in those with the worst underlying lung impairment but is seen even in patients with normal resting pulmonary function.[72]

Ventilatory mechanics probably limit exercise tolerance in many patients with CF.[62] This mechanical limitation is evidenced by the fact that many patients with CF employ a minute ventilation during exercise that approaches or even exceeds their resting maximum voluntary ventilation (MVV),[62] whereas in healthy children and adults, exercise ventilation seldom exceeds 70% of MVV.[78] The patient with CF probably has no reserve beyond what is employed to achieve these high levels of minute ventilation.

Sputum Production. There have been many anecdotes associating exercise sessions with improved sputum production.[73] One study of 10 hospitalized CF patients measured the volume of sputum expectorated during 15 minutes of cycle ergometer exercise and the ensuing 1.75 hours and compared it with the volume expectorated during a comparable 15-minute session of traditional chest physiotherapy.[67] More sputum was expectorated with traditional chest physiotherapy than with cycle exercise (Fig. 34–6), prompting the authors to conclude that "exercise may have a role in aiding sputum expectoration in patients with cystic fibrosis but should not be considered as a replacement for physiotherapy."

Gas Exchange. Even the high minute ventilation used by patients with CF during exercise in an apparent attempt to compensate for a large dead space may be

TABLE 34–2. BREATHING FREQUENCY AT PEAK EXERCISE IN 110 PATIENTS WITH CF: CORRELATIONS WITH DISEASE SEVERITY* AND AGE

	$FEV_1/VC \times 100$		
	>65%	50–64%	<50%
$f_b$max†	55.6 (±12.3)‡	56.9 (±13.7)‡	51.3 (±15.7)‡

	Age		
	<10 yr	10–18 yr	>18 yr
$f_b$max	73.3 (±12.2)§	57.3 (±13.1)§	49.0 (±13.1)§

*Based on FEV_1/VC.
†Maximum breathing frequency.
‡Indicates that differences are not significant.
§Youngest versus intermediate age: $P<.05$; intermediate age versus oldest: $P<.01$; youngest versus oldest: $P<.01$.

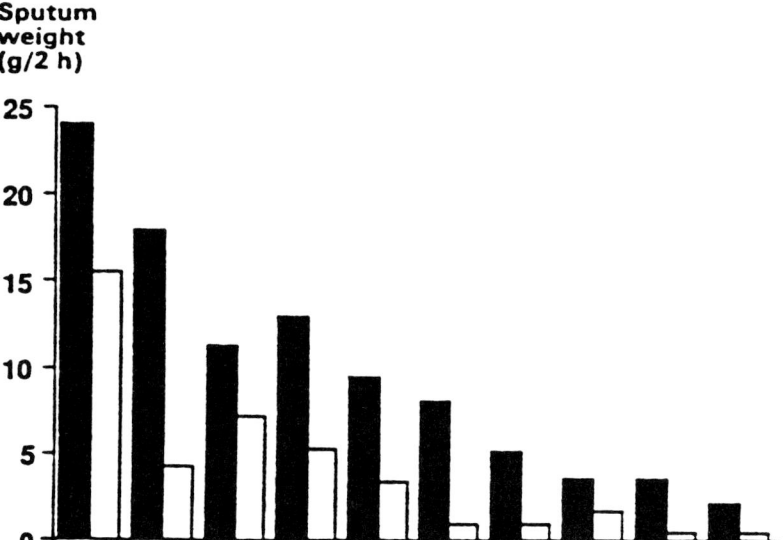

FIGURE 34–6. Sputum production in 10 patients with cystic fibrosis during and 1.75 hours after 15 minutes of standard chest physiotherapy (dark bars) and during and after 15 minutes of cycling exercise at 50% of peak work capacity. Significantly more sputum was produced with standard chest physiotherapy than with exercise ($P<.01$). (From Salh W, Bilton D, Dodd M, Webb AK. Effect of exercise and physiotherapy in aiding sputum expectoration in adults with cystic fibrosis. Thorax 1989; 44:1006–1008.)

inadequate, and some patients may have relative hypoventilation during exercise (with elevated end-tidal carbon dioxide) and hypoxemia.[25, 63, 72] Most patients do not desaturate during exercise, and some even improve their oxygenation.[25, 62] Resting pulmonary function once again does not predict exercise response, but some patterns are recognizable: patients with an FEV_1 greater than 50% of forced vital capacity (FVC) are very unlikely to desaturate[25]; even those with an FEV_1/FVC ratio of less than 50% are just as likely to maintain their oxyhemoglobin saturation at pre-exercise levels or even to increase them as they are to desaturate (Fig. 34–7).[25] In those laboratories capable of carrying out measurements of patients' diffusing capacity for carbon monoxide (D_{LCO}), D_{LCO} can play a predictive role for desaturation during exercise; patients with a D_{LCO} greater than 80% of predicted are at very low risk for desaturation, whereas those whose D_{LCO} is below 65% of predicted are likely to desaturate during exercise.[79] As noted above, although some patients (especially those with relatively severe pulmonary disease) have both sleep-related and exercise-related desaturation,[80] sleep-related desaturation does not correlate with exercise-related desaturation well enough to use either phenomenon to predict the other.[26]

The hypoventilation seen in some patients with advanced lung disease seems to be explained by a ventilatory pattern characterized by a low tidal volume, which in turn is dictated by a short inspiratory time (low respiratory duty cycle [TI/Tt]).[81]

Although most periods of desaturation seen during exercise in patients with CF can be attributed to hypoventilation with decreased oxygen saturation and increased end-tidal carbon dioxide,[72] virtually every combination of changes in oxygenation and carbon dioxide elimination can be seen (Fig. 34–8),[25] indicating complex interactions between pulmonary ventilation and perfusion.

Effect of Desaturation and Oxygen Supplementation on Exercise Tolerance. Despite even profound desaturation in some patients, there is no evidence that oxygenation limits exercise tolerance in CF patients. In fact, there is some evidence that it does not, that is, supplemental oxygen given during exercise effectively blocks desaturation in those who desaturate when exercising in room air, and it decreases heart rate and respiratory rate for submaximum workrates, but it does not increase peak work rate achieved on a progressive test to exhaustion (Fig. 34–9).[82]

Exercise in the Heat. Few studies have examined the response of CF patients to exercise in the heat,[14, 83] despite the fact that these patients have been known for decades to have greater than normal concentrations of sodium and chloride in their sweat.[84] During exercise, children with CF underestimate their fluid needs.[84a] In one controlled study, CF patients had normal temperature, heart rate, hormonal (i.e., renin and aldosterone) and renal responses, but lost more than normal amounts of sodium and chloride when they exercised for 90 minutes in a heat chamber (100° F, 38° C).[14] The sodium and chloride losses were so great that the patients showed decreased concentrations of these ions in serum.[14] However, CF patients have superb homeostatic control; within 24 hours after the 90-minute exercise and heat stress, body weight and serum electrolyte levels were back to baseline when patients were given a free choice of fluid and food.[83]

Other Variables Related to Exercise Tolerance. In addition to resting pulmonary function, three important variables have been found to relate significantly to exercise tolerance independently of the influence of pulmonary function, namely, nutritional status, quality of life, and prognosis. Several different studies have demonstrated that poor nutritional status correlates significantly with exercise tolerance independent of the influence of pulmonary function.[74, 75, 85] In 44 patients with CF, a general scale measuring the quality of well-being (the Quality of Well-being Scale) was found to correlate significantly with exercise test results.[70] Even more intriguing is the observation that fitness was posi-

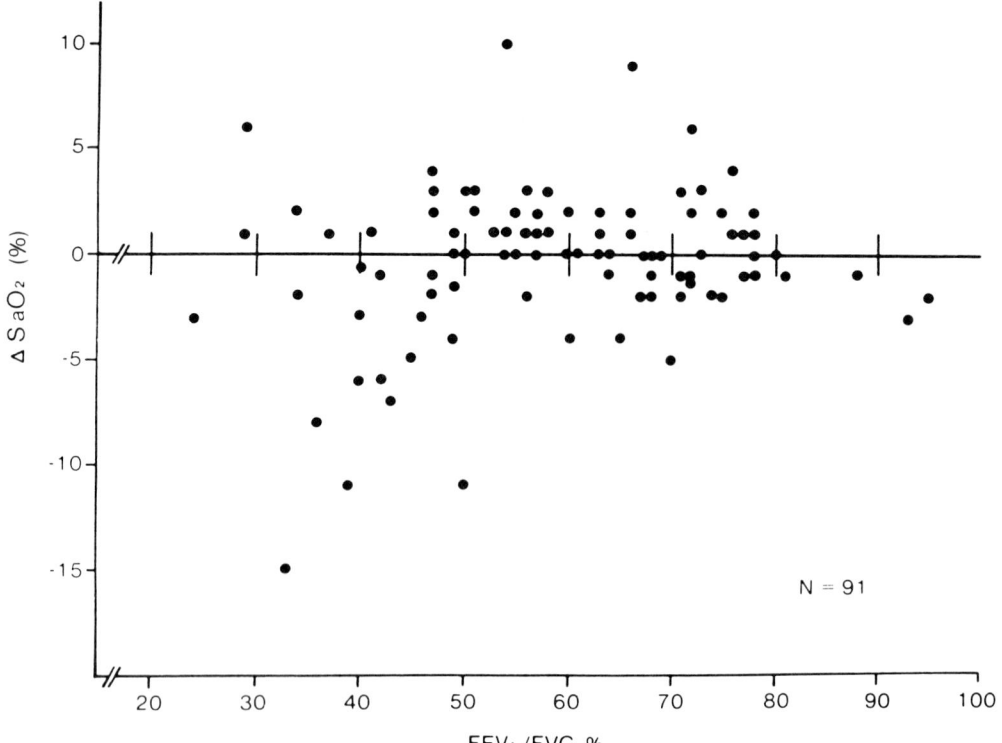

FIGURE 34-7. Changes in oxygen saturation with exercise plotted against FEV_1/FVC for 91 patients with cystic fibrosis. No patient with $FEV_1/FVC > 50\%$ suffered desaturation greater than 5%; of those with $FEV_1/FVC < 50\%$, some desaturated, whereas others did not. (From Henke K, Orenstein D. Oxygen saturation during exercise in cystic fibrosis. Am Rev Respir Dis 1984; 129:708–711.)

tively correlated with survival in 47 patients with CF (Fig. 34–10).[57] In this study, patients with peak oxygen consumption less than 30.2 ml/kg/min were five times less likely to survive 7 years than those with peak oxygen consumption greater than 38 ml/kg/min. Resting pulmonary function tests played a much smaller role in predicting survival than did the exercise tests.

Repeated Bouts of Exercise (Exercise Programs)

In a number of studies published since the late 1970s, exercise programs have been described for patients with CF. The evidence seems to indicate various benefits from these different programs and no obvious harmful effects. However, many of the published studies had design or reporting flaws and included widely varying exercise programs that were sometimes poorly defined as well as patients with very different degrees of underlying pulmonary disease severity. These deficiencies made scientific certainty about the exact effects of these programs difficult. Table 34–3 summarizes studies published between 1977 and 1991.

Published studies of exercise programs for patients with CF have had several different focuses, interventions, and outcome measures. Most have been short, lasting only a few days or weeks.

Types of Exercise. The types of exercise intervention can be roughly divided into ventilatory muscle exercise, jogging and walking, swimming, weight-lifting, cycling, and various exercises.

Ventilatory Muscle Exercise. The first published exercise intervention program in CF was by Keens and colleagues[86] and focused on the ventilatory muscles. This study, although small ($n = 7$) and short (4 weeks' duration), demonstrated unequivocally that daily exercises directed specifically at the ventilatory muscles (25 min/day of eucapnic hyperpnea 5 days/wk) could increase patient endurance as measured by sustained hyperpnea; less-precisely targeted upper body exercise (swimming and canoeing 90 min/day for 4 wk) achieved the same effect.[86] Several years later, Asher and associates[87] similarly demonstrated that 4 weeks of twice daily 15-minute sessions of breathing through an inspiratory resistance device brought about increases in both the strength and endurance of the ventilatory muscles in 11 patients with CF. However, this increased ventilatory muscle performance did not bring about any improvement in overall exercise tolerance (measured by cycle ergometer testing), suggesting that the ventilatory muscles are not the weak link in the exercise tolerance chain.

Jogging and Walking. Aerobic exercise programs are understood to mean programs with adequate frequency, intensity, and duration to bring about an increase in aerobic fitness (usually defined as an increase in maximum oxygen consumption accompanied by a decrease in heart rate for submaximum work rates[88]) in healthy populations. The first study to employ general aerobic exercise in CF rather than exercise targeted specifically at the ventilatory muscles was a 3-month program of supervised jogging and walking with sessions conducted three times per week.[64] The length of time per session devoted to the exercise was gradually increased. Twenty-one CF patients with a wide range of disease severity began with warm-up calisthenics and low-intensity games and then started jogging and walking at an

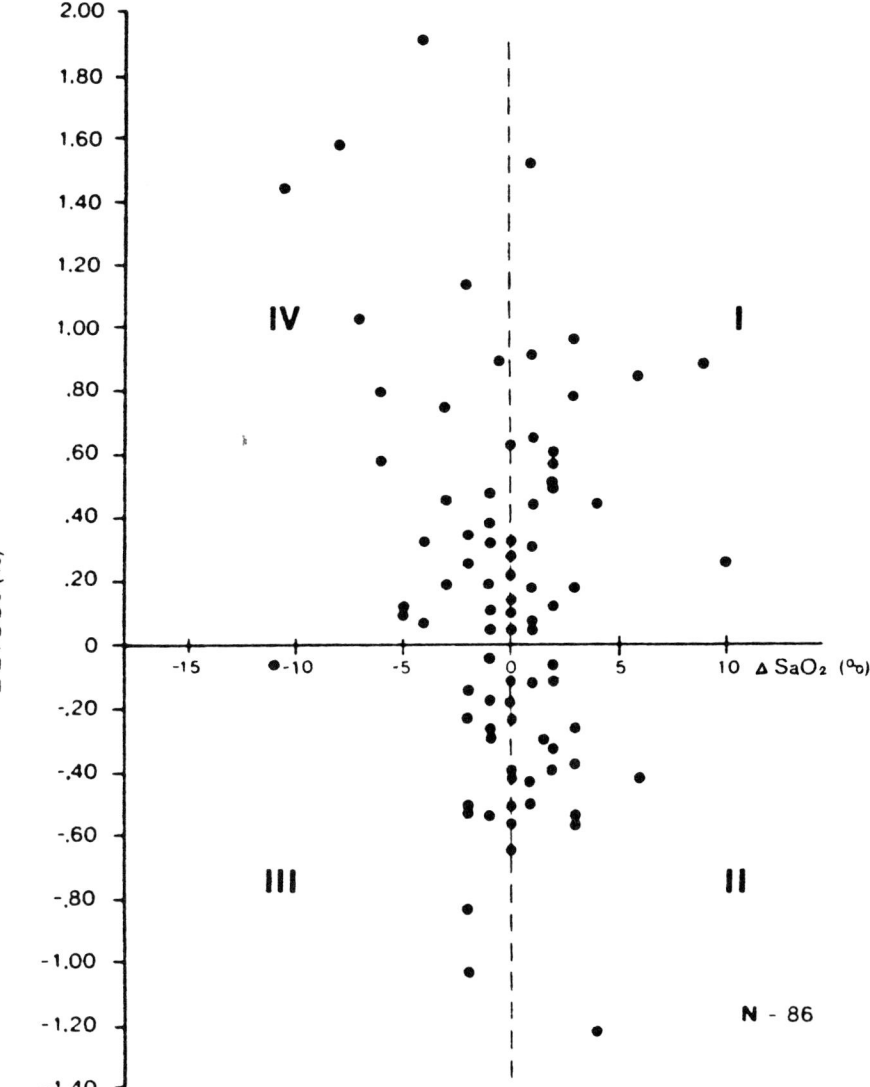

FIGURE 34-8. Changes in end-tidal carbon dioxide fraction (ET$_{CO_2}$) with exercise plotted against changes in Sa$_{O_2}$) with exercise. *Quadrant I* represents those patients whose Sa$_{O_2}$ and ET$_{CO_2}$ increased, *quadrant II*—those patients whose Sa$_{O_2}$ increased and whose ET$_{CO_2}$ decreased, *quadrant III*—those patients whose Sa$_{O_2}$ and ET$_{CO_2}$ both decreased, and *quadrant IV*—those patients whose Sa$_{O_2}$ decreased and whose ET$_{CO_2}$ increased. Some patients fall within each quadrant, indicating complex ventilation-perfusion relationships. (From Henke K, Orenstein D. Oxygen saturation during exercise in cystic fibrosis. Am Rev Respir Dis 1984; 129:708–711.)

intensity sufficient to produce heart rates of 70 to 85% of their own maximum heart rates as determined by progressive tests to exhaustion at the beginning of the program. During the first week of the program, the jogging or walking portion of each session lasted 10 minutes. Two minutes were added to the sessions each week; by the 10th week, patients were jogging steadily for 30 minutes. This study was also the first exercise intervention study in CF to include a control group; this is an important consideration, since the nature of CF is so variable not only among patients but also within patients from time to time. Patients in this study increased their exercise tolerance (i.e., they had a higher work rate on a progressive cycle ergometer test to exhaustion) and their cardiorespiratory fitness (as measured by peak oxygen consumption). They also showed a training bradycardia, with lower heart rates for a given submaximum workload. The control CF patients, who were comparable to those in the exercise group at the onset of the program, did not change their exercise tolerance or fitness. Pulmonary function tests did not change in the exercise group; most pulmonary function values did not change in the control group, but FEV$_1$ did decrease significantly in the controls over the 3-month program. It is unclear whether this represents stabilization of pulmonary function in the intervention group and the expected deterioration in the control group, or if it is a meaningless statistical artifact (with statistical significance defined as $P < .05$ and with about 10 different pulmonary function test variables examined in each of the two groups, one would expect at least one variable to show a statistically significant change).

In another jogging study, conducted in Italy, Braggion and coworkers included a non–CF control group and 10 CF patients with quite mild lung disease in an 8-week program with sessions conducted three times per week.[65] The intensity of exercise was adjusted "so as to produce a heart rate not exceeding 150 beats/min." The length of the exercise sessions was similar to that in the previously mentioned study, starting with 10 minutes and gradually increasing to 25 to 30 minutes by the final week. In this study, virtually no changes were found in

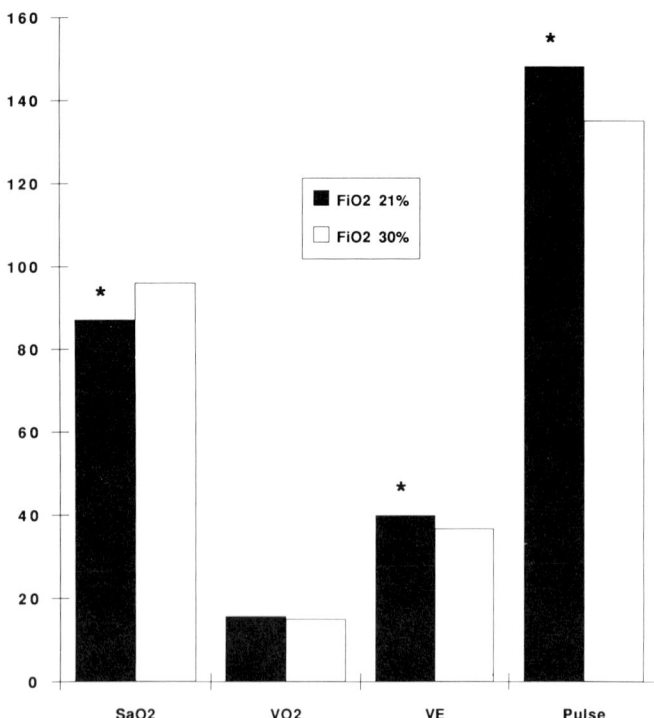

FIGURE 34-9. Oxygen supplementation during submaximal exercise in patients with cystic fibrosis abolishes the desaturation experienced in room air and decreases pulse and minute ventilation; however, it does not improve peak work. Asterisks indicate significant differences between ET_{O_2} of 21% and 30%. (Sa_{O_2} in per cent; $\dot{V}_{O_2}$ in ml/kg/min; $\dot{V}E$ in L/min; pulse in beats/min.) (Drawn based on data from Nixon PA, Orenstein DM, Curtis SE, Ross EA. Oxygen supplementation during exercise in cystic fibrosis. Am Rev Respir Dis 1990; 142:807–811.)

exercise tolerance, cardiorespiratory fitness, or pulmonary function. The authors speculated that the absence of changes might have been a result of the relatively mild degree of lung disease and high initial fitness in these patients or of the low intensity or short duration of the program.

Another study with disappointing results was carried out in Australia by Holzer and coworkers.[89] It included a calisthenics and running program that had an important difference from the previous studies, that is, it was an at-home unsupervised program. Patient compliance was very poor, and no measurable benefits accrued to the patients, forcing the authors to conclude that "there appears limited value in promoting unsupervised home exercise programs for children with CF."

Swimming. In Austria, Zach and colleagues reported a program consisting of 1 hour of swimming two to three times per week for 7 weeks.[90] During the 7-week swimming program, patients continued their usual chest physiotherapy treatments. Exercise tolerance was not measured, but FVC, FEV_1, forced expiratory flow between 25 and 75% of FVC, and peak expiratory flow rate were improved at the end of the 7 weeks, and sputum production was felt to be greater on swimming days than on nonswimming days. By 10 weeks after the swimming program, pulmonary function test results had fallen back to the pre-exercise baseline values.

Edlund and colleagues instituted a 12-week study of a swimming program for 12 CF patients in an exercise group and 11 patients in a control group.[91] Three times per week, the patients warmed up and then swam; each maintained his or her heart rate between 60 and 75% of the previously measured maximum rate. The swimming session lasted 5 minutes in the first week, and 3 minutes were added to each succeeding week's session, resulting in a total of 20 minutes of swimming during the 7th week. Patients' pulmonary function test results were unchanged; time on a treadmill test increased in the exercise group but decreased slightly in the control patients. The Shwachman score, a CF-specific overall clinical scoring system,[92] improved in the swimmers but worsened slightly in the control patients.

Weight Lifting. In one study of nine adults with CF, a 6-month weight training program aimed at upper body conditioning was shown to increase upper body strength and body weight and to decrease hyperinflation (lower RV) compared with baseline values and with values recorded after a 3-month control period.[93] It is unclear how this effect on RV can be explained, except perhaps by an increase in expiratory muscle strength.

Cycling. A British program prescribed 10 minutes of home exercise on a cycle ergometer 5 days per week for 2 months to 19 adults with CF.[67] Only 12 patients (63%) completed the program. Among those who did, significant increases in peak work capacity and fitness (maximum oxygen consumption) were observed. A nonsignificant increase in daily sputum volume at the end of the exercise program compared with the pre-exercise baseline was also noted. FVC and FEV_1 did not change.

Various Exercises. A number of studies have used different kinds of exercise in patients with CF and often presented vague descriptions of which exercise was used for which patients and of the intensity or duration of the exercise sessions. In a small ($n = 7$) but prolonged (30-month) Swedish study, patients were assigned daily exercise sufficient to produce a heart rate of 160 beats/min or more.[94] The exercise mode was jointly selected by the patient and physiotherapist and could include "sit-ups, rope skipping, trampolining, . . . jogging, swimming, and ball games." After 12 months, conventional chest physiotherapy was discontinued. Work capacity did not change in the group as a whole but improved in three of the four sickest patients. Pulmonary function did not change significantly, but thoracic gas volume seemed to decrease, indicating the presence of less trapped gas.

O'Neill and coworkers[66] prescribed an 8-week at-home program for eight CF patients that was based on the Royal Canadian Air Force protocol. Neither pulmonary function nor exercise tolerance changed, but breathlessness during exercise decreased significantly.

Zach and colleagues carried out a 17-day program of astonishingly intense exercise with 12 children with CF during summer holidays at a pediatric rehabilitation hospital in the mountains of Austria.[95] The program included "one hour of swimming and diving twice a day. As the . . . pool was some 2½ km from the paediatric department, the children jogged from one to the other.

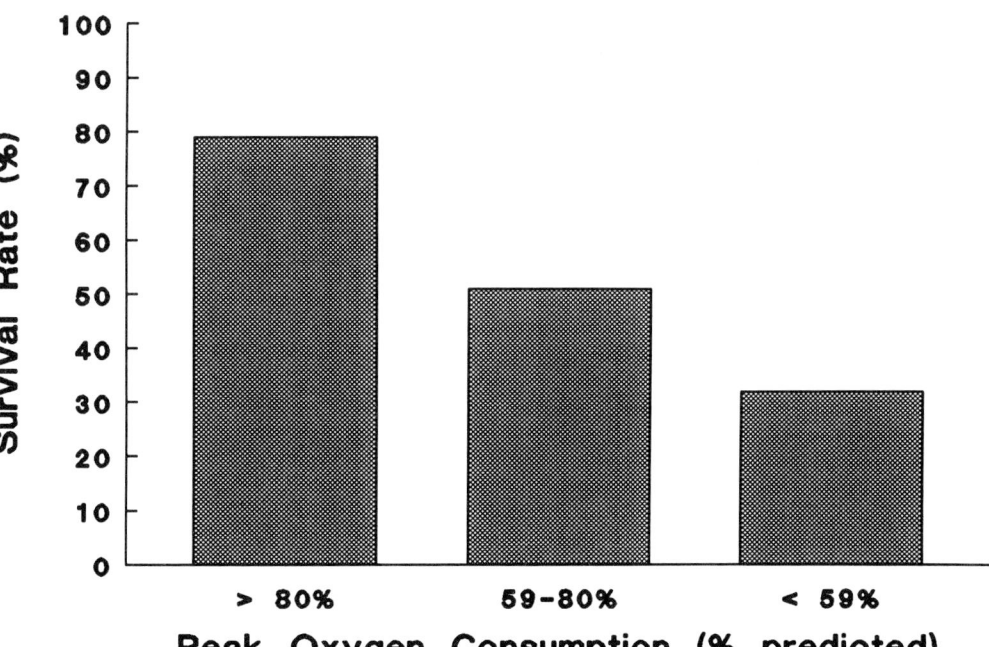

FIGURE 34-10. The relationship between fitness (peak oxygen consumption) and 8-year survival. (Data modified from Pediatric Pulmonology, Nixon P, Orenstein D, Doershuk C. Copyright © 1990. Reprinted by permission of Wiley-Liss, A Division of John Wiley & Sons, Inc.)

The children hiked for several hours through the surrounding forests and mountains, collecting firewood, berries, and mushrooms. In addition, all children took part in gymnastics, skipping, and . . . minigolf, soccer, and table tennis." The children did not perform their regular chest physiotherapy or inhalation treatments during the 17 days. Daily peak flow measurements increased throughout the 17-day program but fell to baseline by 8 weeks later.

Heat Acclimation. Repeated bouts of exercise in the heat can bring about better tolerance to similar stresses in healthy populations. Patients with CF can also improve their tolerance to exercise and heat stress.[83] Eight consecutive days of exercise and heat stress enabled CF patients to withstand exercise in the heat with lower heart rates and lower core body temperatures; however, CF patients did not have a lessening of sweat sodium and chloride concentrations, as was seen in the healthy control subjects.

Lifestyle Change. Studies in the epidemiology of cardiovascular disease in adults without CF suggest that overall physical activity—and not necessarily the intensity of that activity—or levels of aerobic fitness measurable by maximum oxygen uptake changes may be the most important factor influencing outcome.[96] No studies in CF have tried to increase overall physical activity levels throughout the day but instead have tried to prescribe relatively intense exercise for brief periods during the day or week. Furthermore, in adults with heart disease[97] and in overweight children,[98] long-term compliance with aerobic exercise programs is notoriously poor, whereas programs that call for lifestyle changes involving more sustained and perhaps less intense activity throughout the day are better adhered to.[98] Again, no published studies have examined the possible role of lifestyle changes in long-term rehabilitation programs for patients with CF.

Effects of Exercise Programs: Outcome Variables. Exercise programs in CF have not only had varying kinds of intervention but have also focused on different outcome variables, including exercise tolerance and cardiorespiratory fitness, pulmonary function, sputum production, and breathlessness. The influence of exercise programs on life-quality and prognosis is also of interest.

Exercise Tolerance. Most of the exercise programs that have been studied have brought about an increase in exercise tolerance, which might be the most important outcome for a rehabilitation program. The earliest program was our own,[64] which consisted of supervised jogging three times per week (see Table 34-3 for more details on all of the programs). Increased exercise tolerance was documented by improved work rate on the cycle ergometer and by increased peak oxygen consumption. The swimming program of Edlund and colleagues[91] also brought about improved exercise tolerance (measured by time to exhaustion on a treadmill test). Changes in oxygen consumption were less consistent. The varied program described by Andreasson and associates[94] included only seven patients, four of whom had low overall clinical scores; of these four sicker patients, three improved their work capacity on cycle ergometer testing after 12 months. The patients of Stanghelle and coworkers who participated in daily trampoline exercise over an 8-week period[99] showed increased maximum oxygen consumption.

Pulmonary Function. Findings with regard to pulmonary function have been inconsistent, with several studies showing improved pulmonary function and others demonstrating no change or no difference between an exercise group and a control group. Since CF is characterized by progressive decline in pulmonary function, an intervention that prevented that decline would be a very successful intervention, and no change in pulmonary function over time would be a very positive out-

TABLE 34-3. PUBLISHED EXERCISE PROGRAMS IN CF*

	Exercise Program					Study Design			
Reference	Frequency	Intensity	Time per Session	Type of Exercise	Location (Supervised/ Unsupervised)	No. Start/ No. Finish (Age in yr)	Disease Severity	Controls/Randomization	Length of Study
Keens et al.[86] (1977)	5 days/wk	"Maximal"	25 min	Normocapnic hyperpnea	CF summer camp (supervised)	4/4 (16 ± .6)	FEV_1 59 ± 13% pred	Non-CF controls; not randomized	4 wk
	Daily	"Intensive"	1.5 h	Swimming and canoeing	CF summer camp (supervised)	7/7 (13 ± 1)	FEV_1 64 ± 8% pred	Non-CF controls; CF patients undergoing ventilatory muscle training; not randomized	4 wk
Orenstein et al.[64] (1981)	3 times/wk	70–85% of patient's max HR	10 min 1st wk; increased to 30 min by 10th wk	Jogging/walking	Local gymnasium (supervised)	25/21 in exercise group; 10/10 in control group (10–30)	FEV_1 range 32–81% of VC	Not randomized; controls lived far away	3 mo
Zach et al.[90] (1981)	2–3 times/wk		1 h	Swimming	"Teaching pool" (supervised)	10/10	FEV_1 83 ± 24% pred	No controls, not randomized; patients lived within 30 km of hospital	7.5 wk
Zach et al.[95] (1982)	Daily		7.5 hr/day	Swimming, jogging, hiking, gymnastics, soccer, etc.	Pediatric rehab hospital (supervised)	12/10 (12–16)	FEV_1 71 ± 22% pred	No controls, not randomized ("willingness to participate")	17 days
Asher et al.[87] (1982)	Twice daily		15 min	Ventilatory muscle (breathing through an inspiratory resistance device)	Home (supervised by phone and some home visits)	11/11 (9–24)	Severe FEV_1 <50% pred	Patients were their own controls for 4 wk before or after 4 wk of training	4 wk training; 4 wk control
Holzer et al.[89] (1981)	Daily	Graded, increased, depending on capacity	30 min	Various (Royal Canadian Air Force program)	Home (unsupervised)	41/? (8–14)	Mild FEV_1 86 ± 19% pred	No controls, not randomized	3 mo
Blomquist et al.[100] (1986)	Twice daily	HR ≥75% of each patient's max	15 min (at least)	Various (skipping rope, jogging, dance, bowling, etc.)	Home (unsupervised)	14/12 (13–23)	"Moderate to mild"; mean FVC = 77% pred	Patients were their own controls; not randomized	12 mo
Edlund et al.[91] (1986)	3 times/wk	HR 60–75% of patient's max for 5 wk, then 70–85% of max	5 min 1st wk; increased to 20 min by 7th wk	Swimming	University pool (supervised)	12/10 (7–14)	Mild (clinical score = 83/100); initial V_{O_2} = 56 ml/kg/min	Controlled; not randomized (group selection based on proximity to medical center)	12 wk
Strauss et al.[93] (1987)	3 times/wk	Graded increased depending on capacity	?	Weight-lifting with free weights and Universal Gym machine	Home (supervised)	12/9 (16–39)	Moderate to severe; FEV_1 = 42 ± 14% pred	Patients were their own controls; not randomized	3 mo for control group, 6 mo for training group
O'Neill et al.[66] (1987)	Daily		11 min	Various (Royal Canadian Air Force program)	Home (unsupervised)	8/7 (17–27)	Mean FEV_1 1.72 ± .97L	No controls, not randomized	2 mo
Andreasson et al.[94] (1987)	Daily	HR 160 beats/min or greater	30 min	Various (sit-ups, jogging, swimming, ball games, etc.)	Home (unsupervised)	7/7 (6–20)	Mild to moderate; FEV_1 45–106% pred (mean 71%)	No controls, not randomized	30 mo
Braggion et al.[65] (1989)	3 times/wk	HR 150 beats/min or fewer	10 min 1st wk; increased to 30 min by final wk	Jogging (including warm-up and circuit training each session)	Unknown (supervised by physio-therapists/ supervised by physical education teacher)	10/10 in exercise group; 10/10 in control group (11–15)	Mild; FEV_1 43–100% pred (mean 77%)	Patients were their own controls; non-CF control group; not randomized	8 wk
Salh et al.[67] (1989)	5 times/wk	Start at 50% of peak work capacity; increased 5 watts/wk	10 min	Exercise cycle	Home (unsupervised)	19/12 (16–33)	FEV_1 15–94% pred (mean 46%)	No controls, not randomized	2 mo
Cerny[101] (1989)	Twice daily	HR about midway between rest and max HRs	5–10 min for days 1–3; 15–20 min for days 4–14	Exercise cycle	Hospital (supervised)	9/9 in exercise group; 8/8 in control group (15.4 ± 4.9)	Moderate to severe	Random assignment to exercise or standard care (controls)	14 days

*Modified from Shepherd S and Hovell M, personal communication, 1991.
Key: HR: heart rate; max: maximum; rehab: rehabilitation; No. start/No. finish: number of patients who started/finished program; % pred: percent of predicted; Wmax: maximum work; MMEF: maximum midexpiratory flow; PEFR: peak expiratory flow rate; $FEV_{25-75\%}$: forced expiratory flow; Vtg: volume of thoracic gas; PFT: pulmonary function tests.

		Results				
Exercise Tolerance	Ventilatory Muscle Endurance	Peak $\dot{V}O_2$	FEV_1	Other PFT	Sputum Volume	Comments
No change	Increased 53%	No change	No change	No change in MMEF		Ventilatory muscle endurance increased equally in ventilatory muscle training and swimming/canoeing group. Returned to baseline after program
No change	Increased 57%	No change	No change	No change in MMEF		
Improved (exercise group); no change (control group)	Improved (exercise group); no change (control group)	Improved (exercise group); no change (control group)	No change (exercise group); decreased (control group)	No change in either group		Exercise group had training bradycardia (lower submax HR) after program. Fourteen exercise patients who improved began less fit than 7 patients who did not improve
			Improved from 83 to 91% pred	FVC, PEFR, and $FEF_{25-75\%}$ all improved	Greater on swimming days (but difference significant in only 2 patients)	Most patients stopped exercise after program ended; PFT results back to baseline after program ended
No formal testing, but "a gradual increase in performance and endurance was evident"			Improved from 71 to 79% pred	FVC, PEFR, and $FEF_{25-75\%}$ all improved	Reached a max between days 3 and 5, then decreased gradually	Patients stopped regular inhalation and chest physiotherapy for all 17 days. Authors concluded exercise could replace inhalation/physiotherapy for some patients with CF
No change in either max or submax exercise after program	Increased after ventilatory muscle training; ventilatory muscle strength also increased	No change				Ventilatory muscle training did increase ventilatory muscle strength and endurance, but exercise tolerance did not change
No change	No change		No change	No change		Very poor compliance. Authors concluded there appears to be limited value in unsupervised home exercise
No change			No change	Improved PaO_2		No patients did prescribed skipping rope; authors feel self-treatment plus exercise is as good as conventional physiotherapy
Increased treadmill time in exercise group; slight decrease in control group		Measured $\dot{V}O_2$ showed no change; pred $\dot{V}O_2$ increased in exercise group	No change	Clinical scores slightly but significantly better for exercise group; no change in control group		Very fit group. Authors concluded "a swimming program is . . . excellent . . . for improving the clinical status and quality of life in CF"
Increase in strength of all muscle groups			No change	Decreased RV, RV/TLC, and TLC		Body weight increased. Why less hyperinflation? Not clear how many sessions attended. Patients had nonsignificant increase in dates with opposite sex.
No change		No change	No change	Decreased RV from 1.9 to 1.2 L	"In some cases, a decrease in sputum volume"	Breathlessness significantly reduced on submax work, as measured on visual analog scale
No change				No change except for a decrease in Vtg		After 12 mo, usual chest physiotherapy was eliminated, yet PFT values did not decrease. Conclusion: "conventional chest physiotherapy . . . can be replaced by efficient physical training"
Increased (Wmax: from 4.0 to 4.2 watts/kg); improved endurance time, faster obstacle course time in CF; no change in controls		No change in either group	No change	No change		
Increased (Wmax: from 2.7 to 3.1 watt/kg)		Increased from 25.9 to 30.3 ml/gk/min	No change	MVV increased; no change in FVC	Nonsignificant increase in daily sputum volume from 24 to 37 gm (with very large standard deviation)	A separate study reported in same paper compared sputum volume during and after cycle exercise with that during and after standard chest physiotherapy. Significantly more sputum was produced with physiotherapy than with exercise
Increased work load in both groups; no differences between groups			Increased (in both exercise and control groups)	Most PFT results improved in both groups; no differences between groups	No differences between groups in sputum volume	This study was done in a hospital on patients being treated for pulmonary disease exacerbation. Exercise group did 2 cycle sessions and 1 physiotherapy session per day; control group did 3 physiotherapy sessions per day

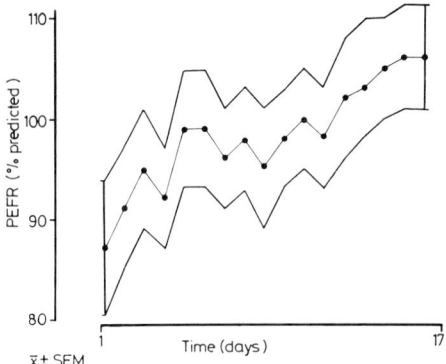

FIGURE 34-11. Daily peak flow recordings in 10 cystic fibrosis patients engaged in a very vigorous 17-day exercise program. (PEFR: peak expiratory flow rate.) (From Zach M, Oberwaldner B, Hausler F. Cystic fibrosis: Physical exercise versus chest physiotherapy. Arch Dis Child 1982; 57:587–589.)

come. Unfortunately, few studies have lasted long enough to confirm that the programs have truly delayed or prevented the expected deterioration. The two studies of Zach and colleagues from Austria—one with 7 weeks of swimming[90] and the other with 17 days of very intense, day-long activity (Fig. 34–11)[95]—showed improved FEV_1 and FVC during the exercise period but deterioration back to baseline values after the exercise programs ended.

Sputum Production. Some investigators point to improved sputum production as the main benefit that CF patients derive from exercise. These studies have been difficult to evaluate; for example, the 7-week swimming program of Zach and colleagues[90] reports that "regular swimming can assist in mucus clearance," but the results indicate a significant difference in only two patients for swimming versus nonswimming days. In the study of Salh and associates,[67] daily cycle ergometer exercise brought about a nonsignificant increase in daily sputum weight by the end of the 2-month intervention.

Breathlessness. One British study focused on the effects of an exercise program on the amount of dyspnea experienced by patients with CF during exercise. O'Neill and coworkers[66] found that a 2-month program significantly reduced breathlessness for a submaximum exercise task even though it did not bring about a measureable increase in exercise tolerance on a maximum exercise test.

Prognosis. None of the studies to date have been long enough or included sufficiently large numbers of patients to be able to examine the influence of exercise programs on prognosis for patients with CF. Certainly, the dual observations that high fitness is a good prognostic sign[57] and that fitness levels can be improved with an aerobic exercise program[64] make it appealing to assume that if an aerobic exercise program could be sustained for long enough, it might improve prognosis.

Comparison with Traditional Chest Physiotherapy. The point of several of the exercise studies was not necessarily to improve pulmonary function but rather to learn whether an exercise program could be a substitute for traditional chest physiotherapy. For these studies, if patients receiving exercise but no chest physiotherapy maintained pulmonary function or sputum production unchanged compared with when they (or control group patients) received traditional treatment, the exercise intervention was usually judged to be a success. Once again, however, most of these studies were too short or too poorly controlled to be able to make these judgments with certainty. Blomquist and colleagues and, in particular, Andreasson and associates felt that the absence of change in pulmonary function seen in their exercise interventions indicated that "self-treatment combined with physical activity is as efficient as conventional physiotherapy"[100] and that "physical exercise in general should be the basis of pulmonary therapy in cystic fibrosis."[94] Cerny[101] substituted cycle exercise for two of three daily chest physiotherapy treatments in nine CF patients hospitalized for intensive intravenous antibiotic treatment of pulmonary disease exacerbation and compared the outcomes with those of eight patients who received the standard three chest physiotherapy sessions. Both groups improved pulmonary function and exercise tolerance to an equal degree, prompting the author to conclude that "in some hospitalized patients with CF, exercise therapy may be substituted for at least part of the standard protocol of bronchial hygiene therapy." It is disappointing that this study did not have a sharp division between the effects of exercise and those of standard treatment. Perhaps the one standard chest physiotherapy treatment that both groups received was the effective part of the treatment, and nothing else—whether exercise or extra chest physiotherapy—made any difference.

Nutritional Rehabilitation

A number of studies of the effects of nutritional supplementation in patients with CF have been published. They report nearly universal agreement that such supplements, whether given orally,[102, 103] by nasogastric tube,[104–106] by gastrostomy tube,[107] by jejunostomy tube,[108] or by the parenteral route[109, 110] can improve patient nutritional status. Several of these studies suggest that such nutritional improvement is associated with better pulmonary function and demonstrate either actual improvement of pulmonary function[109] or less deterioration of pulmonary function than in control subjects[107, 111] or in the same subjects prior to the institution of the nutritional rehabilitation program.[111] Few of the studies employed formal exercise testing or objective, valid, and reliable measurements of physical activity or life-quality. Nonetheless, several studies have included some assessment of these functional outcome measures. General activity has been found to increase with nutritional rehabilitation in a few studies,[102, 103, 107] and well-being has been found to improve in others.[105, 109] A minority of studies have shown no meaningful functional benefit[106] and, one study[110] has even demonstrated worsened oxygenation.

TABLE 34–4. GUIDELINES FOR REHABILITATION IN CF

Aggressive standard treatment program
Frequent evaluation by physician
Regular chest physiotherapy
Antibiotic treatment for pulmonary disease exacerbations
Gastrointestinal/nutritional treatment
    Pancreatic enzyme replacement
    High-calorie diet
Nutritional component (if failure of standard nutritional treatment)
Oral high-calorie supplements
Consider enteral tube feeding (nasogastric, gastrostomy, or jejunostomy)
Consider parenteral feeding
Exercise component
Preprogram exercise test
    Establish baseline for comparison
    Identify desaturation in some and the point at which it occurs
Prescription
    Based on type of exercise patient enjoys or at least can adhere to
    Frequency: 3–5 times/wk
    Intensity: HR 70–85% of patient's own max (patient should try for feeling of pleasant fatigue; he or she must have some fatigue for exercise to be of benefit, but if fatigue unpleasant, exercise should not be continued)
    Duration: Begin with 10 min per session, then increase length of sessions as tolerated (e.g., add 2 min to sessions each wk to achieve a goal of 30 min per session)
    Other: Oxygen administration by nasal cannula to those who develop desaturation when breathing room air

Recommendations for the Rehabilitation of Patients with Cystic Fibrosis

Rehabilitation in patients with CF must be founded on a very solid standard treatment program that includes regular evaluation, chest physiotherapy, aggressive antibiotic treatment of episodes of worsened airways infection, pancreatic enzyme replacement therapy, and careful attention to the maintenance of a high calorie diet. In addition to these basics (but not in place of them), it is likely that some benefit can be gained from specific additional attention to exercise and nutrition.

The nutritional rehabilitation program in CF varies greatly from center to center and from patient to patient. It should be stressed that aggressive intervention, including surgical placement of enteral feeding tubes, may be very helpful. Furthermore, intervention should be initiated relatively early—as soon as a nutritional problem has been identified—and not be delayed until the patient is so wasted and sick that the intervention is of little benefit (Table 34–4).

Preprogram Exercise Test

A graduated test to maximum tolerance with measurement of heart rate and oxygen saturation is helpful in setting up guidelines for an exercise program and for establishing a baseline against which progress or deterioration can be compared. The test is essential for patients whose FEV_1 is less than 50% of FVC or less than 50% of predicted, since these are the patients who are at increased risk for developing desaturation during exercise.[25] If a patient does develop desaturation, it is possible to identify the heart rate at which it occurs and can take this into account, by prescribing exercise below this heart rate. If desaturation occurs even at very low heart rates, it is advisable to prescribe supplemental oxygen to be used with the exercise program.

An exercise prescription in CF, as in any population, should be designed with long-term compliance in mind. Therefore, patient acceptance and even enjoyment must be built in, and the program should be designed with input from the patient and his or her family. Although a swimming program may have theoretical benefits over any other kind of program, for someone who lives in a northern climate and does not have easy access to a pool or dislikes water activities, a swimming prescription is likely to be very unsuccessful. An exercise bike program that is not boring (i.e., does not incorporate television viewing and listening to music) will likewise be unsuccessful. Unless and until further studies indicate the superiority of low-intensity exercise over the now traditional aerobic exercise programs, the following recommendations will be based on an aerobic program.

Once the mode or modes of exercise are selected (e.g., jogging, swimming, and biking), guidelines should be given for the frequency, intensity, and duration of exercise. The frequency of sessions should probably be three to five times per week. Fewer sessions may not be effective, and more sessions may not give adequate musculoskeletal recovery time, making injury more likely. The intensity should generally be great enough to elicit a heart rate that is 70 to 85% of maximum values. In healthy populations and cardiac rehabilitation programs, these "target heart rates" are calculated from population norms based on age. However, patients with CF (or other pulmonary disorders) may be limited by their ventilatory capacity and be at a truly maximum work rate with a heart rate that has not yet reached 70% of their age-predicted maximum.[73] Therefore, in prescribing exercise intensity based on a proportion of maximum heart rate, the maximum heart rate must be the patient's own maximum heart rate as actually measured and not as predicted.

The duration of each session should ideally be 20 to 30 minutes. However, for someone who is unfit, this duration may be too great; it is better to start with whatever the patient can readily tolerate, for example, 10 minutes of exercise, and gradually add time to the individual sessions as exercise tolerance improves. We have found that the addition of 2 minutes to the sessions each week is tolerated by the majority of patients. The overall program should probably be lifelong. Two months of the program are likely to be necessary before a change in maximum oxygen uptake is seen; however, the goal is not to change test results but rather to increase and maintain exercise tolerance and to enable the patient to do more.

Relatively frequent contact between patient and physician or other medical personnel will enable the physician to stay informed as to disease progression. Frequent contact between physician and patient also facilitates patient compliance and helps demonstrate the physician's interest in the program and the patient. Periodic retesting also serves to give the patient positive reinforcement for continuing the program.

SUMMARY

Rehabilitation programs can be useful for patients with CF and must be based on knowledge of the underlying disease process and on a solid foundation of aggressive standard treatment that includes frequent patient-physician contact, attention to nutrition, chest physiotherapy, and intensive antibiotic treatment of episodes of worsened pulmonary infection. Exercise aspects of the program are probably best based on principles of aerobic exercise conditioning, with exercise sessions conducted three to five times per week and lasting 10 to 30 minutes each.

ACKNOWLEDGMENTS

Portions of this chapter were modified with permission from Orenstein DM, "Cystic Fibrosis" (Respiratory Care 1991; 36:746–754). The authors appreciate the kind permission of Steve Shepherd and Mel Hovell to modify their summary of published studies on exercise programs in CF; the modification appears here as Table 34–3.

REFERENCES

1. MacLusky I, McLaughlin F, Levison H. Cystic fibrosis: Part I. Curr Probl Pediatr 1985; 15:1–49.
2. Andersen D. Cystic fibrosis of the pancreas and its relation to celiac disease: A clinical and pathological study. Am J Dis Child 1938; 56:344–399.
3. Knowles M, Stutts M, Yankaskas J, et al. Abnormal respiratory epithelial ion transport in cystic fibrosis. Clin Chest Med 1986; 7:285–297.
4. Klinger K. Genetics of cystic fibrosis. Semin Respir Med 1985; 6:243–251.
5. Riordan J, Rommens J, Kerem B-S, et al. Identification of the cystic fibrosis gene: Cloning and characterization of complementary DNA. Science 1989; 245:1066–1073.
6. Anderson M, Gregory R, Thompson S, et al. Demonstration that CFTR is a chloride channel by alteration of its anion selectivity. Science 1991; 253:202–205.
7. Kerem B-S, Rommens J, Buchanan J, et al. Identification of the cystic fibrosis gene: Genetic analysis. Science 1989; 345:1073–1080.
8. Tsui L-C. International cystic fibrosis genetics consortium update. Bethesda, MD: Cystic Fibrosis Foundation, 1991.
9. Campbell P, Phillips JI, Krishnamani M, et al. Cystic fibrosis: Relationship between clinical status and F508 deletion. J Pediatr 1991; 118:239–241.
9a. Gaskin K, Waters D, Dorney S. Assessment of pancreatic function in screened infants with cystic fibrosis. Pediatr Pulmonol 1991; Suppl 7:69–70.
10. Park R, Grant R. Gastrointestinal manifestations of cystic fibrosis: A review. Gastroenterology 1981; 81:1143–1161.
11. Stern R, Izant RJ, Boat T, et al. Treatment and prognosis of rectal prolapse in cystic fibrosis. Gastroenterology 1982; 82:707–710.
12. Holsclaw D, Rocmans C, Shwachman H. Intussusception in patients with cystic fibrosis. Pediatrics 1971; 48:51–58.
13. Roy C, Weber A, Morin C, et al. Hepatobiliary disease in cystic fibrosis: A survey of current issues and concepts. J Pediatr Gastroenterol Nutr 1982; 1:469–478.
14. Orenstein DM, Henke KG, Costill DL, et al. Exercise and heat stress in cystic fibrosis patients. Pediatr Res 1983; 17:267–269.
15. Beckerman R, Taussig L. Hypoelectrolytemia and metabolic alkalosis in infants with cystic fibrosis. Pediatrics 1979; 63:580–583.
16. Stern R, Boat T, Wood R, et al. Treatment and prognosis of nasal polyps in cystic fibrosis. Am J Dis Child 1982; 136:1067–1070.
17. Corey M, Levison H, Crozier D. Five- to seven-year course of pulmonary function in cystic fibrosis. Am Rev Respir Dis 1976; 114:1085–1092.
18. Pattishall E. Longitudinal response of pulmonary function to bronchodilators in cystic fibrosis. Pediatr Pulmonol 1990; 9:80–85.
19. Thomassen M, Demko C, Doershuk C. Cystic fibrosis: A review of pulmonary infections and interventions. Pediatr Pulmonol 1987; 3:334–351.
20. Marks M. The pathogenesis and treatment of pulmonary infections in patients with cystic fibrosis. J Pediatr 1981; 98:173–179.
21. Wood R, Wanner A, Hirsch J, Farrell P. Tracheal mucociliary transport in patients with cystic fibrosis and its stimulation by terbutaline. Am Rev Respir Dis 1975; 111:733–738.
22. Thomassen M, Boxerbaum B, Demko C, et al. Inhibitory effect of cystic fibrosis serum on pseudomonas phagocytosis by rabbit and human alveolar macrophages. Pediatr Res 1979; 13:1085–1088.
23. Tosi M, Zakem H, Berger M. Neutrophil elastase cleaves c3bi on opsonized pseudomonas as well as CR1 on neutrophils to create a functionally important opsonin receptor mismatch. J Clin Invest 1990; 86:300–308.
24. Francis P, Muller N, Gurwitz D, et al. Hemoglobin desaturation: Its occurrence during sleep in patients with cystic fibrosis. Am J Dis Child 1980; 134:734–740.
25. Henke K, Orenstein D. Oxygen saturation during exercise in cystic fibrosis. Am Rev Respir Dis 1984; 129:708–711.
26. Coffey M, FitzGerald M, McNicholas W. Comparison of oxygen desaturation during sleep and exercise in patients with cystic fibrosis. Chest 1991; 100:659–662.
27. Kaplan E, Shwachman H, Perlmutter A, et al. Reproductive failure in males with cystic fibrosis. N Engl J Med 1968; 279:65–69.
27a. Kopito LE, Kosasky HJ, Shwachman H. Water and electrolytes in cervical mucus from patients with cystic fibrosis. Fertil Steril 1973; 24:512–516.
28. Orenstein D. Diagnosis of cystic fibrosis. Semin Respir Med 1985; 6:252–260.
29. Rosenstein B, Langbaum T, Gordes D, Brusilow S. Cystic fibrosis: Problems encountered with sweat testing. JAMA 1978; 240:1987–1988.
30. Lemna W, Feldman G, Kerem B-S, et al. Mutation analysis for heterozygote detection and the prenatal diagnosis of cystic fibrosis. N Engl J Med 1990; 322:291–296.
31. Wilcken B, Brown A, Urwin R, Brown D. Cystic fibrosis screening by dried spot trypsin assay: Results in 75,000 newborn infants. J Pediatr 1983; 102:383–387.
32. Orenstein DM, Boat TF, Stern RC, et al. The effect of early diagnosis and treatment in cystic fibrosis: A seven-year study of 16 sibling pairs. Am J Dis Child 1977; 131:973–975.
33. Nielsen O, Thomsen B, Green A, et al. Cystic fibrosis in Denmark 1945 to 1985: An analysis of incidence, mortality and influence of centralized treatment on survival. Acta Paediatr Scand 1988; 77:836–841.
34. Reisman J, Rivington-Law B, Corey M, et al. Role of conventional physiotherapy in cystic fibrosis. J Pediatr 1988; 113:632–636.
35. Landau L, Phelan P. The variable effect of a bronchodilating agent on pulmonary function in cystic fibrosis. J Pediatr 1973; 82:863–868.
36. Eggleston P, Rosenstein B, Stackhouse C, et al. A controlled trial of long-term bronchodilator therapy in cystic fibrosis. Chest 1991; 99:1088–1092.

37. Orenstein D. Long-term inhaled bronchodilator therapy in cystic fibrosis (editorial). Chest 1991; 99:1061.
38. Scanlin T. Cystic fibrosis. In: Fishman A (ed). Pulmonary Diseases and Disorders. 2nd ed. New York: McGraw-Hill Book Co., 1988, pp 1273–1294.
39. Knowles M, Church N, Waltner W, et al. A pilot study of aerosolized amiloride for the treatment of lung disease in cystic fibrosis. N Engl J Med 1990; 322:1189–1194.
40. Aitken M, Burke W, McDonald G, et al. Effect of inhaled recombinant human DNase on pulmonary function in normal and cystic fibrosis patients: Phase 1 study (abstract). Am Rev Respir Dis 1991; 143:A298.
41. McElvaney N, Hubbard R, Birrer P, et al. Aerosol alpha-1 antitrypsin treatment for cystic fibrosis. Lancet 1991; 1:392–394.
42. Auerbach H, William M, Kirkpatrick J, Colten H. Alternate day prednisone reduces morbidity and improves pulmonary function in cystic fibrosis. Lancet 1985; 2:686–688.
43. Konstan M, Vargo K, Davis P. Ibuprofen attenuates the inflammatory response to *Pseudomonas aeruginosa* in a rat model of chronic pulmonary infection: Implications for antiinflammatory therapy in cystic fibrosis. Am Rev Respir Dis 1990; 141:186–192.
44. Rosenstein B, Eigen H. Risks of alternate-day prednisone in patients with cystic fibrosis. Pediatrics 1991; 87:245–246.
44a. Szaff M, Hoiby N, Flensborg EW. Frequent antibiotic therapy improves survival of cystic fibrosis patients with chronic *Pseudomonas aeruginosa* infection. Acta Paediatr Scand 1983; 72:651–657.
45. Grenier B. Use of the new quinolones in cystic fibrosis. Rev Infect Dis 1989; 11(Suppl 5):S1245–S1251.
46. Madden BP, Hodson ME, Tsang U, et al. Intermediate-term results of heart-lung transplantation for cystic fibrosis. Lancet 1992; 339:1583–1587.
47. Koletzko S, Stringer D, Cleghorn G, Durie P. Lavage treatment of distal intestinal obstruction syndrome in children with cystic fibrosis. Pediatrics 1989; 83:737–733.
48. Psacharopoulos H, Howard E, Portmann B, et al. Hepatic complications of cystic fibrosis. Lancet 1981; 2:78–80.
49. Mieles L, Orenstein D, Teperman L, et al. Liver transplantation in cystic fibrosis (letter). Lancet 1989; 1:1073.
50. Burke P, Meyer V, Kocoshis S, et al. Depression and anxiety in pediatric inflammatory bowel disease and cystic fibrosis. J Am Acad Child Adolesc Psychiatry 1989; 28:948–951.
51. Finkelstein S, Wielinski C, Elliott G, et al. Diabetes mellitus associated with cystic fibrosis. J Pediatr 1988; 112:373–377.
52. Cystic Fibrosis Foundation Data Registry Report for 1990. Bethesda, MD: Cystic Fibrosis Foundation, 1992.
53. Kerem E, Corey M, Kerem B-S, et al. The relationship between genotype and phenotype in cystic fibrosis: Analysis of the most common mutation (ΔF508). N Engl J Med 1990; 323:1517–1522.
54. MacLusky I, McLaughlin F, Levison H. Cystic fibrosis: Part II. Curr Probl Pediatr 1985; 15:1–39.
55. Stern R, Boat T, Doershuk C. Course of cystic fibrosis in 95 patients. J Pediatr 1976; 89:406–411.
56. Kraemer R, Rudeberg A, Hadorn B, Rossi E. Relative underweight in cystic fibrosis and its prognostic value. Acta Paediatr Scand 1978; 67:33–37.
57. Nixon P, Orenstein D, Doershuk C. Prognostic value of exercise testing in cystic fibrosis (abstract). Pediatr Pulmonol Suppl 1990; 5:254.
58. Thomassen M, Demko C, Klinger J, Stern R. *Pseudomonas cepacia* colonization among patients with cystic fibrosis: A new opportunist. Am Rev Respir Dis 1985; 131:791–796.
59. Drumm M, Pope H, Cliff W, et al. Correction of the cystic fibrosis defect in vitro by retrovirus-mediated gene transfer. Cell 1990; 62:1227–1233.
60. Perry J. Rehabilitation: A definition. In: Nickel V (ed). Orthopedic Rehabilitation. New York: Churchill Livingstone, Inc., 1982, p xi.
61. Stanghelle J, Skyberg D. Cystic fibrosis patients running a marathon race. Int J Sports Med 1988; 9(Suppl 1):37–40.
62. Godfrey S, Mearns M. Pulmonary function and response to exercise in cystic fibrosis. Arch Dis Child 1971; 46:144–151.
63. Cropp GJ, Pullano TP, Cerny FJ, Nathanson IT. Exercise tolerance and cardiorespiratory adjustments at peak work capacity in cystic fibrosis. Am Rev Respir Dis 1982; 126:211–216.
64. Orenstein DM, Franklin BA, Doershuk CF, et al. Exercise conditioning and cardiopulmonary fitness in cystic fibrosis: The effects of a three-month supervised running program. Chest 1981; 80:392–398.
65. Braggion C, Cornacchia M, Miano A, et al. Exercise tolerance and effects of training in young patients with cystic fibrosis and mild airway obstruction. Pediatr Pulmonol 1989; 7:145–152.
66. O'Neill P, Dodds M, Phillips B, et al. Regular exercise and reduction of breathlessness in patients with cystic fibrosis. Br J Dis Chest 1987; 81:62–69.
67. Salh W, Bilton D, Dodd M, Webb AK. Effect of exercise and physiotherapy in aiding sputum expectoration in adults with cystic fibrosis. Thorax 1989; 44:1006–1008.
68. Upton CJ, Tyrrell JC, Hiller EJ. Two minute walking distance in cystic fibrosis. Arch Dis Child 1988; 63:1444–1448.
69. Orenstein D, Nixon P. Exercise performance and breathing patterns in cystic fibrosis: Male-female differences and influence of resting pulmonary function. Pediatr Pulmonol 1991; 10:101–105.
70. Orenstein D, Nixon P, Ross E, Kaplan R. Quality of well-being in cystic fibrosis. Chest 1989; 95:344–347.
71. Cerny FJ, Cropp GJ, Bye MR. Hospital therapy improves exercise tolerance and lung function in cystic fibrosis. Am J Dis Child 1984; 138:261–265.
72. Cerny FJ, Pullano TP, Cropp GJ. Cardiorespiratory adaptations to exercise in cystic fibrosis. Am Rev Respir Dis 1982; 126:217–220.
73. Orenstein D, Henke K, Cerny F. Exercise and cystic fibrosis. Phys Sports Med 1983; 11:57–62.
74. Marcotte JE, Grisdale RK, Levison H, et al. Multiple factors limit exercise capacity in cystic fibrosis. Pediatr Pulmonol 1986; 2:274–281.
75. Marcotte JE, Canny GJ, Grisdale R, et al. Effects of nutritional status on exercise performance in advanced cystic fibrosis. Chest 1986; 90:375–379.
76. Hortop J, Desmond KJ, Coates AL. The mechanical effects of expiratory airflow limitation on cardiac performance in cystic fibrosis. Am Rev Respir Dis 1988; 137:132–137.
77. Benson LN, Newth CJ, DeSouza M, et al. Radionuclide assessment of right and left ventricular function during bicycle exercise in young patients with cystic fibrosis. Am Rev Respir Dis 1984; 130:987–992.
78. Godfrey S, Davies C, Wozniak E, Barnes C. Cardiorespiratory response to exercise in normal children. Clin Sci 1971; 40:419–431.
79. Lebecque P, Lapierre JG, Lamarre A, Coates AL. Diffusion capacity and oxygen desaturation effects on exercise in patients with cystic fibrosis. Chest 1987; 91:693–697.
80. Versteegh FG, Neijens HJ, Bogaard JM, et al. Relationship between pulmonary function, O_2 saturation during sleep and exercise, and exercise responses in children with cystic fibrosis. Adv Cardiol 1986; 35:151–155.
81. Coates AL, Canny G, Zinman R, et al. The effects of chronic airflow limitation, increased dead space, and the pattern of ventilation on gas exchange during maximal exercise in advanced cystic fibrosis. Am Rev Respir Dis 1988; 138:1524–1531.
82. Nixon PA, Orenstein DM, Curtis SE, Ross EA. Oxygen supplementation during exercise in cystic fibrosis. Am Rev Respir Dis 1990; 142:807–811.
83. Orenstein D, Henke K, Green C. Heat acclimation in cystic fibrosis. J Appl Physiol 1984; 57:408–412.
84. di Sant'Agnese P, Darling R, Perera G, Shea E. Abnormal electrolyte composition of sweat in cystic fibrosis of the pancreas. Pediatrics 1953; 12:549–563.
84a. Bar-Or O, Blimkie CJR, Hay JA, et al. Voluntary dehydration and heat intolerance in cystic fibrosis. Lancet 1992; 339:696–699.
85. Coates AL, Boyce P, Muller D, et al. The role of nutritional status, airway obstruction, hypoxia, and abnormalities in serum lipid composition in limiting exercise tolerance in children with cystic fibrosis. Bull Eur Physiopathol Respir 1979; 15:341–342.
86. Keens TG, Krastins IR, Wannamaker EM, et al. Ventilatory

muscle endurance training in normal subjects and patients with cystic fibrosis. Am Rev Respir Dis 1977; 116:853–860.
87. Asher MI, Pardy RL, Coates AL. The effects of inspiratory muscle training in patients with cystic fibrosis. Am Rev Respir Dis 1982; 126:855–859.
88. Saltin B, Blomqvist G, Mitchell J, et al. Response to exercise after bed rest and after training. Circulation 1968; 38(Suppl 7):1–78.
89. Holzer FJ, Schnall R, Landau LI. The effect of a home exercise programme in children with cystic fibrosis and asthma. Aust Paediatr J 1984; 20:297–301.
90. Zach M, Purrer B, Oberwaldner B. Effect of swimming on forced expiration and sputum clearance in cystic fibrosis. Lancet 1981; ii:1201–1203.
91. Edlund LD, French RW, Herbst JJ, et al. Effects of a swimming program on children with cystic fibrosis. Am J Dis Child 1986; 140:80–83.
92. Shwachman H, Kulczycki L. Long-term study of 105 patients with cystic fibrosis. Am J Dis Child 1958; 96:6–15.
93. Strauss G, Osher A, Wang C-I, et al. Variable weight training in cystic fibrosis. Chest 1987; 92:273–276.
94. Andreasson B, Jonson B, Kornfält R, et al. Long-term effects of physical exercise on working capacity and pulmonary function in cystic fibrosis. Acta Paediatr Scand 1987; 76:70–75.
95. Zach M, Oberwaldner B, Häusler F. Cystic fibrosis: Physical exercise versus chest physiotherapy. Arch Dis Child 1982; 57:587–589.
96. LaPorte R, Adams L, Savage D, et al. The spectrum of physical activity, cardiovascular disease and health: An epidemiologic perspective. Am J Epidemiol 1984; 120:507–517.
97. Calmody T, Senner J, Malinow M, Matarazzo J. Physical exercise rehabilitation: Long-term dropout rate in cardiac patients. J Behav Med 1980; 3:163–168.
98. Epstein L, Wing R, Koeske R, et al. A comparison of lifestyle change, aerobic exercise, and calisthenics on weight loss in obese children. Behav Ther 1985; 16:345–356.
99. Stanghelle JK, Hjeltnes N, Bangstad HJ, Michalsen H. Effect of daily short bouts of trampoline exercise during 8 weeks on the pulmonary function and the maximal oxygen uptake of children with cystic fibrosis. Int J Sports Med 1988; 1:32–36.
100. Blomquist M, Freyschuss U, Wiman LG, Strandvik B. Physical activity and self-treatment in cystic fibrosis. Arch Dis Child 1986; 61:362–367.
101. Cerny F. Relative effects of bronchial drainage and exercise for in-hospital care of patients with cystic fibrosis. Phys Ther 1989; 69:633–639.
102. Allan J, Mason A, Moss A. Nutritional supplementation in treatment of cystic fibrosis of the pancreas. Am J Dis Child 1973; 126:22–26.
103. Berry H, Kellogg F, Hunt M, Dietary supplement and nutrition in children with cystic fibrosis. Am J Dis Child 1975; 129:165–171.
104. Moore M, Greene H, Donald W, Dunn G. Enteral-tube feeding as adjunct therapy in malnourished patients with cystic fibrosis: A clinical study and literature review. Am J Clin Nutr 1986; 44:33–41.
105. O'Loughlin E, Forbes D, Parsons H, et al. Nutritional rehabilitation of malnourished patients with cystic fibrosis. Am J Clin Nutr 1986; 43:732–737.
106. Bertrand J, Morin C, Lasalle R, et al. Short-term clinical, nutritional, and functional effects of continuous elemental enteral alimentation in children with cystic fibrosis. J Pediatr 1984; 104:41–46.
107. Levy L, Durie P, Pencharz P, Corey M. Effects of long-term nutritional rehabilitation on body composition and clinical status in malnourished children and adolescents with cystic fibrosis. J Pediatr 1985; 107:225–230.
108. Boland M, Patrick J, Stoski D, Soucy P. Permanent enteral feeding in cystic fibrosis: Advantages of a replaceable jejunostomy tube. J Pediatr Surg 1987; 22:843–847.
109. Shepherd R, Cooksley W, Cooke W. Improved growth and clinical, nutritional, and respiratory changes in responses to nutritional therapy in cystic fibrosis. J Pediatr 1980; 97:351–357.
110. Mansell A, Anderson J, Muttart C, et al. Short-term pulmonary effects of total parenteral nutrition in children with cystic fibrosis. J Pediatr 1984; 104:700–705.
111. Shepherd R, Holt T, Thomas B, et al. Nutritional rehabilitation in cystic fibrosis: Controlled studies of effects on nutritional growth retardation, body protein turnover, and course of pulmonary disease. J Pediatr 1986; 109:788–794.

Chapter 35

Pulmonary Rehabilitation Before and After Lung Transplantation

DOROTHY G. BIGGAR, M.S.N., R.N.
JILL FELDMAN MALEN, M.S., N.S., R.N.
E. P. TRULOCK, M.D.
JOEL D. COOPER, M.D.

The scientific basis for rehabilitation of patients before and after lung transplantation rests on principles of pulmonary rehabilitation and exercise physiology. The pulmonary rehabilitation techniques and practices of the American College of Chest Physician[1, 2] are followed in the pretransplantation phase. Based on studies of pulmonary rehabilitation in patients with advanced restrictive or obstructive lung disease,[3-7] the pretransplantation program is individualized to the patient's underlying disease and is designed to optimize exercise tolerance in preparation for surgery. In the post-transplantation phase, cardiovascular conditioning and musculoskeletal strengthening[8] are emphasized to restore the recipient's lifestyle and functional capacity.

The role of pulmonary rehabilitation in the preoperative and postoperative care of lung transplantation patients has evolved significantly in the past 5 years. In the earliest reports of successful single-lung transplantation for pulmonary fibrosis, pulmonary rehabilitation was identified as an integral part of perioperative care.[9, 10] Initially, it was used only postoperatively, but after the first recipient exhibited considerable muscle weakness and fatigability postoperatively,[9] a program of rehabilitation and muscle training was added preoperatively. Initial reports of pretransplantation rehabilitation in patients with severe pulmonary fibrosis showed that preoperative performance in the 6-minute walking test increased 39% and resulted in an improved postoperative recovery.[10, 11] Since the appearance of these early reports, numerous studies have demonstrated significant improvements in exercise tolerance, as measured by 6-minute walking distance and submaximum exercise test performance, during pretransplantation and post-transplantation rehabilitation in patients with either severe obstructive or restrictive lung disease. Preoperatively, improvements have occurred despite progression of the patients' lung disease.[12-16] Postoperatively, exercise capacity was found to increase for up to 1 year after both unilateral and bilateral transplantation, and this increase has been sustained during longitudinal follow-up.[17]

In this chapter, our lung transplantation rehabilitation program is detailed, and selected results of this program in 55 patients are presented.

OVERALL GOAL AND SPECIFIC OBJECTIVES

The overall goal of the program is to optimize the patient's physical condition both before and after lung transplantation. This goal is achieved through the following objectives:

1. To plan and implement an individualized, comprehensive, graded exercise program that includes en-

durance training as well as strength and flexibility exercises.
2. To continually assess the patient's exercise performance and response.
3. To teach patients about their lung disease and the rehabilitative aspects of their care.
4. To implement and continually assess an optimum pulmonary hygiene program.
5. To assist with monitoring nutritional status and identifying psychologic stress.
6. To recognize and treat early any exacerbations of underlying lung disease (preoperatively).
7. To assess and report signs and symptoms of rejection or infection (postoperatively).

PATIENT POPULATION AND SELECTION CRITERIA

The lung transplantation pulmonary rehabilitation program enrolls patients with severe, end-stage obstructive or restrictive lung disease that has been irreversible and progressively disabling. Virtually all patients require continuous supplemental oxygen, and all have a limited life expectancy without transplantation.[13]

Specific diagnoses have included cystic fibrosis, antitrypsin deficiency emphysema, chronic obstructive pulmonary disease (COPD), pulmonary fibrosis, lymphangioleiomyomatosis, eosinophilic granuloma, bronchiectasis, primary pulmonary hypertension, and selected forms of Eisenmenger's syndrome. Our candidates have been well motivated to prepare for transplantation and are dedicated to life-long care afterwards.[13]

In general, unilateral lung transplantation has been performed for idiopathic pulmonary fibrosis, for COPD or antitrypsin deficiency emphysema in older patients, and for primary pulmonary hypertension or Eisenmenger's syndrome associated with a reparable cardiac defect. Bilateral lung transplantation has been used for antitrypsin deficiency emphysema and COPD in younger patients and for suppurative lung diseases, such as cystic fibrosis or other forms of bronchiectasis.[13] Our recipient selection criteria are summarized in Table 35–1.

TABLE 35–1. SELECTION CRITERIA FOR LUNG TRANSPLANT RECIPIENTS*

- Severe obstructive or restrictive lung disease or severe pulmonary hypertension
- Limited life expectancy
- Adequate cardiac function without significant coronary artery disease
- Ambulatory with rehabilitation potential
- Acceptable nutritional status
- Satisfactory psychosocial profile and emotional support system
- No contraindication to immunosuppression
- No systemic disease with nonpulmonary vital organ involvement
- No significant kidney or liver disease
- No systemic steroid treatment

*From Egan TM, Kaiser LR, Cooper JD. Lung transplantation. Curr Probl Surg 1989; 26:673–752.

PRINCIPLES OF ENDURANCE TRAINING

Aerobic or endurance training utilizes oxygen-dependent pathways to meet energy requirements. Training must focus on frequency (sessions are conducted at least three times per week), intensity (reaching target heart rate range), and duration (20–30 min of exercise per session). The endurance training principles of overload, specificity, and reversibility serve as a framework for the preoperative and postoperative exercise training program.[8] Preoperatively, these principles are applied to condition our patients for the rigors of surgery and to prepare them for early mobilization afterwards. Postoperatively, they guide the patient's recovery to maximum function.

Training normally results in specific anatomic, biologic, and physiologic adaptations,[8] but these generally have not been demonstrable in patients with chronic lung disease.[18, 19] However, despite severe and sometimes worsening impairments of gas exchange, lung mechanics, or both, exercise training prior to lung transplantation has increased submaximum exercise tolerance and maximum tolerable workload, improved functional ability, and allowed performance of a higher workload at the same or lower heart rate and minute ventilation.[9–17] The reasons for these improvements without concomitant, measurable increases in parameters of aerobic fitness have not been fully elucidated. Several theories to explain the increase in submaximum exercise capacity after training have been proposed. They have focused on various causes, including (1) small improvements in aerobic capacity due to very small increases in stroke volume, oxygen pulse, or both; (2) increased motivation; (3) desensitization to dyspnea; and (4) improved ventilatory muscle function and mechanical skill.[18, 19]

More recent reports of aerobic capacity following intensive exercise training in patients with severe or moderately severe COPD have detected improvement in maximum oxygen consumption.[5, 20, 21] Preoperative tests of maximum oxygen uptake have not been done in our patients, but significant improvements in maximum tolerable workload have been demonstrated.

FACILITY AND STAFF

The outpatient facility can accommodate four exercising patients simultaneously. A satellite facility, which is located on the thoracic nursing division, is available for inpatients. Exercise equipment includes treadmills, stationary bicycles, free weights, and an arm ergometer. Monitoring equipment consists of pulse oximeters (portable and stationary), an end-tidal carbon dioxide monitor, and a cardiac rhythm monitor. An emergency cart with defibrillator, emergency drugs, and supplies is also on site. The pulmonary rehabilitation team is an integral component of the transplantation service. It consists of a pulmonary physician who serves as medical director, two pulmonary nurses with masters degrees, three respiratory therapists, and two physical therapists. The rehabilitation team participates in all four stages of the transplantation program: (1) initial evaluation, (2) preoperative rehabilitation, (3) initial post-transplantation care, and (4) long-term rehabilitation and follow-up.

PREOPERATIVE PHASE EVALUATION

The pulmonary rehabilitation team performs a detailed evaluation during the pretransplantation assessment to determine the patient's functional ability and exercise tolerance. Evaluation includes a 6-minute walking test, a stair climb test, and a submaximum treadmill protocol. Oxygen saturation is monitored by pulse oximetry during these tests, and supplemental oxygen is administered and adjusted to maintain arterial blood oxygen saturation (SaO_2) at greater than 90%. Pretransplantation exercise testing in patients with primary pulmonary hypertension or Eisenmenger's syndrome is planned on an individual basis after consultation with the physician. Generally, a 6-minute walking test is performed to assess functional status and to detect desaturation with exercise, but stress testing and stair climbing are usually deferred.

A summary of the pulmonary rehabilitation evaluation is presented at the weekly recipient selection meeting. The exercise data along with the results of other cardiopulmonary, nutritional, and psychosocial tests provide the basis for estimating rehabilitation potential.

The 6-minute walking test is an objective measure of functional status in patients with COPD. This simple exercise test has been loosely correlated with maximum oxygen consumption in patients with chronic bronchitis.[22, 23] The patient is asked to walk as far as possible in 6 minutes. The patient sets the pace and is allowed to rest as many times as necessary. The walk is done twice to eliminate the learning effect.

The stair climb test is performed by having the patient climb as many stairs as possible (usually about two flights), allowing him or her to stop as often as needed. A record is made of the time, the number of flights or steps climbed, the number of stops, and the oxygen used to prevent desaturation.

The submaximum treadmill test protocol is illustrated in Table 35–2. While cardiac rhythm, oximetry parameters, blood pressure, and end-tidal carbon dioxide are monitored, the patient exercises at increasing grade, speed, or both, using a preprogrammed incremental protocol. This test is submaximum or "symptom-limited," that is, it is stopped when the patient can no longer continue (usually because of shortness of breath) or when the patient's heart rate reaches 85% of its age-predicted maximum value. Each increment of speed and grade is assigned a stage number that corresponds to a metabolic equivalent. The test can be repeated periodically, and the stage, metabolic equivalent level, and maximum heart rate that are achieved during the tests can be compared to assess the results of rehabilitation. Arterial blood gases are assessed just prior to terminating the initial stress test to precisely quantify exercise-induced hypercapnia, hypoxemia, and acidemia.

TABLE 35–2. TREADMILL EXERCISE TEST PROTOCOL

Stage	Time (min)	Speed (mph)	Elevation (%)	Metabolic Equivalent
1	2	1.1	1.0	2.0
2	2	2.0	1.0	2.8
3	2	2.0	3.0	3.4
4	2	2.0	7.0	4.5
5	2	2.0	10.0	5.3
6	2	2.5	10.0	6.4
7	2	3.0	10.0	7.4
8	2	3.5	10.0	8.5
9	2	4.0	10.0	9.6
10	2	4.5	10.0	10.7

Patients are monitored with continuous oximetry throughout all exercise testing. Supplemental oxygen is titrated to maintain a saturation that is greater than 90%. If desaturation occurs with a standard 6 L/min cannula, an oxygen reservoir device (e.g., an oxymizer pendant cannula manufactured by Chad Therapeutics, Inc.) is used to increase oxygen delivery during inspiration; up to 12 L/min of oxygen can be delivered using this method. The patient subjectively rates the intensity of each exercise test on the perceived exertion scale. The perceived exertion scale is a Borg Category Scale consisting of 15 numbers from 6 to 20 listed vertically. Next to the odd numbers (7–19) are descriptions characterizing the perceived magnitude of the sensation ranging from "very, very light" to "very, very hard."[24]

In addition to these exercise tests, the patient also completes three dyspnea evaluations to gauge the degree of dyspnea during activities of daily living. The indices currently used are the oxygen cost diagram,[25] the baseline dyspnea index,[26] and the modified Medical Research Council dyspnea scale.[27] The patient is also interviewed to learn about his or her hobbies, previous pulmonary rehabilitation experience, current exercise regimen (if any), smoking history, cough and sputum characteristics, and employment. This information completes the profile of functional impairment and lifestyle changes that are a result of lung disease.

A musculoskeletal assessment is conducted by a physical therapist to determine the presence of (1) musculoskeletal pain syndromes that may limit the patient's exercise tolerance, (2) limitations in normal joint range of motion and strength, and (3) musculoskeletal imbalances and postural faults. An individualized strengthening and flexibility program is then developed. It is modified as needed to treat or prevent musculoskeletal injuries that might occur during endurance training.[28]

The need for chest physiotherapy is also evaluated. Sputum is collected for 24 hours. Based on the volume and nature of the sputum, breath sounds, and chest x-ray changes, a chest physiotherapy program is instituted, if indicated. In addition, support persons are instructed in chest physiotherapy techniques. Patients with cystic fibrosis or other suppurative lung diseases who already use chest physiotherapy routinely have their pulmonary hygiene programs reviewed, and changes are recommended as necessary.[29]

PREOPERATIVE PHASE EXERCISE PROGRAM

The goals of preoperative pulmonary rehabilitation are twofold: (1) to maximize exercise endurance and (2) to optimize pulmonary hygiene (in those patients with mucus hypersecretion). Based on the detailed assessment outlined earlier, an exercise prescription is formulated. It includes strengthening and flexibility exercises in addition to endurance training. The endurance program is carried out 5 days/wk, with the objective of attaining 30 minutes of continuous exercise at a heart rate of 75 to 85% of the predicted maximum heart rate for the patient's age. Patients usually exercise on a treadmill, a bicycle ergometer, or both. Arm ergometry is utilized to condition the upper extremities.

Exercise is monitored with continuous pulse oximetry. End-tidal carbon dioxide monitoring is used in some patients with resting or exercise-induced hypercapnia. The Salter Labs carbon-dioxide–sampling nasal cannula is utilized,[30] but patients using an oxymizer are excluded because the sensor is incompatible with this system. End-tidal carbon dioxide monitoring is used to detect changes in this variable over time. If the trend is upward, an arterial blood gas analysis can be performed to verify changes in Pco_2. Exercise-induced respiratory acidosis may indicate a need for an adjustment in the exercise prescription. The Nellcor N–1000 displays the end-tidal carbon dioxide waveform. Clinically, some patients have been able to change their waveforms. With instruction and coaching, the pattern may become more normal with a lower respiratory rate, higher Sao_2, and lower end-tidal carbon dioxide.

Exercise is terminated in the presence of heart rates exceeding 85% of the predicted maximum for the patient's age, dysrhythmias (other than isolated atrial or ventricular premature beats), bradycardia, blood pressures greater than 180/110, an increase in diastolic pressure of 20 mm Hg or greater, a progressive drop in systolic pressure with increasing workload, chest pain, labored breathing or severe dyspnea, blurred vision, pale or clammy skin, deterioration in coordination, equilibrium, or mental status, or an Sao_2 less than 85% despite maximum oxygen supplementation. Patients with the diagnosis of primary pulmonary hypertension are currently excluded from endurance exercise but may participate in a supervised, monitored stretching program.

The patient is screened for new problems and any medication changes at the daily exercise session. Vital signs, including breath sounds, oximetry, and weight, are recorded prior to exercise. Weekly pulmonary rehabilitation rounds are held to survey progress and chart direction. A 6-minute walking test and submaximum treadmill test are repeated every 6 weeks while the patient awaits transplantation.

Other benefits are derived from integrating pulmonary rehabilitation into pretransplantation care. Symptoms and signs can be monitored regularly, and exacerbations of the underlying lung disease can be diagnosed and treated early. Chest physiotherapy and other pulmonary hygiene measures can be implemented to promote clearance of secretions and to prevent lung infections. Nutritional status and psychosocial situation can be watched and problems can be addressed. Patients can learn about their lung disease and can begin to experience rehabilitative aspects of their care that are so vital to postoperative recovery.

INTRAOPERATIVE PHASE

A complete discussion of donor selection, donor management, lung preservation, and the surgical techniques of lung transplantation are described elsewhere[13, 31] and are beyond the scope of this chapter. Key concepts are briefly summarized. Donor lungs suitable for transplantation are scarce. Optimal pulmonary care of potential donors could increase the number of successful lung retrievals.[13] In our program, the pretransplantation waiting period averages about 8 to 12 weeks but has been increasing. The recipient is matched to the donor according to ABO blood group and lung size. Cytomegalovirus seronegative recipients are matched with seronegative donors whenever possible.

The surgical approach to unilateral lung transplantation has changed little since its original description. The operation is performed through either right or left posterolateral thoracotomy. The main pulmonary artery is encircled and temporarily clamped to assess the impact on hemodynamic stability and gas exchange. If this is not tolerated, the femoral artery and vein are cannulated for venoarterial bypass at the time of extraction; however, bypass is necessary in only a minority of patients. Following the native lung pneumonectomy, the single lung graft is implanted by completing the left atrial anastomosis, the pulmonary artery anastomosis, and the bronchial anastomosis. Then, the omentum, which has been mobilized from the abdomen, is tunnelled retrosternally and wrapped around the airway anastomosis.[32]

The approach to bilateral lung transplantation has evolved substantially during the last few years. As originally developed, the operation was performed through a median sternotomy. The donor lungs were implanted en bloc with a single tracheal anastomosis, and the procedure required a period of total cardiopulmonary bypass. Recently, however, the technique has been revised, and the current bilateral lung transplantation operation is essentially sequential single lung transplants carried out through anterior transverse thoracosternotomy. Using unilateral lung ventilation to the opposite lung, each lung can be completely mobilized. The right lung is then excised and replaced in a fashion similar to that used for single-lung transplantation while the patient is maintained with contralateral lung ventilation. After replacement of the right lung, the recipient's left lung is excised and replaced with the donor left lung. Each bronchial anastomosis is wrapped with an omental pedicle. Partial cardiopulmonary bypass may be necessary, but can be avoided in the majority of cases.

EARLY POSTOPERATIVE COURSE

Early postoperative intensive care focuses on maintaining cardiopulmonary stability and fluid and electrolyte balance. A discussion of management in the intensive care unit is beyond the scope of this chapter; however, it should be emphasized that the rehabilitation team should be familiar with cardiothoracic intensive care monitoring, mechanical ventilation, post-transplantation care, and potential complications. Rehabilitation usually starts during the first or second postoperative day. The transplanted lung is susceptible to pulmonary edema and retention of secretions. Patients are weaned from ventilatory support as early as possible. Preoperative rehabilitation and vigorous postoperative chest physiotherapy facilitate the weaning process.

POSTOPERATIVE REHABILITATION GOALS AND USUAL PROGRESSION

The goals of pulmonary rehabilitation after transplantation are (1) to optimize airway clearance, lung expansion, and chest mobility, (2) wean the patient from supplemental oxygen, (3) improve posture and musculoskeletal strength and flexibility, and (4) restore endurance exercise capacity. In most cases, postoperative pulmonary rehabilitation is integrated into the patient's care within 24 hours after lung transplantation. It begins with chest physiotherapy, patient positioning, and range of motion exercises. Once cardiopulmonary stability is established, usually within the first 2 to 3 postoperative days, the patient sits up in a chair and begins resistance exercises. Ambulation for short distances is begun as soon as tolerated and is facilitated by specially designed walkers (Fig. 35–1). Within the first 2 to 3 weeks after surgery, most patients can walk from 2000 to 3000 ft during the course of a day. They are then advanced to the treadmill room to begin long-term rehabilitation.

POSTOPERATIVE CHEST PHYSIOTHERAPY

Chest physiotherapy is usually needed for 2 to 3 weeks after lung transplantation to promote clearance of secretions, enhance drainage of pleural fluid and air, and prevent postoperative atelectasis and pneumonia.[34–39] In the early postoperative period and prior to discontinuation of mechanical ventilation, several factors can inhibit normal airway clearance. These factors include pain, the use of analgesics, impaired cough, tracheal intubation, infection, and decreased mobility.[33] In addition to these postoperative factors, the transplanted lung has inherent characteristics that may contribute to airway clearance problems. These include denervation, loss of cough reflex, and diminished mucociliary clearance.[34] For 24 to 48 hours after extubation, chest physiotherapy is even more crucial because deep breathing and coughing are often further impaired by fatigue, altered glottic function, and the effects of analgesia and pain.

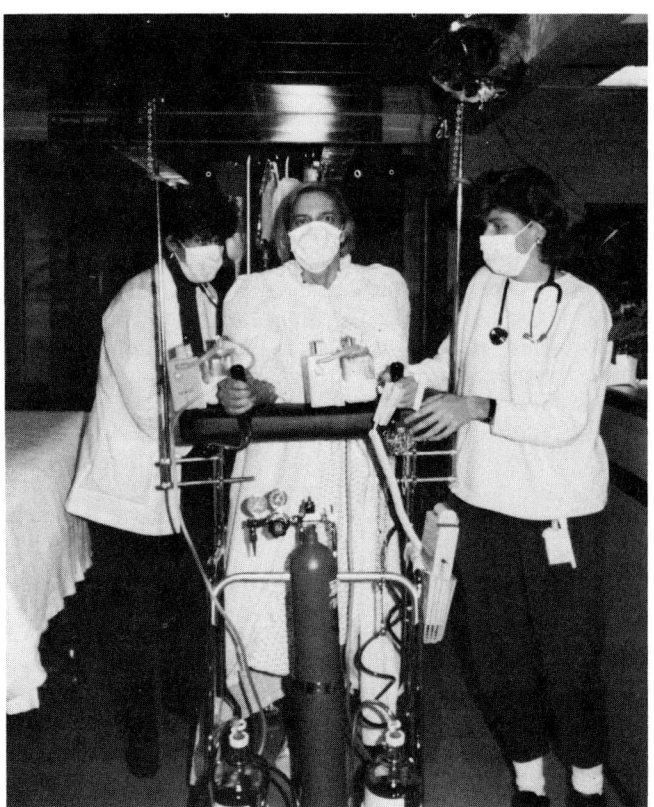

FIGURE 35–1. Ambulation for short distances is begun as soon as it is tolerated, and it is facilitated by specially designed walkers.

Chest physiotherapy is administered every 2 to 4 hours while the patient is awake. It is usually preceded by inhalation of aerosolized albuterol. Physiotherapy usually includes (1) 5 to 10 minutes of postural drainage to all lobes of the transplanted lung, (2) vibration, (3) deep breathing, and (4) coughing. During the first few days and while the patient is intubated, sterile suctioning with saline lavage is performed after each drainage position and as needed. Incentive spirometry is used after extubation to encourage deep breathing and coughing. Due to loss of cough reflexes in the denervated lung, patients are verbally coached to cough and expectorate their mucus. Daily assessments of chest x-ray changes, breath sounds, blood gases, and sputum characteristics guide the physiotherapy regimen.

Careful positioning of the patient is important in the postoperative period. After single lung transplantation, the allograft should be in a nondependent position as much as possible. In general, the patient is kept in the lateral decubitus position with the nonoperative side down. This reduces edema, facilitates gravitational drainage of the airway, and decreases mediastinal shift toward the operative side. After bilateral lung transplantation, the patient is turned from side to side every 1 to 2 hours. The supine position is avoided to minimize retention of secretions.

In the first few days after surgery, physiotherapy should be initiated gradually. Oxygen saturation and blood pressure may drop rapidly when repositioning, percussing, or suctioning the patient. Increased concentrations of inspired oxygen may be required just before and during repositioning and suctioning and when the patient is sitting and getting out of bed for the first several times. Patients who have undergone single lung transplantation for pulmonary hypertension are more labile during the early postoperative period, and their therapy is usually advanced more slowly.

Adequate rest and pain management are integrated with rehabilitation. A daily schedule that allows for frequent rest periods and uninterrupted sleep at night is provided for each patient. Before each physiotherapy session, pain control measures are assessed and adjusted. Intravenous or epidural narcotics are used for the first few days; thereafter, oral analgesics are prescribed.

PROGRESSIVE AMBULATION AND AEROBIC CONDITIONING

After transfer from intensive care, ambulation is progressed as rapidly as tolerated. A specially designed wheeled walker is used to assist ambulation. The walker provides support for the patient and can hold an oxygen tank, two to four chest tube bottles, a portable chest tube suction device, an oximeter, several intravenous fluid bags, and a bladder catheter drainage bag. Patients can usually walk 50 to 150 ft on their first attempt. By ambulating three to four times per day and increasing the distance each time, most patients can walk a total distance of 1 mile per day by the third postoperative week. Oxygen therapy is usually necessary initially and is adjusted to keep SaO_2 above 90% during exercise.

Exertional dyspnea and tachypnea usually persist for several weeks postoperatively. In unilateral lung transplant recipients with pulmonary fibrosis, the native, diseased lung is still innervated and presumably can send feedback to the respiratory center. Many emphysema patients continue pursed-lip breathing for some time after transplantation. Some patients still associate dyspnea with the need for oxygen therapy. Use of the pulse oximeter for positive reinforcement along with support and encouragement facilitates gradual weaning from oxygen therapy. Supplemental oxygen can be withdrawn from the majority of recipients by the second or third postoperative week.

Once the patient can walk from 2000 to 3000 ft per day and chest tubes have been removed, endurance training is started in the treadmill room, and an individualized strengthening and flexibility program is added. Principles of aerobic training are applied in this phase of the program.[8] With the ventilatory limitations to exercise removed, the goal of exercise training is aerobic conditioning. The primary limitation to exercise at this point appears to be deconditioning. For the first 3 months, the patient exercises 5 days/wk. The goal is to perform 30 to 40 minutes of continuous treadmill walking or stationary cycling at 75 to 85% of the age predicted maximum heart rate. SaO_2, heart rate, distance, speed, grade, and perceived exertion are closely monitored.

Declines in exercise performance, in desaturation, or both during exercise sometimes precede episodes of infection or rejection. Other indicators include low-grade fever, fatigue, general malaise, cough, shortness of breath, and decreases in spirometric values. The rehabilitation staff screens the patients daily for symptoms and signs of rejection and infection so that diagnosis and treatment can be started early and exercise conditioning can continue.

HOME EXERCISE PROGRAM AND FOLLOW-UP

After 3 months of supervised post-transplantation rehabilitation, patients are given a home exercise program. The prescription is based on the patient's postoperative exercise regimen. Consideration is given to the availability of exercise equipment in the patient's home. Patients are instructed in how to measure and achieve their target heart rate and are told to exercise 30 minutes daily. Follow-up includes the 6-minute walking test and cardiopulmonary stress test, both of which are done at completion of the post-transplantation rehabilitation program and during subsequent routine follow-up visits.

LONG-TERM RESULTS

Between July 1, 1988, and April 19, 1991, 78 lung transplants were performed at our institution in 75 recipients with an overall survival rate of 77%. The results of pretransplantation and post-transplantation pulmonary rehabilitation have been analyzed in 55 of these recipients with adequate follow-up. A profile of the 55 patients analyzed is presented in Table 35–3. The mean time spent in pretransplant rehabilitation for all patients (excluding those with primary pulmonary hypertension) was 14.3 weeks. For all patients receiving transplants, the mean time in the intensive care unit was 6.1 days, and the average hospital stay was 23.6 days.

Pulmonary Function

FEV_1 showed no significant change during pretransplantation pulmonary rehabilitation in any of the groups (Tables 35–4 and 35–5). By the third to sixth week after transplantation, significant increases in FEV_1 were seen in all groups (except primary pulmonary hypertension patients undergoing single-lung transplantation [Group 5]) compared with pretransplantation values. The FEV_1 of all groups (except of Group 5) also increased significantly at 12 weeks compared with that at 6 weeks. These increases were maintained throughout the 6-month period. The two bilateral transplantation groups had significantly greater improvement in FEV_1 than the 3 unilateral transplantation groups.

Mean PaO_2 showed significant increases at 3 weeks compared with the pretransplantation period in all groups (except Group 5). The cystic fibrosis group had

TABLE 35–3. PATIENT PROFILE IN LUNG TRANSPLANTATION

Group	Diagnosis	Type of Transplant	Age* (yr)	Sex (male:female)	Time in Rehabilitation* (wk)		Oxygen Requirements* (L/min)	
					Pretransplant	Post-transplant	Pretransplant	Post-transplant
1	COPD	bilateral	45	11:6	15	12.4	5.5	0
2	COPD	single	53	5:13	11.5	12	4.0	0
3	Cystic fibrosis	bilateral	25	3:3	26.5	12.3	7.7	0
4	Idiopathic pulmonary fibrosis	single	48	2:5	8.2	12.0	9.9	0
5	Primary pulmonary hypertension	single	32	1:7	0.0	12.0	1.5	0

*Mean values.

TABLE 35–4. FEV_1 BEFORE AND AFTER TRANSPLANTATION

	FEV_1 (L)				
Group	Pretransplantation	Post-transplantation			
		3 wk	6 wk	12 wk	24 wk
1	0.49	2.37	2.71	2.94	3.13
2	0.49	1.31	1.31	1.49	1.48
3	0.63	2.35	2.83	3.22	3.57
4	1.25	1.68	1.79	1.75	1.91
5	2.45	2.27	2.22	2.69	2.55

TABLE 35–5. MEAN ROOM AIR Pao_2

	Pao_2 (mm Hg)				
Group	Pretransplantation	Post-transplantation			
		3 wk	6 wk	12 wk	24 wk
1	55	78	82	85	89
2	57	74	71	76	78
3	48	77	72	87	98
4	47	71	83	83	82
5	64	75	73	79	74

TABLE 35–6. HEMODYNAMICS

Parameter	Pretransplantation	Post-transplantation
Mean pulmonary artery pressure (mm Hg)	58 ± 6	18 ± 5
Cardiac index (L/min/m^2)	2.15 ± 0.37	2.75 ± 0.50
Pulmonary vascular resistance (Wood units)	14 ± 4	2 ± 1
Right ventricular ejection fraction (%)	20 ± 8*	58 ± 14†
Left ventricular ejection fraction (%)	62 ± 16	63 ± 12

*$n = 5$; all others, $n = 7$.
†$P = .06$ pre-versus post-transplantation.

TABLE 35-7. MEAN SIX-MINUTE WALKING DISTANCE

Group	Distance (m)					
	Pretransplantation		Post-transplantation			
	At Evaluation	After Rehabilitation	3 wk	6 wk	12 wk	24 wk
1	240	306	317	486	560	627
2	219	308	259	428	494	491
3	355	524	408	696	741	750
4	236	296	280	454	554	535
5	246	—	293	434	514	571

further significant increases in mean PaO_2 at 12 and 24 weeks after transplantation. The other groups maintained their mean PaO_2 values throughout the 6-month period. All patients but two were freed from supplemental oxygen by 2 to 3 weeks after transplantation.

Hemodynamics

The patients with primary pulmonary hypertension had markedly elevated pulmonary artery pressures and pulmonary vascular resistance before transplantation (Table 35-6). Right ventricular function was moderately to severely impaired. After transplantation, the pulmonary artery pressures and vascular resistance returned to normal or nearly normal values, and cardiac function recovered significantly.

Exercise Tolerance

Pretransplantation pulmonary rehabilitation was associated with an improvement in 6-minute walking distance in Groups 1 to 4 (Tables 35-7 and 35-8); as previously discussed, Group 5 did not participate in pretransplantation rehabilitation. Following transplantation, the 6-minute walking distance again improved in all groups. By 6 weeks after transplantation, the mean values exceeded the pretransplantation results, but further gains occurred at 12 to 24 weeks.

The mean metabolic equivalent level achieved on the submaximum exercise stress test increased in all groups over time. The longest increase occurred in the cystic fibrosis group. Improvements occurred preoperatively despite little change or a decline in lung function.

TABLE 35-8. MEAN MET* LEVEL ON SUBMAXIMUM EXERCISE STRESS TEST

Group	MET Level			
	Pretransplantation		Post-transplantation	
	At Evaluation	After Rehabilitation	6 wk	12 wk
1	2.69	4.44	6.09	7.46
2	1.94	3.72	3.95	4.63
3	3.77	5.45	7.95	9.97
4	2.70	—	6.15	6.63

*MET: Multiple of resting metabolic rate.

REFERENCES

1. Petty TL. Pulmonary rehabilitation. Basics of R.D. New York: American Thoracic Society, 1975.
2. Hodgkin JE (ed). Chronic Obstructive Pulmonary Disease. Current Concepts in Diagnosis and Comprehensive Care. Park Ridge, IL: American College of Chest Physicians, 1979.
3. Foster S, Lopez D, Thomas HM. Pulmonary rehabilitation in COPD patients with elevated PCO_2. Am Rev Respir Dis 1988; 138:1519–1523.
4. Foster S, Thomas HM. Pulmonary rehabilitation in lung disease other than chronic obstructive pulmonary disease. Am Rev Respir Dis 1990; 141:601–604.
5. Holle RH, Williams D, Vandree J, et al. Increased muscle efficiency and sustained benefits in an outpatient community hospital-based pulmonary rehabilitation program. Chest 1988; 94:1161–1168.
6. Mall WR, Medeiros M. Objective evaluation of results of a pulmonary rehabilitation program in a community hospital. Chest 1988; 94:1156–1160.
7. Pineda H, Hass F, Axen K. Treadmill exercise training in chronic obstructive pulmonary disease. Arch Phys Med Rehabil 1986; 67:155–158.
8. McArdle WD, Katch FI, Katch VL. Exercise physiology, energy, nutrition, and human performance. Philadelphia: Lea & Febiger, 1990.
9. The Toronto Lung Transplant Group. Unilateral lung transplantation for pulmonary fibrosis. N Engl J Med 1986; 314:1140–1150.
10. The Toronto Lung Transplant Group. Experience with single-lung transplantation for pulmonary fibrosis. JAMA 1988; 259:2258–2262.
11. Dear CL, Grossman PD, Maurer JR. Pre-operative rehabilitation of patients awaiting single lung transplant (abstract). Chest 1989; 96:163S.
12. Malen JF, Biggar DG, Trulock EP. Pre and post operative rehabilitation of single and double lung transplant patients (abstract). Am Rev Respir Dis 1990; 141:762A.
13. Egan TM, Kaiser LR, Cooper JD. Lung transplantation. Curr Probl Surg 1989; 26:673–752.
14. Craven JL, Bright J, Dear CL. Psychiatric, psychosocial and rehabilitative aspects of lung transplantation. Clin Chest Med 1990; 11:247–257.
15. Williams T, Grossman RF, Maurer JR. Long-term functional follow-up of lung transplant recipients. Clin Chest Med 1990; 11:347–358.
16. Frost A, Dear CL, Grossman RF et al. Exercise tolerance in patients undergoing double lung transplant for end stage pulmonary disease (abstract). Am Rev Respir Dis 1988; 137:336A.
17. de Hoyos A, Ramirez J, Dear CL, et al. Late results after single and double lung transplantation (abstract). Am Rev Respir Dis 1991; 143:467A.
18. Belman MJ. Exercise in chronic obstructive pulmonary disease. Clin Chest Med 1986; 7:585–597.
19. Wasserman K, Whipp BJ. Exercise physiology in health and disease. Am Rev Respir Dis 1975; 112:219–247.
20. Make BJ, Buchholz J. Exercise training in COPD patients improves cardiac function (abstract). Third International Conference

on Pulmonary Rehabilitation and Home Ventilation, Colorado, 1991.
21. Carter R, Nicotra N, LeMon C. Exercise conditioning in the rehabilitation of patients with chronic obstructive pulmonary disease. Arch Phys Med Rehabil 1988; 69:118–122.
22. Butland RJ, Pang J, Gross ER, et al. Two-, six-, and 12-minute walking tests in respiratory disease. BMJ 1982; 284:1607–1608.
23. McGavin CR, Gupta SP, McHardy GJR. Twelve-minute walking test for assessing disability in chronic bronchitis. BMJ 1976; 1:822–823.
24. Borg G. Perceived exertion as an indicator of somatic stress. Scand J Rehabil Med 1970; 2:92.
25. McGavin CR, Artvinli M, Naoe H, et al. Dyspnea, disability and distance walked: Comparison of estimates of exercise performance in respiratory disease. BMJ 1978; 2:241–243.
26. Mahler DA, Weinberg DH, Wells CK, et al. The measurement of dyspnea: Contents, interobserver agreement, and physiologic correlates of two new clinical indexes. Chest 1984; 85:751–758.
27. Altose MD. Assessment and management of breathlessness. Chest 1985; 88(Suppl):77–78.
28. Kendall FP, McCreary EK. Muscle testing and function. Baltimore, MD: Williams & Wilkins, 1983.
29. Reisman JJ, Rivington-Law MC, Marcotte J, et al. Role of conventional physiotherapy in cystic fibrosis. J Pediatr 1988; 113:632–636.
30. Feaster WM, Jost KA, Swedlow DB. Capnography: A quick reference. Hayward, CA: Nellcor, Inc., 1988.
31. Cooper JD. The evolution of techniques and indications for lung transplantation. Ann Surg 1990; 212:249–255.
32. Egan TM, Cooper JD. Surgical aspects of single lung transplant. Clin Chest Med 1990; 11:195–205.
33. Breslow MJ, Mill CF, Rogers M. Perioperative management. St. Louis: C.V. Mosby, 1990.
34. Maurer JR. Unilateral lung transplant. Pulm Perspect 1987; 4:1–3.
35. Bartlett RH, Gazzaniga AB, Geraghty T. Respiratory maneuvers to prevent post-operative pulmonary complications. Surg Forum 1971; 22:196–201.
36. Jaworshi A, Goldberg SK, Waklenstein MD, et al. Utility of immediate post lobectomy fiberoptic bronchoscopy in preventing atelectasis. Chest 1979; 94:971–978.
37. Marini JJ, Pierson DJ, Hudson LD. Acute lobar atelectasis: A prospective comparison of fiberoptic bronchoscopy and respiratory therapy. Am Rev Respir Dis 1979; 119:971–978.
38. Stein M, Cassera EL. Pre-operative pulmonary evaluation and therapy for surgery patients. JAMA 1970; 211:787–791.
39. Thoren L. Post-operative pulmonary complication: Observations on their prevention by means of physiotherapy. Acta Chir Scand 1954; 107:193–197.

Chapter 36

The Ventilator-Dependent Patient

THOMAS L. PETTY, M.D.

Ventilator dependence may occur in patients with chronic respiratory insufficiency because of progressive disease or complications of therapy. It commonly occurs in states of chronic obstructive pulmonary disease (COPD), fibrotic lung disease, kyphoscoliosis, progressive myopathies, and neuropathies. This chapter addresses the systematic approach to the ventilator-dependent patient and focuses on patients with COPD. The principles of management of patients with COPD are largely applicable to other disease states associated with prolonged ventilator dependence.

NUTRITION

A major component in ventilator dependence is malnutrition.[1] Malnutrition adversely affects respiratory muscle function and lung function itself, since micronutrients are important in surfactant formation and function.[2] The presence of hypoalbuminemia was closely correlated with the development of new infections and ventilator dependence in intensive care unit patients.[3] The rapid normalization of the serum albumin via exogenous albumin replacement as a part of total parenteral nutrition has been advocated to restore the serum oncotic pressure.[4] It is not the purpose of this chapter to deal with all of the details of the impact of malnutrition on ventilator dependence, but it must be understood by all in the field that the correction of malnutrition is the key to recovery in many patients who are ventilator-dependent. Various approaches to the correction of malnutrition exist. These include total parenteral nutrition,[5, 6] nasogastric feeding,[7] needle catheter jejunostomy,[8] and patient-oriented feeding with normal food.[9] Each method of nutritional support is useful and applicable to certain clinical situations. In general, the gastrointestinal tract, when intact and functional, is the preferable route for nutrition because it is more physiologic and less costly and helps protect the integrity of the gastrointestinal mucosa. Self-feeding of all necessary nutrients is the ultimate goal and is achievable in the majority of ventilator-dependent patients.

The key to restoration of a normal nutritional state is to allow and encourage patients to eat normal food. This is possible with the use of a tracheostomy, which is the only airway that can be used in the long-term in the recovering patient. In fact, a tracheostomy should probably be performed after 1 week of mechanical ventilation if it is anticipated that the needs for ventilatory assistance will be prolonged for even a few more days. The advantage of the tracheostomy is that it is comfortable and facilitates mouth care. A tracheostomy allows the patient to eat without the impediment of an endotracheal tube, which usually interferes with swallowing. Suctioning of small amounts of aspirated food via a tracheostomy is usually not a problem. A tracheostomy is a superior airway with respect to suctioning. It is also a far superior airway when weaning attempts are initiated because of its low resistance to airflow.

Patients should be given a tray with an attractive selection of food at each mealtime. They should be allowed to feed themselves. Family members can also participate in feeding. After all, patients have all day to eat each meal. It is best if they eat throughout the day.[10] Normal food provides fiber, which helps to restore the integrity of the gastrointestinal mucosa. Normal food also contains every micronutrient needed by the body. If the patient is capable of managing his or her own feeding, the wisdom of the body can select the nutrients for the restoration of tissue and organ integrity, including that of the gastrointestinal tract itself. Enteral nutrition preserves the gastrointestinal mucosa and promotes immunocompetence. Thus, migration or bloodstream invasion of organisms across the gut wall is reduced by enteral nutrition.

DEPRESSION

The great majority of ventilator-dependent patients suffer from profound depression. They often feel trapped, feeling that they can neither live nor die. This is indeed a dilemma for the desperately ill.

Patients need to be in a comfortable environment and near a window. They require orientation with the daytime and nighttime cycle and should be awakened at sunrise and allowed to sleep shortly after sunset. Patients often experience "intensive care delirium" if day–night orientation is disrupted. Placement of the patient's head near a window has a salutary effect on this transient condition.[11] Ventilator-dependent patients should not be sedated except in rare instances. The excessive use of sedatives may interfere with physiologic sleep. Patients also need other input from life and society. The television should be on during specific periods, whether or not the patient appears to be sleeping. A transistor radio can be placed near the pillow. Friends and family should be allowed unrestricted visiting hours. If there are times when no friends or family are present, the nurse, respiratory therapist, or physician should read to the patient or visit for a meaningful period of time on a regular basis. Those with religious orientation should have an opportunity to read religious texts, such as the Bible, or have such texts read to them. The clergy should be encouraged to visit. A cheery and positive attitude should be present at all times. It is rare that antidepressant drugs are useful in this setting, but they may be judiciously employed.

ACTIVITY

Eating, of course, is a major activity; contact with the outside world is also extremely important. The patient should be allowed to sit upright in a chair at least twice daily. The upright posture improves gastrointestinal motility; it mitigates the possibility of aspiration and improves bladder drainage. Patients should also be assisted in walking even if they require mechanical ventilatory support (Fig. 36–1). Walking and breathing are related, that is, our respiratory system has been trained to accept input from the skeletal muscles in order to coordinate breathing with the activities of exercise. Walking with associated deep breathing also strengthens the muscles of respiration and the extremities. Walking also improves venous return from the extremities, thus lessening the risk of thromboembolism. Every patient should ambulate at least once per day and should sit in a chair at least twice per day at appropriate times.

EFFORTS IN WEANING

Many so-called ventilatory dependent patients can ultimately be weaned. Periods of simple T-tube (Fig.

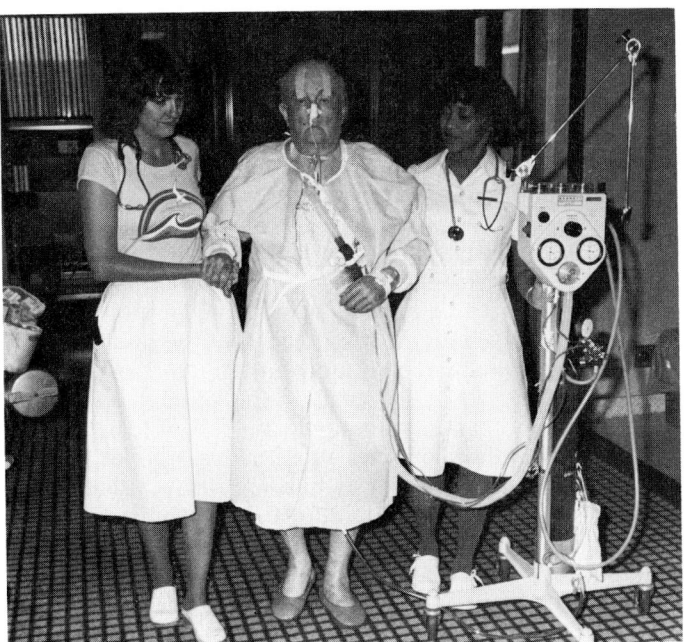

FIGURE 36–1. A method of ambulating the ventilator-dependent patient using a pressure-cycled ventilator on wheels and powered by an E-cylinder.

36–2) or tracheostomy collar weaning conducted according to strictly systematized schedules should be employed. The greatest mistake in weaning is exhausting the patient. There is no simple recipe for weaning. The intermittent mandatory ventilation method and the pressure support ventilation effort are primarily gimmicks. These techniques can be successful if applied in a systematic, physiologically oriented manner that allows for appropriate exercise of the respiratory muscles *without producing fatigue*. It is the system and discipline of weaning and the avoidance of fatigue that are critical to success. Neither the intermittent mandatory ventilation

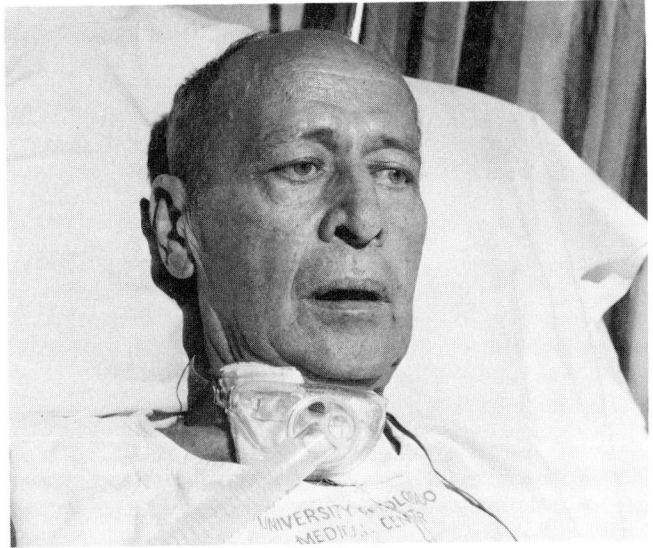

FIGURE 36–2. The method of tracheal collar weaning via a tracheostomy. This method is equivalent to T-piece weaning.

nor pressure support ventilation methods of so-called weaning can predict whether the patient will become fatigued. Respiratory muscle fatigue guarantees failure. Respiratory muscle fatigue is evidenced by a rising respiratory rate of more than 25 breaths per minute, use of accessory muscles of the chest, and paradoxical abdominal breathing. Strict criteria for weaning patients do not apply to the so-called ventilator-dependent patient. While attempting to wean, patients should either breathe on their own or should rest. Sometimes, weaning begins with 1 minute without respirator support followed by 1 hour of rest. The time without support can be approximately doubled each day, or at least improved by 50%, as long as the patient is not exhausted. The patient should always rest at least 1 hour, as the respiratory muscles require this amount of time to rest. Signs of weaning failure are tachycardia, tachypnea, diaphoresis, and paradoxical breathing. Observation of the patient's struggle to breathe along with diaphoresis and tachycardia is a clear indication of exhaustion. Our success in weaning mechanically ventilated patients with apparent ventilation dependence has been previously described.[12] Basic criteria for weaning a broad spectrum of patients who require short-term mechanical ventilation were also reported.[13]

TRANSTRACHEAL HIGH-FLOW OXYGEN

Recent studies have shown that carbon dioxide homeostasis can be improved by high-flow oxygen mixtures delivered via a transtracheal catheter (Figs. 36–3 and 36–4). Inspired oxygen fractions of 0.4 to 0.6 are controlled by a blender and delivered at 8 to 10 L/min. Normoxia is conveniently monitored by pulse oximetry.[14] Many patients feel relief of dyspnea with this new method of oxygen delivery. A reduction in acutely elevated carbon dioxide has already been observed in a pilot study of two patients with acute retention of carbon dioxide superimposed on chronic compensated carbon

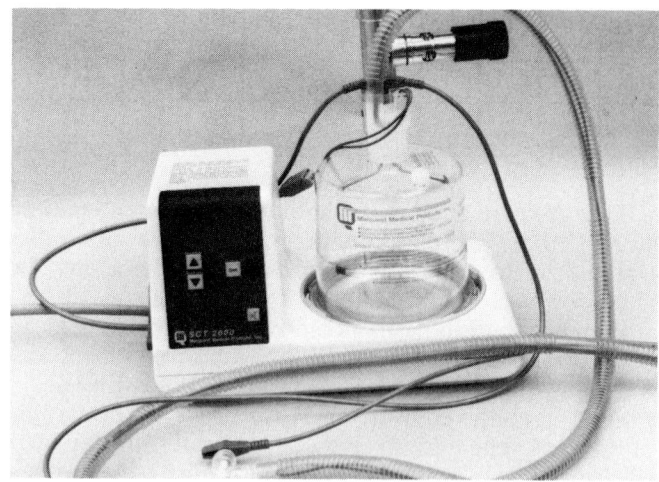

FIGURE 36–4. Close-up view of a humidifier for high-flow transtracheal oxygen delivery.

dioxide retention.[14] This was done to avoid repeated intubation and mechanical ventilation in the hospital during an exacerbation of disease with respiratory muscle fatigue. Both patients were selected to continue receiving high-flow transtracheal oxygen at home. They experienced a 50 to 60% reduction in minute ventilation, which was mainly due to a reduction in tidal volume. P_{CO_2} decreased by 7% in spite of a marked reduction in minute ventilation.[14] Both patients lived at home with this novel method of "ventilatory support" for 9 and 10 months, respectively. Post mortem evaluations revealed no significant airway mucosal changes as a result of high-flow transtracheal oxygen administration.

The possibility that this method could be useful in weaning some patients who have borderline ventilatory ability is currently being investigated. An oxygen catheter can be placed in the tracheostomy stoma during periods when the patient is off the ventilator. At the time of this writing, this has already been found to be successful in one patient. Its effectiveness probably lies in the reduction of the work of breathing provided by high-flow oxygen or perhaps in the reduction of dyspnea via the stimulation of tracheal flow receptors.

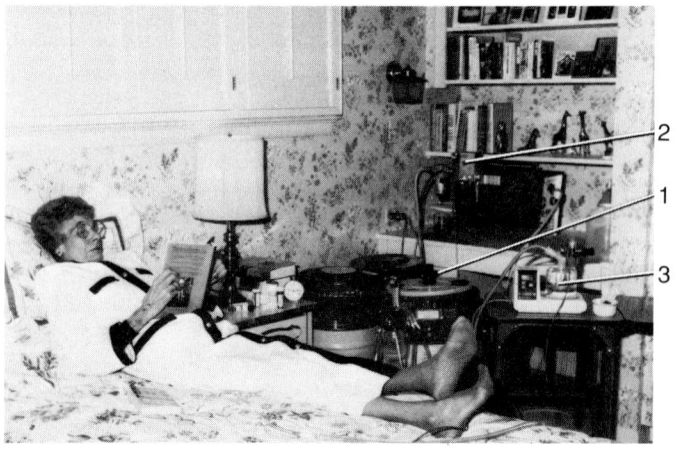

FIGURE 36–3. Patient receiving high-flow oxygen at an inspired fraction of 0.5. Transtracheal delivery is not shown. (1, liquid oxygen cylinders; 2, air compressor with oxygen air blender; 3, humidifier.)

SPECIAL FACILITIES

The need for special facilities for the ventilator-dependent patient has been cited.[15] Some larger hospitals have developed ventilator weaning units. A new chain of special-purpose hospitals for catastrophically ill ventilator-dependent patients is rapidly growing in this country. "Vencor" hospitals accept patients from other hospitals for the purpose of completing the weaning process or for preparation for the transition to home care. Seventeen such hospitals are now in existence, including one in Denver, Colorado (Figs. 36–5 to 36–7). The author is involved in the development of the Denver unit and in developing an organization of all

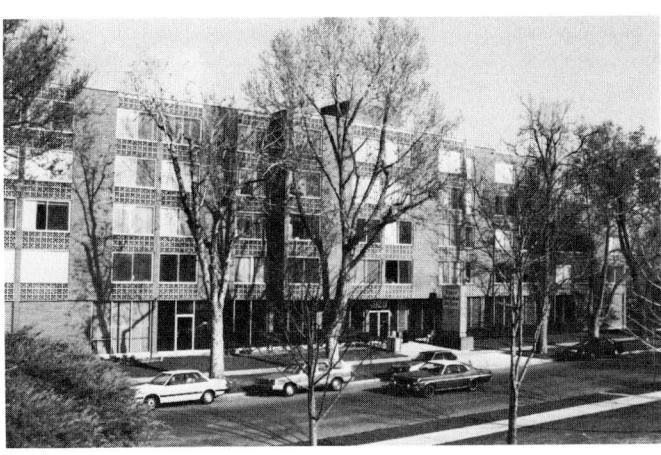

FIGURE 36–5. A picture of Vencor Hospital in Denver, CO. The hospital is able to care for 30 ventilator-dependent patients. It is equipped with a four-bed intensive care unit.

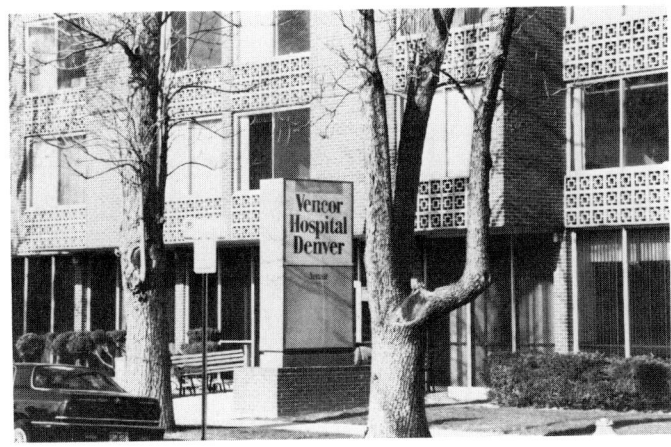

FIGURE 36–6. Close-up view of the entrance to Vencor Hospital in Denver, CO.

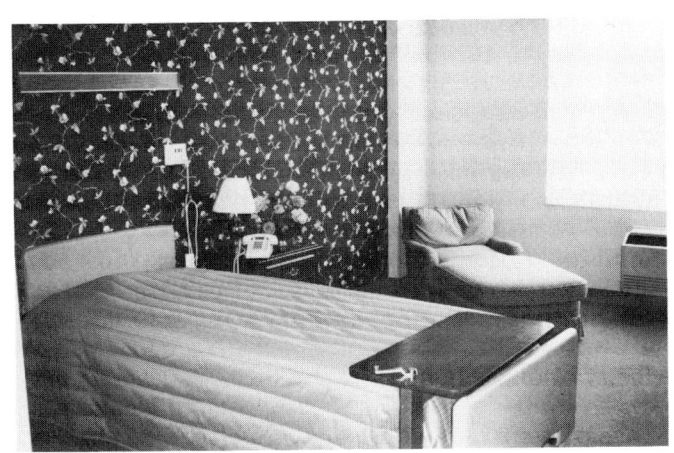

FIGURE 36–7. A large patient room equipped to provide oxygen, suction, and air. There is ample space for visitors.

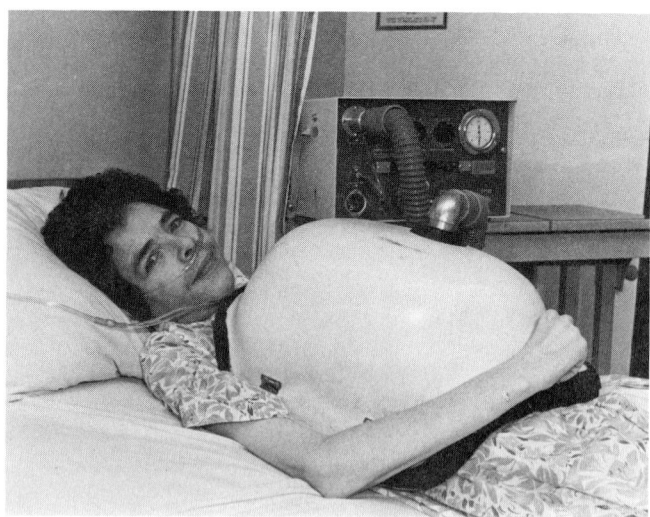

FIGURE 36-8. Cuirass-type ventilator used at home for a patient with residual of polio and chronic obstructive pulmonary disease.

Vencor Hospital medical directors in order to establish research protocols.

In the future, we will be able to study the impact of facilities dedicated to the treatment of this special population of ventilator-dependent patients. Many individuals who are chronically ventilator-dependent are victims of their disease as well as of their treatment. For example, they are commonly malnourished, fatigued, depressed, and discouraged. Most are septic due in large part to malnutrition and numerous invasive procedures—many of which, such as urinary catheterization, are not necessary. These patients need a new approach to "rehumanization." They need food, activity, care, and hope in order to get well. Most of all, they need time.

Some ventilator-dependent patients will die of progressive disease or of the complications of multiorgan failure, which are commonly mediated by sepsis. Many other patients will be successfully "emancipated" from their preoccupation with the details of ventilatory care cited in this chapter. Others can be transferred home to continue ventilator care.[16] Even some who continue to require home mechanical ventilation will eventually recover sufficient ventilatory capacity to be able to have progressively prolonged periods off the ventilator. Some will continue to require nocturnal mechanical ventilation via a tracheostomy tube, which is plugged during the daytime.

Most of these patients live comfortable lives for months or years following discharge. External ventilation without a tracheostomy and with supplemental oxygen is successful in selected patients with marginal ventilatory compatibility (Fig. 36–8). Most of these patients die at home. In all cases, these patients require the care of dedicated physicians, respiratory therapists, home care nurses, and suppliers.

REFERENCES

1. Driver AG, LeBrun ML. Iatrogenic malnutrition in patients receiving ventilatory support. JAMA 1980; 244:2195–2196.
2. Branson RD, Hurst JM. Nutrition and respiratory function: Food for thought. Respir Care 1988; 33:89–92.
3. Murray MJ, Marsh HM, Wochos DN, et al. Nutritional assessment of intensive-care unit patients. Mayo Clin Proc 1988; 63:1106–1115.
4. Kaminski MV, Williams SD. Review of the rapid normalization of serum albumin with modified total parenteral nutrition solutions. Crit Care Med 1988; 18:327–335.
5. Grant JP. Handbook of Parenteral Nutrition. Philadelphia: W.B. Saunders Co., 1980.
6. Goodgame JJ. A critical evaluation of the results of total parenteral nutrition in various disease states: Cost and benefit. In: Fischer JE (ed). Surgical Nutrition. Boston: Little, Brown & Co., Inc., 1983, pp 779–793.
7. Heymesfield SB, Bethel RA, Ansley JD, et al. Enteral hyperalimentation: An alternative to central venous hyperalimentation. Ann Intern Med 1978; 90:63–71.
8. Ryan JA Jr, Page CP. Intrajejunal feeding: Development and current status. J Parenter Enteral Nutr 1984; 8:187–198.
9. Nett LM, Petty TL (ed). Intensive and Rehabilitative Respiratory Care. 3rd ed. Philadelphia: Lea & Febiger, 1982, pp 170–171.
10. Jenkins DJA, Wolever TMS, Vuksan V, et al. Nibbling versus gorging: Metabolic advantages of increased meal frequency. N Engl J Med 1989; 321:929–934.
11. Wilson LM. Intensive care delirium: The effect of outside deprivation in a windowless unit. Arch Intern Med 1972; 130:225–226.
12. Morganroth ML, Morganroth JL, Nett LM, et al. Criteria for weaning from prolonged mechanical ventilation. Arch Intern Med 1984; 144:1012–1016.
13. Sahn SA, Lakshminarayan S. Bedside criteria for discontinuation of mechanical ventilation. Chest 1973; 63:1002–1005.
14. Schaten MA, Christopher KL, Goodman S, et al. High-flow transtracheal oxygen: A promising technique for the management of hypercarbic respiratory failure (abstract). Chest 1990; 98(Suppl):22S.
15. Bone RC. Long-term ventilator care: A Chicago problem and a national problem. Chest 1987; 92:536–539.
16. Peters SG, Viggiano RW. Home mechanical ventilation. Mayo Clin Proc 1988; 63:1208–1213.

5

Special Environments for Pulmonary Rehabilitation, and the Aspects of Care Reimbursement

RICHARD CASABURI, Ph.D., M.D.

In this final section of this text, the practical aspects of operating and financing a pulmonary rehabilitation program are stressed. We asked the directors of four prominent pulmonary rehabilitation programs who operate in a variety of settings to share their experiences. These chapters should be a helpful resource for those setting up new programs or attempting to optimize the function of existing programs.

In the first chapter, Judy Tietsort, a registered nurse and respiratory therapist, describes an approach for the operation of a rehabilitation program with minimal overhead and complexity. Referral patterns and marketing strategies for a well-established program are discussed. The program content and the interaction of the members of the therapeutic team are considered in detail.

Dr. Frank Sutton of Birmingham, Alabama, describes a chain of pulmonary rehabilitation programs that are operated in an independent mode. He provides an instructive review of how the laws dictating reimbursement for pulmonary rehabilitation developed. The concept of the Comprehensive Outpatient Rehabilitation Facility (or CORF) is introduced. How such a facility is established and the organizations with oversight responsibilities are described. Dr. Sutton presents results of 202 consecutive patients treated in his facility. As others have found (see Chapter 16), pulmonary rehabilitation programs do not generally improve lung mechanics or gas exchange but can yield impressive increases in exercise tolerance.

Dr. Howard Kravetz, a private pulmonary practitioner, describes his extensive experience in operating an office-based pulmonary rehabilitation program. A step-by-step approach to the work-up necessary to evaluate the prospective candidate is given. The components of the program, including patient activities and patient education, are covered. The facilities necessary for operation of the program are described. Revenue strategies are also briefly considered.

Dr. Wayne Mall and Margaret Mederios operate a rehabilitation program in a community hospital in Fremont, California. In their contribution, they reveal the pitfalls in obtaining reimbursement for rehabilitation, particularly from Medicare. Techniques for proper documentation of services, which is a necessary prerequisite for reimbursement, are extensively discussed. Methods for constructing treatment plans are described. Particularly helpful are the inclusion of specific sample forms for assessing progress and documenting services.

Chapter 37

A Storefront Program for Pulmonary Rehabilitation

JUDY TIETSORT, R.N., R.R.T.

WHY A STOREFRONT SETTING?

Successful pulmonary rehabilitation programs can be provided in a variety of locations, most commonly in a hospital setting and less commonly in a medical office setting. But an even more nontraditional setting, which we have found to be very successful in our area, is the shopping center storefront. Here, we provide an effective and efficient fee-for-service program.

The storefront facility has two main advantages over a traditional hospital or medical office setting. First, it usually has ample parking space and is close to other services, such as drug and grocery stores. Second and more important, it is economical. If the program is run in an acute care setting within a hospital's budget, certain costs are allocated to that program to cover hospital expenses. These are called *indirect costs;* some examples are depreciation, cafeteria costs, payroll costs for non-revenue–producing departments, and maintenance/public service costs, which are usually based on square footage. When a program is operated outside the hospital, those costs directly related to square footage (rent) are no longer allocated as indirect costs in the department's budget. Instead, rent for the space becomes a new *direct cost.* Commonly, the indirect amount charged to a program to cover rent in a hospital is approximately $20 to $30 per square foot. In contrast, in 1992, rent in a storefront setting is commonly $8 to $12 per square foot. Thus, in a storefront facility, a savings of $2000 to $2500 per month is possible.

PROGRAM HISTORY

Prior to 1970, most pulmonary rehabilitation education programs were begun at the end of an acute phase of illness while the patient was still considered an inpatient. In the late 1960s, a number of groups in the United States began studying the effects of outpatient pulmonary rehabilitation programs. These programs included patient education and exercise with the use of home supplemental oxygen supplies. In Colorado, Petty and associates did a number of early studies with outpatients and showed that with a formalized education/exercise program, the number of hospital admissions could be decreased. In 1972, our hospital began looking at such a program and designed its own using the guidelines set forth by Petty and associates.[1-4]

Our program started as a one-to-one teaching program for inpatients prior to their hospital discharge. Soon after beginning the program, we realized that an outpatient program would be more convenient and more cost-effective than a hospital-based service. However, at that time, there was no third-party payer reimbursement for outpatient pulmonary rehabilitation. We began working closely with Blue Cross/Blue Shield (the fiscal intermediary for Medicare) in an attempt to justify our outpatient program economically. We used data collected by a number of outpatient programs that had done research on the subject and, with the help of Blue Cross/Blue Shield, arrived at charges that would be reimbursed regularly.

In 1972, these charges were based on physical therapy codes for outpatient exercise classes and patient instructions. Development of our program proceeded slowly, and we provided only a small number of outpatient classes prior to 1980. From 1980 to 1987, we conducted six outpatient education classes per year; each class consisted of four patients. We provided education as well as demonstrations of selected exercises. Patients were then given the option of joining a 6-week outpatient exercise class that was reimbursed by most carriers. We held only one or two classes per week due to the limited space available in our hospital setting.

REFERRALS

At Lutheran Medical Center, 95% of our inpatients have their respiratory therapy ordered by "respiratory protocol." A respiratory therapist first evaluates the patient and then adjusts or discontinues therapy based on the criteria established by a consensus of our pulmonary physicians. The respiratory protocol also allows our pulmonary rehabilitation therapist to interview selected patients for our pulmonary rehabilitation program, entitled Project M.O.V.E. (Motivation for Oxygen and Ventilation through Exercise). Once a suitable candidate is identified, the pulmonary rehabilitation therapist then calls the patient's physician to obtain a physician's order for the patient to be interviewed and possibly enrolled in the program.

In the early years of our program, physician referrals were minimal. Most of our referrals were for patients from acute care facilities who had been recruited by the pulmonary rehabilitation therapist. The majority were patients of pulmonary physicians.

OUR CURRENT PROGRAM

As hospital space became limited, we took a serious look at our entire pulmonary rehabilitation program and made three basic changes: we (1) rented storefront space at a shopping center close to the hospital, (2) redesigned the class format, and (3) developed a comprehensive marketing plan.

Marketing

Our current experience shows that patient referrals come from three sources: medical workers within the hospital system, physicians, and patients and their families. We worked closely with our hospital's Community Relations/Marketing Department to develop a marketing plan. By interviewing many hospital staff physicians, we determined that, although our program had been available for many years, many of the physicians had either "forgotten" about it or had not realized it was still available. Based on this finding, we developed a marketing strategy.

To promote our program to physicians, we presented basic information to a number of medical subspecialty groups in the hospital; we followed this up with letters and copies of our redesigned program pamphlets. In addition, we placed articles in different hospital newsletters sent to physicians, former patients and employees, as well as the Senior Services Network. In these publications, we described the program and compared its cost with that of other pulmonary rehabilitation programs in the area.

Sending information to patients and their families followed. We designed marketing material that basically described the program, and this material was delivered to the offices of physicians who saw large numbers of appropriate patients. The material was oriented toward patients and their families in the hope that requests would be made to the physician for a referral to the program.

Periodically throughout the year, we offer educational sessions for the community. These include lectures on exercise that are given by our pulmonary rehabilitation staff as well as a number of lectures that are presented by doctors from pulmonary physician groups. Furthermore, one of our pulmonary rehabilitation therapists, who also serves as an educator of the hospital's transtracheal oxygen program, encourages appropriate patients receiving transtracheal oxygen to enroll in our pulmonary rehabilitation program.

Other items we consider to be marketing tools are our monogramed T-shirts, tote bags, and water bottles that are given to patients enrolling in the education and exercise classes.

Space Rental

We began to see a major improvement in attendance for our program as soon as we leased the store space. Currently, we offer 18 exercise classes per week, with 9 groups of patients that each meet twice per week (approximately 100 patients). Exercise classes, as well as formal education classes, are conducted in the storefront setting. The space is divided so that warm-up and floor mat work can be done in one room while workouts on exercise equipment can proceed in another room. In addition, we have a cushioned aerobic floor that provides comfort and safety for our patients. Best of all, a popular yogurt store is located only four doors away.

Format Change

We underwent a significant change in program format when we added 6 weeks of conditioning (covered by insurance) to follow the patients' initial education classes. Rather than allowing the patients to choose the conditioning classes as an option after completion of the classes, we automatically enrolled them in the 6-week program. When the 6 weeks of insurance-covered classes were completed, patients had the option of continuing in the self-pay conditioning classes. Since we changed the program and all patients were introduced to "conditioning," 75% of them have continued with the self-pay conditioning program. We currently have approximately 100 patients enrolled in 18 to 20 classes per week.

We interviewed former patients to learn which hours they felt were most desirable not only to attend class but also to allow for assimilation of the educational materials. Based on the interviews, we now offer a 12-hour class program, which is broken down into 2-hour sessions twice weekly for 3 weeks. Once the 12 hours of education are completed, the patients begin 6 weeks of insurance-covered exercise sessions, which include two sessions per week.

We also added other hospital services to the revised program. An occupational therapist teaches a class on activities of daily living, and a psychiatric nurse (who also sees inpatients with COPD) presents a formal session within the education program on coping with chronic disease. These optional unstructured classes are offered free of charge each month on an "as-needed" basis.

THE PROGRAM

Our program title, Project M.O.V.E., stands for motivation, oxygen, ventilation, and exercise. It has five components: interview, evaluation, education, exercise, and follow-up. Patients can refer themselves to the program or be referred by their primary physicians. The primary physician is contacted by the rehabilitation therapist prior to a patient's entering the program so that instructions about restrictions, medications, or other aspects of patient care are clear. Once the patient has begun the exercise program, the physician receives progress reports on a regular basis. The physician is always called if there are questions or concerns about the patient; we emphasize that the primary physician is always in charge of the patient and that at no time do hospital physicians who are involved in the respiratory therapy department either treat or take over the care of a patient.

When a new patient enters the program, a respiratory therapist interviews him or her and family members to help them establish realistic goals and to let them know from the outset what to expect of the program. During the educational sessions, patients learn about pulmonary diseases and their effects. Staff therapists provide information on breathing techniques, medications, bronchial hygiene, nutrition, psychologic aspects of pulmonary disease, early warning signs, and infection control. We also recommend certain daily activities and inform patients about community resources.

The exercise sessions focus on the patients' endurance with walking, stationary bicycling, or both. Patients learn to coordinate better breathing techniques with exercise and relaxation techniques. They also are taught how to avoid panic.

Following the initial 6 weeks of exercise classes, each patient receives an individualized pulmonary rehabilitation program to continue at home. However, we encourage them to continue in one of the many exercise classes (on a self-pay basis) with their peers. The primary physician continues to receive reports of each patient's progress.

We now offer one to two education classes per month, each of which includes six to eight patients. The exercise classes are more frequent, with 26 sessions per week that include about 100 patients, the majority of whom self-pay at a cost of $40 per month. Each patient comes twice per week and has the option of attending a third session.

Our staff for the program currently consists of a full-time respiratory therapist, a part-time exercise physiologist, and a number of volunteers who assist during exercise classes. These volunteers are patients' spouses who began coming to class when the patients were first enrolled in the education program.

Table 37–1 shows the number of patients per year that have been enrolled in the formal education classes and self-pay exercise classes. The storefront facility opened in August 1988.

TABLE 37–1. PARTICIPANTS IN THE M.O.V.E. PULMONARY REHABILITATION PROGRAM

Number of Participants in Initial Education and Exercise Program	
1991	110 (Extrapolated)
1990	84
1989	75
1988	44
1987	40
1986	24
1985	15
Number of Participants in Self-pay Exercise Classes	
1991	320 (Extrapolated)
1989	47 to 62
1990	62 to 72

REIMBURSEMENTS

Procedures for reimbursement to hospitals by third-party payers as payment for services rendered have changed a number of times over the past 20 years. These changes will probably continue to occur as the cost of delivery of medical care continues to increase. Prior to the advent of prospective payment reimbursement, that is, Medicare's Diagnosis Related Groups (DRGs), services for outpatient care were reimbursed according to the written description of charges that was submitted. Since 1985, reimbursement for outpatient services offered to Medicare patients has been based on various coding schemes, including the International Classification of Diseases 9th Revision Clinical Modification (ICD-9-CM) coding, Current Procedural Terminology 4th Edition (CPT IV) coding, and revenue codes; these codes are recorded on a Medicare claim form by coders and billers once the patient is discharged. Since the majority of patients who receive pulmonary rehabilitation have their services reimbursed by Medicare, we have paid particular attention to the billing process necessary to receive payment.

"5.2.5.7. Respiratory Therapy"

The Hospital Intermediary 10th Edition Manual (HIM 10), in the section entitled "Hospital and Patient Rehabilitation," clearly defines in section 5.2.5.7. how Medicare interprets pulmonary rehabilitation:

> "Respiratory therapy (respiratory care) is defined as those services that are prescribed by a physician for the assessment, diagnostic evaluation, treatment, management, and monitoring of patients with deficiencies and abnormalities of cardiopulmonary function.
>
> "Respiratory therapy services include but are not limited to pulmonary rehabilitation techniques that include a) exercise conditioning; b) breathing retraining; and c) patient education regarding the management of the patient's respiratory problems."

When coding the outpatient records of patients receiving pulmonary rehabilitation, three separate codes need to be utilized. Two of these codes are called "diagnosis codes," and the third is a revenue code, as follows:

1. "V codes" (nonspecific diagnosis codes) explain the services being rendered. For example, V65.4 is for counseling or investigation, and V57.0 is for breathing exercises.
2. Specific diagnosis codes explain why a particular V-code is necessary. These include 492.8 for emphysema and 496 for chronic airway obstruction.
3. Revenue codes are used for billing Medicare on VB82 claim forms to define specific services and charges. For example, the code 410 is used for respiratory services.

Billing occurs after each section of the program is completed; that is, after interviews and goal setting are completed, a bill is submitted for "complete pulmonary patient status evaluation." Once the education is completed, a bill for "pulmonary rehabilitation" follows. Two additional bills are also submitted for the "introduction to pulmonary rehabilitation physical conditioning" and the "6 weeks of pulmonary rehabilitation physical conditioning."

PROGRAM COST TO PATIENTS

The cost of the Project M.O.V.E. program is just over $1000 for each patient. It includes the individual patient interview, 12 hours of education, and 12 hours of exercise. The majority of our patients are covered by Medicare, which pays 80% of the cost. About 82 to 86% of the patients at Lutheran Hospital are covered by a secondary insurance policy, which pays the remaining 20%. The additional self-pay exercise sessions cost $40 per month.

EVIDENCE OF IMPROVEMENT

Our patients' enthusiastic response and continued participation at their own expense attest to the practical effect of their increased capabilities. Probably as a result of the individual attention given to our patients, we have seen dramatic subjective improvement, even in those patients whose objective improvement has been minimal. With any chronic disabling disease process, evaluation of psychologic factors can be among the most important in assessing therapy outcome.[5]

Preliminary analysis of our patients' progress indicates that most are able to tolerate higher levels of exercise (and are able to tolerate a given level of exercise longer) after the rehabilitation program. Therefore, we feel that a storefront pulmonary rehabilitation program can achieve the same end result—both subjectively and objectively—as do more costly inpatient programs.

THE INGREDIENTS FOR SUCCESS

We believe that a pulmonary rehabilitation program can flourish both fiscally and clinically in a storefront location. Success requires determination, hard work, a good comprehensive program, willing patients, and—most important—dedicated staff members.

REFERENCES

1. Petty TL, Nett LM, Finigan MM, et al. A comprehensive care program for chronic airflow obstruction. Ann Intern Med 1969; 70:1109–1120.
2. Petty TL. Pulmonary rehabilitation basics. Respir Dis 1975; 4:1–6.
3. Petty TL, Cherniack RM. Comprehensive care of COPD. Clin Notes Respir Dis 1981; 20:3–12.
4. Sahn SA, Petty TL. Results of a comprehensive rehabilitation program for severe COPD. In: Petty TL. Chronic Obstructive Pulmonary Disease. New York: Marcel Dekker, Inc., 1978.
5. Fishman DB, Petty TL. Physical symptomatic and psychological improvement in patients receiving comprehensive care for chronic airway obstruction. J Chron Dis 1971; 24:775–785.

Chapter 38

The Proprietary Pulmonary Rehabilitation Program

FRANK D. SUTTON, M.D.

In its widest application, rehabilitation has been known to be of great social, economic, and medical benefit. Pulmonary rehabilitation has been documented to improve lifestyle and activity levels, to have enormous educational value for patients and families, and to reduce morbidity and the frequency of hospitalization. Insurers have slowly become believers in the rehabilitation of patients with chronic disease, who can be improved yet not "fixed" or cured. Naturally, the last to accept and fund effective cardiac and pulmonary rehabilitation has been Medicare. Requirements and standards are, however, sufficiently clearly and strictly defined as to be of general benefit to those interested in establishing a proprietary outpatient pulmonary rehabilitation program. This appendix has been prepared with this perspective, and it is hoped that it will be informative and encourage others to continue efforts to help their patients return to a more normal and healthy lifestyle.

BACKGROUND

After more than a decade of effort by the National Association of Rehabilitation Facilities (NARF), Section 933 of the Omnibus Reconciliation Act of 1980 (P.L. 96–499) was passed. This act established comprehensive outpatient rehabilitation facilities (CORFs) as Medicare providers.

Since the advent of the Medicare program in 1965, services have been covered under the Supplemental Medical Insurance Program (Part B) when they were provided by hospitals either on an inpatient or outpatient basis. However, the same services have not been covered when they were provided by a freestanding outpatient facility. Formerly, outpatient facilities were limited to providing only a portion of physical and speech therapy services to Medicare recipients. Section 933 did not add new benefits to Medicare but simply permitted these benefits to be received in another setting. A full range of services were covered, including physician's services, physical and occupational therapy, speech pathology services, respiratory therapy services, prosthetic and orthotic services, social and psychologic services, nursing care, and drugs, biologicals, oxygen supplies, appliances, and equipment medically necessary and ordinarily provided by rehabilitation facilities.

The inclusion of these "services" naturally required the recruitment of a wide variety of health care professionals who could coordinate the care of disabled, deconditioned, and debilitated individuals with a wide variety of diagnoses. Thus, both cardiac and pulmonary rehabilitation now had access to alternative, out-of-hospital sites where they could follow a truly multidisciplinary approach to care. For example, the elderly patient with combined heart and lung disease who had an orthopedic injury could be referred to a CORF for physical therapy until he or she was sufficiently mobile to be studied by a pulmonologist or cardiologist to determine whether a prescription for an approved 8- to 12-week fully monitored and supervised exercise rehabilitation program should be implemented.

The advent of diagnostic-related groups, the aging of the population of the United States, and consumer awareness of exercise and preventive measures combined with the experience of business and industry in salvaging workers previously disabled by heart disease, lung disease, or both, have helped establish a clear market for the comprehensive outpatient rehabilitation center. Cost savings of approximately $14 for every $1 spent on rehabilitation were another important factor in the transfer of health care services to facilities that have the additional attractions of an upbeat atmosphere away from the "dreaded" hospital, level parking, single-story access, and assured insurance coverage as well as the use of lower cost facilities and the absence of the economic restraints of diagnostic-related groups.

Although the final regulations for CORFs were not completed until late in 1983, as of May 1986, 89 facilities had been certified as CORFs, and requests for certification from another 100 facilities were pending in regional offices.

CERTIFICATION OF COMPREHENSIVE OUTPATIENT REHABILITATION FACILITIES under the Medicare Act, Section 1861 (cc) Title XVIII, Social Security Act (42 US 1395x)

Any facility seeking to become a CORF first must thoroughly review the statute and regulations[1] to be certain that it meets all requirements. The law states that at a minimum a facility must:

1. primarily engage in the provision of diagnostic, therapeutic, and restorative services (by or under the supervision of physicians) on an outpatient basis for the rehabilitation of injured, disabled, or sick persons;
2. at least provide the services of physicians who are available at the facility on a full-time or part-time basis; physical therapy; and social or psychologic services;
3. maintain clinical records on all patients;
4. have policies established by a group of professionals who are associated with the facility, including one or more physicians who govern the comprehensive outpatient rehabilitation services furnished, and provide for the carrying out of these policies by a full- or part-time physician, referred to in paragraph (B)(i) of the law;
5. ensure that every patient has been referred by and is under the care of a physician;
6. comply with state or local laws that provide for the licensing of facilities of this nature;
7. have in effect a utilization review plan that is in accordance with regulations prescribed by the Secretary;
8. have in effect an overall plan and budget; and
9. meet such other conditions of participation as the Secretary may find necessary in the interest of the health and safety of individuals who are furnished services by such facilities, including conditions concerning the professional qualifications of personnel in these facilities.

Before proceeding with the application process, a facility must also check with the state agency responsible for the state health plan and certificate of need (CON) program to determine if a CON is required for a CORF. Some states do not require a CON for a CORF, whereas others do. For example, California requires a CON for outpatient rehabilitation centers. However, in Pennsylvania, whether a CON is required by a CORF is a function of its corporate structure. If a CORF is being established "by or on behalf of an existing health care facility," the state department of health requires that a letter be sent to it that outlines the plan for the facility; the department of health then determines if CON review is required. Tennessee also requires a CON for "rehabilitation facilities" and "all outpatient facilities" not otherwise excluded as private professional practices.

Finally, if a hospital is considering establishing a CORF, it should perform a complete financial analysis of the advantages and disadvantages of being a certified CORF or of simply modifying its outpatient department. However, a hospital *is not* paid for social services or nursing or counseling services as are CORFs. Rehabilitation services rendered by hospitals on an outpatient basis are covered as "medical and other health services" under 42 CFR 405.231.[1]

THE REVIEW PROCESS

Although the Joint Commission on Accreditation of Health Care Organizations has no jurisdiction over outpatient rehabilitation facilities, the Health Care Financing Administration nonetheless requires ongoing medical review of claims "to assure that all services provided by the CORF are required because the beneficiary needs skilled rehabilitation services."[1]

Thus, all claims are reviewed as submitted, and periodic on-site inspections of facilities are carried out by the Commission on Accreditation of Rehabilitation Facilities.[2] This agency has a lengthy check list to ensure that:

1. the patient is physician-referred;
2. a physician or physicians are provided for medical direction of the CORF and that all treatment plans are reviewed at least every 60 days by this physician or these physicians;
3. the staff is fully certified or accredited in their area of care or are graduates of a program accredited by The American Medical Association (e.g., in occupational therapy);
4. specific written requirements for entrance/admission are met;
5. policies and procedures are established that ensure that the services provided to each patient are coordinated and integrated and address defined goals;
6. services are not continued once a functional plateau has been achieved by the patient and no evidence of continuing functional improvement is apparent;
7. progress is evaluated on a weekly basis (e.g., at staff

conferences), with timely mid-term reports and conclusive reports sent to the referring physician; and
8. a follow-up plan is established prior to discharge.

REIMBURSEMENT

The majority of third party insurers exclusive of Medicare recognize and reimburse pulmonary rehabilitation, including the associated diagnostic testing (e.g., metabolic stress testing, exercise gas exchange assessment, pulmonary function testing, and exercise electrocardiograms) even when such testing is done at the rehabilitation center.

Medicare, however, reimburses only 80% of the charges directly related to the program, including those for oxygen and inhaled bronchodilator therapy. It does not reimburse for procedures that are deemed "diagnostic" and, therefore, best delivered in the hospital or physician's office prior to referral to the program. During the Medicare review procedure, if documentation is either missing or questionable in that (1) it is not clear why the patient was referred; (2) the description of therapy is limited or absent; (3) therapy is not being delivered by skilled nurses (i.e., registered nurses or licensed practical nurses) or respiratory therapists; (4) the program is continued after a functional plateau has been achieved; or (5) the patient fails to show achievement with respect to his or her treatment goals; then "reasonable costs" are adjusted downward to below the 80% reimbursement level or are rejected entirely. An appeal can then be initiated; the appeal process almost always requires direct physician involvement if the adjustment or rejection has been capricious.

PROGRAM EXPERIENCE IN BIRMINGHAM, ALABAMA

HealthSouth Rehabilitation Corporation is a Birmingham-based company that provides one of the nation's largest networks of comprehensive medical rehabilitation services in 22 states. Forty-three of their fifty-four facilities are outpatient centers and are qualified as CORFs. Pulmonary rehabilitation programs were among the initial services designed and operated in many of the company's first facilities, which were built in the mid-1980s. The program description that follows is based on the experience of one of HealthSouth's center's in Birmingham, Alabama, and reflects proprietary pulmonary rehabilitation conducted under CORF guidelines. This description satisfies a wide variety of payers, including Medicare.

Referral Criteria

A licensed physician in the state of record was required to refer the patient with historical documentation of the following:

1. dyspnea on effort,
2. limitation of activity level,
3. desire for rehabilitation, and
4. proven or suspected static or dynamic lung function abnormalities.

Testing

Simple spirometry or a full pulmonary profile either accompanied the patient referral or was performed at the rehabilitation center. If no exercise data was provided on referral, the Medical Director for pulmonary rehabilitation or the referring physician performed one of three entry exercise studies to

1. assess functional capacity;
2. determine the presence of exercise-related arrhythmia, hypertension, signs of myocardial ischemia, or any combination of these; and
3. determine the presence of exercise-related hypoxemia, hypercarbia, right-sided heart strain, or any combination of these.

If a patient had mild pulmonary function abnormalities, a simple metabolic stress test with oximetry was performed to determine maximum oxygen consumption, maximum minute ventilation, and oxygen pulse, double product, and saturation.

Patients with moderately severe* obstructive or restrictive ventilatory abnormalities were uniformly studied using metabolic stress testing employing an indwelling arterial line. Such testing was also performed on patients with severe functional abnormalities who were not significantly hypoxic (i.e., they had a PaO_2 greater than 60 mm Hg) at rest and who had an FEV_1 greater than 600 ml. Both program entry test data and exit test data were obtained; consecutive results of the first 202 patients were recorded and analyzed and are shown in Tables 38–1 and 38–2.

Patients with an FEV_1 of less than 600 ml or resting hypoxemia underwent graded exercise testing with electrocardiography and oximetry while receiving oxygen sufficient to raise their resting PaO_2 to approximately 75 mm Hg.

Prescription

All patients received a total of 36 hours of aerobic exercise training (3 sessions/wk). Sessions were fully supervised with cardiac monitoring if the need was indicated by the testing physician. Oxygen supplementation during exercise allowed 22 patients to be effec-

---

Moderately severe obstruction is defined as the presence of a forced expiratory capacity in 1 second (FEV_1) of less than 2.5 L but greater than 1.0 L; *moderately severe restriction* is defined as the presence of a forced vital capacity (FVC) that is less than 60% but greater than 40% of predicted. In contrast, *severe obstruction* is characterized by an FEV_1 less than 1.0 L with or without hypoxemia, and *severe restriction* is characterized by an FVC of 40% of predicted or less.

tively rehabilitated; 7 of these patients were able to discontinue oxygen use before completion of the 12-week program.

Classroom instructors worked with patients for a minimum of 1 hour per week to inform patients about:

1. airway anatomy and physiology;
2. energy conservation techniques and proper nutrition;
3. body mechanics and diaphragmatic strengthening exercises;
4. the management of airway secretions;
5. pursed-lip breathing and panic control;
6. the proper use of oral and nebulized/aerosolized bronchodilators;
7. the timely use of steroids, antibiotics, and mucolytics;
8. travel arrangements; and
9. stress, sexuality, and chronic disease.

Vital signs and baseline oxygen saturation were checked prior to each class, and repeat measurement of blood pressure, pulse, and oxygen saturation was performed at peak exercise workloads. Symptoms were also assessed briefly every week. No patients who continued to smoke were allowed to enter the program. Unless the testing physician specifically limited exercise time or pulse rate, all patients started with 2 to 5 minutes of exercise with 2 minutes of rest and progressed individually using six work stations until they were exercising at 80 to 85% of the heart rate achieved in the graded exercise test, which usually corresponded to 70 to 80% of maximum oxygen consumption.

Results

Total exercise time per session was able to be advanced progressively to 30 minutes in over 90% of all

TABLE 38–1. 202 CONSECUTIVE PATIENTS, BIRMINGHAM'S HEALTHSOUTH CORF: CHANGES IN TREADMILL PERFORMANCE BEFORE VERSUS AFTER REHABILITATION PROGRAM

	COPD	CRPD	Mixed COPD and CRPD
Mean Age (y)	64.4	57.1	63.8
% Δ TT			
Female	70.3 (80.1)	46.0 (45.7)	82.5 (96.5)
Male	64.9 (137.3)	37.9 (36.9)	85.4 (91.8)
		$P < .0001$*	
DP			
Pretreatment	20067	20709	20770
Post-treatment	18015	17467	18248
		$P < .002$	
% Δ $\dot{V}O_2$ max			
Female	8.90 (23.01)	7.25 (21.96)	9.25 (23.46)
Male	8.17 (19.05)	5.25 (10.66)	32.27 (33.04)
		$P = NS$	

*Significance of changes produced by rehabilitation judged by MANOVA analysis.
Key: COPD: Chronic obstructive pulmonary disease; CRPD: Chronic restrictive pulmonary disease; %Δ TT: Per cent change in total treadmill time; DP: Double product, peak pulse × peak systolic blood pressure (mm Hg × beats/min); %Δ$\dot{V}O_2$max: Per cent changes in maximum oxygen consumption. Values in parentheses are ±1 standard deviation.

TABLE 38–2. 202 CONSECUTIVE PATIENTS, BIRMINGHAM'S HEALTHSOUTH CORF: PULMONARY FUNCTION AND OXIMETRY RESULTS BEFORE AND AFTER REHABILITATION PROGRAM

	COPD	CRPD	Mixed COPD and CRPD
FEV_1 (L)			
Pretreatment	1.42 (0.74)	1.85 (0.65)	1.45 (0.75)
Post-treatment	1.44 (0.77)	1.84 (0.66)	1.48 (0.77)
Δ	0.02	−0.01	0.03
FVC (L)			
Pretreatment	2.52 (0.88)	2.40 (0.99)	2.25 (0.87)
Post-treatment	2.52 (0.84)	2.34 (0.99)	2.29 (0.90)
Δ	0.0	−0.06	0.04
Oxygen Saturation (%)			
Pretreatment	92.3 (4.9)	92.0 (5.6)	92.4 (4.7)
Post-treatment	92.1 (5.0)	91.4 (7.2)	90.3 (6.4)
Δ	−0.2	−0.6	−0.1

Values in parentheses are ±1 standard deviation; none of the changes produced by rehabilitation is significant by MANOVA analysis.

patients participating in the program. Work stations included a rowing machine, arm crank machine, stairs, exercycle, treadmill, and track.

Personal activity goals set at the beginning of the program were met by 94% of the participants. Ten per cent of the patients had delays of at least 1 week in the program because of intercurrent medical illness, and only 4% did not complete the 12-week program as outlined.

Fifty patients were followed to obtain repeat exercise data 1 year after the program; all of these patients had been prescribed a home program and had been encouraged to "stay active and in shape." One of these patients was hospitalized for carotid artery surgery, one for coronary artery bypass grafting, and three for exacerbations of their lung disease, with these last three having a mean hospitalization time of 3 days in the year of follow-up.

As seen in Table 38–1, patients with all forms of lung disease—obstructive, restrictive, and mixed obstructive and restrictive—can be effectively rehabilitated, with improvement in activity levels, exercise treadmill time, and double product and a trend toward improvement in maximum oxygen uptake. In keeping with a large body of literature, these changes occur without a significant change in static pulmonary function (Table 38–2); however, they do have a beneficial effect on patient oxygen use and personal independence and facilitate a lifestyle that leads to a decrease in morbidity and the amount of time spent in hospitals.

Summary

Reimbursement for pulmonary rehabilitation is currently better than that for cardiac rehabilitation in many states. In the HealthSouth program, private insurers paid over 90% of billed charges incurred over a 5-year period, and Medicare paid a full 80% on greater than 95% of submitted claims. Both private insurers and Medicare did allow pre-entry or baseline exercise testing and spirometry to be done at the rehabilitation center in Alabama but denied requests for payment of any testing except simple spirometry at the conclusion of the program. This seems incongruous, since the medical literature clearly indicates that factors other than static pulmonary function should be tested and should show improvement from rehabilitative efforts in patients with lung disease. Despite established guidelines, reimbursement may vary from state to state, depending on the Medicare intermediary, and information regarding reimbursement should be individually determined by submission of a certification and funding request from locale to locale for a proprietary, comprehensive outpatient facility.

REFERENCES

1. Comprehensive Outpatient Rehabilitation Facilities: The New Medicare Providers. National Association of Rehabilitation Facilities, Washington, D.C., June 1986.
2. Standards Manual for Organizations Serving People with Disabilities. Alabama State Board of Health, Bureau of Licensure and Certification, Chapter 420-5-11, Accreditation of Rehabilitation Facilities, Montgomery, Alabama, June 1990.

Chapter 39

How the Office-based Pulmonary Rehabilitation Program Works

HOWARD M. KRAVETZ, M.D., F.C.C.P.

"To preserve a man alive in the midst of so many diseases and hostilities, is as great a miracle as to create him."

Jeremy Taylor, M.D., 1774

This chapter is intended to provide a working model for an office-based pulmonary rehabilitation program operated by a pulmonologist working alone or by a small specialty practice. A front office person and a nurse can work together with a physician as a team that is able to deliver a fully functional pulmonary rehabilitation program on a day-to-day basis. This primary unit can be expanded to include all of the other members of a traditional pulmonary rehabilitation team, but only as dictated by the needs of the patient population and community setting of the practice. In this manner, effective long-term rehabilitation can be provided by the members of a basic outpatient unit in a simple and cost-effective environment.

Pulmonary rehabilitation involves strong commitments from both chronic obstructive pulmonary disease (COPD) patients and health care providers. If you wish to develop an office-based pulmonary rehabilitation program for your practice, it is best to incorporate rehabilitation into the acute and chronic care of your patients from the beginning. In a private practice setting, pulmonary rehabilitation should be an important component of each office visit. Patients can be conditioned to expect rehabilitation as a part of office visits and of their home routine.

In our model, initiation of an office-based pulmonary rehabilitation program begins when the patient first contacts the practice. Brochures, booklets, and questionnaires that are sent to patients emphasize that the practice is committed to improving their health through education and exercise as well as by means of more conventional treatments. Since the pulmonologist usually represents the "last court of appeals" for many COPD patients, a detailed general medical questionnaire is sent to patients before their first visit. The brochures, booklets, literature, and the questionnaire provide a starting point for patients to learn that all aspects of their health are involved in the rehabilitative process.

In the model program described here, the first office visit is with a nurse. During this visit, the patient's answers to the questionnaire are reviewed, and a basic database is established with results from routine blood work (complete blood count and SMAC), urinalysis, radiography, chest electrocardiography, appropriate skin tests for granulomatous disease, pulmonary function testing, and arterial blood gas analysis. This first visit usually takes 1 to 1½ hours of a nurse's time. The nurse also explains to patients how the next visit with the physician and the rehabilitation program will be conducted.

The next 1½-hour appointment is with the physician. During this visit, a history is abstracted from the questionnaire with help from the patient and, perhaps, from a spouse. A complete physical exam is given, and the previously obtained laboratory data are reviewed with the patient. From all of the information collected, the physician formulates a working diagnosis, treatment plan, and exercise prescription for the patient in a stable condition. For the acutely ill patient, the severely malnourished patient, or the severely depressed patient, the rehabilitative process is delayed.

If clinically appropriate, between the first and second visits to the physician, patients undergo an exercise oxygen evaluation on a treadmill to determine whether oxygen is needed during exercise. The measurement of distance covered and oxygen required during a 12-minute walking test provides the basis for the initial exercise prescription. Digital blood pressure units enable the staff to monitor blood pressures while patients are in motion. A basic, handheld oximeter provides exercise oxygen data.

Three months later, patients are retested to determine whether they still need supplemental oxygen. This makes possible an objective comparison between the patient's initial and present status. The physician can then determine whether each patient is capable of walking an increased distance as a result of the exercise program.

A large room (e.g., 12 ft × 15 ft) can be converted into an exercise room. Exercise room equipment includes a treadmill to conduct the 12-minute walking test, which evaluates the patients' need for oxygen and helps them realize that they can walk, if only at a slow pace.

> "Few people know how to take a walk. The qualifications . . . are endurance, plain clothes, old shoes, an eye for nature, good humor, vast curiosity, good speech, good silence, and nothing too much."
> Ralph Waldo Emerson, 1803–1882

Each patient is given a walking log or diary, a list of exercise tips, and a suggested walking schedule that establishes realistic goals. (If patients are chair-bound or bed-bound, an excellent reference is Bob Anderson's book *Stretching*. The book explains stretching, strengthening, and flexibility exercises for the patient who is not ready to walk.) Patients are encouraged to walk on a daily basis, either by themselves or with a spouse or special friend, a dog, a neighbor, or someone from a list of walking partners in their neighborhood. They are also encouraged to join a Brisk Walking Group in their community. Such groups are often sponsored by city programs, YWCAs and YMCAs, shopping malls, and other organizations specifically designed to offer various kinds of walking experiences. The organized hospital rehabilitation programs or storefront programs are usually oriented toward the use of specific exercise equipment and structured, timed exercise. Our model program focuses more on mileage or on the distances achieved. Typical walking parameters for patients without acute problems are 1/4 mile per day (even if they are using oxygen), with the goal of walking up to 1 mile per day by the end of 4 weeks. Eventually, patients should be encouraged to walk 3 to 4 miles per day, even if they need 3 to 4 months to reach this goal. Suggested routes with mileage distances are provided by the physician's office. For example, three times around the town square might equal 1 mile; alternatively, four circuits of a middle school track might also equal 1 mile.

At the next visit (usually after 1–3 wk), the physician reviews the patient's progress, assesses the walking log, and encourages even minimal gain in strength and endurance. Some perspective is important here. The total distance walked during the 1 to 3 weeks may only be a couple of miles. However, when considered from the viewpoint that the patient was formerly confined to his or her house and inactive and had only sporadic exercise, the daily walking regimen is a major first step in a return to a more active lifestyle. Patients are praised for their efforts and accomplishments. They are also encouraged to treat themselves to a good pair of walking shoes and clothing appropriate for this kind of routine. On subsequent visits, a portion of the medication summary always includes a review of the exercise program. Patients are advised that in the event of bad weather they are not to stop exercising; instead, they should be prepared to walk in the house, a supermarket, a shopping mall, or the local YMCA. At times, we suggest that an exercycle, such as a Schwinn Airdyne, be rented or purchased. The purchase of a treadmill is discouraged because of expense and boredom and because it does not exercise the upper body.

Involvement in walking programs can take many forms. Some organized walking groups invite patients to walk with them on special occasions. Physicians and nurses can invite patients to go along with them on personalized group walks. Bird-watching groups, such as the Audubon Society, can serve those who desire a more leisurely walk. These kinds of experiences not only keep patients interested but also keep them in contact with healthy people and involved in their community.

Following the second visit with the physician, the educational segment of the office-based rehabilitation program is begun after normal office hours. Generally speaking, such a program consists of 1-hour sessions that are conducted two times per week for 6 weeks. The program is part of a continuous lecture-discussion series that allows patients to enter the cycle at any time. Topics that are covered in this series include medications, the use of oxygen and aerosol devices, the use of home exercise equipment, chest physiotherapy at home, energy-saving techniques and devices, home physical therapy for flexibility and strengthening, psychosocial adaptation to chronic disease, nutrition, and travel. In addition to the physician and the office staff, community people can also be used as resources; they might include social service workers (from hospitals or social service agencies), occupational therapists (from hospitals or private practices), pharmacists, respiratory therapists (from hospitals or private practices), patient-teachers (explained later in this chapter), "telephone tree" volunteers, and aerobic instructors.

In a typical small community, a office-based pulmonary rehabilitation program might enlist the support of local resources, such as the county or city health department (to provide nutritional counseling), public or private adult centers (to provide classroom space or space indoors for brisk walking in inclement weather), local social service agencies (to provide financial assistance or service information and referral), YMCAs or YWCAs (to provide an adult exercise program), a local hospital (to provide classrooms or an adult fitness program), local schools (to provide track and gym facilities or classrooms in the evening), or the American Lung Association (to provide educational materials). The booklets "Help Yourself to Better Breathing" and "The Asthma Handbook," which are both published by the American Lung Association, are used as informal texts for the program.

Once the educational component of the program is completed, patients can be introduced to a volunteer "patient-teacher" who has gone through the rehabilitation process for 6 months to 1 year. Such a patient is recognized for his or her successes with exercise and rehabilitation, but most of all for his or her obvious enthusiasm. The patient-teachers are informal mentors who can give help and informal counseling and can "coach" their "students" through difficult times during their treatment program. Collectively, they can serve as an informal support network. Health care professionals are resources for more technical information. It is important to note that if a patient must be admitted to a hospital for an acute problem, some of these professionals (e.g., pharmacists, respiratory therapists, social workers, physical therapists, and occupational therapists) are a part of the hospital treatment team. Thus, the same person who taught the patient in evening educational sessions is also involved in his or her hospital care.

In our model program, patients are usually seen by the physician once per month for 3 months, and then once every 3 months on an ongoing basis. Keeping the patient involved and encouraged between office visits can be a problem. This problem can be solved by newsletters aimed at keeping patients informed and interested in their rehabilitation program. Awards for walking certain distances, such as certificates, pins, T-shirts, magazine subscriptions, books, pedometers, and walking sticks, make patients feel good about themselves and the progress they make in walking and exercise. Support groups and patient-teachers can help patients feel that they do not have to deal with their pulmonary problems alone. Other patients can call sicker patients in a "telephone tree" system to check on their well-being and progress and to lessen feelings of depression and isolation.

SPACE

With careful planning, even a relatively small setting (1000–1500 ft^2) can accommodate an office-based pulmonary rehabilitation program. Space can often be used for multiple purposes.

For example, a reception area can be used for small classes. In our office-based program, the reception area not only doubles as a classroom but also contains a small but well-used patient library operated on the honor system. The shelves are filled with books on walking, exercising, nutrition, humor, and philosophic approaches to chronic diseases.

A large treatment room is used as an audiovisual viewing room (for video and slide presentations), a place where pamphlets and booklets are read, and a place to demonstrate the various kinds of aerosol equipment and oxygen.

Examination room walls are used to exhibit photographs of patients engaged in various activities, such as walking, bicycling, exercising, horseback riding, and swimming. The purpose of this is to demonstrate to new patients models of a more active lifestyle.

If the office site permits, a small outdoor walking course could be constructed at a modest cost; such a course might incorporate some existing walkways and paths. Rest stations could be designed and outfitted with simple sturdy outdoor benches. High school tracks, tennis courts, shopping malls, and parking lots located in close proximity to an office site can also serve as level areas for patients to walk.

REIMBURSEMENT AND FUNDING SOURCES

The reimbursement and cost effectiveness of any office-based pulmonary rehabilitation program have become a paramount issue in the care of patients with chronic pulmonary disease. A primary assumption that must be made is that such a program is *not* a "money maker." Medicare and most third-party payers are not yet ready to reimburse services provided by office-based pulmonary rehabilitation programs.

The easiest and least frustrating way to fund a rehabilitation program in the office setting is to incorporate the rehabilitation concept in the initial evaluation of every patient and at each succeeding visit. For example, if regular office visits are 30 minutes long, perhaps 5 to 10 minutes can be devoted to the discussion of rehabilitation and exercise. Thus, charges can be interwoven into the regular office visit. Charges for spirometry, arterial blood gas analysis, and oxygen evaluations with exercise are billed as separate procedures.

There are several other approaches that may be used to help fund an office-based pulmonary rehabilitation program. Creativity should be used to develop approaches that are most applicable to individual practices. For example, a not-for-profit foundation might be established. Such a foundation can be used (1) for payment of professional teachers in the lecture/discussion component, (2) to subsidize the activities of the support group, (3) to purchase educational materials, (4) to produce or publish audiovisual teaching materials, (5) to underwrite free group forums, (6) to subsidize scholarships to train patient-teachers and health care professionals to increase their effectiveness with patients in an outpatient setting, (7) to purchase equipment for an exercise room, and (8) to sponsor special activities such as outings and social events.

Certain professionals can help such organizations to comply with Internal Revenue Service requirements and develop the necessary not-for-profit structure. Be advised that not-for-profit foundations require nurturing and time from you and your staff. If possible, patients and their spouses can be asked to assume major or supportive roles in establishing and maintaining a foundation. Ideally, these people are included on the Board of Directors.

Patients and their families should be made aware that

the not-for-profit foundation welcomes contributions in the form of cash, trusts, and memorial contributions. Contribution information may be given directly in a description of the foundation or put in a special publication that explains the benefits and tax advantages of making such contributions, both to the foundation or rehabilitation program and to patients and their families. Most professional charitable fund raisers can assist with the legality and the language of your appeal.

Direct educational grants can be solicited from pharmaceutical companies. The budgets of such companies often include monies earmarked for this purpose. Requests for funding should be well conceived and well communicated, as companies direct funds to where they feel they will be best used.

While not bringing in direct revenue, free group forums, which might be conducted by the physician, office staff, and community resource people, generate support and goodwill for the foundation. Held every 2 to 3 months, these forums are open to all patients in the practice and to the community. Such forums explain the rehabilitation concept, serve as educational tools, and generate interest in the foundation.

SUMMARY

In today's rapidly changing medical world, office-based pulmonary rehabilitation provides a new dimension for enhanced patient care. This approach to rehabilitation is in its infancy and is not, at the present time, acknowledged or accepted by third-party payers. It is open to each clinician's experimentation and creativity. The ideas suggested here have been tested in real life but are still only suggestions. The greatest source of information on program development, resources, and sources of revenue can come from your own patient population. These patients have lived with their disease for many years and often know what they need and want in order to return to a more normal lifestyle and how to get it.

Office-based pulmonary rehabilitation is challenging if it is done on a day-to-day basis. If you want to prevent the so-called "burn-out" syndrome, give office-based pulmonary rehabilitation a try.

> I would rather be ashes than dust,
> I would rather my spark should burn out in a brilliant blaze
> Than it should be stifled in dry-rot.
>
> I would rather be a superb meteor,
> Every atom of me in magnificent glow,
> Than a sleepy and permanent planet.
>
> Man's chief purpose is to live, not to exist.
> I shall not waste my days trying to prolong them.
> I shall use my time.
>
> Jack London, 1876–1916

Chapter 40

Reimbursement for a Community Hospital-Based Program

R. WAYNE MALL, M.D.
MARGARET MEDERIOS, R.C.P.

Pulmonary rehabilitation (PR) provides patients with individualized instruction and training to reduce and control the symptoms of pulmonary disease and to make possible the performance of daily activities within the limitations of disease. Many components of a typical PR program are reimbursable under the Medicare insurance program.

Because of the disability and age of most PR patients, Medicare is the usual insurance carrier. PR is also covered by many private insurance carriers, although some carriers require prior authorization. The cost savings of PR can be reported when documenting the medical necessity in a prior authorization request. Many Health Maintenance Organizations (HMOs) cover costs when they are associated with services provided by a contracting hospital. PR is not a benefit provided by some insurance carriers, including Medi-Cal in California.

As fiscal intermediary for Medicare, Blue Cross of California has developed PR guidelines based on Medicare policy and California state law. It should be noted, however, that there may be variations in the interpretation of Medicare policy by other fiscal intermediaries across the nation. At Blue Cross of California, physical therapy, occupational therapy, and respiratory therapy consultants review the documentation within the outpatient medical records and use the PR guidelines to evaluate the services provided to Medicare beneficiaries. The PR documentation should show that the services rendered are tailored to the individual's specific needs, are reasonable and necessary for his or her diagnosis, reflect individualized goals that can be accomplished in a predictable amount of time, and are a benefit of the Medicare insurance program.

Several technical errors occur routinely; so that such errors can be avoided, certain guidelines should be followed. First, since physician orders must be complete and specific, a blanket order for PR or as-needed care is not acceptable. Orders need to match the specific services rendered. All orders and certifications must be signed and dated by the physician; a physician's signature stamp is not valid. Second, all daily notes of the physical therapy or occupational therapy aides must be cosigned by the licensed clinician, as required by state law. Third, the itemized services billed on the financial ledger must match the daily documentation. Finally, services rendered must be a benefit of the Medicare insurance program. For example, biofeedback for relaxation training is not reimbursable because it is not a medicare benefit. Other services (e.g., nutritional counseling, social services, physician or pharmacist lectures, team conferences, documentation time, and discharge summary) are not specifically stated as Part B Medicare benefits and therefore are considered administrative functions. Bills for these services should not be submitted for reimbursement.

The fiscal intermediary evaluates the claim for medical necessity. A reviewer looks for documentation that reflects that services are individualized, reasonable, and necessary; that services provided are of a skilled level of care and not of a maintenance nature; that delineation of services rendered is evident in multidisciplinary programs (i.e., there is no duplication of services); and that the patient has rehabilitation potential.

The treatment, activity, or instruction provided must be tailored to the individual's needs and directly related to the specific problems identified in the assessment. The established treatment plan should be flexible to meet individual needs, and the plan should be modified as necessary.

Documented progress toward the stated goals should be seen in a reasonable and predictable amount of time. If the patient is at the same functional level week after week, then progress has not been shown, and care is considered to be of a maintenance nature. Also, if progress is made in a "sawtooth pattern," (i.e., gains are seen only while the patient is with the clinician), but the patient is unable to sustain these gains between sessions, then no overall improvement is realized, and again, the care is considered maintenance therapy. Services for a chronic baseline condition in which the patient is stable are also considered maintenance care (e.g., if a patient with chronic bronchitis has finished a PR program and is still in need of bronchodilators, it is not reasonable for a therapist to continue to administer them). Many PR programs utilize a multidisciplinary approach and employ registered nurses, respiratory therapists, physical therapists, and occupational therapists, or any combination of these. A duplication of services occurs when more than one provider administers similar care when a single service could provide the care. For example, if the occupational therapy program is only for upper extremity exercises and these exercises are not related to functional activity training unique to occupational therapy and if the physical therapy program consists of lower extremity exercises and treadmill use, then only the physical therapy program would be covered because the physical therapy is able to provide upper extremity exercises as well. If, however, the occupational therapist's program, the physical therapist's program, and the respiratory therapist's program all include compensatory breathing techniques related to their own area of expertise (i.e., occupational therapy with activities of daily living, physical therapy with exercises, and respiratory therapy with medications), then there is no duplication of services, as each program reflects the unique skills of the individual therapists. This is critical in establishing that services provided by various disciplines are necessary and distinct from one another.

During the initial assessment, many problems may be identified that indicate whether a person is a poor candidate for rehabilitation. These problems may include low motivation, poor memory, medical complications, and an unwillingness to be committed to the program and to the changes that are required. Some patients may warrant a brief trial in rehabilitation, but this should be discontinued if they prove to be poor rehabilitation candidates.

Once the provider understands how the medical review process proceeds and that the medical records are used to determine medical necessity, then it is clear how valuable the provider's documentation becomes. It is essential to note that the format in which the documentation is written is not as important as the content of what is documented. The entire PR team is responsible for compiling a complete medical record that (1) documents clearly the rationale for skilled intervention and the progress toward individualized goals and that (2) meets the technical requirements for full Medicare reimbursement.

DOCUMENTATION GUIDELINES

The PR programs must be under the supervision and guidance of a physician to qualify for Medicare reimbursement. This means that the initial referral or order for PR services must also come from a physician. A specific order includes the treatment, instruction, procedure, or activity to be performed and the frequency and duration of the service.

A physician's certification is also required for physical therapy and occupational therapy services. After receiving a specific order, each clinician must document a clear, concise, and objective record of the patient's problems. The problems identified should be as specific and measurable as possible. An example of the explanation of a problem might be the following: "Patient was interviewed regarding aerosol medications (meds). Patient using metered-dose inhaler (MDI) with Proventil and Vanceril. Patient demonstrated poor technique using MDI with placebo. Patient knew 'heart problems' could result from his meds, but was unable to recognize complications that may occur." Another clinician assessing the same patient may document the following problems: "(1) Endurance limited to ambulation (amb) on treadmill (TM) at 1.0 mph for 5 min with 8/10 shortness of breath (SOB) level; (2) inefficient breathing pattern (3:1) and excessive use of accessory muscles during amb; and (3) absence of home exercise program to maintain fitness." Both examples show clear problems that are appropriate for skilled intervention.

Individualized treatment goals are then established to address the problems identified. The goals need to be as objective, measurable, and functional as possible. An example of appropriate goals related to the first set of problems identified might state the following: "(1) Patient to demonstrate appropriate technique for use of MDI; and (2) patient to identify complications of Proventil/Vanceril and the signs that would indicate their occurrence." A sample of goals related to the second set of problems identified might state: "(1) Amb on TM at 2.0 mph at 0% grade × 20 min with 2/10 SOB utilizing compensatory breathing techniques; and (2) patient will incorporate home exercise program into daily routine."

It is clear that these goals are individualized to the specific problems identified initially. They are written objectively and functionally so that it is an easy task to detect in the daily documentation whether progress is being made toward accomplishing the goals.

An individualized treatment plan to accomplish goals should then be established along with an anticipated overall frequency and duration of service. This reflects that the program is tailored to meet the individual's specific needs. Using the previous examples, the first clinician might establish the following as part of his or her plan of treatment: "(1) Instruction in proper use of MDI; and (2) instruction in recognition of complications of Vanceril and Proventil," whereas the second clinician might establish a plan as follows: "(1) TM exercise training using compensatory breathing techniques; and (2) instruction in home exercise program." Whether a registered nurse or respiratory therapist establishes this treatment plan or whether the physician has written a specific plan of treatment that differs from the recommendations of the clinician (registered nurse, respiratory therapist, physical therapist, or occupational therapist), the treatment plan must be signed by the physician before treatment is initiated (Fig. 40–1).

Once the specific problems, goals, and therapeutic plan of treatment have been established, the treatment phase of PR begins. Documentation of each session is important to demonstrate progress toward the stated goals (Figs. 40–2 and 40–3). The daily documentation should reflect the individualized activity or instruction given and note the patient's response to the skilled service. The date and duration of the session must correspond to the itemized bill, and the clinician's signature must complete the record. An example of the daily documentation of one treatment session corresponding to the aforementioned problems, goals, and treatment plan is as follows: "6/17/88 — 45 min. Patient again demonstrated technique of MDI. Reminded to emphasize breathholding at end of inspiration. Patient now demonstrates proper MDI technique utilizing a spacer. Patient questioned about complications of meds and was able to answer all key questions. Weekly summary: This week, patient received instruction on proper MDI use and medication complications. Goals on MDI use and medication complications achieved. [signed] John Doe, Registered Clinician." With respect to the second example of problems and goals and adhering to the specific plan of treatment, documentation might be as follows: "6/17/88 — 30 min. S: Patient reports he has a stationary bike at home that he would like to incorporate into his exercise program. Patient reports increased endurance on home walking program to 1/4 mile twice each day, with SOB level decreased to 5/10. O: Patient ambulated on TM at 1.6 mph at 0% grade with 2 L of supplemental oxygen. Patient instructed in compensatory breathing techniques with amb. A: Patient required 50% verbal cuing with breathing techniques during amb. SOB level decreased to 4/10. Minimal accessory muscle use noted. P: Continue TM exercise and add bike ergometer next session. [Signed] Jane Doe, Skilled Clinician."

Notice how each example followed the documented plan of treatment. Both clinicians addressed the individual's specific problems and progress toward the goals established initially. The documentation states the treatment or activity rendered, the patient's response to the service, and the measurable progress made. It is important to note that the documentation does not have to follow any particular format (i.e., it can consist of a narrative, SOAP [subjective, objective, assessment, and plan] notes, grids, or flow sheets); however, it must reflect the content discussed earlier. The documentation also reflects an individualized program; this is necessary if Medicare coverage is sought, since prepackaged programs are not a benefit. The outpatient rehabilitation services are generally of an intermittent rather than a continuous nature because this allows for effective self-practice and carry-over of various learned techniques into each patient's own lifestyle.

If these guidelines are used for the initial assessment and for each daily session, then the fiscal intermediary's medical reviewers have a clear, accurate, objective, and concise picture of each patient's PR program. The reviewer is looking for complete records, demonstration of the need for skilled intervention, and the clinician's sound judgment and clinical reasoning when evaluating the billed charges.

The California Blue Cross concurrent review of outpatient PR services is presented in Figure 40–4.[1]

DOCUMENTATION OF PROGRESS

Documentation of all activities is required. Team conferences held at least biweekly should be documented. At these conferences, the patient's progress toward achieving his or her short-term goals should be assessed, and, if indicated, the patient's treatment plan should be modified to better achieve these goals.

LONG-TERM FOLLOW-UP

Ongoing care is generally the responsibility of the primary care physician. If the patient's condition changes, the physician may order additional retraining or new components of the program for the patient. Routine "screening" for possible needed care is not considered a Medicare program benefit.

BILLING

Each therapy session must be verifiable by documentation in the progress notes. Team conferences, family conferences, and mileage are not billable. Billing on the UB-82 billing form may be itemized by revenue code for each discipline or combined under revenue code 419. Refer to Bulletins 218 S–1 and 219 S–1 for other billing information.

A discharge summary of changes from start of care is required and not billable. Which goals were or were not achieved and why should be documented. A discharge plan should be recorded.

Outpatient physician certification for physical therapy and occupational therapy is required when billing for physical therapy (Revenue Code 420) or occupational therapy (Revenue Code 430) separately (see Bulletins 218 and 218 S–1).[2]

Name: _____ Tx Dx: _____ Onset: _____

Patient will come to pulmonary rehabilitation 2 to 3 times per week for 4 to 6 weeks approximately 2 hours at a time to a maximum of 12 sessions.

During this time the patient is to be demonstrated and instructed in the performance of proper breathing techniques in the following categories:

_____	Pursed lip breathing	_____	Diaphragmatic breathing
_____	Segmental breathing	_____	Basal expansion
_____	Breathless positions	_____	Panic control for fear of dyspnea
_____	Inspiratory Muscle Trainer	_____	Oxygen therapy

_____ Use of respiratory care equipment

_____ Proper use of medications

_____ Peak flow meter

_____ Proper and effective utilization of a bronchial hygiene therapy program, including: cough techniques, identification of signs of infection, and PD & P.

_____ Exercise of activities of daily living with breathing retraining and energy conservation.

_____ Physical conditioning program utilizing proper breathing techniques with mobility, strengthening exercises, and body mechanics for a home exercise program.

EXERCISE PRESCRIPTION:

1) _____ graded exercise
2) Symptom - limited maximal exercise
3) Monitor ECG: yes/no
4) Monitor O_2 saturation: yes/no
5) Exercise limited to THR of: _____
6) Exercise limited to: _____
7) _____

_____
Physician's Signature   Date

OUTPATIENT PULMONARY REHAB
PHYSICIAN'S ORDERS

FIGURE 40–1. An example of a form to be used for designing a patient's individualized treatment program.

ASSESSMENT:

Patient has moderate obstructive disease with an inefficient breathing pattern (3:2) and the moderate use of accessory muscles.

GOALS:

Patient is to demonstrate the basic proper breathing technique.

PLANS:

Patient is to be taught pursed lip, diaphragmatic, segmental breathing, and basal expansion.

Patient is to start on IMT at #1 x 15 minutes.

Date: _____   Total Tx Time: _____
       mm/dd/yy   minutes

Patient is instructed on the basic proper breathing techniques. Patient demonstrates average technique with diaphragmatic use, depth of excursion, strength of contraction, and coordination. Patient demonstrates average technique on the increase of segmental expansion. Demonstrates the moderate use of accessory muscles. Patient demonstrates pursed lip breathing with a pattern of (___ : ___) at rest. Patient will coordinate these breathing techniques with the exercise program. The verbal cuing percentage is documented daily. IMT at #1 x 15 minutes is to be used at home and prior to TM workouts.

_____
Signature   RCP

Weekly Summary: _____
_____
_____
_____

PULMONARY REHABILITATION
PLB/DB BREATHING RETRAINING

FIGURE 40-2. An example of a form used to document the patient's status and to establish the goals of his or her treatment program.

A PR program must follow the fiscal intermediary Medicare Bulletins for proper reimbursement. The right codes must be used or reimbursement amounts will be denied or reduced. Good rapport with billing personnel is important.

An outpatient PR patient is registered as a "continuous patient." Each one-hour session is billed separately on a daily basis and is verified with each progress note in the patient's chart. Once per month, the billing office receives the itemized charges of all continuous (PR) patients. The bills are not processed until each patient has completed the 6-week PR program (i.e., when the Uniform Bill-82 [UB-82] is submitted). Billing personnel time is saved when the complete itemized bill is entered on the Direct Data Entry (DDE) screen at those hospitals that bill electronically. A special note on the UB-82 field marked 94, labeled "REMARKS," states "end of treatment." This may prevent the hospital from being subjected to medical review or audit.

Additional patient information may be required by the Medicare fiscal intermediary. This patient information is found on Form 5097. The PR coordinator completes this form, and the business office enters this information on the Therapy Information Entry (TIE)

Medications taken today: _____

Breath sounds: _____

Problems since last exercise session: _____

IMT: x _____ minutes at # _____ , Mobility exercise: x _____ minutes,

Strengthening exercise: x _____ minutes, THR: _____ _____ _____

MPH/%Grade	Time	RR	HR	B/P	%SAT	Comments
						Total Distance:

Relaxation exercise: x _____ minutes

Daily Tx Note: Patient exercised and ambulated on TM as noted above. Patient instructed in PLB/DB with mobility, strengthening, ambulation, and relaxation exercise. Required ____% verbal cuing, SOB level ____/____. Plan to continue increasing the workload.

Weekly summary: Patient increased TM from ____ to ____ MPH @ ____% grade x a total of ____ minutes.

Verbal cues for PLB/DB with exercise decreased from ____% to ____% of the time. Distance ____

to ____. _____

_____

_____   _____
Date Signature   Total Treatment Time

PULMONARY REHABILITATION
EXERCISE PROGRESS RECORD

FIGURE 40–3. An example of a form used to document a patient's progress or problems at each therapeutic session.

1. Review Period: _____

2. Treatment Diagnosis: _____   Onset Date: _____

3. Secondary Diagnosis: _____   Onset Date: _____

4. Start of Care Date: _____

5. Orders and certification
   A. Written Order states the specific therapeutic intervention/activity
   B. Specific frequency and duration of treatment

	RT	PT	OT	RN

   C. Certification is timely   YES   NO
      (For PT/OT billed under
      Revenue Codes 420/430)   FROM: _____ TO: _____ DATE: _____

6. Prior history of pulmonary rehabilitation: YES   NO   COMMENTS: _____
7. Initial evaluation present for each discipline involved?

	RT	PT	OT	RN	MD

   A. Were the following addressed during the assessment?
      1. Medical history
      2. Prior functional level
      3. Psychosocial status
      4. Current status
         a. Pulmonary function tests
         b. Treadmill stress tests
         c. Baseline ABG's
         d. Medications
         e. Cough/sputum history
         f. Breathing pattern
         g. Bronchial hygiene/therapy
         h. Oxygen therapy
         i. Exercise endurance
         j. Dyspnea level
         k. Functional activities
         l. PT/OT assistive devices
         m. Other
   B. Are there objective functional goals stated related to the patient's specific problems?
   C. Is there an individualized plan of treatment that addresses the stated problems?
8. Daily documentation
   A. States actual treatment/activity
   B. Reflects patient's response to treatment
   C. Was treatment individualized to stated problems?
   D. Treatment time/unit value corresponding to financial ledger
   E. PR team members signature and date

9. Are there weekly objective measures of the patients progress (or problems interfering with achieving treatment goals?) Comments: _____
10. Biweekly conferences documenting changes from beginning of treatment? Comments: _____

11. Is there a discharge plan?   YES   NO

12. Was the patient discontinued from pulmonary rehabilitation when one of the following criteria was met?
    ____ A. Achieved goals.
    ____ B. Has reached a plateau in progress (slow or no progress).
    ____ C. Unable to participate in the treatment program because of medical, psychologic, or social complications.
    ____ D. Treatment no longer requires skilled therapeutic intervention (*i.e.*, can be continued by patient or caregivers).
    ____ E. Goals no longer realistic and no new goals established.
    ____ F. Has patient reached maximum benefit?
13. Is the provider billing for services that are not a Medicare benefit?
    A. Nutritional assessment and treatment   YES   NO
    B. Case conferences   YES   NO
    C. Social service assessment and treatment   YES   NO
    D. Biofeedback for relaxation or stress/tension reduction   YES   NO
    E. Documentation/paperwork time/discharge summary   YES   NO

FIGURE 40–4. The California Blue Cross concurrent review of outpatient pulmonary rehabilitation services. (Published by permission of Blue Cross of California.)

screen. After this information is keyed, it is stored for medical review. Once reviewed, the claim is released for payment consideration.

A community hospital that electronically bills on the DDE can ideally be reimbursed in 14 days, but reimbursement may take up to 3 months.

A community hospital can establish its own cost center for PR. Such a center makes it possible for physical therapists, occupational therapists, social service providers, and nutritional support staff to charge for their time only. It prevents the need for an "outpatient physician certification" for separate billing charges for physical and occupational therapy.

REFERENCES

1. Elkousy NM, Komorowski PT, Foto M, et al. Outpatient pulmonary rehabilitation: A Medicare fiscal intermediary's viewpoint. Cardiopulmon Rehabil 1988; 8:492–498.
2. Blue Cross of California. Pulmonary Rehabilitation Guidelines: Medicare Bulletin No. 224. 1987, pp 1–4.

Index

Note: Page numbers in *italics* refer to illustrations; page numbers followed by t refer to tables.

Abdominal breathing, for relaxation, 371–372
Abdominal muscles, electromyography of, in chronic obstructive pulmonary disease, 43–44
Abdominal pressure, 43
Absorption atelectasis, from long-term oxygen therapy, 199
Abstinent violation effect, 297
Acetazolamide, for hypoventilation, 61
　for nocturnal hypoxemia, in chronic obstructive pulmonary disease, 98–99
　respiratory muscle function and, 161
Acetylcholine, pathophysiology of hypoxic syndromes and, 89–90
N-Acetylcysteine, for chronic airflow obstruction symptom exacerbations, 145, 145t
Acid-base balance, derangements of, diagnosis of, 125, *125*
　in chronic obstructive pulmonary disease, 29–30
　ventilatory response and, 55, *55*
Active tension, 34
Activities of daily living training, for pulmonary rehabilitation programs, 311, *313*
Acute treatment model, 252–253
Adaptive ability, use of, 255
Adherence. See *Compliance.*
Aerobic conditioning, for postoperative lung transplantation, 464
Aerosol therapy, for cystic fibrosis, 442
Age, chronic illness incidence and, 366
　exercise prescription and, 324–325
　exercise program efficacy and, 209
　in chronic airflow obstruction, mortality and, 139
　　prediction of disease course and, 142
　interest in sex and, 383, 384t
　rehabilitation candidate selection and, 318
　sexual response and, 386, 386t
Air, transtracheal administration of, 132
Air travel, by hypoxemic patients, oxygen therapy for, 190–191

Air travel *(Continued)*
　oxygen therapy and, 403
Airflow limitations, chronic forms of, dyspnea in, 108, 110–112, *110–112*
　leg effort in, 108, 110–112, *110–112*
　emphysema severity and, 31
　in chronic obstructive pulmonary disease, 23–24, *24*
Airflow obstruction, chronic form of, 31
　course of, prediction of, 142t, 142–144, *143–144*
　diagnosis of, problems in, 138–139, *139*
　exacerbation of symptoms of, by N-acetylcysteine, 145, 145t
　forced expiratory volume in 1 second and, 138
　　improvement with bronchodilators, 145–146
　　need for long-term prospective studies of, 148–149
　　predictors of mortality for, 139–142, 140t, *140–141*, 144
　　prognostic predictors for, 144–147, 145t, 146t
　rehabilitation for, 147–148
　survival rates for, in IPPB and NOT trials, 144, *144*
　symptoms of, forced expiratory volume in 1 second improvement and, 144–145
　treatment goals for, 144
　in chronic obstructive pulmonary disease, 22–26, *23–26*
　reversibility of, mortality from chronic airflow obstruction and, 141–142
Airway conductance (Gaw), 26
Airway hyperresponsiveness, in chronic airflow obstruction, mortality and, 140–141
　prediction of disease course and, 143
　in chronic obstructive pulmonary disease, 28
Airway inflammation, treatment of, in cystic fibrosis, 442

Airway obstruction, chronic, diaphragmatic breathing exercises for, 171–172, *173*, 174
　reduction in load as treatment for, 132
　reversibility of, prediction of disease course and, 143, *143*
Airway resistance (Raw), 25–26, *26*
Airway responsiveness. See also *Airway hyperresponsiveness.*
　definition of, 27
　in chronic obstructive pulmonary disease, 27, 27–28
Alarm phase, of General Adaptation Syndrome, 367, *368*
Alcohol, for nocturnal hypoxemia in chronic obstructive pulmonary disease, 99
Alcoholism, skeletal muscle strength and, 162
Allergy, in chronic airflow obstruction, 139–140
　forced expiratory volume in 1 second and, 143
Allied health clinical assessments, in candidate assessment for rehabilitation, 320
All-or-nothing concept, 367
Almitrine, for hypoventilation, 61
　for nocturnal hypoxemia, in chronic obstructive pulmonary disease, 98
　respiratory muscle function and, 161–162
Alpha-motor neuron activity, intramuscular homeostasis and, 111
Altitude, ventilatory responses to, 56–57
Alveolar filling disorders, exercise tolerance in, 121
Alveolar partial oxygen pressure mechanisms, in lung disease, 116t, 116–117
Alveolar ventilation, alveolar partial carbon dioxide and, 52–54, *53*
　oxygen therapy and, 185
Amantadine, for respiratory infection prophylaxis, 160
Ambulation. See also *Walking.*
　for ventilator-dependent patients, 469, *469*

495

Ambulation *(Continued)*
  progressive, after lung transplantation, 464
Ambulatory care, for chronic obstructive pulmonary disease, 262–263
Aminophylline, for chronic obstructive pulmonary disease, 155–156
Amyotrophic lateral sclerosis, 129
Anthropometry assessment, description of, 338
  in cystic fibrosis, 346
Antibiotics, for respiratory infections, 158, 158t
  in cystic fibrosis, 442–443
Anticholinergics, bronchodilation effects of, 154, *154*
  for chronic obstructive pulmonary disease, 154, 393
  mechanism of action of, 153–154
  psychosis due to, 268
Anticipatory rehearsal technique, 374–375
Antidepressant hypothesis of exercise, 242, 243
Antidepressants, for psychiatric disease, 267t, 267–268, 269t–270t
Antipsychotics. See *Neuroleptics.*
Antitussives, 157
Anxiety, disorders of, as cause for referral, 379–380
  dyspnea and, 352
Anxiolytic agents, for psychiatric disease, 268, 271–272, 272t
Apnea, definition of, 103
Apneustic respiration, 51
Arm exercise training, 328
Arrhythmias, in exercise therapy, 329
Arterial blood gases. See *Blood gases, arterial.*
Arterial partial oxygen pressure mechanisms, in lung disease, 116t, 116–117
Assisted breathing therapy, for emotional stress, 259
Asthma, 18–19, 424
  cardiorespiratory performance characteristics in, 425–428, 427t, *428*
  chest physiotherapy for, 178
  death rates for, 12, *12*
    regional patterns of, 14
    time trends in, 13–14
  definition of, 18–19, 424
  dyspnea in, 427, *427*
    exercise tolerance and, 425
  exercise-induced form of, cardiorespiratory performance and, 425–426
    severity and, 431t, 432–433
  exercise testing in, 426
  exercise training for, 424–425
    external work performance and, 248, 248t
    heart rate response to, 248, 248t
    physiologic outcome and, 428–433
  interpatient variability in, 424
  intrapatient variability in, 424
  prevalence rates for, 12–13, 13t, *14*
  pulmonary rehabilitation for, 434–435, *436*
  P-V curve in, 22
  severity of, exercise and, 431t, 432–433
  treatment of, by reduction in load, 132
  vs. emphysema, 31
Asthmatic bronchitis, chronic, 141
Atelectasis, absorption form of, from long-term oxygen therapy, 199
  obstructive form of, chest physiotherapy for, 179
Atropine, bronchodilating effects of, 154
Autogenic or autosuggestion relaxation technique, 370–371, 372t
Auto-positive end-expiratory pressure (AUTO-PEEP or intrinsic-PEEP), 127, *127*
Aversive stimulus, psychophysical assessment and, 257–258

Balchum, Oscar, 4, *5*
Barach, Alvan, 1, *3*, 183
Beclomethasone, 156
Behavior, change in, 357–358
  evaluation of obstacles in, 356–357, 357t
  goal setting and, 357
  rationale for, 356
  self-monitoring and, 357
  self-reward and, 357
  social support and, 357–358
  counseling on, for smoking cessation, 294
  interventions in, 356–358, 357t, 363
  relationships of, brain and, 79–80
  seductive, of patient, 388–389, 389t
  target, definition of, 356
  techniques for smoking relapse prevention and, 297–299, 298t
Bending forward posture, as controlled breathing technique, 169–171, *171*
Bereavement states, 258
Beta-adrenergic agonists, advantages of, 153
  classes of, 152–153
  disadvantages of, 152–153
  exercise tolerance and, 332
  for advanced chronic obstructive pulmonary disease, 393
  mechanism of action of, 152
  metered-dose inhalers of, 153, 153t
  side effects of, 153
Beta-endorphins, for dyspnea, 245–248, 247t
  release of, exercise and, 248
    genetically determined mechanism for, 248
Beta-lipotropin release, exercise and, 248
BIA (bioelectrical impedance analysis), of lean body mass, 338, *338*
Bias, sexual, 389
Bicycle ergometer testing, 326
Billing, for community hospital pulmonary rehabilitation program, 489, 491, 494
Biochemical testing, in candidate assessment for rehabilitation, 319–320
Bioelectrical impedance analysis (BIA), of lean body mass, 338, *338*
Biofeedback, in pulmonary rehabilitation programs, 308–309
  relaxation therapy and, 375–376
Biologic tests, as motivation for smoking cessation, 290–291
Blacks, obstructive pulmonary disease in, 12
Blood, oxygen-carrying capacity of, 185
Blood gases, arterial, for monitoring of oxygen therapy, 196
  in advanced chronic obstructive pulmonary disease case histories, 395–396, 396t
  in respiratory failure, 130–131
Blue bloaters, beta-endorphin levels of, 247, 247t
  characteristics of, 59
  dyspnea sensitivity and, 247–248
  eucapnia in, 30
  exercise and, 248
  nocturnal oxygen desaturation and, 88
  ventilation-perfusion mismatch in, 28

Body composition, 337–338
Body fluids, biochemical parameters for, 338–339
Body image alteration, in chronic obstructive pulmonary disease, 258
Body plethysmography, of functional residual capacity, 21
Body position, dyspnea relief from, 44–45
Body space, in psychophysical assessment, 257
Body weight, ideal, concept of, 338
  management of, smoking and, 344–345
  prevention of gain in, interventions for, 344
  standards for, 337
Borg scaling, 107
Bowel obstruction, in cystic fibrosis, 439–440
Bradypnea, 130
Brain, behavior relationships and, 79–80
  hypoxemia-induced dysfunction of, mechanisms of, 89–90
Breathing. See also *Work of breathing.*
  during sleep, in chronic obstructive pulmonary disease, clinical value of studies on, 97, 97–98
  dyssynchronous, with arm exercise, 328
  exercises for, 1, *2*, 4
  pathologic derangements in chronic obstructive pulmonary disease and, 322, *322*
  pattern of, in chronic obstructive pulmonary disease, 30, 60
  resting form of, in chronic obstructive pulmonary disease, 42–44, *44*
  retraining of. See *Controlled breathing techniques.*
  work of. See *Work of breathing.*
Breathlessness. See *Dyspnea.*
British Medical Research Council Study. See *Medical Research Council Study (MRC Study).*
Bronchial challenge, of chronic obstructive pulmonary disease patient, 27–28
Bronchiectasis, chest physiotherapy for, 177
  cystic fibrosis nutritional interventions and, 345–346
Bronchitis, chronic, 18
  death rates for, regional patterns of, 14
  definition of, 18
  etiology of, 18
  prevalence rates for, 12–13, 13t, *14*
  pulmonary pressure in, 67
  P-V curve in, 22
Bronchodilators, anticholinergic, mechanism of action of, 153–154, *154*
  for cystic fibrosis, 442
  for forced expiratory volume in 1 second improvement in chronic airflow obstruction, 145–146
  inhalation of, response of COPD patient to, 27, *27*
  sympathomimetic, 152–153
Bronchopulmonary dysplasia, in infants receiving oxygen therapy, 199
Bullous emphysema, functional residual capacity in, 21
Bus trips, continuing care programs and, 403
Buspirone, respiratory muscle function and, 161

Caffeine, respiratory muscle function and, 160–161

CAO. See *Airflow obstruction, chronic form of.*
Captopril, cough syndrome of, 163–164
Carbimazole, exercise tolerance and, 332
Carbon dioxide. See also *Hypercapnia.*
  arterial set-point of, 116
  elimination of, in chronic obstructive pulmonary disease, 29–30
  in ventilatory control system, 58, *58*
  production of, nutrition interventions and, 341
  respiratory stimulation and, 52–54, *53*
  retention of, in exercise, 331
  sensitivity response to, 53
    hypnosis and, 244
    inspired oxygen and, *53*, 53–54
Carbon monoxide, diffusing capacity of, 30, 110
  exhaled levels of, in smokers, 290
Carboxyhemoglobin, increased levels of, exercise intolerance in lung disease and, 122, 122t
  ventilatory response to exercise and, 117
  oxygen-carrying capacity of blood and, 185
  pulse oximetry and, 196
Cardiac output, pulmonary hypertension and, 110
Cardiac reflexes, 57
Cardiodynamic hyperpnea, 56
Cardiorespiratory system, fitness of, in asthma, 425–426, 427t, *428*
  performance characteristics in asthma and, 425–428, 427t, *428*
Cardiovascular system, exercise response of, in asthma, 431
  in cystic fibrosis, 445–446
  fitness of, program efficacy and, 209, 210
  ventilatory response to exercise and, 117
Caregiver-patient relationship, sexuality and, 387–388
Carotid body, bilateral resection of, for dyspnea desensitization, 249
  inhibition of, 55
    for dyspnea control, 63
Catecholamines, blood levels of, after exercise, 206
  disadvantages of, 152–153
  pharmacologic effects of, 152
Category scaling, 107
Central chemoreceptor stimulation, dyspnea and, 105
Central fatigue, in progressive ventilatory failure, 125–126
  of respiratory muscles, 231–232
Central pattern generator, 50
Central receptors, dyspnea and, 105–106
Central respiratory depressants, for dyspnea, 63
Certificate of need (CON), 479
CF. See *Cystic fibrosis.*
C-fibers, 52, 105
cGMP (guanosine 3′,5′-cyclic monophosphate), 154
Chemical respiratory stimuli, responses to, 52–55, *53–55*
Chemoreceptors, respiratory, 51, 105
Chest physiotherapy, complications of, 179–180
  for asthma, 178
  for bronchiectasis, 177
  for chronic obstructive pulmonary disease, 176–180
  for cystic fibrosis, 177–178, 442, 454
  for lung transplantation, 463–464
  for obstructive atelectasis, 179

Chest physiotherapy *(Continued)*
  for pneumonia, 178
  for postoperative care, 178–179
  for preoperative care, 178–179
  for pulmonary rehabilitation programs, 309
  for specific lung disorders, 176
  goals of, 174–175
  metabolic effects of, 179–180
  sputum expectoration in, 176
  techniques for, definition of, 175–176
Chest wall, in end-expiration, 35, *35*
  motion of, in chronic obstructive pulmonary disease, 42–46, *44*
  in hyperinflation, 37
  structural alterations of, in chronic obstructive pulmonary disease, 39–40
  in experimental emphysema, 38
Chest wall receptors, 52
Chlorpromazine, for dyspnea, 63
Cholinergic drugs, hypoxia-induced behavioral deficits and, 89
Chronic Obstructive Pulmonary Disease: Current Concepts, 7
Chronic obstructive pulmonary disease (COPD), activity level in, downward spiral of, 204, *205*
  acute form of, chest physiotherapy for, 177
  advanced form of, case histories of, 395–396, 396t
  counseling for, 394–395
  definition of, 392–393
  dyspnea management in, 393–394
  pharmacologic therapy for, 393
  airflow obstruction in, 22–26, *23–26*
  airway hyperresponsiveness in, 28
  breathing during sleep and, 97, 97–98, 100
  breathing pattern in, 60
  bronchial challenge response in, 27–28
  cardiac dysfunction in, 66–69
  chest physical therapy in, 176–180
  chest wall motion in, 42–46, *44*
  chest wall structural alterations in, 39–40
  continuous positive airway pressure for, *237–238*, 238–239
  cough in, 174
  death rates for, 11–13, *12*, 13t
    age-adjustment of, *14–15*
    regional patterns of, 14
    time trends in, 13–14
  definition of, 18
  diaphragm length in, 41
  diaphragmatic breathing exercises for, 171–172, *173*, 174
  diffusing capacity in, 30
  exercise for, effects of, 242
    limitations, pathophysiologic mechanisms of, 117–119, 118t, *119–120*
    oxygen consumption in, 68
    physiologic disadvantages of patient and, 204–205
    psychological effects of, 242
    responses to, *60*, 60–61, 218–220, 219t
    tolerance limitations in, 204–205, *205*
    training programs for upper extremities and, 220–221
  flow-volume loop in, 23–25, *24–25*
  functional residual capacity in, 225–226, *226*
  gas exchange in, 28–30, *29*, 31
  genetic predisposition of, 60
  heart dysfunction in, 66–69
    hemodynamic evidence of, 67–68
    pathologic evidence of, 66–67
    treatment of, 69–71
  heart rate reserve of, 119

Chronic obstructive pulmonary disease *(Continued)*
  hypercapnia of, respiratory muscle weakness and, 232
  hypercapnic sensitivity in, 59, 59–60
  hypoxemia of, 119
  intermittent negative-pressure ventilation for, 234–236, 235t, *236*
  left ventricular dysfunction in, hemodynamic evidence of, 68–69
  life quality in, heuristic model of, 89, *89*
  lung hyperinflation in, 31
  lung volumes in, 19–22, *19–22*
  morbidity of, 10, 11t
  mortality of, 11t, 11–12, *12*
  mucociliary clearance in, 174
  neurobehavioral impairment in, predictors of, 89
  neurocognitive functioning in. See *Neurocognition.*
  neuropsychiatric evaluation in, multicenter investigations for, 81–83, *82, 84, 85–87, 86–87*
  neuropsychology of, brain hypoxemia dysfunction mechanisms of impairment in, 89–90
    clinical implications of deficits in, 90
    studies on, 80–81
  nocturnal hypoxemia in, 88
    mechanisms of, 92–95, *94*
    sleep consequences of, 95, 95–96
    treatment of, 98–100, *99*
    ventilation/perfusion imbalance and, 94
  nocturnal oxygenation prediction in, 96, 96–97
  noninvasive ventilatory support in, 234–236, 235t, *236*
  oxygen saturation in, during sleep, 92, *93*
  oxygenation in, 28–29, *29*
  pathologic correlates of, 30–31
  pathologic findings of, in diaphragm, 40
  pharmacotherapy for, 155–156, 163t, 163–164. See also specific drugs.
    drugs to avoid in, 163t, 163–164
  physiologic correlates of, 30–31
  postural relief of dyspnea in, 44–45
  psychophysiology of, issues in, 253–259
    treatment and, 259–263
  psychosocial issues in, 253–259
  psychosocial treatment of, 259–263
  pulmonary vascular resistance in, 68
  respiratory muscle function in, 42–46, *44*, 225–226, *226*
    during acute hyperinflation, 33–38, *34–37*
    exercise and, 45–46
    length of muscles and, 41
  response to bronchodilator inhalation in, 27, *27*
  resting breathing in, 42–44, *44*
  severity of obstruction in, 59, *59*
  smoking and, 15
  stable form of, chest physiotherapy for, 176–177
  survival rates for, 7, 392, *393*
  treatment of. See also specific treatment modalities.
    ambulatory vs. stationary oxygen for, 6–7
    conference on, 4
  heart function and, 69–71
  model for, 253
  type A. See *Pink puffers.*
  type B. See *Blue bloaters.*
  ventilation in, 29–30
  ventilatory control in, 58–60, *59*

Chronic obstructive pulmonary disease *(Continued)*
   ventilatory drive of, 118, *118*
   with sleep apnea/hypopnea syndrome, 94
     consequences of, 96
     oxygen therapy for, 98
     treatment of, *99*, 100
   work of breathing in, *26*, 26–27, 55
Chronic pulmonary disease, vicious cycle of, 185, *185*
Chronic Respiratory Questionnaire (CRQ), 359–360
   for assessment of rehabilitation candidate, 321
Chronic treatment model, 253
Cigarette advertising, 293, *293*
Cigarette smoking. See *Smoking.*
Circulation, respiration interaction and, 57–58
Class Method of Treatment, 261
Clinical studies. See also specific studies.
   control groups for, 406–407
   design aspects of, 405–406
   longevity of benefits and, 407
   patient numbers and, 406
   patient selection and, 406
   randomization and, 407
CO_2. See *Carbon dioxide.*
Coefficient of elastic retraction, 19–20
Cognitive techniques, to prevent smoking relapse, 297–299, 298t
Cognitive-behavioral treatment, for relaxation therapy, 377–378, 378t
Community hospital rehabilitation program, billing and, 489, 491, 494
   documentation for, 488–489, *490–493*
   fiscal intermediary and, 487–488
   long-term follow-up and, 489
   reimbursement documentation guidelines for, 488–489
Compliance, lung, definition of, 19
   dynamic form of, 20
   frequency dependence of, 20, *20*
   specific form of, 19
   patient, improvement of, for COPD drug regimens, 163
     in exercise therapy, 353–354
     in medical regimens, 354
     overadherence in, 354–355
     suggestions for, 357t
     terminology in, 352–353
Comprehensive outpatient rehabilitation facilities (CORFs), background of, 478–479
   certification of, 479
   program experience in Birmingham, Alabama and, 480–482, 481t
   reimbursement for, 480, 481–482
   review process for, 479–480
CON (certificate of need), 479
Continuing care programs, committees for, 401–402
   exercise in, 398–400, *399*
   newsletters and, 402
   patient clubs and, 400–401
   respiratory rally for, 402
   travel and, 402–404
Continuous positive airway pressure (CPAP), *237–238*, 238–239
Control groups, for clinical studies, 406–407
   for exercise therapy programs, 216
Controlled breathing techniques, diaphragmatic breathing exercises and allied maneuvers, 171–174, 172t, 173t
   goals of, 168

Controlled breathing techniques *(Continued)*
   historical aspects of, 168
   in pulmonary rehabilitation programs, 308
   instruction for, 167–168
   of bending forward posture, 169–171, *171*
   of head down posture, 169–171, *171*
   of pursed-lip breathing, 167, 168–169, *169*
   quality of life and, 167
COPD. See *Chronic obstructive pulmonary disease (COPD).*
Coping ability, use of, 255
CORFs. See *Comprehensive outpatient rehabilitation facilities (CORFs).*
Corticosteroids, for advanced chronic obstructive pulmonary disease, 393
   for forced expiratory volume in 1 second improvement in chronic airflow obstruction, 146t, 146–147, 147t
   indications for, 156–157
Cost benefit analysis, of pulmonary rehabilitation, 412
Cost-effectiveness of health care programs, evaluation of, 360–362, 361t
Costs, of long-term oxygen therapy, 197–198
   of storefront rehabilitation program, 474, 477
COT. See *Oxygen therapy, continuous form of.*
Coughing, as sign of underlying disease, 157
   captopril and, 163–164
   for mucus expulsion, 175–176
   in chronic obstructive pulmonary disease, 175
   in ventilatory failure, 130
Counseling, for advanced chronic obstructive pulmonary disease, 394–395
   for sexual problems, 384–387, 385t, 386t
   on behavior, for smoking cessation, 294
Countertransference, 390
CPAP (continuous positive airway pressure), *237–238*, 238–239
Creatinine, urinary, 339
Critical knowledge, for pulmonary rehabilitation programs, 307–308
CRQ (Chronic Respiratory Questionnaire), 359–360
   for assessment of rehabilitation candidate, 321
Cruises, continuing care programs and, 403–404
Cyanosis, 196
Cycling, for cystic fibrosis, 450
Cystic fibrosis, chest physiotherapy for, 177–178, 442
   clinical manifestations of, 439–441, *441*
   diagnosis of, 441, 442t
   exercise for, guidelines for programs of, 455t, 455–456
     in rehabilitation program, 444–451, *445–451*, 446t, 452t–453t, *454*, 454–456, 455t
     outcome variables of, 451
     prognosis and, 454
     published programs of, 452t–453t
     exercise tolerance in, oxygen desaturation and supplementation and, 447, *450*
   gastrointestinal tract in, 439–440
   genetics of, 439
   hyperglycemia in, 444
   lung transplantation for, 443
   nutrition in, 439–440
     assessment for, 346
     interventions for, 345–346
     clinical investigations of, 346
     needs for, 347, 348t

Cystic fibrosis *(Continued)*
   rehabilitation programs for, 454
   prevalence of, 439
   prognosis for, 444, *444*
   rehabilitation in, 444–451, *445–451*, 446t, 452t–453t, *454*, 454–456, 455t
   respiratory tract in, 440, *441*
   sweat glands in, 440
   treatment of, 441–444
     gastrointestinal therapy for, 443
     hyperglycemia and, 444
     psychologic considerations for, 443
     pulmonary therapy in, 442–443

DDE (Direct Data Entry), 491, 494
Death, during sleep, in chronic obstructive pulmonary disease, 96
Death rates, for asthma, 12, *12*
   for chronic obstructive pulmonary disease (COPD), 11–12, *12*
Dejour switch technique, 55
Denison, Dr. Charles L., 1
Depression, as cause for referral, 379–380
   exercise and, 242, *243*
   in chronic obstructive pulmonary disease, 258–259, 352
   of ventilator-dependent patients, 469
Diagnosis Related Groups (DRGs), 476
Diaphragm, breathing exercises for, benefits of, 172, *173*, 174
   candidates for, 171–172
   controlled breathing techniques and, 171–172, 172t, 173t, 174
   breathing from, for relaxation, 371–372
   in chronic obstructive pulmonary disease, 43
   in head down and bending forward postures, 170–171, *171*
   length of, in chronic obstructive pulmonary disease, 41
   length-tension relationship of, in active hyperinflation, 34–35, *35*, *36*
   in experimental emphysema, 38–39, *39*
   paresis of, 130
   pathologic findings of, in chronic obstructive pulmonary disease, 40
   zone of apposition of, 35, *35*
     in chronic obstructive pulmonary disease, 43
Diary form, for smoking cessation, 292, 292t
Diazepam, for dyspnea, 63, 245
Diet history, in nutritional assessment, 339–340
Dietary Guidelines for Americans, 338
Dietitian, as pulmonary rehabilitation team member, 304, *305*
Diffusing capacity, emphysema severity and, 31
   in chronic obstructive pulmonary disease, 30
   measurement of, 30
Diffusion block, 117
Direct Data Entry (DDE), 491, 494
Discharge planning, for long-term mechanical ventilation, 279–281, 281t
Distal intestinal obstruction syndrome, 440
Distraction hypothesis, of exercise, 243–244, *244*
Dorsal respiratory group, 50
Doxapram, for hypoventilation, 61
   for ventilatory drive improvement, 133
   respiratory muscle function and, 161
Doxepin, for chronic obstructive pulmonary disease, 267

DRGs (Diagnosis Related Groups), 476
Drugs. See *Pharmacotherapy*; specific drugs.
Duchenne muscular dystrophy, 128, 129
Dyspnea, anxiety and, 352
  as end-point symptom for exercise, 322
  definition of, 103
  description of, 103
  desensitization to, 204, 241, 249–250
    bilateral carotid body resection for, 249
    by exercise training, 242–244, *243–244*
    by hypnosis, 244–245, 245t, *246*
    by neurochemical methods, 245–248, *246–247*, 247t, 248t
    by peripheral source, 248–250, 249t
    by pharmacological methods, 245–248, *246–247*, 247t, 248t
  exercise training and, 242
  historical aspects of, 103–104
  in acute respiratory failure, 129
  in asthma, 427, *427*
  in chronic airflow limitation, 108, 110–112, *110–112*
  in chronic obstructive pulmonary disease, factors in, 118, *118*
  in chronic respiratory failure, 129–130
  in cystic fibrosis, exercise program outcome and, 454
  in exercise, 327
  management of, 241
    by pursed-lip breathing, 168–169
    in advanced chronic obstructive pulmonary disease, 393–394
  mechanisms of, 104–106
    factors in, 241, *243*
    historical aspects of, 104
  oxygen therapy for, 188
  paroxysmal nocturnal, in ventilatory failure, 129
  physical deconditioning of, 241, *242*
  physiologic cues on, 241
  postural relief of, in chronic obstructive pulmonary disease, 44–45
  psychophysics and, 106–108
  relief of, by head down and bending forward postures, 169–171, *171*
  symptoms of, during exercise in normal subjects, *107–109*, 108
  therapy for, 62
  vs. pain, 256
Dyspnea index, definition of, 408
Dyspneic stimulus, 241
Dysrhythmias, hypoxemia during sleep in chronic obstructive pulmonary disease and, 95

Ear oximetry, for oxygen therapy monitoring, 196
Education, of family, 262–263
  of patient. See *Patient education.*
Eighth Aspen Emphysema Conference, 4
Elastic recoil, definition of, 19
  in chronic obstructive pulmonary disease, exercise limitation and, 118, *118*
  loss of, in emphysema, 31
Elastic resistance, 55
Elderly, sexual abuse of, 389–390
Electrolytes, in nutritional assessment, 339
Emphysema, death rates for, regional patterns of, 14
  definition of, 18
  differentiation of, from chronic severe asthma, 31

Emphysema *(Continued)*
  experimental model of, chest wall structural alterations in, 38
    diaphragm length-tension relationship in, 38–39, *39*
  loss of elastic recoil in, 31
  predictors of, 31
  prevalence rates for, 12–13, 13t, *14*
  P-V curve in, *2*, 22
  severity of, 31
  ventricular hypertrophy and, 66–67
Encephalopathy, metabolic, increased ventilatory drive and, 125
Endogenous opioids, for dyspnea, 245–248, 247t
Endurance training principles, in rehabilitation for lung transplantation, 460
Energy demands, in chronic obstructive pulmonary disease, 226
Environment, exposures from, obstructive pulmonary disease risk and, 17
  relationship of, to chronic obstructive pulmonary disease, 253
Epinephrine, 152
Equal pressure point (EPP), 24, *24*
ERV, 22
Ethical issues, in sexual health care, 388–390
Eucapnia, in chronic obstructive pulmonary disease, 30
Euthyroid sick syndrome, 131
Exercise, antidepressant hypothesis of, 242, *243*
  benefits of, 210–211, 212t–215t, 216–218
  beta-endorphin release and, 248
  beta-lipotropin release and, 248
  blue bloaters and, 248
  body weight gain prevention and, 344
  cellular respiration of, *116*, 1115
  critical training intensity for, 328
  diary of, 398–399, *399*
  distraction hypothesis of, 243–244, *244*
  drugs and, 332
  dyspnea symptoms of, in normal subjects, *107–109*, 108
  endurance in, improvement of, 217
  for rehabilitation therapy, adherence to, 353–354
    benefits of, 210–211, 212t–215t, 216–218, 332
    characteristics of, 207–210, 328
    control groups for, 216
    desensitization to dyspnea and, 242–244, *243–244*
    easing patient into, 328
    effective program for, 207–210
    goals for, 329, 330t
    in chronic obstructive pulmonary disease, 218–220, 219t
    maintenance programs of, 329
    oxygen supplementation in, 210, 216
    patient characteristics in, 210
    program characteristics in, 210–211
    program duration for, efficacy and, 209
    program results for, 212t–215t, 216–218
    rationale for, 308
    risks in, 329, 331
    session of, 328–329
      duration and, 209
    setting and supervision for, 216
    for upper and lower extremity, 313–314, *314*
  in asthma, heart rate response to, 248, 248t

Exercise *(Continued)*
  in chronic obstructive pulmonary disease, *60*, 60–61
    effects of, 242
    limitations of, 117–119, *118*
    oxygen consumption and, 68
    responses to, 218–220, 219t
  in continuing care programs, 398–400, *399*
  in cystic fibrosis, programs for, 448–451, 452t–453t, 454, *454*
    responses to single bouts of, 445–448, *445–451*, 446t
  in healthy individuals, physiologic responses of, 206, *207*
    structural adaptations of, 205–206
  in heat, cystic fibrosis and, 447
  in interstitial pulmonary fibrosis, pathophysiologic mechanisms of limitations in, 120–121, 121t
  in obstructive lung disease, abnormal responses to, 119t, 119–120, *120*
  in respiratory failure treatment, 132
  in restrictive lung disease, limitations in, physiology of, 421–422
  intensity of, 227
    in effective programs, 207–209
  maximum performance of, in program evaluation, 408–409
  modalities of, 327–328
    for training programs, 210
    program efficacy and, 209
  nutrition and, 332
  options for, 400
  overload principle of, 227
  peripheral muscular effort intensity in, during dyspnea, *107–109*, 108
  prescription of. See *Exercise prescription.*
  programs for, 327–328
    before lung transplantation, 462
    characteristics of, 210–211
    effective types of, 207–210
    efficacy of, 209
    duration and, 209
    for upper extremities, 220–221
    session frequency for, 209
  psychologic factors in, 332
  respiratory muscle function in, chronic obstructive pulmonary disease and, 45–46
    homeostasis of, 110, *111*
    stress and, 331
  reversibility, principle of, 227
  social interaction hypothesis of, 242–243
  specificity, principle of, 227
  submaximum form of, endurance effect from rehabilitation and, 409, 409t
  tolerance of, after lung transplantation, 466, 466t
    in alveolar filling disorders, 121
    in chronic airflow obstruction, 142
    in cystic fibrosis, 445, *446*, 447–448, *450–451*, 451
    in pulmonary vascular occlusive disease, 121t, 121–122
    noncardiopulmonary factors in, 122, 122t
    oxygen therapy and, 187–188, *188*
    pathophysiologic processes in, 115–116
    types of, for cystic fibrosis, 448–451, 452t–453t
  ventilatory requirements for, 117t
  ventilatory responses in, 56, *57*
Exercise for Pulmonary Invalids, 1, *2*
Exercise prescription, evaluation for, 325–327, *327*

Exercise prescription *(Continued)*
 formulation of, problems with, *322*, 322–323
 in comprehensive outpatient rehabilitation facilities, 480–481
 lung function of patient and, 323
 motivation of patient and, 323
 obstacles to, 207–208
 practical steps in, 328–329
 selection criteria for, 323–325, *324*
Exercise testing, for assessment of rehabilitation candidate, 321
 for evaluation of pulmonary rehabilitation, 408t, 408–410, 409t
 for exercise prescription evaluation, 324, *324–325*
 improvements in responses from exercise training and, 217–218
 in lung transplantation candidates, 461, 461t
 measurements for, 326–327
 modalities for, 325
 preprogram, for cystic fibrosis, 455–456
 protocols for, 325–326, *327*
 vs. resting pulmonary function measurements, 116–117
Exercise therapy. See *Exercise, for rehabilitation therapy.*
Exhaled carbon monoxide test, 290
Exhaustion stage, of General Adaptation Syndrome, 367, *368*
Expectorants, 157
Expiratory flow, effort-independent type of, 24
Extracorporeal membrane oxygenation, for hypoxemia, 132

Face masks, 193
Facial expression, in psychophysical assessment, 257
Fagerstrom Nicotine Tolerance Score, 293–294
Failure of force development, 106
Family education, 262–263
Family support, for overwhelmed patient, 379
Family training, in pulmonary rehabilitation programs, 314
Fatigue, role of, in dyspnea, 106
FET (forced exhalation time), 23
FEV_1. See *Forced expiratory volume in 1 second (FEV_1).*
Fiduciary relationship, 388
Fight or flight reaction, 367
Finger oximetry, for oxygen therapy monitoring, 196
FIO_2 (fractional concentration of inspired oxygen), home positive-pressure ventilators and, 285
 oxygen therapy and, 185
Fiscal intermediary, 304, 487–488
Flenley, David, 7
Flow-volume loop, in chronic obstructive pulmonary disease, 23–25, *24–25*
Flunisolide, 156
Focal biliary fibrosis, 440
Forced exhalation time (FET), 23
Forced expiratory technique (huffing), 176
Forced expiratory volume in 1 second (FEV_1), 116
 chronic airflow obstruction mortality and, 139, *140*
 exercise and, 323

Forced expiratory volume in 1 second *(Continued)*
 improvement of, corticosteroids and, 146t, 146–147, 147t
 in chronic airflow obstruction treatment, 144–145
 with bronchodilators, 145–146
 in chronic airflow limitation, 108, 110, *111–112*
 in chronic airflow obstruction, 138, 142
 in chronic obstructive pulmonary disease, 22–23, *23*
 severity of chronic obstructive pulmonary disease and, 392–393
 smoking cessation and, 142–143
Forced vital capacity (FVC), in chronic obstructive pulmonary disease, 22–23, *23*
Fractional concentration of inspired oxygen (FIO_2), home positive-pressure ventilators and, 285
 oxygen therapy and, 185
FRC. See *Functional residual capacity (FRC).*
Frequency dependence of compliance, 20, *20*
Frictional resistance, 55
Functional residual capacity (FRC), body plethysmography of, 21
 definition of, 19, 20–21, *21*
 diaphragm length-tension relationship and, 34
 emphysema prediction and, 31
 exercise and, 323
 in chronic obstructive pulmonary disease, 42, 225–226, *226*
 in nocturnal hypoxemia of chronic obstructive pulmonary disease, 94
 in obstructive pulmonary disease, 22, *22*
Funding sources, for office-based pulmonary rehabilitation program, 485–486

Gas cylinders, compressed, 191, 192t
Gas exchange, in chronic obstructive pulmonary disease, 28–30, *29*, 31
 exercise limitation and, 118, *118*
 pathologic derangements and, 322, *322*
 in cystic fibrosis during exercise, 446–447, *448–449*
Gastrografin (meglumine diatrizoate), 443
Gastrointestinal tract, in cystic fibrosis, 439–440
Gaw (airway conductance), 26
General Adaptation Syndrome, phases of, 367–368, *368*
Glaser, Dr. Edward, 4, *5*
Glucocorticoid agents, 156–157
Golgi tendon organs, 52, 105
GoLytely bowel prep, 443
Group psychotherapy, for chronic obstructive pulmonary disease, 260–262
 variables affecting participation in, relation of, 261
Group trips, continuing care programs and, 403
Guanosine 3′,5′-cyclic monophosphate (cGMP), 154
Guanyl cyclase, 154
Guided imagery technique, for relaxation, 373, 373t
Guillain-Barré syndrome, 128, 131

Haas, Albert, 1, *3*, 4

Halstead-Reitan Neuropsychological Battery (HRB), 80
Handshake, in psychophysical assessment, 257
Head down posture, as controlled breathing technique, 169–171, *171*
Health care professionals, boundary violations of, 388
 role in sexual health care of patient and, 384
 seductive behavior of patient and, 388–389, 389t
 sexual bias of, 389
 sexuality of patient and, 387–388
Health maintenance organizations (HMOs), 304, 487
Heart rate, as descriptor for exercise intensity, 208
 response to exercise training in asthma and, 248, 248t
Heart rate reserve, in chronic obstructive pulmonary disease, 119
Heat acclimation, in exercise for cystic fibrosis, 451
Hematology, in candidate assessment for rehabilitation, 319–320
 oxygen therapy and, 187
Hemodynamics, after lung transplantation, 465t, 466
 exercise training and, 331
 hypoxemia during sleep and, 95, *95*
 in chronic obstructive pulmonary disease, evidence of cardiac dysfunction and, 67–68
 oxygen therapy and, 186
Hemoglobin, oxygen-carrying capacity of blood and, 185
Hemoglobin saturation, 28
Hering-Breuer reflex, 52, 55
Heterocyclic antidepressants. See *Antidepressants.*
Hill, Leonard, 183
Histamine bronchial challenge, in chronic obstructive pulmonary disease, 27–28
HMOs (Health Maintenance Organizations), 304, 487
Hodgkin, John E., 6
Home, assessment of, for home ventilator care, 281
 care for ventilatory-dependent patients and, 472, *472*
 exercise program in, for post–lung transplantation patient, 464
 pulmonary rehabilitation program for, 314–315
Home care team, 280–281, 281t
Home ventilator care, determination to leave hospital and, 277–279, 280t
 equipment for, 281–286, 282t, *283*, 284t, 285t, *286*
 in approaches other than positive-pressure ventilation, 281–284, 282t, *283*
 in negative-pressure ventilation, 282, 282t, *283*
 in positive-pressure ventilation, 284t, 284–285, 285t, *286*, 287
 pneumobelts as, 282, *283*
 rocking bed as, 282–284, *283*
 patient selection for, 279, 280t
 positive-pressure ventilators for, modes of ventilation of, 284–285, *286*
Hoover's sign, 226
Hospital Intermediary 10th Edition Manual (HIM-10), 477

Hospitals, special facilities for ventilator-dependent patients and, 470, 471, 472
HRB (Halstead-Reitan Neuropsychological Battery), 80
Humidification systems, for home positive-pressure ventilators, 285, 286, 287
Hydrogen ion, ventilatory response and, 55, 55
Hyperbaric oxygen therapy, duration of, cognitive functioning and, 88
Hypercapnia, chemoreceptor response and, 51
   from long-term oxygen therapy, 199
   hypoxemia development and, 29
   mediation of, 103–104
   sensitivity to, in chronic obstructive pulmonary disease, 59, 59–60
Hyperglycemia, in cystic fibrosis, 444
Hyperinflation, acute form of, vs. chronic obstructive pulmonary disease, 38
   in chronic obstructive pulmonary disease, respiratory muscles and, 225–226, 226
Hypertension, pulmonary, cardiac output and, 110
   chronic obstructive pulmonary disease and, 67
   oxygen therapy for, 69–70, 183–184
   pulmonary vascular impedance in, 71–74, 72–75
Hypnosis, desensitization to dyspnea and, 244–245, 245t, 246
Hypnotics, for nocturnal hypoxemia in chronic obstructive pulmonary disease, 99
Hypoglycemia, 331
Hypoventilation, nocturnal hypoxemia in chronic obstructive pulmonary disease and, 92–94, 94
   therapy for, 61–62
Hypoxemia, acute effects of, on neurocognitive functioning, 80
   chronic, expected prevalence of, long-term oxygen therapy for, 188–189
   detection of, 196
   from chest physiotherapy, 179–180
   heart function and, 69–71
   in chronic obstructive pulmonary disease, exercise limitation and, 118, 118
   hypoventilation in sleep and, 92–94, 94
   low ventilation-perfusion mismatch and, 28–29, 29
   mechanisms of, 124–125, 125t
   in lung disease, 116t, 116–117
   nocturnal, in chronic obstructive pulmonary disease, 92–95, 94
      consequences of, 95, 95–96
      functional residual capacity decreases in, 94
      mechanisms of, 92–95, 94
      treatment of, 98–100, 99
      ventilation/perfusion imbalance and, 94
   oxygen therapy for, during air travel, 190–191
   pulmonary vascular impedance and, 71–74, 72–75
Hypoxia, chemoreceptor response and, 51
   heart function and, 69–71
   mediation of, 103–104
   ventilatory response to, 54, 54–55
Hypoxia-Altitude Simulation Test, 190–191

IC (inspiratory capacity), 21, 21

ICD (International Classification of Disease), 11, 11t
Imagination, stimulation of, in relaxation therapy, 372–373, 373t
Immunoreactive trypsin (IRT), 441
Impersonal factors, as obstacles to sexual functioning, 383–384
IMV/SIMV mode (intermittent mandatory ventilation/synchronized intermittent mandatory ventilation mode), 284
Inappropriateness, role of, in dyspnea, 106
Individualized treatment program, documentation of, 488–489, 490
Indomethacin, for dyspnea, 63
Inertial force, 55
Inflammation therapy, for cystic fibrosis, 442
Information, limited, in PLISSIT model for sexual counseling, 385t, 385–386, 386t
Inotropic agents, respiratory muscle function and, 161
Inpatient pulmonary rehabilitation programs, 304
Insomnia, relaxation methods for, 313, 313
Inspiration, elastic and resistive loads in, 55–56
Inspiratory capacity (IC), 21, 21
Inspiratory loads, types of, 126t, 126–127
Inspiratory muscles. See Respiratory muscles.
Inspiratory reserve volume (IRV), measurement of, 21, 22
Inspiratory resistive loading technique, 228, 228–230, 229, 229t
Inspiratory resistive training and weaning, 230
Inspiratory threshold loading technique, 230, 230t, 231
Insurance, for ventilator-dependent patients, 279
Insurance companies, reimbursement for pulmonary rehabilitation and, 304
Intensive care unit (ICU), incentives for moving patient out of, 274–275
   psychophysiologic treatment in, 259–260
   psychosocial treatment in, 259–260
   staff of, 259–260
   reduction of patient stress and, 260
Intermittent mandatory ventilation/synchronized intermittent mandatory ventilation (IMV/SIMV) mode, 284
Intermittent negative-pressure ventilation, for chronic obstructive pulmonary disease, 234–236, 235t, 236
Intermittent Positive-Pressure Breathing Clinical Trial (IPPB Trial), data combined with NOT Trial, results of, 85–86, 86
   life quality assessment results for, 85
   methodology of, 83, 85
   neuropsychologic findings of, 85
   prediction of disease course and, 143, 143
   purpose of, 83
   smoking effects and, 142–143
   survival rates for chronic airflow obstruction and, 142, 144, 144
Intermittent positive-pressure ventilation, via nasal mask, for nocturnal hypoxemia in chronic obstructive pulmonary disease, 99
Intermittent ventilatory support, as rest therapy, 232, 234
Internal oblique muscles, lengthening of, 36
International Classification of Disease (ICD), 11, 11t

International Conference on Pulmonary Rehabilitation and Home Mechanical Ventilation, 7
International conferences, 7
Interpersonal factors, as obstacles to sexual functioning, 384
Interstitial pulmonary fibrosis, exercise limitations in, 120–121, 121t
Intrapersonal factors, as obstacles to sexual functioning, 384
Intrinsic positive end-expiratory pressure (PEEPi), 20, 237
Ipratropium bromide, bronchodilating effects of, 154, 155
Iron-lung, 274
Irritant receptors, 52, 105
IRT (immunoreactive trypsin), 441
IRV (inspiratory reserve volume), measurement of, 21, 22
Isoetharine, 152
Isoproterenol, 152
Isovolume pressure-flow curves, 24

JAMA (Journal of the American Medical Association), 4, 6
Jogging programs, for cystic fibrosis, 448–450
Joint Commission on Accreditation of Health Care Organizations, 479
Journal of the American Medical Association (JAMA), 4, 6

Katz Adjustment Scale, 83
Kinesthetic sensory system, 104–105
Kyphoscoliosis, respiratory loads in, 126–127

Lactate, blood, airway obstruction and, 118, 118t
   in exercise training, 206
   chronic obstructive pulmonary disease and, 218–219, 220–221
Lactic acidosis, in chronic obstructive pulmonary disease, exercise and, 118, 118, 218–219, 219t
   in interstitial pulmonary fibrosis, 121
   in obstructive lung disease, 120
   in oxygen therapy monitoring, 197
   work rate associated with, training effect for chronic obstructive pulmonary disease and, 324, 324
Laplace's equation, 35
Laplace's law, 225
Lean body mass (LBM), anthropometric measurements of, 337–338
   bioelectrical impedance analysis of, 338, 338
Left ventricular dysfunction, in chronic obstructive pulmonary disease, hemodynamic evidence of, 68–69
Leg effort, in chronic airflow limitation, 108, 110–112, 110–112
   in normal subjects, dyspnea symptoms of, 107–109, 108
Level of function, after rehabilitation for chronic airflow obstruction, 148
Life change units, 254
Life quality. See Quality of life.
Lifestyle of patient, active, pulmonary rehabilitation and, 307
   change in, for cystic fibrosis, 451

Liquid oxygen supply, 191, 192t
Lithium, for psychiatric disease, 268, 271t
Long-term mechanical ventilation (LTMV),
　　as elective therapy, clinical experience with, 277, 277
　　to rest ventilatory muscles, 276–277, 278
　　as life support, 274–276, 275, 276t, 277, 278t
　　　clinical experience with, 275–276, 277, 278t
　　　coexisting medical conditions, considerations for, 275, 276–277
　　definition of, 274
　　diagnostic categories for, 275, 276t, 276–277
　　discharge planning for, 279–281, 281t
　　historical aspects of, 274
　　initiation of, 274, 275
　　placement alternatives outside hospital and, 277–279. See also *Home ventilator care*.
Long-term oxygen therapy (LTOT), assessment of oxygenation in, 196–197
　　clinical indications for, 188–191, 189t, 190
　　clinical stability of, 189
　　compliance with, 197
　　complications of, 198–200
　　economic considerations for, 197–198
　　efficacy of, 189–190, 190
　　equipment for, 191–196, 192t, 193t, 194, 194t
　　　fire hazards of, 198–199
　　future directions for, 200
　　guidelines for, adherence to, 191
　　in special situations, 190–191
　　monitoring of, 196–197
　　Nocturnal Oxygen Therapy Trial and, 184, 184–185
　　prescription criteria for, 189, 189t
　　reimbursement issues in, 198
　　smoking and, 190
　　toxicity of, 199–200
Longevity. See *Survival rates*.
Loss, in chronic obstructive pulmonary disease, 258–259
Low-frequency fatigue, 232, 233
LTMV. See *Long-term mechanical ventilation (LTMV)*.
LTOT. See *Long-term oxygen therapy (LTOT)*.
Lung(s), elastic recoil of, 19
　　parenchymal injury of, from long-term oxygen therapy, 199
　　resting function of, assessment of, in evaluating rehabilitation, 407
　　in prescribing exercise therapy, 323–324
Lung age concept, 290
Lung compliance. See *Compliance, lung*.
Lung disease. See also specific lung diseases.
　　acute obstructive form of, treatment model for, 252–253
　　adaptations to, 58–59, 58–60
　　chronic forms of, challenge of, 366
　　　sexuality and, 383–384, 384t
　　　treatment of, 366
　　chronic obstructive form of. See *Chronic obstructive pulmonary disease (COPD)*.
　　exercise tolerance and, 115, 122, 122t
　　interstitial form of, nutrition intervention in, 348
　　nonobstructive forms of, 416, 417t
　　　characteristics of, 416–417
　　　clinical presentation of, 419–420

Lung disease *(Continued)*
　　　rehabilitation case histories for, 420t, 420–422
　　　rehabilitation results vs. results for chronic obstructive pulmonary disease, 418–419, 420t
　　obstructive forms of. See *Obstructive pulmonary disease(s)*.
　　prevalence of, 11
　　restrictive form of, pathophysiologic responses to exercise in, 120–121, 121t
　　　physiology of exercise limitation in, 421–422
　　social indicators of, 255–258
Lung elasticity, measures of, 19–20
Lung hyperinflation, in chronic obstructive pulmonary disease, 19, 31
Lung transplantation, chest physiotherapy following, 463–464
　　early rehabilitation course following, 463
　　exercise program preceding, 462
　　follow-up for, 464
　　for cystic fibrosis, 443
　　home exercise program following, 464
　　intraoperative approach for, 462
　　long-term results of, 464, 465t, 466, 466t
　　nutrition intervention in, 347–348
　　progressive ambulation and aerobic conditioning following, 464
　　pulmonary rehabilitation for, endurance training principles and, 460
　　　facility for, 460–461
　　　goals of, 459–460
　　　objectives of, 459–460
　　　patient population and, 460
　　　preoperative phase evaluation and, 461, 461t
　　　selection criteria for, 460, 460t
　　　staff for, 460–461
　　recovery from, goals following, 463, 463
Lung volumes, abnormalities of, emphysema predictions and, 31
　　in obstructive pulmonary disease, 21, 22
　　definitions of, 20–22, 21
　　determinants of, 20–22, 21. See also specific determinants.
　　in chronic obstructive pulmonary disease, 19–22, 19–22
　　maximum mouth pressure and, 37–38
　　measurement of, 20–22, 21
Lymphocyte count, total, 338–339

Major tranquilizers. See *Neuroleptics*.
Malnutrition, in chronic obstructive pulmonary disease, 332, 340–341, 342t, 343
　　in cystic fibrosis, 439
Manic-depressive agents, for psychiatric disease, 268, 271t
Marketing, of storefront rehabilitation program, 475
Maximum expiratory pressure (PEmax), at mouth, 37
Maximum inspiratory pressure (PImax), 21
　　at mouth, 37–38
Maximum inspiratory pressure test, 131
Maximum oxygen consumption, exercise intensity and, 208–209
Maximum power output, in chronic airflow limitation, 108, 110, 111–112
Maximum sustained ventilatory capacity (MSVC), 227, 229
Maximum voluntary ventilation (MVV), 25

Maximum voluntary ventilation (MVV) *(Continued)*
　　in exercise, 323
MDI (metered-dose inhalers), 153, 153t
Mechanical chest percussors, for cystic fibrosis, 178
Mechanical ventilation, for oxygenation failure, 132
　　for respiratory failure, 134
　　long-term. See *Long-term mechanical ventilation (LTMV)*.
　　patients dependent on. See *Ventilator-dependent patients*.
Mechanoreceptors, respiratory, 51–52
Meconium ileus, 443
Medical conditions, coexisting, selection of rehabilitation candidates and, 319
Medical director, as pulmonary rehabilitation team member, 304, 305
Medical history, in candidate assessment for rehabilitation, 319
Medical personnel, on pulmonary rehabilitation team, 305, 305–306, 306t
Medical regimens, adherence to, 354
Medical Research Council Study (MRC Study), survival from long-term oxygen therapy and, 70, 184, 184–185, 392
Medicare, comprehensive outpatient rehabilitation facilities and, 478–479
　　fiscal intermediary for, 487
　　interpretation of pulmonary rehabilitation and, 477
　　reimbursement for pulmonary rehabilitation, 303–304
Medicine chart, for pulmonary rehabilitation programs, 308, 310
Medicine list, for pulmonary rehabilitation programs, 308, 309
Medroxyprogesterone, for nocturnal hypoxemia, in chronic obstructive pulmonary disease, 98
Meglumine diatrizoate (Gastrografin), 443
Mellaril (thioridazine), 265t, 266, 266t
Membrane component of diffusing capacity, 30
Membrane separator oxygen enrichers, 192–193
Mental preparation, for smoking cessation, 291–293, 292t
Metabolic acidosis, chronic, exercise intolerance in lung disease and, 122, 122t
Metabolism, responses to exercise in asthma and, 431, 431t, 432
Metaproterenol, exercise tolerance and, 332
Metered-dose inhalers (MDI), 153, 153t
Methacholine bronchial challenge, in chronic obstructive pulmonary disease, 27–28
3-Methyl histidine, 339
Methylxanthines, for chronic obstructive pulmonary disease, 154–155
　　respiratory muscle function and, 160–161
Metropolitan Life Insurance Tables, 338
Miller, Dr. William F., 4
Minnesota Multiphasic Personality Inventory (MMPI), 81, 83, 84
Minute ventilation, reduction of, treatments for, 132
　　respiratory workload and, 127
Mitchell, Dr. Roger, 4
Mixed venous oxygen tension, for oxygen therapy monitoring, 197
MMPI (Minnesota Multiphasic Personality Inventory), 81, 83, 84
Modes of ventilation, for home positive-pressure ventilators, 284–285, 286

Molecular sieve oxygen concentrators, 191–192
Morphine, for dyspnea, 245, *246*
Mortality predictors, for chronic airflow obstruction, 139–142, 140t, *140–141*
Motivation, patient, for exercise therapy, 323
Mouth, maximum inspiratory pressure of, lung volume and, 37–38
M.O.V.E. pulmonary rehabilitation program, 474–477, 476t
MRC Study (Medical Research Council Study), survival from long-term oxygen therapy and, 70, *184*, 184–185, 392
MSVC (maximum sustained ventilatory capacity), 227, 229
Mucolytics, 157, 442
Mucus clearance, in chronic obstructive pulmonary disease, 175
  in normal airway, 175
Multicenter investigations, for neuropsychiatric evaluation of chronic obstructive pulmonary disease, 81–83, *82*, *84*, 85–87, *86–87*
  IPPB trial. See *Intermittent Positive-Pressure Breathing Clinical Trial (IPPB Trial)*.
  Medical Research Council Study, 70, *184*, 184–185, 392
  NOT trial. See *Nocturnal Oxygen Therapy Trial (NOT Trial)*.
Multiple inert gas elimination technique, 28
Muscle cramps, 331
Muscle function testing, in nutritional assessment, 339
Muscle spindles, 52, 105
Muscles. See also specific muscles.
  conditioning of, ventilatory response to exercise and, 117
  peripheral, effort intensity of, during dyspnea in normal subjects, *107–109*, 108
    in chronic airflow limitation, 108, 110–112, *110–112*
Muscular receptors, dyspnea and, 105
Musculoskeletal system, assessment of, in preoperative lung transplantation patient, 461
  response of, in chronic obstructive pulmonary disease, 253
Music, for relaxation, 373–374
MVV (maximum voluntary ventilation), 25
Myasthenia gravis, 128, 131
Myxedema, ventilatory failure in, 133

Naloxone, for dyspnea, *247*, 247–248
  for hypoventilation, 61–62
  pain sensitivity and, *247*, *247*
Nasal cannulas, 193, 193t
National Health Interview Survey (NHIS), 11
Navane (thiothixene), 265t, 266, 266t
Nebulizers, hand-held, 153, 153t
Negative-pressure ventilation (NPV), 274
  for home care, 282, 282t, *283*
  for nocturnal hypoxemia, in chronic obstructive pulmonary disease, 99
  via iron-lung, 274
Neurochemical methods, desensitization to dyspnea and, 245–248, *246–247*, 247t, 248t
Neurocognition, acute effects of hypoxemia and, 80

Neurocognition *(Continued)*
  in chronic obstructive pulmonary disease, sleep findings and, 88
  oxygen therapy and, amount of, 87–88
    duration of, 87–88
Neuroleptics, contraindications for, 265t
  dosage of, 265t
  for psychiatric disease, 264, 265t, 266t, 266–267
  properties of, 265t
  receptor blocking properties of, 266t
  side effects of, 265t
Neuromuscular diseases, ventilatory failure in, 129
Neuropsychiatry, oxygen therapy and, 187
Neuropsychology, assessment of, goal of, 80
  test batteries for, 80
  brain-behavior relationships and, 79–80
  of chronic obstructive pulmonary disease, 80–81
  clinical implications of deficits in, 90
Newsletters, for continuing care programs, 402
NHIS (National Health Interview Survey), 11
Nicotine addiction, criteria for, 289
  treatment of. See *Smoking, cessation of*.
Nicotine dependence, diagnostic criteria for, 293–294, 294t
  diagnostic notation for, 293, 296t
  evaluation of, 293–294, 295t
Nicotine polacrilex, for nicotine addiction treatment, 294–297, 296t
Nicotine withdrawal, diagnostic criteria for, 293–294, 294t
  evaluation of, 293–294, 295t
Nitrogen, dietary form of, for malnutrition in chronic obstructive pulmonary disease, 340–341
  dietary intake of, 339
  urinary output of, 339
Nocturnal desaturators, 96
Nocturnal Oxygen Therapy Trial (NOT Trial), choice of inspired oxygen concentrations in, 98
  continuous oxygen therapy reevaluation results for, 86–87, *87*
  data combined with IPBB Trial, results of, 85–86, *86*
  life quality assessment results of, 83, *84*
  long-term oxygen therapy and, 184, *184*
  methodology of, 81–82
  neuropsychologic findings of, *82*, 82–83
  pulmonary hemodynamics and cardiac function in, 69–70
  pulmonary rehabilitation and, 6–7
  purpose of, 81
  survival in, oxygen therapy and, 392
  survival rates for chronic airflow obstruction and, 144, *144*
Nonadherence, rational form of, 355–356
Noncompliance, patient, 353
Noninvasive intermittent ventilatory support, 232, 234
  methods for, *234*, 234–237, 235t, *236*
Nonverbal communication, in psychophysical assessment, 257
NOT Trial. See *Nocturnal Oxygen Therapy Trial (NOT Trial)*.
NPV. See *Negative-pressure ventilation (NPV)*.
Nurse, as pulmonary rehabilitation team member, 304, *305*
Nursing evaluation, in candidate assessment for rehabilitation, 320

Nutrition, assessment of, 336–340, *338*
  for cystic fibrosis, 346
  condition-specific concerns for, 340–348, 342t, 343t, *345*, 348t
  counseling for, 340, 341
  exercise and, 332
  for ventilator-dependent patients, 468–469
  in cystic fibrosis, 439–440
  interventions in, 348–349
    for cystic fibrosis, 345–346
    for interstitial lung disease, 348
    for lung transplantation, 347–348
    for malnutrition in chronic obstructive pulmonary disease, 340–341, *343*
    for obesity treatment, 343–344, *345*
    for pulmonary rehabilitation programs, 308
    for weight gain prevention, 344
  needs for, in cystic fibrosis, 347, 348t
Nutritional support, for respiratory failure, 133

Obesity, exercise intolerance in lung disease and, 122, 122t
  identification of, 341–342
  in chronic obstructive pulmonary disease, 341–344
  lower-body form of, 342–343
  morbid, definition of, 342
  treatment of, 343–344, *345*
  upper-body form of, 342
Obstructive pulmonary disease(s), abnormal responses to exercise in, 119t, 119–120, *120*
  asthma as. See *Asthma*.
  chronic. See *Chronic obstructive pulmonary disease (COPD)*.
  chronic bronchitis as. See *Bronchitis, chronic*.
  death rates for, regional patterns of, 14
    time trends in, 13–14
  definition of, 10–11
  emphysema as. See *Emphysema*.
  epidemiology of, 10
  frequency of, 11t, 11–13
  lung volume abnormalities in, *21*, 22
  P-V curve in, *2*, 22
  risk factors for, 15, 16, *16*
  transpulmonary pressure in, *19*
Occupational exposures, obstructive pulmonary disease risk and, 17
Occupational therapist, as pulmonary rehabilitation team member, 304, *305*
  assessment of candidate for rehabilitation and, 320
Office-based program, for pulmonary rehabilitation, 483–486
Ohm's law, 24
Omnibus Reconciliation Act of 1980, 478
Open magnitude scaling, 107
Opioids, endogenous forms of, for dyspnea, 245–248, 247t
  exogenous forms of, exercise tolerance and, 332
  for dyspnea, 245
Osteoarthropathy, hypertrophic pulmonary, in cystic fibrosis, 441
Outcome analyses, for pulmonary rehabilitation, 410–412
Outcome measures, 359–360
Outpatient pulmonary rehabilitation programs, 304

Overadherence, in patient compliance, 354–355
Oxygen, inspired, carbon dioxide sensitivity response and, 53, 53–54
  uptake of, per heart beat in chronic obstructive pulmonary disease, 119–120
  ventilatory response and, 54, 54–55
Oxygen desaturation, in cystic fibrosis, exercise tolerance and, 447, 450
  in exercise therapy, 329, 331
  nocturnal form of, 88
    in chronic obstructive pulmonary disease, prediction of, 96, 96–97
    long-term oxygen therapy for, 190
Oxygen dissociation curve, chronic exposure to high altitude and, 57
Oxygen pulse, in chronic obstructive pulmonary disease, 119–120, 120
  in mitral valve disease, 120
Oxygen saturation, in chronic obstructive pulmonary disease, during sleep, 92, 93
  in exercise, 326–327
  pursed-lip breathing and, 168
Oxygen therapy, adherence to, 354
  ambulatory vs. stationary, clinical trial of, 6–7
  amount of, neurocognitive functioning and, 87–88
  continuous form of, benefits of, 70–71
    vs. nocturnal oxygen therapy, 86–87, 87
  delivery of, equipment for, 193t, 193–196, 194, 194t
  duration of, neurocognitive functioning and, 87–88
  equipment for, adapters for, 403
    fire hazards of, 198–199
  for chronic obstructive pulmonary disease, 69, 205
  for nocturnal hypoxemia, in chronic obstructive pulmonary disease, 98
  for pulmonary hypertension, 69–70
  for supplementation, in cystic fibrosis, exercise tolerance and, 447, 450
  in exercise therapy, 210, 216
  heart function and, 69–71
  history of, in modern era, 183–185, 184
    origins of, 183
  in pulmonary rehabilitation, 187–188, 188, 309, 311
  long-term administration of. See Long-term oxygen therapy (LTOT).
  monitoring of, 196–197
  nocturnal form of, vs. continuous oxygen therapy, 86–87, 87
  physiologic mechanisms of, 185–187
  supplemental form of, for exercise training, 331
  supply of, equipment for, 191–193, 192t, 195–196
  transtracheal administration of, 132
  transtracheal form of, 193–195, 194, 194t
  transtracheal high-flow technique of, for ventilator-dependent patients, 470, 470
  traveling with, 403
Oxygenation, assessment of, in long-term oxygen therapy, 196–197
  during sleep, in chronic obstructive pulmonary disease, clinical value of studies on, 97, 97–98
  failure in, clinical manifestations of, 124
    management of, 132
  in chronic obstructive pulmonary disease, 28–29, 29

Oxygenation (Continued)
  of tissues, monitoring of, in long-term oxygen therapy, 196, 197
    oxygen therapy and, 186–187
Oxyhemoglobin dissociation curve, 28

Pace race, 402
Pain, vs. dyspnea, 256
Pain sensitivity, naloxone and, 247, 247
Palm breathing device, 195
Pancreatic insufficiency, exocrine, in cystic fibrosis, 439–440
Parasternal intercostal muscles, electrical activity of, in chronic obstructive pulmonary disease, 43
  inspiratory activation of, 37
  length-tension relationship of, 36
    in experimental emphysema, 39
  primary action of, 35
Passive tension, 34
Patient(s), attitudes of, pulmonary rehabilitation and, 307
  motivation of, pulmonary rehabilitation and, 307
Patient clubs, board of directors for, 401
  committees for, 401–402
  formation of, 400
  membership of, stimulation of, 400–401
Patient compliance. See Compliance, patient.
Patient education, active participation in, 263
  adequacy of program objective and, 263
  evaluation process in, effectiveness of, 263
  for ambulatory care, 262–263
  identification of resources in, 263
  long-term oxygen therapy compliance and, 197
Patient support groups, for pulmonary rehabilitation programs, 315
Peak expiratory flow rate (PEFR), in chronic obstructive pulmonary disease, 23–24, 24
PEEPi (intrinsic positive end-expiratory pressure), 20, 237
Pentoxifylline, 332
Perceived exertion, in asthma during exercise, 431–432, 433
Percussion, with postural drainage, 175
Peripheral airways disease, 18
Peripheral chemoreceptors, discovery of, 104
  oxygen therapy and, 188
  stimulation of, dyspnea and, 105
Peripheral densensitization, for dyspnea, 248–250, 249t
Peripheral fatigue, of respiratory muscles, 232
  low-frequency type of, 232, 233
Peripheral receptor inhibitors, for dyspnea, 63
Permission-giving, in PLISSIT model for sexual counseling, 385, 385t
Pharmacotherapy. See also specific drugs and drug classes.
  adherence to, 354
  adverse effects of, 162t, 162–163
  antitussives in, 157
  desensitization to dyspnea and, 245–248, 246–247, 247t, 248t
  exercise and, 332
  expectorants in, 157
  for advanced chronic obstructive pulmonary disease, 393
  for chronic obstructive pulmonary disease, 163t, 163–164
  for respiratory infections, 157–169

Pharmacotherapy (Continued)
  maximum use of, selection of rehabilitation candidates and, 319
  mucolytics in, 157
  of respiratory muscles, 160–163, 162t
  sexual dysfunction and, 386, 386t
  side effects of, rational nonadherence and, 355–356
Physical appearance, in psychophysical assessment, 257
Physical examination, in candidate assessment for rehabilitation, 319
Physical stressors, 367
Physical therapist, as pulmonary rehabilitation team member, 304, 305
  assessment of candidate for rehabilitation and, 320
Physical therapy, chest. See Chest physiotherapy.
Physician, as aversive stimulus, 257–258
  as pulmonary rehabilitation team member, 304, 305
  for pulmonary rehabilitation programs, follow-up of, 315
  office-based pulmonary rehabilitation program of, 483–486
  patients in pulmonary rehabilitation programs and, 313
Physostigmine, for anticholinergic psychosis, 268
Pink puffers, beta-endorphin levels of, 247, 247t
  characteristics of, 59
  dyspnea sensitivity and, 247–248
  minute ventilation failure in, 30
  ventilation-perfusion mismatch in, 28
PLB. See Pursed-lip breathing (PLB).
Pleural pressure, fall in, 36
PLISSIT model, for sexual counseling, 385t, 385–387, 386t
Pneumobelts, 282, 283
Pneumococcal pneumonia, mortality for, 159
Pneumonia, chest physiotherapy for, 178
  management of, 159
  pneumococcal, mortality for, 159
Pneumotaxic center, 51
Polycythemia, altitude and, 57
  hypoxemia in chronic obstructive pulmonary disease during sleep and, 95, 95–96
  in chronic hypoxia, 131
Polysomnography, for assessment of rehabilitation candidate, 321
  in chronic obstructive pulmonary disease, clinical value of, 97, 97–98
Pontine respiratory group, 50–51
Positive end-expiratory pressure/continuous positive airway pressure (PEEP/CPAP), home positive-pressure ventilators and, 285
Positive expiratory pressure physiotherapy, 176
Positive-pressure ventilation, for home care, clinical status of, 276, 278t
  elective nasal type of, 284
  equipment for, 284t, 284–285, 285t, 286, 287
  invasive type of, 284, 284t
  noninvasive form of, 236, 236–237
Postoperative care, chest physiotherapy for, 178–179
Postural drainage, technique for, 175
  with percussion, 175
  with vibration, 175

Prednisolone, for forced expiratory volume in 1 second improvement in chronic airflow obstruction, 146t, 146–147
Preoperative care, chest physiotherapy for, 178–179
Pressure-volume curve (P-V curve), 19, 19–20, 31
   in obstructive pulmonary disease, 2, 22
Pressure-volume relationships, static, of lung, 19, 19–20
Profile of Mood Scale, 83
Progesterone, for hypoventilation, 61
   for ventilatory drive improvement, 133
   respiratory muscle function and, 161
Progressive muscle relaxation methods, 370, 371t
   for insomnia, 313, 313
Protriptyline, for nocturnal hypoxemia, in chronic obstructive pulmonary disease, 98
Psychiatric disease, antidepressants for, 267t, 267–268, 269t–270t
   anxiolytic agents for, 268, 272t
   dealing with, 263–264, 265t, 266t, 266–268, 267t, 269t–272t, 271–272
   lithium for, 268, 271t
   manic-depressive agents for, 268, 271t
   neuroleptics for, 264, 265t, 266t, 266–267
   psychoactive medications and, 264
      general guidelines for, 264
         neuroleptics for, 264, 265t, 266t, 266–267
   vs. psychophysiologic disorders, 264
   vs. psychosocial disorders, 264
Psychoactive medications, for psychiatric disease, 264, 265t, 266t, 266–268, 267t, 269t–272t, 271–272
Psychologic stressors, 367
Psychologist, as pulmonary rehabilitation team member, 304, 305
Psychology, considerations for cystic fibrosis treatment and, 443
Psychophysical assessment, 256–258
Psychophysics, dyspnea and, 106–108
Psychophysiology, chronic obstructive pulmonary disease and, 253–259
   disorders of, vs. psychiatric disease, 264
   vs. psychosocial disorders, 264
   exercise evaluation methods for, 327
   intensive care unit treatment and, 259–260
Psychosocial factors, adherence or compliance and, 352–356
   assets, use of, 254–255
   behavioral interventions and, 356–358, 357t
   disorders of, vs. psychiatric disease, 264
   vs. psychophysiologic disorders, 264
   in chronic obstructive pulmonary disease, 253–259, 352
   intensive care unit treatment and, 259–260
   interventions in, methodologic issues in evaluation of, 359–362, 361t, 362t
   pulmonary rehabilitation programs and, 311, 313
   social indicators of disease and, 255–258
   social support and, 358–359
Pulmonary arterial pressure, hypoxemia during sleep in chronic obstructive pulmonary disease and, 95
Pulmonary function tests, after lung transplantation, 464, 465t, 466
   at rest, vs. exercise tests, 116–117
   for comprehensive outpatient rehabilitation facilities, 480

Pulmonary function tests (Continued)
   in advanced chronic obstructive pulmonary disease case histories, 395–396, 396t
   in candidate assessment for rehabilitation, 320
   in cystic fibrosis, exercise outcome and, 451, 454
   on hospital admissions, for chronic obstructive pulmonary disease, 420, 420t
      for nonobstructive pulmonary disease, 420, 420t
   pathologic correlates of, in chronic obstructive pulmonary disease, 30–31
   physiologic correlates of, in chronic obstructive pulmonary disease, 30–31
   smoking cessation and, 290–291
Pulmonary oxygen toxicity, from long-term oxygen therapy, 199
Pulmonary patient, exercise tolerance of, pathophysiologic processes in, 115–116, 122
Pulmonary receptors, dyspnea and, 105
Pulmonary rehabilitation. See Rehabilitation, pulmonary.
Pulmonary Rehabilitation from Hospital to Home, O'Ryan, 7
Pulmonary Rehabilitation (Guidelines to Success), Hodgkin, Zorn and Connors, 7
Pulmonary therapy, in cystic fibrosis treatment, 442–443
Pulmonary vascular impedance, hypoxemia and, 71–74, 72–75
Pulmonary vascular occlusive disease, exercise tolerance in, 121–122
Pulmonary vascular resistance, increase of, ventilatory response to exercise and, 117
Pulse oximetry, for oxygen therapy monitoring, 196
Pulse oxygen delivery, 195
Pursed-lip breathing (PLB), benefits of, 168–169
   mechanism of action of, 132
   technique for, 167, 168–169, 169
P-V curve (pressure-volume curve), 19, 19–20, 31
   in obstructive pulmonary disease, 2, 22

Quality-Adjusted Life Years (QALYs), 360
Quality of life, assessment of, in Intermittent Positive-Pressure Breathing Clinical Trial, 85
   in Nocturnal Oxygen Therapy Trial, 83, 84
   in chronic airflow obstruction, 148
   in chronic obstructive pulmonary disease, heuristic model of, 89, 89
   measurement of, from pulmonary rehabilitation, 411
Quality of Well-Being system (QWB system), 361t, 362, 362t

Randomization, for clinical studies, 407
Rapid-eye movement sleep (REM), hypoventilation in, hypoxemia of chronic obstructive pulmonary disease and, 92–94, 94
Ratio scaling, 107
Raw (airway resistance), 25–26, 26
Red blood cell residence time, shortening of, 117
Red blood cell resistance, 30

Reflex control, of respiration, 104
Rehabilitation, pulmonary, 1, 6
   candidates for, 317
      assessment of, 319–321
      clinical factors of, 318–319
      comprehension of, 318
      expectations of, 318
      home situation of, 318
      preprogram motivation of, 318
      reasons for admission of, 317–318, 318t
      reasons for referral of, 317
      selection of, 318–319
         asthmatic patients and, 434
      sources for referral of, 317
      symptoms of, 318
   components of program for, 307–309, 309–314, 311, 313–315
   conferences for, 306
   contract for, 306
   coordination of program and, 306
   cost benefit analysis of, 412
   daily instructions for, 308, 311
   definition of, 1, 6
   documentation for, 304
   endurance and strength training in, 313–314
   evaluation of, 405, 406t
      exercise testing for, 408t, 408–410, 409t
      outcome analyses for, 410–412
      study design for, 405–407
   exercise for. See Exercise, for rehabilitation therapy.
   expectations of, 302–303, 303t
   facilities for, 303, 303t
   family training in, 314
   follow-up for, 315
   for asthmatic patients, 434–435, 436
   for chronic airflow obstruction, 147–148
   for chronic obstructive pulmonary disease, anxiety and, 352
      as basis for nonobstructive rehabilitation, 417, 417–420, 419, 420t
      depression and, 352
      dyspnea and, 352
      vs. results for nonobstructive lung disease, 418–419, 420t
   for nonobstructive lung disease, basis for, 417, 417–420, 419, 420t
      case histories for, 420t, 420–422
      program guidelines for, 422
      vs. results for chronic obstructive pulmonary disease, 418–419, 420t
   goals of, 204, 302–303, 303t, 315, 351
      physiologic achievement of, analysis of failure in, 411–412
   home program in, 314–315
   in cystic fibrosis. See Cystic fibrosis, rehabilitation in.
   in lung transplantation, 459
      endurance training principles and, 460
      facility for, 460–461
      goals for, 459–460
      intraoperative phase approach for, 462
      objectives for, 459–460
      postoperative chest physiotherapy for, 463–464
      postoperative goals for, 463, 463
      preoperative phase evaluation and, 461, 461t
      preoperative phase exercise program for, 462
      staff for, 460–461
   marketing of, 303

Rehabilitation *(Continued)*
    Medicare interpretation of, 477
    medicine chart for, 308, *310*
    medicine list for, 308, *309*
    M.O.V.E. program of, 474–477, 476t
    nutrition intervention for, 308
    office-based program for, 483–486
    organization of, 302, 304
        inpatient vs. outpatient forms of, 304
    oxygen therapy in, 187–188, *188*
    patient daily charting for, 308, *312*
    patient guidebook for, 306–307, 307t
    patient support groups for, 315
    patients in, acceptance of disease and, 307
        active lifestyle and, 307
        attitudes of, 307
        critical knowledge for, 307–308
        feelings of, 313
        insomnia of, 313, *313*
        motivation of, 307
        physician and, 313
        sexuality of, 313
    personal historical perspective of, 1, *2–3, 4, 6*, 6–7
    physician for, follow-up of, 315
    presentation of information in, 304
    program components of, for smoking cessation, 298t
    program selection for, asthmatic patients and, 434–435, *436*
    proprietary program for. See *Comprehensive outpatient rehabilitation facilities (CORFs)*.
    psychosocial factors of, 311, 313
    psychosocial issues in, 351
    referrals for, comprehensive outpatient rehabilitation facilities and, 480
        in storefront program, 475
    reimbursement for, 303–304
    reporting for, 304
    respiratory muscle effects of, 409–410
    rounds and, 306
    skeletal muscle effects of, 410
    skills and techniques for, 308–309, 311, *311–312*. See also specific skills and techniques.
    smoking and, 307–308
    storefront program for, cost to patient and, 477
        current program of, 475–476, 476t
        history of, 474–475
        improvement evidence of, 477
        rationale of, 474
        referrals of, 475
        reimbursements of, 476–477
        success of, 477
    survival rate of, 6, *6*
    team for, *305*, 305–306, 306t
        follow-up of, 315
Reimbursement, for community-based hospital program, billing and, 489, 491, 494
    documentation guidelines for, 488–489, *490–493*
    fiscal intermediary role and, 487–488
    long-term follow-up and, 489
    for comprehensive outpatient rehabilitation facilities, 480, 481, 482
    for office-based pulmonary rehabilitation program, 485–486
    for pulmonary rehabilitation programs, 303–304
    for storefront pulmonary rehabilitation program, 476–477

Relaxation therapy, biofeedback technique and, 375–376
    cognitive-behavioral approach for, 377–378, 378t
        alteration of negative thinking and, 378, 378t
        problem clarification in, 377–378
        problem solving in, 378
        self-talk and, 378
    for insomnia, 313, *313*
    generalizing and maintaining ability to relax in, 376–377
    goals of, 368–369
    identifying appropriate patients for, 369
    intrusive thoughts and, 369–370
    overwhelmed patient and, 379
    positioning of patient for, 369
    preparation of patient for, 369
    problems in, anticipation of, 376
    properties of, 368
    referral decision and, 379–380
    sensations in, 369
    tapes for, 370
    techniques for, 370–375, 371t–373t
REM (rapid-eye movement sleep), hypoventilation in, hypoxemia of chronic obstructive pulmonary disease and, 92–94, *94*
Reproductive system, in cystic fibrosis, 440–441
Reservoir oxygen-conserving devices, 195
Residual volume (RV), *21*, 21–22
    in obstructive pulmonary disease, 22, *22*
Resistance stage, of General Adaptation Syndrome, 367–368, *368*
Respiration, circulation interaction and, 57–58
    elastic and resistive loads of, 55–56
    reflex control of, 104
Respiration patterns, abnormalities of, in respiratory failure, 130
Respiratory acidosis, chronic, in chronic obstructive pulmonary disease, 29
Respiratory center, 50–51
Respiratory chemostat, 58, *58*
Respiratory compensation point, 56
Respiratory control, abnormalities of, therapy for, 61–62
    physiology of, 50–58, *53–55, 57*
    structures of, 50–52
Respiratory cycle, phases of, 51
Respiratory failure, chronic form of, 134–135
    clinical characteristics of, 129–131
    definition of, 124
    laboratory findings in, 130–131
    management of, 131–134
    signs of, 130
    symptoms of, 129–130
    types of, 124. See also *Oxygenation, failure in; Ventilatory pump failure.*
Respiratory infections, antibiotics for, 158, 158t
    in cystic fibrosis, 440
        treatment of, 442–443
    pathogens of, 157–158
        antibiotic selection and, 158
    pharmacotherapy for, 157–169
    prophylaxis for, 159–160
    severe, management of, 158–159
Respiratory muscles. See also *Diaphragm.*
    during acute hyperinflation, 33–38, *34–37*
    endurance of, respiratory workload and, 129, *129*
        training for, 133
    energy expenditure of, 127–128

Respiratory muscles *(Continued)*
    fatigue of, 231
        central source for, 231–232
        definition of, 231
        historical aspects of, 276
        peripheral source for, 232
        relieving, to achieve dyspnea desensitization, 248–249
        vs. weakness, 232, 234
    function of, in head down and bending forward postures, 170–171, *171*
        pursed-lip breathing and, 169, *169*
    functional improvement of, for respiratory failure treatment, 132–133
    homeostasis of, in exercise, 110, *111*
    in chronic obstructive pulmonary disease, 42–46, *44*, 225–226, *226*
        exercise and, 45–46
    in dyspnea, 110
    length of, in chronic obstructive pulmonary disease, 41
    length-tension relationship of, during acute hyperinflation, 33–34, *34*
        in experimental emphysema, 38–39, *39*
    peripheral fatigue of, low-frequency type of, 232, *233*
    pharmacotherapy of, 160–163, 162t
    pulmonary rehabilitation effects on, 409–410
    rest therapy for, 234, *234*
        intermittent ventilatory support as, 232, 234
        long-term mechanical ventilation as, 276–277, *278*
        rationale of, 231–232, *233*, 234
        ventilatory muscle training and, 231
    strength of, 21, 37–38
        in chronic obstructive pulmonary disease, 41–42, *42*
    stress on, exercise and, 331
    training of. See *Ventilatory muscle training (VMT).*
    unloading of, 237–238
    visible contractions of, in respiratory failure, 130
    weakness of, 128–129, 129t
        metabolic factors and, 128
Respiratory phased demand oxygen delivery, 195
Respiratory rally, 402
Respiratory rate, oxygen therapy and, 186
Respiratory sensation, quality of, dyspnea and, 106
Respiratory stability, selection of rehabilitation candidates and, 318–319
Respiratory stimulants, respiratory muscle function and, 161–162
Respiratory stimuli, responses to, 52–58, *53–55, 57*
Respiratory system, in cystic fibrosis, 440, *441*
    mechanics of, oxygen therapy and, 186
    response of, in chronic obstructive pulmonary disease, 253
    to exercise in asthma, 431, 431t, *432*
    volume-pressure curves of, *37*, 37–38
Respiratory therapist, as pulmonary rehabilitation team member, 304, *305*
    assessment of candidate for rehabilitation and, 320
Respiratory workload, excessive, in ventilatory pump failure, 126t, 126–128
    inspiratory muscle endurance and, 129, *129*
Respironics BiPAP unit, 284–285

Resting breathing, in chronic obstructive pulmonary disease, 42–44, *44*
Retrolental fibrodysplasia, 200
Rib cage, parasternal region of. See *Parasternal intercostal muscles.*
Right-to-left shunt, through patent foramen ovale, 117
Right ventricular ejection fraction, 74–75
Right ventricular mass, hypoxemia during sleep in chronic obstructive pulmonary disease and, 95, *95*
Rocking bed, for home ventilator care, 282–284, *283*
RV (residual volume), *21*, 21–22
  in obstructive pulmonary disease, 22, *22*

SAHS. See *Sleep apnea/hypopnea syndrome (SAHS).*
Sarcomere, 38
Scalene muscles, electrical activity of, in chronic obstructive pulmonary disease, 43
  length-tension properties of, 36
  in experimental emphysema, 39
  primary function of, 35
Scaling methods, 107
Schedule of Recent Experience, 254
Secretion clearing techniques, for pulmonary rehabilitation programs, 309
Sedative-hypnotics. See *Anxiolytic agents.*
Self-efficacy, evaluation of, 357
Self-efficacy tool, for smoking cessation program, 297–298, 298t
Self-talk, 297, 377, 378
Sex, interest in, age and, 383, 384t
  vs. sexuality, 382t, 382–383
Sexual abuse, 389–390
Sexual activity, level of, 383
Sexual bias, 389
Sexual counseling, 384–387, 385t, 386t
Sexual functioning, obstacles to, 383–384
Sexual health care, definition of, 383
  ethical issues in, 388–390
  health provider role in, 384
Sexual interactions, between patient and caregiver, 390
Sexual problem(s), definition of, 383
  intensive therapy for, 387, 387t
  nonorganic causes of, 387, 387t
Sexuality, as lifetime activity, 383
  caregiver-patient relationship and, 387–388
  chronic illness and, 383–384, 384t, 390
  patients in pulmonary rehabilitation programs and, 313
  suggestions for lovemaking and, 386t, 386–387
  vs. sex, 382t, 382–383
Shoulder girdle muscles, dual postural and respiratory functions of, 45
Sickness Impact Profile (SIP), for assessment of rehabilitation candidate, 321
  for chronic obstructive pulmonary disease patients, 83, *84*, 85
  functional outcome and, 360
  in chronic airflow obstruction, 148
SIDS (sudden infant death syndrome), 248
SIP. See *Sickness Impact Profile (SIP).*
"Six-Point Plan," 198
Skeletal muscle, fiber types of, 226
  pulmonary rehabilitation effects on, 410
  strength of, alcoholism and, 162
  structural changes of, exercise training and, 205–206

Skeletal muscle *(Continued)*
  training, response to, 226–227
Sleep, arterial oxygen saturation in COPD and, 92
  death during, in chronic obstructive pulmonary disease, 96
  disturbances of, relaxation therapy for, 378–379
  fear of, 394
  neurocognitive impairments from nocturnal oxygen desaturation and, 88
  nocturnal hypoxemia of chronic obstructive pulmonary disease and, 94–96, *95*
  quality of, hypoxemia in chronic obstructive pulmonary disease during sleep and, 96
Sleep apnea syndrome, 88
Sleep apnea/hypopnea syndrome (SAHS), with chronic obstructive pulmonary disease, 94
  consequences of, 96
  detection of, 97
  treatment of, *99*, 100
Smoking, cessation of, behavioral techniques to prevent relapse and, 297–299, 298t
  benefits of, 289t, 289–290
  cognitive techniques to prevent relapse and, 297–299, 298t
  encouragement of efforts for, 291
  forced expiratory volume in 1 second and, 144–145
  mental preparation for, 291–293, 292t
  motivation and, biologic tests for, 290–291
  pharmacologic therapy for, 293–297
  preparation for, 289–290
  pulmonary function testing and, 290–291
  selection of rehabilitation candidates and, 318
  cigarette advertising and, 293, *293*
  exercise intolerance in lung disease and, 122, 122t
  habit smoker and, 294
  in chronic airflow limitation, 18
  in chronic airflow obstruction, 138–139, *139, 141*
    prediction of disease course and, 142–143
  in chronic obstructive pulmonary disease, 15
  long-term oxygen therapy and, 190
  mortality data for obstructive pulmonary disease and, 14
  obstructive pulmonary disease risk and, 15, *16*, 17
  pulmonary rehabilitation programs and, 307–308
  sick smoker and, 293
Social indicators of disease, 255–258
Social interaction hypothesis, of exercise, 242–243
Social Security Act, 479
Social support, behavior change and, 357–358
  functional effects of, 358–359
  health outcomes and, 358
  suggestions for, 359t
  use of, 254–255
Social worker, as pulmonary rehabilitation team member, 304, *305*
  assessment of candidate for rehabilitation and, 320–321
Sodium bicarbonate, 132
Space, for office-based pulmonary rehabilitation program, 485

Specific compliance, 19
Spirometry, exercise performance and, 323–324
  improvement on, from exercise, 216
  in differentiation of restrictive and obstructive conditions, 131
Spirometry testing, of smokers, 290
Sputum, expectoration of, in chest physiotherapy, 176
  production of, in cystic fibrosis, during exercise, 446, *447*
    exercise program outcome and, 454
  in ventilatory failure, 130
Stair climb test, for lung transplantation candidates, 461
Standard Gamble, for assessment of rehabilitation candidate, 321
Sternocleidomastoid muscle diameter, in chronic obstructive pulmonary disease, 40
Steroids, 156–157
Stress, assisted breathing therapy for, 259
  definition of, 367
  reduction of, by intensive care unit staff, 260
Stress buffering channel, 358–359
Stress response, 366–368, *367–368*
Stressors, 367, 377
Stretch receptors, dyspnea and, 105
  pulmonary, 52
Stroke volume, reduction of, in obstructive lung disease, 120
Sudden infant death syndrome (SIDS), 248
Survival rates, after rehabilitation for chronic airflow obstruction, 148
  for chronic obstructive pulmonary disease, 392, *393*
  for pulmonary rehabilitation, 6, *6*, 410–411
Sweat glands, in cystic fibrosis, 440
Sweat testing, for cystic fibrosis, 441, 442t
Swimming programs, for cystic fibrosis, 450
Sympathomimetic agents, 152–153, 153t, 161
Symptomatic improvement, oxygen therapy and, 188
Systematic desensitization technique, 374

Teaching skills, for patient and family education, 262–263
Team concept, pulmonary rehabilitation team and, 305–306, 306t
Theophylline, bronchodilation from, 155t
  for chronic obstructive pulmonary disease, 155–156, 393
  for hypoventilation, 61
  for nocturnal hypoxemia, in chronic obstructive pulmonary disease, 99
  half-life of, 155t
  mechanism of action of, 155
  respiratory muscle function and, 160–161
Therapy Information Entry (TIE), 491
Thioridazine (Mellaril), 265t, 266, 266t
Thiothixene (Navane), 265t, 266, 266t
Thomas L. Petty Aspen Lung Conference, 4
Thoracentesis, 132
Thought Control Clinic, 261
Threshold load, 127
TIE (Therapy Information Entry), 491
Time constant, concept of, 20, *20*
  prolonged, 21
Tissue oxygenation, monitoring of, in long-term oxygen therapy, 196, *197*
  oxygen therapy and, 186–187
TLC. See *Total lung capacity (TLC).*

Total lung capacity (TLC), definition of, 19, 21, *21*
  diaphragm length-tension relationship and, 34–35
  emphysema prediction and, 31
  in chronic obstructive pulmonary disease, 42
  in obstructive pulmonary disease, 22, *22*
  measurement of, 21, *21*
Touch, boundaries for, 388
Tranquilizers, for dyspnea, 245
  major. See *Neuroleptics*.
  minor. See *Anxiolytic agents*.
Transcutaneous oxygen tension, for oxygen therapy monitoring, 196–197
Transference, 390
Transpulmonary pressure, in obstructive pulmonary disease, *19*
Transtracheal high-flow oxygen, for ventilator-dependent patients, 470, *470*
Transtracheal oxygen therapy (TTOT), 193–195, *194*, 194t
Transversus abdominis muscle, contraction of, in chronic obstructive pulmonary disease, 44
  lengthening of, 36
Trapped gas, 1
Travel, continuing care programs and, 402–404
Treadmill exercise testing, for lung transplantation candidates, 461, 461t
  vs. bicycle ergometer testing, 409, 409t
Trendelenburg position, for postural drainage, 175
  in controlled breathing technique, 169–171, *171*
Tricyclic antidepressants. See *Antidepressants*.
TTOT (transtracheal oxygen therapy), 193–195, *194*, 194t
Type A patients. See *Pink puffers*.
Type B patients. See *Blue bloaters*.
Type J receptors, 52

Uniform Bill-82 (UB-82), 489, 491
Unloading, of respiratory muscles, 237–238
Upper airway receptors, dyspnea and, 106
Upper extremities, exercise training programs for, 220–221

Vaccines, for respiratory infection prophylaxis, 159–160
Vasoconstrictors, for cystic fibrosis, 442
VC (vital capacity), measurement of, *21*, 22
Ventilation, in chronic obstructive pulmonary disease, 29–30
  mechanical. See *Mechanical ventilation*.

Ventilation *(Continued)*
  oxygen therapy and, 186
  requirements for, at different levels of exercise, 117t
  responses to exercise in cystic fibrosis and, 446, 446t
Ventilation-perfusion relationship, *29*
  mismatch of, hypoxemia of chronic obstructive pulmonary disease during sleep and, 94
    in chronic obstructive pulmonary disease, 28
    in interstitial pulmonary fibrosis, 121
    in type A patients, 28
    in type B patients, 28
    low, arterial hypoxemia and, 28–29, *29*
    ventilatory requirements and, 116
  normal, *29*
  oxygen therapy and, 185
Ventilator-dependent patients, activity of, 469, *469*
  characteristics of, for home ventilator care, 279, 280t
  depression of, 469
  factors determining hospital discharge and, 279, 280t
  insurance for, 279
  nutrition for, 468–469
  special facilities for, 470, *471*–*472*, 472
  transtracheal high-flow oxygen and, 470, *470*
  weaning efforts for, 469, 469–470
Ventilatory demands, in chronic obstructive pulmonary disease, 226
Ventilatory drive, adjustments of, in respiratory failure treatment, 133–134
  inadequate, in ventilatory pump failure, 125–126
Ventilatory failure. See *Respiratory failure*.
Ventilatory-limited patients, determination of, 323
  exercise tolerance limitations in, 204–205, *205*
Ventilatory muscle training (VMT), continuous positive airway pressure and, 237–238, *238*–*239*
  for asthma, 435, *436*
  for chronic obstructive pulmonary disease, 225
  for cystic fibrosis, 448
  for dyspnea desensitization, 248–249
  in pulmonary rehabilitation, 314
  methods of, 227–231, *228*, 228t, *229*, 229t, 230t, *231*
    inspiratory resistive loading technique for, *228*, 228–230, *229*, 229t
    inspiratory resistive training and weaning for, 230
    inspiratory threshold loading for, 230, 230t, *231*
  respiratory muscle rest and, 231
  respiratory muscle unloading and, 237–238

Ventilatory muscle training (VMT) *(Continued)*
  rest therapy for, 234, *234*
    intermittent ventilatory support as, 232, 234
    long-term mechanical ventilation as, 276–277, *278*
    rationale of, 231–232, *233*, 234
    ventilatory muscle training and, 231
  skeletal muscle response to, 226–227
Ventilatory pump failure, clinical manifestations of, 124–129, 125t, *125*–*128*, 126t, 128t
Ventral respiratory group, 50–51
Vibration, with postural drainage, 175
Visual analog scaling, 107
Visualization technique, for relaxation, 372–373, 373t
Vital capacity (VC), measurement of, *21*, 22
VMT. See *Ventilatory muscle training (VMT)*.
Volume-pressure curves, of respiratory system, *37*, 37–38
Volume-time curve, in chronic obstructive pulmonary disease, 22–23, *23*
Voluntary isocapneic hyperpnea technique, 227, 228t

Walking, 6-minute test of, 326
  for chronic obstructive pulmonary disease, 420, 420t
  for lung transplantation candidates, 461
  for nonobstructive pulmonary disease, 420, 420t
  in evaluation of rehabilitation programs, 409
  12-minute test of, 326, *327*
  in evaluation of rehabilitation programs, 409
  as group activity, 398–400
  programs of, for cystic fibrosis, 448–450
Weaning, of ventilator-dependent patients, *469*, 469–470
Weight lifting, for cystic fibrosis, 450
Wheezing, in ventilatory failure, 130
White blood cell counts, elevated, pulmonary function and, 17
Work of breathing, definition of, 26
  in chronic obstructive pulmonary disease, 26, 26–27, 55
  pursed-lip breathing and, 169
  resistance and, 55
World Congress on Oxygen Therapy and Home Care, 7
World Health Organization International Classification of Disease, 11, 11t

Zone of apposition, in chronic obstructive pulmonary disease, 43